Neonatal-Perinatal Medicine

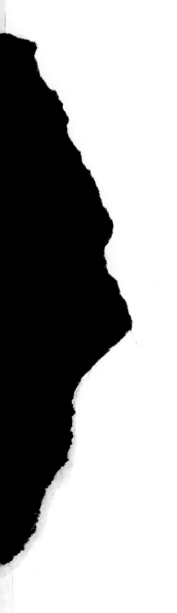

Neonatal-Perinatal Medicine

Diseases of the Fetus and Infant

7THedition

Volume One

Avroy A. Fanaroff, MB, FRCP (Edinburgh), DCH

Eliza Henry Barnes Chair in Neonatology
Professor of Pediatrics and Neonatology in Reproductive Biology
Case Western Reserve University School of Medicine
Co-Director of Neonatology
Rainbow Babies and Children's Hospital
Cleveland, Ohio

Richard J. Martin, MB, FRACP

Professor of Pediatrics, Neonatology in Reproductive Biology, Physiology, and Biophysics
Case Western Reserve University School of Medicine
Director of Neonatology
Rainbow Babies and Children's Hospital
Cleveland, Ohio

 Mosby

An Imprint of Elsevier Science

St. Louis   London   Philadelphia   Sydney   Toronto

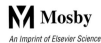

Acquisitions Editor: Judith Fletcher
Developmental Editor: Jennifer Shreiner
Manuscript Editor: Robin E. Davis
Production Manager: Mary Stermel
Illustration Specialist: Walt Verbitski

SEVENTH EDITION

NOTICE

Neonatology is an ever-changing field. Standard safety precautions must be followed, but as new research and clinical experience broaden our knowledge, changes in treatment and drug therapy may become necessary or appropriate. Readers are advised to check the most current product information provided by the manufacturer of each drug to be administered to verify the recommended dose, the method and duration of administration, and contraindications. It is the responsibility of the treating physician, relying on experience and knowledge of the patient, to determine dosages and the best treatment for each individual patient. Neither the publisher nor the editor assumes any liability for any injury and/or damage to persons or property arising from this publication.

Mosby, Inc.
An Imprint of Elsevier Science
11830 Westline Industrial Drive
St. Louis, Missouri 63146

Printed in the United States of America.

Library of Congress Cataloging-in-Publication Data

Neonatal-perinatal medicine: diseases of the fetus and infant / [edited by] Avroy A. Fanaroff, Richard J. Martin.—7th ed.

p.; cm.

Includes bibliographical references and index.

ISBN 0–323–00929–8

1. Infants (Newborn)—Diseases.   2. Fetus—Diseases.   I. Fanaroff, Avroy A.
II. Martin, Richard J.
[DNLM: 1. Fetal Diseases.   2. Infant, Newborn, Diseases.   3. Perinatal
Care.   4. Pregnancy Complications.

WS 420 N438 2002]
RJ254.N456 2002
618.92'01—dc21   2001030256

Last digit is the print number: 9   8   7   6   5   4   3   2

To our wives
Roslyn and Patricia,

the Fanaroff children and grandchildren
Jonathan, Amanda, Jodi and Peter, Austin,
and Morgan,
and the Martin children
Scott and Sonya

with love, admiration, and deep appreciation
for their continued support and inspiration

Contributors

Heidelise Als, PhD
Associate Professor of Psychology (Psychiatry),
Harvard Medical School; Senior Associate,
Department of Psychiatry, Director, Neurobehavioral
Infant and Child Studies, Children's Hospital,
Boston, Massachusetts
Neurobehavioral Development of the Preterm Infant

Jacob V. Aranda, MD, PhD
Professor of Pediatrics and Pharmaceutical Sciences,
Department of Clinical Pharmacology/Toxicology,
Wayne State University School of Medicine; Chief
and P.I., Division of Clinical Pharmacology/
Toxicology NIH-NICHD Pediatric Pharmacology
Research Unit Network, Children's Hospital of
Michigan, Detroit, Michigan
Developmental Pharmacology

James E. Arnold, MD
Professor and Chair of Otolaryngology–Head and
Neck Surgery, Professor of Pediatrics, Case Western
Reserve University School of Medicine; Pediatric
Otolaryngology and Director, Otolaryngology—Head
and Neck Surgery, Rainbow Babies and Children's
Hospital, Cleveland, Ohio
*Hearing Loss in the Newborn Infant; The Respiratory
System (Part Six)*

Ellis D. Avner, MD
Gertrude Lee Chandler Tucker Professor and Chair
of Pediatrics, Case Western Reserve University
School of Medicine; Chief Medical Officer, Rainbow
Babies and Children's Hospital, Cleveland, Ohio
*Fluid, Electrolytes, and Acid-Base Homeostasis (Parts
One and Two); The Kidney and Urinary Tract*

Jill E. Baley, MD
Associate Professor of Pediatrics, Case Western
Reserve University School of Medicine; Medical
Director, NICU Stepdown Nursery, Rainbow Babies
and Children's Hospital, Cleveland, Ohio
The Immune System (Part Four)

William F. Balistreri, MD
Dorothy M. M. Kersten Professor of Pediatrics,
Director, Division of Pediatric Gastroenterology,
Hepatology, and Nutrition, Medical Director, Liver
Transplantation, Children's Hospital Medical Center
and University of Cincinnati Medical Center,
Cincinnati, Ohio
*The Neonatal Gastrointestinal Tract (Parts One through
Three and Five)*

Eduardo H. Bancalari, MD
Professor of Pediatrics, Director of Neonatology,
University of Miami School of Medicine; Chief of
Newborn Services, Department of Pediatrics, Jackson
Memorial Medical Center, Miami, Florida
The Respiratory System (Part Seven)

David A. Bateman, MD
Associate Professor of Clinical Pediatrics, Columbia
University; Director of Neonatology, Harlem
Hospital Center, New York, New York
Infants of Addicted Mothers

Michael D. Bates, MD, PhD
Assistant Professor of Pediatrics, Division of
Pediatric Gastroenterology and Nutrition, Children's
Hospital Medical Center, Cincinnati, Ohio
The Neonatal Gastrointestinal Tract (Part One)

Françoise Baylis, PhD
Associate Professor of Medicine and Philosophy,
Department of Bioethics, Dalhousie University,
Halifax, Nova Scotia, Canada
Ethics in Perinatal and Neonatal Medicine

Cynthia F. Bearer, MD, PhD
Assistant Professor of Pediatrics and Neurosciences,
Case Western Reserve University School of
Medicine; Assistant Professor, Division of
Neonatology, Department of Pediatrics, Rainbow
Babies and Children's Hospital, Cleveland, Ohio
Occupational and Environmental Risks to the Fetus

Richard E. Behrman, JD, MD
Clinical Professor of Pediatrics, Stanford University
School of Medicine and University of California, San
Francisco School of Medicine; Senior Vice President
of Medical Affairs, Lucile Packard Foundation for
Children's Health, Stanford, California
Neonatal Risk Factors

David A. Benaron, MD
Assistant Professor of Pediatrics, Stanford University
School of Medicine, Stanford, California
Biomedical Engineering Aspects of Neonatal Monitoring

Ronald S. Bloom, MD
Professor, University of Utah School of Medicine,
Salt Lake City, Utah
Delivery Room Resuscitation of the Newborn

Jeffrey L. Blumer, PhD, MD
Professor of Pediatrics and Pharmacology, Case
Western Reserve University School of Medicine;
Chief, Division of Pediatric Pharmacology and
Critical Care, Rainbow Babies and Children's
Hospital, Cleveland, Ohio
*Fetal Therapy (Part One); Appendix A: Therapeutic
Agents*

Olaf Bodamer, MD, PhD
Assistant Professor of Human and Molecular
Genetics, Baylor College of Medicine; Geneticist,
Texas Children's Hospital, Houston, Texas
The Central Nervous System (Part Seven)

Waldemar A. Carlo, MD
Edwin M. Dixon Professor of Pediatrics, Director,
Division of Neonatology, Director of Nurseries,
University of Alabama at Birmingham, Birmingham,
Alabama
The Respiratory System (Parts Two and Four)

Suzanne B. Cassidy, MD
Professor of Clinical Pediatrics, University of
California, Irvine, Irvine, California; Chief, Division
of Human Genetics and Birth Defects, UCI Medical
Center, Orange, California
Congenital Anomalies

Mitchell B. Cohen, MD
Professor of Pediatrics, University of Cincinnati;
Attending Physician, Division of Pediatric
Gastroenterology and Nutrition, Children's Hospital
Medical Center, Cincinnati, Ohio
The Neonatal Gastrointestinal Tract (Part Three)

Daniel R. Cooperman, MD
Associate Professor of Orthopedic Surgery, Case
Western Reserve University School of Medicine,
Cleveland, Ohio
Neonatal Orthopedics

James M. Coticchia, MD
Assistant Professor of Pediatrics, Case Western
Reserve University School of Medicine; Division of
Pediatric Otolaryngology, Rainbow Babies and
Children's Hospital, Cleveland, Ohio
Hearing Loss in the Newborn Infant

Tracy A. Cowles, MD
Associate Professor, University of Missouri, Kansas
City, Kansas City, Missouri
Perinatal Infections

Timothy M. Crombleholme, MD
Associate Professor of Surgery and Obstetrics and
Gynecology, University of Pennsylvania School of
Medicine; Fetal Surgeon, Center for Fetal Diagnosis
and Treatment, The Children's Hospital of
Philadelphia, Philadelphia, Pennsylvania
Fetal Therapy (Part Two)

William T. Dahms, MD
Professor of Pediatrics, Case Western Reserve
University School of Medicine; Division of Pediatric
Endocrinology and Metabolism, Rainbow Babies and
Children's Hospital, Cleveland, Ohio
Metabolic and Endocrine Disorders (Part Four)

Robert K. Danish, MD
Associate Professor of Pediatrics, College of
Medicine, University of Tennessee Health Center;
Division of Endocrinology and Metabolism,
Le Bonheur Children's Medical Center, Memphis,
Tennessee
Metabolic and Endocrine Disorders (Part Four)

Utpala (Shonu) G. Das, MD
Assistant Professor of Pediatrics, Medical College of
Wisconsin; Neonatologist, Department of Pediatrics,
Children's Hospital of Wisconsin, Milwaukee,
Wisconsin
Intrauterine Growth Retardation

Ira D. Davis, MD
Associate Professor of Pediatrics, Case Western
Reserve University School of Medicine; Chief,
Division of Pediatric Nephrology, Rainbow Babies
and Children's Hospital, Cleveland, Ohio
*Fluid, Electrolytes, and Acid-Base Homeostasis (Parts
One and Two)*

Sergio DeMarini, MD
Director, Division of Neonatology, Ospedale S.
Croce, Cuneo, Italy
Metabolic and Endocrine Disorders (Part Two)

Scott C. Denne, MD
Professor of Pediatrics, Indiana University School of
Medicine; Staff Neonatologist, James Whitcomb
Riley Hospital for Children, Indianapolis, Indiana
*Nutrition and Metabolism in the High-Risk Neonate
(Parts One and Two)*

Lois H. Dickerman, PhD
Retired Professor of Genetics, Pediatrics, and
Environmental Health Science, Case Western Reserve
University School of Medicine; Retired Director,
Prenatal Screening Laboratory, Cleveland, Ohio
*Genetic Aspects of Perinatal Disease and Prenatal
Diagnosis*

Juliann M. Di Fiore, BSEE
Research Engineer, Rainbow Babies and Children's
Hospital, Cleveland, Ohio
The Respiratory System (Part Two)

Beth A. Drolet, MD
Associate Professor of Dermatology, Medical College
of Wisconsin; Children's Hospital of Wisconsin,
Milwaukee, Wisconsin
The Skin

David J. Edwards, PharmD
Associate Professor of Pharmacy Practice, College of
Pharmacy and Allied Health Professions, Wayne
State University; Clinical Pharmacologist, Division of
Clinical Pharmacology/Toxicology, Children's
Hospital of Michigan, Detroit, Michigan
Developmental Pharmacology

Morven S. Edwards, MD
Professor of Pediatrics, Baylor College of Medicine;
Active Staff, Texas Children's Hospital and Ben Taub
General Hospital, Houston, Texas
The Immune System (Parts Two and Three)

Judith A. Ernst, DMSc, RD
Associate Professor of Nutrition and Dietetics,
School of Allied Health Sciences, Indiana University
School of Medicine, Indianapolis, Indiana
*Nutrition and Metabolism in the High-Risk Neonate
(Part One)*

Nancy B. Esterly, MD
Professor of Dermatology and Pediatrics, Medical
College of Wisconsin; Medical Director, Pediatrics
Dermatology, Children's Hospital of Wisconsin,
Milwaukee, Wisconsin
The Skin

Avroy A. Fanaroff, MB, BCh, FRCP(E), DCH
Eliza Henry Barnes Chair in Neonatology, Professor
of Pediatrics and Neonatology in Reproductive
Biology, Case Western Reserve University School of
Medicine; Co-Director of Neonatology, Rainbow
Babies and Children's Hospital, Cleveland, Ohio
*Perinatal Services and Resources; The Respiratory
System (Parts Three, Four, and Five)*

Susan E. Gerber, MD
Fellow, Maternal-Fetal Medicine, Northwestern
University Medical School, Chicago, Illinois
Estimation of Fetal Well-Being (Part Two)

Robert L. Goldenberg, MD
Professor of Obstetrics-Gynecology, University of
Alabama at Birmingham, Birmingham, Alabama
Obstetric Management of Prematurity

Bernard Gonik, MD
Professor and Associate Chair of Obstetrics and
Gynecology, Wayne State University School of
Medicine; Chief, Department of Obstetrics and
Gynecology, Sinai-Grace Hospital, Detroit, Michigan
Perinatal Infections

Jeffrey B. Gould, MD, MPH
Professor of Maternal and Child Health, Division of
Public Health Biology and Epidemiology, School of
Public Health, University of California, Berkeley,
Berkeley, California; Clinical Professor of
Neonatology, Lucile Packard Children's Hospital,
Stanford University Medical Center, Stanford,
California
*Evaluating and Improving the Quality of Neonatal Care
(Part One)*

Andrée M. Gruslin, MD, FRCS
Associate Professor of Obstetrics and Gynecology,
Division of Maternal-Fetal Medicine, University of
Ottawa; Ottawa Hospital, General Campus, Ottawa,
Ontario, Canada
Erythroblastosis Fetalis

Balaji K. Gupta, MD
Assistant Professor of Ophthalmology, Department
of Ophthalmology and Visual Sciences, University of
Illinois at Chicago, Chicago, Illinois
The Eye (Parts One and Two)

Maureen Hack, MB, ChB
Professor of Pediatrics and Reproductive Biology,
Case Western Reserve University School of
Medicine; Director, High Risk Follow-up, Rainbow
Babies and Children's Hospital, Cleveland, Ohio
Follow-up for High-Risk Neonates

Louis P. Halamek, MD
Assistant Professor of Pediatrics, Division of
Neonatal and Developmental Medicine, Stanford
University School of Medicine; Attending
Neonatologist, Lucile Packard Children's Hospital,
Stanford University Medical Center, Stanford,
California
Neonatal Jaundice and Liver Disease

Barbara F. Hales, PhD
Professor of Pharmacology and Therapeutics, McGill University, Montreal, Quebec, Canada
Developmental Pharmacology

Nancy A. Hamming, MD
Assistant Professor of Ophthalmology, Rush-Presbyterian-St. Luke's Medical Center, Chicago, Illinois
The Eye (Parts One and Two)

Jonathan Hellmann, MB.BCh, FCP(SA), FRCPC
Associate Professor of Paediatrics, University of Toronto; Clinical Director, Neonatal Intensive Care Unit, Division of Neonatology, Hospital for Sick Children, Toronto, Ontario, Canada
Ethics in Perinatal and Neonatal Medicine

Susan R. Hintz, MD
Assistant Professor of Pediatrics, Stanford University School of Medicine, Stanford, California
Biomedical Engineering Aspects of Neonatal Monitoring

Jeffrey D. Horbar, MD
Professor of Pediatrics, University of Vermont College of Medicine; Chief Executive and Scientific Officer, Vermont Oxford Network, Burlington, Vermont
Evaluating and Improving the Quality of Neonatal Care (Part One)

Louanne Hudgins, MD
Associate Professor of Pediatrics, Stanford University School of Medicine; Director, Perinatal Genetics, Lucile Packard Children's Hospital, Stanford University Medical Center, Stanford, California
Congenital Anomalies

Susan D. Izatt, MD
Assistant Professor of Pediatrics, Case Western Reserve University School of Medicine, Cleveland, Ohio
Physical Examination and Care of the Newborn (Part Two)

Jay J. Jacoby, MD, PhD
Clinical Professor of Anesthesiology, The Ohio State University College of Medicine, Columbus, Ohio
Anesthesia for Labor and Delivery

Alan H. Jobe, MD, PhD
Professor of Pediatrics, University of Cincinnati; Professor of Neonatology/Pulmonary Biology, Children's Hospital Medical Center, Cincinnati, Ohio
The Respiratory System (Part One)

Nancy E. Judge, MD
Assistant Professor of Reproductive Biology, Case Western Reserve University School of Medicine; Director, Reproductive Imaging, Faculty, Division of Maternal-Fetal Medicine, University MacDonald Women's Hospital, Cleveland, Ohio
Perinatal Ultrasound

Satish C. Kalhan, MBBS, DCH, FRCP
Professor of Pediatrics and Reproductive Biology, Case Western Reserve University School of Medicine; Director, Robert Schwartz Center for Metabolism and Nutrition, Staff Neonatologist, MetroHealth Medical Center, Cleveland, Ohio
Metabolic and Endocrine Disorders (Part One)

Reuben Kapur, PhD
Assistant Scientist, Department of Pediatrics, Indiana University School of Medicine, Indianapolis, Indiana
The Immune System (Part One)

John Kattwinkel, MD
Charles Fuller Professor of Neonatology, Professor of Pediatrics, University of Virginia; Director of Neonatology, University of Virginia Hospital, Charlottesville, Virginia
Perinatal Outreach Education

Ajay Kaul, MBBS, MD
Assistant Professor of Clinical Pediatrics, Division of Pediatric Gastroenterology and Nutrition, Children's Hospital Medical Center, Cincinnati, Ohio
The Neonatal Gastrointestinal Tract (Part Five)

John H. Kennell, MD
Professor of Pediatrics, Case Western Reserve University School of Medicine; Division of Behavioral Pediatrics and Psychology, Rainbow Babies and Children's Hospital, Cleveland, Ohio
Care of the Mother, Father, and Infant

Marshall H. Klaus, MD
Adjunct Professor of Pediatrics, University of California, San Francisco School of Medicine, San Francisco, California
Care of the Mother, Father, and Infant

Robert M. Kliegman, MD
Professor and Chair of Pediatrics, Medical College of Wisconsin; Pediatrician-in-Chief, Pamela and Leslie Muma Chair in Pediatrics, Children's Hospital of Wisconsin, MACC Fund Research Center, Milwaukee, Wisconsin
Intrauterine Growth Retardation

Neil K. Kochenour, MD
Professor of Obstetrics and Gynecology, University of Utah School of Medicine; Medical Director, University of Utah Hospitals and Clinics, Salt Lake City, Utah
Fetal Effects of Autoimmune Disease; Obstetric Management of Multiple Gestation; Post-term Pregnancy

John R. Lane, MD
Assistant Professor of Pediatrics, Case Western Reserve University School of Medicine; Pediatric Cardiologist, Rainbow Babies and Children's Hospital, Cleveland, Ohio
The Cardiovascular System (Part Five)

Michael H. LeBlanc, MD
Professor of Pediatrics, University of Mississippi School of Medicine, Jackson, Mississippi
The Physical Environment

Catherine A. Leitch, PhD
Associate Scientist, James Whitcomb Riley Hospital for Children, Indianapolis, Indiana
Nutrition and Metabolism in the High-Risk Neonate (Parts One and Two)

James A. Lemons, MD
Hugh McK. Landon Professor of Pediatrics, Indiana University School of Medicine; Director, Section of Neonatal-Perinatal Medicine, Indiana University Medical Center, Indianapolis, Indiana
Nutrition and Metabolism in the High-Risk Neonate (Part One)

Pamela K. Lemons, RN, MSN, CNNP
Adjunct Assistant Professor of Nursing, Indiana University School of Nursing; Neonatal Nurse Practitioner, James Whitcomb Riley Hospital for Children, Indianapolis, Indiana
Nutrition and Metabolism in the High-Risk Neonate (Part One)

Carol Andrea Lindsay, MD
Assistant Professor of Reproductive Biology, Case Western Reserve University School of Medicine; Perinatologist, Department of Obstetrics-Gynecology, Division of Maternal-Fetal Medicine, MetroHealth Medical Center, Cleveland, Ohio
Pregnancy Complicated by Diabetes Mellitus

Tom Lissauer, MB, BChir, FRCPCH
Senior Clinical Lecturer, Imperial College School of Medicine; Consultant Neonatologist, St. Mary's Hospital, London, England
Physical Examination and Care of the Newborn (Part One)

Lori Luchtman-Jones, MD
Assistant Professor of Pediatrics, Clinical Director of Hematology-Oncology, Washington University School of Medicine; Assistant Professor of Pediatrics, St. Louis Children's Hospital, St. Louis, Missouri
The Blood and Hematopoietic System

Henry H. Mangurten, MD
Professor of Pediatrics, Acting Chairman, Department of Pediatrics, Finch University of Health Sciences/The Chicago Medical School, North Chicago, Illinois; Chairman, Department of Pediatrics, Lutheran General Children's Hospital, Park Ridge, Illinois
Birth Injuries

Richard J. Martin, MB, BS, FRACP
Professor of Pediatrics, Neonatology in Reproductive Biology, Physiology, and Biophysics, Case Western Reserve University School of Medicine; Director of Neonatology, Department of Pediatrics, Rainbow Babies and Children's Hospital, Cleveland, Ohio
The Respiratory System (Parts Three, Four, and Five)

John S. McDonald, MD
Professor of Obstetrics and Gynecology, University of California, Los Angeles School of Medicine; Professor and Chair of Anesthesiology, Harbor-UCLA Medical Center, Los Angeles, California
Anesthesia for Labor and Delivery

Geoffrey Miller, MA, MD, FRCP, FRACP
Professor of Pediatrics and Neurology, Baylor College of Medicine; Chief, Developmental Pediatrics Section, Texas Children's Hospital, Houston, Texas
The Central Nervous System (Part Seven)

Marilyn T. Miller, MD
Professor of Ophthalmology, Director of Pediatric Ophthalmology and Adult Strabismus, Department of Ophthalmology and Visual Sciences, University of Illinois at Chicago, Chicago, Illinois
The Eye (Parts One and Two)

Martha J. Miller, MD, PhD
Associate Professor of Pediatrics, Division of Neonatology, Case Western Reserve University School of Medicine; Associate Professor of Pediatrics, Rainbow Babies and Children's Hospital, Cleveland, Ohio
The Respiratory System (Part Five)

Thomas R. Moore, MD
Professor and Chair of Reproductive Medicine, University of California, San Diego School of Medicine, San Diego, California
Erythroblastosis Fetalis; Amniotic Fluid and Nonimmune Hydrops Fetalis

Stuart C. Morrison, MB, ChB, MRcP
Staff Radiologist, Cleveland Clinic Foundation,
Cleveland, Ohio
Perinatal Ultrasound; Diagnostic Imaging

Kevin Muise, MD
Assistant Professor of Reproductive Biology, Case
Western Reserve University School of Medicine,
Cleveland, Ohio
Perinatal Ultrasound

Nancy S. Newman, RN
Research Coordinator, Rainbow Babies and
Children's Hospital, Cleveland, Ohio
Appendix B: Tables of Normal Values

Charles Palmer, MB, ChB
Professor of Pediatrics (Neonatology), Pennsylvania
State University College of Medicine, Milton S.
Hershey Medical Center, Hershey, Pennsylvania
The Central Nervous System (Part Three)

Lu-Ann Papile, MD
Professor of Pediatrics and Obstetrics and
Gynecology, University of New Mexico Health
Sciences Center, Albuquerque, New Mexico
The Central Nervous System (Part Five)

Barbara V. Parilla, MD
Associate Professor, Northwestern University
Medical School, Chicago, Illinois; Director, Fetal
Diagnostic Center, Evanston Hospital, Evanston,
Illinois
Estimation of Fetal Well-Being (Part One)

Prabhu S. Parimi, MBBS, DM
Assistant Professor of Pediatrics, Case Western
Reserve University School of Medicine; Staff
Neonatologist, MetroHealth Medical Center,
Cleveland, Ohio
Metabolic and Endocrine Disorders (Part One)

Chandrakant R. Patel, MBBS
Assistant Professor of Pediatrics, Case Western
Reserve University School of Medicine; Director,
Pediatric Echocardiography Laboratory, Rainbow
Babies and Children's Hospital, Cleveland, Ohio
*The Cardiovascular System (Parts Three, Six, and
Seven)*

Dale L. Phelps, MD
Professor of Pediatrics and Ophthalmology,
University of Rochester School of Medicine and
Dentistry, Rochester, New York
The Eye (Part Three)

Brenda B. Poindexter, MD
Assistant Professor of Pediatrics, Indiana University
School of Medicine; Neonatologist, James Whitcomb
Riley Hospital for Children, Indianapolis, Indiana
*Nutrition and Metabolism in the High-Risk Neonate
(Parts One and Two)*

Richard A. Polin, MD
Professor of Pediatrics, Columbia University College
of Physicians and Surgeons; Director, Division of
Neonatology, Babies and Children's Hospital, New
York, New York
The Immune System (Part One)

Tonse N. K. Raju, MD
Professor of Pediatrics and Obstetrics and
Gynecology, University of Illinois, Chicago, Illinois
*From Infant Hatcheries to Intensive Care: Some
Highlights of the Century of Neonatal Medicine*

Patrick S. Ramsey, MD
Fellow/Instructor of Maternal-Fetal Medicine,
Department of Obstetrics-Gynecology, University of
Alabama at Birmingham, Birmingham, Alabama
Obstetric Management of Prematurity

Raymond W. Redline, MD
Associate Professor of Pathology and Reproductive
Biology, Case Western Reserve University School of
Medicine; Pediatric Pathologist, University Hospitals
of Cleveland, Cleveland, Ohio
Placental Pathology

Michael D. Reed, PharmD
Professor of Pediatrics, Case Western Reserve
University School of Medicine; Director, Pediatric
Clinical Pharmacology and Toxicology, Rainbow
Babies and Children's Hospital, Cleveland, Ohio
Fetal Therapy (Part One)

Michael J. Rieder, MD, PhD, FRCPC
Professor of Pediatrics, Pharmacology and
Toxicology, and Medicine, University of Western
Ontario; Counseling Staff, Children's Hospital of
Western Ontario, London, Ontario, Canada
Developmental Pharmacology

Ricardo J. Rodriguez, MD
Assistant Professor of Pediatrics, Case Western
Reserve University School of Medicine; Attending
Neonatologist, Department of Pediatrics, Rainbow
Babies and Children's Hospital, Cleveland, Ohio
The Respiratory System (Part Three)

Susan R. Rose, MD
Professor of Pediatric Endocrinology, University of Cincinnati; Professor of Endocrinology, Children's Hospital Medical Center, Cincinnati, Ohio
Metabolic and Endocrine Disorders (Part Three)

Tove S. Rosen, MD
Professor of Clinical Pediatrics/Neonatology, Columbia University; Attending Pediatrician, New York-Presbyterian Hospital, New York, New York
Infants of Addicted Mothers

Frederick C. Ryckman, MD
Associate Professor of Surgery/Pediatric Surgery, University of Cincinnati; Children's Hospital Medical Center, Cincinnati, Ohio
The Neonatal Gastrointestinal Tract (Parts Two and Four)

Denver Sallee, MD
Assistant Professor of Pediatrics, Division of Pediatric Cardiology, Case Western Reserve University School of Medicine; Pediatric Cardiologist, Rainbow Babies and Children's Hospital, Cleveland, Ohio
The Cardiovascular System (Part Three)

Harvey B. Sarnat, MD, FRCPC
Professor of Neurology, Pathology (Neuropathology), and Pediatrics, University of Washington School of Medicine; Pediatric Neurologist and Neuropathologist, Children's Hospital and Regional Medical Center, Seattle, Washington
The Central Nervous System (Part Two)

Alan L. Schwartz, MD, PhD
Harriet B. Spoehrer Professor and Chair of Pediatrics, Washington University School of Medicine; Professor of Pediatrics, St. Louis Children's Hospital, St. Louis, Missouri
The Blood and Hematopoietic System

Stuart Schwartz, PhD
Professor of Genetics and Oncology, Case Western Reserve University School of Medicine; Laboratory Director, Center for Human Genetics, University Hospitals of Cleveland, Cleveland, Ohio
Genetic Aspects of Perinatal Disease and Prenatal Diagnosis

Dinesh M. Shah, MD
Associate Professor of Reproductive Biology, Case Western Reserve University School of Medicine; Director, Division of Maternal-Fetal Medicine, Department of Obstetrics/Gynecology, University MacDonald Women's Hospital, Cleveland, Ohio
Hypertensive Disorders of Pregnancy

Patricia H. Shiono, MA, PhD
Director of Research and Grants for Epidemiology, Center for the Future of Children, David and Lucile Packard Foundation, Stanford, California
Neonatal Risk Factors

John C. Sinclair, MD
Emeritus Professor of Pediatrics and Clinical Epidemiology and Biostatistics, McMaster University, Hamilton, Ontario, Canada; Adjunct Professor, School of Epidemiology and Public Health, Yale University, New Haven, Connecticut
Evaluating and Improving the Quality of Neonatal Care (Part Two)

Bonnie S. Siner, RN
Research Nurse, Division of Neonatology, Rainbow Babies and Children's Hospital, Cleveland, Ohio
Appendix B: Tables of Normal Values

Robert C. Sprecher, MD
Assistant Professor of Otolaryngology—Head and Neck Surgery and Pediatrics, Case Western Reserve University School of Medicine; Chief, Division of Pediatric Otolaryngology, Rainbow Babies and Children's Hospital, Cleveland, Ohio
The Respiratory System (Part Six)

David K. Stevenson, MD
Professor and Associate Chair of Pediatrics, Chief, Division of Neonatal and Developmental Medicine, Stanford University; Director, Charles B. and Ann L. Johnson Center for Pregnancy and Newborn Services, Director of Nurseries, Lucile Packard Children's Hospital, Stanford University Medical Center, Stanford, California
Biomedical Engineering Aspects of Neonatal Monitoring; Neonatal Jaundice and Liver Disease

Eileen K. Stork, MD
Associate Professor of Pediatrics, Director, ECMO Center, Case Western Reserve University School of Medicine; Rainbow Babies and Children's Hospital, Cleveland, Ohio
The Respiratory System (Part Eight)

John E. Stork, MD
Assistant Professor of Anesthesiology and Pediatrics, Case Western Reserve University School of Medicine; Departments of Anesthesiology and Pediatrics, Rainbow Babies and Children's Hospital, Cleveland, Ohio
Anesthesia in the Neonate; Fluid, Electrolytes, and Acid-Base Homeostasis (Part Two)

George H. Thompson, MD
Professor of Orthopedic Surgery and Pediatrics, Case Western Reserve University School of Medicine; Director, Pediatric Orthopedics, Rainbow Babies and Children's Hospital, Cleveland, Ohio
Neonatal Orthopedics

Philip Toltzis, MD
Associate Professor of Pediatrics, Case Western Reserve University School of Medicine; Attending Physician, Rainbow Babies and Children's Hospital, Cleveland, Ohio
The Immune System (Part Four)

Reginald C. Tsang, MBBS
Professor of Pediatrics, University of Cincinnati; Children's Hospital Medical Center, Cincinnati, Ohio
Metabolic and Endocrine Disorders (Part Two)

George F. Van Hare, MD
Associate Professor of Pediatrics, Stanford University School of Medicine; Director, Pediatric Arrhythmia Center at Stanford and UCSF, Lucile Packard Children's Hospital, Stanford University Medical Center, Stanford, California
The Cardiovascular System (Part Eight)

Robert C. Vannucci, MD
Professor of Pediatrics (Pediatric Neurology), Pennsylvania State University School of Medicine, Milton S. Hershey Medical Center, Hershey, Pennsylvania
The Central Nervous System (Parts One, Three, Four, Six, and Eight)

Beth A. Vogt, MD
Assistant Professor of Pediatrics, Case Western Reserve University School of Medicine; Attending Physician, Pediatric Nephrology, Rainbow Babies and Children's Hospital, Cleveland, Ohio
The Kidney and Urinary Tract

Michele C. Walsh-Sukys, MD, MS
Associate Professor of Pediatrics, Case Western Reserve University School of Medicine; Co-Director, Neonatal Intensive Care Unit, Rainbow Babies and Children's Hospital, Cleveland, Ohio
Perinatal Services and Resources

Michiko Watanabe, PhD
Associate Professor, Case Western Reserve University School of Medicine; Associate Professor, University Hospital Research Institute, Rainbow Babies and Children's Hospital, Cleveland, Ohio
The Cardiovascular System (Part One)

David B. Wilson, MD, PhD
Chief of Pediatric Hematology-Oncology, Associate Professor of Pediatrics and Molecular Biology and Pharmacology, Washington University School of Medicine; Associate Professor of Pediatrics, St. Louis Children's Hospital, St. Louis, Missouri
The Blood and Hematopoietic System

Deanne E. Wilson-Costello, MD
Assistant Professor, Case Western Reserve University School of Medicine; University Hospitals of Cleveland, Cleveland, Ohio
Follow-up for High-Risk Neonates

Richard B. Wolf, DO, FACOG
Adjunct Assistant Professor of Obstetrics and Gynecology, Uniformed Services University of the Health Sciences School of Medicine, Bethesda, Maryland; Attending Perinatologist, Division of Maternal-Fetal Medicine, Charette Health Care Center, Naval Medical Center, Portsmouth, Virginia
Amniotic Fluid and Nonimmune Hydrops Fetalis

Jerome Y. Yager, MD, FRCP(C)
Professor of Pediatrics (Pediatric Neurology), University of Saskatchewan College of Medicine, Royal University Hospital, Saskatoon, Saskatchewan, Canada
The Central Nervous System (Parts One and Six)

Mervin C. Yoder, MD
Professor of Pediatrics, Biochemistry, and Molecular Biology, Indiana University School of Medicine; Attending Physician, James Whitcomb Riley Hospital for Children, Indianapolis, Indiana
The Immune System (Part One)

Kenneth G. Zahka, MD
Professor of Pediatrics, Case Western Reserve University School of Medicine; Director, Pediatric Cardiology, Rainbow Babies and Children's Hospital, Cleveland, Ohio
The Cardiovascular System (Parts Two through Seven and Nine)

Arthur B. Zinn, MD, PhD
Associate Professor of Genetics and Pediatrics, Case Western Reserve University School of Medicine; Attending Physician, Center for Human Genetics, University Hospitals of Cleveland, Cleveland, Ohio
Inborn Errors of Metabolism

Preface

It is with a sense of awesome relief that the Seventh Edition of this book can finally be called complete. The metamorphosis of a textbook is painfully slow, but the satisfaction of knowing that the final product reflects our stated goals and aspirations serves as more than adequate compensation for the long wait. Eleanor Roosevelt said, "The future belongs to those who believe in the beauty of their dreams." We do. There have been many changes and many new authors, all of whom have graciously given their time and knowledge to ensure that the book contains the most up-to-date information and recommendations for practice based on the best available evidence.

The foundation for success in *Neonatal-Perinatal Medicine* has been the ability to apply knowledge of the fundamental pathophysiology of the various neonatal disorders to safe interventions. Molecular, biologic, and technologic advances have facilitated the diagnosis, monitoring, and therapy of these complex disorders. Advances at the bench have been transformed to the bedside, and survival statistics reveal steady improvements. Nonetheless, whereas the survival rates may be reasons to rejoice, the high early morbidity and persistent neurodevelopmental problems remain causes for concern. These problems include chronic lung disease, nosocomial infections, necrotizing enterocolitis, hypoxic-ischemic encephalopathy, cerebral palsy, and the inability to sustain the intrauterine rate of growth when infants are delivered prematurely. These problems need to be addressed in addition to the complex birth defects and genetic disorders that now loom as major problems in the intensive care unit.

In this millennium we must enhance our efforts to ensure intact survival. We need to learn from each other and attempt to decipher why and how there is such great intercenter and international variability in practice and outcomes. Through techniques of benchmarking and quality improvement we must determine the factors that are important at the centers with the best individual results for a particular problem and be able to apply them to all centers. We must renew our efforts to avoid medication errors and unnecessary complications that may lead to irreparable harm for our patients. Only the highest standards of care, based on the best available evidence, are acceptable.

We are truly grateful to all of the behind-the-scenes contributors, as well as all of our colleagues who continue to willingly contribute their time and knowledge so that we may all benefit from their expertise. Once again we have been blessed with an in-house editor, Bonnie Siner, to whom we cannot adequately express our thanks. She is the glue behind the binding in the book. Harcourt Health Sciences and Mosby have once again provided the resources to accomplish this mammoth task. We acknowledge, especially, the help of Lisette Bralow and Judith Fletcher.

Avroy A. Fanaroff, MB, BCh, FRCP(E), DCH
Richard J. Martin, MB, BS, FRACP

Contents

I

The Field of Neonatal-Perinatal Medicine

1

From Infant Hatcheries to Intensive Care: Some Highlights of the Century of Neonatal Medicine

Tonse N. K. Raju

We trust we have been forgiven for coining the words, "neonatology" and "neonatologist." We do not recall ever having seen them in print. The one designates the art and science of diagnosis and treatment of disorders of the newborn infant, the other the physician whose primary concern lies in the specialty . . . We are not advocating now that a new subspecialty be lopped from pediatrics . . . yet such a subdivision . . . [has] as much merit as does pediatric hematology . . .

A. J. SCHAFFER, 1960[71]

The American Board of Pediatrics offered the first examination in the subspecialty of *neonatal-perinatal medicine* in 1975. Through February 2000, the board had certified 3708 men and women as neonatologists —practitioners of a discipline that had no formal name 40 years ago. The 1950 *Index Medicus* listed 218 annual publications under the *Infant, Newborn* subject heading. In 1967, the number had increased to 6365, and in 1999, to 10,102.[59] Dr. Schaffer need not have apologized for his visionary understatement—the specialty and the physicians he christened proved him immensely prophetic. Although it was not "lopped" from pediatrics, this *final frontier* (another Schaffer term) carved a niche of its own, bridging obstetrics with pediatrics and intensive care with primary care.

The formal birth of neonatology may appear to be recent, but its roots extend into the 19th century, when systematic and organized care began for groups of premature infants. This chapter traces the origins and growth of modern perinatal and neonatal medicine, with a brief perspective on its promises and failures. The reader may consult scholarly monographs and review articles on specific topics for in-depth analyses.*

---

*References 6, 7, 22, 24, 61, 73, and 77.

PERINATAL PIONEERS

Many scientists played key roles in developing the basic concepts in neonatal-perinatal medicine that helped rationalize the evolving clinical care and inspired further research. For the sake of brevity, only a few are shown in Figure 1–1.

Medicinal chemistry (later called biochemistry) and classical physiology gained popularity and acceptance toward the end of the 19th century, leading to studies on biochemical and physiologic problems in the fetus and the newborn. Sir Joseph Barcroft[8, 34] and Jeffery Dawes in England (gas exchange and nutritional transfer across the placenta and oxygen carrying in fetal and adult hemoglobin); Arvo Ylppö in Finland (neonatal nutrition, jaundice, and thermoregulation); John Lind in Sweden (circulatory physiology); and Clement Smith[75] (fetal and neonatal respiratory physiology), Joseph DeLee[26, 27] (who founded the first lying-in hospital in Chicago and who researched incubators and high-risk obstetrics), Richard Day (temperature regulation, retinopathy of prematurity, and jaundice), Harry Gordon[38] (nutrition), and others in the United States made numerous basic contributions and trained scores of scientists from around the world. Dr. Clement Smith once said, "If you were interested in babies and liked Boston, I was the only

2

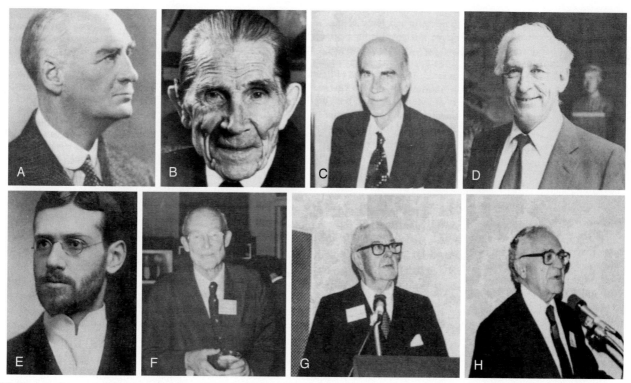

FIGURE 1–1. Some pioneers in perinatal and neonatal physiology and medicine. *A,* Joseph Barcroft; *B,* Arvo Ylppö; *C,* John Lind; *D,* William Liley; *E,* Joseph DeLee; *F,* Richard Day; *G,* Clement Smith; *H,* Harry Gordon. (*A,* From Barcroft J: Research on Pre-natal Life, vol 1, Oxford, Blackwell Scientific, 1977, courtesy Blackwell Scientific; *B–D, F–H,* From Smith GF, Vidyasagar D [eds]: Historical Review and Recent Advances in Neonatal and Perinatal Medicine. Vol 1, Neonatal Medicine. Evansville, IN, Ross Publication, 1984, pp ix, xix, xxii, xvi, xii, xiv, respectively, courtesy Mead Johnson Nutritional; *E,* Courtesy of Mrs. Nancy DeLee Frank, Chicago, IL.)

wheel in town!"[60] Table 1–1 highlights some of the milestones in perinatal medicine.

HIGH-RISK FETUS AND PERINATAL OBSTETRICS

Because so many deaths occurred during early infancy, many cultures adopted remarkably innovative methods to deal with the tragedies. According to a Jewish tradition, full, yearlong mourning is not required for infants who die before 30 days of age.[40] In some Asian ethnic groups, infant-naming ceremonies are held only after several months, until which time the baby is simply called *it*. In India, the first infant who survives after the death of a previous newborn sibling is often given an odd or coarse-sounding name, to prevent evil spirits from repeating their deeds. In her book on the history of the Middle Ages, Barbara Tuchman notes that infants were seldom depicted in medieval artworks.[83] When they were shown (e.g., the infant Jesus), women in the pictures looked away from the infant, ostensibly conveying a sense of respect, but in fact suggesting fearful aloofness.

Since antiquity, the care of pregnant women has been the purview of midwives, grandmothers, and experienced female elders in the community. Wet nurses helped when mothers were unavailable or unwilling to nurse their infants. Little or no assistance

was generally needed for normal or uncomplicated labor and delivery. For complicated deliveries, however, male doctors were summoned, but they could do little, for many of them lacked expertise or interest in treating women. Disasters were therefore common, rendering labor and delivery the most dreaded period in the lives of pregnant women.[43] As recently as the early 1900s, *accidents of childbirth*—unexpected intrapartum complications—accounted for 50% to 70% of all maternal deaths in England and Wales.[17, 56] Because the immediate concern during most high-risk deliveries was saving the mother, sick newborn infants were naturally ignored, and their death rates remained very high.

Rarely, however, happy outcomes did occur. In one of the oldest works of art depicting labor and delivery (Fig. 1–2*A*), a bearded man and his assistant are standing behind a woman in labor, holding devices remarkably similar to the modern obstetric forceps. The midwife has delivered an evidently live infant. In Figure 1–2*B*, three infants from a set of quadruplets, nicely swaddled, have been placed on the mother, as the unwrapped fourth infant is being handed to her for nursing. A divine figure in the background is blessing the newcomers.

Cesarean sections were seldom carried out on living women before the 13th century. Even subsequently, the procedure was performed only as a final act of desperation. Contrary to popular belief, Julius Caesar's birth was not likely by cesarean section.

TABLE 1–1   SOME MILESTONES IN PERINATAL MEDICINE

CATEGORY	YEAR(S)	DESCRIPTION
Antenatal aspects	1752	Queen Charlotte's Hospital, the world's first maternity hospital, is founded in London.[57]
	1915–1924	Dame Janet Campbell introduces outlines of regular prenatal visits, which become a standard.
	1923–1925,	Estrogen and progesterone are discovered.
	1928	First pregnancy test is described in which women's urine is shown to cause changes in mouse ovaries.
Fetal assessment	1543	Vesalius observes fetal breathing movements in pigs.
	1634	Ambroise Paré teaches that absence of movement suggests a dead fetus.
	1819, 1821	René Laënnec introduces the stethoscope in 1819, and his friend Kergaradec shows that fetal heart sounds can be heard using it.
	1866	Forceps are recommended when there is "weakening of the fetal heart rate."
	1903	Einthoven publishes his work on the electrocardiogram.
	1906	The first recording of fetal heart tracings is taken.
	1908	The term *fetal distress* is introduced.
	1948–1953	There are developments in the external tocodynamometer.
	1953	Virginia Apgar describes her scoring system.[3]
	1957–1963	Systematic studies are conducted on fetal heart rate monitoring.
	1970	Dawes reports studies on breathing movement in fetal lambs.
	1980	Fetal Doppler studies begin.
	1981	Nelson and Ellenberg report that Apgar scores are poor predictors of neurologic outcome.
Labor and delivery	c 1000–500 BC	In Ayurveda, the ancient Hindu medical system, doctors describe obstetric intruments.
	98–138	Soranus develops the birthing stool and other instruments.
	1500s	There are isolated reports of cesarean sections on living women.
	1610	The first intentional cesarean section is documented.
	1700s	The Chamberlene forceps are kept as a family secret for three generations.
	1921	The lower segment cesarean section is reported.
	1953	The modern vacuum extractor is introduced.
Fetal physiology	1900–1950	Sir Joseph Barcroft, Dawes, Lind, Liley, and others study physiologic principles of placental gas exchange and fetal circulation.

See references 2, 41, 43, 61, and 77 for primary citations.

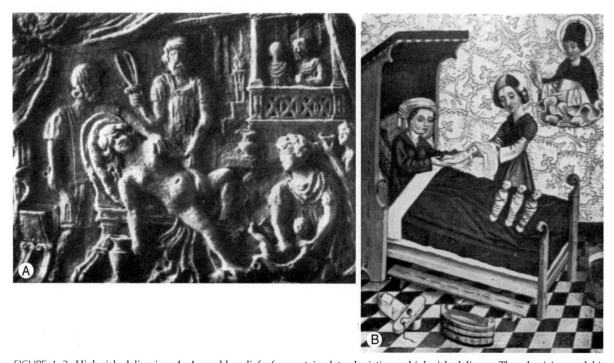

FIGURE 1–2. High-risk deliveries. *A*, A marble relief of uncertain date depicting a high-risk delivery. The physician and his assistant in the background are holding devices similar to the modern obstetric forceps. A midwife has just helped deliver a live infant while two people are looking through the window. *B*, Delivery of quadruplets. (From Graham, H: Eternal Eve: The History of Gynecology & Obstetrics. New York, Doubleday, 1951, pp 68, 172.)

Because Caesar's mother was alive during his reign, historians believe that she probably delivered him vaginally. The term probably originated from *lex caesarea*, in turn from *lex regia*, the "royal law" prohibiting burial of corpses of pregnant women without removal of their fetuses.[11, 89] The procedure allowed for baptism (or a similar blessing) if the child was alive, or burial otherwise. Infants surviving the ordeal of cesarean birth were assumed to possess special powers, as supposedly did Shakespeare's Macduff, "not of a woman born," but of a corpse, thus able to slay Macbeth.[54]

Soranus of Ephesus (38–138 AD) influenced obstetric practice for 1600 years like no other physician from antiquity. His *Gynecology*, perhaps the first formal textbook of perinatal medicine, was rediscovered in 1870 and translated into English in 1956.[82] In it are superb chapters on podalic version, obstructed labor, multiple gestations, fetal malformations, and other maternal and fetal disorders. In an age of magic and the occult, Soranus insisted that midwives must be educated and free from superstitions, and he forbade wet nurses from drinking alcohol lest it render the infant "excessively sleepy." The chapter "How to Recognize the Newborn that Is Worth Rearing" may be one of the earliest accounts on the viability of sick newborn infants—a topic of great concern even today.

MIDWIVES AND PERINATAL CARE

In spite of an occasional caricaturing (Fig. 1–3), the midwife bore the burden of the obstetric care of the entire community for thousands of years. Men disliked obstetrics and women shied away from male

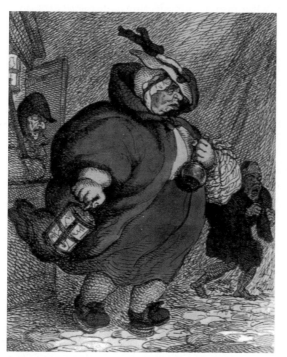

FIGURE 1–3. On call. *A Midwife Going to a Labour* caricature by Thomas Rowlandson, 1811. (Courtesy of The British Museum, London.)

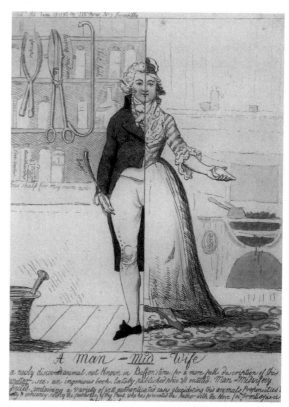

FIGURE 1–4. Man-Midwife. (Courtesy of Clements C. Fry Print Collections, Harvey Cushing/John Hay Whitney Medical Library, New Haven, CT.)

doctors because of modesty. Good midwives were therefore always in great demand, and many of them held important social and political positions in European courts.[43, 61, 86]

The emergence of man-midwives (Fig. 1–4) in England had a major effect on high-risk obstetric practice. Peter Chamberlene the elder (1575–1628) is usually credited for inventing the modern obstetric forceps.[43, 61, 63] However, for 150 years, the instrument remained a trade secret through three generations in his family. By then, others had developed similar devices, and patients had been associating good obstetric outcomes with male doctors—a key factor in transforming midwifery to a male-dominated craft.[43] Some historians also argue that the shift from female midwifery to male midwifery was the result of a culmination of changing social values and gender relationships that led women to make voluntary choices about their bodies.[86] Today's high rates of home deliveries and increasing roles for female midwives are interesting reversals of trends seen in the late 18th century—albeit originating from women's personal choices and subtle pressures from the health insurance industries.

NEONATAL RESUSCITATION: TALES OF HEROISM AND DESPERATION

Popular artworks and centuries-old medical writings provide accounts of the miraculous revival of apparently dead adults and children.[66] These are tales of successes, for the failures were buried. Attempts to "stimulate" and revive apparently dead newborn infants included such practices as beating, shaking, yelling, fumigating, dipping in ice-cold water, and dilating and blowing smoke into the rectum.[25, 30, 66] Oxygen administration through an orogastric tube to revive asphyxiated infants persisted well into the mid-1950s, when James and Apgar showed conclusively that the therapy was useless.[1, 52]

APGAR AND THE LANGUAGE OF ASPHYXIA

Few scientists this century influenced the course of neonatal resuscitation like Dr. Virginia Apgar (1909–1974). A surgeon, she chose obstetric anesthesia as a career, and her scoring system inaugurated the modern era of assessing infants at birth based on simple clinical examination.[3] Right or wrong, the Apgar score became the language of asphyxia. Whereas "giving the Apgar" often became a ritual, its profound effect was on formalizing the process of "seeing" and assessing infants at birth and communicating the findings in a consistent way. This process led to the formal steps of resuscitation at birth based on the score. Few people know that it was also Dr. Apgar who introduced umbilical artery catheterization.[16] A woman of enormous energy, talent, and compassion, Apgar was honored with her depiction on a 1994 U.S. postage stamp (Fig. 1–5).

FOUNDLING ASYLUMS AND INFANT CARE

In its early days, the Roman Empire faced a trend of decreasing population growth. The emperors taxed bachelors and rewarded married couples to encourage procreation.[76] In 315 AD, Emperor Constantine decreed that all "foundlings" would become slaves of those raising them, and he had hoped to encourage the raising of orphans and to curb infanticide. Similar humanitarian efforts by kings and the Council of the Roman Church led to the institutionalization of infant care by establishing *foundling asylums* for abandoned infants,[76] also called *hospitals for the innocent*—the world's first children's hospitals.

Parents of unwanted infants "dropped off" their babies into a revolving receptacle at the door of such asylums, rang the doorbell, and disappeared into the night (Fig. 1–6). Such accounts are poignant reminders of the contemporary problem of child abandonment. The states of Alabama, Minnesota, and Texas have now begun programs to save "dumpster babies," abandoned newborn infants. Fourteen other states are planning to implement similar programs.[69]

Founded with altruistic motives, foundling asylums adopted pragmatic techniques for fundraising. In 18th century France, lotteries were held and souvenirs were sold. In May 1749, George Frederick Handel gave a concert to support London's Hospital for the Maintenance and Education of Exposed and Deserted Young Children. The final item of the program was the playing of "The Foundling Hymn."[76]

SAVING BABIES TO MAN THE ARMY

Around the period of the French Revolution, the infant mortality rate in France was appallingly high, exceeding 50%. In 1789, the Revolutionary Council enacted a remarkable decree, proclaiming that working-class parents "have a right to the nation's succors at all times."[76] The postrevolutionary zeal regarding equality and fraternity stimulated such reforms, heralding an idealistic welfare state. In that era in France began the notion of collecting valid statistics on children, creating the world's first national databases.[76]

By the late 1800s, however, France faced a problem similar to that of ancient Rome—a negative population growth. The birth rate had declined and infant mortality remained high, alarming the military brass that was deeply engaged in battles with Prussia. Calling for remedial action, commissions were set up to study "depopulation," and programs were implemented to improve maternal and neonatal care.[6, 7, 22, 24, 76] Young parents were exhorted to uphold their patriotism and bear more children to "man the future French Armies." It is the irony of our times that such noble actions as saving babies were motivated by such brutal needs as enhancing military might.

AN INGENIOUS CONTRIVANCE, THE *COUVEUSE,* AND PREMATURE STATIONS

A popular story of the origin of modern incubator technology is that upon seeing the poultry section during a casual visit to the Paris zoo in 1878, Stéphane Tarnier (1828–1897), a renowned obstetrician, conceived the idea of "incubators" similar to the "brooding hen" or *couveuse*.[6, 7, 22, 24] He then asked M. Odile

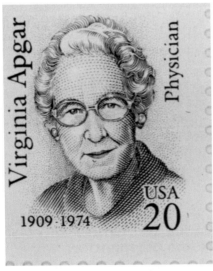

FIGURE 1–5. Virginia Apgar U.S. postage stamp. (Courtesy of the United States Postal Service.)

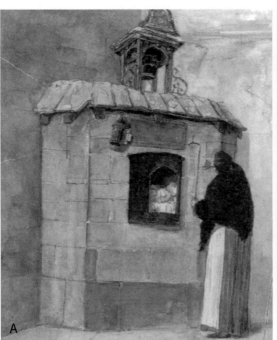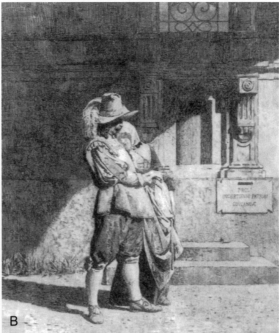

FIGURE 1–6. Foundling homes. *A, Le Tour*—Revolving receptacle. Mother ringing a bell to notify those within that she is leaving her baby in the foundling home (watercolor by Herman Vogel, France, 1889). *B, Remorce* (Remorse)—Parents after placing their infant in a foundling home (engraving and etching by Alberto Maso Gilli, France, 1875). (*A and B*, Courtesy of the Museum of the History of Medicine, Academy of Medicine, Toronto, Ontario, Canada; From Spaulding M, Welch P: Nurturing Yesterday's Child. A Portrayal of the Drake Collection of Pediatric History. Philadelphia, B.C. Decker, 1991, p 110 and p 119, respectively.)

Martin, an instrument maker, to construct similar equipment for use with babies. With a "thermo-syphon" method to heat the outside with an alcohol lamp, Martin devised a sufficiently ventilated, one-cubic-meter, double-walled metal cage, spacious enough to hold two premature babies. The first couveuses were installed at the Paris Maternity Hospital in 1880. Tarnier documented dramatic improvements in the survival of premature infants.

Perhaps Tarnier knew of other incubators before his famous visit to the zoo.[7] Yet, it is Tarnier, and Piérre Budin (1846–1907) and Alfred Auvard, two of his students and associates, that we credit for institutionalizing care of premature babies. By using several incubators side by side, they developed the concept of caring for groups of premature infants in geographically identified units in their hospital.[6, 7, 80] Budin and Auvard also improved the original couveuse by replacing its walls with glass and using simpler methods for heating it. Their combined efforts had a major influence on the evolution of incubator technology during the first half of the 20th century in Europe and the United States (Fig. 1–7 and Table 1–2).

In 1884, Tarnier made another major invention. He developed a small, flexible rubber tube, introducing it through the mouth and extending it into the stomach of premature infants, so that milk could be directly dripped into the stomach. He called this method of nutritional support the *gavage feeding*. A large number of premature infants had been surviving by then, enabling implementation of gavage feeding into clinical practice immediately; the two Tarnier innovations soon gave impressive results.[15, 21] Tarnier

also made a bold recommendation that the legal definition of viability should be 180 days of gestation; this was opposed by contemporary obstetricians.[7]

THE INCUBATORS ON THE ROAD AND PREMATURE BABY SHOWS

In the late 1890s, a bizarre set of episodes led to an era of "premature baby side shows"—a clever, if dubious undertaking that lasted nearly 50 years.[6, 7, 73, 80] About 15 years into using incubators in Paris, Budin had gained an international reputation as an expert on premature infants. According to a later account by one Dr. Martin Couney (a Budin associate of doubtful medical credentials), Budin had felt a need to popularize the French technology abroad and show the world the value of "conserving" premature infants. It seems that Budin asked Couney to organize a special pavilion for exhibiting incubators at the 1896 Berlin Exposition. (There is some doubt about the accuracy of this account.[7]) To add a sense of drama, Couney brought six premature infants from Rudolph Virchow's maternity unit in Berlin and exhibited the infants inside the six incubators he had brought from Paris. Couney coined a catchy phrase for the show—*kinderbrutanstalt* or *child hatchery*—igniting the imagination of the public that was thirsty for sensational scientific breakthroughs.

The premature baby exhibit was an astounding success. Comic songs and gags were constructed in its honor; at one German mark per visit, the child

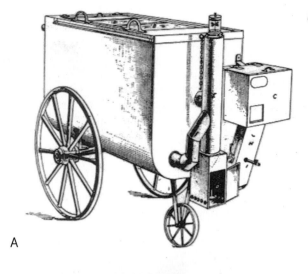

A

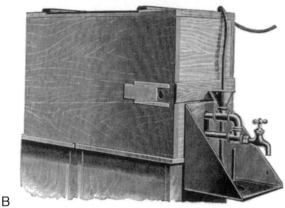

B

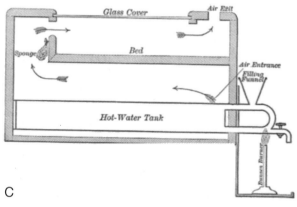

C

FIGURE 1–7. Early incubators. Rotch incubator (*A*), circa 1893. Holt incubator (*B*) and schematics of the Holt incubator (*C*). (*A*, From Cone TE Jr: History of American Pediatrics. Boston, Little Brown, 1979, pp 57 and 58, courtesy of Little Brown; *B* and *C*, From Holt LE: The Diseases of Infants & Children. New York. Appleton, 1897, pp 12 and 13, courtesy of Appleton.)

hatchery outdrew the Congo Village, sky riders, and Tyrolean yodelers. Thousands delighted in seeing the marvel of human infants being incubated inside heated cages, similar to chicks in hatcheries. Fortunately for Budin, all six premature infants survived,

probably because he had chosen "healthy-looking" babies, who had survived for at least 5 days.

Spurred by the Berlin success, Couney convinced Budin to continue such exhibitions and took the incubators to Great Britain's 1897 Victorian Era Exhibition. However, things were not so simple in Britain, for there he met with British pride: No self-respecting Londoner would let *his* premature infant be placed inside a *French* incubator! Thus, Couney requested that Budin provide him with babies, and Budin complied. "A bunch of Parisian premature infants" were transported across the English Channel in wash baskets warmed with hot-water bottles and pillows and exhibited in London's Fair.[6, 7, 73]

On May 29, 1897, an editorial in *The Lancet* welcomed the incubator show.[36] Concern was expressed, however, that a majority of the public might not benefit from the incubator technology, because the middle class was "not poor enough to go to the hospital, nor rich enough to purchase" the incubators. The journal proposed establishing large "incubator stations" similar to "fire stations," from which the incubators could be loaned to the needy families. Thus, the origin of the phrase "premature infant station" has its roots in the pages of *The Lancet*.

Within 8 months of the show at Earl Court, the incubator craze was all over Britain, prompting another *Lancet* editorial.[37] This time it complained about "copycat exhibitions" organized by "all sorts of showmen . . . just as they might have exhibited marionettes, fat women, or other such catch-penny monstrosity." In many of the shows, the infants in incubators had to breathe cigar smoke and the exhaled air from thousands of visitors. Often, obnoxious odors emanated from the live leopards kept in cages next to the baby incubators to provide a dramatic contrast. Fraud was common. Some show owners brought term infants, claiming that the infants were growing, premature babies. An indignant *Lancet* asked, "Is it in keeping with the dignity of science that incubators and living babies should be exhibited amidst the aunt-sallies, merry-go-rounds, five-legged mules, wild animals, clowns, and penny peep-shows, along with the glare and noise of a vulgar fair?"

Within a year of gaining popularity at Earl Court, Couney set sail to New York, and in 1898 he organized the first U.S. incubator show at the Omaha Trans Mississippi Exposition. Having made the United States his home by 1903, Couney began the saga of premature baby shows that lasted for nearly 40 years. He took the shows to state fairs, traveling circuses, and science expositions all over the United States (Fig. 1–8). He also established a permanent annual exhibit at New York's Coney Island.

Academic physicians were uncomfortable with making a spectacle of babies—but they grudgingly recognized the value of publicity and accepted those benefits. It is estimated that about 80,000 "Couney babies" were raised in all of the Couney exhibits. The last of the baby shows was held during the 1939–1940 season—at its site in Atlantic City there now stands a Holiday Inn. A bronze plaque has been placed on the

TABLE 1–2 THE EVOLUTION OF INCUBATORS

YEAR(S)	DEVELOPER/PRODUCT	COMMENTS
1835, c1850	George von Ruehl (1769–1846)	A physician to Czarina Feodorovna, wife of Czar Paul I, Ruehl develops the first known incubator for the Imperial Foundling Hospital in St. Petersburg. About 40 of these "warming tubs" are installed in the Moscow Foundling Hospital in 1850.
1857	Jean-Louis-Paul Denucé (1824–1889)	The first *published* account of introducing an incubator is a 400-word report by Denucé. This is a "double-walled" cradle.
1880–1883	Stéphane Tarnier (1828–1897)	The Tarnier incubator is developed by M. Odile Martin, installed in 1880 at the Port-Royal Maternité.
1884	Carl Credé (1819–1892)	Credé reports the results of 647 infants treated over 20 years using an incubator similar to that of Denucé.
1887	John Bartlett	Bartlett reads a paper on a "warming-crib" based on Tarnier's concept, but uses a "thermo-syphon."
1893	Piérre Budin (1846–1907)	Budin popularizes the Tarnier incubator and establishes the world's first "special care unit for premature infants" at Maternité and Clinique Tarnier in Paris.
1893	Thomas Morgan Rotch (1849–1914)	The first American incubator with a built-in scale, wheels, and fresh-air delivery system is developed; the equipment is very expensive and elaborate.
1897	The Holt Incubator	A simplified version of the Rotch incubator is developed. In this double-walled wooden box, hot water circulates between the walls.
1897–1920s	Edward Brown, John Lyons, Joseph DeLee, Frank Allin	Many modifications are made to the early incubators by American and European physicians. These are called "baby-tents," "baby boxes," "warming beds," and other names.
1922	Julius Hess	Hess introduces his famous incubator with an electric heating system. For transportation, he develops special boxes that can be plugged into the cigarette lighters in Chicago's taxicabs.
1930–1950s	Large-scale commercial incubators	There is worldwide distribution of Air Shields and other commercial ventilators.
1970–1980	Modern incubators	Transport incubators with built-in ventilators and monitoring equipment are developed—mobile intensive care units.

See references 6, 7, 22–24, 73, and 74 for primary citations.

wall next to the entrance to the hotel, commemorating the Couney shows.[73]

In the early 1920s in Chicago, Dr. Julius Hess and his nurse Ms. Evelyn Lundeen (Fig. 1–9) developed an incubator built on the concept of a double-walled metallic "cage," with warm water circulating between the walls. Hess used electricity for heating, and he devised a system to administer free-flow oxygen. The only extant Hess incubator known to this author is now on display at the Spertus Museum in Chicago (Fig. 1–10).

In May 1922, Hess founded the first Premature Infant Station in the United States at Sarah Morris Children's Hospital (of the Michael Reese Medical Center) in Chicago. With meticulous attention to environmental control, aseptic practices, and a regimental approach to feeding schedules using the "hands-free" method of caring, Hess and Lundeen achieved spectacular survival rates.[47, 67] Hess made Couney's acquaintance in 1922; the particulars of their relationship are not clear, but Hess respected Couney for his contributions to popularizing infant care. In fact, Hess and Ms. Lundeen helped Couney organize an exhibition at the 1933–1934 Chicago World's Fair, which was also a great hit.[67]

What of incubators in general and baby shows in particular in today's context? That the incubators were able to save babies who would otherwise die became a powerful symbol of the might of the machine. In that heroic age of mechanical revolution, this notion was all too appealing to the public and to professionals, leading to a euphoric hope that any and all human problems could be solved by machines. Such tunnel vision is quite prevalent even in today's neonatal intensive care units (NICUs). Thus, the incubator stands as the most enduring symbol of the spectacular success of modern intensive care as well as (paradoxically) its glaring failures.

The baby incubator shows of the past, on the other hand, also evoke hauntingly familiar contemporary themes. Today's news media's clamoring for stories of medical breakthroughs and the public's voyeuristic curiosity about such intensely personal events as the birth of quintuplets or sextuplets are similar to the spectacle of premature baby exhibitions. The shows are also symbolic of the difficulty in preserving a delicate balance between information and education and public awareness and sensationalism. Traveling baby shows were similar to traveling moon rock exhibits, which exploited the popularity of man's landing on the moon and helped increase NASA's annual budgets.

SUPPORTIVE CARE AND OXYGEN THERAPY

In a single-page note in 1891, Bonnaire referred to Dr. Tarnier's use of oxygen in treating "debilitated"

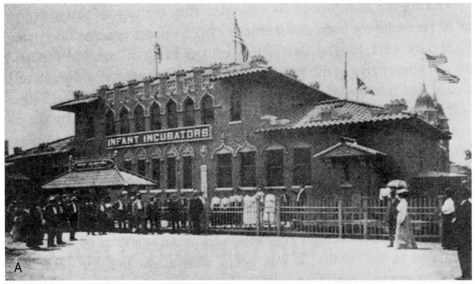

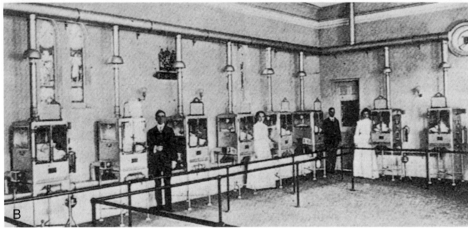

FIGURE 1-8. Incubator baby shows. *A,* People lined up to see the Infant Incubator Show, Buffalo, New York. *B,* Interior of an incubator baby show, Buffalo, New York. (*A* and *B,* From Silverman WA: Incubator-baby side shows. Pediatrics 64:127, 1979, courtesy of the American Academy of Pediatrics, 1979.)

premature infants two years earlier[14]—this was the first published reference to the administration of supplemental oxygen in premature infants for a purpose other than resuscitation.

However, the use of oxygen in premature infants did not become routine until the 1920s. Initially, a mixture of oxygen and carbon dioxide—instead of oxygen alone—was employed to treat asphyxia-induced narcosis. It was argued that oxygen relieved hypoxia, whereas carbon dioxide stimulated the respiratory center[80]; however, oxygen alone was reserved for "pure asphyxia" (whatever that meant). Only after mobile oxygen tanks became available for general use by the mid-1940s did the use of oxygen during delivery become possible on a routine basis.[51, 74]

The success of incubator care brought new and unexpected challenges.[68] Innovative methods had to be developed to feed the increasing number of premature infants who were surviving for longer periods than ever before. Their growth needed to be moni-

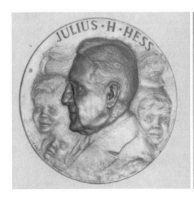

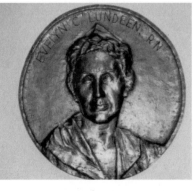

FIGURE 1-9. Hess and Lundeen medallions at the Michael Reese Hospital, Chicago. (Photo courtesy of Tonse N.K. Raju)

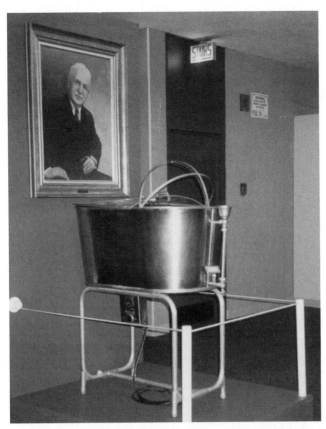

FIGURE 1–10. The only known extant Hess incubator on display at the Spertus Museum in Chicago. (Courtesy of the International Museum of Surgical History, Chicago, and the Spertus Museum, Chicago).

tored, and illnesses related to prematurity, such as sepsis, apnea, anemia, jaundice, and respiratory distress, had to be studied and treated. Of all of these, providing ventilatory assistance became the most urgent necessity.

VENTILATORY CARE: "EXTENDED RESUSCITATION"

The first mechanical instrument used for intermittent positive pressure ventilation in newborn infants was *aerophore pulmonaire,* a simple device developed by French obstetrician Dr. Gairal.[65, 66] It was a rubber bulb attached to a J-shaped tube. By placing the bent end of the tube into the infant's upper airway, one could pump air into the lungs. Holt recommended its use for resuscitation in his influential 1897 book[48].

Before starting mechanical ventilation, however, one needed to *cannulate* the airways, a task nearly impossible without a laryngoscope and an endotracheal tube. James Blundell (1790–1878), a Scottish obstetrician, was the first to use a mechanical device for tracheal intubation in living newborn infants.[13, 32] Introducing two fingers of his left hand over the infant's tongue, he would feel the epiglottis and then guide a silver pipe into the trachea with his right hand. His *tracheal pipe* had a blunt distal end and two

side holes. By blowing air into the tube about 30 times a minute until the heartbeat began, Blundell saved hundreds of infants with birth asphyxia, as well as those with laryngeal diphtheria. His method of tracheal intubation is practiced in many countries even today.[85]

In the late 19th century, a wide array of instruments evolved to provide longer periods of augmented or extended ventilation for those infants who had been resuscitated in the labor room. Most of the early instruments, however, were designed for use in adults and were used later in newborns and infants, particularly to treat paralytic polio and laryngeal diphtheria.[45, 78, 79]

The *iron lung* (or "man-can") was one of the earliest mechanical ventilatory devices (Fig. 1–11), and a U.S. patent had been issued for it in 1876.[42] In other ventilatory equipment, varying methods for rhythmic inflation and deflation of the lungs were used for prolonged ventilation.* Among those, the Fell-O'Dwyer apparatus used a unique foot-operated bellows system connected to an implement similar to the aerophore bulb.[25, 65, 66]

Between 1930 and 1950 there were sporadic but important reports of providing prolonged assisted ventilation in the newborn.[62, 78, 79] Only since the late 1950s through the 1960s, however, did more NICUs begin providing such ventilatory assistance regularly (Table 1–3), and not until the early 1970s, when continuous positive pressure was incorporated into ventilatory devices, did ventilatory care become predictably successful.[44, 58, 62, 78]

SUPPORTIVE CARE: INTRAVENOUS FLUID AND BLOOD TRANSFUSIONS

When it comes to intravenous therapy, our legacy is one of bloodletting, not of transfusing. Blundel (of intubation fame) also made a major contribution to

---

*References 12, 19, 20, 30, 39, 45, 46, 49, and 79.

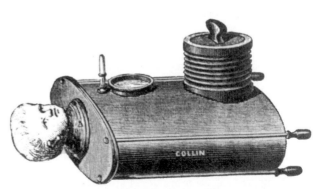

FIGURE 1–11. The Man-Can, circa 1873 to 1875. A hand-held negative-pressure ventilatory device for which a patent was applied in 1876. (From DeBono E: Eureka: How and When the Greatest Inventions Were Made: An Illustrated History of Inventions from the Wheel to the Computer. New York, Holt, Rinehart and Winston, 1974, p 159.)

TABLE 1–3 VENTILATORY CARE AND RESPIRATORY DISORDERS

CATEGORY	APPROXIMATE TIME SPAN	PROCEDURES AND TECHNIQUES
Resuscitation and oxygen	From antiquity to early 1970s	Mouth-to-mouth breathing (although it fell from favor in the late 18th century, because many influential physicians declared it as a "vulgar method" of revival)
	1878	Tarnier uses oxygen in debilitated premature babies
	1900–1930s	The Schultz, Sylvester, and Laborde methods of resuscitation involve various forms of swinging babies, traction of the tongue, and compression of the chest, respectively
	1930–1960s	O_2 administration to the oral cavity through a rubber catheter
	1930s–1940s	Tight-fitting tracheal tube and direct tracheal O_2 administration
	1913–1920s	Byrd-Dew method: while immersed in warm water, alternate flexing and extending the pelvis to help the "lungs open"
	1850–1930s	Dilatation of the rectum
	1930–1950s	Inhalation of O_2 and 7% CO_2 mixture (for morphine-induced narcosis)
	1940–1950s	Positive pressure air-lock (Bloxsom method)
	1940–late 1950s	The concept that "air in the digestive tract is good for survival" is promoted; administration of O_2 to the stomach
	1950–late 1960s	Hyperbaric oxygen in Vickers Pressure Chamber
	1950–1960s	Mouth-to-mouth or mouth-to-endotracheal tube breathing
Assisted ventilation	1930s–1980s	Alexander Graham Bell develops a negative-pressure jacket
	1930–1950	Negative pressure ventilators and iron lungs, used rarely in infants
	1960s	Positive pressure respirators used for prolonged ventilatory support
	1971	Continuous positive airway pressure introduced for use in newborns
	1973	Intermittent mandatory ventilator
	1970–1980s	High-frequency ventilators; continuous monitoring of pulmonary function
Surfactant	1903	Hochheim reports "hyaline membranes" noted in the lungs of infants with respiratory distress syndrome (RDS)
	1940–1950s	Clinical descriptions and pathology studied
	1955–1956	Pattle discovers surfactant in pulmonary edema foam and lung extracts
	1959	Avery and Mead demonstrate absence of surfactant in infants with hyaline membrane disease[4]
	1971	Gluck introduces the lecithin-sphingomyelin ratio
	1973	Liggins suggests that antenatal steroid helps mature the pulmonary surfactant system
	1980	First effective clinical trial of postnatal surfactant therapy (bovine, Fujiwara)
	1989–1991	Commercial surfactants become available
	1995	Widespread antenatal steroid leads to drops in rates for RDS and improves survival rates for infants with a birth weight below 1000 gm, heralding a new era of epidemics of bronchopulmonary dysplasia and retinopathy of prematurity

See references 5, 18, 25, 46, 49, 58, 61, and 88 for primary citations.

transfusion science. Having believed that "only human blood should be employed for humans," he developed instruments, syringes, and funnels for this purpose. In 1818, Blundel carried out the first direct transfusion from a healthy donor into a recipient; 5 of his first 10 patients survived.

Human-to-human transfusions gradually became accepted, but the 19th-century doctor was puzzled about unexpected disasters among blood transfusion recipients. It took 15 more years after Karl Landsteiner's discovery of blood groups in 1901 for the general acceptance and understanding of the scientific basis for blood group incompatibility.[87]

Adult transfusions were rare, but newborn transfusions were rarer still. On March 8, 1908, a 4-day-old term infant who had hemorrhagic disease of the newborn made history. "As the child's skin became waxen white and mucous membranes without color, it was decided to attempt transfusion of blood obtained from the infant's father," wrote Dr. Samuel Lambert from New York.[55] Surgeon Alexis Carrel from Rockefeller University Hospital performed an end-to-end anastomosis of the right popliteal vein of the baby with the left radial artery of the father. No anesthetic was given to either patient. "The amount of blood transfused could not be measured, but enough blood was allowed to flow into the baby to change her color from pale transparent whiteness to brilliant red . . . [and] as soon as the wound was sutured, the infant fed ravenously and immediately went to sleep," according to Dr. Lambert. Incidentally, Carrel was the first surgeon to develop innovative methods of suturing blood vessels—a contribution for which he received the 1912 Nobel Prize.

Despite Lambert's dramatic report, direct father-to-infant transfusion did not become routine. Because of unexpected reactions among the recipients, blood transfusions continued to be risky, in spite of proper matching of the donors' blood for major blood types. The mystery was understood only after the discovery of Rh subtypes by Landsteiner and Wiener in 1940.[87, 90]

The discovery of the Rh blood types and the conquest of erythroblastosis fetalis remains a rare phenomenon in science, in which an orderly progression of accumulating knowledge led to the near eradication of a disease. First came the clinical descriptions of erythroblastosis, then evolved its treatment, followed by efforts to prevent it. These stages are superbly told in monographs and review articles.[28, 29, 87, 90]

TOOLS AND SUPPLIES FOR NICUs

It is perhaps impossible for today's generation to realize how hard it was to perform such simple and mundane chores as the collection of blood or insertion of catheters. For intravenous therapy in children, one needed ultra-small needles, pumps, and tubing, but none were available until the 1930s. In 1912, Blackfan (1883–1941) developed an ingenious suction device for blood collection.[9] Parenteral fluid therapy was laborious, performed through venous cut-downs or subcutaneous routes. Well into the early 1970s, only a handful of laboratories in Chicago performed blood gas analyses on microsamples, using up to 5 mL of arterial blood.

Often, the intraperitoneal route was used to infuse fluids, and the sagittal sinus or the anterior fontanelle was punctured to draw blood from newborn infants.[10, 91] In 1923, Sidbury introduced umbilical venous catheterization for neonatal blood transfusions,[72] and in the 1950s Diamond and colleagues began using this route for exchange transfusions.[28, 29] Only in 1951 were indwelling polyethylene tubes introduced for gastric feeding.[70]

PEDIATRIC SURGERY—NOT FOR RABBITS ANYMORE

As the trend of specialization among surgical subspecialties became popular, the generalist surgeons resisted the change. Dr. Edward Churchill, a famous surgeon, once remarked that his surgical residents at Massachusetts General Hospital "were quite proficient at operating on rabbits" and, therefore, there was no need for a subspecialty in pediatric surgery.[35] Despite those objections, Harvard Medical School founded the first department of Pediatric Surgery in 1941 and named William E. Ladd as its chair. Ladd and his pupils (among others) went on to show that

pediatric and neonatal surgery was not the same as operating on rabbits.

NEONATOLOGY EDUCATION AND RESEARCH

Of all the advances in the 20th century, none has made a greater impact than the publication and dissemination of scientific information through journals and books. Duncan has compiled an impressive list of classic papers in neonatal and perinatal medicine.[31] The impact of current computer technology, the Internet, and the electronic age on neonatal education remains to be assessed.

GLOBAL NEONATAL CARE

By the middle of the 20th century, scores of neonatal units were built using the Hess model in a number of European countries (Fig. 1–12), including the United Kingdom.[33, 61] During the final decades of the 20th century, Asian countries developed indigenous means of improving neonatal resuscitation and intensive care of sick newborn infants. The collective impact of these international initiatives on global neonatal care has yet to be assessed.[84]

THE SHAPE OF FUTURE NICUs AND SOME REMAINING PROBLEMS

Although today's NICU is a technological marvel, conceptually it remains a miniaturized version of the adult intensive care unit (ICU). Recent interest in environmental influences on brain growth may change the shape of future NICUs. The Neonatal Indi-

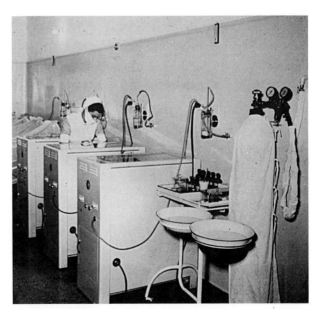

FIGURE 1–12. The first Preterm Infant Unit in Athens, Greece, using incubators with oxygen flowed into them (circa 1947). (Courtesy of John Sofatzis, MD, Athens, Greece.)

vidualized Developmental Care and Assessment Program (NIDCAP)[2] promises to transform the noisy, technical, and impersonal intensive care environment into a baby-friendly unit. Several ultra-modern NICUs have now been built on the concepts of NIDCAP. Such "kind and gentle" NICUs may be what Tarnier, Budin, Hess, and others conceived of some 100 years ago. (See Chapter 41.)

Despite incredible advances in the care of premature infants, today's scientists are facing many unresolved issues: limits of viability, cost of care, quality of life for intensive care "graduates," and an ever-increasing battle against opportunistic, nosocomial microorganisms. These and similar concerns also vexed the early pioneers of our subspecialty. Future historians may assess this century of neonatal medicine with the same sense of surprised wonder and awe that we now feel when remembering the days of infant hatcheries and baby incubator shows.

SOME FAMOUS HIGH-RISK INFANTS

Shakespeare's King Henry VI offers one of the most poignant musings on the burdens of disability and

TABLE 1-4 OMINOUS BEGINNINGS OF SOME FAMOUS PERSONALITIES

CATEGORY	NAME	DESCRIPTION*
Religious	Moses	Jewish tradition holds that Moses was born "6 months and 1 day" after he was conceived; thus, he could be hidden for 3 months from Pharoah's soldiers who were looking to find and kill the liberator of Jews.[50, 60]
Historical personalities and characters	Duke of Glouchester (later Richard III) (1452–1485)	Footling presentation, possibly premature; might have had cerebral palsy (hemiplegia?).[54]
	Macduff (Scottish nobleman in Shakespeare's *Macbeth*)	Delivered by cesarean section after his mother's death, thus "not of a woman born" but of a corpse.[54]
Artists and writers	Jonathan Swift (1667–1745)	Quoted by Cone.[24]
	Licetus Fortunio (1577–1657)	"A fetus no more than five and one-half inches" at birth. His father, a doctor, raised him in an oven, "similar to chicken hatching method used in Egypt."[81] The boy becomes scholar, writing 80 books.
	Pablo Picasso (1881–1973)	Left on the table as a stillbirth; his uncle, Don Salvador, a doctor, resuscitated him.
	Voltaire (1694–1778)	Premature and asphyxiated, the "puny little boy" was not expected to live and was hurriedly baptized; he was raised in the attic to keep him warm.
	Samuel Johnson (1709–1784)	A huge baby, he was "strangely inert" at birth, required slapping and shaking. With persuasion, he made a few whimpers and lived.
	Johann Wolfgang von Goethe (1749–1823)	After 3 days of labor, his mother delivered him; he was "lifeless and miserable" and thought to be stillborn at birth.
	Anna Pavlova (1882–1931)	Famous Russian ballerina, "a premature, so puny and weak," she was wrapped in cotton wool for 3 months.
	Thomas Hardy (1840–1928)	He was thrown aside as dead at birth. "A good slapping" from the midwife revived him.
	Sidney Poitier (born 1927)	Being 3 months premature, he was so small that his father "could place him in a shoebox." His grandmother said that despite prematurity, he would "walk with the kings." He did, when he became Bahamian ambassador to Japan in the 1990s.†
Scientists	Johannes Kepler (1571–1630)	German astronomer: a "seven-month" baby; estimated IQ, 161.
	Christopher Wren (1632–1723)	Quoted by Cone.[24]
	Isaac Newton (1642–1727)	Thought to be "as good as dead" at birth. He was such a "tiny mite" that he could be placed in a quart mug.
Politicians	Franklin D. Roosevelt (1882–1945)	Weighed 10 pounds at birth, but was "blue and limp with a death like respiratory standstill" from too much chloroform given to his mother, Sara Roosevelt.
	Winston Churchill (1874–1965)	His early birth "upset the ball." Later a duchess remarked that the baby had such a lusty "earth-shaking" cry as she had ever heard. Recent historians doubt his premature birth.

*The biographical notes are derived mostly from anecdotal statements of historians or family members or are from later recollection by the characters themselves; thus, we cannot be certain of the scientific validity of these stories.
†Quoted by Sidney Poitier in the television show "Biography," CNN, Spring 2000.

the difficult birth (owing to footling presentation) of his brother, Duke of Glouchester, who later became Richard III. Henry says to the Duke,[54] who was supposedly born premature (not confirmed by other historians), "Thy mother felt more than a mother's pain, yet brought forth less than a mother's hope." King Richard himself in a different Shakespeare play bemoans his misfortune.[54] "Deformed, unfinish'd, sent before my times/Into this breathing world scarce half made up . . ."

Did King Richard suffer from hemiplegic cerebral palsy as a consequence of prematurity? We cannot be sure. The list of leaders, celebrities, and famous persons supposed to have been regarded as high risk at birth (Table 1–4), however, is impressive,[64] although the authenticity of those stories is difficult to confirm, because most of them were derived from anecdotal statements.

ACKNOWLEDGMENTS

I sincerely thank Kristine M. McCulloch, MD, for helping during the preparation of the manuscript, and I thank all of the copyright holders for permission to reproduce the illustrations used in this chapter.

A NOTE ON REFERENCES: I have restricted my citations to mostly secondary sources and scholarly reviews. Readers interested in the original references can find them in many of the major secondary references noted in the following list.

■ R E F E R E N C E S

1. Akerrén Y, Fürstenberg N: Gastro-intestinal administration of oxygen in treatment of asphyxia in the newborn. J Obstet Gynaecol (British Empire) 57:705, 1950.
2. Als H, et al: Individualized developmental care for the very low-birth-weight preterm infant. Medical and neurofunctional effects. JAMA 272:853,1994.
3. Apgar V: A proposal for a new method of evaluation of the newborn infant. Anesth Analg 32:260, 1953.
4. Avery ME, Mead J: Surface properties in relation to atelectasis and hyaline membrane disease. Am J Dis Child 97:517, 1959.
5. Avery ME: Surfactant deficiency in hyaline membrane disease: The story of discovery. Am J Respir Crit Care Med 161:1074, 2000.
6. Baker JP: The incubator controversy: Pediatricians and the origins of premature infant technology in the United States, 1890–1910. Pediatrics 87:654,1991.
7. Baker JP: The Machine in the Nursery: Incubator Technology and the Origins of Newborn Intensive Care. Baltimore, Johns Hopkins University Press, 1996.
8. Barcroft J: Research on Pre-natal Life, vol 1, Oxford, Blackwell Scientific, 1977.
9. Blackfan KD: Apparatus for collecting infant's blood for Wassermann reaction. Am J Dis Child 4:33, 1912.
10. Blackfan KD, Maxcy, KF: The intraperitoneal injection of saline solution. Am J Dis Child 15:19, 1918.
11. Blumfeld-Kusinski R: Not of a Woman Born: Representation of Childbirth in Medieval and Renaissance Culture. Ithaca, NY, Cornell University Press, 1990.
12. Bloxsom A: Resuscitation of the newborn infant: Use of positive pressure oxygen-air lock. J Pediatr 37:311, 1950.
13. Blundell J: Principles and Practice of Obstetrics. London, E. Cox, 1834, p 246.
14. Bonnaire E: Inhalations of oxygen in the newborn. Arch Pediatr 8:769, 1891.
15. Budin P, Maloney WJ (translator): The Nursling: The Feeding and Hygiene of Premature and Full-Term Infants. London, Caxton Publishing Co, 1907.
16. Butterfield LJ: Virginia Apgar, MD, MPhH. Neonatal Netw 13:81, 1994.
17. Campbell DJ, et al: High maternal mortality in certain areas: Reports on public health and medical subjects. Ministry of Health and Department of Health Publications. London, UK. No. 68, 1932.
18. Clements JA, Avery ME: Lung surfactant and neonatal respiratory distress syndrome. Am J Respir Crit Care Med 157:S59, 1998.
19. Comroe JH Jr: Retrospectroscope: Man-Cans. Am Rev Resp Dis 116:945, 1977.
20. Comroe JH Jr: Man-Cans (Conclusion). Am Rev Resp Dis 116:1011, 1977.
21. Cone TE Jr: 200 Years of Feeding Infants in America. Columbus, Ohio, Ross Laboratories, 1976.
22. Cone TE Jr: History of American Pediatrics. Boston, Little Brown, 1979, p 57.
23. Cone TE Jr: The first published report of an incubator for use in the care of the premature infants (1857). Am J Dis Child 135:658, 1981.
24. Cone TE Jr: Perspective in neonatology. In Smith GF, Vidyasagar D (eds): Historical Review and Recent Advances in Neonatal and Perinatal Medicine. Vol 1, Neonatal Medicine, Evansville, Ind, Ross Publication, 1984 p 9.
25. DeBard ML: The history of cardiopulmonary resuscitation. Ann Emerg Med 9:273, 1980.
26. DeLee J: A Brief History of the Chicago Lying-In Hospital. Chicago, Alumni Association Lying-In Hospital and Dispensary Souvenir, 1895, p 1931.
27. DeLee JB: Infant incubation, with the presentation of a new incubator and a description of the system at the Chicago Lying-in-Hospital. Chicago Medical Recorder 22:22, 1902.
28. Diamond LK, et al: Erythroblastosis fetalis and its association with universal edema of the fetus, icterus gravis neonatorum, and anemia of the newborn. J Pediatr 1:269, 1932.
29. Diamond LK, et al: Erythroblastosis fetalis, VII: Treatment with exchange transfusion. N Engl J Med 244:39, 1951.
30. Donald I, Lord J: Augmented respiration: Studies in atelectasis neonatorum. The Lancet 1:9, 1953.
31. Duncan RG: Neonatology on the Web. Available at: http://www.neonatology.org/diversions/classics
32. Dunn PM: Dr. James Blundell (1790–1878) and neonatal resuscitation. Arch Dis Child Fetal Neonatal Ed 64:494, 1988.
33. Dunn PM: The development of newborn care in the UK since 1930. J Perinatol 18:471, 1998.
34. Dunn PM: Sir Joseph Barcroft of Cambridge (1872–1947) and prenatal research. Arch Dis Child Fetal Neonatal Ed 82:F75, 2000.
35. Easterbrook G: Surgeon Koop. Knoxville, Tenn, Whittle Direct Books, 1991.
36. Editorial. The Victorian Era Exhibition at Earl's Court. Lancet 2:161, 1897.
37. Editorial. The danger of making a public show of incubator for babies. Lancet 1:390, 1898.
38. Gartner LM: Dr. Harry Gordon. In Smith GF, Vidyasagar D (eds): Historical Review and Recent Advances in Neonatal and Perinatal Medicine. Vol 1, Neonatal Medicine, Evansville, Ind, Ross Publication, 1984, p xiv.
39. Gilmartin ME: Body ventilators. Equipment and techniques. Respir Care Clin N Am 2:195, 1996.
40. Ginzberg L: The Legend of the Jews, II: Bible Times and Characters from Joseph to the Exodus. (Translated from the German manuscript by Henrietta Szold.) Philadelphia, The Jewish Publication Society of America, 1989, p 262.
41. Goodlin R: History of fetal monitoring. Am J Obstet Gynecol 133:323, 1979.
42. Gould D: Iron lung. In DeBono (ed): Eureka! An Illustrated History of Invention from the Wheel to the Computer. New York, Holt, Rinehart and Winston, 1974, p 160.
43. Graham H: Eternal Eve: The History of Gynecology and Obstetrics. Garden City, NY, Doubleday, 1951.
44. Gregory GA, et al: Treatment of idiopathic respiratory distress

syndrome with continuous positive pressure. N Engl J Med, 284:1333, 1971.

45. Henderson AR: Resuscitation experiments and breathing apparatus of Alexander Graham Bell. Chest 62:311, 1972.
46. Henderson Y: The inhalation method of resuscitation from asphyxia of the newborn. Am J Obst Gynecol 21:542, 1931.
47. Hess JH: Premature and Congenitally Diseased Infants. Philadelphia, Lea & Febiger, 1922.
48. Holt LE: The Diseases of Infants & Children. New York, Appleton, 1897, p 12.
49. Hutchison JH, et al: Controlled trials of hyperbaric oxygen and tracheal intubation in asphyxia neonatorum. Lancet 1:935, 1966.
50. Isaiah AB, Sharfman B: The Pentatueuch and Rashi's Commentary: A Linear Translation into English. Exodus. New York, S.S.& R. Publishing, 1960, p 9.
51. Jacobson RM, Feinstein AR: Oxygen as a cause of blindness in premature infants: "Autopsy" of a decade of errors in clinical epidemiologic research. J Clin Epidemiol 11:1265, 1992.
52. James LS, et al: Intragastric oxygen and resuscitation of the newborn. Acta Pediatr 52:245,1963.
53. James LS, Lanman JT: History of oxygen therapy and retrolental fibroplasia. Supplement. Pediatrics 57:59, 1976.
54. Kail AC: The Medical Mind of Shakespeare. Balgowhas, Australia, Williams & Wilkins, 1986, p 101.
55. Lambert SW: Melaena neonatorum with report of a case cured by transfusion. Medical Record. 73:22, 1908.
56. Loudon I: Deaths in Childbed from the 18th Century to 1935. Med Hist, 30:1, 1986.
57. Morton LT, Moore RJ: A Chronology of the Diseases & Related Sciences. Aldershot, UK, Scolar Press, 1997, p 84.
58. Murphy D, et al: The Drinker respirator treatment of the immediate asphyxia of the newborn: With a report of 350 cases. Am J Obstet Gynecol 21:528, 1931.
59. National Library of Medicine: Available at: http://igm.nlm.nih.gov/
60. Nelson NM: An appreciation of Clement Smith. In Smith GF, Vidyasagar D (eds): Historical Review and Recent Advances in Neonatal and Perinatal Medicine. Vol 1, Neonatal Medicine, Evansville, Ind, Ross Publication, 1984, p xii.
61. O'Dowd MJ, Phillipp AE: The History of Obstetrics and Gynecology. New York, Parthenon, 1994.
62. Papadopoulos MD, Swyer PR: Assisted ventilation in terminal hyaline membrane disease. Arch Dis Child 39:481, 1964.
63. Radcliffe W: The Secret Instrument. London, William Heinemann Medical Books Ltd, 1947.
64. Raju TNK: Some famous "high-risk" newborn babies. In Smith GF, Vidyasagar D (eds): Historical Review and Recent Advances in Neonatal and Perinatal Medicine. Vol 2, Perinatal Medicine, Evansville, Ind, Ross Publication, 1984, p 187.
65. Raju TNK: The principles of life: Highlights from the history of pulmonary physiology. In Donn SM (ed): Neonatal and Pediatric Pulmonary Graphics: Principles and Clinical Applications. Armonk, NY, Futura Publishing, 1998, p 3.
66. Raju TNK: The history of neonatal respiration: Tales of heroism and desperation. Clinics in Perinatology. 1999; 26:629–40.
67. Rambar AC: Julius Hess, MD. In Smith GF, Vidyasagar D (eds): Historical Review and Recent Advances in Neonatal and Perinatal Medicine. Vol 2, Perinatal Medicine, Evansville, Ind, Ross Publication, 1984, p 161.
68. Ransom SW: The care of premature and feeble infants. Pediatrics 9:322, 1890.
69. Roche T: A refuge for throwaways: The spate of "Dumpster babies" stirs a movement to provide a safe space for unwanted newborns. Time 155:50, 2000.
70. Royce S, et al: Indwelling polyethylene nasogastric tube for feeding premature infants. Pediatrics 8:79, 1951.
71. Schaffer, AJ: Diseases of the Newborn. Philadelphia, Saunders, 1960, p 1.
72. Sidbury JB: Transfusion through the umbilical vein in hemorrhage of the newborn. Am J Dis Child 25:290, 1923.
73. Silverman WA: Incubator-baby side shows. Pediatrics 64:127, 1979.
74. Silverman WA: Retrolental fibroplasia: A modern parable. New York, Grune & Stratton, 1980.
75. Smith CA: Physiology of the Newborn Infant. Springfield, Charles C. Thomas, 1945.
76. Spaulding M, Welch P: Nurturing Yesterday's Child. A Portrayal of the Drake Collection of Pediatric History. Philadelphia, B. C. Decker, 1991, p 110.
77. Speert H: Obstetrics and Gynecology in America: A History. Baltimore, Waverly Press, 1980.
78. Stalhman MT: Assisted ventilation in newborn infants. In Smith GF, Vidyasagar D (eds): Historical Review and Recent Advances in Neonatal and Perinatal Medicine. Vol 2, Perinatal Medicine, Evansville, Ind, Ross Publication, 1984, p 21.
79. Stern L, et al: Negative pressure artificial respiration: Use in treatment of respiratory failure of the newborn. Can Med Assn J, 102:595, 1970.
80. Stern L: Thermoregulation in the newborn. Historical, physiological, and clinical considerations. In Smith GF, Vidyasagar D (eds): Historical Review and Recent Advances in Neonatal and Perinatal Medicine. Vol 1, Neonatal Medicine, Evansville, Ind, Ross Publication, 1984, p 35.
81. Sterne L: The Life and Opinions of Tristram Shandy, Gentleman. New York, Penguin, 1997, p 231.
82. Tempkin O: On the care of the newborn. In Soranus' Gynecology. Baltimore, Johns Hopkins Press, 1956, p 79.
83. Tuchman BU: A Distant Mirror: The Calamitous 14th Century. New York, Balantine Books, 1978, p 49.
84. Vidyasagar D, et al: Evolution of neonatal and pediatric critical care in India. Crit Care Cin 13:331, 1997.
85. Wijesundera CD: Digital intubation of the trachea. Ceylon Med J 35:81, 1990.
86. Wilson A: The Making of Man-midwifery: Childbearing in England 1660–1770. Cambridge, Mass, Harvard University Press, 1995, p 1.
87. Winthrobe MM: Blood: Pure and Eloquent. New York, McGraw-Hill, 1981.
88. Wrigley M, Nandi P: The Sparklet carbon dioxide resuscitator. Anaesthesia 49:148, 1994.
89. Young JH: Caesarean Section, The History and Development of the Operation From Earliest Times. London, H.K. Lewis, 1994.
90. Zimerman DA: Rh. New York, MacMillan Publishing, 1973.
91. Zimmerman JJ, Strauss RH: History and current application of intravenous therapy in children. Pediatr Emerg Care 5:120, 1989.

2 Neonatal Risk Factors

Richard E. Behrman

Patricia H. Shiono

OVERVIEW

The neonatal-perinatal period is a time when the mother and fetus experience a period of rapid growth and development. At birth, the fetus makes an abrupt transition from the protective environment of the uterus to the outside world; the newly born baby must undergo extreme physiologic changes to survive this transition. Therefore, it is not surprising that the highest risk of infant death occurs during the first 24 hours after birth. Increased rates of mortality and morbidity continue during the *neonatal period*, from birth to the 28th day of life. Mortality and morbidity rates are high early in life because the fetus and baby are vulnerable to numerous metabolic, genetic, physiologic, social, economic, and environmental injuries. These diverse factors influence the gestation, delivery, and neonatal period and have a major impact on the health of the fetus and the infant.

The high incidence of mortality and morbidity during the *perinatal period*, which starts at the 28th week of pregnancy and extends to the 28th day after birth, makes it important to identify, as early as possible, the mothers, fetuses, and infants who are at greatest risk. Of equal importance is the need to lower the risk of morbidity, especially for handicapping conditions such as mental retardation. There is increasing evidence that early recognition of women with high-risk pregnancies, and of high-risk infants, followed by appropriate prenatal, intrapartum, and postpartum care, can reduce the incidence of handicapping conditions and will reduce the incidence of infant mortality.

Infants who die are a source of anguish and grief to their parents and relatives for a period, which is usually relatively brief. Those infants who survive with disabilities and disease must endure personal suffering and may be a continuing source of pain, anguish, and loss of resources for their parents and society. They may also impose a biologic burden on future generations by increasing the frequency of maladaptive genes in the population. In addition to the human tragedy, the fiscal impact of these problems on our society is estimated to be in the billions of dollars each year.[5]

Infants who are born before attaining normal intrauterine growth and development are at greatest risk of dying during infancy and are at significant risk of morbidity during childhood.[8] Infants with a *low birth weight* (LBW), weighing less than 2500 gm, are 40 times more likely to die than infants of normal birth weight. The relative risk of neonatal death is almost 200 times greater for infants with a very low birth weight (VLBW), weighing less than 1500 gm. Infants with LBW are at a much higher risk of being born with cerebral palsy, mental retardation, and other sensory and cognitive impairments, compared with infants of normal birth weight. Surviving infants with LBW also have an increased incidence of disability for a broad range of conditions, including various neurodevelopmental handicaps, respiratory illness, and injuries acquired as a result of neonatal intensive care. Moreover, these infants often have a diminished ability to adapt socially, psychologically, and physically to an increasingly complex environment. The risk factors for high-risk pregnancies that are often associated with LBW are listed in Box 2–1.

It is becoming evident that important antecedents of many adult diseases, such as coronary artery disease, chronic renal and liver disease, and obesity, may have roots in early childhood, which implies that there may be very early opportunities for the prevention of adult chronic diseases. Further improvement in longevity and decreased morbidity are likely to result from a better understanding of the origins of adult disease in fetal life and infancy and from the prevention and early treatment of these diseases.

Advances in neonatal-perinatal medicine have focused attention on a number of legal and ethical issues. There is a continuing concern about life-and-death decision making in neonatal intensive care units. New and complex physician-patient-family-nursing-societal relationships are evolving, which will make more exacting demands on the physician's ability to perceive what is meant from what is said by family members about neonatal management decisions.

■ **BOX 2–1**

FACTORS ASSOCIATED WITH HIGH-RISK PREGNANCY

Economic

Poverty
Unemployment
Uninsured, underinsured health insurance
Poor access to prenatal care

Cultural-Behavioral

Low educational status
Poor health care attitudes
No care or inadequate prenatal care
Cigarette, alcohol, drug abuse
Age <16 or >35 yrs
Unmarried
Short interpregnancy interval
Lack of support group (husband, family, religion)
Stress (physical, psychological)
African American race
Abusive partner

Biologic-Genetic

Previous LBW infant
Low maternal weight at her birth
Low weight for height
Poor weight gain during pregnancy
Short stature
Poor nutrition
Inbreeding (autosomal recessive?)
Intergenerational effects
Hereditary diseases (inborn error of metabolism)

Reproductive

Previous cesarean section
Previous infertility
Prolonged gestation
Prolonged labor
Previous infant with cerebral palsy, mental retardation, birth trauma, congenital anomalies
Abnormal lie (breech)
Abruption
Multiple gestation
Premature rupture of membranes
Infections (systemic, amniotic, extra-amniotic, cervical)
Preeclampsia or eclampsia
Uterine bleeding (abruptio placentae, placenta previa)
Parity (0 or more than 5)
Uterine or cervical anomalies
Fetal disease
Abnormal fetal growth
Idiopathic premature labor
Iatrogenic prematurity
High or low levels of maternal serum α-fetoprotein

Medical

Diabetes mellitus
Hypertension
Congenital heart disease
Autoimmune disease
Sickle cell anemia
TORCH infection
Intercurrent surgery or trauma
Sexually transmitted diseases
Maternal hypercoagulable states

LBW, low birth weight; TORCH, toxoplasmosis, other agents, rubella, cytomegalovirus, herpes simplex.

From Stoll JB, Kliegman RM: Section 1: Noninfectious disorders. In Behrman RE, et al (eds): Nelson Textbook of Pediatrics, 16th ed. Philadelphia, WB Saunders Co, 2000, p 461.

HIGH-RISK INFANTS

To decrease infant morbidity and mortality, pregnant women and infants at high risk should be identified as early as possible. High-risk infants should be under close observation by experienced physicians and nurses. Although it is usually needed for only a few days, such intensive care may range from a few hours to several weeks or more. Some institutions find it advantageous to provide a special or transitional care nursery for high-risk infants, which is often located in the labor and delivery suite. This special nursery should be equipped and staffed similarly to a neonatal intensive care area so that well but high-risk infants can be observed and cared for immediately after birth. This special nursery should also allow special care without causing extended periods of mother-infant separation (see Chapter 3).

The factors that define high-risk infants are listed in Box 2–2. Many of these factors are also related to the risk of LBW (see Box 2–1). Examination of a fresh placenta, cord, and membranes may alert the physician to a newborn infant at high risk. However, many high-risk infants are born preterm, are small for gestational age, have significant perinatal asphyxia, or are born with life-threatening congenital anomalies, but they do not have any identifiable risk factors.

INFANT MORTALITY

Infant mortality is a critical measure of the health and welfare of a population. In 1998, 3.94 million infants were born in the United States, and nearly 28,486 died before reaching age 1, resulting in an *infant mortality* rate of 7.2 deaths per thousand live births.[3] Rates of infant deaths in the United States have been dropping steadily for at least 30 years and reached an all-time low in 1998 (Fig. 2–1).[3] In spite of the constant

■ **BOX 2–2**

HIGH-RISK INFANTS

Demographic Social Factors

Maternal age <16 or >40 yrs
Illicit drug, alcohol, cigarette use
Poverty
Unmarried
Emotional or physical stress

Past Medical History

Genetic disorders
Diabetes mellitus
Hypertension
Asymptomatic bacteriuria
Rheumatologic illness (SLE)
Long-term medication

Prior Pregnancy

Intrauterine fetal demise
Neonatal death
Prematurity
Intrauterine growth retardation
Congenital malformation
Incompetent cervix
Blood group sensitization, neonatal jaundice
Neonatal thrombocytopenia
Hydrops
Inborn errors of metabolism

Present Pregnancy

Vaginal bleeding (abruptio placentae, placenta previa
Sexually transmitted diseases (colonization: herpes simplex, group B streptococcus), chlamydia, syphilis, hepatitis B
Multiple gestation
Preeclampsia
Premature rupture of membranes
Short interpregnancy time
Polyoligohydramnios
Acute medical or surgical illness
Inadequate prenatal care
Familial or acquired hypercoagulable states

Labor and Delivery

Abruptio placentae
Premature labor (<37 wks)
Postdates (>42 wks)
Fetal distress
Immature L/S ratio: absent phosphatidylglycerol
Breech presentation
Meconium-stained fluid
Nuchal cord
Cesarean section
Forceps delivery
Apgar score <4 at 1 min
Vacuum extraction

Neonate

Birthweight <2500 or >4000 gm
Birth before 37 or after 42 wks of gestation
SGA, LGA growth status
Tachypnea, cyanosis
Congenital malformation
Pallor, plethora, petechiae

LGA, large for gestational age; *SGA,* small for gestational age; *SLE,* systemic lupus erythematosus.
From Stoll JB, Kliegman RM: Section 1: Noninfectious disorders. In Behrman RE, et al (eds): Nelson Textbook of Pediatrics, 16th ed. Philadelphia, WB Saunders Co, 2000, p 474.

improvement in national infant mortality rates, the United States ranks only 23rd in the world in infant mortality, well behind Sweden, Japan, Singapore, and Hong Kong.[3] Paradoxically, the birth weight–specific mortality in the United States is relatively low. That is, at each birth weight level, the infant mortality in the United States is very low. This low rate of birth weight–specific mortality is due to advances in neonatal care systems; the majority of extremely tiny infants who weigh as little as 750 gm at birth are now surviving.[10, 13]

Most notable in the United States is the large disparity between African-American and white infant mortality. The mortality rate for African-American infants is more than double that for white infants (Fig. 2–2).[3] In recent years, this ethnic and racial disparity has widened because the rate of decline in infant mortality has been higher among white infants than among African-American infants. The five leading causes of infant death in 1997 were congenital anomalies, short gestation and low birth weight, sudden infant death syndrome, respiratory distress syndrome, and maternal complications of pregnancy (Fig. 2–3).[6] Of the five leading causes of infant deaths, those that African-American infants are much more likely to die from than infants of other races are being born too soon or too small and maternal complications of pregnancy.

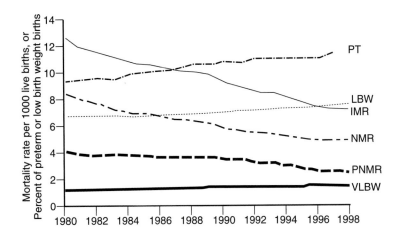

FIGURE 2–1. Infant (IMR), neonatal (NMR), and post-neonatal (PNMR) mortality rates are shown annually from 1980 to 1998 in the United States. Total preterm (PT) births, low birth weight (LBW) births, and very low birth weight (VLBW) births are also shown. IMR has declined more than 40% since 1980. NMRs declined more rapidly during the 1980s, whereas PNMRs declined more rapidly during the 1990s. (From Guyer B, et al: Annual summary of vital statistics 1998. Pediatrics 104:1229, 1999. Used with permission of the American Academy of Pediatrics.)

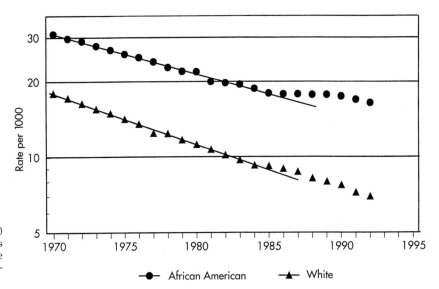

FIGURE 2–2. Infant mortality rates by race, 1970 to 1995. The infant mortality rate is defined as the number of infant deaths per 1000 live births. (From National Center for Health Statistics, Hyattsville, MD.)

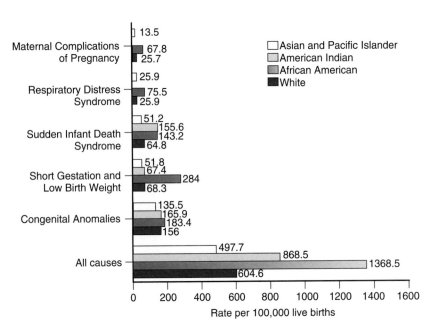

FIGURE 2–3. Infant death and mortality rates for the five leading causes of death by race of mother, United States, 1997 linked file. Where data are missing, there were too few deaths in the category to calculate reliable rates. (From MacDorman MF, et al: Infant mortality statistics from the 1997 period linked birth/infant death data set. National Vital Statistics Reports 47:23, 1999.)

Infant deaths are divided into two categories according to age: *neonatal* (deaths of infants younger than 28 days) and *postneonatal* (deaths of infants between the ages of 28 days and 1 year). A decline in infant mortality rates was observed for both neonatal deaths (4.8 per 1000) and postneonatal deaths (2.4 per 1000).[3] Infant mortality numbers have declined by over 40% since 1980. Neonatal death rates declined more steeply in the 1980s, whereas postneonatal death rates declined more steeply in the 1990s.[3] Neonatal deaths are generally attributable to factors that occur during pregnancy, such as congenital malformations, LBW, maternal toxic exposures (smoking or other forms of drug abuse), and lack of appropriate medical care. In contrast, postneonatal deaths are generally associated with the infant's environmental circumstances, such as poverty, which often results in inadequate food, housing, sanitation, and medical care.

The decline in neonatal deaths among infants with LBW in the 1990s may be because of increased survival in neonatal intensive care units, healthier babies with LBW, or both.[10] It is estimated that two thirds of the decline in severity-adjusted mortality was due to increased survival in neonatal intensive care and that one third was due to healthier babies with LBW. Increased survival in neonatal intensive care is attributed to the more aggressive use of respiratory and cardiovascular treatments. The improved health of infants with LBW is attributed to improvements in obstetric and delivery room care.

Generally, for any given gestational age, the lower the infant birth weight, the higher the neonatal mortality; and for any given birth weight, the younger the gestational age, the higher the neonatal mortality. Infant death rates drop steeply with increasing infant birth weight. The lowest risk of infant death occurs among infants with birth weights of 3000 to 4000 gm, and risk increases slightly for infants over 4000 gm (Fig. 2–4) and for those whose gestational age is older

than 42 weeks. Infants who survive past the first 28 days of life have a vastly better prognosis.

PRETERM, LOW BIRTH WEIGHT, AND SMALL FOR GESTATIONAL AGE INFANTS

Live-born infants born before 37 completed weeks of gestation (less than 259 days after the date of the mother's last menstrual period) are defined as *preterm*. Measures of live-born infant size include *low birth weight* (infants weighing less than 2500 gm) and two subgroups of LBW, *moderately low birth weight* (infants weighing between 1500 and 2499 gm) and *very low birth weight* (infants weighing less than 1500 gm). Other measures take into consideration both gestational age and weight, such as *small for gestational age* (SGA), defined as live-born infants weighing less than the 10th percentile for gestational age; *appropriate for gestational age*, defined as infants weighing between the 10th and the 90th percentiles for gestational age; and *large for gestational age*, defined as infants weighing above the 90th percentile for gestational age. The health of a baby with LBW is directly related to its gestational age. An 1800-gm infant born at term is very different from an 1800-gm infant born at 32 weeks. An 1800-gm infant born at term is defined as LBW and SGA, but an 1800-gm infant born at 32 weeks is defined as LBW, preterm, and appropriate for gestational age. Two 1800-gm infants of unequal gestational ages would obviously require very different care (see Chapter 13).

In the United States today, infants with LBW account for a relatively greater proportion of infant deaths than in the past. Early in the 20th century, two thirds of infant deaths occurred in the postneonatal period, primarily from infectious diseases. However, by 1950, 7.5% of live-born infants weighed less than 2500 gm, and two thirds of all infant deaths occurred in the neonatal period. The causes of these deaths

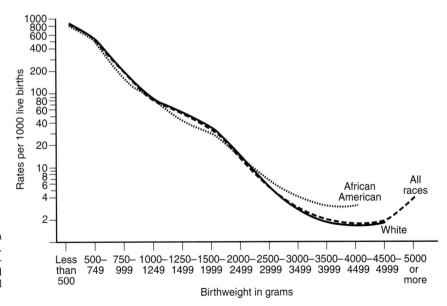

FIGURE 2–4. Infant mortality rates by birth weight, United States, 1997 linked file. (From MacDorman MF, et al: Infant mortality statistics from the 1997 period linked birth/infant death data set. National Vital Statistics Reports 47:23, 1999.)

were related to antenatal and intrapartum events, such as birth injury, asphyxia, congenital malformations, and "immaturity." Advances in the development of perinatal care in the 1950s and 1960s came as a result of the awareness of the increased morbidity in surviving infants with LBW coupled with a greater understanding of fetal and infant nutrition, pharmacology, and pathophysiology. The infant mortality rate decreased 47% from 1965 to 1980, primarily because of the increased survival of high-risk infants with LBW. The regionalization of neonatal intensive care has brought perinatal intensive care to most families in need and has contributed significantly to the increase in the proportion of infants with LBW and VLBW who are cared for in tertiary centers. Decreased rates of neonatal mortality also were observed after the introduction of regionalized care.[7] (See Chapter 3).

At the beginning of the 1980s, despite their increased survival rates, infants with LBW still accounted for two thirds of the neonatal deaths, whereas infants with VLBW accounted for half. Surviving infants with LBW also remained three times as likely as infants of normal birth weight to have adverse neurologic sequelae. The risk of adverse sequelae increases with decreasing birth weight. Lower respiratory tract problems, particularly infections, are more common, as are complications of neonatal care.

National rates of LBW have been essentially stable for the past four decades. The seemingly contradictory decline in infant mortality without parallel declines in LBW or preterm birth is due to the increasing survival of infants with LBW, not to prevention of LBW and preterm birth. Improvements in neonatal intensive care and new therapies such as surfactant have resulted in measurable decreases in infant mortality and morbidity. A slight unexplained increase in LBW was observed among African-American infants in the late 1980s. The risk of having a baby with LBW is increased among African-American women, women who smoke during pregnancy, unmarried women, women with low educational attainment, women who have no or inadequate prenatal care, and women who have had a previous infant with LBW (see Box 2–1).

There is a substantial and persistent difference between African-American and white infants in the risk of LBW and preterm delivery.[11, 12] African-American women are 2 times more likely to have a baby with LBW than white women and 2.6 times more likely than Chinese-American women (Fig. 2–5). The higher LBW rates among African-American women has been observed for over 20 years. African-American infants are more likely to die of preventable causes than are white infants. In addition, African-American infants have significantly higher rates of mortality for every cause of infant death, except for congenital anomalies and sudden infant death syndrome.

Decades of research about the disparities between LBW rates and infant mortality between African-American and white infants have not been able to explain the racial disparities in birth outcomes. Scientists have studied the impact of education, maternal age, vaginal infection, exposure to cigarette smoke, use of alcohol, stress, socioeconomic status, and many other risk factors. None of these factors explain the racial disparities in death or LBW rates. Compounding the widening gap between African-American and white rates of LBW is the increasing number of women at high risk in the population. Increases during the 1980s in AIDS, poverty, use of illicit drugs such as crack cocaine, syphilis, and births to unmarried women are additional factors that are associated with further increases in infant mortality and LBW.

Conditions that make the uterus unable to retain the fetus, interference with the course of pregnancy, premature separation of the placenta, or a stimulus to produce uterine contractions before term are generally associated with preterm infants with an appropriate weight for gestational age. Medical conditions

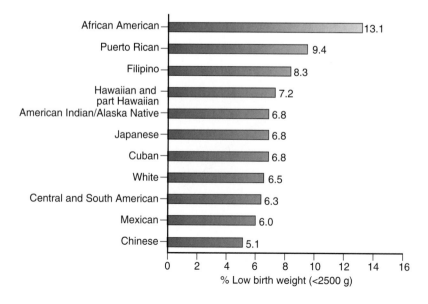

FIGURE 2–5. Low birth weight rates by race, 1997. Infants who are considered to be of low birth weight weigh less than 2500 gm at birth (about 5.5 pounds). (From Centers for Disease Control and Prevention, National Center for Health Statistics, National Vital Statistics System, Ventura SJ, et al: Births: Final data for 1997, National Vital Statistics Reports 47:18, 1999, and Ventura SJ, et al: Report of final natality statistics, Monthly Vital Statistics Report, 46:11, Suppl, 1998.)

that interfere with the circulation and efficiency of the placenta, the development or growth of the fetus, or the general health and nutrition of the mother are associated with infants who are SGA (Table 2-1).

DISEASE IN LOW BIRTH WEIGHT INFANTS

Although substantial overlap exists, the incidence of certain neonatal risks varies with birth weight, gestational age, and birth weight for gestational age. Problems of major clinical significance associated with preterm birth include respiratory distress (hyaline membrane disease, pulmonary hemorrhage, transient tachypnea, congenital pneumonia, pneumothorax, bronchopulmonary dysplasia), recurrent apnea, hypoglycemia, hypocalcemia, hyperbilirubinemia, anemia,

edema, cerebral anoxia, circulatory instability, hypothermia, bacterial sepsis, and disseminated intravascular coagulopathies. In addition, preterm infants frequently have a weak or uncoordinated ability to feed and prolonged failure to gain weight.

Infants who are SGA are a heterogeneous population, even when those with congenital anomalies and infections are excluded. They tend to have problems related more to their gestational age than to their birth weight. Preterm infants who are SGA have a lower incidence of respiratory distress syndrome than is expected for their birth weight. Problems encountered in infants who are SGA include perinatal asphyxia, hypoglycemia, hypothermia, meconium aspiration, necrotizing enterocolitis, polycythemia, and illnesses related to congenital anomalies, syndromes,

TABLE 2-1 MATERNAL NONINFECTIOUS DISEASE AFFECTING THE FETUS OR NEONATE

DISORDER	EFFECTS	MECHANISM
Cholestasis	Preterm delivery	Unknown; possibly hepatitis E
Cyanotic heart disease	Intrauterine growth retardation	Low fetal oxygen delivery
Diabetes mellitus		
Mild	Large for gestational age, hypoglycemia	Fetal hyperglycemia—produces hyperinsulinemia; insulin promotes growth
Severe	Growth retardation	Vascular disease, placental insufficiency
Drug addiction	Intrauterine growth retardation, neonatal withdrawal	Direct drug effect, plus poor diet
Endemic goiter	Hypothyroidism	Iodine deficiency
Graves disease	Transient neonatal thyrotoxicosis	Placebo immunoglobin passage of thyroid-stimulating antibody
Herpes gestationalis	Bullous rash	Unknown
Hyperparathyroidism	Neonatal hypocalcemia	Maternal calcium crosses to fetus and suppresses fetal parathyroid gland
Hypertension	Intrauterine growth retardation, intrauterine fetal demise	Placental insufficiency, fetal hypoxia
Idiopathic thrombocytopenic purpura	Thrombocytopenia	Nonspecific maternal platelet antibodies cross placenta
Isoimmune neutropenia or thrombocytopenia	Neutropenia or thrombocytopenia	Specific antifetal neutrophil or platelet antibody crosses placenta after sensitization of mother
Malignant melanoma	Placental or fetal tumor	Metastasis
Myasthenia gravis	Transient neonatal myasthenia	Immunoglobulin to acetylcholine receptor crosses placenta
Myotonic dystrophy	Neonatal myotonic dystrophy, congenital contractures, respiratory insufficiency	Genetic anticipation
Obesity	Macrosomia, hypoglycemia	Unknown
Phenylketonuria	Microcephaly, retardation	Elevated fetal phenylalanine levels
Preeclampsia, eclampsia	Intrauterine growth retardation, thrombocytopenia, neutropenia, fetal demise	Uteroplacental insufficiency, fetal hypoxia, vasoconstriction
Renal transplant	Intrauterine growth retardation	Uteroplacental insufficiency
Rhesus or other blood group sensitization	Fetal anemia, hypoalbuminemia, hydrops, neonatal jaundice	Antibody crosses placenta directed to fetal cells with antigen
Sickle cell anemia	Preterm birth, intrauterine growth restriction	Maternal sickling producing fetal hypoxia
Systemic lupus erythematosus	Congenital heart block, rash, anemia, thrombocytopenia, neutropenia	Antibody directed to fetal heart, red and white blood cells, and platelets
Thrombophilia (familial)	Stillborn, growth retardation	Thrombosis of uteroplacental circulation

Modified from Stoll JB, Kliegman RM: Section 1: Noninfectious Disorders. In Behrman RE, et al (eds): Nelson Textbook of Pediatrics, 16th ed. Philadelphia, WB Saunders Co, 2000, p 462.

or infections.[14] The prognosis depends in part on the cause of their growth retardation (see Chapter 13). Head circumference that is less than the 10th percentile at birth and abnormal results from a newborn neurologic examination are associated with poor growth, later microcephaly, and neurologic deficits.

Hemorrhage is frequent and often severe in infants with LBW. Subcutaneous ecchymosis and subependymal and intraventricular hemorrhage are frequent. Contributing causes may be increased capillary fragility (including arterial and venous networks in friable periventricular germinal tissue) and increased vascular pressure. Sudden shock during the first few days of life often is due to massive intraventricular hemorrhage, which occurs predominantly in very small preterm infants. Less severe degrees of hemorrhage may be associated with lethargy, seizures, apnea, and an acute fall in hematocrit level. Pulmonary hemorrhage has a similar pattern of increased incidence and high mortality in preterm infants.

Respiratory distress syndrome (hyaline membrane disease) occurs most frequently and mortality is highest in infants of shortest gestation, and incidence and mortality fall progressively with increasing gestational age (see Chapter 42, Part Three).

There is a higher *congenital malformation rate* in both preterm infants with LBW and term infants who are SGA than in term infants of normal birth weight. Those with the slowest intrauterine growth rates have the highest incidence of malformations. The incidence of *patent ductus arteriosus* is much higher in infants with LBW and in those whose gestational age is less than 34 weeks than among larger or older infants (see Chapter 43).

Hypoglycemia may occur in 15% of preterm infants and in up to 65% of infants who are SGA. Hyperglycemia is common in extremely small infants who receive high concentrations of glucose or develop sepsis (see Chapter 47, Part One).

Recurrent apnea, necrotizing enterocolitis, and *retinopathy of prematurity* occur most commonly in infants with VLBW and in those with shorter gestations.

FUTURE PROGRESS

PREVENTION OF INFANT MORTALITY AND LOW BIRTH WEIGHT

Although we do not know all the precise causes of infant mortality and LBW, prevention efforts can make substantial progress toward decreasing infant mortality and LBW.[13] In the United States, much of the progress in reducing infant mortality has been a result of improvements in neonatal and perinatal care. As evidenced by the stable rates of LBW and preterm birth in the United States, there has been little or no progress in preventing LBW or preterm birth. However, there are things that can be done to prevent LBW. If smoking during pregnancy was eliminated, the infant mortality rate would decrease by 10%, and

the LBW rate would decrease by 25%. Decreasing the incidence of unplanned pregnancies, decreasing the abuse of alcohol and other illicit drugs, increasing enrollment in the Special Supplemental Food Program for Women, Infants, and Children (WIC), and providing prenatal care in a comprehensive and coordinated manner also could reduce infant mortality and LBW.[2, 4]

Preventing pediatric mortality and morbidity associated with LBW requires a broad range of activities that involve the family, health care professionals, and community groups. These activities include identifying prepregnancy risks; counseling for risk reduction; implementing school health and related educational programs; increasing accessibility of early, high-quality prenatal care services; expanding the content of prenatal care to meet the variable needs of individual women and selected high-risk groups; and developing, implementing, and supporting a long-term public information program with a few well-chosen messages targeted at LBW risks (e.g., smoking cessation).

FETAL DEVELOPMENT, PHYSIOLOGY, AND BIOCHEMISTRY

The continuing expansion of our understanding of and ability to measure embryonic and fetal physiologic and biochemical homeostasis is likely to advance the practice of neonatal-perinatal medicine. In addition, as our appreciation of the mechanisms controlling labor, the protective circulatory adjustments of the fetus to hypoxia, and our understanding of pharmacology increases, we can develop new means to successfully detect high-risk pregnancies, treat the fetus, and prevent preterm labor.

In 1960 our ability to detect *fetal asphyxia* consisted of auscultation of the fetal heart rate during labor and observation of the amniotic fluid for meconium staining when the membranes ruptured. We now know the sequence of events in the fetus that occurs in response to maternal hypotension or hypoxia.[1] The heart rate and blood pressure initially increase; then, with the rapid onset of fetal bradycardia and hypotension, the fetus develops a mixed metabolic and "placental" respiratory acidosis. The cardiac output and umbilical blood flow decrease sharply. A greater portion of the oxygenated umbilical vein blood is shunted past the liver into the inferior vena cava and returned to the heart. The cardiac output to the brain, heart, and adrenal glands is preferentially maintained so that tissue perfusion of these organs initially does not decrease significantly, although oxygenation decreases. In contrast, the fetal lungs and cortex of the kidneys have a decreased perfusion. The oxygen consumption of the fetus decreases by over 50%. When this sequence of events becomes far enough advanced in the rhesus monkey and baboon, and probably in the human, the problem is detectable by continuous monitoring of the fetal heart rate and uterine pressure curves.

Characteristic high-risk patterns such as those for cord occlusion or placental insufficiency can be identified (see Chapter 9). Nevertheless, the treatments for fetal asphyxia that are currently available are limited to surgical intervention, oxygen, or position changes. Improved understanding of the hormonal and neural regulation of labor and the patterns of fetal pathophysiologic response, especially in the brain, may broaden our pharmacologic approach to treatment before birth. Our ability to diagnose and treat some diseases before birth, such as erythroblastosis, respiratory distress syndrome (hyaline membrane disease), and a large number of genetic defects, has changed dramatically in recent years.

Investigation of the cellular and molecular levels of development and pharmacology of the uterus, placenta, and fetus may be critical to understanding the control of labor.[9] This understanding would enable us to decrease the incidence of preterm infants or those with LBW. Prenatal diagnosis and biochemical and ultrasonic fetal monitoring may be only the first steps toward the development of future treatments. These future treatments may include hybridization of cells in the early blastocyst or embryo to correct inborn errors of metabolism, the stimulation of embryogenesis of organs, gene therapy, the acceleration of organ maturation, and pharmacologic interventions to ameliorate hypoxic injury to the central nervous system.

LEGAL AND ETHICAL ISSUES

Advances in the field of neonatal-perinatal medicine have focused attention on a number of legal and ethical issues. There is continuing concern about life-and-death decision making in neonatal intensive care units. New and complex physician-patient-family-nursing societal relationships exist in these units, and this development has had an enormous impact on the process of making medical decisions. As a result of regionalization, we now have nearly universal access to care in neonatal intensive care units, and this has brought these ethical issues into a sharper and more demanding focus. Specific criteria must now be formulated for making decisions that previously were made on the basis of access to the health system, which was strongly influenced by the economic position of a family. For example, should a 500-gm infant with a poor prognosis for intact survival be accepted to a neonatal intensive care unit when it means one cannot accept a 2000-gm infant who is at high risk but has a good prognosis if he or she survives, just because the referring physician in the case of the 500-gm infant calls first or because the infant is born in the same hospital where the intensive care unit is located?

The nature of the evolving customs or legal restraints differs in some important respects from those impinging on the traditional physician-patient relationship outside neonatal intensive care centers. Discussions before decision making will involve a variety of people, will be more explicitly informative, and

will make more exacting demands on the physician's ability to perceive what is meant from what is said. Ironically, but not surprisingly, as the technology of care increases in these units, the difficult choices for the physician are not the technical medical decisions but rather the matters of judgment that require evaluating, analyzing, and interpreting the complex human interests and concerns of the relatives, their friends and advisors, the staff, and the various consequences for the people involved. These decisions have always been the most challenging and demanding ones for physicians because they cannot be delegated to others. The new elements are the frequency and complexity of these judgments in regional neonatal intensive care centers (see Chapter 4).

QUALITY OF CARE

Whatever decision-making process is used to improve the quality of care, certain principles are important but often not easy to apply. The fundamental responsibility of all who are concerned is to do no harm or, at least, no harm without a reasonable expectation of a compensating benefit for the patient. A corollary principle is that there must be continuous, objective, critical, and scientific evaluation of the care being provided and of proposed innovations. Activities should not be initiated or continued that on balance do harm to the well-being of a newborn infant. The definition of *well-being* is a major problem, because the varying ethical values, religious commitments, and life experiences of all those who care for and about the infants, as well as legal restraints, must be taken into consideration. In general, the minimum elements of well-being include a life prolonged beyond infancy, without excruciating pain, and with the potential of participating in human experience to at least a minimal degree.

Awareness of these considerations has contributed to the impetus for further clinical specialization within pediatrics and obstetrics and gynecology, resulting in the formation of a field of clinical medicine for the fetus and neonatal infant called *neonatal-perinatal medicine*. This field has already expanded to encompass the developing embryo before and after organ formation and to encompass older infants whose immaturity or disease process makes them best cared for in neonatal intensive care centers.

■ REFERENCES

1. Behrman RE, et al: Distribution of the circulation in the normal asphyxiated fetal neonate. Am J Obstet Gynecol 108:956, 1970.
2. Caring for our future: The content of prenatal care. Washington, DC, U.S. Department of Health and Human Services, Public Health Service, Panel on the Content of Prenatal Care, 1988.
3. Guyer B, et al: Annual summary of vital statistics—1998. Pediatrics 104:1229, 1999.
4. Institute of Medicine: Prenatal Care: Reaching Mothers, Reaching Infants. Washington, DC, National Academy Press, 1985.
5. Lewit GM, et al: The financial cost of low birth weight. Future Child 5:35, 1995.

6. MacDorman MF, et al: Infant mortality statistics from the 1997 period linked birth/infant death data set. National Vital Statistics Reports 47:23, 1999.
7. McCormick M, et al: Access to neonatal intensive care. Future Child 5:162, 1995.
8. National Commission to Prevent Infant Mortality: Troubling trends: the health of America's next generation. Washington, DC, NCPIM, February 1990.
9. Report and recommendation for research on the fetus. Washington, DC, The National Commission for the Protection of Human Subjects of Biomedical and Behavioral Research, Department of Health, Education, and Welfare 1975, publ No (05)76-127.
10. Richardson DK, et al: Declining severity adjusted mortality: Evidence of improving neonatal intensive care. Pediatrics 102:893, 1998.
11. Shiono PH, et al: Birth weight among women of different ethnic groups. JAMA 255:48, 1986.
12. Shiono PH, et al: Ethnic differences in preterm and very preterm delivery. Am J Public Health 76:1317, 1986.
13. Shiono PH, Behrman RE: Low birth weight: Analysis and recommendations. Future Child 5:4, 1995.
14. Stoll BJ, Kliegman R: Section 1: Noninfectious disorders. In Behrman RE, et al (eds): Nelson Textbook of Pediatrics, 16th ed., Philadelphia, WB Saunders Co, 2000.

Perinatal Services and Resources

3

Michele C. Walsh-Sukys

Avroy A. Fanaroff

The successful delivery of high-quality care to perinatal patients requires not only excellence from physicians, nurses, and other health professionals but also community involvement and a system of organization that permits the health professionals to function as cohesive teams. *Regionalization* is the term used to define one such care system. In a regionalized perinatal care system, all physicians and hospitals providing maternal and perinatal care coordinate services based on the needs of the population. Some systems are organized by mutual cooperative agreements, whereas others are mandated by regulatory agencies. Regardless of the mechanism, the sophistication of maternal and perinatal care each hospital can provide is identified and made available to consumers to accomplish the following objectives: quality care to all pregnant women and newborns, maximum use of highly trained perinatal personnel and intensive care facilities, and assurance of cost-effectiveness.

The major push toward regionalization in the United States began in the 1970s. At present, regionalization is threatened with increased competition among institutions, disrupting the mutual agreements on which regionalization was based. However, the objectives of regionalization are still desirable. Therefore, a review of the historic complex in which they were developed is instructive.

BACKGROUND AND HISTORICAL PERSPECTIVE

Before 1940, perinatal care services were delivered in the United States, Canada, and Europe without any particular organization or structure. Most of the care was provided by an individual physician or midwife. In many areas the majority of the deliveries occurred in the home. A number of maternity hospitals developed in larger urban areas, usually serving as teaching hospitals. These maternity hospitals often had home delivery services and neighborhood clinics serving a geographic area.

During the 1940s and early 1950s a number of U.S. cities developed centers for the care of premature infants. Many European countries, particularly Scandinavia and the Netherlands, developed systems of care for perinatal patients based on the development of primary prenatal care clinics staffed largely by midwives, with district and regional hospitals for the care of mothers with complications.

From 1964 to 1968 studies were undertaken in Massachusetts, Wisconsin, and Arizona to analyze the causes of neonatal mortality and morbidity.[4, 8, 15, 23, 28] These studies spurred the development of the earliest regional systems to give perinatal and neonatal care. In 1976, the report of the Joint Committee on Perinatal Health of the American Medical Association, the American College of Obstetricians and Gynecologists, the American Academy of Family Physicians, and the American Academy of Pediatrics, entitled "Toward Improving the Outcome of Pregnancy" (TIOP) was released.[36]

In the 1970s and 1980s, many different states regionalized perinatal care with the goal of reducing both neonatal and maternal morbidity and mortality. In some areas this was highly successful, whereas in others a superficial attempt at organization was never enforced, and therefore little progress was made. In the early 1990s, state by state, the regionalized systems were weakened as numerous factors put pressure on the system (Table 3–1).

In 1993, the March of Dimes convened the second TIOP conference and re-examined the theory supporting regionalization.[7] The conference participants concluded that even in the era of the 1990s, regionalization continued to be the best option for reducing perinatal morbidity.

KEY PRINCIPLES OF REGIONAL CARE

There are general principles that form the basis for the development of regional health care services for perinatal patients.[1, 27] These principles are derived from an understanding of the care needs of the mother, fetus, and family during pregnancy and of the mother, newborn, and family after birth.

27

TABLE 3–1 FACTORS THREATENING
REGIONALIZED PERINATAL
CARE

PHYSICIAN RELATED	INSTITUTION RELATED
Oversupply and maldistribution of physicians	Use of "high-tech" procedures as a marketing tool
Desire to perform all services for which they were trained, regardless of level of care designated	Desire to perform all services to allow contractual arrangements with provider
Lack of incentive to improve care at other hospitals and potential decrease in patient referrals	Lack of incentive to improve care at other hospitals and potential decrease in patient referrals
Fear of loss of patients	Institutional ego
Failure to recognize problems deserving of referral	

Modified from Institute of Medicine: Prenatal Care: Reaching Mothers, Reaching Infants. Washington, DC, National Academy Press, 1988.

ACCOUNTABILITY OF POPULATION

A region denotes a geographic area or population with definable care needs. The regional center and the network of related institutions are accountable for the overall perinatal health care for the region. Data on mortality and morbidity, frequency of problems, and quality of care are assessed for the entire population in the area. The availability and quality of care in any given institution become the responsibility of all the institutions, including the perinatal center.

ONE STANDARD OF QUALITY

Regionalization is based on the premise that there should be a single standard of quality perinatal care. Any mother or infant should have equal access to all the components of a functioning perinatal system (Table 3–2).

DIFFERING CARE CAPABILITIES OF INSTITUTIONS

Institutions operating within a region differ in their capability for providing perinatal care. These differences reflect the number of patients, educational background and experience of medical and nursing staff, and availability of equipment and facilities. Each institution is expected to deliver high-quality care up to the level of its capability. When care requirements exceed its capability, the patient is referred to the closest facility that has the required capability.

Sixty to eighty percent of problems associated with increased risk for the mother, fetus, or newborn are detectable sufficiently in advance of the crises to permit either the appropriate care resources to be made available locally or to transfer the patient to where appropriate resources are available.[14] Even under ideal circumstances, certain patients have to move from one facility to another during the course of care. Thus, institutions within a region must be effectively linked to permit ease of patient movement.

MINIMAL PATIENT MOVEMENT

The organization of the regional care network should be designed to make it possible for patients to receive care appropriate to their needs as close to their homes as possible. Only those patients with care needs exceeding the resources of their community facility should need to be referred to another institution. Through outreach education (see Chapter 5) and consultation programs, efforts should be made to continually develop and expand the care capabilities of each institution to minimize the number of patients who must be dislocated while receiving care.

OPTIMAL USE OF FACILITIES AND PERSONNEL

The concept of regionalization is designed to permit optimal use of both facilities and personnel. With the use of a regional perinatal center, it is possible to have sufficient numbers of high-risk mothers and neonates concentrated in a single location to justify economically the staffing and equipment necessary to meet their care needs.[10] In addition, personnel who have frequent opportunities to use their skills are able to maintain and enhance these skills. Institutions with smaller numbers of high-risk patients avoid the expense of developing services that are infrequently used.

DIFFERING CARE NEEDS FOR DIFFERENT GROUPS

Groups within a population have differing care needs by virtue of socioeconomic conditions, education, ethnic background, personal health care practices, age, and other factors. The organization of facilities and personnel involved in perinatal care must reflect these varying needs.

PERINATAL CARE: A TEAM SERVICE

The health care needs of the perinatal patient require a close working relationship among the various disciplines involved to prevent fragmentation and gaps in care.

CURRENT RECOMMENDATIONS ON ORGANIZATION

Those countries with better perinatal mortality and morbidity statistics have carefully organized and universally made available primary care for all pregnant mothers and have established mechanisms for referral of mothers and infants from primary care institutions to district or center hospitals when needed. They have placed less emphasis on tertiary care or intensive care because of the relatively low demand for such

TABLE 3–2 DEFINITIONS OF CARE AT PERINATAL CENTERS

SERVICE	BASIC	SPECIALTY	SUBSPECIALTY
Care Provided			
Basic inpatient care for women and newborns without complications	√	√	√
High-risk pregnancies with moderate complications		√	√
Neonatal intensive care including ventilation			√
Inpatient care for critically ill neonates			√
Follow-up medical care of NICU grads			√
Follow-up developmental assessment			√
Consultation and referral arrangements			√
Transport service			√
Personnel			
Physician and nursing staff to care for uncomplicated pregnancy	√	√	√
Obstetrician		√	√
Pediatrician		√	√
OB anesthesia			√
Neonatologist			√
Perinatal social worker			√
Genetic counselor			√
Pediatric subspecialists			√
Pediatric Surgery, Subspecialties, and Support Services			
Laboratories to assess fetal well-being and maturity		√	√
Level III ultrasound capability			√
Laboratories with microspecimen capability		√	√
Blood gases available on a 24-hour basis			√

NICU, neonatal intensive care unit; OB, obstetric.
From March of Dimes Birth Defects Foundation: Toward Improving the Outcome of Pregnancy: The 1990s and Beyond. White Plains, NY, March of Dimes, 1993.

services. By contrast, the perinatal health services of the United States and Canada place great emphasis on the specialized hospital services for the perinatal patient, but the primary care services available to the mother during her pregnancy are disorganized and inconsistent. The number of perinatal patients requiring intensive in-hospital care is inversely related to the quality and availability of primary services, as well as to the general health status of the mother before pregnancy.

An organized system for perinatal care begins with a well-integrated ambulatory care system that emphasizes early risk assessment. The prenatal care may be delivered by basic providers (family practice or nurse practitioners), specialty providers (obstetricians and experienced family practitioners), or subspecialty providers (maternal-fetal medicine specialists) as appropriate to the level of risk. As women's risk status changes during pregnancy, so may the level of care needed. No care system is effective if it is not used. TIOP II has emphasized that "early and continuous prenatal care is an important and effective means to improve the outcome of pregnancy."[7] However, in the 1980s, virtually no progress was made in increasing the number of women receiving early prenatal care, and the number of women receiving late or no care increased. Therefore, more work needs to be done to better understand the barriers to prenatal care. The Institute of Medicine described the following six barriers to adequate prenatal care: (1) financial, (2) inadequate capacity in care systems used by low-income

women, (3) services that are difficult to navigate (unfriendly), (4) lack of awareness and acceptance of unintended pregnancy, (5) personal beliefs about prenatal care, and (6) social isolation.[3, 19] TIOP II proposed solutions to ameliorate each of these barriers (Table 3–3).[7]

An organized system for providing care to the maternity patient and her neonate consists of the following types of units or facilities: physicians' offices and clinics, basic perinatal facilities, specialty perinatal facilities, subspecialty perinatal facilities, regional perinatal centers, and specialized units such as children's hospitals and cardiac centers.

PHYSICIANS' OFFICES AND CLINICS

The basic units for care during pregnancy as well as for care of the mother and infant after delivery are physicians' offices and general clinics. These units need to have the capability for obtaining a complete health history, careful physical assessment of the mother or infant, systematic risk assessment (using one of the available risk scoring systems), and laboratory resources for determination of hematocrit or hemoglobin concentration and urinalysis.

BASIC PERINATAL FACILITIES (LEVEL I)

Basic perinatal facilities are those designed primarily for the care of the maternal and neonatal patients who have no complications. Since even uncompli-

TABLE 3–3 REDUCING BARRIERS TO PRENATAL CARE THROUGH SYSTEM CHANGE

BARRIERS	RELATED COPH RECOMMENDATIONS
Financing	Health care coverage for all pregnant women
	Mechanisms to ensure adequate provider payment
Capacity	More efficient use of existing providers
	Improved linkages between public and private as well as ambulatory and inpatient providers
Lack of user-friendly services	Matching provider capabilities and expertise to individual need and risks
	Risk assessment to identify medical, personal, and cultural barriers
Unintended pregnancy	Reproductive awareness among all women
	Greater emphasis on preconception and interconception care, including family planning
Personal beliefs and attitudes	Health promotion and health education for all children
	Reproductive awareness among all women
Social isolation	Outreach programs

COPH, Committee on Perinatal Health.
From March of Dimes Birth Defects Foundation: Toward Improving the Outcome of Pregnancy: The 1990s and Beyond. White Plains, NY, March of Dimes, 1993.

cated maternal and neonatal patients have a potential for unexpected complications, basic units must have the resources to provide competent emergency services when the need arises. The necessary services for a basic perinatal facility are shown in Table 3–2 and include a normal newborn nursery.

SPECIALTY PERINATAL FACILITIES (LEVEL II)

Specialty perinatal facilities are those hospitals that have larger maternity and newborn services. These hospitals are located in urban and suburban areas serving larger communities. In addition to providing a full range of maternal and newborn services for perinatal patients who have no complications, they provide services for some of the obstetric and neonatal patients who have one or more complications. The range of obstetric and neonatal complications that a given institution offers depends on the resources available. The services available in specialty units are presented in Table 3–2 and include both a normal newborn nursery and a transitional care nursery. Care of neonates who are high risk should be provided by appropriately qualified physicians. A board-certified pediatrician with special interest, experience, and in some situations, subspecialty certification in neonatal-perinatal medicine should be chief of the neonatal care services.

SUBSPECIALTY PERINATAL FACILITIES (LEVEL III)

In addition to the resources and capabilities of a specialty unit, subspecialty facilities are able to provide for a full range of maternal complications and newborn intensive care. The neonatal intensive care unit needs to have a full range of services for the neonate, with the possible exception of an occasional infant with congenital heart disease or other complex congenital anomaly who requires a specialized unit. The services offered by subspecialty facilities are listed in Table 3–2 and include the capacity to provide intensive care for both mother and infant. The director of a subspecialty unit should be a full-time, board-certified pediatrician with subspecialty certification in neonatal-perinatal medicine.

REGIONAL PERINATAL CENTER

A regional perinatal center is a subspecialty facility that also has responsibility for the coordination and management of special services, including transportation, that are needed for the region. In areas where there is only one subspecialty facility, it is expected to function as the regional perinatal center. In areas where there is more than one unit with subspecialty capabilities, one of the units would serve as the regional perinatal center. The regional perinatal center must offer outpatient and inpatient consultation and diagnostic services for basic and specialty facilities within the region, including ultrasonography, laboratory analysis of amniotic fluid, gestational age assessment, genetic studies, and other studies of fetal health. It also should provide specialized nursing services and consultation in nutrition, social services, respiratory therapy, and laboratory and radiology services. The center is responsible for carrying on an active outreach education program for the institutions, health professionals, and public within the region.

A regional perinatal center has unique personnel needs. It should be directed by a full-time physician with extensive training and experience in perinatal medicine as well as administration. There also should be a director of obstetric services and a director of neonatal services. The director of obstetric services should be a full-time physician with training and experience in fetal-maternal medicine, including maternal intensive care. The director of neonatal services should be a full-time neonatologist with training and experience in neonatal care, including newborn intensive care. The perinatal nursing services should be directed by a clinical nurse specialist with advanced experience in maternal and neonatal nursing and in administration. The center also may require a full-time director of the outreach education program to coordinate the active participation of physicians in obstetrics and newborn care, nurses in obstetrics and newborn care, nutritionists, social workers, and other specialized personnel. The obstetric and newborn care units, including the newborn intensive care, should have clinical nurse specialists in obstetrics and neonatal care, respectively, responsible for organizing the nursing program and coordinating the patient care needs.

It is important to estimate the number of pregnant women who may need specialized obstetric and neonatal services within the area of a given regional perinatal center. The percentage of pregnancies at increased risk may vary from 10% for general populations, such as an entire state or country, to more than 90% in some urban hospitals. In an Ontario perinatal study, 32% of pregnancies had some increased risk factor that resulted in 60% of the neonatal problems.[29] In the Nova Scotia Fetal Risk Project, 11% of 9483 patients accounted for 50% of the stillbirths and 75% of the neonatal deaths.[41]

The number of neonatal care beds and neonatal intensive care days needed for a given population are most influenced by the frequency of premature birth and low birth weight (LBW). There are great differences in these frequencies among countries and among populations within a country. Infants with LBW account for less than 5% of the births in the Scandinavian countries and 6% to 9% of infants in some states in the United States; in some institutions the frequency may run as high as 15% to 20%.[31]

Swyer and associates calculated a need for neonatal intensive care beds at 0.7 beds per 1000 live births on the basis of a 7% LBW rate.[43] Transitional or intermediate and convalescent bed needs were approximately 4 per 1000 live births. The Wisconsin Perinatal Care Program predicted a need for 12 intensive care beds for 6000 live births (7% LBW rate). Data from Utah indicate a need for 2 beds per 1000 annual live births in special care facilities. The estimated breakdown was 0.5 level I beds, 0.5 level II beds, and 1 bed per 1000 annual live births at level III.[21] Field and colleagues, in the United Kingdom, reported that the demand for neonatal intensive care was 1.1 beds per 1000 deliveries.[13] This was a minimum estimate, and factors such as increased survival of extremely immature infants would increase the demand for beds.

MATERNAL AND NEONATAL TRANSPORT SERVICES

Despite the proliferation of neonatal coverage for specialty nurseries, efficient maternal-fetal and neonatal transport services form a key component of regional perinatal care. Ideally, the delivery of an infant of less than 32 weeks' gestation or weighing less than 1.5 kg should occur at a perinatal center. Although comparisons of mortality statistics after maternal transfer versus neonatal transfer suffer from many confounding variables, several studies have demonstrated a lower morbidity and shorter neonatal hospitalization after maternal-fetal transport.[5, 32]

Paneth and associates analyzed all singleton births and deaths with known birth weight and gestational age in New York City from 1976 through 1978.[30] Mortality rates for full-term, appropriately grown infants were not influenced by the hospital of birth. However, preterm and LBW infants were at a 24% higher risk of death if birth occurred at either a level I or level II unit. These small infants constituted only a small percentage of the births but accounted for 70% of the deaths. Fanaroff and others analyzed the outcomes of neonates delivered between 24 and 28 weeks at a National Institute of Child Health and Human Development network level III unit with neonates of similar gestational age who were transported to the centers after birth.[12] "Outborn" infants had significantly more respiratory distress syndrome (88% versus 81%), more grade III or IV intraventricular hemorrhages (24% versus 17%; odds ratio 1.61, 1.12 to 2.16), and greater mortality (32% versus 22%; odds ratio 1.63, 1.15 to 2.30). Yeast and colleagues compared neonatal mortality in two 5-year periods (1982 to 1986 versus 1990 to 1994) in Missouri. They found that in both periods the relative risk of neonatal mortality in level II centers was 2.28 compared with level III centers and that no substantial improvement had occurred in those 10 years.[45] Similar data have been reported from California.[32] Thus, there are compelling reasons for preterm deliveries to occur at tertiary centers.

It is estimated that antenatal maternal transfer is not possible in up to 50% of high-risk pregnancies. In these situations neonatal transport must be performed by specially trained teams skilled in adequate stabilization before, and effective management during, transport. Hood and associates have documented a 60% greater mortality rate when neonates were transferred by an untrained versus a trained neonatal transport team.[18] Hypothermia and acidosis, in particular, were more common after transfer by an untrained team. The transport team from the referral hospital also serves an important educational function and can influence and improve methods of stabilization at the referring center, which in turn may influence mortality statistics (see Chapter 5).

In many areas, limited regional perinatal resources have hampered referrals and required the referring physician to make multiple calls until an available bed can be located. Central telephone operator systems have partially alleviated this problem. A computer-based coordination of telecommunications has been developed in North Carolina. The system, which is linked to the state's nine tertiary centers and provides updates every 2 hours on neonatal and maternal bed availability, appears cost-effective.[2]

An effective means of managing overcrowding at the perinatal referral center is to encourage reverse transport of previously ill neonates to levels I and II nurseries for intermediate care.[20] Transfer can include not only babies with resolved acute medical problems but also those with chronic problems such as bronchopulmonary dysplasia. However, the tertiary center must be familiar with the capabilities, facilities, and resources of the hospitals to which reverse transport is occurring so that quality of care can be ensured. This evaluation can be combined with an outreach education program. Apart from the obvious cost-effectiveness of reverse transport, it can encourage family bonding and greater involvement of the pediatrician who will be offering continuing care to the infant.

The outcome of infants transported back from tertiary centers to community hospitals (level II units staffed by skilled personnel) was compared with that of infants convalescing in the tertiary center. Lynch and colleagues documented that the infants received appropriate care, were less likely to need readmission to the intensive care unit (7% versus 14%), and required fewer transfusions.[24] Major new health problems developed in 27% of the patients during convalescence. However, the overall complication rate was lower for the reverse transfers. The current medical economic climate is mandating that tertiary units establish criteria for reverse transfer, and many health maintenance organizations and preferred provider organizations are demanding early reverse transport. Tertiary units are obliged to ensure that there are appropriately trained personnel and adequate facilities so as not to compromise the medical needs or care of the neonates requiring reverse transfer.

In the late 1990s, the desire to constrain runaway medical costs led to the proliferation in health maintenance organizations and to consolidation in the health systems. Both are characterized by contractual arrangements with "preferred providers." These events have led to an increased frequency of transports of fragile neonates between level III institutions that are solely driven by the demands of the insurer rather than the health care needs of the infant. The impact of these transfers on the care of the neonates and their families is largely unassessed. However, there are some data to suggest that these transfers disproportionately affect uninsured and publicly insured infants.

OTHER SERVICES IN A REGIONAL CARE SYSTEM

An effective public health nursing system and an availability of public health services are essential ingredients for effective perinatal care. Home visits during pregnancy and after birth provide a dimension of care not met by physicians' offices or community hospitals. Their importance is increasing in an era where discharge of mothers and infants at 24 to 36 hours of age is becoming the norm. Finally, a perinatal center must develop close working relationships with regional blood banks and state or regional laboratories that provide special diagnostic services to meet the needs of the perinatal patient.

PROBLEMS OF REGIONALIZATION

One of the most common disorders of regionalization is centralization in place of regionalization. This is the end product of a regional center that operates with no outreach education program or other mechanisms for continuing the development and improvement of services in the other hospitals of the region. With such a system, the central hospital continues to receive the referrals of high-risk mothers or high-risk neonates but makes no effort to help the referring hospital develop programs for preventing the problems. This may be particularly true in university medical centers, where outreach education and service are not considered a regular academic or hospital activity. This problem improved with increased use of reverse transports, in which neonates no longer requiring tertiary level care are transported back to their community hospitals.[6] However, this progress is threatened because some third-party and government payers will not reimburse the expense of the reverse transport, even when the result is to relocate care to a less expensive institution.

A second common disorder of regionalization is unnecessary duplication of units. This includes the unnecessary duplication of both basic and specialty units within rural or urban areas and competing subspecialty units, particularly in urban areas. The duplication results in difficulties in recruiting and maintaining the necessary personnel for such care units as well as an increased cost per patient for such care. Such duplication invariably is a result of competing institutions and competing medical staffs, who view maternal intensive care and neonatal intensive care units as important to their business, income, or institutional image.

Many regional centers are staffed with inadequate or inappropriately trained personnel. One of the most common problems is the staffing of infant intensive care nurseries with inadequately supervised and inexperienced house staff as the primary responsible physicians, particularly during night hours and weekends. This practice seems to be changing. Denson and others found 23% of academic centers with 24-hour, in-house coverage by attending neonatologists.[9] An equally serious problem of medical supervision is seen in those intensive care units that operate with no full-time staff. The coverage and time commitment available from busy pediatric general practitioners do not permit the attention necessary for intensive care or the development of expertise. Inadequate or inappropriate staffing also is often manifested in the use of licensed practical nurses by hospitals in place of experienced professional nurses in the care of high-risk mothers and high-risk neonates. This is usually done as a cost-saving measure with inadequate understanding of the value of experienced professional nurses in the delivery of high-risk perinatal care. There is, likewise, a reluctance to use clinical nurse specialists and nurse clinicians because of the cost and lack of understanding of their role in patient care.

A keystone of an effective perinatal regional system is an integrated system for transport. In the 1970s these systems flourished with well-trained and well-equipped coordinated systems, which frequently were based in a single hospital but served a geographic region by sharing patients among level III centers in a cooperative fashion. In the 1980s these systems became dysfunctional when the transport systems, themselves, were used as marketing tools by hospital administrators and were designed to attract and retain paying customers. Duplication of expensive transport services and overutilization of helicopter transport resulted. Then, as the rush to control health care costs in the 1990s began, transport services were often the first victims. Elimination of or severe reductions in staff limited the availability of services. The impact of this has not yet been adequately assessed.

Finally, in most regions there are some institutions and physicians who consistently fail to use the resources of a regional center appropriately when the care of the patient clearly indicates such a need. The hospitals that make least use of the center may be located closest to the center. Fear of loss of patients, physician ego, and failure to recognize problems promptly were the major inhibitors to appropriate use of perinatal center resources in the past. Increasing problems in the 1990s include the constraints of preferred providers placed by payers on physicians and patients. The appropriate regional subspecialty center may not be a member of the payer's network, creating pressure to retain a patient in a specialty center rather than transfer her to a subspecialty center.

IS REGIONALIZATION OF PERINATAL CARE NEEDED?

In the 1970s a spirit of altruism drove the development of regionalized systems. At the dawn of the new millennium the realities of health care reform, competition, and cost constraints have dimmed that spirit. More hospitals are merging and forming networks that then jointly contract with payers to supply complete health services to a population of "covered lives." These forces lead every network to wish to provide all levels of service in a given area so that covered lives stay within that system. This leads to duplication of services that runs counter to the principles of regionalization. In addition, the availability of a large supply of highly trained neonatologists created a physician oversupply that led to diffusion of intensive level III services down to level II nurseries, and the creation of new levels of care termed, somewhat tongue-in-cheek, *level IIB*, or *level II plus*. Some authors have argued that mortality is similar in these smaller units when compared with level III units. However, comparison of these populations is difficult because the sickest newborns with the highest expected mortality are transferred out of the level II units, reducing the expected mortality in these units. The work by Fanaroff, Paneth, and Yeast with their associates clearly documents that outcomes are better in subspecialty centers.[12, 30, 42, 45]

Despite two decades of work and a steady decline in infant mortality (see Fig. 2–1 in previous chapter), more progress can be made.[16] As shown in Table 3–4, in 1998 infant mortality rate nationwide was 7.2 deaths per 1000 live births, and infant mortality among black infants was 2.4 times higher than that in white infants. The disparities in infant mortality by race remain a major public health concern (see Chapter 2). In addition, there is substantial geographic variation in mortality. The District of Columbia and five states had infant mortality rates in excess of 10%.

TABLE 3–4 INFANT AND NEONATAL MORTALITY RATES BY BIRTH WEIGHT AND RACE OF MOTHER, UNITED STATES, 1997 LINKED FILE

BIRTH WEIGHT (gm)	INFANT MORTALITY RATE				NEONATAL MORTALITY RATE			
	All Races*	Non-Hispanic White	Black	Hispanic	All Races*	Non-Hispanic White	Black	Hispanic
Total	7.2	6.0	13.7	6.0	4.8	3.9	9.2	4.0
<2500	61.7	56.0	75.8	58.4	50.3	46.0	61.3	47.6
<1500	252.8	240.7	270.1	250.1	223.8	215.7	236.1	218.3
<500	883.9	899.7	875.2	864.1	869.2	886.0	861.1	838.9
500–749	492.7	510.7	456.9	506.3	437.5	461.0	396.2	446.5
750–999	161.3	172.5	140.4	174.6	122.4	136.6	96.8	137.4
1000–1249	75.9	75.8	72.3	84.9	53.7	58.4	42.5	61.7
1250–1499	48.6	51.7	38.9	56.0	34.3	39.3	22.6	38.2
1500–1999	30.2	31.1	26.6	33.4	18.8	20.2	14.0	22.2
2000–2499	12.4	12.5	12.3	12.0	6.5	7.0	5.2	7.1
≥2500	2.7	2.5	4.1	2.3	1.0	1.0	1.1	0.9
2500–2999	4.9	5.0	5.8	4.3	2.0	2.1	1.8	2.0
3000–3499	2.6	2.5	3.7	2.1	0.9	0.9	0.9	0.8
3500–3999	1.9	1.8	2.9	1.6	0.6	0.6	0.7	0.5
4000–4499	1.7	1.5	3.0	1.6	0.7	0.6	1.0	0.7
≥4500	2.2	1.9	5.1	2.1	1.0	0.8	†	†

*Includes races other than white and black.
†Figure does not meet standards of reliability or precision.
Note: Infant and neonatal mortality rates by race from the linked file differ slightly from those based on unlinked data because the linked file uses the self-reported race of mother from the birth certificate, whereas the unlinked data uses the race of child as reported by the funeral director on the death certificate. Births are tabulated separately by race and Hispanic origin; persons of Hispanic origin may be of any race.
Adapted from MacDorman MF, Atkinson JO: Infant mortality statistics from the 1997 period linked birth/infant death data set. Natl Vital Stat Rep 47:1, 1999.

Short gestation and LBW increased as a cause of mortality. In 1997, 65% of all infant deaths occurred among the 7.5% of infants born weighing less than 2500 gm. Maine, New Hampshire, Massachusetts, Rhode Island, and Connecticut ranked highest for early utilization for prenatal care, had half the national average for late or no prenatal care, and had the lowest infant mortality rates. Overall, the United States continues to rank poorly in international comparisons of infant mortality. Some states are making an impact.

Richardson and colleagues have published a case study of one community that illustrates the continued benefits of regionalization in the 21st century.[38] When two independent pediatric services proposed a merger into a full-service children's hospital, community hospitals reacted with plans to upgrade their obstetric-neonatal units to level II or II plus neonatal intensive care units. The fear that unrestricted competition would drive up overall health care costs led the U.S. Chamber of Commerce to retain consultants to analyze the number and location of neonatal intensive care unit beds needed. The consultants found that the existing system worked well with high levels of patient and provider satisfaction. Interviews with parents of infants and providers emphasized the care provided. In contrast, hospital administrators emphasized competitive threats and the financial disincentives to support existing regionalization, whereas business leaders emphasized the need to control costs. Consultants found that the number of neonatal intensive care unit beds in the community was adequate and that substantial cost savings could be realized through using reverse transport of convalescent infants.

Pollack has also reported a similar cooperative, voluntary implementation of a regional system of care among a network of level IIs staffed by private practice neonatologists working collaboratively with existing university-based level III facilities and staff.[34] The implementation of the guidelines resulted in a reduced number of neonates with LBW and very LBW born at the community hospitals, increased maternal transports, increased reversed transports of neonates from level III to level II centers, and, most important, decreased neonatal mortality.

Is regionalization part of the solution to reduce infant mortality and reduce morbidity? These studies argue that it is.

MEASUREMENTS OF EFFECTIVENESS OF CARE ORGANIZATION

When the effectiveness of any care system as well as its individual components is measured, it is essential to analyze data for the entire region. There are many examples of dramatic changes in mortality or morbidity statistics for a given hospital in the course of a single year, not as a result of improvement of care but as a result of movement of patients with particular problems to another institution. If the geographic

boundaries of a region are well designed, there will be limited patient movement from region to region. This permits consistent year-to-year evaluation of the care within the region.

Maternal mortality has declined to the point that it is no longer a satisfactory index of quality of care. Fetal and neonatal mortality are still reasonable indicators of perinatal care. In evaluating a region, the data must link the hospital in which the death is recorded with the institution and the community in which the birth occurred or the care was initiated. Fetal and neonatal mortalities should also be divided by weight groups. The weight groups should be in 500-gm increments or less, beginning with 500 gm. If possible, the gestational age distribution and cause of death for the fetal or neonatal deaths should be established. Finally, both sex and transport status (maternal or neonatal) have been shown to affect mortality.[11, 39] Such practices make it possible to identify those areas or institutions within a region in which there are major problems with care. Any comparison of mortality is most useful if a risk adjustment tool is applied, such as the Clinical Risk Index for Babies (CRIB) or Score for Neonatal Acute Physiology (SNAP)[37, 44] (see Chapter 6.) Such scores correct for the inherent bias of subspecialty centers that receive only the sickest neonates and therefore experience the highest mortality.

When maternal, fetal, or neonatal mortality or morbidity rates are used, certain other information is necessary to permit useful interpretation. For maternal mortalities, it is essential to separate those maternal deaths that occurred during or as a result of pregnancy associated with other maternal disease, such as severe cardiac disease or malignancy, from those deaths associated primarily with the pregnancy. This requires analysis of each death and assignment to preventable or nonpreventable categories. For evaluation of neonatal programs and regionalization, the frequency of 1-minute Apgar scores of 3 or under and 5-minute Apgar scores of 5 or under should be recorded. Also helpful in assessing effectiveness of care are the frequency of sepsis, traumatic delivery, respiratory distress syndrome, and neurologic problems; the number of intensive care days; and the number of patient transfers from community institutions to institutions of greater care capability.

All high-risk mothers and neonates should have systematic follow-up care. Those infants with a birth weight of less than 1500 gm are at high risk for developmental, neurologic, or learning problems and should be followed into school age with careful neurologic and educational testing.[17, 25] (see Chapter 39). The incidence of child abuse and failure to thrive may also reflect parenting disorders having antecedents in the perinatal period.

FINANCIAL IMPACT OF REGIONALIZATION

The facilities within a regional network, including a regional perinatal center, financially depend on a combination of patient revenue and public support to care for neonatal patients. With carefully coordinated use of resources and facilities, the cost of care delivery can be contained.[40] It is essential that health insurance programs provide adequate coverage for obstetric and neonatal conditions and that charges reflect the cost of delivering the services. Medical assistance and other forms of payment, as well as direct support of state and county hospitals, must be adequate for the care needs. There must be adequate nursing staff, physician coverage, equipment, and supplies to achieve an acceptable quality of care. The reimbursement schemes should provide for patient transfer between institutions without multiplication of deductibles or major financial hardship to the patient. The cost of emergency transport of high-risk maternal and newborn patients should be covered. Financial incentives should promote, rather than discourage, the use of resources appropriate to patient care needs.

Diagnostic-related grouping has been implemented as the basis for federal reimbursement, and other third-party payers have followed suit. The limited initial database used to determine the reimbursement level did not take into account many variables that influence length of stay, particularly at a tertiary center.[22, 26, 33, 35] If the guidelines are not modified, major tertiary centers will be at a distinct financial disadvantage, particularly when providing care for extremely complicated problems and infants with LBW. The system may also discourage transport of infants from both primary and specialty units if the referring hospitals perceive financial gain; hence, the quality of care may be compromised.

IMPLICATIONS FOR EDUCATION

In the organization of most perinatal regions, the educational needs of health care professionals must be carefully integrated with the needs of the patient and family (see Chapter 5). It is essential that the patient's needs for privacy, care, professional attention, and time for personal interactions among infant, family, and other important caretakers be recognized by those participating in patient care, for example, nurses, medical students, and house staff. However, quality care, in large part, depends on undergraduate and graduate education programs that are an integral part of the responsibilities of a regional perinatal center. Senior staff physicians and nurses must accept direct responsibility for patient care and major management decisions, while fulfilling their educational responsibilities toward those in training or in practice in the community.

FUTURE CONSIDERATIONS

Centers for newborn care have expanded at the specialty (level II) institutions with large delivery services so that many have developed capabilities similar to those at subspecialty centers. In many geographic areas the subspecialty and specialty units compete; in others the two centers work hand in hand. In all communities it is essential that mutually productive relationships be re-established between the academic and community hospitals. A majority of board-certified neonatologists in the United States now practice outside the traditional academic settings. These personnel needs are being met by the university-based training programs. However, with fewer training programs accredited and more trainees completing a third fellowship year, it is conceivable that in the near future there will not be enough trained neonatologists to staff the ever-expanding specialty units. At present, the major strategies are to provide cost-effective medical care, to comply with regulations that dictate standards required for reimbursement and, above all, to prevent LBW and prematurity.

■ REFERENCES

1. Aubrey RH, et al: High-risk obstetrics: I. Perinatal outcome in relation to a broadened approach to obstetrical care for patients at special risk. Am J Obstet Gynecol 105:241, 1969.
2. Bostick JS, et al: A minicomputer-based perinatal/neonatal telecommunications network. Pediatrics 71:272, 1983.
3. Brown SS, et al: Barriers to access to prenatal care. In Kotch JB, et al (eds): A Pound of Prevention: The Case for Universal Maternity Care in the United States. Washington, DC, American Public Health Association, 1992.
4. Callon HF: Regionalizing perinatal care in Wisconsin. Nurs Clin North Am 10:263, 1975.
5. Campbell MK, et al: Is perinatal care in Southwestern Ontario regionalized? Can Med Assoc J 144:305, 1991.
6. Chiu T, et al: University neonatal centers and level II centers capability: The Jacksonville experience. J Fla Med Assoc 79:464, 1992.
7. Committee on Perinatal Health, March of Dimes Birth Defects Foundation: Toward Improving the Outcome of Pregnancy: The 1990s and Beyond. White Plains, NY, March of Dimes, 1993.
8. Committee on Perinatal Welfare: Report on perinatal and infant mortality in Massachusetts, 1967 and 1968. Boston, Massachusetts Medical Society, 1971.
9. Denson SE, et al: Twenty-four hour in-house coverage for NICUs in academic centers: Who, how and why? J Perinatol 10:257, 1990.
10. Erickson S: Infant ICUs save lives, but too many units may add cost and hamper growth. Mod Hosp 15:80, 1970.
11. Fanaroff AA, et al: Very low birthweight outcomes of the National Institute of Child Health and Human Development Neonatal Research Network, May 1991–December 1992. Am J Obstet Gynecol 173:1423, 1995.
12. Fanaroff AA, et al: Deliveries between 24 and 28 weeks' gestation should occur at tertiary centers [abstract]. Pediatr Res 35:224A, 1994.
13. Field DS, et al: The demand for neonatal intensive care. BMJ 299:1305, 1989.
14. Goodwin JW, et al: Antepartum identification of the fetus at risk. Can Med Assoc J 101:458, 1969.
15. Graven SN, et al: Perinatal health care studies and program results in Wisconsin, 1964–1970. In Stetson JB, et al (eds): Neonatal Intensive Care. St. Louis, Warren H. Green, 1975, p 1.
16. Guyer B, et al: Annual summary of vital statistics, 1998. Pediatrics 104:1229, 1999.
17. Hack M, et al: Effect of VLBW and subnormal head size on cognitive abilities at school age. N Engl J Med 325:231, 1991.
18. Hood JL, et al: Effectiveness of the neonatal transport team, Crit Care Med 11:419, 1983.
19. Institute of Medicine: Prenatal Care: Reaching Mothers, Reaching Infants. Washington, DC, National Academy Press, 1988.

20. Jung AL, et al: Back transport of neonates: Improved efficiency of tertiary nursery bed utilization, Pediatrics 71:918, 1983.

21. Jung AL, et al: Total population estimate of newborn special care bed needs. Pediatrics 75:993, 1985.

22. Lagoe RJ, et al: Impact of selected diagnosis-related groups on regional neonatal care. Pediatrics 77:627, 1992.

23. Leonard T: History of the Wisconsin Maternal Mortality Study Survey Committee. Wis Med J 69:75, 1970.

24. Lynch T, et al: Neonatal back transport: Clinical outcomes. Pediatrics 82:845, 1988.

25. McCormick MC, et al: The health and developmental status of VLBW children at school age, JAMA 267:2204, 1992.

26. Merenstein GB, et al: Personnel in neonatal pediatrics: Assessment of numbers and distribution. Pediatrics 76:454, 1985.

27. Merkatz IR, et al: The regional perinatal network. In Caplan RM, et al (eds): Advances in Obstetrics and Gynecology. Baltimore, Williams & Wilkins, 1978, p 1.

28. Meyer HBP: Regional perinatal care in Arizona: Paper presented at Sixty-Sixth Ross Conference on Pediatric Research, Columbus, Ohio, 1974.

29. Ontario Perinatal Mortality Study Committee: Second report of perinatal mortality study in ten university teaching hospitals in Ontario, Canada. Ontario Canadian Department of Health, 1967.

30. Paneth N, et al: The choice of place of delivery. Effect of hospital level on mortality in all singleton births in New York City. Am J Dis Child 141:60, 1987.

31. Paneth NS: The problem of low birthweight. Future Child 5:19, 1995.

32. Phibbs CS, et al: The effects of patient volume and level of care at the hospital of birth on neonatal mortality, JAMA 276:1054, 1996.

33. Poland RL, et al: Analysis of the effects of applying federal diagnosis-related grouping (DRG) guidelines to a population of high-risk newborn infants, Pediatrics 76:104, 1985.

34. Pollack LD: An effective model of reorganization of perinatal services in a metropolitan area. J Perinatology 16:3, 1996.

35. Pomerance JJ, et al: Cost of living for infants weighing 1.5 kilograms or less at birth. Pediatrics 61:908, 1978.

36. Report of the Committee on Perinatal Health of the American Medical Association, American College of Obstetricians and Gynecologists, American Academy of Pediatrics, and American Academy of Family Physicians: Toward Improving the Outcome of Pregnancy. New York, March of Dimes National Foundation, 1975.

37. Richardson DK, et al: Score for Neonatal Acute Physiology: A physiologic severity index for neonatal intensive care. Pediatrics 91:617, 1993.

38. Richardson DK, et al: Perinatal regionalization versus hospital competition: The Hartford example. Pediatrics 96:417, 1995.

39. Roth J, et al: Changes in survival patterns of VLBW infants from 1980 to 1993. Arch Pediatr Adolesc Med 149:1311, 1995.

40. Sandhu B, et al: Cost of neonatal intensive care for very-low-birthweight infants. Lancet 1:600, 1986.

41. Scott KE: Report of the Committee on Maternal and Perinatal Health of the Province of Nova Scotia. Nova Scotia Med Bull 49:81, 1970.

42. Stevenson DK, et al: Very low birth weight outcomes of the National Institute of Child Health and Human Development Neonatal Research Network, January 1993 through December 1994. Am J Obstet Gynecol 179:1632, 1998.

43. Swyer PR, et al (eds): Regional Services in Reproductive Medicine. Toronto, Joint Committee of the Society of Obstetricians and Gynaecologists of Canada and the Canadian Paediatric Society, 1973.

44. Tarnow-Mordi W, et al: The CRIB (Clinical Risk Index for Babies) score: A tool for assessing initial neonatal risk and comparing performance of NICUs. Lancet 342:193, 1993.

45. Yeast JD, et al: Changing patterns in regionalization of perinatal care and the impact on neonatal mortality. Am J Obstet Gynecol 178:131, 1998.

Ethics in Perinatal and Neonatal Medicine

Françoise Baylis

Jonathan Hellmann

Moral problems and uncertainties abound in perinatal and neonatal medicine: a pregnant patient abuses alcohol and drugs but refuses offers of treatment for substance abuse; a routine prenatal ultrasound identifies a minor fetal anomaly that is amenable to treatment, but the couple asks to terminate the pregnancy; the parents of an infant with extremely low birth weight insist on continuing intensive care treatment, against the medical team's recommendation.

In the clinical setting, these types of problems are frequently experienced as moral dilemmas. A physician faces a *moral dilemma* when he or she believes that two (or more) conflicting courses of action carry a moral obligation. Because both courses cannot be pursued, a value-based choice must be made. A classic example of a moral dilemma in health care is a conflict between a course of action required by the principle of autonomy and one required by the principle of beneficence. Consider, for example, the case of a pregnant woman acting in a manner that is potentially harmful to her fetus: her physician may believe that he or she has an obligation to intervene to protect the fetus from harm (principle of beneficence) but is obligated to respect the competent wishes of the pregnant patient (principle of autonomy).

Two other common types of moral problems in health care are moral uncertainty and moral distress.[28] *Moral uncertainty* typically arises when the presenting issue is unclear. For example, parents whose fetus has a major congenital anomaly are presented with the options of termination of pregnancy or postnatal surgery. They are unwilling to end the pregnancy but are underinsured and cannot afford the surgery. They are then informed about a clinical trial for in utero surgery, the cost of which would be absorbed by the institution. In this situation, whereas the physician might experience some uneasiness about the research intervention being more likely to attract those without adequate health insurance, he or she might remain unclear about the principles and values that are in conflict.

Moral distress arises when the presenting problem is clear and there is certainty on the part of the person regarding the morally "right" thing to do, but the perceived "right" course of action is precluded because of institutional or financial constraints or a lack of decision-making authority. When the parents of a newborn with a hopeless prognosis insist on resuscitation and continued aggressive treatment that the physician believes is not in the infant's best interests, the physician may experience moral distress. Similarly, when neonatal nurses who have intense hands-on contact with newborn infants feel powerless regarding their treatment decisions, they too may experience moral distress.[26]

The complexity of these types of moral problems is explored in this chapter. First, it gives an overview of the broader context in which these problems arise. Next, it discusses three specific ethical issues: maternal-fetal dilemmas, fetal therapy, and withholding or withdrawing life-sustaining treatment in the newborn infant. In each instance, ways in which members of the health care team can provide ethical care to pregnant women and their partners, fetuses, and newborn infants are explored. A collaborative framework for ethical decision making is then described and its limits identified, and finally, the physician's ethical responsibility in perinatal and neonatal care is outlined.

THE CONTEXT

The climate in which medicine has been practiced during the late 20th century has changed significantly, marked by a profound shift toward a more democratic, participatory process of health care decision making. The predominant view now is that patients' values, beliefs, and preferences should be incorporated into the decision-making process and that medical technical expertise should not dominate the many value considerations that are implicit in health care. This shift in perspective ushered in important changes in the patient-physician relationship and the communication of health care information.

THE PATIENT-PHYSICIAN RELATIONSHIP

A sound patient-physician relationship is a sine qua non of good medicine. It is within this relationship that physicians exercise their humanity, understanding, and respect for the values of others. Over the years a number of patient-physician models have been described.[19, 36, 58–60] These are briefly outlined in the following paragraphs.

PATERNALISTIC (OR PARENTALISTIC) MODEL. In this model the physician acts as the patient's guardian, articulating and implementing what the physician believes will best promote the patient's welfare. This model assumes both limited patient participation and the physician's ability to discern the patient's best interests. The literature draws distinctions between "strong" paternalism, "weak" paternalism, and "invited" paternalism. With strong paternalism, a course of action is pursued without the competent patient's consent. With weak paternalism, the physician acts for the good of an incompetent patient who cannot participate in decision making (e.g., a newborn). With invited paternalism, the patient asks the physician to make health care decisions on his or her behalf because the patient is too ill to do so.[59, 60]

INFORMATIVE (OR CONSUMER) MODEL. In this model the physician provides the patient with the relevant medical information, and the patient decides what interventions are appropriate. This model is patient driven: The patient makes the decisions and the physician implements them.

INTERPRETIVE MODEL. In this model the physician not only provides the patient with necessary information but also assists the patient with the elucidation, articulation, and realization of the patient's values in making health care choices. This approach moves beyond the informative model insofar as the physician's legitimate role includes recommending medical interventions that are consistent with the patient's value system.

DELIBERATIVE-INTERACTIVE OR BENEFICENCE-IN-TRUST MODEL. In this model the physician not only helps the patient with values clarification but also strives to make his or her professional reasoning transparent for the patient to appreciate the many factors that inform the recommendation.[10] In this type of interaction the physician may sometimes prod the patient to re-examine and possibly revise or reaffirm his or her own values, in an attempt to harmonize patient autonomy and physician beneficence. This model is most respectful of patient autonomy and attentive to the physician's obligation to "do good." In the context of perinatal medicine, therefore, it is the preferred model for interactions between competent pregnant patients and their physicians.

THE PARENT-PHYSICIAN RELATIONSHIP

In perinatal and neonatal medicine, the patient is a fetus* or a newborn, unable to participate in a patient-physician relationship. The physician's relationship is thus with the pregnant woman (and her partner) or the parents of the newborn. These are the persons legally and morally responsible for making health care decisions on behalf of the fetus or child.

The state confers this legal responsibility on parents for several reasons. The most important is the recognition of the parents' moral authority and the belief that they will normally act to promote their children's best interests. In the neonatal context, therefore, a relationship between the *parents* and the physician replaces the patient-physician relationship. Communication and decision making rests with the patient's parents. Here again, optimal interaction appears to take place within the deliberative model. Two factors in particular argue strongly for this mode of interaction: the diminishing acceptance of medical paternalism by parents who want to be part of the decision-making process for their infants, and the fact that better outcomes result when there is consensual decision making involving both parents and physicians.[16, 24] With this model, the expectations are that parents will identify their values and treatment preferences and physicians will provide parents with accurate and timely information, as much medical certainty as possible, and a professional recommendation. In conversation with the physician, parents may be invited to re-examine their values and treatment preferences, which on reflection they may either affirm or alter. On the basis of the available medical information and an understanding of the parents' values and preferences, the physician will explain the reasons for his or her professional recommendation. The goal, through dialogue and negotiation, is to reach a harmonious decision that respects parental authority and promotes physician beneficence.

EFFECTIVE AND RESPECTFUL COMMUNICATION

Common understanding and mutual trust must be established to ensure effective and respectful communication. When these background conditions are satisfied, several decisions must then be made regarding the disclosure of information. What information is needed for pregnant women and parents to make an informed choice? When is the best time to share this information? How can it be conveyed most effectively? And, who is the best person to do this?

WHAT INFORMATION IS NEEDED FOR PREGNANT WOMEN AND PARENTS TO MAKE AN INFORMED CHOICE? Pregnant patients and parents require complete and truthful information about the diagnosis and prognosis, the available treatment options (including the option of no treatment), the benefits and harms associated with each option, and the limits of available technology. Sometimes this is relatively easy information to provide; however, as medicine advances, patients, parents, and physicians must struggle with difficult decisions that are often at the limits of medical knowledge. The manner in which medical uncertainty is (or is not) communicated to parents is extremely im-

---

*When a pregnant woman pursues treatment for her fetus, the physician has two patients in one body—the pregnant woman and her fetus.

portant: it will influence decision making when the prognosis becomes more certain with increasing manifestation of disease or progressive damage over time. Although an unwillingness (and perhaps even an inability) to deal with uncertainty is understandable, it is not commendable. Pregnant patients and parents need to fully appreciate the complexity and uncertainty of much of medical information. On their part, physicians must be aware of patients' and parents' concerns and appreciate that what *they* want to know may not correspond with what *physicians* believe they need to tell.[31, 48, 49]

WHEN IS THE BEST TIME TO SHARE THIS INFORMATION? The timing of any communication with pregnant patients and parents is of crucial importance. Ideally, their readiness to receive information and their coping resources should be ascertained, so that appropriate information is shared with due consideration of their acculturation to the medical setting. In acute situations, however, the time available to establish a trusting relationship is limited. Frequently, when pregnant women are transferred to the delivery room of a referral center, or the parents of a sick newborn unexpectedly find themselves in a tertiary neonatal intensive care unit (NICU), the patient-parents and the physicians are "moral strangers"—persons who share no common history or moral framework.[35] If an urgent decision is required, the physician needs to move the relationship rapidly from one of strangers to one in which moral issues can be discussed openly. In these situations it is important that physicians recognize the vulnerability of pregnant patients and parents. For example, in the immediate postpartum period, when there may be shock and grief (and possibly even denial), it may be extremely difficult for parents to carefully weigh all of the relevant considerations, particularly if there is prognostic uncertainty. The problem for the physician is that while effective communication is not something that can be rushed, the urgent context in which the interaction is taking place exerts its own demands.

HOW CAN INFORMATION BE CONVEYED MOST EFFECTIVELY? The manner in which important information is communicated to pregnant patients and parents influences their understanding of the situation and their ability to make sound decisions. It also affects their ability to discuss moral issues and values openly. Information communicated in an honest and respectful manner is likely to foster trust. In contrast, information that is confusing, incomplete, evasive, or conveyed in a hurried or dismissive way is unlikely to do so. Effective communication entails more than mere disclosure of information: it means encouraging the patient's and parents' active participation in discussion and assuring them that their views are fundamental to the decision-making process.

WHO IS THE BEST PERSON TO PROVIDE IMPORTANT INFORMATION? Responsibility for communication must be clearly defined and not fragmented. Fragmentation is a risk in perinatal and neonatal medicine where care is provided by many individuals with expertise in different fields. Although the responsibilities of each discipline are generally known, in certain situations boundaries may be difficult to define and patterns of responsibility and communication may be affected. There is the potential not only for team members but also for pregnant patients and parents to be confused or unsure as to who is responsible for what.

The role and responsibilities of the team leader are to unite the team into an effective common cause, with a clear understanding of the differences in responsibility between conveying day-to-day information versus information about severe diagnoses and the prognostic significance of specific findings. Ideally, the responsible physician is able to integrate all the important information and maintain a consistent pattern of communication with patients or parents. His or her leadership role becomes particularly important when difficult ethical negotiations have to be undertaken in the care of a sick fetus or newborn. Even more critical is that there be leadership or guidelines for junior staff when emergencies require decisions to be made in morally uncertain situations.

"BEST INTERESTS" STANDARD OF JUDGMENT

Parents are expected to make health care choices that are in the best interests of their liveborn infant. If they do not do so, the state (at the request of the physician) may intervene and exercise its *parens patriae* authority to override the parents' decision. To say the least, situations in which there is conflict between parents and physicians regarding the best interests of an infant are both emotionally charged and ethically challenging.

What does it mean to say that health care decisions should reflect the best interests of the newborn? *Best interests* is an inherently subjective concept whereby surrogates employ this standard to maximize benefits and minimize harms to newborn infants. It is shorthand for the following statement:

> On balance, taking into consideration both the nature and probability of occurrence of the benefits and harms of various courses of action, the anticipated benefits of the proposed course outweigh the anticipated harms, and the proposed course also has a more favorable benefit/harm ratio than other possible courses of action.

But who decides, and on what basis, what constitutes a benefit and what constitutes a harm? That is, who decides what is in the best interests of the patient? This procedural question is of pivotal importance because "benefits" and "harms" often lie "in the eyes of the beholder" (e.g., the parents, the physician, or the nurse), whose perceptions are influenced by personal values and experiences.

For both legal and moral reasons, the parents are the first to determine what is in their child's best interests. As noted earlier, this authority is not absolute, and their assessment can be challenged. But doing so is often controversial, particularly when conflicting assessments of what is in the child's best interests result from conflicting values. For example, a parent who believes in the sanctity of life will perceive the benefits and harms of aggressive intervention differently from a physician who places greater value on quality of life and relief of suffering. Can the physician authoritatively assert that his or her values are better than those of the parents, and thus should be the ones that inform the assessment of the best interests of the newborn? To be sure, the physician may better understand the medical facts and doubtless has considerably more expertise and experience in dealing with sick newborns. This medical expertise, however, does not necessarily confer moral expertise.

Another complicating factor is that the best interests of the newborn may conflict with the *family's* interests (possibly including the interests of other children). Although the current wisdom is that the child's best interests must be pursued, some question this narrow perspective, arguing that it is legitimate for both physicians and parents to consider *family* interests in making health care decisions for a sick family member.[23] Despite the potential tension between the interests of the individual and those of the family, and other criticisms, Kopelman argues that the best-interests standard "is an important moral and legal guide. It has three related meanings: as a threshold for intervention and judgment, as an ideal or to establish prima facie duties, and as a standard of reasonableness."[33]

ETHICAL ISSUES

MATERNAL-FETAL DILEMMAS

Physicians may encounter a moral dilemma when they believe a conflict exists between their obligation to respect a pregnant patient's wishes and their obligation to promote fetal health and well-being. This conflict may arise because of the pregnant woman's personal health care choices, her lifestyle, or her occupational situation. On occasion, the physician's experience of conflict is so acute that efforts will be made to have the state intervene to protect the fetus.

IS STATE INTERVENTION IN THE LIVES OF PREGNANT WOMEN EVER JUSTIFIED? When there is a serious risk of harm to the developing fetus, some argue that state intervention, including forced treatment, detention, or incarceration, is morally justified. Others maintain that such interventions violate the woman's personal autonomy and undermine the principle of reproductive freedom.[20] The principle of autonomy recognizes the right of competent women to make their own health care choices. The principle of reproductive freedom stipulates that women have the right to make reproductive choices and that the state should foster conditions under which this can occur.

Those who advocate state intervention consider

the principle of reproductive freedom to be morally unsound. In their view, whatever rights a pregnant woman may have to direct the course of her pregnancy, they do not override the fetus' right to life or include the right to harm the fetus. This counterclaim is problematic, however, for two reasons. First, it ignores the fetus' contested moral status. The fetus-to-be-born, unlike the child or the pregnant woman, is not uniformly recognized as a person with full moral standing, which includes the right to life. Second, it suggests that the pregnant woman intentionally seeks to harm her fetus, which is generally false. All things being equal, pregnant women want healthy children and accept considerable inconvenience and risk to ensure a healthy birth.

Other participants in this debate readily acknowledge that the fetus does not have the same rights as a person and that the pregnant woman may not intend to harm her fetus. They maintain, however, that the woman has obligations to the fetus that include a duty of care. In "choosing" to continue her pregnancy, the woman is said to have incurred an obligation to do what is necessary (within reasonable limits) to ensure that the fetus is born healthy.[39] Should she violate this obligation, the state is entitled or obliged to intervene to protect the fetus. This argument, however, misunderstands the context in which women continue their pregnancy and ignores the overlapping interests of the fetus and the pregnant woman. The relationship between the pregnant woman and her fetus is characterized as adversarial: the woman is cast in the role of aggressor and the fetus in that of innocent victim, although in fact the situation is far more complex.

There is no doubt that pregnant women sometimes make unfortunate choices about their own health care and the management and continuation of their pregnancy. These may be choices made in ignorance or constrained by social and psychological factors, such as fear and denial. They may also be choices informed by past experience, a bias toward the present and near future, or a lack of trust in the medical profession.[9] Sometimes, however, choice is not the issue. In the case of addictions, for example, the behaviors that ultimately harm the fetus cannot properly be described as choices. Acknowledging this contextual factor, however, does not lessen the moral uncertainty for the people confronted with the dilemma—to respect the autonomy of their pregnant patient or to intervene in an effort to promote the best interests of the fetus. This moral dilemma is particularly acute for those who believe that they have conflicting responsibilities to two patients in one body.[25, 57]

Considered from a policy perspective, professional bodies have commonly resolved the dilemma in favor of respecting the principle of autonomy. According to the American College of Obstetricians and Gynecologists, "The maternal-fetal relationship remains a unique one, requiring a balance of maternal health, autonomy, and fetal needs. Every reasonable effort should be made to protect the fetus, but the pregnant woman's autonomy should be respected."[2] Similarly, the Society of Obstetricians and Gynecologists of Canada Ethics Committee "opposes involuntary intervention in the lives of pregnant women. . . . The primary objective of physicians who work with pregnant women should be to promote women's health and well-being while respecting their autonomy."[56]

The prevailing ethical view regarding state intervention in the lives of pregnant women is that the autonomy of competent women should be respected. The reasoning underlying this view is multifaceted. First is the principled commitment to respect personal autonomy. Second is the belief that state intervention harms the pregnant woman without any benefit necessarily accruing to her fetus (e.g., when the court intervenes after the fetal harm has occurred). Third is the pragmatic concern that a policy of state intervention may discourage the women whose fetuses are most at risk from seeking appropriate care, for fear of being prosecuted.[3, 38] Fourth are concerns about oppression and gender discrimination. State intervention is disproportionately oppressive of poor and minority women. It also typically ignores paternal actions that are hazardous to the fetus.[37, 55] Fifth, state intervention in pregnancy is an intrusion into the lives of pregnant women in excess of anything that would be tolerated to protect nonfetal lives.[20]

For these compelling reasons, caring, compassionate health care providers who are confronted with a maternal-fetal dilemma are well advised to educate and attempt to persuade, but never to coerce, pregnant women.

FETAL THERAPY

Prenatal diagnosis frequently confirms a healthy pregnancy and a healthy fetus. On occasion, however, the fetus is diagnosed with a serious genetic disease or a major congenital anomaly. If the woman chooses treatment (see Chapter 11) and there is a dietary, pharmacologic, surgical, or genetic intervention that might benefit the fetus, a number of ethical concerns arise.

ETHICAL ISSUES UNIQUE TO FETAL MEDICINE. What obligation is there to treat the developing human fetus? Considered from another perspective, when does the human fetus become a patient? These are difficult questions to answer, given the conflicting views about the moral status of the fetus. What is uncontroversial, however, is that when a woman chooses to pursue treatment for her fetus, she confers on the fetus the status of patient.[39]

Another difficult question for health care providers arises in situations where there is no established therapy for the fetal patient. In such circumstances, is there an obligation to recommend a novel, nonvalidated practice or participation in a clinical trial? This question may present the physician with ethical uncertainty. To minimize the risk of exploitation, it has been suggested that when a pregnant woman is desperate to save her fetus and thus is vulnerable to the lure of unproven claims of success, health care providers should temper their enthusiasm for nonroutine care and research.[11]

In anticipation of increasing pressure by some researchers to begin clinical trials for in utero human gene transfer, some of the ethical issues raised by this prospect are briefly considered in the following paragraphs.

RESEARCH IN HUMAN FETAL GENE TRANSFER. Worldwide, there are more than 400 approved clinical trials for somatic cell gene transfer in children and adults.[69] These involve the transfer of an exogenous "corrective" gene into the research participant's somatic cells in the hope of treating the genetic disease. The success of these interventions so far has been limited because of problems with the transfer of the corrective gene to the appropriate target cell, as well as problems with gene expression.

Arguments in support of in utero gene transfer—using either a gene-engineered cell transfer or a direct injection of vector approach—suggest that in utero transfer will improve on some of the current technical problems. For example, it is argued that the uptake and permanent integration of foreign DNA should be more efficient in the developing fetus than in more mature organisms. As well, there are the potential benefits to the developing fetus, because prenatal gene transfer may prevent irreversible disease manifestation. For these reasons, the proponents of in utero gene transfer argue that prenatal studies should not be delayed until gene transfer in adults has been proved clinically successful.[54, 69]

In deciding whether to proceed with clinical trials involving the fetus, researchers need to consider the potential benefits and harm to the fetus, the pregnant woman, and the society at large. With in utero gene transfer, potential harms to the fetus vary with the technique used: with gene-engineered human stem cell transplantation, harms are associated with the removal and reinjection of blood; with a direct-injection approach, harms are associated with insertional mutagenesis, which could affect the developmental process or lead to tumor formation. In addition, if the intervention is successful, there are potential psychological and other harms associated with an unchosen, life-long role as research participant, resulting from the continuing need for scientific and medical follow-up.

Potential harms to the pregnant woman include those associated with the procedures used to gain access to the fetus; the risk of premature delivery and cesarean section; the risk of reduced future reproductive capacity; the risk of accidental transfer of vector into the woman's blood stream; and the risk that a fetus with a lethal disease will be kept alive but in critical condition, thus inducing toxicity in the woman.[21, 69] Furthermore, because of the timing of the prenatal intervention, an accurate and safe prenatal diagnostic test may not be available to confirm the effectiveness of the gene transfer. The woman, therefore, would not have the option of abortion if the transfer failed.

Finally, there is the risk of inadvertent germline alteration. This has serious implications not only for the individual but for the society as a whole. Other societal concerns are the possible impact of the technology on current attitudes to screening for genetic disease[14] and the possibility that this technology might be used for enhancement purposes.

If in utero gene transfer trials are eventually approved by the Recombinant DNA Advisory Committee of the National Institutes of Health,[50] individual physicians who may be involved in recruiting research participants will have to resolve for themselves the moral uncertainty of a number of difficult questions. For example, in terms of resource allocation, what priority should be given to this research? Is there a sufficiently good reason to develop and use this technology instead of developing and using pre-implantation genetic diagnosis and selective transfer, or promoting adoption or child-free living? In addition, considered from an individual patient's perspective, when should this research option be presented to parents, and what information and advice should they be given? Clearly, technological possibilities in fetal therapy and research have to be extremely carefully and thoughtfully pursued.

WITHHOLDING OR WITHDRAWING LIFE-SUSTAINING MEDICAL TREATMENT IN THE NEWBORN

The report that first brought the issue of withholding or withdrawing life-sustaining treatment in neonatal intensive care to the fore was that of Duff and Campbell in 1973.[17] Their seminal report noted that 14% of 299 NICU deaths were related to withholding of therapy. More recent studies confirm that decisions to limit or forgo life-sustaining treatment are made in the majority of NICU deaths.[13, 53, 65, 66] The marked increase in this practice relates in part to the increased number of infants with extremely low birth weight who are resuscitated and given trials of intensive early management. As well, changes in social attitudes and a greater appreciation of the burdens of intensive care in survivors, together with a greater expression of parental authority in decision making, help explain the increase in the discontinuation of life-sustaining medical treatment in the NICU.

Withholding life-sustaining medical treatment involves a choice to omit a form of treatment that is not considered beneficial. Withdrawal, on the other hand, entails a choice to remove treatment that has not achieved its beneficial intent. Is there an important moral difference? Viewed from an individual perspective, some will perceive failure to initiate treatment likely to be ineffective as a greater moral wrong than stopping such treatment when it has proved unsuccessful. If the question is viewed from a moral perspective, however, there is no inherent difference in terms of the praiseworthiness or blameworthiness of either action. If it is morally right (or wrong) to withhold treatment deemed ineffective or even futile by the parents and the physician, it is equally right (or wrong) to withdraw this same treatment once started, should it later become evident that it is ineffective.

DEALING WITH UNCERTAINTY

In dealing with prognostic uncertainty, particularly for the infant with extremely low birth weight, physicians frequently adopt one of three strategies: a *statistical* approach in which decisions are made on birth weight or gestational age, an *individualized prognostic* approach, and a *wait-until-certainty* approach.[51]

The first strategy bases decisions on the statistical analysis of the outcomes of infants with extremely low birth weight or gestational age. Concerns about resource allocation may also be factored into the decision making. The primary objective is to avoid the survival of severely impaired infants, even at the cost of the death of some potentially viable infants.

With the individualized prognostic approach, treatment is initiated for all infants who have a reasonable chance of survival. Decision making framed solely by biomedical factors is avoided, and the ongoing moral responsibility of the decision makers is emphasized, because it seeks to involve parents and family members in navigating ensuing prognostic uncertainty. This approach avoids the extremes of withholding treatment from all infants who fall below a minimum threshold and treating all infants until the outcome is certain.[30]

The wait-until-certainty approach is one in which *medical* events play the determining role. Treatment is actively pursued in almost every infant who is believed to have any chance of survival, and consideration of the "right thing to do" is undertaken only when severe, adverse medical findings become unequivocally evident. Its most significant drawbacks are that it creates a momentum in favor of treatment that may be difficult to stop, that it tends to relegate parents (and often nurses) to the role of bystanders, and that it denies the ethical complexity of situations by failing to address moral as well as medical uncertainty. A further problem with this strategy is that frequently, even with the passage of time, uncertainty still remains. There may be a high probability of a specific outcome, but the outcome is nonetheless uncertain. The issue is thus not certainty per se but rather the degree of certainty required by physicians and parents to facilitate decision making.

Diffusion of medical responsibility for care in the NICU may compound the difficulties of dealing with prognostic uncertainty. Two emerging trends are worth highlighting in this regard: First is the increasing involvement of subspecialists in the care of the complex infant in the NICU. Organ-specific specialization may result in individual medical problems being treated and managed separately, (a "patchwork" strategy), almost without any consideration of long-term sequelae.[44] Second is the designation of the neonatologist as an intensivist, with responsibility limited to immediate care in the NICU and longer-term issues left to developmentalists (individuals involved in the developmental follow-up of NICU graduates). Both these trends tend to diffuse the responsibility and concerns for the patient as a whole and for their long-term outcomes. This compartmentalization of care, particularly in combination with a wait-until-certainty approach, establishes a momentum in favor of continuing treatment and risks alienating parents from the decision-making process.

Prognostic uncertainty has tended to preclude the use of generalized definitions of nonviability, or identification of situations in which resuscitation should *not* be offered. In the delivery room, for example, apart from the birth of a fetus who is younger than 23 weeks' gestation or the definitive diagnosis of anencephaly, most newborns receive full initial support, unless an antenatal decision to the contrary has been agreed on. And in the NICU, although an integrated individualized prognostic strategy may be the ethically preferred model, a more technologically driven wait-until-certainty approach still tends to dominate most North American practice.[30]

CRITERIA FOR WITHHOLDING OR WITHDRAWING LIFE-SUSTAINING MEDICAL TREATMENT: FUTILITY AND QUALITY-OF-LIFE CONSIDERATIONS

Recent studies in North America suggest that decisions to withhold or withdraw life-sustaining treatment are generally based on an assessment of the inevitability of death or the futility of continued medical treatment.[53, 66] Although the prediction of a poor quality of life for infants who may survive with significant impairment is certainly a factor in decisions, it is not usually the determining factor. There is hesitation in using quality of life alone as a decisive criterion because this assessment clearly involves a value judgment—a subjective determination of the value of limited well-being, self-awareness, relational capacity, and pleasure.

It is also true to say that the "Baby Doe" regulations of the early 1980s have influenced the criteria for end-of-life decision making. These regulations include the 1984 amendments to the U.S. Child Abuse Prevention and Treatment Act[63] and the regulations issued by the Department of Health and Human Services.[64] A survey conducted in 1988 showed that the Baby Doe regulations directly influenced the way that physicians justified their decisions on the withholding of treatment.[32] The more recent evidence presented by Wall and Partridge suggests that physicians' actual decision making may be less influenced by the Baby Doe proscriptions than previously.[66] There may, in fact, not be a clear demarcation line between decisions based on futility, and those based on a prediction of poor quality of life, because quality-of-life considerations are often included in futility determinations. (In the study by Wall and Partridge,[66] 51% of the decisions included quality-of-life concerns; these were also the major criterion in 23% of the deaths attributable to the withholding or withdrawal of treatment.) Clearly, different societal contexts play an important role in whether quality-of-life considerations are explicitly documented and accepted in decision making.[12, 15, 27, 40]

But what constitutes "futile" treatment? In the last few years the meaning of futility has been extensively debated but without clear resolution.[5, 29, 41, 61] In brief, a life-sustaining treatment is considered physiologically futile when there is no probability of medical benefit. Mechanical ventilation, for example, is physiologically futile when it will not maintain adequate ventilation and oxygenation. In practice, however, few interventions are physiologically futile. More common are interventions of which the probable effectiveness is low and the anticipated quality of life for the patient, from the perspective of some observers, is unacceptable.

In addition to debate about the meaning of the term *futility*, arguments have emerged about the authority of the physician to determine when an intervention is futile. Some contend that this is a medical decision to be made by the physician alone; others believe that the decision is value laden and that patients or family members should be involved in this determination. The Appleton International Conference on Developing Guidelines for Decisions to Forgo Life-Prolonging Medical Treatment proposed the following approach:

> Where a doctor considers a life-prolonging treatment not to be physiologically futile, but nonetheless 'futile' in another sense of the word, because of the low probability of success or because of the low quality of life that would remain, then decisions about the withholding or withdrawal of such treatments should be made in the context of full and open discussion of the nature and extent of the 'futility' of the treatment with the patient or the patient's representative.[4]

When futility is determined solely on the basis of medical factors (a rare occurrence unless death is imminent), unilateral decision making by the physician based on sound medical knowledge and expertise may be appropriate. When subjective elements form part of the determination, however, the physician has no unique claim to moral expertise. Further, as Frader and Watchko observed, attempts by physicians to "truncate and trump medical decisions through futility claims . . . do not seem to be the best way to return to a trusted position in the doctor-patient-family relationship."[22]

PARENTAL PARTICIPATION IN DECISION MAKING

Parents are authorized, both morally and legally, to make decisions for their young children. How this authority is enabled in the delivery room or the NICU, however, is clearly influenced by the validity ascribed to the parents' preferences and the physician's interpretation of the infant's best interests. In general, the greater the doubts about prognosis and outcome, the greater the moral weight given to parents' views.

Generally, in North American NICUs the decision to withhold or withdraw life-sustaining medical treatment is based on a medical recommendation, and a consensual decision-making process is undertaken with the parents. A recent study provides strong evidence to support this approach: where parental wishes with regard to delivery room resuscitation for extremely premature infants could be ascertained prior to birth, and decision-making responsibility was shared, the infants had the lowest mortality.[16] Those infants who died did so at less than 1 day of age. The study also makes the case for physicians to express *their* views: when the amount of resuscitation coincided with physicians' preferences, fewer infants for whom treatment was initiated ultimately died.

Other studies have shown that parental participation in decision making in the NICU did not intensify their grief, interfere with mourning, or burden them with guilt.[7, 67] Rather, parents tended to accept responsibility for the decision to withdraw support and to believe that they had made the right decision. There is also a strong perception that parental involvement in end-of-life decision making may even ameliorate their subsequent grieving process. These findings demonstrate that parental involvement in decision making should be encouraged. The more open, informed, and collaborative the process, the more likely it is that the quality of decisions and the comfort with which they are made will improve.[44]

FRAMEWORK FOR ETHICAL DECISION MAKING

A procedurally defined, collaborative framework for ethical decision making should facilitate the management and resolution of ethical problems in a consistent and compassionate manner. The process should include the following steps:

1. *Create an optimal environment for discussion*, one in which ethical issues and values can be thoroughly explored despite the demands on the time and energy of staff. Creating such an environment requires anticipating and responding to parental expectations. For example, parents may rightfully expect that physicians, nurses, and other care providers will put the good of the patient first. They may also expect the physician to serve as advocate for their child when there is a perceived need to balance inequities within the health care system.
2. *Establish that the presenting issue is indeed an ethical problem*, one in which concepts such as the "good" of the patient and quality of life require consideration. An ethical problem is one in which moral values conflict or moral uncertainty exists. Ethical deliberation is always complicated by subjective and psychological factors that are integral to severe illness and require disentangling from the ethical issue.[34]
3. *Identify the rightful decision makers*, including, at the least, the patient or the parents, the most responsible physician, and other members of the health care team directly involved in providing care. More generally, those who bear the greatest burden of care and conscience, those with special knowledge, and the health professionals with the most continuous, committed, and trusting relationship with the patient or parents should be involved in making decisions.[43]
4. *Establish the relevant facts*. It is a truism that good ethics begin with good facts. Medical facts include the diagnosis, the prognosis (and the estimated certainty of outcomes), past experience on the unit, relevant institutional policies, and relevant professional guidelines. Nonmedical facts include information about any legal and financial constraints on decision making* and information about the patient or parents (and family). In particular, it is important to gather information about family relationships, language barriers, cultural and religious beliefs, and past experiences with the health care system. It is also important to ascertain the pregnant woman's or parents' understanding of the medical facts, their expectations of the technology involved, the quality of communication between the parents themselves, and the degree of trust in physicians and the medical system. The willingness of the physician to discuss personal views and beliefs may enhance the gathering of nonmedical information.
5. *Explore the options*. This entails an explicit discussion of treatment options and their known and potential short- and long-term consequences. The options available to parents are limited in two ways:
   (a) their choice should not deny life-sustaining measures that would be beneficial for their child and
   (b) the limitations imposed by the therapeutic options presented by the responsible physician. For physicians, an often troubling element at this stage is whether they should describe *all* possible options or only those they consider legitimate. Different physicians perceive their obligations differently. If the physician feels morally obliged to inform the pregnant woman or parents of all possible options, then he or she should not hesitate, at the same time, to offer a professional recommendation on the course of action he or she considers medically and ethically most appropriate.
6. *Derive consensus*. All participants in the decision-making process need to take into account the professional and personal beliefs, values, and preferences of the various persons involved and,

---

*Although approaching issues in a "letter-of-the-law" manner is potentially harmful to all the parties concerned, there is the conviction that practice must be medically and ethically sound as well as legally bound. Similarly, there ought to be a general reluctance to invoke arguments about cost-effective use of resources; these should be less of a priority to the physician at the bedside than treating the individual patient and family.[8]

on this basis, attempt to reach a consensual decision. Open, compassionate discussion of the goals and consequences of treatment usually results in a harmonious decision.

7. *Implement the decision.* Once a decision has been reached, typically a number of issues have to be addressed to ensure its effective implementation.

Two ethical issues that may arise with implementation of a decision to withdraw life-sustaining medical treatment in the newborn are (1) the use of drugs for pain relief and (2) the withdrawal of nutrition and hydration.

1. *The use of drugs to relieve pain and discomfort.* Although there are difficulties in determining whether infants perceive pain at the time of impending death, use of analgesic agents may be considered part of the provision of comfort care. Their use might be justified by concern not only about potential pain at the time of discontinuing life support but also about future pain and suffering should the infant survive. Partridge and Wall have shown that in most cases of withholding or withdrawing life support from critically ill infants, neonatologists provided opioid analgesia to these infants at the end of life, despite the potential respiratory depression of these agents.[47] The *intent* of the action—to alleviate pain and promote comfort—distinguishes the use of analgesics from the use of paralyzing agents, whose intent is to *ensure* death. The introduction of the latter neuromuscular blocking agents at the time of withdrawal of life-sustaining medical treatment is considered ethically inappropriate.[52, 62]

2. *The withdrawal of hydration and nutrition.* After other, more obviously invasive forms of life-sustaining treatment have been withdrawn, the withdrawal of hydration and nutrition may, rarely, become an issue. The practice may be philosophically defensible when an infant with a hopeless prognosis cannot be fed orally, and feeding via other routes is perceived to be a burdensome life-sustaining technological support.[46] However, it creates great stress for caregivers who view the practice as withholding basic comfort care that is morally obligatory and symbolic of their relationship with the most vulnerable and dependent members of society. Withdrawal of hydration or nutrition is in fact seldom entertained and would generally be considered only at the specific request of parents.[42] The implementation of such decisions is extremely difficult and requires intensive attention to the child's comfort. Support of the family and members of the health care team is essential.

Following a structured decision-making process such as that outlined here, that carefully explores reasoned arguments for and against various options, has a twofold purpose: It is most likely to result in a decision that maximizes patient and family interests, and it is most likely to promote harmonious decision making, because all the participants in the process understand the reasons and values underlying a particular choice.

WHEN CONSENSUS CANNOT BE REACHED

In most instances, participants in the decision-making process can arrive at a morally sound decision regarding the best course of action in a particular situation. Attempts at consensual decision making, however, are sometimes unsuccessful and may result in a degree of intractability. Occasionally, in the care of infants and children, this intractability is between the parents who disagree with each other regarding what is in the best interests of their child. Although the responsible physician may be able to proceed legally with the authorization of only one parent, it would be unwise to do so.[6] More frequently, intractability is between the patient or parents and the health care providers.

In the NICU, there is no ready or comfortable resolution to the tension between the physician's assessment of what is in the best interests of the newborn and the parents' authority in decision making; this is probably rightly so. Nonetheless, disagreements between parents and health care providers should not be taken at face value. Early expressions of preference by parents, such as "do everything possible" or "stop everything," need to be re-examined with fuller disclosure over time. On occasion, physicians deal with parental insistence on a course of action by deferring entirely to the parents' decision, despite their own ethical reservations. Doing so without exploring and possibly challenging parental preferences, however, is inconsistent with good medical practice and the physician's professional duty to the infant whose interests (in his or her assessment) are not being served.

Guidelines to promote continuing discussion and negotiation are the following[1, 8, 45, 52]:

1. *Allow time for further clinical observation.* In the specific case of parental objections to forgoing treatment that the physician believes is not beneficial, it may be unrealistic to expect agreement from the parents the first time this option is raised. Prudence suggests moving as fast as the slowest member of the decision-making group, provided that the infant is not thereby further compromised.

2. *Ensure full parental comprehension of the medical information.* This may require a formal interdisciplinary case conference and the identification of differing viewpoints that have been expressed to parents. (In our experience this is best achieved with all the subspecialists and other health professionals directly involved, without the parents present, but with full disclosure of the content of the meeting thereafter.) Further discussion is then required to

deal with any incorrect or incomplete information.

3. *Continue to discuss and explore the underlying reasons for the differences in choice.* Health care providers must understand the pregnant patient's or the parents' views, beliefs, and preferences. Specifically, physicians must recognize that the patient's or parents' beliefs and values are informed by ethnic and cultural traditions, customs, and institutions and that these influences may be significantly divergent from their own.[18]

4. *Continue to negotiate toward consensus.* Parents may have great difficulty in making an unassisted decision. The consensual nature of the decision-making process and the shared burden of the decision must be reinforced.

5. *Broaden the parents' "moral community."* This may involve inclusion of additional family members, significant others, and religious or spiritual advisors.

6. *Share the attending physician's "moral load" by his or her actively seeking opinions from colleagues.* Although the physician responsible for the case bears the final responsibility for the approach taken with the parents, for both personal as well as legal reasons, it is important to establish that the physician is supported in his or her actions by a responsible body of medical opinion.

7. *Involve a bioethicist or ethics committee, as appropriate* (see "Ethics Consultations").

ETHICS CONSULTATIONS

When broadening the moral community does not resolve the presenting ethical problem, there may be some benefit in involving a multidisciplinary institutional ethics committee, provided that it has experience in case consultation and review. Most hospitals in North America have an ethics committee that includes experts in medicine, nursing, philosophy, law, religion, and social services. The functions of these committees vary widely, but some are particularly skilled at case consultation. The ethics committee's multidisciplinary approach should help ensure consideration of all relevant concerns; in turn this should help with the elucidation of the ethical issues. However, committee members may disagree among themselves, and some members may dominate others. Also, the committee may not be qualified to deal with the subject matter or may be overly concerned with the institutional impact of a decision rather than with the specifics of the case. In our experience, consultation with individual bioethicists or individuals with expertise in moral matters has been of greater benefit to decision makers than the practice of "ethics by committee."

Removing communication barriers, expanding the consultation process, encouraging religious rituals, and involving a bioethicist all are important steps in overcoming conflict. Despite such efforts, in the final analysis, the moral problem may not be amenable to consensual resolution: rational people of good will may hold views that are irreconcilable. In the effort to reach a consensus, however, at least the relevant ethical dimensions of the problem will have been explored. Nonetheless, individuals involved in a failed attempt at deriving consensus may experience what Webster and Baylis term *moral residue*—"that which each of us carries with us from those times in our lives when in the face of moral distress we have seriously compromised ourselves or allowed ourselves to be compromised."[68]

THE LAW

As a last resort, when all else fails to resolve the conflict, it is sometimes possible (or necessary) to use the judicial system. Generally, however, this course of action is inherently unsatisfactory, for a number of reasons: it invariably destroys the patient-parent–physician relationship, it increases anguish for everyone involved (especially the families), and it can be extremely costly and time consuming. The legal system may also not help physicians or health care organizations when parents or other guardians dissent from the medical recommendations.[22]

A FINAL WORD: THE PHYSICIAN'S ETHICAL RESPONSIBILITY

The physician's responsibility to the competent pregnant patient is well defined and well established—to respect the patient's wishes regarding treatment. So, too, the physician's traditional responsibility to the neonatal patient is well defined and well established—a right and good action within the best-interests standard of judgment. In the broadest terms, this responsibility, at minimum, requires the development of a constructive and mutually respectful patient-parent–physician relationship so that the patient's and family's values and beliefs are incorporated into the decision-making process.

The attending physician is also responsible for developing relationships with other members of the health care team to promote open discussion of the ongoing negotiations with pregnant patients and parents. This is not a responsibility that arises only after stressful conflicts but forms an integral part of routine care. The health care team's willingness to explore value issues, the general culture, and mode of communication within a unit can be strongly influenced by the responsible physician's sensitivity to these issues. The physician also has an obligation to foster the ethical experience and education of the interdisciplinary team, as well as that of junior staff and trainees. The physician leader and the team have a responsibility to develop and implement guidelines for their practice. These should emphasize the importance of relevant ethical principles and concepts and include a procedural framework for decision making and conflict resolution.

By setting a standard of ethical responsibility for

the care of vulnerable fetuses, newborns, pregnant women, and families, physicians working in perinatal and neonatal care send a message to society that will ensure public confidence and trust in their professional practice. The perinatal high-risk unit or NICU team should be more than a group of physicians, nurses, and many others working in an isolated area of the hospital, trying to master new technology and break new ground. It should ideally be an open, analytic, self-critical, and responsive group providing ethically responsible care to pregnant women, newborn infants, and their families.

■ REFERENCES

1. American Academy of Pediatrics, Committee on Fetus and Newborn Pediatrics: The initiation or withdrawal of treatment for high-risk newborns. Pediatrics 96:362, 1995.
2. American College of Obstetricians and Gynecologists, Committee on Ethics: Patient choice: Maternal-fetal conflict. Washington DC, American College of Obstetricians and Gynecologists, 1987, Committee Opinion No. 55.
3. American Medical Association, Board of Trustees: Legal interventions during pregnancy: Court-ordered medical treatment and legal penalties for potentially harmful behavior by pregnant women. JAMA 264:2663, 1990.
4. Appleton International Conference. In Stanley JM (ed): Developing guidelines for decisions to forgo life-prolonging medical treatment. J Med Ethics 18(Suppl):6, 1992.
5. Avery GB: Futility considerations in the neonatal intensive care unit. Semin Perinatol 22:216, 1998.
6. Baylis F, Caniano D: Medical ethics and the pediatric surgeon. In Oldham KT, et al (eds): Surgery of Infants and Children: Scientific Principles and Practice. Philadelphia, Lippincott-Raven, 1997, p 381.
7. Benfield DG, et al: Grief response of parents to neonatal death and parent participation in deciding care. Pediatrics 62:171, 1978.
8. Benitz WE: A paradigm for making difficult choices in the intensive care nursery. Camb Q Healthc Ethics 2:281, 1993.
9. Brock DW, Wartman SA: When competent patients make irrational choices. N Engl J Med 322:1595, 1990.
10. Brody H: Transparency: Informed consent in primary care. Hastings Cent Rep 19:5, 1989.
11. Caniano D, Baylis F: Ethical considerations in prenatal surgical consultation. Pediatr Surg Int 15:303, 1999.
12. Caniano DA, et al: End-of-life decisions for surgical neonates: Experience in the Netherlands and United States. J Pediatr Surg 30:1420, 1995.
13. Cook LA, Watchko JF: Decision making for the critically ill neonate near the end of life. J Perinatol 16:133, 1996.
14. Coutelle C, et al: The challenge of fetal gene therapy. Nature Med 1:864, 1995.
15. De Leeuw R, et al: Forgoing intensive care treatment in newborn infants with extremely poor prognoses. J Pediatr 129:661, 1996.
16. Doron MW, et al: Delivery room resuscitation decisions for extremely premature infants. Pediatrics 102:574, 1998.
17. Duff RS, Campbell AGM: Moral and ethical dilemmas in the special care nursery. N Engl J Med 289:890, 1973.
18. Elliott C: Where ethics come from and what to do about it. Hastings Cent Rep 22:28, 1992.
19. Emanuel EJ, Emanuel LL: Four models of the physician-patient relationship. JAMA 267:2221, 1992.
20. Flagler E, et al: Bioethics for clinicians: XII. Ethical dilemmas that arise in the care of pregnant women: Rethinking "maternal-fetal conflicts." Can Med Assoc J 156:1729, 1997.
21. Fletcher JC, Richter G: Human fetal gene therapy: Moral and ethical questions. Hum Gene Ther 7:1605, 1996.
22. Frader JE, Watchko J: Futility issues in pediatrics. In Zucker

MB, Zucker HD (eds): Medical Futility. Cambridge, UK, Cambridge University Press, 1997.
23. Hardwig J: What about the family? Hastings Cent Rep 20:5, 1990.
24. Harrison H: The principles for family-centered neonatal care. Pediatrics 92:643, 1993.
25. Harrison MR, Golbus MS, Filly RA: The Unborn Patient. New York, Grune & Stratton, 1984.
26. Heffernan P, Heilig S: Giving "moral distress" a voice: Ethical concerns among neonatal intensive care unit personnel. Camb Q Healthc Ethics 8:173, 1999.
27. Jacobs S, et al: The practice of withdrawal of life-sustaining medical technology (LSMT) in a neonatal intensive care unit (NICU) [abstract]. Pediatr Res 45:34A, 1999.
28. Jameton A: Nursing Practice: The Ethical Issues. Englewood-Cliffs, NJ, Prentice-Hall, 1984.
29. Jecker NS, Schneiderman LJ: Medical futility: The duty not to treat. Camb Q Healthc Ethics 2:151, 1993.
30. Kinlaw K: The changing nature of neonatal ethics in practice. Clin Perinatol 23:417, 1996.
31. Kirschbaum MS: Life support decisions for children: What do parents value? Adv Nurs Sci 19:51, 1996.
32. Kopelman LM, et al: Neonatologists judge the "Baby Doe" regulations. N Engl J Med 318:677, 1988.
33. Kopelman LM: The best-interests standard as threshold, ideal, and standard of reasonableness. J Med Philos 22:271, 1997.
34. Lederberg MS: Disentangling ethical and psychological issues. Acta Oncol 38:771, 1999.
35. Loewy EH: Physicians, friendship, and moral strangers: An examination of a relationship. Camb Q Healthc Ethics 3:52, 1994.
36. Loewy EH: Textbook of Medical Ethics: Doctors and Their Patients, Patients and Their Doctors. New York, Plenum, 1989.
37. Losco J, Shublack M: Paternal-fetal conflict: An examination of paternal responsibilities to the fetus. Polit Life Sci 13:63, 1994.
38. Mahowald MB: Women and Children in Health Care: An Unequal Majority. New York, Oxford University Press, 1993.
39. McCullough LB, Chervenak FA: Ethics in Obstetrics and Gynecology. New York, Oxford University Press, 1994.
40. McHaffie HE, et al: Withholding/withdrawing treatment from neonates: Legislation and official guidelines across Europe. J Med Ethics 25:440, 1999.
41. Meadow W, et al: Putting futility to use in the NICU: Ethical implications of non-survival after CPR in very low-birth-weight infants. Acta Paediatr 84:589, 1995.
42. Miraie ED, Mahowald MB: Withholding nutrition from seriously ill newborn infants: A parent's perspective. J Pediatr 113:262, 1988.
43. Mitchell C: Care of severely impaired infant raises ethical issues. Am Nurse 16:9, 1984.
44. Muraskas J, et al: Neonatal viability in the 1990s: Held hostage by technology. Camb Q Healthc Ethics 8:160, 1999.
45. Nelson LJ, Nelson RM: Ethics and the provision of futile, harmful, or burdensome treatment to children. Crit Care Med 20:427, 1992.
46. Nelson LJ, et al: Forgoing medically provided nutrition and hydration in pediatric patients. J Law Med Ethics 23:33, 1995.
47. Partridge JC, Wall SN: Analgesia for dying infants whose life support is withdrawn or withheld. Pediatrics 99:76, 1997.
48. Perlman NB, et al: Informational needs of parents of sick neonates. Pediatrics 88:512, 1991.
49. Pinch WJ, Spielman ML: The parents' perspective: Ethical decision-making in neonatal intensive care. J Adv Nurs 15:712, 1990.
50. RAC—Recombinant DNA Advisory Committee: In utero statement, March 11, 1999. Available at http://www4.od.nih.gov/oba/racinutero.htm.
51. Rhoden NK: Treating Baby Doe: The ethics of uncertainty. Hastings Cent Rep 16:34, 1986.
52. Royal College of Paediatrics and Child Health: Withholding and Withdrawing Life-Saving Treatment in Children: A Framework for Practice. London, Royal College of Paediatrics and Child Health, 1997.
53. Ryan CA, et al: No resuscitation and withdrawal of therapy in

a neonatal and a pediatric intensive care unit in Canada. J Pediatr 123:534, 1993.

54. Schneider H, Coutelle C: In utero gene therapy: The case for. Nature Med 5:256, 1999.
55. Schroedel JR, Peretz P: A gender analysis of policy formulation: The case of fetal abuse. J Health Polit Policy Law 19:335, 1994.
56. Society of Obstetricians and Gynaecologists of Canada (SOGC): SOGC Clinical Practice Guidelines, Policy Statement No. 67: Involuntary intervention in the lives of pregnant women. J Soc Obstet Gynaecol Can 19:1200, 1997.
57. Steinbock B: Maternal-fetal conflict and in utero fetal therapy. Albany Law Rev 57:782, 1994.
58. Szasz TS, Hollender MH: A contribution to the philosophy of medicine: The basic models of the doctor-patient relationship. Arch Intern Med 97:585, 1956.
59. Thomasma DC: Models of the doctor-patient relationship and the ethics committee: II. Camb Q Healthc Ethics 3:10, 1994.
60. Thomasma DC: Models of the doctor-patient relationship and the ethics committee: I. Camb Q Healthc Ethics 1:11, 1992.
61. Truog RD, et al: The problem with futility. N Engl J Med 326:1560, 1992.
62. Truog RD, et al: Pharmacologic paralysis and withdrawal of mechanical ventilation at the end of life. N Engl J Med 342:508, 2000.
63. U.S. Child Abuse Protection and Treatment Amendments of 1984: Public Law 98–457.
64. U.S. Department of Health and Human Services: Child abuse and neglect prevention and treatment program 50. Fed Reg 14878, 1985.
65. Van der Heide A, et al: Medical end-of-life decisions made for neonates and infants in the Netherlands. Lancet 350:251, 1997.
66. Wall SN, Partridge JC: Death in the intensive care nursery: Physician practice of withdrawing and withholding life support. Pediatrics 99:64, 1997.
67. Walwork E, Ellison PH: Follow-up of families of neonates in whom life support was withdrawn. Clin Pediatr 24:14, 1985.
68. Webster G, Baylis F: Moral residue. In Rubin S, Zoloth L (eds): Margin of Error: The Ethics of Mistakes in the Practice of Medicine. Hagerstown, MD, University Publishing Group, 2000, p 217.
69. Zanjani ED, Anderson WF: Prospects for in utero human gene therapy. Science 285:2084, 1999.

Perinatal Outreach Education

5

John Kattwinkel

The basic tenet of regionalized perinatal care is that all fetuses and newborn infants should receive optimum care consistent with their degree of illness or risk and regardless of their place of residence. Since more than 80% of pregnancies are managed outside of regional perinatal centers, the main responsibility for early identification of the high-risk patient resides with community-based practitioners. Thus, if perinatal statistics are to improve, the community-based perinatal professionals should be the main target population for learning optimum perinatal principles and techniques.

CLASSIC APPROACHES

The original perinatal regionalization plan, "Toward Improving the Outcome of Pregnancy,"[16] charged the regional perinatal center with the responsibility of developing an outreach education program and identified the community inpatient perinatal professional as the primary student. Although the regional concept called for high-risk pregnancies to be referred antenatally to regional centers for delivery, it was recognized that nearly half of fetuses who would die in utero, or were destined to become at-risk or sick newborns, were not identifiable early enough to make antenatal referral practical. Therefore, primary care practitioners must be prepared not only to identify the high-risk case appropriate for referral but also to provide optimum resuscitation and stabilization of newborns not identified as high-risk prior to delivery. In rural areas the number of babies requiring such stabilizing care is even higher because of the inadvisability of transporting a woman in advanced labor over long distances.

Most of the traditional programs of continuing education have been based on the regional center's perception of the community hospital's needs. The most familiar of these is the 1- to 3-day *lecture series* organized for referring physicians and held at the regional center or at some remote site. Content often covers those subject areas that are appealing to the program

director or that are particularly current in the medical literature. Usually the mistaken assumption is that the audience has a significant and uniform background fund of knowledge on which the speakers can build fairly complex concepts. There is frequently little attempt made to evaluate the practitioners' needs and then to design a program around those needs.

Another form of continuing education has been the *miniresidency*, in which practicing physicians and community hospital nurses visit the regional center for several days or even weeks to function as short-term staff members.[17] Although this format gives the practitioner more "hands-on" experience than does the lecture approach, generally the patients at the regional center have more complex problems, and the equipment used is more sophisticated than is encountered or needed in the participant's local environment.

Many regional centers have developed a *traveling outreach program* in which a neonatologist, perinatologist, and perinatal nurse spend several hours in each of their referring hospitals giving lectures, critiquing the hospital's perinatal facilities, and reviewing the patients recently referred to the regional center. This format is often more successful than the others because it makes a significant attempt to tailor the educational experience to the unique needs of the community hospital. Disadvantages to the single-visit program are that it is a relatively brief educational experience, it tends to attract the least busy individuals who often need the teaching the least, it is viewed with skepticism by many busy practitioners, and it is relatively time consuming for regional center personnel.

In general, each of these classic approaches is structured after the traditional teaching model of medical education (e.g., classroom lectures, apprentice training, education of each professional group separately). However, modern perinatal medicine does not function in a classic format of a single physician treating a single patient. The obstetrician relies on consultation from the pediatrician; the practicing physician cannot prescribe rational therapy for the infant without the expertise of the nurse at the bedside; and the perinatal patient with complex problems requires an intricate interdigitation of respiratory therapist, laboratory technician, social worker, nutritionist, and perinatal nurses and physicians to receive quality care. Community hospital perinatal medicine may rely on a smaller team, but the same interdigitation of medical, nursing, and support disciplines is essential. There is also recent evidence that passive learning experiences result in far less change in performance than do programs that encourage active hands-on participation by the learner.[6] Thus, although many of the classic teaching methods may be quite well received, they are not likely to have a significant effect on altering care practices unless they are incorporated as part of a comprehensive program that is team oriented, uses local resources, and employs participation rather than passive learning techniques.

IDENTIFYING THE EDUCATORS, COURSE CONTENT, AND STUDENTS

The following three major changes in perinatology and neonatology have resulted in a substantial evolution of the regionalization concept and the population of health care professionals who need continuing education in perinatal and neonatal medicine (see Chapter 3):

1. Significant improvements in technology have resulted in more opportunities for in utero diagnosis and management and thus fewer surprise crises occurring in ill-prepared facilities.
2. Financial pressures and health care reform have resulted in a dramatic shift of care from the inpatient to the outpatient arena. Hospitalization of the uncomplicated baby born at term has decreased from 3 to 4 days in the 1970s to 24 hours or less in the 2000s; preterm babies are being back-transported to their community hospitals sooner and discharged home at lower weights; babies with chronic illnesses such as bronchopulmonary dysplasia, short bowel syndrome, and congenital heart disease are being returned earlier to their primary care practitioners in the community rather than remaining for long periods in regional centers.
3. Competition among hospitals and an increase of neonatology staff have led to more and more smaller hospitals marketing full-service obstetric programs, thus leading to a deregionalization movement.

These changes have created new challenges for perinatal outreach education. First, the educational target population must broaden considerably from captive inpatient nurses and physicians to a more diversified spectrum that includes outpatient perinatal providers (Fig. 5–1). Outpatient perinatal professionals often have less well-defined interdisciplinary relationships; are more geographically scattered; and

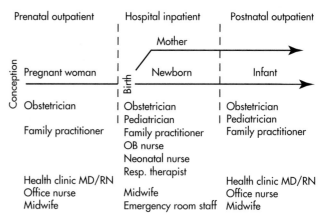

FIGURE 5–1. Outpatient and inpatient continuum of perinatal care. Note that some health care workers (e.g., family practitioners) may be involved throughout the period, whereas others may be involved at only discrete times. Because comprehensive perinatal care depends greatly on interaction of health care workers throughout the time continuum, it is important that educational programs also reach all members of the team. Thus, perinatal outreach education must be multidisciplinary and include both outpatient and inpatient providers as students.

have varied responsibilities, depending on the individual structure of the health care systems in various locales. For example, in some areas, prenatal care for the indigent population is provided by public health nurses with little input from obstetricians until risk factors are identified or delivery is imminent, whereas in other locales, indigent care is absorbed into private obstetric offices. New categories of professionals requiring education have been created. The early discharge movement, for example, has stimulated the development of new standards of care, which include home visits conducted by visiting nurses[1]; home health care agencies must be prepared to deal with infant oxygen administration, monitoring, and even ventilator management in the home[3]; primary care physicians must be prepared to manage patients who previously were in the exclusive domain of regional neonatal centers.

Second, the subject matter must be expanded to include outpatient management subjects such as first-trimester identification of prenatal risk factors, identification of early neonatal disorders in the home environment, and acute and chronic management of neonatal conditions that persist after discharge from intensive care nurseries.

Third, responsibility for providing education may require change. Although the original perinatal regional plan assigned this task to regional perinatal centers, in some localities competitive forces have resulted in relative isolation of some level II hospitals and a deterioration in their formal relationship with a regional perinatal center. Thus, although this chapter describes educational responsibilities as belonging primarily to regional centers, there may be instances where some of these responsibilities have been assumed by state government or perhaps by managed care organizations. In some urban areas, large groups of neonatologists have assumed primary care of neonates throughout a network of hospitals. In this situation, the responsibility for education will generally fall on the group practice.

PRINCIPLES OF OUTREACH EDUCATION

COMMUNITY-BASED PROGRAM

It is important that program participants be able to relate what they learn to their available resources for new knowledge to be translated into altered care practices. Also, because of the nature of community hospital staffing patterns, health clinic schedules, and private practice demands, it is virtually impossible for more than several individuals to leave their jobs at one time. Therefore, for a program to be effective in changing patient care and to reach the most individuals, it should require a minimum of off-the-job travel time. A program based in the community hospital or clinic or in the private practice office is ideal for this purpose.

MULTIDISCIPLINARY ORIENTATION

The most successful perinatal educational program is aimed at the same multidisciplinary team that is involved with taking care of the patient in the clinical setting. Thus pediatricians, obstetricians, perinatal nurses, and supporting professionals such as respiratory therapists must be exposed to the same concepts simultaneously. A program aimed at only nurses or only physicians generally is not reflected in clinical practice without the endorsement of the other team members. Likewise, for maximum acceptability and practicality of subject matter, it is just as important that the program be developed and introduced to the community by the same type of multidisciplinary group. The minimum components of a regional center outreach education team include a perinatal physician and nurse. Optimally, all the disciplines just mentioned should be represented on this team.

LOCAL PARTICIPATION IN TEACHING PROCESS

It is extremely beneficial to have some of the program's activities coordinated by local personnel. This is particularly valuable if the program is expected to last several weeks or months or, preferably, to be a continuous experience. In most regional systems, geography and staffing limitations prohibit frequent interaction between center and community personnel. Also, in general, new concepts and skills are more readily accepted and adapted to local care practices if first introduced by local community professionals. Therefore, the most efficient and useful program will use selected local physicians and nurses as teachers and coordinators.

CONTENT MATCHED TO PATIENT CARE GOALS

Program content should be selected to match the complexity of care anticipated. If, for example, it is hospi-

tal practice and consistent with the state's regional plan for babies with very low birth weight or babies requiring mechanical ventilation to be referred to another center, then these subjects should be deleted from the program for that specific hospital. There are certain basic topics, such as resuscitation of the newborn, that are appropriate for all perinatal professionals; however, the overall content should be flexible to meet each community's specific patient care goals. In some regions these goals will have already been determined through the regionalization planning process. In others a process of identification of goals and

---

■ **BOX 5-1**

PERINATAL OUTREACH EDUCATION CONTENT OUTLINE

The following is not intended to constitute a complete list of fetal, maternal, and neonatal subjects but rather to identify those areas most appropriate for perinatal continuing education of the primary care provider.

For Inpatient Providers

Fetal Evaluation
  Identifying high-risk pregnancies
  Evaluating fetal age, growth, and maturity
  Evaluating fetal well-being
  Identifying and managing high-risk deliveries

Maternal and Fetal Care
  Peripartum hypertension
  Obstetric hemorrhage
  Perinatal infections
  Abnormal rupture of membranes
  Preterm labor
  Inducing and augmenting labor
  Abnormal labor progression
  Difficult deliveries

Immediate Newborn Assessment
  Resuscitation
  Gestational age and size assessment

Newborn Care
  Temperature control
  Oxygen therapy and monitoring
  Respiratory distress
  Apnea
  Umbilical catheters
  Blood pressure
  Hypoglycemia
  Intravenous therapy
  Feeding
  Hyperbilirubinemia
  Infections
  Preparation for transport
  Continuing care for infants at risk

For Outpatient Providers

Prenatal Care
  Identifying the high-risk pregnancy
  Medical complications of pregnancy
  Prenatal evaluation of the fetus
  Perinatal infections
  Woman at risk for preterm delivery
  Diabetes in pregnancy
  Hypertension in pregnancy

At-Risk Infant after Discharge
  Identifying healthy, at-risk, and sick infants
  Resuscitation
  Early postpartum discharge and follow-up care
  Hyperbilirubinemia
  Infant with a nutritional disorder
  Neonatal infections
  Congenital heart disease
  Neurologic disease (seizures)

Preterm Infant after Discharge
  Well-child care of the preterm infant
  Development of the preterm infant
  Postdischarge complications of prematurity
  Apnea
  Chronic lung disease

resources must precede the educational program. An outline of the content for perinatal outreach education is presented in Box 5–1.

COMPONENTS OF A COMPREHENSIVE PROGRAM

The following items should be included in any comprehensive outreach education program. Each step builds on the accomplishments of the preceding one and anticipates the existence of the subsequent step. Therefore, a regional center should have organized an entire plan (including provisions for funding, personnel, and educational materials) before the potential participants are approached. Model programs include the Perinatal Continuing Education Program developed at the University of Virginia,[13] the Neonatal Resuscitation Program of the American Heart Association and the American Academy of Pediatrics,[2] the Perinatal Education Programme in South Africa,[20] a perinatal education program developed for rural China,[11] the Canadian Neonatal Resuscitation Program,[19] and the STABLE program.[9]

INITIAL CONTACT

Unless a close rapport has already been developed between the community facilities and the regional center, the proposed program often is viewed with skepticism at this stage. Physicians are concerned about the regulation of care practices, nurses anticipate unrealistic demands on staff time, and administrators predict that the program will impose an unneeded expense on the hospital budget. Therefore, community leaders from all three groups (medicine, nursing, and administration) should be contacted simultaneously to prevent misconceptions from developing.

COMMITMENT

Some general commitment to participate should be secured from the hospital, clinic, or office practice and signed by the individuals just noted. At this time the commitment should be no more than an agreement between the organization and the regional center to devote the staff time and funds (if any) to the program. Issues such as referral contracts or patient care agreements should be avoided or at least postponed until after the educational program is completed. By that time a much closer working relationship will have developed, and all parties will be aware of the resources required for delivery of various intensities of care.

INVENTORY PROCESS

Before any education is provided, it is important to define goals and identify resources. It is pointless to teach procedures or concepts that will never be used, either because the appropriate type of patient will not be managed locally or because the necessary equipment will not be available to the practitioner. Therefore, local practitioners should be encouraged to define their patient care goals, and hospital personnel should be asked to define the facilities, staffing, and equipment available for patient care before any educational intervention begins. There should then be an attempt to compare the goals and resources so that the facilities can be expanded to accommodate the stated goals. In some cases the practitioners may elect to change their goals rather than acquire the recommended resources. Inasmuch as possible, this process of goal setting and resource identification should take place at the local level with regional center personnel acting as advisors rather than prescribers.

REGIONAL CENTER WORKSHOP

At this point it is beneficial to have selected nurses and physicians visit the regional center to learn the new concepts and skills that will be introduced to the entire local staff during the upcoming program. This type of workshop differs from the classic miniresidency in that the participants should learn through structured sessions oriented toward community medicine rather than through focus on care practices appropriate for a tertiary care center.

COGNITIVE PROGRAM

Educational content areas for the program vary, depending on the organization's patient care goals (see Box 5–1). However, several areas (e.g., resuscitation of the newborn) are basic for any perinatal service. Several different formats have been developed (e.g., self-instructional books, mediated programs, programmed texts, organized lecture series), and several are available commercially. Although direct comparative studies of different formats have not been performed, there is evidence that programs that are interactive and that encourage participant activity and skills practice are more likely to result in changes of practice and patient outcome.[6]

SKILLS ACQUISITION

Many of the new concepts introduced in the cognitive program require the performance of newly acquired skills before they can be translated into altered care practices. Teaching of new skills often requires hands-on practice sessions in addition to a written or mediated lesson. Models such as mannequins, sections of human umbilical cords, and anesthetized or preserved animal specimens can provide subjects for the practice of certain complex skills, such as umbilical catheterization, endotracheal intubation, and chest tube insertion.[5, 12]

PROGRAM AND POLICY REVIEW

Acquisition of new knowledge by perinatal professionals does not necessarily translate into improved care practices. Long-standing inappropriate routines are difficult to break and often require specific discussion before change occurs. Therefore, it may be helpful for regional center personnel to meet with the local leadership to highlight local care practices and policies that should be considered for change.[4, 11, 14, 15] When such meetings occur before the educational process, they are often viewed as threatening by local practitioners. However, if a meeting is scheduled soon after completion of the educational program, the rationale for change is usually evident.

CONTINUATION

All hospitals, clinics, and other patient care organizations should have a comprehensive basic educational program available for orientation of new staff. The local professionals who have visited the regional center are appropriate staff for organizing such basic in-service education. The regional center should periodically update the basic program as well as provide a mechanism for teaching new concepts and skills to the individuals who have previously completed the basic program.

One format, which I have found effective, is the mortality and morbidity review, in which physicians and nurses from the regional center and community meet to discuss the management of previously jointly managed patients.[18] For hospitals, such patients may include all those who were transported or died. For both outpatient and inpatient practices, patients identified by local personnel as particularly controversial or illustrative of a new care practice may be selected. These conferences are particularly valuable after the community participants have been exposed to the basic program but may prove overly controversial and threatening if sufficient background knowledge has not been acquired.

Periodically, personnel in the community hospital or practice should be exposed to another comprehensive educational experience, even though update activities may have been taking place frequently. Evaluation of performance in the hospital environment has shown that knowledge within the institution does not deteriorate significantly with time following an initial comprehensive educational experience (Fig. 5–2). However, evidence suggests that staff turnover is significant, even in rural locales, and reintroduction of a comprehensive program will result in further improvement of institutional performance.[14] My colleagues and I have found that communities have responded well to a cycle of intensive educational activities for inpatient facilities occurring every 4 years, with a program for outpatient practices taking place midway in the 4-year cycle.

EVALUATION*

The type of evaluation process used should depend on the following: the purpose of the evaluation, the

*References 7, 8, 10, 13–15.

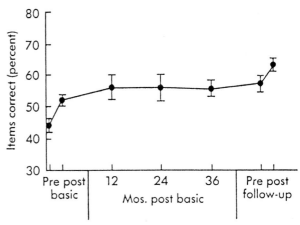

FIGURE 5–2. Patient care as determined by a review of 1435 neonatal charts from 10 community hospitals whose staffs had participated in the perinatal continuing education program. Evaluations performed at predetermined intervals revealed higher preprogram test scores by new participants before the follow-up program when compared with results of similar tests administered before the basic program, a plateau of patient care quality between programs, and a further improvement in patient care quality after the follow-up program. All results suggest an "institutionalization" of knowledge and care practices. Data are expressed in terms of percentage of optimum care delivered for the 30 care practices analyzed. (From Kattwinkel J, et al: Perinatal outreach education: A continuation strategy for a basic program. Am J Perinatol 1:335, 1984.)

size of the population being evaluated, and the extent of the evaluation resources. Measurements can be made of ultimate outcomes (such as changes in perinatal mortality and morbidity) or of intermediate outcomes (such as changes in patient care practices or referral patterns). Ultimate outcomes require longer periods of analysis and larger populations and are therefore affected by more variables than are intermediate outcomes. On the other hand, if intermediate outcomes are used as a measure of effectiveness, one must make the assumption that a change in intermediate outcome will lead to a corresponding change in ultimate outcome. In general, ultimate outcomes are of particular value for analyzing the effects of multifactorial programs on large populations (such as the statewide effects of a perinatal regionalization program), whereas intermediate outcomes are more valuable for measuring specific changes in a small population (such as the effects of an educational program on the perinatal care delivered by a specific hospital).

BASELINE PREPROGRAM MEASUREMENTS

There are two purposes in obtaining baseline measurements. First, it is helpful to determine which communities are in greatest need of an educational program. Second, to measure the effects of a program, preintervention data must be collected for comparison with data obtained after program activities.

The perinatal mortality data are probably the simplest and most accessible data for determining which communities are in greatest need of an educational program. However, as just mentioned, mortality data are not reliable for small populations; therefore, one should be extremely cautious about interpreting mortality data collected from individual hospitals, particularly if the birth rate is low. Therefore, for the purposes of determining educational need, only perinatal mortality trends occurring over several years should be examined. Estimates of educational need may also be derived from an analysis of patient status at the time of referral or by preprogram administration of one of the instruments listed in Table 5–1.

MEASURES OF PROGRAM EFFECTIVENESS

For an educational program to be truly effective, it must be used by the community professionals and result in improved knowledge; the facilities required for delivery of optimum care must improve; the care delivered to patients must change; and, ultimately, the number of babies dying or damaged must decrease (see Table 5–1). Only two of these measures (changes in cognitive knowledge and facilities) require that prospective, preprogram measurements be made. The others (e.g., changes in patient records or referral patterns) are best analyzed retrospectively to avoid having the evaluation process directly affect the outcome.

Program use is easily assessed by comparing the number of program participants with the total number of available personnel in each professional group. Most programs also include an evaluation form asking for the participants' assessment of the program's format and appropriateness.

Cognitive knowledge change is classically measured by a written test administered before and after the program. However, good test questions are difficult to prepare and require extensive validity analysis before one can be confident of the results. Tests can also be threatening to the participants, particularly if administered on a pass-fail basis. If possible, answers should be returned to the participants so that the test becomes part of the learning process. A particularly valuable form of testing is the patient management problem of the branching tree, or algorithm, format, which is amenable to interactive computerization. However, again, it is difficult to prepare such problems without ambiguity, and considerable validation testing of large populations is advisable.

Changes in facilities can be measured by a simple postprogram repetition of the self-inventory process suggested for analysis of baseline resources.

Changes in care practices are the most important of the intermediate outcomes to measure. Unfortunately, they also require the most time-consuming and expensive evaluation techniques. Also, they generally are among the slowest to show change as the result of an educational effort. It is not unusual for perinatal professionals to know intellectually the appropriate clinical action but then not to practice it in the field. For example, although a physician may answer a test question correctly regarding the increased incidence of hypoglycemia in infants who are large for gestational age, considerable time may pass before a change in hospital policy will result in all babies who are large for gestational age receiving a blood glucose screen. A hospital or office chart review or analysis of patient status at the time of transport can be used to document various care practices.

Once new knowledge has been translated into altered care practices, such practices tend to become "institutionalized" and show little evidence of deterioration over time. Then when knowledge from repeat or new educational experiences also becomes institutionalized, patient care improves even further (see Fig. 5–2). Thus, effective ongoing educational interaction between a regional center and community facility can become an even more satisfying activity than may be experienced with the traditional teacher–new student relationship. Because there is a constant improvement of performance by primary care practitioners, overall patient care and outcome throughout the region tend to show parallel progressive improvement.

Changes in patient outcome cannot be measured reliably on a short-term basis and therefore are of limited value for assessing the results of a specific educational intervention. A reflection in mortality statistics requires many thousands of births to occur, and true morbidity cannot be tested reliably in neonates. However, with appropriate resources, large populations, and sufficient follow-up time, these ultimate outcomes provide the most convincing evidence of true change.

■ REFERENCES

1. American Academy of Pediatrics and American College of Obstetricians and Gynecologists: Guidelines for Perinatal Care, 4th ed. Elk Grove Village, IL, American Academy of Pediatrics, 1997.
2. American Academy of Pediatrics and American Heart Association: Textbook of Neonatal Resuscitation, 4th ed. Elk Grove Village, IL, American Academy of Pediatrics, 2000.
3. Bailey C: Education for home care providers. J Obstet Gynecol Neonatal Nurs 23:714, 1994.
4. Bailey C, et al: Establishing a neonatal resuscitation team in community hospitals. J Perinatol 10:294, 1990.
5. Clarke TA, et al: Use of the placenta as a teaching model. Pediatrics 62:23, 1978.
6. Davis D, et al: Impact of formal continuing medical education:

TABLE 5–1 MEASURES OF PROGRAM EFFECTIVENESS

EVALUATION MEASURE	INSTRUMENT
Program use and acceptance	Completion rate Evaluation forms
Changes in cognitive knowledge	Preprogram versus postprogram test scores
Changes in facilities	Preprogram versus postprogram inventory survey
Changes in care practices	Chart review Patient status at transport Referral patterns
Changes in patient outcome	Mortality Morbidity

Do conferences, workshops, rounds, and other traditional continuing education activities change physicians' behavior or health care outcomes? JAMA 282:867, 1999.

7. Farley J: Does continuing nursing education make a difference? J Cont Educ Nurs 18:184, 1987.

8. Friedman CP, et al: Charting the winds of change: Evaluating innovative medical curricula. Acad Med 65:8, 1990.

9. Gaus J: Program educates community hospital caregivers about pretransport stabilization. Neonatal Network 18:61, 1999.

10. Harlan RH, et al: Impact of an education program on perinatal care practices. Pediatrics 66:893, 1980.

11. Hesketh TM, et al: Improvement of neonatal care in Zhejiang Province, China, through a self-instructional continuing education programme. Med Educ 28:252, 1994.

12. Jennings PB, et al: A teaching model for pediatric intubation utilizing ketamine-sedated kittens. Pediatrics 53:283, 1974.

13. Kattwinkel J, et al: Improved perinatal knowledge and care in the community hospital through a program of self-instruction. Pediatrics 64:451, 1979.

14. Kattwinkel J, et al: Perinatal outreach education: A continuation strategy for a basic program. Am J Perinatol 1:335, 1984.

15. Kattwinkel J, et al: A regionalized perinatal continuing education program: Successful adaptation to a foreign health care system and language. Med Educ 31:210, 1997.

16. March of Dimes National Foundation, Committee on Perinatal Health: Toward Improving the Outcome of Pregnancy: Recommendations for the Regional Development of Maternal and Perinatal Health Services. White Plains, NY, March of Dimes National Foundation, 1977.

17. Rosner F, et al: Reviewing the Long Island Jewish Medical Center's experience with "miniresidencies." Acad Med 66:628, 1991.

18. Shenai JP, et al: Neonatal transport: Outreach educational program. Pediatr Clin North Am 40:275, 1993.

19. Walker DE, et al: A practical program to maintain neonatal resuscitation skills. Can Med Assoc J 151:299, 1994.

20. Woods DL, et al: The perinatal education programme. S Afr Med J 84:61, 1994.

6

Evaluating and Improving the Quality of Neonatal Care

part one

DATABASES FOR THE EVALUATION OF NEONATAL AND PERINATAL CARE

Jeffrey D. Horbar and Jeffrey B. Gould

The systematic evaluation of the effectiveness and efficiency of clinical care has become an integral part of medical practice. Physicians, hospitals, and large health care organizations are all under increasing pressure to monitor, report, and continuously improve the quality and cost-effectiveness of their services. Relman has described this as the "era of assessment and accountability."[63] In this new era, neonatologists must learn how to evaluate themselves and how they will be evaluated by others, including policy makers, hospital administrators, regulators, payers, and consumers. Most importantly, they must learn how to use available information to continuously improve the quality of medical care. In this section of the chapter, we review the ways in which information can be collected, evaluated, and applied to improve the quality of medical care for newborn infants and their families. We discuss the available sources of such data for neonatology and describe how these data can be used to evaluate and improve the processes, outcomes, and costs of medical care for newborn infants. We focus primarily on neonatal intensive care and address how data can be collected and used to answer four basic questions: (1) Whom do we care for? ("Case Mix"); (2) What do we do for them? ("Medical Practices"); (3) How efficiently do we provide care? ("Costs and Resource Use"); and (4) How do we evaluate and improve the quality of care that we provide? ("Quality of Care").

DATABASES

In this discussion, we distinguish between primary databases, those designed specifically for the evaluation of neonatal care, and secondary databases, those designed originally for other purposes. We also outline two basic approaches to constructing a database. One approach attempts to create a "virtual patient." This approach is exhaustive, and it retains a detailed description of all aspects of a patient's hospital stay, such as what would be included in the medical record. The advantage of the virtual approach is that factors that may be of importance in the future will be available. The disadvantage of the virtual approach is that data collection, entry, and quality control are resource intensive.

The alternative is to collect a minimal data set. This approach begins with the notion of creating an information base. The information base is founded on the premise that information is data that inform decision making and improvement efforts.[92] Therefore, the first task in constructing a minimal database is to determine what questions need to be answered. Only data items that are needed to answer these questions are included. Achieving the proper balance between detail and simplicity is difficult but crucial. It involves making tradeoffs between costs/resource use and the number of data items.

Regardless of how many data elements are included in a database, the elements must be clearly defined. System users should have access to standardized definitions in a printed manual of operations to facilitate both the coding and the interpretation of data. Access to standardized definitions is particularly important with regard to diagnostic information. Because physicians and nurses rarely use precise definitions in their daily notes, the medical record may not provide a reliable source of clinical information. The importance of uniform definitions cannot be overstated. Without them, valid comparisons and inferences cannot be made from a database. A few well-defined data items are far more valuable than an extensive list of poorly defined items.

Paper forms, which are used to record data, must be simple and easy to use. Several revisions may be necessary in the first months of data collection. Additional strategies are essential to improve the quality of data. The computer-user interface must be well designed. Entry flow should match the paper form, entry screens should be easy to read, and there should be a clear distinction between a null response, such as "0" or "not present," and a missing value. Methods to minimize data entry errors, such as double entry or visual verification, should be used.[6, 34] Logic, range, and consistency checks should be applied to each data element in the database so that errors in coding or transcription can be detected during the process of data entry. Finally, data reports must be available in a timely manner. Data that are too old cannot reliably inform decision making. Because of the lengthy hospitalization of the very premature infant, it is often useful to enter data at the end of the first 28 days as well as at discharge. This strategy allows one to perform an analysis of neonatal outcomes in a timely fashion. To be of optimal use, reports should be produced at least biannually. Quarterly reports are even more effective in identifying emerging clinical trends and correcting data collection and processing problems. Furthermore, reports must be clear and concise, focusing on information that is appropriate to the decision-making task. An ideal place to start when designing a neonatal database is to consider what routine reports are desired as end products and how often they are needed. Appropriate data items can then be chosen for inclusion in the database, the best sources for these data items can be identified, and an effective timetable for report generation can be established.

SOURCES OF DATA

Data regarding neonatal patients are available from a variety of sources (Box 6-1). Vital statistics for newborn infants are maintained by government agencies at the state, federal, and international levels.[1, 14, 22, 83] Birth and death data are usually available within 12 months of the close of a calendar year, but data derived from a primary nursery database tend to be more timely. In the past, the usefulness of birth certificate data has been limited by variability in the quantity and quality of sociodemographic and health data. The development of a standardized national birth certificate and its adoption by many states has greatly improved the potential usefulness of information derived from birth certificates.[86] The scope of, timeliness of, specific definitions for, and quality of state birth certificate data still vary considerably.[7, 56, 59] Information about birth certificates can be obtained by consulting one's state Department of Maternal and Child Health and the state Department of Vital Statistics.

Death certificates are a second important source of vital information for neonates. The major limitation of the death certificate is that it does not contain the birth weight or other important sociodemographic and health data that are included on a birth certificate. For example, one cannot calculate birth weight–

■ **BOX 6-1**

DATA SOURCES FOR EVALUATING NEONATAL CARE

Vital Statistics
Federal and state data
Birth certificates
Death certificates

Hospital Information Systems
Clinical information systems
Administrative information systems
Decision support systems

Claims Data
Medicaid
Other insurers

Neonatal Databases
Locally designed databases
Commercial databases

Neonatal Networks
Australian and New Zealand Neonatal Network
British Association of Perinatal Medicine
Canadian NICU Network
International Neonatal Network
National Perinatal Information Center
NICHD Neonatal Research Network
Vermont Oxford Network

NICHD, National Institute of Child Health and Human Development; NICU, neonatal intensive care unit.

---

specific mortality without first linking birth and death certificates. Fortunately, most states now routinely link birth certificate and death certificate data. The only drawback to this approach is the lack of timeliness. To report on death during the first year of life (infant mortality) for a calendar year cohort requires the observation of the last born infant of the calendar year for an additional year. Most state vital statistics based on a linked birth certificate and death certificate cohort cannot begin to be assembled until 12 months from the end of the cohort calendar year. Despite this limitation, these databases provide a unique and important resource for population-based evaluations of neonatal care. At the national level this process has been accelerated by using period-linked infant birth and death certificates (all infant deaths in a specific year are linked to their birth certificates using the number of births during the period year as the denominator). Infant mortality statistics for 1997, based on this technique, were published in July 1999.[47]

Data are available within individual hospitals and multi-institutional hospital systems from several different sources. These include clinical or medical information systems designed to support direct patient care; administrative information systems used to assist organizational managers in areas such as finance, payroll, and inventory; and executive decision support systems intended to address strategic policy concerns, such as long-range planning and evaluation of institutional performance.[3] These systems are likely to become highly integrated in the future.

Patient records contain extensive data concerning the practices and outcomes of care. Currently, data must be abstracted from these records for entry in a database. As electronic medical records are used more widely, aggregated patient-level data will be more readily available. As with off-line databases, electronic clinical records must contain uniformly defined and accepted sociodemographic, diagnostic, treatment, and outcome elements in order to be useful for evaluation purposes.

Government agencies and private payers maintain extensive databases of claims data, which include information regarding neonates. Although such databases were not originally intended to be used in the evaluation of medical care, their data increasingly will be applied to this purpose.

PRIMARY DATA

Neonatal Intensive Care Unit Data

Primary patient-level databases for neonatal patients can be developed locally, acquired commercially, or obtained as part of a multihospital neonatal network. In a 1989 survey of 305 level III neonatal intensive care units (NICUs), 78% had a database. Of these, 74% were developed locally.[79] For example, Escobar and colleagues have described a minimal data set developed for Northern Kaiser Permanente Hospitals in order to identify clusters of preventable adverse outcomes in a timely manner and to assess the feasibility of specific research trial designs.[17, 18] The advantage of a locally developed custom database is that it can contain items that may be extremely important in the local environment (e.g., details of transport could be essential in a facility with a high proportion of regional transports). The disadvantage of a locally developed custom database is that definitions, quality control methods (such as automated analysis for range, logic, and internal consistency), or routine review for entry accuracy may not be comparable with those used in other databases. In building a custom database, the major problems are not software or hardware. The availability of highly efficient personal computers, an abundance of inexpensive storage options, and extremely user-friendly database programs greatly facilitate this option. The major difficulties are designing the database, deciding what questions will be asked, and ensuring that accurate and reliable data needed to answer the questions and generate the desired reports are included.

The survey on NICU databases revealed that databases that included a lot of data and that were available for multiple purposes gave the most satisfaction. It is not clear, however, that satisfaction reflects the actual utility of the database. The finding that almost 33% of the respondents had tried one or two databases previously and that 18% were contemplating either abandoning or making major modifications to their present database speaks to the difficulties of database design. Our personal recommendation (with software and hardware being readily available) is to choose an existing database with set quality control and system management protocols with the intention of making the custom modifications needed to design it to your specific needs. One important consideration, even for those who choose to design a customized database system of their own, is to create the option for exporting core data electronically to a large neonatal network. Doing this requires collection of data using the standard definitions and procedures adhered to by all members of that network and developing the capability for exporting the data in an accepted format. For example, the Vermont Oxford Network has recently published standards for electronic data submission by its members.[90] The advantage of this approach is that it allows an institution to maintain a customized database while permitting it to compare its performance on a core set of well-defined measures with a large cohort of other hospitals.

In a recent review, Slagle provides an overview and blueprint for perinatal information systems (Figure 6–1).[80] The development of these systems should be guided by three important premises. First, the highest quality data can be achieved with real-time entry by clinicians who use standardized terms and definitions. Second, the effort expended in data entry must have clear benefits to the clinician (save time, improve the care of the patient). Third, the data, entered once, must be put to multiple uses (routine outputs include admission, progress, and discharge reports; billing information; exports to national networks; and quality of care analyses).

Medical Data Systems (NeoKnowledge, www.mdsinfo.com), MetaSoft (NeoData, www.ms-systems.com), MacNICU, and Site of Care Systems (The Daily Baby, www.siteofcare.com) are examples of commercially available systems that have been specifically developed for the perinatal environment.[80, 84] Each system is a step toward creating an electronic medical record for neonatology. In addition to electronically producing clinical, statistical, cost, and outcome data, some have utilities such as practice guidelines or parental nutrition orders calculators to facilitate clinical management. These systems use keyboard data entry facilitated by structured pull-down menus. Several systems (e.g., MetaSoft Systems Inc. or Computer Voice Dictation Solutions [www.cvds.com]) also allow the data to be voice entered.

When evaluating commercial systems, one must consider not only the ease of data entry and the extent and quality of the reports that are routinely generated from the database but also the extent to which the system is capable of capturing information from other hospital data systems (e.g., laboratory and x-ray reports). The extent to which obstetric data can be incorporated into the neonatal database and reports is especially important. Systems that have an integrated obstetric module greatly facilitate a more comprehen-

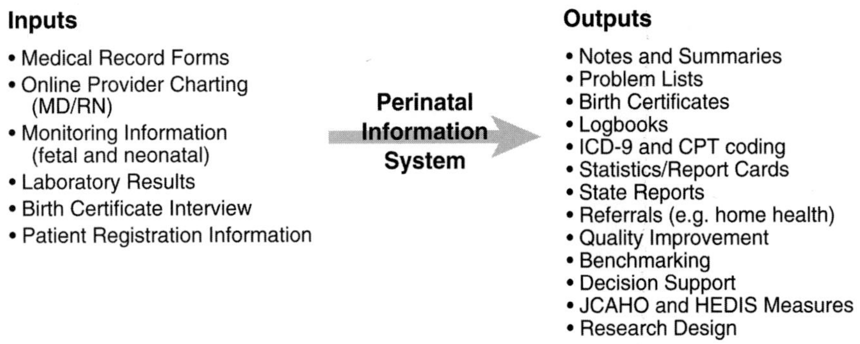

Inputs

- Medical Record Forms
- Online Provider Charting (MD/RN)
- Monitoring Information (fetal and neonatal)
- Laboratory Results
- Birth Certificate Interview
- Patient Registration Information

Perinatal Information System →

Outputs

- Notes and Summaries
- Problem Lists
- Birth Certificates
- Logbooks
- ICD-9 and CPT coding
- Statistics/Report Cards
- State Reports
- Referrals (e.g. home health)
- Quality Improvement
- Benchmarking
- Decision Support
- JCAHO and HEDIS Measures
- Research Design

FIGURE 6–1. Blueprint for the ideal perinatal information system design. (From Slagle TA: Perinatal information systems for quality improvement. Pediatrics 103:268, 1999. Used with permission of the American Academy of Pediatrics.)

sive perinatal approach to improving neonatal outcomes. Finally, one must also evaluate the extent to which the system allows comparison with other hospitals across the nation. Site of Care Systems, MacNICU, and MetaSoft approach this by generating data forms for submission to the Vermont Oxford Network.

Neonatal Networks

Several NICU networks that maintain databases have been formed to evaluate the effectiveness and efficiency of neonatal intensive care. Examples include the Australian and New Zealand Neonatal Network,[15] the Canadian NICU Network,[64] the International Neonatal Network,[41] the National Institute of Child Health and Human Development (NICHD) Neonatal Research Network,[19, 25, 26, 85, 87] and the Vermont Oxford Network (see Box 6–1).[32, 33, 34, 42, 89] Medical Data Systems has established a network (National NeoKnowledge Network and Obstetric Information System) in order to facilitate comparison and benchmarking among its users.

The NICHD Neonatal Research Network is a group of 14 academic NICUs whose government-funded activities include randomized trials and observational studies. Participants in the network are chosen based

on competitive application to the NICHD. The NICHD Neonatal Research Network maintains a database for infants with birth weights of 401 to 1500 gm who were treated at participating NICUs. Uniform definitions for data items and attention to maintenance of data quality make the NICHD Neonatal Research Network database a valuable resource for neonatologists. The published reports from the database can be used by other NICUs for comparison. An example of the type of data produced by the NICHD Neonatal Network is shown in Table 6–1. The validity of making comparisons with these data depends on the definitions of data items used by an individual NICU and the similarity of their patient populations to those treated at NICUs in the NICHD Network.

The Vermont Oxford Network is a collaborative network of neonatologists and other health care professionals, representing over 350 institutions from North America and around the world.[32, 33] Membership is voluntary and open to all who are interested. The nonprofit network is supported by membership fees, research grants, and contracts. The primary philosophy of the Vermont Oxford Network is to improve the effectiveness and efficiency of medical care for newborn infants and their families through a coordinated program of research, education, and quality improvement projects. In support of all three aspects

TABLE 6–1 BIRTH WEIGHT–SPECIFIC SURVIVAL AND SELECTED NEONATAL MORBIDITY AMONG SURVIVORS BORN IN THE NICHD NEONATAL RESEARCH NETWORK BETWEEN 1/1/95 AND 12/31/96*

SURVIVORS	501–750 gm (n = 1002)	751–1000 gm (n = 1084)	1001–1250 gm (n = 1053)	1251–1500 gm (n = 1299)	501–1500 gm (n = 4438)
Total	540 (53.9)	935 (86.3)	992 (94.2)	1257 (96.8)	3724 (83.9)
Survived without morbidity	199 (36.9)	540 (57.8)	766 (77.2)	1132 (90.1)	2637 (70.8)
Survived with morbidity	341 (63.1)	395 (42.2)	226 (22.8)	125 (9.9)	1087 (29.2)
CLD†	189 (35.0)	245 (26.2)	121 (12.2)	71 (5.6)	626 (16.8)
Severe ICH‡	33 (6.1)	47 (5.0)	46 (4.6)	22 (1.8)	148 (4.0)
NEC§	22 (4.1)	30 (3.2)	32 (3.2)	23 (1.8)	107 (2.9)
CLD/Severe ICH	56 (10.4)	39 (4.2)	19 (1.9)	6 (0.5)	120 (3.2)
CLD/NEC	25 (4.6)	26 (2.8)	6 (0.6)	3 (0.2)	60 (1.6)
NEC/Severe ICH	9 (1.7)	5 (0.5)	2 (0.2)	0 (0.0)	16 (0.4)
CLD/Severe ICH/NEC	7 (1.3)	3 (0.3)	0 (0.0)	0 (0.0)	10 (0.3)

*Data expressed as number of infants with percentages in parentheses.
†Chronic lung disease as O_2 at 36 weeks' postmenstrual age.
‡Grade III-IV intraventricular hemorrhage.
§Necrotizing enterocolitis (Bell's classification stage ≥2).
Courtesy of Linda L. Wright, MD, National Institute of Child Health and Human Development Neonatal Research Network, November 1999.

of this program, the network maintains a database for infants with birth weights of 401 to 1500 grams who were born at participating centers or admitted to them within 28 days of birth. Members of the Vermont Oxford Network complete brief data forms using standardized definitions.[32, 33, 42, 89] Strict attention is paid to maintenance of data quality.[34] The database provides core data for network clinical trials, is used for observational studies and outcomes research, and generates reports for members that compare their performance with that of other NICUs in the network. These reports are produced quarterly and are intended for use in local quality management efforts.

In 1999, the Vermont Oxford Network database enrolled over 25,000 infants weighing 401 to 1500 gm; in the 9-year period from 1990 to 1999, over 125,000 infants were enrolled in the database. A major advantage of participating in a network database is that comparisons among NICUs based on uniform definitions are then possible. Members of the Vermont Oxford Network receive standardized reports that document their performance, track changes over time, and compare the individual NICU with the Network as a whole and with a group of similar institutions. An example of the type of data available in these confidential reports is shown in Figure 6–2, which shows the proportion of infants weighing 501 to 1500 gm who were treated with high frequency ventilation at one participating NICU, referred to as "NICU X," compared with all Vermont Oxford Network centers for the years 1990 to 1998. The proportion of infants treated with high-frequency ventilation has increased dramatically during this time period in the overall Network, whereas at NICU X, high frequency ventilation was not introduced until 1995. Similar data are available for a wide range of neonatal outcomes and interventions. These data, which provide comparisons with overall network reference rates as well as identification of trends over time, are available to all NICUs participating in the Vermont Oxford Network database. A limitation of the databases maintained by the NICHD and the Vermont Oxford Network is that they are currently limited to infants with birth weights of 1500 gm or less. The Vermont Oxford Network is

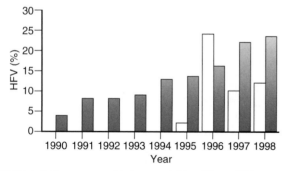

FIGURE 6–2. Percentage of infants weighing 501 to 1500 gm who were treated with high frequency ventilation (HFV) at anonymous NICU X (white bars) and at all NICUs in the Vermont Oxford Network (shaded bars) from 1990 to 1998. The figure is based on a total of 448 infants from NICU X and 95,569 infants in the total Network for the years 1990 to 1998. (Courtesy of the Vermont Oxford Network, Burlington, Vermont.)

now expanding data collection to include infants over 1500 gm.

In addition to national and international networks, there are several statewide efforts in the United States that are focused on monitoring and improving newborn care. For example, New York is in the process of implementing a Statewide Perinatal Data System (SPDS) that will consist of a core birth certificate, birth log, and modules for neonates and mothers who are at high risk. Data, which will be entered via the Internet, will allow performance of basic analyses online and serve numerous reporting needs, including those of vital records, birth logs, newborn screening, and immunization registry. The system will provide outcomes data for hospitals, integrated health care systems, and perinatal regions for use in quality improvement efforts.[2]

Another example is the California Perinatal Quality Care Collaborative (CPQCC), a statewide outgrowth of an initiative proposed by the California Association of Neonatologists (CAN) and supported by the David and Lucile Packard Foundation and the California Department of Health Services, Maternal and Child Health Branch. The collaborative exists to improve the health of pregnant women, infants, and children by collecting high-quality information on perinatal outcomes and resource use and using these data for performance improvement and benchmarking processes in perinatal care and NICUs throughout California. The CPQCC forms a public and private alliance of stakeholders, including the Maternal and Child Health Branch, California Children's Services, and the Office of Vital Records (all within the California Department of Health Services); the Office of Statewide Health Planning and Development; the Hospital Council; Regional Perinatal Programs of California; the Health Insurance Plan of California; the American College of Obstetricians and Gynecologists; the California Association of Neonatologists; the Pacific Business Group on Health; the David and Lucile Packard Foundation; and the Vermont Oxford Network. The goals of the collaborative are to (1) provide a timely analysis of perinatal care, outcomes, and resource use based on a uniform statewide database; (2) provide mechanisms for benchmarking and continuous quality improvement (CQI); and (3) serve as a model for other states. The Vermont Oxford Network has provided major input to the development of the database and CQI activities. The Vermont Oxford Network database for infants weighing less than 1500 gm has provided the foundation for the CPQCC database. In 2000, this was expanded to include a subset of the sickest infants weighing over 1500 gm. The large-baby data will be processed by the CPQCC data center, and special reports will be developed for inborns, outborns, and infants readmitted to an NICU during the first 28 days of life. In the future, the database will be expanded to include individual state birth certificate and death certificate data (which are now used to audit the completeness of CPQCC hospital data submission) and hospital discharge summary data. Currently, there are almost 50 member hospitals with NICUs admitting nearly 70% of California's newborn infants who require critical care. Timely high-quality data fuel the project, but the major purpose of the CPQCC is to improve the quality of care.

SECONDARY DATA

Secondary data sources that are frequently used are the birth certificate, the hospital discharge abstract, and hospital billing data. The major advantage to using secondary data is that someone else maintains the data system. The major disadvantages are that the secondary data sources may not have all of the necessary data items; that the definitions may not be appropriate or the same as those used in other NICUs; and that the accuracy may not be adequate. For example, demographic information, prenatal care, mode of delivery, and birth weight tend to be fairly reliable on birth certificates.[7, 56, 59] However, the presence of congenital anomalies, an important item because of the high degree of complexity and mortality in this group, is markedly underreported on both birth certificates and death certificates.[30, 36, 81] A recent review describes both the advantages and disadvantages of using vital records for quality improvement.[22] Linked birth and death certificate files are an important source of population-based studies of factors that affect perinatal outcomes. These studies span a wide range of areas (e.g., the effect of the increase in multiple births on infant mortality,[39] factors associated with the birth of infants with very low birth weight [VLBW] at non-NICU hospitals,[23] and quality assessment of perinatal regionalization[16])· However, to maximize the potential usefulness of vital records, clinicians must become actively involved in ensuring their uniformity of definition, accuracy, and completeness.

The hospital discharge abstract may be a useful data source for evaluating neonatal care.[38, 76] The U.S. Department of Health and Human Services mandates that a Uniform Hospital Discharge Data Set (UHDDS) that includes 14 core data items be submitted for each acute patient whose care is paid for by Medicare or Medicaid. The most widely used format for these submissions is the Uniform Bill, introduced in 1992 (UB-92).[72, 76] UB-92 contains data items for patient identification, insurance coverage, total charges, and entries for up to five diagnostic and three procedural codes. These codes are assigned based on the International Classification of Diseases, Ninth Revision, Clinical Modification (ICD-9-CM).[37] UB-92 is required for hospitals submitting claims to Medicare, Medicaid, Blue Cross, and other commercial insurers. Although hospitals are not required to submit UB-92 for all neonates, most hospitals do complete this form. The Uniform Bill can provide useful information on procedures, diagnoses, and charges. The major advantage of this data source is its widespread use at a large number of institutions and its ready availability as a computer data set at many hospitals.

There are several weaknesses, however, that must be considered. The Uniform Bill was designed for reimbursement, not for monitoring institutional performance or for clinical research. As a result, distortions in the data may result from attempts by hospitals to code diagnostic and procedural data with the goal of maximizing reimbursement.[20] Significant errors in diagnostic coding may occur. Studies of the reliability of hospital discharge abstracts have found that the principal diagnosis identified in the discharge abstract agrees with the actual diagnosis based on chart review only 65% of the time.[40] The accuracy of coding for neonatal conditions has not been studied in detail. However, neonatal discharge abstracts tend to contain less reliable data on race than do birth certificates. Another problem with hospital discharge abstract data is the absence of birth weight as a data item. It is not included on UB-92. Because of the powerful predictive relationship of birth weight to both resource use and neonatal outcomes, recommendations to revise the UHDDS to include birth weight have been made.[38] This addition would greatly increase the value of discharge abstract data for the care of newborns.

It is also possible to use linkage strategies to enhance the usefulness of secondary data sources for quality improvement. Highly successful links can be established without using personal data such as names, hospital numbers, or social security numbers, by employing virtual identifiers such as ZIP code of residence, clinical factors, and sociodemographic factors. California's Office of State Health Planning and Development sponsored a project to link the state-linked infant birth and death file and a modification of the UB-92 file.[29] This database allows one to select outcomes from the ICD-9 and procedure codes available on the discharge billing file and adjust these outcomes based on the birth weight and clinical, demographic, and socioeconomic information from the birth certificate. Further links to this database have included the mother's discharge file for the current pregnancy as well all infant readmission discharge files during the first year of life. Examples of population-based studies using this linked database include the relationship between discharge timing after birth and infant readmission,[13] shoulder dystocia, risk factors and neonatal outcomes,[52] and neonatal outcomes in childbearing beyond the age of 40.[21] In a project sponsored by the Pacific Business Group on Health with the technical oversight of the California Perinatal Quality Care Collaborative, this database was used to perform a risk-adjusted analysis of primary cesarean section rates in California hospitals (www.healthscope.org). The technical details of the analysis are available at the CPQCC website (www.CPQCC.org).

CASE MIX

The resources that are required to run a neonatology program and the degree of morbidity and mortality that patients served by that program can expect to experience depend on the volume of patients as well as the complexity and severity of their diseases. For example, the very low neonatal mortality rates and costs per neonate that are observed in level I facilities

TABLE 6–2 ALTERNATIVE DIAGNOSIS-RELATED GROUP CLASSIFICATION SYSTEMS

DRG SYSTEM	DEVELOPER	USERS
HCFA-DRG	Medicare	Medicare and some Medicaid programs
PM-DRG	NACHRI	No longer maintained
AP-DRG	New York State	New York and other states
CHAMPUS-DRG	Department of Defense	CHAMPUS
R-DRG	HCFA	Ohio Health Department
APR-DRG	3M Health Information Systems	State Health Departments
	NACHRI	Health Data Commissions

AP, all patients; APR, all patients refined; CHAMPUS, Civilian Health and Medical Program of the Uniformed Services; DRG, diagnosis-related group; HCFA, Health Care Financing Administration; NACHRI, National Association of Children's Hospitals and Related Institutions; PM, pediatric modified; R, refined.

From John Muldoon, The National Association of Children's Hospitals and Related Institutions, Inc, December 1994.

reflect low neonatal acuity, not medical practices that are more effective or efficient than those in level III facilities.[28] Therefore, from a practical perspective, it is important to define exactly whom we care for, in order to plan for and justify resource allocation and to make meaningful comparisons between other institutions and our own over time. The data needed for these comparisons must include factors that reflect complexity and influence both morbidity and mortality. Because birth weight and gestational age are the most important determinants of both the level of intervention required and the outcome,[77] they are crucial items in any neonatal database. Because it may be difficult to assign accurate gestational ages, birth weight is often used as the primary variable. Sex, prenatal care, the administration of antenatal steroids, condition at birth as reflected by the Apgar scores, and location of birth are also important in specifying the complexity of neonatal patients. Factors that reflect ethnicity and socioeconomic status, such as maternal age, education, and payer source, have important implications in terms of both morbidity and discharge planning.

DIAGNOSIS-RELATED GROUPS

Diagnosis-related group (DRG) systems are classification schemes that use data that are routinely available in hospital discharge abstracts to group patients into relatively homogeneous categories. They provide one method for describing the answer to the question *Whom do we care for?* Because of the widespread use of DRGs, it is important for neonatologists to be familiar with these systems. Ideally, each DRG category should contain patients who are clinically similar, whose care requires the same resource intensity, and who are at similar risk for adverse events, mortality, and morbidity. These systems, which were originally developed to guide prospective payment to hospitals, are used increasingly to classify patients for risk stratification in analyses of outcomes and costs. Several alternative DRG classification systems have been developed (Table 6–2). They are updated periodically and exist in different versions. Individual DRGs are grouped into major diagnostic categories that contain related DRGs. The following discussion is limited

to the DRGs in major diagnostic category 15, which includes "normal" newborns and neonates with conditions originating in the perinatal period.

The Health Care Financing Administration DRG system (HCFA-DRG), which is used by Medicare, includes only seven DRG categories for neonates (Table 6–3). The HCFA-DRG categories are heterogeneous, explaining only 16% to 22% of the variation in costs and length of stay for neonates.[49, 50, 58, 61] Because of the limitations of the HCFA-DRG system, alternatives have been developed. The first version of the Pediatric Modified DRG (PM-DRG) system, developed by the National Association of Children's Hospitals and Related Institutions (NACHRI) in the late 1980s, explained 46% of the variation in the costs of caring for neonates.[46, 57] The New York State Health Department and several other states adopted the All Patient DRG (AP-DRG) system in the late 1980s, which includes most, but not all, of the categories in the PM-DRG. The AP-DRG (version 12.0) now includes 28 base categories for newborns.[50]

The All Patient Refined DRG (APR-DRG) system (version 15.0), the most recent alternative DRG system, developed by 3M Health Information Systems and the NACHRI, contains 35 base neonatal categories (Table 6–4). These categories are further subdivided into four subclasses of complexity (minor, moderate, major, and extreme), resulting in a total of 140 categories. Muldoon has compared the structural and

TABLE 6–3 HEALTH CARE FINANCING ADMINISTRATION DIAGNOSIS-RELATED GROUP (HCFA-DRG) CATEGORIES FOR MAJOR DIAGNOSTIC CATEGORY 15

HCFA-DRG NUMBER	CATEGORY
385	Neonate, died or transferred
386	Neonate, extreme immaturity
387	Prematurity with major problems
388	Prematurity without major problems
389	Full-term neonate with major problems
390	Neonates with other significant problems
391	Normal newborn

TABLE 6–4   ALL PATIENT REFINED DIAGNOSIS-RELATED GROUP (APR-DRG) CATEGORIES,
VERSION 15.0*

APR-DRG NUMBER	CATEGORY
580	Neonate, transferred <5 days old, not born here
581	Neonate, transferred <5 days old, born here
582	Neonate, with organ transplant
583	Neonate, with extracorporeal membrane oxygenation
590	Neonate, birth weight <750 gm, with major OR procedure
591	Neonate, birth weight <750 gm, without major OR procedure
592	Neonate, birth weight 750–999 gm, with major OR procedure
593	Neonate, birth weight 750–999 gm, without major OR procedure
600	Neonate, birth weight 1000–1499 gm, with major OR procedure
601	Neonate, birth weight 1000–1499 gm, with major anomaly or hereditary condition
602	Neonate, birth weight 1000–1499 gm, with respiratory distress syndrome
603	Other neonate, birth weight 1000–1499 gm
610	Neonate, birth weight 1500–1999 gm, with major OR procedure
611	Neonate, birth weight 1500–1999 gm, with major anomaly or hereditary condition
612	Neonate, birth weight 1500–1999 gm, with respiratory distress syndrome
613	Neonate, birth weight 1500–1999 gm, with congenital/perinatal infection
614	Other neonate, birth weight 1500–1999 gm
620	Neonate, birth weight 2000–2499 gm, with major OR procedure
621	Neonate, birth weight 2000–2499 gm, with major anomaly or hereditary condition
622	Neonate, birth weight 2000–2499 gm, with respiratory distress syndrome
623	Neonate, birth weight 2000–2499 gm, with congenital/perinatal infection
624	Neonate, birth weight 2000–2499 gm, not born here, with PDX of other significant condition or other problem
625	Neonate, birth weight 2000–2499 gm, born here, with other significant condition
626	Neonate, birth weight 2000–2499 gm, born here, normal newborn and newborn with other problem
630	Neonate, birth weight >2499 gm, with major cardiovascular OR procedure
631	Neonate, birth weight >2499 gm, with other major OR procedure
632	Neonate, birth weight >2499 gm, with other OR procedure
633	Neonate, birth weight >2499 gm, with major anomaly or hereditary condition
634	Neonate, birth weight >2499 gm, with respiratory distress syndrome
635	Neonate, birth weight >2499 gm, with aspiration syndrome
636	Neonate, birth weight >2499 gm, with major congenital/perinatal infection
637	Neonate, birth weight >2499 gm, not born here, with PDX of other significant condition
638	Neonate, birth weight >2499 gm, not born here, with PDX of other problem
639	Neonate, birth weight >2499 gm, born here, with other significant condition
640	Neonate, birth weight >2499 gm, born here, normal newborn and newborn with other problem

*APR-DRG, version 15.0 developed by 3M Health Information Systems and the National Association of Children's Hospitals and Related Institutions.
OR, operating room; PDX, principal diagnosis.
From Muldoon JH: Structure and performance of different DRG classification systems for neonatal medicine. Pediatrics 1999; 103:302.

statistical performance of the major DRG systems for neonates.[50] He concludes that Medicare DRG categories are the least developed structurally and yield the poorest overall statistical performance and that the AP-DRG categories are intermediate in performance, rating somewhere between the Medicare DRG system and the APR-DRG system.

A difficulty with analyses based on DRGs is the validity of the ICD-9 diagnostic codes from which they are derived. In evaluations of charts coded by medical records personnel, error rates for some adult[10] and neonatal[78] diagnoses and procedures are as high as 20% to 40%. The practice of "upcoding" for the purpose of obtaining higher reimbursements has been cited as a potential source of these errors.[44]

Even detailed classification schemes such as the newer DRG systems may not adequately provide data that can be used to answer the question *Whom do we care for?* Alternative approaches to classifying patients

according to their underlying risk for morbidity or mortality are discussed later (see "Risk Adjustment").

MEDICAL PRACTICES

The second major question to be answered by data collected from neonatal databases, *What do we do for them?*, relates to the interventions and procedures used in routine medical and nursing practice. Again, two approaches may be taken. The virtual patient approach attempts to capture all activities and the diagnoses they address. Detailed electronic medical record, billing, and cost accounting systems used by hospitals can be used to create a virtual patient. As more hospitals develop sophisticated cost accounting systems in response to the monitoring requirements of managed care settings, these databases should allow detailed description of treatment input by diagnostic category and by specific caregiver. Such databases, developed as components of administrative hospital information systems, are relatively new to pediatrics and neonatology. Because these databases were designed primarily for financial analysis, coding of clinical data and procedures may not be accurate. Another drawback of using the systems that are currently available is that physician procedures often are not included in hospital billing systems. To be effective for evaluating clinical care, cost accounting data sets must be customized to the local environment. This process requires clinical input and provides the neonatologist with an opportunity to build in appropriate safeguards to more accurately reflect clinical status and procedures. Although administrative information systems promise important possibilities for the future, primary neonatal databases now offer the best approach to recording what doctors and nurses do for their patients.

Primary neonatal databases vary in terms of how detailed they are with respect to specific interventions. Most databases include certain key interventions, such as surgery, ventilation, and the use of oxygen at 28 days, or 36 weeks adjusted gestational age. There is little consensus, however, regarding what elements to include or at what level of detail to include them.

The Neonatal Therapeutic Intervention Scoring System (NTISS) is a measure of neonatal therapeutic intensity.[24] This score, based on a modification of the adult Therapeutic Intervention Scoring System (TISS),[12] assigns 1 to 4 points for each of 62 intensive care therapies in eight categories (respiratory, cardiovascular, drug therapy, monitoring, metabolic/nutrition, transfusion, procedural, vascular access). Data for the score are abstracted from the medical record. The NTISS score is highly correlated with markers of illness severity and a measure of nursing acuity, and it is predictive of NICU length of stay and total hospital charges for survivors. If scores such as NTISS can be simplified and validated in a large number of NICUs, they will be valuable tools for measuring the scope and intensity of therapeutic interventions. Ideally, the data items needed to measure therapeutic intensity should be available in either primary or secondary data sets already being collected. Future neonatal database systems should attempt to incorporate measures of therapeutic intensity so that chart review will not be necessary to collect the required data items. Patients inherently differ in the therapeutic intensity that they will require, so a perinatal service's outcomes must be measured within the context of its case mix.

RISK ADJUSTMENT

Because evaluating the quality of care involves comparison among NICUs, the documented outcomes of an individual NICU must be considered in the context of the severity and complexity of that NICU's case mix, using an appropriate analytic approach to measure and adjust for differences in risk. A simple ap-

proach is to compare outcomes for relatively homogeneous categories of patients, such as individual DRGs, discharge categories, or birth weight groupings. The outcomes and interventions for infants at a given NICU in a particular category are then compared with those for infants in that category at all other NICUs in the network. This is one approach used by the Vermont Oxford Network, which provides members with reports that compare birth weight and gestational age–specific outcomes and intervention rates at their NICUs with those at network hospitals. It is also used by the National Perinatal Information Center. Reports such as these are useful to focus attention on specific outcomes or interventions that deserve further analysis and study.

More sophisticated multivariate methods can also be used to adjust for differences in case mix, illness severity, and patient risk.[27, 69, 70] Williams and associates pioneered this type of approach to assess the objective outcomes of fetal, neonatal, perinatal, postneonatal, and infant mortality in all California hospitals.[93, 94] The analysis uses secondary data from linked birth and death certificates. It is based on all births to California residents. The basic paradigm is that to make valid interpretations of the observed mortality rate, one must account for the following components that affect its variability: (1) risk, (2) chance, and (3) quality of care. The risk component reflects differences in observed outcome that solely are due to differences in case mix. Williams considers the primary risk factors to be birth weight, race, ethnicity, sex, and plurality, because these factors have been shown to be important predictors of neonatal mortality and are available from birth and death certificates. His strategy is to use indirect standardization. Using all California births, the mortality rate for each combination of the four risk factors is calculated. For a given hospital, the overall observed mortality is compared with an expected mortality calculated by applying the overall California mortality rates to each of the hospital's neonates and summing the results. To account for the chance component, Williams offers two statistical assessments (Z score and Bayesian) to test for a significant difference between a hospital's observed and expected mortality rates. A hospital with poor performance would have a higher observed mortality rate than what would be expected on the basis of its birth weight, race, ethnicity, sex, and plurality case mix. A major criticism of the Williams approach is that it may exclude important predictors of risk for poor outcome, such as disease severity.

Severity of illness scores for both adult and pediatric intensive care patients have been developed and validated.[27, 62] These scores, based on multivariate modeling techniques, can be used to adjust for case mix differences among intensive care units when comparing patient outcomes. Similar physiology-based severity scores have been developed for use in neonatal intensive care.[69] The *Clinical Risk Index for Babies* (CRIB) was developed by the International Neonatal Network under the leadership of W. O. Tarnow-Mordi to predict mortality risk for infants with birth weights less than 1500 gm or gestational ages younger than 31 weeks.[41] Using a process that includes univariate and multiple logistic regression analyses, six prognostic variables were selected from among 40 candidates. The CRIB score was then constructed by converting into integers the regression coefficients for the six prognostic variables in a logistic model for predicting hospital death (Table 6–5). The variables are birth weight, gestational age, maximum and minimum fraction of inspired oxygen, maximum base excess during the first 12 hours, and the presence of congenital malformations. The CRIB score correlates with both mortality risk and the risk for major cerebral abnormality on cranial ultrasound. A major strength of the CRIB score is its simplicity; a limitation is that it was designed specifically for infants weighing less than 1500 grams or those younger than 31 gestational weeks.

The *Score for Neonatal Acute Physiology* (SNAP), developed by Richardson and coworkers, is a physiology-based illness severity score originally based on measurements of 26 routine clinical tests and vital signs.[67, 68] Birth weight and SNAP are independent predictors of mortality. An additive score that is based on birth weight, 5-minute Apgar score, size for gestational age, and SNAP, called the *SNAP-PE* (SNAP–Perinatal Extension), has been shown to be superior to either birth weight or SNAP alone.[66] The more recent version of the score, SNAP II, uses only six laboratory and clinical parameters (lowest mean blood pressure, lowest temperature, lowest pH level, lowest PaO_2/FiO_2 ratio, urine output, and seizures), collected during the first 12 hours after admission. A recent abstract based on 4864 admissions (2052 infants over 31 weeks' gestation) concludes that the new score is compatible with SNAP I, is valid for infants of all birth weights, and takes only 5 minutes to collect.[65] Both CRIB score and SNAP are potentially useful for comparing mortality rates and other outcomes at different NICUs. The limited number of data elements required for both CRIB score and SNAP II makes them compatible with a minimal data set approach.

One drawback of both scores is their use of variables, which are measured during the first 12 hours after NICU admission. This raises two potential problems. The first problem relates to the 12-hour period of observation. The authors state that the longer the period of observation, "the more contaminated it becomes with the effects of successful (or unsuccessful) treatment and thus no longer reflects admission severity."[70] Because their values may be influenced by treatments provided after admission, these illness severity scores are not truly independent of the effectiveness or quality of care. The second problem is that the observed severity of illness in the first hours of life may differ from the observed severity of illness in the very same infant in the first 6 hours following transfer and admission to another unit. Further studies will be required to determine the extent to which these potential problems limit the usefulness of CRIB and SNAP II for case mix adjustment.

An alternative to severity of illness adjustment is prediction based on variables measured before NICU admission. Williams' risk adjustment technique, discussed earlier, based on birth weight, ethnicity, sex, and plurality, is an example of a prediction model based on data that are independent of the quality of clinical care. The model does not include several factors, such as 1-minute Apgar, congenital abnormalities, and inborn/outborn status, that have been shown to be associated with the risk of neonatal mortality.

A mortality prediction model based on variables measured before NICU admission that are routine components of a minimal neonatal database was developed by the Vermont Oxford Network and has been used in routine annual reporting to members since 1991. The logistic regression model on which the predictions are now based includes terms for gestational age (birth weight had been used in some years), gestational age squared, race (African American, Hispanic, white, other), sex, location of birth (inborn or outborn), multiple birth (yes or no), 1-minute Apgar score, size for gestational age (<10th percentile, >10th percentile), major birth defect (yes

---

TABLE 6–5 CLINICAL RISK INDEX FOR BABIES (CRIB)

FACTOR	SCORE
Birth Weight (gm)	
>1350	0
851–1350	1
701–850	4
≤700	7
Gestation (wks)	
>24	0
≤24	1
Congenital Malformations*	
None	0
Not acutely life-threatening	1
Acutely life-threatening	3
Maximum Base Excess in First 12 Hours (mmol/L)	
>−7.0	0
−7.0 to −9.9	1
−10.0 to −14.9	2
≤−15.0	3
Minimum Appropriate FiO_2 in First 12 Hours	
≤0.40	0
0.41–0.60	2
0.61–0.90	3
0.91–1.00	4
Maximum Appropriate FiO_2 in First 12 Hours	
≤0.40	0
0.41–0.80	1
0.81–0.90	3
0.91–1.00	5

*Excludes lethal malformations.

From The International Neonatal Network: The CRIB (Clinical Risk Index for Babies) Score: A tool for assessing initial neonatal risk and comparing performance of neonatal intensive care units. Lancet 342:193, 1993.

or no, added in 1994), and mode of delivery (vaginal or cesarean). The model is calibrated each year. Using this model, the expected number of deaths at each NICU for infants weighing 501 to 1500 gm can be determined based on the characteristics of infants treated at that NICU. The ratio of the observed number of deaths to the expected number of deaths, called the *Standardized Neonatal Mortality Ratio* (SNMR), can then be calculated.

An SNMR value of greater than 1 indicates that an NICU has more deaths than would be expected based on the characteristics of infants treated there, whereas an SNMR value of less than 1 indicates that an NICU has fewer deaths than expected. The SNMRs and their 95% confidence intervals for 290 NICUs participating in the Vermont Oxford Network during 1998 are shown in Figure 6–3. The data points are plotted in order of increasing SNMR. It is apparent that the point estimates of the SNMR vary substantially among the NICUs, with some values being less than 1 and others being greater than 1. The 95% confidence intervals are very wide because of the relatively small number of infants who are treated at each individual NICU in a given year. Thus, the statistical power to detect quality of care outliers using multivariate risk-adjustment methods such as this may be low. Even very accurate predictive models cannot overcome the problem of a small sample at each NICU.[31] Despite this shortcoming, multivariate risk models may be useful for identifying individual infants who died despite having a low predicted probability of death. The medical records of such infants can then be chosen for detailed review and audit. It is important to recognize that although multivariate prediction models that are based on admission variables will perform well for infants with very low birth weights for whom gestational age or birth weight is highly predictive of mortality, physiologic measures of disease severity will be necessary to achieve similar predictive performance for larger, more mature infants.

Further research is required to identify the best models for predicting neonatal risk and to determine whether such models are in fact of value in identifying individual cases or institutions with poor quality of care.[55] However, even without a firm foundation in research, risk-adjusted comparisons of NICUs will become more common. The public release of risk-adjusted comparisons of mortality rates for U.S. hospitals by the Health Care Financing Administration[48] and the publication of hospital-specific and surgeon-specific mortality rates for cardiovascular surgery by the New York State Department of Health[8] are two examples of this phenomenon. An example in the field of perinatology is the Pacific Business Group on Health's publication of risk-adjusted primary cesarean section rates for California hospitals (www.healthscope.org). This analysis is unique in that technical oversight was provided by neonatologists, perinatologists, and researchers who are members of the California Perinatal Quality Care Collaborative. The public release of comparative performance data and the use of such data for contracting and performance-based reimbursement will become increasingly common over the next few years. Neonatologists must understand the strengths and weaknesses of different methods for making risk-adjusted comparisons of neonatal outcomes as they attempt to assist the public in understanding these data and to use the data themselves to monitor, evaluate, and improve the quality of care that they provide.

COSTS AND RESOURCE USE

The next question, *How efficiently do we provide care?*, refers to the costs and resource use for neonatal care. Although a detailed discussion of this topic is beyond the scope of this chapter, it is important for neonatologists to understand that they will be under increasing pressure to justify and reduce the costs of neonatal

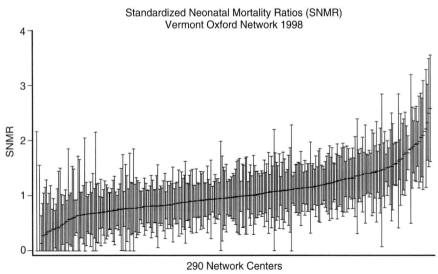

Standardized Neonatal Mortality Ratios (SNMR)
Vermont Oxford Network 1998

290 Network Centers
Vertical bar represents 95% confidence interval

FIGURE 6–3. Standardized neonatal mortality ratios (SNMRs) and 95% confidence intervals for 290 NICUs participating in the Vermont Oxford Network in 1998. The SNMR is the ratio of observed-to-predicted deaths for infants weighing 501 to 1500 gm. Predicted deaths are calculated using a logistic regression equation that includes terms for gestational age, gestational age squared, race (African American, Hispanic, white, other), sex, location of birth (inborn or outborn), multiple birth (yes or no), 1-minute Apgar score, size for gestational age (<10th percentile, >10th percentile), major birth defect (yes or no), and mode of delivery (vaginal or cesarean). (Courtesy of the Vermont Oxford Network, Burlington, Vermont.)

care. Neonatal intensive care is among the most expensive types of hospital care,[54, 72] and it has come under increasing scrutiny by both public and private insurers seeking to contain health care costs. Insurers seek to compare treatment costs across institutions to determine whether costs at a given institution are excessively high.

Meaningful comparisons of neonatal intensive care treatment costs across institutions are difficult to make. Most insurers have access to data from only a small set of hospitals, whose case mix may vary considerably. If case mix adjustments are made at all, they are typically based on the Medicare DRGs. As previously discussed, the Medicare DRGs contain only seven categories for newborn infants and explain only 22% of variation in costs.[50, 58] Thus, the Medicare DRGs do not provide a good method for adjusting for case mix. This fact underscores the need for information systems that use alternative DRG systems to collect more detailed information on clinical aspects of care for infants treated in the NICU.

Comparisons of treatment costs across institutions are not straightforward, even in the absence of case mix differences. Because of the wide variation in pricing policies across hospitals, comparisons of charged amounts may be misleading. To compare treatment costs across institutions, costs must be computed. Data from hospital billing systems or UB-92s are typically used to generate measures of treatment costs. These data contain information on charges for hospital services, which are converted to costs using information on the internal pricing structure of hospital services. Standard methods exist for such conversions.[11, 71, 72] Calculating conversions based on detailed hospital bills can be a daunting task because of the volume of services (tens of thousands) that must be converted. Those based on the Uniform Bill forms are more easily performed because of the aggregation of charges on them. Cost conversion methodologies must allocate both direct and indirect costs to each hospital service. Direct costs, such as the cost of a

prescription medication, are relatively easy to identify. However, decisions about how to allocate indirect costs, which include facility costs and services such as administrative salaries, security services, laundry, housekeeping, and individual services, are more difficult to make. There are many ways these assignments can be made. How indirect costs are allocated has a major effect on the ultimate calculated costs.[4] If costs at different institutions are to be compared, it is crucial that these assignments be made in a uniform manner.[72]

Computerized hospital discharge abstracts can be used to create hospital-specific reports that address perinatal care and its costs.[76] The nonprofit National Perinatal Information Center (Providence, Rhode Island) uses data from UB-92 supplemented with birth weight submitted by over 50 participating hospitals with approximately 180,000 yearly births to create detailed reports that document and compare hospital performance and costs.[75, 76] Figure 6–4 is an example of this type of report, comparing average length of stay (ALOS) and hospital charges for infants in two birth weight categories at a sample hospital (labeled "your hospital"), a subgroup of similar hospitals, and all 37 hospitals in the database. Unadjusted and case mix–adjusted data are provided to participating institutions in tabular and graphic formats.

ALOS is often used as a proxy for cost. In making ALOS comparisons, it is essential that one adjust for differences in case mix. The Vermont Oxford Network has developed multivariate risk models for predicting length of stay that are used in routine reporting to members. As with mortality, there is substantial variation among the Network hospitals even after adjusting for case mix, with adjusted total length of stay for surviving infants 501 to 1500 gm ranging from less than 40 days at some institutions to over 75 days at others.[33]

Documenting comparative outcomes in the context of comparative costs is extremely important to managed care organizations with respect to selecting cost-

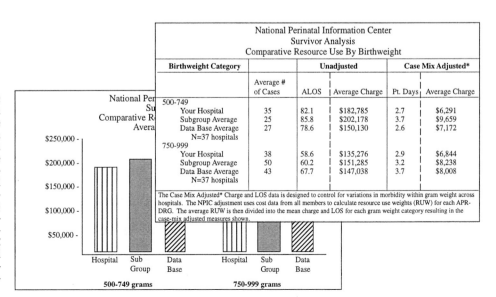

FIGURE 6–4. Tabular and graphic report comparing average length of stay (ALOS) and average charges for survivors in two birth weight categories (500 to 749 gm and 750 to 999 gm) at a sample hospital *(Your Hospital),* a subgroup of similar hospitals, and all 37 hospitals in the National Perinatal Information Center (NPIC) database. This report is an example of the data available to institutions participating in the NPIC database. (Courtesy of Rachel Schwartz, MPH, National Perinatal Information Center, Providence, Rhode Island.)

National Perinatal Information Center
Survivor Analysis
Comparative Resource Use By Birthweight

Birthweight Category	Average # of Cases	ALOS	Average Charge	Pt. Days	Average Charge
		Unadjusted		**Case Mix Adjusted***	
500-749					
Your Hospital	35	82.1	$182,785	2.7	$6,291
Subgroup Average	25	85.8	$202,178	3.7	$9,659
Data Base Average	27	78.6	$150,130	2.6	$7,172
N=37 hospitals					
750-999					
Your Hospital	38	58.6	$135,276	2.9	$6,844
Subgroup Average	50	60.2	$151,285	3.2	$8,238
Data Base Average	43	67.7	$147,038	3.7	$8,008
N=37 hospitals					

The Case Mix Adjusted* Charge and LOS data is designed to control for variations in morbidity within gram weight across hospitals. The NPIC adjustment uses cost data from all members to calculate resource use weights (RUW) for each APR-DRG. The average RUW is then divided into the mean charge and LOS for each gram weight category resulting in the case-mix adjusted measures shown.

effective hospitals and negotiating reimbursement rates. However, as indicated in the preceding discussion, valid comparisons across institutions are difficult to make. The financial modules of generic hospital information systems are intended for application in all clinical areas of a hospital; therefore, these systems will have broad appeal to hospital managers and yet may not have the granularity, clinical precision, or reporting flexibility to meet the needs of the perinatal unit. Neonatologists must become familiar with the management tools in use at their hospitals. They must understand their analytic shortcomings and their interpretation, because decisions regarding resource allocations within hospitals increasingly will be based on these tools.

QUALITY OF CARE

The final question, *How do we evaluate and improve the quality of care that we provide?*, is the most important. To address quality of care requires the ability to specify outcomes. Outcomes may be objective or subjective. Typically, objective outcomes consist of mortality, morbidity, and long-term neurodevelopmental status. The most important morbidities to record are those that could be influenced by the quality of care, for example, nosocomial infection. In some cases, we presume that certain morbidities can be minimized by optimal care, although the specifics of what constitutes optimal care have not been defined. Conversely, it is clear that suboptimal practices can increase morbidity. For example, excessive ventilation can lead to pneumothorax or bronchopulmonary dysplasia; fluid overload may increase the risk for patent ductus arteriosus; and inadequate maintenance of thermal environment and suboptimal nutritional practices may result in prolonged hospitalization as a result of poor weight gain. In addition to the traditional clinical outcomes, subjective outcomes, such as parent satisfaction and quality of life, will become increasingly important measures of the quality of neonatal care.[9, 74, 91]

Specifying and measuring the practices and outcomes of care are only the starting point for improvement. The information must be analyzed, synthesized, and presented so that opportunities for improvement can be identified and the results of improvement efforts can be monitored and evaluated. However, information and performance feedback alone cannot cause the profound changes in care processes and in the behavior of caregivers that are necessary to improve the quality of medical care. These will occur only when all members of the care team have the knowledge, skills, motivation, and organizational support required to make continuous quality improvement an integral and ongoing component of their work.

Multidisciplinary collaborative quality improvement has been applied successfully in a number of health care settings.[60] The management of quality in the field of health care has borrowed heavily from the techniques of quality management science in use in general industry. Berwick has pioneered the application of these techniques to medical care and applied them to a number of clinical problems in the Breakthrough Series of the Institute for Health Care Improvement.[5, 43] O'Connor has shown that multidisciplinary collaborative improvement based on feedback of performance data, quality improvement training, and collaborative learning through site visiting can reduce mortality for cardiovascular surgery.[53] Many health care organizations are now using these general methods to improve the quality of medical practice. The CPQCC and the Vermont Oxford Network provide two examples of how quality improvement is being applied to neonatal care.

The CPQCC, discussed earlier, has established a permanent subcommittee made up of neonatologists, perinatologists, perinatal nurses, state and hospital representatives, and health outcomes researchers with experience in quality improvement and outcomes measurement to review the statewide data and recommend quality improvement objectives, to provide models for performance improvement, and to assist providers in transforming data into information that can help to improve care. This Perinatal Quality Improvement Panel has selected two measures for first-cycle improvement: antenatal steroid administration and chronic lung disease prevention and management. Figure 6–5, derived from a Vermont Oxford Network analysis of CPQCC and all Network hospitals in 1998, demonstrates the variability of practice and potential for improvement in this important area. An extensive CQI tool kit has been developed for antenatal steroids. This tool kit is an all-inclusive package that, when put in the hands of committed physicians and other health care providers, promotes and facilitates improved clinical outcomes, more efficient resource allocation, and superior patient care. It is the first of a comprehensive set of tool kits, each to focus on a key topic related to perinatal care. A second tool kit on chronic lung disease prevention and management is nearing completion. For both measures, performance standards are established during an observation year. Following dissemination of the tool kits, statewide educational activities, and an appropriate period for CQI, performance will be reassessed and the results will be prepared for public release. The program is being structured to improve the performance of all hospitals, and it is CPQCC's goal that all participating hospitals meet the established goals at the conclusion of the initial period of CQI.

The Vermont Oxford Network has been working since the early 1990s to adapt collaborative quality improvement methods and apply them to neonatal intensive care.[32, 33, 35] The Network's initial collaborative improvement project, known as the NIC/Q Project, involved multidisciplinary teams from 10 institutions. Teams consisting of neonatologists, neonatal nurses, administrators, allied professionals, and quality improvement coaches from the institutions worked closely together to set common improvement

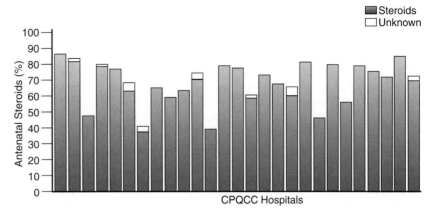

FIGURE 6–5. Proportion of infants weighing 501 to 1500 gm who were born in 1998 and whose mothers received antenatal steroids. Each bar represents 1 of 27 hospitals in the California Perinatal Quality Care Collaborative (CPQCC) for that year. (Courtesy of the CPQCC Executive Committee.)

goals, to identify "potentially better practices" for achieving those goals, and to implement the practices in their own NICUs. The clinical improvement goals included reductions in nosocomial infection and chronic lung disease for infants of very low birth weight; resource-related goals included reductions in length of stay and more appropriate use of blood gas testing and x-ray procedures. The teams received training in quality improvement from a professional quality improvement trainer and held discussions in a series of facilitated large group and small focus group meetings and conference calls. The "potentially better practices" were identified based on review and evaluation of the evidence in the literature, detailed analysis of the processes of care, and site visits to other participating institutions and benchmark units with superior performance outside the project. The Vermont Oxford Network database was used to provide performance feedback to participants and to monitor the results. The preliminary results of the project demonstrated significant reductions in nosocomial infections (six institutions) and chronic lung disease (four institutions) in the subgroups that focused on those goals, both when compared with themselves over time and when compared with a comparison group of 66 nonparticipating units that were members of the Vermont Oxford Network during the same time period.[35] In addition, the costs of care for infants of very low birth weight at the 10 NIC/Q sites decreased over the course of the project. This project demonstrated the potential for a multifaceted intervention of training in evidence-based collaborative quality improvement, feedback of performance data, and site visiting to improve the quality of neonatal intensive care.

As a result of this initial experience, the Vermont Oxford Network has now organized an expanded Evidence-Based Quality Improvement Collaborative for Neonatology, NIC/Q 2000.[33] This collaborative, composed of multidisciplinary teams from 34 member institutions, applies four key improvement habits to a broad range of clinical, operational, and organizational improvement goals.[33, 60] As in the original NIC/Q Project, participants receive training in quality improvement; work together closely in facilitated large group meetings, focus groups, and conference

calls; and use data from the Vermont Oxford Network database for feedback to monitor performance.

The four key habits are shown in Figure 6–6. The first is the *Habit for Change*. Change is extremely difficult both for individuals and for organizations, yet without change, there cannot be improvement. Participants in NIC/Q 2000 are taught to use a simple model for change, developed by Langley, Nolan, and colleagues.[45] The model is based on three questions: What are we trying to improve? (measurable improvement goal); How will we know that a change is an improvement? (measurement); and What changes can we make that will lead to improvement? (better practices). Multidisciplinary NICU teams answer these questions and test their proposed changes in a series of Plan-Do-Study-Act (PDSA) cycles within their institution. The focus is on rapid trial and learning cycles with measurable improvement goals. Improvements are applied to a broad range of clinical, operational, and organizational domains of performance. The second key habit is the *Habit for Evidence-Based Practice*. Participants learn to evaluate the strength and quality of the evidence for different practices and to apply the principles of evidence-

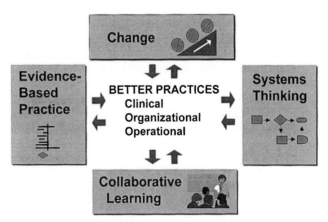

FIGURE 6–6. The four key habits for clinical improvement are applied by participants in the Vermont Oxford Network NIC/Q Evidence-Based Quality Improvement Collaborative for Neonatology to identify and implement better clinical, operational, and organizational practices for the care of newborn infants and their families. (Courtesy of the Vermont Oxford Network, Burlington, Vermont.)

based medicine in their daily practice.[73, 82] The third key habit is the *Habit for Collaborative Learning*. This process involves collaboration among the disciplines and specialties within an institution and among multidisciplinary teams from different institutions. One example of this habit is the Vermont Oxford Network Collaborative Learning Directory, a compendium of self-reported areas of excellence contributed by Network members.[88] The directory can be used by members to identify and contact institutions that have achieved excellence in some area of neonatal care. The fourth key habit is the *Habit for Systems Thinking*. This habit involves systems thinking and the understanding that neonatal intensive care involves complex processes involving many people and organizational subsystems. NICUs are complex adaptive systems. By analyzing these systems and the processes of care, it is possible to redesign them to be more effective and efficient. Furthermore, monitoring the implementation of and adherence to evidence-based processes of care within an institution provides a powerful method for quality improvement that in many instances is quicker, more practical, and more efficient than monitoring outcomes alone.

The participants in NIC/Q 2000 contribute the results of their learning to a growing archive of improvement knowledge maintained by the Vermont Oxford Network. This archive is currently being organized into an Internet site (NICQ.org) that will provide the neonatal community with unique resources and tools for collaborative evidence-based quality improvement.

CONCLUSION

The recognition that there is widespread variation among physicians and hospitals in clinical practice and patient outcomes and the growing pressure to increase the cost-effectiveness of medical care have resulted in unprecedented interest in assessing, evaluating, and improving medical practice. If health professionals are to function successfully in this environment, they must understand both how to evaluate their own performance and how their performance will be evaluated by others. These evaluations require accurate and reliable information. Most importantly, neonatologists and other health care professionals will have to learn how to use the information to improve the quality of the medical care that they provide. In this section of the chapter we reviewed some of the available data sources and discussed a number of issues related to their use for improvement. Although neonatologists should not be expected to become experts in databases and evaluation methods, they do need to develop a basic understanding that will allow them to work effectively with other professionals in the changing health care environment. In this "era of assessment and accountability," we must all develop the knowledge, skills, and motivation necessary to assume leadership roles in multidisciplinary collaborative quality improvement

within our institutions, in larger health care organizations, and across regions. Only then can the potential benefits of modern databases and information systems be translated into better medical care for newborn infants and their families.

ACKNOWLEDGMENTS

We thank Mr. John Muldoon from the National Association of Children's Hospitals and Related Institutions, Inc; Jeannette Rogowski, PhD, from RAND; Rachel Schwartz, MPH, from the National Perinatal Information Center; Linda L. Wright, MD, from the National Institute of Child Health and Human Development Neonatal Research Network; and Terri A. Slagle, MD, from California Pacific Medical Center and Site of Care Systems for providing material used in this chapter.

part two
PRACTICING EVIDENCE-BASED NEONATAL-PERINATAL MEDICINE

John C. Sinclair

This section of the chapter focuses on five key processes in practicing evidence-based neonatal-perinatal medicine: (1) asking a focused clinical question; (2) searching MEDLINE, the Cochrane Library, and other sources for high-quality evidence (both primary reports and systematic reviews); (3) critically appraising the retrieved evidence for its validity; (4) extracting the data; and (5) applying the results to patient care. The role of the Cochrane Collaboration in the preparation, dissemination, and timely updating of systematic reviews of evidence from randomized clinical trials is highlighted. Strategies for promoting evidence-based clinical practice are presented.

Evidence-based medicine has been described as "the conscientious, explicit, and judicious use of current best evidence in making decisions about the care of individual patients."[118] The practice of evidence-based medicine requires efficient access to the best available evidence that is applicable to the clinical problem.

It is essential, however, to make two disclaimers. First, not every clinical decision can be based on strong evidence, because such evidence may not exist. Regarding a general internal medicine inpatient service in England, Ellis and coworkers estimated that principal treatments prescribed for patients' primary diagnoses were based on strong evidence from randomized controlled trials (RCTs) in about 50% of cases; treatment was based on convincing non-RCT evidence in about 30% of cases; and there was no substantial evidence available in about 20% of cases. In a similar study in the neonatal intensive care unit (NICU) at McMaster University Medical Centre, there was strong evidence from RCTs to support the choice of the prescribed treatment in a similar proportion of cases.[98] Second, evidence provides a necessary but not sufficient ground for clinical decisions. Clinical expertise is no less important under the evidence-based approach; indeed, an accurate history, physical examination, and clinical diagnosis are critical to a properly directed search for evidence that is directly applicable to the patient's problem. In addition, it is essential to consider the values and preferences of parents with respect to the probable clinical outcomes of the treatments being considered for their baby.

With this background, we now consider, in turn, the five elements in making an evidence-based clinical decision.

ASKING A FOCUSED CLINICAL QUESTION

A focused clinical question should contain the following elements:

- in whom (the patients of interest)
- the treatment or exposure of interest
- the nature of any comparisons to be made
- the primary outcome of interest and other important outcomes

The exact form of a focused clinical question depends on whether the question concerns treatment or prevention, etiology, diagnosis, or prognosis.[119] For questions concerning treatment or prevention, a focused question has the following form:

In . . . (patient, problem, or risk factor)
. . . does . . . (treatment A)
. . . compared with . . . (control, or treatment B)
. . . reduce . . . (adverse outcome[s])

For example: In women carrying babies of 24 to 34 weeks' gestation who are threatening to deliver, does corticosteroid (dexamethasone or betamethasone) compared with no treatment reduce the incidence of respiratory distress syndrome (RDS) in their babies? Another example: In babies of 24 to 30 weeks' gestational age, does prophylactic surfactant, given immediately at birth in the delivery room, compared with selective use of surfactant in those who develop moderate or severe RDS reduce neonatal death or chronic lung disease?

Armed with a focused clinical question based on an accurate delineation of the clinical problem, the treatment alternatives being considered, and the important clinical outcomes, you can now target your search for valid evidence that is applicable to the problem.

FINDING EVIDENCE

SOURCES OF EVIDENCE

Clinical evidence that is relevant to problems in neonatal-perinatal medicine is appearing at an accelerating rate and can be found in a vast number of journals, books, conference proceedings, and other sources. Many published reports provide only weak evidence, because strong research designs were not used. Evidence is constantly changing as new evidence becomes available. The challenge for the busy clinician, then, is to be able to detect evidence that is valid, up-to-date, and applicable to the clinical problem using strategies that are comprehensive and yet efficient. These strategies may be directed to retrieving both primary reports and reviews. Because most reviews do not use explicit review methods, there is a special need for the efficient retrieval of *systematic* reviews (discussed later). Although textbooks can provide valid evidence that is based on systematic methods of review,[100, 122] most textbooks do not require their contributors to use explicit and systematic methods when reviewing evidence and making treatment recommendations. Moreover, there tends to be a long time gap between the appearance of new evidence and its impact on therapeutic recommendations found in textbooks.[96] Thus, in neonatal-perinatal medicine and other fields in which new evidence is rapidly accumulating, it is especially important to be able to access systematic reviews that are continuously updated.

EFFICIENT STRATEGIES FOR SEARCHING FOR EVIDENCE

Primary Reports

Primary reports that are relevant to neonatal-perinatal medicine are published in a large number of journals. Most of these journals are indexed in MEDLINE, but additional reports may appear in journals indexed in other computerized databases, including CINAHL, EMBASE, and HealthSTAR. If you have access to the Internet, you can now search MEDLINE for clinical evidence using either PubMed or Internet Grateful Med. PubMed can be accessed at http://www.ncbi. nlm.nih.gov/pubmed/; Internet Grateful Med can be accessed at http://igm.nlm.nih.gov/ (this site also provides access to databases other than MEDLINE).

To define the topic of your search, use Medical Subject Headings (MeSH terms), text words, or a combination, combining them appropriately in a Boolean search with "AND" or "OR" (your medical librarian can quickly teach you the logic of this).

Often, you will find that a MEDLINE search based only on topic descriptors yields a long list of reports that you do not have time to scan or, certainly, to read. The busy clinician needs to prune this potentially cumbersome list by incorporating into the search a strategy for limiting the retrieval to reports that are likely to be of high methodological quality and, therefore, more likely to provide valid evidence. Such a

TABLE 6–6 SEARCHING MEDLINE FOR SOUND CLINICAL STUDIES USING METHODOLOGICAL FILTERS

TYPE OF QUESTION	CRITERION STANDARD FOR METHODOLOGIC QUALITY
Treatment/ prevention	Random or quasi-random allocation of participants to treatment and control groups
Etiology	Formal control group using random or quasi-random allocation; nonrandomized concurrent controls; cohort analytic study with matching or statistical adjustment; or case control study
Diagnosis	Provision of sufficient data to calculate the sensitivity and specificity of the test, or likelihood ratios
Prognosis	A cohort of subjects who, at baseline, have the disease of interest but not the outcome of interest

Table derived from Haynes RB, et al: Developing optimal search strategies for detecting clinically sound studies in MEDLINE. J Amer Med Inform Assoc 1:447, 1994.

strategy is provided by using methodological "filters" that have been validated against "hand-searching"[107] to detect articles that, depending on the type of focused question posed, have the attributes shown in Table 6–6. These methodological filters are used together with your topic descriptors (through the use of "AND"), so that only articles that both are on topic in clinical terms and that satisfy the methodological criteria are retrieved. Furthermore, by choosing different methodological filters, you can maximize either the sensitivity (for comprehensiveness) or specificity (for fewest methodological false-positive results) of your search. To do this, use PubMed's Clinical Queries using Research Methodology Filters page (www.ncbi.nlm.nih.gov/pubmed/clinical.html). There you will be asked to click on the category type of the question you are asking (therapy, diagnosis, etiology, or prognosis) and on whether you want the methodological filters to emphasize sensitivity or specificity. If, for example, you are reviewing a topic and want to be comprehensive in your retrieval of sound clinical studies, you would click on "sensitivity." If you have limited time and want urgent access to perhaps only one or two reports that are likely to be methodologically sound, you would click on "specificity."

Reviews

Systematic reviews[99, 123] are distinguished from other types of reviews by the rigor of the review methods. The objectives and methods are explicitly spelled out a priori, and they are documented in the review. A review without a "Methods" section is unlikely to be a systematic review.

Systematic reviews of the results of randomized controlled trials attempt to identify all trials that have tested a defined therapy against an alternative in a defined population. If the populations and the contrasting interventions are similar, the results may be summarized quantitatively by calculating a typical effect based on the results of all eligible trials. This latter step, called a meta-analysis, increases the precision of the estimates of treatment effect. A meta-analysis, however, is not a necessary part of a systematic review; indeed, if there is clinical or statistical heterogeneity across trials, it may be inappropriate to calculate a typical effect. Systematic reviews can be detected in MEDLINE by searching with the appropriate topic descriptors and using the word "AND" to join them to the terms shown in Table 6–7.

For example: You wish to find a systematic review, with meta-analysis, of studies of women with threatened preterm delivery that assess the effect of antenatal corticosteroids on the incidence of respiratory distress syndrome in their babies. Using PubMed, enter your search terms: corticosteroid AND respiratory distress syndrome. Limit your search by publication type to meta-analysis. Alternatively, you could add to your topic descriptors one or more of the methodological text words shown in Table 6–7: corticosteroid AND respiratory distress syndrome AND (systematic review OR meta-anal*).

COCHRANE SYSTEMATIC REVIEWS. The Cochrane Collaboration is an international organization that prepares, maintains, and disseminates up-to-date systematic reviews of health care interventions. The reviews are prepared by members of collaborative review groups, including the Pregnancy and Childbirth Review Group and the Neonatal Review Group. The reviews are published electronically in The Cochrane Library,[108] which is published every 3 months and allows the reviews to be updated continuously as new evidence appears. The reviews prepared by the Neonatal Review Group can also be found at a website maintained by the National Institute of Child Health and Human Development (http://www.nichd.nih.gov/cochraneneonatal/).

TABLE 6–7 USEFUL TERMS FOR SEARCHING MEDLINE FOR SYSTEMATIC REVIEWS

MeSH	PUBLICATION TYPE	TEXT WORDS
Meta-analysis	Meta-analysis	meta-anal* metaanal* quantitative* review* or quantitative* overview* systematic* review* or systematic* overview* medline

*Asterisk placed at end of term directs search for all variations of a truncated term.

TABLE 6–8 READERS' GUIDES FOR APPRAISING THE VALIDITY OF CLINICAL STUDIES

THERAPY

Was the assignment of patients to treatments randomized?
Were all patients who entered the trial accounted for and attributed at its conclusion?
Were outcomes assessed "blindly," without knowledge of treatment group?
When possible, were patients and caretakers blind to treatment?

ETIOLOGY

Were there clearly defined comparison groups, similar with respect to important determinants of outcome, other than the one of interest?
Were the outcomes and exposures measured in the same way in the groups being compared?
Was follow-up sufficiently long and complete?
Is the temporal relationship correct?

DIAGNOSIS

Was there an independent, blind comparison with a criterion standard?
Did the patient sample include the kinds of patients to whom the diagnostic test will be applied in practice?
Were the test results prevented from influencing the decision to perform the criterion standard (workup bias avoided)?
Can the test be replicated on the basis of the method reported?

PROGNOSIS

Was there a representative, well-defined sample of patients at a uniform point in the course of the disease (inception cohort)?
Was follow-up sufficiently long and complete?
Were objective and unbiased outcome criteria used?
Was there adjustment for important prognostic factors?

Criteria from references 105, 109, 111, and 112.

CRITICALLY APPRAISING EVIDENCE FOR ITS VALIDITY

The fundamental goal of clinical research is to obtain an unbiased answer to the question posed. Bias leads to an answer that is systematically different from the truth.

Guides to assessing the validity of clinical research in the realms of therapy, etiology, diagnosis, prognosis, and reviews are available.[105, 112, 109, 111, 116] A simple distillation of the major methodological issues to be considered is provided in Table 6–8. More comprehensive guides, with specific applicability to therapeutic studies in neonatal-perinatal medicine, have been published.[125, 117]

Most studies on treatment or prevention use designs that can be classified into one of four categories, listed in order of increasing methodological rigor:

1. case series without controls
2. nonrandomized studies using historical controls
3. nonrandomized studies using concurrent controls
4. randomized controlled trials

The randomized trial is the strongest design for evaluating the effect of treatment. It offers maximum protection against selection bias that can invalidate comparisons between groups of patients. The allocation process should be truly random (not quasi-random, e.g., alternate) and blinded so that it is impervious to tampering or code breaking. In addition, follow-up should be complete, with all randomized patients being accounted for in the primary analysis, and outcome measurements should made by observers who are blinded to the treatment allocation. When feasible, blinding of the caretakers, the patient, and the patient's family to the treatment allocation should be accomplished. When reading reports of therapeutic studies, you should scan the "Methods" section to assess validity using these criteria.

EXTRACTING THE DATA AND EXPRESSING THE EFFECT OF TREATMENT

Table 6–9 displays the structure of a typical study that assesses the effectiveness of a treatment. There are two exposure groups (labeled as *treated* or *control*) and two possible outcome categories (labeled as *event* or *no event*). An event is a categorical adverse outcome such as occurrence of disease, adverse neurodevelopmental outcome, treatment side effect, or death. The effect of treatment is given by comparing the event rate in the treated and control groups, which can be accomplished using either relative or absolute treatment effect estimators. The relative risk (RR), $a/(a + b) \div c/(c + d)$, indicates the relative, but not absolute, size of reduction in the event rate. The complement of the relative risk (1-RR) is the relative risk reduction (RRR). Thus, a relative risk of 0.75 represents a 25% RRR. The risk difference (RD), $a/(a + b) - c/(c + d)$, indicates the absolute magnitude of reduction in risk. For example, a risk difference of -0.05 represents an absolute 5 percentage point reduction of the event rate in the treated group. The

TABLE 6–9 STRUCTURE OF A STUDY TO ASSESS THE EFFECT OF A TREATMENT AND MEASURES OF TREATMENT EFFECT

	OUTCOME	
	Event	**No Event**
EXPOSURE		
Treated	a	b
Control	c	d
TREATMENT EFFECT MEASURES		
Relative Risk (RR)	$a/(a+b) \div c/(c+d)$	
Relative Risk Reduction (RRR)	1-RR	
Odds Ratio	ad/bc	
Risk Difference (RD)	$a/(a+b) - c/(c+d)$	
Number Needed to Treat (NNT)	1/RD	

reciprocal of the risk difference (1/RD) indicates the number of patients who must be treated to expect to prevent the event in one patient. In the example, 20 patients (1/0.05) need to be treated to prevent the event in 1. The number needed to treat (NNT) is particularly relevant when deciding whether to use a treatment that is effective but causes important clinical side effects or results in an important increase in economic costs. Discussed later, the patient's expected event rate in the absence of treatment may be a critical determinant of this decision.

When outcome data are reported on a continuous scale (e.g., blood pressure measured in mm of mercury), a different measure of effect, the mean difference, is computed.

APPLYING THE RESULTS TO PATIENT CARE

The results of randomized trials of therapy indicate the likely effects of the therapy, beneficial and adverse, on important clinical outcomes. However, these effects are average effects in the patients who are entered in the trials, and they may or may not accurately predict the net benefit to be expected in specific subgroups or in individual patients.[102, 104] This problem becomes especially important when a treatment has been shown to produce both benefits and harm. Often, those patients at high risk of the primary outcome are more likely than those at low risk to be the ones that actually benefit from an effective therapy. However, both patients at high risk and those at low risk who receive a treatment are exposed to the adverse side effects of that treatment; thus, the balance between likely benefits and harm will shift. This problem is compounded because individual patients may value differently the relative importance of benefits and harm caused by treatment.

In deciding whether to use an effective therapy in the individual patient, particularly when that therapy results in important clinical side effects, one must consider the relative likelihood that the therapy will actually prevent the adverse target event, or cause adverse aside effects, in that individual patient. One way of approaching this is to determine whether the report of the relevant trial, or systematic review of trials, described the size of risk reduction for the primary outcome, and risk increases for any side effects caused, according to patient subgroups defined by patient characteristics at entry. If so, it may be possible to derive a relative likelihood of being helped or harmed from the subgroup most similar to your patient. More often, however, either RRR across subgroups is not clearly different or you cannot judge this because data by subgroups are not presented. Assuming that RRR is indeed constant across the range of baseline risk, you can calculate a patient-specific absolute risk reduction (ARR) using the formula ARR = RRR × PEER, where PEER is your patient's expected event rate in the absence of treatment. In neonatal-perinatal medicine, such information may often be available from estimates of risk

based on gestational age, birth weight, and postnatal age. Using this approach, ARR (and its inverse, NNT) commonly will be shown to vary with PEER: In patients at high risk, ARR will be high and NNT will be low, whereas in patients at low risk, the reverse will occur.[106]

An example of this form of analysis is shown in Figure 6–7. A systematic review of randomized trials of antenatal corticosteroid for the prevention of RDS in mothers who threaten to deliver prematurely showed that this therapy was effective in reducing the incidence of RDS, with an RRR of 41%.[101] RRR was fairly constant across subgroups based on gestational age. Because the expected risk for RDS is high at short gestation but decreases markedly with increasing gestation, NNT to prevent one case of RDS is low when gestation is less than 30 weeks, but it rises sharply after 34 weeks. Although the trials did not demonstrate short-term toxic effects, few of them undertook the assessment of long-term effects. Given the uncertain balance at gestation periods beyond 34 weeks between the small likelihood of short-term benefits at that gestational age and the undocumented but not well-studied possibility of long-term risks, the National Institutes of Health (NIH) Consensus Conference on prenatal corticosteroids recommended that women carrying babies of 34 weeks' gestation or

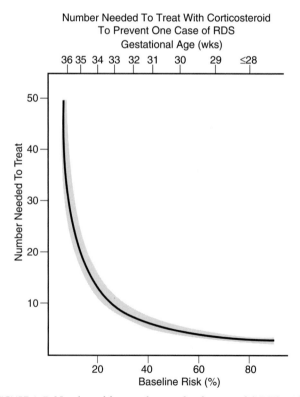

FIGURE 6–7. Number of fetuses that need to be treated (NNT) with antenatal corticosteroid to prevent one case of respiratory distress syndrome (RDS), as a function of baseline risk. The NNT is derived from the typical relative risk reduction (RRR) of 41% calculated from the data of the trials included in the systematic review of Crowley.[101] The shaded zone indicates the 95% confidence interval. As the gestational age increases, baseline risk for RDS decreases, and NNT increases.

less who threaten to deliver prematurely be considered as candidates for steroid treatment.[115] (See Chapter 42.)

PROMOTING EVIDENCE-BASED CLINICAL PRACTICE

The evidence-based practice paradigm places responsibility on the physician to develop and maintain the skills needed to efficiently find relevant evidence, critically appraise it for its validity, and apply it to the clinical problem. The development of these skills should begin in undergraduate education, and there is evidence that teaching critical appraisal skills can be incorporated successfully into clinical clerkships.[97] A useful tool for both acquiring critical appraisal skills during residency and enabling evidence-based care is the critically appraised topic,[121] which comprises asking a focused question about a patient, finding and appraising relevant articles quickly, and synthesizing the evidence into a one- or two-page summary.

Attainment of the required skills by individual practitioners, however, poses a challenge. A survey of English general practitioners[114] revealed that although they were favorably disposed to the concept of evidence-based clinical practice, they believed they lacked the necessary knowledge and skills to carry it forward. For example, only 16% had formal training in searching for evidence, and only about 33% believed they had sufficient understanding of key terms, such as *relative risk* and *number needed to treat*, that they could explain them to others. Most believed that the best way to promote evidence-based practice was the introduction of evidence-based practice guidelines or protocols.

The preparation and dissemination of practice guidelines or consensus recommendations, however, does not ensure their use in practice. Several strategies aimed at promoting change of behavior among clinicians have been tested, and some have been found to be successful. Two of these strategies—introducing guidelines through opinion leaders and providing audit and feedback—were included in an intervention package designed to encourage the use of antenatal corticosteroids in eligible women, in accordance with the NIH Consensus recommendations.[115] In a randomized trial in which this package was compared with a control intervention consisting of usual dissemination of the recommendations, the evidence-based use of antenatal corticosteroids was found to be increased in the experimental group.[113] Thus, randomized trials are being used not just to test the effectiveness of new therapies but also to evaluate competing strategies for promoting the use of evidence in clinical practice.

There is also a need for the further development of practical methods for measuring the importance or value that patients attach to clinical outcomes.[124] In neonatal-perinatal decision making, these values are usually sought from the parents, by using informal and unsystematic approaches. More formal and systematic methods for measuring preferences,[110] including rating scales and the standard gamble, were used by teenage survivors of extremely low birth weight and their parents in a study of the quality of life of the adolescents.[120] Such methods for rating health outcomes may be used increasingly in the future to assess the importance that parents attach to the probable outcomes of neonatal-perinatal treatment alternatives and, thus, to help guide evidence-based decision making.

■ REFERENCES

Part One: Databases for the Evaluation of Neonatal and Perinatal Care

1. Annual Summary of Births, Deaths, Marriages and Divorces, United States, 1993. Monthly Vital Statistics Report. Washington, DC, National Center for Human Statistics, Oct 11, 1994.
2. Applegate M: personal communication, January 28, 2000.
3. Austin CJ: Information systems for health services administration, 4th ed. Ann Arbor, Mich, AUPHA Press/Health Administration Press, 1992.
4. Berman JH, et al: The Financial Management of Hospitals, 8th ed. Chicago, Health Administration Press, 1994.
5. Berwick DM, et al: Curing Health Care: New Strategies for Quality Improvement. San Francisco, Jossey-Bass, 1990.
6. Blumenstein BA: Verifying keyed medical research data. Stat Med 12:1535, 1993.
7. Buescher, et al: The quality of the new birth certificate data: A validation study in North Carolina. Am J Pub Health 83:1163, 1993.
8. Cardiac Surgery in New York State. Albany, NY, New York State Department of Health, Dec 1993.
9. Conner J, Nelson E: Neonatal intensive care satisfaction measured from a parent's perspective. In Horbar JD, Gould JB (eds): Evidence-Based Quality Improvement in Neonatal and Perinatal Medicine [Pediatrics electronic pages, Suppl]. Pediatrics 103:336, 1999.
10. Corn RF: Quality control of hospital discharge data. Med Care 18:416, 1980.
11. Cotterill P, et al: Comparison of alternative relative weights for diagnosis-related groups. Health Care Financing Review 7:37, 1986.
12. Cullen DJ, et al: Therapeutic intervention scoring system: A method for quantitative comparison of patient care. Crit Care Med 2:57, 1974.
13. Danielsen B, et al: Newborn discharge timing and readmissions: California, 1992–1995. Pediatrics 106:31, 2000.
14. Demographic Yearbook, 1992. New York, United Nations, 1994.
15. Donoghue D: Australia and New Zealand Neonatal Network 1996–1997. Sydney, Australian Institute of Health and Welfare National Perinatal Statistics Unit, 1999, Neonatal Network Series, no 3 (AIHW catalogue no PER 11).
16. Dooley SL, et al: Quality assessment of perinatal regionalization by multivariate analysis: Illinois 1991–1993. Obstet Gynecol 89:193, 1998.
17. Escobar GJ, et al: Rapid retrieval of neonatal outcomes data: The Kaiser Permanente neonatal minimum data set. Qual Manag Health Care 5:19, 1997.
18. Escobar GJ: The neonatal "sepsis work-up": Personal reflections on the development of an evidence-based approach toward newborn infections in a managed care organization. In Horbar JD, Gould JB (eds): Evidence-Based Quality Improvement in Neonatal and Perinatal Medicine [Pediatrics electronic pages, Suppl]. Pediatrics 103:360, 1999.
19. Fanaroff AA, et al: Very-low-birth-weight outcomes of the National Institute of Child Health and Human Development Neonatal Research Network. May 1991 through December 1992. Am J Obstet Gynecol 173:1423, 1995.

20. Gardner E: UB-82 forms offer wealth of information, misinformation. Modern Healthcare 20:18, 1990.

21. Gilbert WM, et al: Childbearing beyond 40: Pregnancy outcomes in 24,032 cases. Obstet Gynecol 93:9, 1999.

22. Gould JB: Vital records for quality improvement. In Horbar JD, Gould JB (eds): Evidence-Based Quality Improvement in Neonatal and Perinatal Medicine [Pediatrics electronic pages, Suppl]. Pediatrics 103:278, 1999.

23. Gould JB, et al: Very low birth weight births at non-NICU hospitals: The role of sociodemographic, perinatal, and geographic factors. J Perinatol 19:197, 1999.

24. Gray JE, et al: Neonatal therapeutic intervention scoring system: A method for quantitative comparison of patient care, Crit Care Med 2:57, 1974.

25. Hack MB, et al: Very low birth weight outcomes of the National Institute of Child Health and Human Development Neonatal Network, Pediatrics 87:587, 1991.

26. Hack M, et al: Very-low-birth-weight outcomes of the National Institute of Child Health and Human Development Neonatal Network. November 1989 to October 1990. Am J Obstet Gynecol 172:457, 1995.

27. Hadorn DC, et al: Assessing the Performance of Mortality Prediction Models. Santa Monica, Calif, RAND, 1993.

28. Hein HA, et al: Neonatal mortality review: A basis for improving care. Pediatrics 68:504, 1981.

29. Herrchen B, et al: Vital statistics linked birth/infant death and hospital discharge record linkage for epidemiological studies. Comput Biomed Res 30:290, 1997.

30. Hexter, et al: Evaluation of the hospital discharge diagnoses index and the birth certificate as sources of information on birth defects, Public Health Rep 105:296, 1990.

31. Horbar JD: Birthweight-adjusted mortality rates for assessing the effectiveness of neonatal intensive care. Med Decis Making 12:259, 1992.

32. Horbar JD: The Vermont Oxford Neonatal Network: integrating research and clinical practice to improve the quality of medical care, Semin Perinatol 19:124, 1995.

33. Horbar JD: The Vermont Oxford Network: Evidence-based quality improvement for neonatology. In Horbar JD, Gould JB (eds): Evidence-Based Quality Improvement in Neonatal and Perinatal Medicine [Pediatrics electronic pages, Suppl]. Pediatrics 103:350, 1999.

34. Horbar JD, Leahy KA: An assessment of data quality in the Vermont-Oxford Trials Network Database, Control Clin Trials 16:51, 1995.

35. Horbar JD, et al: Collaborative quality improvement for neonatal intensive care [abstract]. Pediatr Res 43: 177A, 1998.

36. Hudome, et al: Contribution of genetic disorders to neonatal mortality in a regional intensive care setting. Am J Perinatol 11:100, 1994.

37. ICD-9-CM: International classification of diseases: Clinical modification, 4th ed. Los Angeles, Practice Management Information Corporation, 1995.

38. Iezzoni LI: Data sources and implications: Administrative databases. In Iezzoni LI (ed): Risk Adjustment for Measuring Health Care Outcomes. Ann Arbor, Mich, Health Administration Press, 1994, p. 119.

39. Impact of Multiple Births on Low Birthweight—Massachusetts, 1989. MMWR Morb Mortal Wkly Rep 48:289, 1999.

40. Institute of Medicine: Reliability of Hospital Discharge Abstracts. Washington, DC, National Academy of Sciences, 1977.

41. International Neonatal Network: The CRIB (clinical risk index for babies) score: A tool for assessing initial neonatal risk and comparing performance of neonatal intensive care units. Lancet 342:193, 1993.

42. Investigators of the Vermont Oxford Trials Network Database Project: The Vermont Oxford Trials Network: Very low birth weight outcomes for 1990. Pediatrics 91:540, 1993.

43. Kilo CM: Improving care through collaboration. In Horbar JD, Gould JB (eds): Evidence-Based Quality Improvement in Neonatal and Perinatal Medicine [Pediatrics electronic pages, Suppl]. Pediatrics 103:384, 1999.

44. Lagnado L: Hospitals profit by "upcoding" illness. Wall Street Journal, Apr 27, 1997:B1.

45. Langley GJ, et al: The Improvement Guide: A Practical Approach to Enhancing Organizational Performance. San Francisco, Jossey-Bass. 1996.

46. Lichtig LK, et al: Revising diagnosis-related groups for neonates. Pediatrics 84:49, 1989.

47. MacDorman MF, Atkinson JO: Infant Mortality Statistics from the 1997 Period Linked Birth/Infant Death Data Set. Natl Vital Stat Rep 47:1, 1999.

48. Medicare Hospital Information 1988, 1989, 1990, vol 55, Technical Supplement. Washington, DC, U.S. Government Printing Office, 1992.

49. Muldoon, JH: personal communication, April 1995.

50. Muldoon JH: Structure and performance of different DRG classification systems for neonatal medicine. In Horbar JD, Gould JB (eds): Evidence-Based Quality Improvement in Neonatal and Perinatal Medicine [Pediatrics electronic pages, Suppl]. Pediatrics 103:302, 1999.

51. Neonatal Information System II: Medical Data Systems [promotional brochure]. Wayne, Pa.

52. Nesbitt TS, et al: Shoulder dystocia and associated risk factors with macrosomic births in California. Am J Obstet Gynecol 172:476, 1998.

53. O'Connor GT, et al: A regional intervention to improve the hospital mortality associated with coronary artery bypass grafting. JAMA 275:841, 1996.

54. Office of Technology Assessment: Neonatal intensive care for low birthweight infants: Costs and effectiveness. Washington, DC, Congress of the United States, Dec 1987, Health Technology Case Study 38.

55. Park RE, et al: Explaining variations in hospital death rates. JAMA 264:484, 1990.

56. Parrish KM, et al: Variations in the accuracy of obstetric procedures and diagnoses on birth records in Washington State, 1989. Am J Epidemiol 138:119, 1993.

57. Payne SMC, et al: An evaluation of pediatric-modified diagnosis-related groups. Health Care Financing Review 15:51, 1993.

58. Phibbs CS, et al: Alternative to diagnosis related groups for newborn intensive care. Pediatrics 78:829, 1986.

59. Piper JM, et al: Validation of 1989 Tennessee birth certificates using maternal and newborn hospital records. Am J Epidemiol 137:758, 1993.

60. Plsek P: Quality improvement methods in clinical medicine. In Horbar JD, Gould JB (eds): Evidence-Based Quality Improvement in Neonatal and Perinatal Medicine [Pediatrics electronic pages, Suppl]. Pediatrics 103:203, 1999.

61. Poland RL, et al: Analysis of the effect of applying federal diagnosis-related grouping (DRG) guidelines to a population of high-risk newborn infants. Pediatrics 76:104, 1985.

62. Pollack MM, et al: Accurate prediction of the outcome of pediatric intensive care: A new quantitative method, N Engl J Med 316:134, 1987.

63. Relman AS: Assessment and accountability: The third revolution in medical care [editorial]. N Engl J Med 319:1220, 1988.

64. Report of the Canadian NICU Network 1996 to 1997. Vancouver, BC, Canadian NICU Network, 1999.

65. Richardson DK, Escobar GJ: Simplified and revalidated score for neonatal acute physiology (SNAP II) maintains excellent predictive performance [abstract]. Pediatr Res 43:227A, 1998.

66. Richardson DK, et al: Birthweight and illness severity: Independent predictors of neonatal mortality. Pediatrics 91:969, 1993.

67. Richardson DK, et al: Score for acute neonatal physiology: A physiologic severity index for neonatal intensive care. Pediatrics 91:617, 1993.

68. Richardson DK, et al: Score for neonatal acute physiology (SNAP): Validation of a new physiology-based severity of illness index. Pediatrics 91:617, 1993.

69. Richardson DK, et al: Measuring illnesses severity in newborn intensive care, Journal of Intensive Care Medicine 9:20, 1994.

70. Richardson D, et al: Risk adjustment for quality improvement. In Horbar JD, Gould JB (eds): Evidence-Based Quality Improvement in Neonatal and Perinatal Medicine [Pediatrics electronic pages, Suppl]. Pediatrics 103:255, 1999.

71. Rogowski J, et al: Comparison of alternative weight recalibration methods for diagnosis-related groups, Health Care Financing Review 12:87, 1990.

72. Rogowski JA: Measuring the cost of neonatal and perinatal care. In Horbar JD, Gould JB (eds): Evidence-Based Quality Improvement in Neonatal and Perinatal Medicine [Pediatrics electronic pages, Suppl]. Pediatrics 103:329, 1999.

73. Sackett DL, et al: Evidence-Based Medicine. How to Practice and Teach EBM. London, Churchill Livingstone, 1997.

74. Saigal S, et al: Comparison of the health-related quality of life of extremely low birth weight children and a reference group of children at eight years, J Pediatr 125:418, 1994.

75. Schwartz, R: personal communication, April 1995.

76. Schwartz RM, et al: Administrative data for quality improvement. In Horbar JD, Gould JB (eds): Evidence-Based Quality Improvement in Neonatal and Perinatal Medicine [Pediatrics electronic pages, Suppl]. Pediatrics 103:291, 1999.

77. Shapiro S, et al: Relevance of correlates of infant deaths for significant morbidity at 1 year of age. Am J Obstet Gynecol 136:363, 1980.

78. Slagle TA, Le HA: Database information: Fact or fiction [abstract]. Pediatr Res 29:266A, 1991.

79. Slagle TA, et al: Database use in neonatal intensive care units. Pediatrics 90:959, 1992.

80. Slagle TA: Perinatal information systems for quality improvement: Visions for today. In Horbar JD, Gould JB (eds): Evidence-Based Quality Improvement in Neonatal and Perinatal Medicine [Pediatrics electronic pages, Suppl]. Pediatrics 103:266, 1999.

81. Snell, et al: Reliability of birth certificate reporting of congenital anomalies. Am J Perinatol 9:219, 1992.

82. Soll RF, Andruscavage L: The principles and practice of evidence-based neonatology. In Horbar JD, Gould JB (eds): Evidence-Based Quality Improvement in Neonatal and Perinatal Medicine [Pediatrics electronic pages, Suppl]. Pediatrics 103:215, 1999.

83. Statistical Papers: Population and vital statistics reports, ser A, vol 46, New York, United Nations, 1994.

84. Stavis R: Neonatal databases part 3: Physicians' programs: Products and features. Perinatal Section News 25:17, 1999.

85. Stevenson DK, et al: Very-low-birth-weight outcomes of the National Institute of Child Health and Human Development Neonatal Research Network. January 1993 through December 1994. Am J Obstet Gynecol 179:1632, 1998.

86. Tolson GC, et al: The 1989 revision of the U.S. Standard Certificates and Reports. Vital Health Stat 4 28:14, 1991.

87. Tyson JE, et al: Viability, morbidity and resource use among newborn infants 501- to 800-g birth weight. The National Institute of Child Health and Human Development Neonatal Research Network. JAMA 276: 1645, 1996.

88. Vermont Oxford Network: Vermont Oxford Network Collaborative Learning Directory, Draft Edition 1999. Burlington, Vt, Vermont Oxford Network, 1999.

89. Vermont Oxford Network: Vermont Oxford Neonatal Network Database Manual of Operations. Release 4.0. Burlington, Vt, Vermont Oxford Neonatal Network, 1999.

90. Vermont Oxford Network: Member Instructions for Submitting Electronic Data, Version 1.24. Vermont Oxford Network, Burlington, Vt, 1999.

91. Ware JE, et al: Patients' assessment of their care. The quality of medical care information for consumers. Washington, DC, Congress of the United States, Office of Technology Assessment, 1988, p 229.

92. Weed LL: Knowledge Coupling, New Premises and Tools for Medical Care and Education. Springer-Verlag, New York, 1991.

93. Williams RL, et al: Identifying the sources of the recent decline in perinatal mortality rates in California. N Engl J Med 306:207, 1982.

94. Williams RL: Measuring the effectiveness of perinatal care. Medical Care 17:95, 1979.

95. Worthman LG: Review of the literature on diagnosis related groups; prepared by the Health Care Financing Administration: a Rand Note; N-2492-HCFA. Santa Monica, Calif, Department of Health and Human Services, 1986.

Part Two: Practicing Evidence-Based Neonatal-Perinatal Medicine

96. Antman EM et al: A comparison of results of meta-analyses of randomized control trials and recommendations of clinical experts. JAMA 268:240, 1992.

97. Bennett KJ, et al: A controlled trial of teaching critical appraisal of the clinical literature to medical students. JAMA 257:2451, 1987.

98. Cairns PA, et al: Is neonatal care evidence-based [abstract]? Pediatr Res 43:168A, 1998.

99. Chalmers I, Altman DG (eds): Systematic Reviews. London, BMJ Publishing Group, 1995.

100. Chalmers I, et al: Effective Care in Pregnancy and Childbirth. Oxford, Oxford University Press, 1989.

101. Crowley P: Antenatal corticosteroid therapy: A meta-analysis of the randomized trials. Am J Obstet Gynecol 173:322, 1995.

102. Dans AL, et al: Users' guides to the medical literature. XIV. How to decide on the applicability of clinical trial results to your patient. JAMA 279:545, 1998.

103. Ellis J, et al. In-patient general medicine is evidence-based. Lancet 346:407, 1995.

104. Glasziou P, et al: Applying the results of trials and systematic reviews to individual patients. ACP J Club 129:A15, 1998.

105. Guyatt GH, et al: Users' guides to the medical literature. II. How to use an article about therapy or prevention. A. Are the results of the study valid? JAMA 270:2598, 1993.

106. Guyatt GH, et al: Users' guides to the medical literature. IX. A method for grading health care recommendations. JAMA 274:1800, 1995.

107. Haynes RB, et al. Developing optimal search strategies for detecting clinically sound studies in MEDLINE. J Amer Med Inform Assoc 1:447, 1994.

108. Information on obtaining The Cochrane Library: Available at: http://www.update-software.com/cochrane.htm

109. Jaeschke R, et al: Users' guides to the medical literature. III. How to use an article about a diagnostic test. A. Are the results of the study valid? JAMA 271:389, 1994.

110. Kaplan RM, et al: Methods for assessing relative importance in preference based outcome measures. Qual Life Res 2:467, 1993.

111. Laupacis A, et al: Users' guides to the medical literature. V. How to use an article about prognosis. JAMA 272:234, 1994.

112. Levine M, et al: Users' guides to the medical literature. IV. How to use an article about harm. JAMA 271:1615, 1994.

113. Leviton LC, et al: Methods to encourage the use of antenatal corticosteroid therapy for fetal maturation: A randomized controlled trial. JAMA 281:46, 1999.

114. McColl A, et al: General practitioners' perceptions of the route to evidence-based medicine: A questionnaire survey. BMJ 316:361, 1998.

115. NIH Consensus Development Panel: Effect of corticosteroids for fetal maturation on perinatal outcomes. JAMA 273:413, 1995.

116. Oxman AD, et al: Users' guides to the medical literature. VI. How to use an overview. JAMA 272:1367, 1994.

117. Reisch JS, et al: Aid to the evaluation of therapeutic studies. Pediatrics 84:815, 1989.

118. Sackett DL, et al: Evidence-based medicine: what it is and what it isn't. BMJ 312:71, 1996.

119. Sackett DL, et al: Evidence-based Medicine. How to practice and teach EBM. 2nd ed. New York, Churchill Livingstone, 2000, p 13.

120. Saigal S, et al: Self-perceived health status and health-related quality of life of extremely low-birth-weight infants at adolescence. JAMA 276:453, 1996.

121. Sauve S, et al: The critically appraised topic: A practical approach to learning critical appraisal. Annals of the Royal College of Physicians and Surgeons of Canada 28:396, 1995.

122. Sinclair JC, Bracken MB: Effective Care of the Newborn Infant. Oxford, Oxford University Press, 1992.

123. Sinclair JC, et al: Introduction to neonatal systematic reviews. Pediatrics 100:892, 1997.

124. Straus SE, McAlister FA: Evidence-based medicine: Past, present, and future. Annals of the Royal College of Physicians and Surgeons of Canada 32:260, 1999.

125. Tyson JE, et al: An evaluation of the quality of therapeutic studies in perinatal medicine. J Pediatr 102:10, 1983.

II The Fetus

7 Genetic Aspects of Perinatal Disease and Prenatal Diagnosis

Stuart Schwartz

Lois H. Dickerman

Although specific genetic diseases and congenital malformations are rare occurrences, as a whole, they are significant causes of perinatal mortality and morbidity. Approximately 3% of all infants are born with genetic disorders or congenital anomalies that lead to mental or physical handicaps or early death.[24] Minor malformations are found in an additional 7% to 8% of newborns (see Chapter 28). If the genetic disorders that are expressed later in childhood and in adolescence are included, the burden of genetic disease is substantial. A Canadian study assessing genetic load in individuals from birth to age 25 ascertained through the Health Surveillance Registry found that approximately 12% of all individuals suffered health problems related to recognized genetic syndromes, diseases with genetic influences, or congenital disorders. Roughly half of the congenital disorders had a genetic etiology.[2]

Genetic disorders and birth defects generally fall into three major categories: chromosomal abnormalities, single gene mutations inherited primarily in a mendelian fashion, and multifactorial defects that may result from a combination of genetic or environmental factors. New projections based on the increased diagnostic accuracy of modern techniques suggest that approximately 1% of newborns have a recognizable chromosomal abnormality; earlier newborn screening studies found an incidence of about 0.5%.[28] Genetic disorders caused by single gene mutations, regardless of the mode of inheritance, were found in 0.4% of the population in the Canadian study, and the incidence of multifactorial genetic disease was approximately 10-fold higher, at 4.6%.[2] Unfortunately, many birth defects have no obvious or likely explanations, a situation that contributes to the mental and emotional anguish of the parents and other family members who must cope with the birth and subsequent care of an infant with a severe handicap.

CHROMOSOMAL ABNORMALITIES

With the advent of chromosome banding in 1970, it became possible to identify each chromosome conclusively on the basis of individual banding properties. Since then, the resolution with which chromosomes can be analyzed has improved. Abnormalities fall into two categories: *numerical* abnormalities, in which the modal number varies from normal, and *structural* abnormalities, in which physical changes occur in the chromosome's structure. In humans, each normal somatic cell contains 46 chromosomes (*diploid state*). Twenty-two pairs of chromosomes, the *autosomes,* are identical in both sexes. In women, the *sex chromosomes* constitute a homologous pair, designated X *chromosomes;* men have a nonhomologous pair, the X and Y *chromosomes.*

CHROMOSOME STRUCTURE

Each chromosome is composed of a linear molecule of deoxyribonucleic acid (DNA) complexed with proteins to form chromatin. This complex becomes a highly compact structure during cell division, reducing the length of the DNA molecule approximately 10,000-fold. Each chromosome may be defined structurally on the basis of telomeres, a centromere, and a long and short arm. *Telomeres,* the tips of chromosomes, contain tandemly repeated copies of the sequence TTAGGG. The telomere is critical to maintaining the integrity and stability of the chromosome. It is also important in replication and localization of the chromosome in the nucleus. In dividing cells, the *centromere* appears as a primary constriction; it is here that the microtubules attach to the chromosome to effect chromosome movement during cell division. The centromere is essential for proper segregation of the chromosomes in both mitosis and meiosis. The centromere's position divides the chromosome into two arms—the *p* (or short) arm and the *q* (or long) arm.

The relative position of the centromere determines whether the chromosomes are *metacentric* (having arms of approximately equal length), *submetacentric* (having the centromere nearer to one end), or *acrocentric* (having a greatly shortened p arm). In humans, the acrocentric chromosomes are pairs 13, 14, 15, 21, and 22. The ends of the p arms of these chromosomes contain specialized structures, called *stalks* and *satellites*, where the ribosomal ribonucleic acid (rRNA) genes and other repetitive sequences are located (Fig. 7–1).

Chromosome analysis involves production of a karyotype, in which the chromosomes are paired and placed in roughly decreasing size order with the p arms oriented upward. A standard nomenclature has been developed that allows a karyotype to be described by dividing each chromosome into regions, bands, and sub-bands. The present version of this nomenclature, the International System for Human Cytogenetic Nomenclature (ISCN 1995),[44] includes the incorporation of fluorescence in situ hybridization (FISH) technology (see later). A karyotype designation includes the modal chromosome number and the sex chromosome constitution, followed by standard abbreviations and band designations for abnormalities and variants. A chromosomally normal woman is denoted as 46,XX, and a chromosomally normal man as 46,XY (Fig. 7–2).

NUMERICAL ABNORMALITIES

Abnormalities in the number of chromosomes generally arise from a mistake in cell division (*nondisjunction*) in which aberrant segregation leads to the loss or gain of one or more chromosomes by a daughter cell (Fig. 7–3). The resulting cell is called *aneuploid*, because its modal number is not an exact multiple of the haploid (n) number. Nondisjunction can occur during either meiosis or mitosis, but it more commonly occurs during meiosis.

In meiosis I, homologous chromosomes synapse (because DNA replication occurs before meiosis, each chromosome consists of two sister chromatids), undergo recombination, and segregate, with one homologue migrating to each daughter cell. The chromosome number has been reduced by half. Then, during meiosis II, sister chromatids separate, and one chromatid migrates to each daughter cell. The genetic content has been reduced by half to the haploid state in the resulting gamete. Errors in nondisjunction in either meiosis I or meiosis II may lead to aneuploid gametes.

Fertilization of an aneuploid gamete with a normal gamete forms a conceptus with an extra (*trisomy*) or missing (*monosomy*) chromosome. Because nondisjunction can involve any chromosome, most resulting aneuploidies are nonviable. Almost all conceptions with autosomal monosomy and most with autosomal trisomy are spontaneously aborted. Even the "viable" trisomies (21, 13, and 18) are associated with a high rate of pregnancy loss. Approximately 70% of fetuses with trisomy 21 spontaneously abort, and the pregnancy loss figures for trisomy 13 and trisomy 18 are as high as 95%.

Numerical abnormalities of the sex chromosomes form a special class. The more common sex chromosome aneuploidies are 47,XXY (Klinefelter syndrome); 47,XYY; 47,XXX; and 45,X (Turner syndrome). Unlike most sex chromosome aneuploidies, Turner syndrome is associated with a very high rate of fetal loss. It is estimated that 98% of 45,X conceptions are lost as spontaneous abortions. Compared with the autosomal aneuploidies, the phenotypic effects of sex chromosome aneuploidies seen in living children are relatively mild. Many sex chromosome abnormalities are not apparent until puberty, and a large percentage (especially XYY and XXX) are underdiagnosed.

Although the fundamental causes of meiotic nondisjunction are not well understood, there is a clear association between advanced maternal age and nondisjunction (Fig. 7–4). The most common chromosomal abnormality seen in newborns, trisomy 21 (Down syndrome), has long been recognized as an increased risk in pregnancies of older mothers. Molecular studies have demonstrated that in approximately 95% of patients with trisomy 21, the meiotic error was maternal in origin.[50] Most errors occurred during the first meiotic division. It is believed that a reduced frequency of recombination between homologous chromosomes (crossing over) leads to an increase in nondisjunction.[60] Other aneuploidies correlated with advanced maternal age include trisomy 18, trisomy 13, Klinefelter syndrome, and triple X syndrome. The principal features of the autosomal trisomies are shown in Figure 7–5.

Numerical abnormalities that involve multiples of the haploid number are found primarily in material from spontaneous abortions. *Triploidy* (modal number of 69) usually arises from simultaneous fertilization

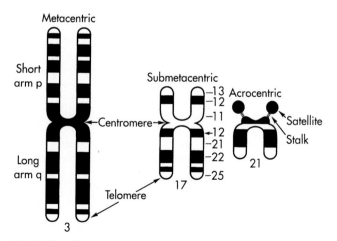

FIGURE 7–1. Human chromosome types with designated structural landmarks and diagrammatic banding representing the pattern seen with standard Giemsa staining, or G banding. The arrow on chromosome 17 points to a specific position on the chromosome that would be designated as 17q12 under the International System for Human Cytogenetic Nomenclature.[44]

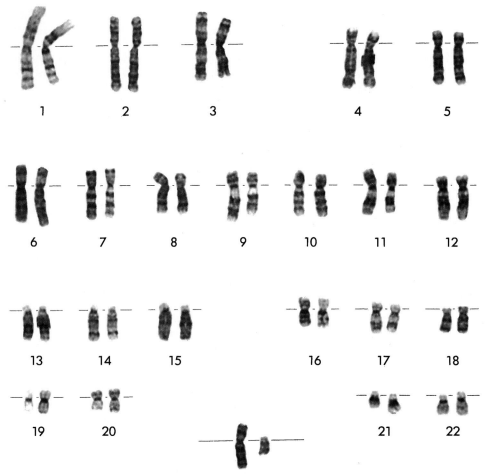

1

2

3

4

5

6

7

8

9

10

11

12

13

14

15

16

17

18

19

20

21

22

Sex chromosomes

FIGURE 7–2. G-banded normal male karyotype.

of a normal ovum by two sperm *(dispermy)*, yielding a conceptus with three haploid chromosome sets. Although most (99.9%) triploid fetuses spontaneously abort (seen in approximately 15% of chromosomally abnormal spontaneous abortuses), they occasionally survive to term. However, this condition is incompatible with long-term survival. *Tetraploidy* (modal number of 92) occurs in about 6% of the chromosomally abnormal spontaneous abortions and is incompatible with survival.[13, 17, 68]

Nondisjunction that occurs during mitosis results in *mosaicism*, which is the presence of more than one cell line in an individual. Most often, both a cytogenetically abnormal cell line and a cytogenetically normal cell line are present. Mosaicism is more often encountered in abnormalities of the sex chromosomes. For example, in Turner syndrome, approximately 15% of diagnosed patients have a normal female cell line in addition to a cell line with monosomy X. In the karyotypic designation, the cell lines in a mosaic individual are separated by a forward slash (/), and the number of cells in each is placed in brackets (e.g., mos 45,X [8]/46,XX [12]). Autosomal abnormalities such as trisomy 21 are also seen in mosaic form. In general, the phenotypic effects are similar to but less severe than those observed when

there is no normal cell line present.[53] However, gross generalizations should not be made.

Because the distribution of mosaic cell lines may vary from tissue to tissue in an affected individual, the diagnosis depends on the level of the abnormal cell line in the specimen sent for analysis. For example, in Pallister-Killian syndrome, tetrasomy 12p has been identified as an abnormal mosaic cell line in affected individuals {mos 46,X- [ ]/47,X-, + i(12) (p10) [ ]}. However, the diagnosis is usually made by chromosomal analysis of skin fibroblasts, because peripheral blood contains predominantly chromosomally normal cells. In some cases of fetal mosaicism, a chromosomally abnormal cell line appears to be confined to extraembryonic tissue (confined placental mosaicism).[32] This may be a complicating factor in prenatal diagnosis.

STRUCTURAL ABNORMALITIES

Structural abnormalities are the result of chromosome breakage that is improperly repaired. Chromosome rearrangements may maintain the diploid genetic content *(balanced)*, or they may result in the loss or gain of one or more chromosome segments *(unbalanced)*. Structural rearrangements may segregate

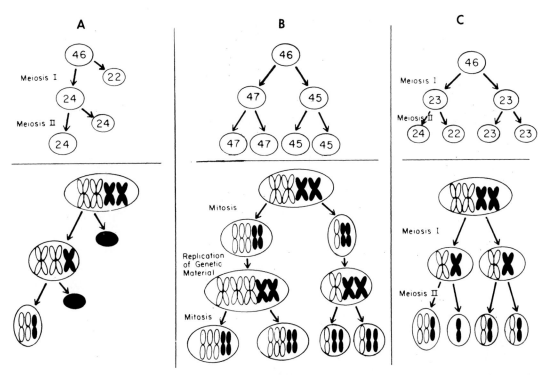

FIGURE 7–3. *A*, Nondisjunction in female meiosis I, resulting in an ovum with 24 chromosomes. Blackened circles represent the first and second polar bodies. *B*, Nondisjunction in mitosis, demonstrating development of mosaicism, with one cell line having 45 chromosomes and the other cell line having 47 chromosomes. *C*, Nondisjunction in male meiosis II, resulting in spermatozoa having 22, 23, and 24 chromosomes.

within a family *(familial)*, or they may arise as a new "mutation" *(de novo)*.

Translocation involves the exchange of segments between two chromosomes. There are two major types of translocations: *reciprocal* and *Robertsonian*. In reciprocal translocation, breakage occurs within two chromosome arms, with exchange of the distal segments (Fig. 7–6*A*). The derivative chromosomes are hybrids of the chromosomes involved, containing parts of both chromosomes. Although most balanced

translocation carriers are phenotypically normal, they are at risk of producing unbalanced gametes. Meiotic segregation of the chromosomes involved in a translocation is complex, and many segregation patterns are possible, but there are four major patterns. Alternate segregation of a reciprocal translocation gives rise to either chromosomally normal gametes or gametes carrying the balanced translocation (see Fig. 7–6*B*). In adjacent-1 segregation, the centromeres segregate appropriately (homologous centromeres to opposite poles), but the gamete receives the normal homologue of one chromosome and the derived homologue of the second chromosome (see Fig. 7–6*C*), with the risk of producing unbalanced gametes. In this situation, there is duplication of one translocated segment and deletion of the other.[17] Adjacent-2 segregation is similar to adjacent-1, except that the homologous centromeres go to the same pole. In 3:1 segregation, either three chromosomes segregate together, or one by itself, resulting in a fetus with 45 or 47 chromosomes.

Although a normal phenotype is seen in most individuals with a balanced translocation, there is an increased incidence of both congenital anomalies and mental retardation in translocations that are de novo. There is an approximate 8% chance of a phenotypic abnormality in de novo rearrangements detected prenatally.[72] These abnormalities may result from position effects, a break within a gene, a subtle deletion or duplication, or uniparental disomy.[34]

Robertsonian translocations are the most common structural abnormality, occurring in about 1 of 1000 live births. They involve two acrocentric chromo-

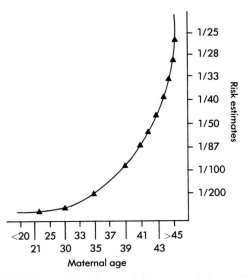

FIGURE 7–4. Observed incidence of chromosomal abnormalities in live births relative to maternal age at the time of delivery.

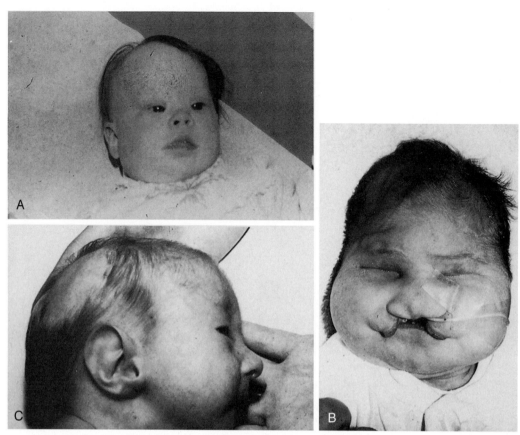

FIGURE 7–5. *A*, Trisomy 21. Prominent features of the syndrome noted during the neonatal period and the system or organ involved are as follows: central nervous system—abnormal neurologic examination (hypotonia); head—mild microcephaly, flat occiput, midfacial hypoplasia; eyes—Brushfield spots, epicanthal folds, upslanting palpebral fissures; mouth—protuberant tongue; ears—anomalous auricles; hands—simian crease, distal triradius, increased ulnar loops, short metacarpals and phalanges; fingers—dysplasia of midphalanx of fifth finger; cardiac—cardiac defects (approximately 40%); genitalia—hypogonadism; pelvis—hypoplasia, shallow acetabular angle; other—redundant skin at nape of neck, wide space between first and second toes. *B*, Trisomy 13. Prominent features of the syndrome noted during the neonatal period and the system or organ involved are as follows: central nervous system—severe malformations, holoprosencephaly; head—microcephaly, sloping forehead; eyes—microphthalmia, colobomata; mouth—cleft lip, cleft palate; ears—abnormal auricles, low-set ears; hands—distal triradius, simian crease; fingers—polydactyly; chest wall—thin or missing ribs; cardiac—cardiac defects (over 80%); genitalia—cryptorchidism, abnormal scrotum; pelvis—hypoplasia; other—apneic spells, seizures, persistence of fetal hemoglobin, increased nuclear projection in neutrophils. *C*, Trisomy 18. Prominent features of the syndrome noted during the neonatal period and the system or organ involved are as follows: central nervous system—malformations; head—narrow biparietal diameter, occipital prominence; eyes—short palpebral fissures; mouth—micrognathia, small mouth; ears—malformed auricles, low-set ears; hands—increased arches, hypoplastic nails; fingers—overlapping fingers; chest wall—short sternum; cardiac—cardiac defects (over 50%); genitalia—cryptorchidism; pelvis—small pelvis, limited hip abduction; other—growth deficiency, thrombocytopenia.

somes and arise from exchanges within the pericentromeric region of the short arm. Most of the short arm segments normally present on the involved chromosomes are lost as a result of these exchanges. Because the short arms of acrocentric chromosomes contain redundant genetic material, loss of a portion of this material has no phenotypic effect. Although the translocation involving chromosomes 14 and 21 is the most common Robertsonian rearrangement, any acrocentric chromosomes can be involved, including homologous chromosomes [e.g., der (21;21) (q10;q10)]. Because a Robertsonian rearrangement is a fusion between two chromosomes, a balanced carrier has a modal number of 45, whereas an individual with an unbalanced karyotype has 46 chromosomes.

As in reciprocal translocations, alternate segregation of a Robertsonian translocation gives rise either to chromosomally normal gametes or to balanced gametes that carry the translocation (Fig. 7–7*B*). Adjacent-1 segregation leads to duplication or deletion of an entire long arm, and most segregants are nonviable. However, if the aberrant segregant gives rise to a viable trisomy (e.g., trisomy 21), unbalanced offspring may result. For example, a woman who carries a 14/21 translocation [der (14;21) (q10;q10)] has a 10% to 15% risk of having a child with Down syndrome who carries two normal copies of chromosome 21 in addition to the Robertsonian translocation [46,X-,der (14;21) (q10;q10), +21]. For a man carrying the same translocation, the risk is considerably lower (less than

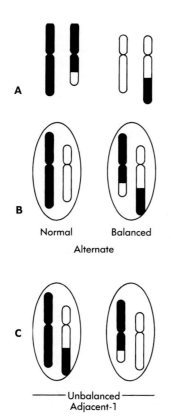

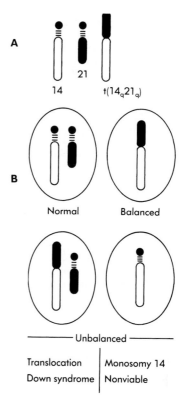

FIGURE 7–6. Reciprocal translocation. *A*, Reciprocal translocation between two nonhomologous chromosomes. In addition to the derivative chromosomes, each cell contains a normal copy of each chromosome. *B*, The meiotic products of alternate segregation. *C*, The meiotic products of adjacent-1 segregation.

FIGURE 7–7. Robertsonian translocation. *A*, Robertsonian translocation between two acrocentric chromosomes [t(14;21)(q10;q10)]. *B*, Four of the possible segregants of a Robertsonian translocation. Only the "normal" and "balanced" products are genetically balanced.

5%). Approximately 3% of live-born infants with Down syndrome carry an unbalanced form of a Robertsonian translocation. Half of these are inherited, so there is a significant risk of recurrence in those families. De novo cases of translocation Down syndrome carry a negligible risk of recurrence.[17, 25]

Other types of structural abnormalities include inversions, deletions, and duplications (Fig. 7–8). A chromosome inversion is the result of two breaks in a single chromosome, with the resulting interstitial segment assuming a reversed orientation during repair of the breaks. In a *pericentric* inversion, each arm of the chromosome has one breakpoint, and the inverted segment contains the centromere. In a *paracentric* inversion, both breakpoints are in a single arm—either the long or the short one—and the centromere is not included in the rearrangement. Although most carriers of inversions are phenotypically normal, there is a reproductive risk. Meiotic recombination within the inverted segment may lead to formation of an unbalanced recombinant chromosome.[17, 68] These recombinations and resultant unbalanced offspring are more likely to occur with carriers of pericentric rather than paracentric inversions. The recombinant chromosomes formed by both paracentric and pericentric carriers have both deletions and duplications; however, the recombinant chromosomes from paracentric carriers are dicentric (two centro-

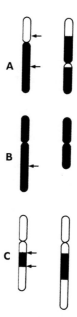

FIGURE 7–8. Structural chromosome abnormalities. In each panel, the normal chromosome is illustrated on the left, and the abnormal chromosome is on the right. Breakpoints are indicated by arrows. *A*, Pericentric inversion. *B*, Terminal deletion. *C*, Tandem duplication.

meres) or acentric (no centromere) and less likely to be viable.

Chromosome deletions may be either terminal or interstitial. In a terminal deletion, a segment of varying size is missing from the end of a chromosome; in an interstitial deletion, two breaks occur within a single chromosome, with loss of the central segment before repair. In either type of deletion, the genetic constitution is unbalanced, and the individual is monosomic for the deleted segment. A specific subgroup of deletions—the microdeletion (or contiguous gene deletion) syndromes—has become extremely important in clinical genetics. The diagnosis of these disorders is facilitated by FISH and is explained in greater detail later.

In chromosome duplications, a chromosome segment of varying size is duplicated within the chromosome. Because the homologous chromosome is normal (contains one copy of the relevant segment), an individual with a duplication is trisomic for a specific segment (i.e., he or she has three copies of the duplicated segment). In tandem duplications, the additional segment may be in the normal orientation with respect to the centromere (direct duplication), or it may be in an inverted orientation (inverted duplication).

The nature and effects of structural abnormalities can be summarized as follows. Because chromosome breakage is apparently a random event, the variety of potential abnormalities is infinite with respect to breakpoints, type of rearrangement, and chromosome segments involved. Therefore, in most cases, each rearrangement is unique (unless the disorder is familial). In terms of effect on phenotype, the critical issue is not the type of rearrangement but whether it is balanced. Most individuals with balanced rearrangements are phenotypically normal. With a de novo rearrangement that apparently is balanced, there is an 8% empiric risk that the rearrangement will be associated with adverse phenotypic consequences.[72] The implication is that a subset of rearrangements that appears to be balanced is actually unbalanced at a submicroscopic level (presumably, a submicroscopic duplication or deletion) or may involve breakage within a gene. More complex explanations, such as position effects on gene expression, also may be involved.

The vast majority of autosomal imbalances that can be detected microscopically have associated phenotypic abnormalities, including mental retardation. An imbalance that constitutes more than 4% to 5% of the haploid autosomal genome is nonviable, regardless of the chromosome segment involved. In fact, many smaller imbalances are nonviable. In general, for a given chromosome segment, trisomy is better tolerated than monosomy.[17, 68]

FLUORESCENCE IN SITU HYBRIDIZATION

Advances in DNA technology that have been applied to the field of cytogenetics have bridged the resolution gap between light microscopy and the molecular level. Using specially labeled DNA probes, we can now determine the presence or absence of specific genes or gene sequences along a chromosome's length. Changes in DNA structure in the range of 2 kb to 2 Mb along the length of the chromosome can be pinpointed by the process of FISH. Furthermore, this technology can be applied to interphase cells as well as to metaphase chromosomes, thus expanding the possibilities of diagnosing chromosomal abnormalities in nondividing cells.

FISH technology depends on two factors: the intrinsic ability of single-strand DNA to bind and anneal to complementary DNA sequences, and the generation of DNA probes that have been modified by incorporating biotin-dUTP or digoxigenin-UTP in place of thymine in the probe DNA sequence or, more recently, probes that are directly labeled with a fluorochrome. The labeled DNA probe is denatured and hybridized in the cells of interest to the native DNA, which also has been denatured to the single-strand state. After the probe has annealed to the complementary DNA sequence (or sequences) of the cells, the newly formed DNA complex can be detected directly or indirectly by adding fluorochrome-tagged avidin, which binds to biotin, or fluorochrome-tagged antidigoxigenin. The signal of the fluorescent complex can be amplified by layering antiavidin (antibody to avidin) that has also been biotinylated, to provide additional sites for binding of fluorochrome-tagged molecules. The cell DNA–probe DNA–biotin-avidin-fluorochrome sandwich, or directly labeled probe, is visualized by analysis with epifluorescence microscopy using a light source with appropriate excitation wavelengths. Imaging also may be enhanced by using a digital imaging microscope. Using different fluorochromes tagged to two or more different DNA probes allows simultaneous visualization of multiple chromosome sites within a single cell.

DNA probes for FISH may be formulated to detect specific genes or gene sequences or to anneal to chromosome-specific centromere sequences. In addition, there is a National Institutes of Health–supported project whose aim is to generate bacterial artificial chromosome (BAC) probes for every 1 Mb of DNA in the genome.[47] This would facilitate the overall examination of chromosomes by FISH by providing a detailed physical map. Other available types of probes for FISH include whole chromosome "paints" or libraries that have been derived by flow cytometry or single-cell human hybrids, region-specific probes made by microdissection, and centromere-specific probes. The utility of the probe used depends on the type of cytogenetic abnormality being evaluated and the type of tissue being analyzed. For example, centromeric probes, from unique α-satellite DNA sequences, have been widely used to detect aneuploidy in interphase cells (Fig. 7–9A). However, because of the sequence similarity of centromeric α-satellite DNA of chromosomes 13 and 21, specific identification of a trisomic 13 or trisomic 21 condition in interphase cells is not possible if only an α-satellite–

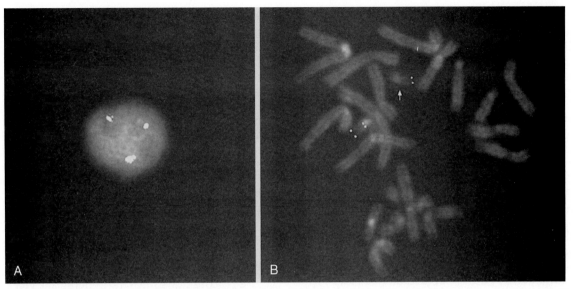

FIGURE 7–9. *A*, Fluorescence in situ hybridization (FISH) analysis of an interphase nucleus (using a chromosome X pericentromeric α-satellite DNA probe) reveals three signals consistent with three copies of chromosome X. *B*, FISH analysis of metaphase chromosomes, using the DiGeorge chromosome region probe (22q11.2), reveals the absence of the DiGeorge locus on one of the two chromosomes 22, indicated by an arrow. A specific probe (22q13.3) for the telomeric region of chromosome 22 is used as a control to show hybridization to each chromosome 22.

based probe is used. Therefore, specific single-copy probes for these chromosomes are used.

The ability to use FISH to detect specific gene sequences that may be duplicated or deleted in specific chromosomes has greatly enhanced our ability to diagnose contiguous gene syndromes, also known as microdeletion syndromes. Microdeletion syndromes are patterns of abnormality that arise because of loss of a continuous segment of DNA, usually involving multiple genes. The affected individual thus has only one copy of the gene present per cell, a condition also called segmental aneusomy. Approximately 20 of these syndromes have been defined by the association of a region of a chromosome with characteristic physical and developmental problems. Some of the more common microdeletion syndromes and their critical chromosomal regions are aniridia–Wilms tumor association (11p13), DiGeorge syndrome and velocardiofacial (VCF) syndrome (22q11.2), Miller-Dieker syndrome (17p13.3), and Prader-Willi and Angelman syndromes (15q11–13, discussed later). FISH technology allows unequivocal delineation of these syndromes by identifying a deletion at the submicroscopic level; this can be visualized as the loss of a binding site of a region-specific probe in the cells of the affected individual. In VCF-DiGeorge syndrome, for example, only about 30% of cases can be identified by a deletion seen with high-resolution cytogenetics. With FISH techniques, almost all patients can be shown to have the deletion (see Fig. 7–9B).

Another major application of FISH is the increased ability to identify marker chromosomes, which occur in about 1 in 750 prenatal diagnoses and in about 1 in 2500 newborns. By definition, marker chromosomes are chromosome fragments that lack distinctive banding patterns, making identification by standard staining methods virtually impossible. Although many patients with marker chromosomes may be asymptomatic, identifying the source of a marker is always important for clinical management. Patients with 45,X/46,X, + mar, for example, may be at risk for gonadoblastoma if the marker is of Y chromosome origin. Using FISH techniques, it can usually be determined whether the marker is derived from an X or a Y chromosome and whether removal of streak gonads is indicated. Studies of marker chromosomes have demonstrated that about half of satellited markers are derived from chromosome 15, and many nonsatellited markers originate from chromosomes 15, 18, and X.[11, 43] Although this information is not always clinically useful, the presence or absence of specific genes or these markers may be associated with an abnormal or normal phenotype. For example, the presence of SNRPN in a chromosome 15–derived marker is associated with an abnormal phenotype.

Of similar diagnostic importance is the use of FISH to identify cryptic chromosomal rearrangements that might go undetected by standard banding techniques. For example, through FISH methodology, children affected with Miller-Dieker syndrome, with ostensibly normal karyotypes, have been identified as carriers of an unbalanced translocation involving 17p.[35] This technology has been used to detect the presence of deleted material in presumed "balanced" translocations and to detect the presence or absence of specific genes in cytologically visible deletions.[34, 64]

Other FISH techniques are available to better characterize structural abnormalities. These include comparative genomic hybridization (CGH), reserve painting, spectral karyotyping (SKY), and multicolor FISH (M-FISH). CGH is a technique that uses DNA from the individual (or cell line) with an abnormal karyotype.[31] This test DNA is labeled green, and a control (normal) DNA is labeled red. These are mixed and hybridized to normal chromosomes. The red-green ratio is analyzed by computer software, allowing for detection of gain or loss of chromosomal material from the test DNA.[31] Both SKY and M-FISH are techniques that use combinational or ratio-labeled probes to create a distinct "color" for each chromosome.[56, 65] These probes are all applied simultaneously, and specialized computer software is used to detect the probes and pseudo-color the chromosomes. The metaphase can then be visualized and analyzed, with a distinct pseudo-color for each chromosome. In reserve painting, the unidentified chromosome is either flow-sorted away from the other chromosomes or scraped off a microscope slide.[7] The DNA is extracted, amplified, and labeled and is then used as a probe on normal metaphases to identify the origin of the chromosomal material. Future applications of FISH technology appear to be limited only by the development, definition, and availability of specific diagnostic probes; this technology will continue to progress, along with the delineation of the human genome.

SINGLE GENE DISORDERS

Human genetic disorders caused by mutations within single genes that lead to recognizable and predictable expression in the individual (phenotype) and that segregate within families in generally predictable proportions are called mendelian genetic traits.[41] These disorders follow the classic laws of inheritance established by Gregor Mendel for all diploid organisms. These laws state that genes from nonhomologous chromosomes assort independently during gamete formation and that pairs of genes (alleles) from homologous chromosomes segregate during gamete formation.

In humans, as in all diploid organisms, genes exist in pairs on homologous chromosomes (with the exception of the sex chromosomes in men). Thus, single gene disorders are classified on the basis of the interaction between a specific pair of alleles—the *genotype*—leading to an expressed, observable genetic effect—the *phenotype*. An individual with nonidentical alleles at any specific genetic locus is called a *heterozygote*, or is said to have a *heterozygous* genotype. If the alleles at a specific genetic locus are identical, the individual is *homozygous* for this genetic characteristic and may be called a *homozygote*. If the interaction of a single mutant allele with a normal gene leads to expression of the disorder in the individual, the genetic disorder is expressed in the heterozygous state and is considered to be *dominant*. A *recessive* genetic disease can occur only when both alleles are mutant or homozygous. Single gene disorders are further categorized as to whether they are transmitted on the autosomes or the sex chromosomes; thus, there are four major patterns of mendelian inheritance in humans: autosomal dominant, autosomal recessive, X-linked dominant, and X-linked recessive.

For most genetic disorders in humans, the specific genetic defect is unknown. In addition, there are many instances of genetic heterogeneity or different genes mutations leading to the same phenotype. A good example is retinitis pigmentosa, a disorder leading to hyperpigmentation within the retina and eventual blindness. Retinitis pigmentosa may be inherited as an autosomal dominant, autosomal recessive, or X-linked recessive disorder. When the biochemical or molecular basis for genetic diseases with similar phenotypes is unknown, the principal means of discriminating between heterogeneous mutations and determining the pattern of inheritance is by analysis of the family history, or pedigree.[15, 26, 57, 69]

AUTOSOMAL DOMINANT INHERITANCE

The example of an autosomal dominant pedigree in Figure 7–10 demonstrates the general rules for autosomal dominant inheritance:

1. There is a *vertical* pattern of transmission, with the genetic disorder appearing in each successive generation.
2. Affected individuals are equally likely to be male or female.
3. Affected children have at least one affected parent, except in cases of new mutations.
4. Affected individuals, if reproductively fit, transmit the abnormal gene to their progeny with a 50:50 probability. Within any one family, about half the children of an affected parent are normal and about half are expected to be affected.
5. Affected men may transmit the gene to sons as well as to daughters; this is called male-to-male transmission.
6. An individual within the family who is not affected in most cases will not transmit the gene to progeny.

Other characteristics of autosomal dominant genetic diseases in humans are frequently noted. In the homozygous state, autosomal dominant diseases or disorders are rare and generally lethal. For example, matings between individuals with autosomal dominant achondroplastic dwarfism lead to families with approximately two thirds of children affected and one third normal, rather than three fourths affected and

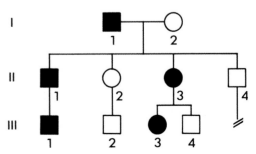

FIGURE 7–10. Example of an autosomal dominant pedigree. Note the vertical pattern of transmission. ○, male; □, female; ●, ■, affected.

one fourth normal. The homozygous children with achondroplasia either do not survive to delivery or die shortly after birth. Another characteristic often associated with autosomal dominant disorders is *variable expressivity.* Not all the individuals who inherit the mutant gene are affected to the same degree. In *neurofibromatosis,* a relatively common autosomal dominant genetic disorder affecting about 1 in 3000 individuals, the range of expression may vary from mild (with minimal café-au-lait spots and few if any tumors) to severe (with numerous café-au-lait spots and massive neurofibromata covering the entire body). *Penetrance* is another concept used in the characterization of autosomal dominant diseases. Not every individual carrying the gene may manifest the disorder overtly. In a "fully penetrant" disorder, the person with the dominant gene always demonstrates phenotypic expression. If the disorder has "reduced penetrance," there may be individuals within the pedigree who transmit the gene but ostensibly do not have the disease. Penetrance is often confused with variable expressivity, but penetrance is a statistical concept indicating the percentage of individuals within the pedigree at risk for the disorder (i.e., having the mutant gene) and affected by it. Variable expressivity refers to the degree to which the gene is expressed within a single individual.

Finally, one of the problems in differentiating an autosomal dominant genetic disease from other patterns of inheritance is new mutation. Any dominant mutation carried in the gamete at conception leads to the appearance of the dominant disorder for the first time in the kindred. *Achondroplasia,* for example, is a new mutation in approximately 80% of occurrences.[30] For the normal parents of a child with achondroplasia, there is little likelihood of recurrence in future pregnancies, but for the affected child, the mutation will be transmitted to 50% of his or her offspring. In many dominant genetic disorders affecting humans, there is a positive correlation between increased rate of new mutations and paternal age. Examples include achondroplasia, Apert syndrome, Marfan syndrome, and myositis ossificans. This correlation is thought to reflect the accumulation of DNA replicative errors during spermatogenesis throughout the long period of male reproductive life. The primary germ cells in the female population have a finite period of replication of approximately 22 to 26 cell divisions, as opposed to continuous mitotic replenishment of sperm precursor cells in the male population once puberty begins.

As previously described, somatic nondisjunction can give rise to chromosomal mosaicism. Mutational mosaicism can arise as the result of postfertilization errors in replication or repair of nucleotide sequences in somatic cells or germ cells at any stage in development. In rare cases in which two *unaffected* parents have two or more affected offspring with a completely penetrant dominant condition (e.g., osteogenesis imperfecta, neurofibromatosis, or achondroplasia), germline mutation mosaicism of one parent can be inferred. When there are new cases of dominant disorders in offspring of normal parents, the implications for genetic counseling are that recurrence risks must be revised upward by a few percentage points to account for the possibility of germline mosaicism in one of the parents.[26, 69]

AUTOSOMAL RECESSIVE INHERITANCE

Because they occur only in the homozygous state, recessive disorders are much rarer than autosomal dominant disorders. An example of a typical autosomal recessive pedigree is shown in Figure 7–11. The primary features of an autosomal recessive pattern of inheritance are:

1. The disorder most often occurs in siblings in a *horizontal* pattern within a generation.
2. Both male and female populations are affected.
3. Parents usually are unaffected, and affected individuals rarely have affected children.
4. The recurrence risk in each subsequent pregnancy to known carriers is one in four (25%).
5. Consanguinity is often observed in pedigrees of extremely rare recessive disorders.

For some of the known recessive genetic diseases in which the specific defective gene product has been identified, biochemical tests can confirm the absence or deficiency of that product in the affected individual. Carrier status, signified by reduced levels of gene product, can be determined in the parents. A well-known example of such biochemical diagnosis is found in *Tay-Sachs disease,* in which affected individuals have deficient or greatly reduced levels of hexosaminidase A in serum and lymphocytes. Carriers of this disorder can be identified by their reduced levels of hexosaminidase A activity—approximately 50% of that found in the tissues of noncarriers. As an increasing number of genetic diseases are identified at the DNA level by alterations in the nucleotides making up the gene itself, rather than at the level of the gene

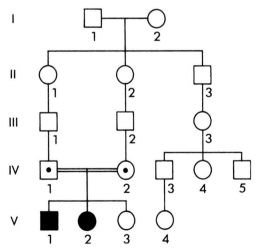

FIGURE 7–11. Example of an autosomal recessive pedigree. Note the horizontal pattern of affected individuals. =, consanguinity; ⊙, ⊡, obligate carriers; ○, male; □, female; ●, ■, affected.

product, more carriers will be identified by molecular analysis, and an increased number will be identified as the human genome is delineated.[18, 26, 69]

SEX-LINKED INHERITANCE

Because relatively few genes associated with abnormal phenotypes have been identified on the Y chromosome in humans (see later), sex-linked disorders are often considered synonymous with X-linked genetic diseases. There are proportionally more recognized genetic diseases linked to the X chromosome than to any of the autosomes. This reflects the fact that men, with only one X chromosome, are *hemizygous* for X-linked genes and therefore are affected by any mutant gene located on the X chromosome. X-linked diseases, such as hemophilia A, were among the earliest recognized human genetic diseases because of this differential expression rate in the male population. Women, with two X chromosomes, may be either homozygous or heterozygous for any X-linked gene. An example of an X-linked recessive pedigree is shown in Figure 7–12. The features of an X-linked recessive mode of inheritance are:

1. Men are more frequently affected than women.
2. Male-to-male transmission of the mutant gene is never seen.
3. The daughters of affected men are obligate carriers for the disorder.
4. Carrier mothers of X-linked disorders transmit the disorder to half of their sons; half of their daughters are carriers. Therefore, in an X-linked pedigree, all affected male members are related to one another through the female members.

An interesting association between sporadic cases of known X-linked disorders, such as hemophilia A and Lesch-Nyhan syndrome, and the age of the maternal grandfather has been observed. Just as there appears to be an increase in the risk for new dominant mutations with paternal age, there is an increased risk for new mutations of X-linked disorders in the sons of mothers whose fathers were older. It is speculated

that a well-known historical example of a new mutation—that of hemophilia A in the descendants of Queen Victoria—may be a consequence of an X-linked mutant gene inherited from her unaffected father, who was older than 50 years of age when she was born.

X-linked dominant disorders in humans are relatively rare diseases. The best-described example is vitamin D–resistant rickets (hypophosphatemia). X-linked dominant disorders can be distinguished from X-linked recessive diseases by the following criteria (Fig. 7–13):

1. Affected women are twice as common in the pedigree as affected men. In some disorders, the mutation may be lethal in men.
2. Affected men have affected daughters but no affected sons.
3. Affected women transmit the disorder to half of their daughters and to half of their sons. There is a 50% chance of having an affected child.

X CHROMOSOME INACTIVATION IN THE FEMALE POPULATION

A unique mechanism that has evolved to regulate gene expression in mammalian females, including humans, is random inactivation of one X chromosome in the somatic tissues. Although both X chromosomes must be "turned on" for genetic transcription to occur in ovarian tissues to ensure normal oogenesis and secondary sexual development, only one entire X chromosome remains accessible for genetic transcription in somatic cells. This is necessary because the two X chromosomes in women must be compensated for, to be equivalent to the one X chromosome in men. This hypothesis of dosage compensation was initially espoused by Mary Lyon in the 1960s. The Lyon hypothesis, which has been proved correct in most aspects, states that the following occurs in the somatic cells of chromosomally normal women:[27, 38, 39]

1. Only one of the two X chromosomes is transcriptionally active.
2. The inactivation of one X chromosome occurs early in embryonic life.
3. The inactivation of one X chromosome occurs

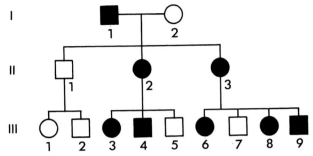

FIGURE 7–13. X-linked dominant pedigree. Approximately twice as many women as men are affected. ○, male; □, female; ●, ■, affected.

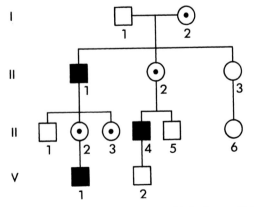

FIGURE 7–12. X-linked recessive pattern of inheritance. Note that sons of affected men are not affected. ⊙, ⊡, obligate carriers; ○, male; □, female; ●, ■, affected.

randomly, and either the maternal or the paternal X chromosome in a cell is inactivated.

4. The inactivation is irreversible and clonally propagated, such that all the descendants of a given cell have the same X chromosome inactivated.

More recent studies indicate that there are some exceptions to the original Lyon hypothesis. Random X inactivation does not always occur, whether due to stochastic effects, mutations, or the presence of structurally abnormal X chromosomes. Not every gene is inactivated on the inactive X chromosome. At least 16 genes are known to escape inactivation, and it is estimated that possibly up to one third of all the genes on the X chromosome are not inactivated.[5] Lastly, X inactivation is not irreversible; it is reversible in the development of the germ cells.

The inactive X chromosome can be visualized in nondividing cells as the Barr body (sex chromatin body), a densely compacted, heterochromatic structure within the nucleus associated with the nuclear membrane. In dividing cells, the inactive X chromosome can be identified by special techniques that demonstrate DNA replication and the late replication pattern of the inactive X chromosome during the S phase of mitosis.[27, 38, 39]

Because only one X-linked gene is functionally active in the somatic tissues of women, a woman who is heterozygous for an X-linked disorder is a mosaic for cells expressing either the normal or the abnormal gene. For this reason, carrier women themselves may manifest some signs of X-linked recessive diseases if, by chance, the X chromosome carrying the normal gene is inactive in most cells in critical tissues. For example, a woman who is a carrier of Duchenne muscular dystrophy may demonstrate mild muscle weakness, and a carrier of hemophilia A may have diminished clotting activity. This variability in X chromosome expression also makes it extremely difficult to identify female carriers of X-linked recessive disorders, even when the biochemical defect or marker is known (e.g., hypoxanthine guanine phosphoribosyltransferase activity in Lesch-Nyhan syndrome). The measurable levels of X chromosome gene product in carriers may overlap the normal range of gene products found in noncarrier women. When the mother of an affected son does not have other affected sons, brothers, or maternal uncles, it may be difficult to determine whether the X-linked disorder represents a new mutation or is an inherited defect. Molecular genetic diagnostic techniques play an important role in distinguishing between these two possibilities.[18, 58, 69]

Y CHROMOSOME INHERITANCE

As stated earlier, few genes associated with abnormal phenotypes have been identified on the Y chromosomes in humans. The best examples of genes localized to the Y chromosome are those involved in dimorphic traits, sexual development, or sperm pro-

duction. SRY, the testis-determining factor, is localized to the Y chromosome short arm. A mutation in this gene leads to a sex-reversed fetus. The DAZ gene is localized to the long arm of the Y chromosome. A mutation in this gene leads to azoospermia and infertility. The features of a Y-linked mode of inheritance are:

1. Only the male population is affected.
2. All sons of an affected father are affected.
3. Male-to-female transmission of the mutant gene is never seen.

NONTRADITIONAL PATTERNS OF INHERITANCE

Although Mendel's laws have withstood the test of time, recent studies have revealed some remarkable exceptions. Nontraditional forms of inheritance have been identified that are not predicted by Mendel's laws. There are three major types of nontraditional inheritance: mitochondrial inheritance, imprinting, and trinucleotide repeats.

Mitochondrial Inheritance

As described earlier, most genes located on chromosomes within the cell nucleus follow mendelian patterns of inheritance. However, another source of DNA within mammalian cells is the circular molecule of DNA located within mitochondria and thus confined to the cell's cytoplasm. Although many of the proteins controlling mitochondrial function and the respiratory enzyme complex are coded by nuclear genes, some of the mitochondrial proteins are the translation products of mitochondrial DNA. The mitochondria contain circular DNA, consisting of 16,569 base pairs. This DNA contains a unique genetic code, which differs from the nuclear DNA. There are no introns, and the DNA sequence codes for 2 ribosomal RNA (rRNA) genes and 22 transfer RNA (tRNA) genes.

An example of mitochondrial inheritance is shown in Figure 7–14. The general rules for such inheritance are:

1. Genes encoded by mitochondrial DNA follow a matrilineal inheritance. All the functional mitochondria are derived from the cytoplasm of the oocyte. At fertilization, the mitochondria

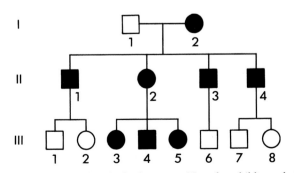

FIGURE 7–14. Mitochondrial inheritance. Note that children of affected men are not affected. ○, male; □, female; ●, ■, affected.

within the sperm head are not transferred to the ovum.

2. An affected woman passes the trait to *all* her children.
3. An affected man *never* passes the trait to his children.
4. There is significant tissue and organ variability owing to *heteroplasmy* (see later).
5. The phenotype may vary over time.

Because mitochondria are the cellular organelles with the key function of energy production, mitochondrial genetic diseases fundamentally affect the processes of oxidative phosphorylation. The phenotype of a specific mitochondrial genetic disorder may vary considerably, depending on both the nature of the mutation and a unique property of mitochondrial genetics known as heteroplasmy. At the time of fertilization, the cytoplasm of the human ovum contains thousands of mitochondria. In addition, each mitochondrion may contain multiple copies of DNA. Mitochondrial inheritance, therefore, may involve the distribution of both mutant and normal mitochondrial DNA within the cytoplasm of cells. If a mitochondrial genetic variant is present, the ovum probably contains both normal and variant genotypes. Furthermore, as mitochondrial DNA replicates, the possibility of mitochondrial DNA mutation means that multiple copies of DNA within the single organelle may not be genetically identical. Depending on the replication and distribution patterns of the mutant mitochondria in developing tissues, as well as the tissues' specific energy requirements, the clinical phenotype in mitochondrial disorders may be highly unpredictable and may change over a lifetime. A single family may have widely different manifestations of the same mitochondrial disease, and in a single individual, the manifestations may change with age.

Predictably, in disorders of energy metabolism, the tissues most affected are those with the highest energy demands. Myopathies are a common expression of mitochondrial genetic diseases. External ophthalmoplegia, or paralysis of the muscles of the eye and eyelid, is found in Kearns-Sayre syndrome; cardiac arrhythmia may be a clinical feature of this syndrome as well. Hypertrophic cardiomyopathy may be another presenting feature of mitochondrial genetic disease, and disorders of the central nervous system are likely to be cardinal features. Myoclonic epilepsy with ragged red fibers is characterized by ataxia, hearing loss, and generalized central nervous system dysfunction, as well as by myoclonic seizures. The hallmark clinical feature of Leber hereditary optic neuropathy is acute or subacute onset of blindness in late childhood or adolescence, resulting from isolated involvement of the optic nerve and retinal degeneration.

Because there are nuclear genes coding for proteins, structural components, and enzymes of the mitochondria, as well as mitochondrial genes, defining the particular genetic defects leading to a problem with energy metabolism can be exceedingly difficult. Diagnosis of mitochondrial disorders requires specialized investigations. DNA-based diagnostic procedures are now available for many mitochondrial diseases, because the DNA sequence of the mitochondrial chromosome has been delineated, and many mutations have been detected. Therapy for individuals with mitochondrial disease is limited to attempting to increase adenosine triphosphate production or efficiency by replacing cofactors involved in energy metabolism.[12, 62]

Imprinting

Genomic imprinting refers to the differential modification of the paternal and maternal contributions to the zygote, resulting in the differential expression of parental alleles (for some genes, paternal and maternal alleles function differently). This is a clear departure from typical mendelian inheritance and applies to only a small number of genes.

Pronuclear transplantation experiments in mice have revealed that the parent's sex may reversibly affect the genetic contribution to the embryo. Mouse embryos have been conceived with both haploid chromosomal complements coming from either the mother or the father. Mouse zygotes with all *paternally* derived genes had placental development with arrested embryonic development; zygotes with all *maternally* derived genes had embryonic development but arrested placental development. Neither embryo developed normally beyond an early stage. This phenomenon, genomic imprinting, leads to the concept that some genes or chromosome segments are expressed differently in the embryo, depending on whether they were inherited from the mother or the father. Human examples of genomic imprinting include *hydatidiform moles* or *complete moles*, which are placental tumors with no embryonic tissue and a genome derived from two paternal sets of haploid chromosomes. *Ovarian teratomata* are benign tumors consisting of disorganized masses of differentiated embryonic tissue but devoid of placental tissue. These teratomata contain two maternally derived sets of haploid chromosomes.[23]

As the molecular dissection of human genetic syndromes has advanced, genomic imprinting has been demonstrated to play an important role in specific syndromes. The best-known examples are *Prader-Willi syndrome* and *Angelman syndrome*. Prader-Willi syndrome is characterized by hypotonia at birth, obesity and uncontrolled appetite with age, and moderate mental retardation. In most cases (70%), it is associated with a deletion of chromosome 15 [del (15) (q11–q13)]. Angelman syndrome is characterized by severe mental retardation, inappropriate laughter, and characteristic ataxic movements. It also is associated with a deletion of 15q11–q13, the same region deleted in Prader-Willi syndrome. The problem of explaining two distinct genetic conditions caused by the same cytogenetic deletion was unresolved until it was demonstrated that the deletion in Prader-Willi syndrome was always *paternally* derived and that the deletion in Angelman syndrome was *maternally* derived.[33] Infants who inherit a 15q11–q13 deletion from their fathers have Prader-Willi syndrome, because a critical region on maternal chromosome 15 required for normal development is imprinted or inactivated during the normal process of maternal meiosis. The corresponding region on the paternal chromosome 15, which normally must remain active in embryonic development, is lost with the paternal 15q11–q13 deletion. Infants develop Angelman syndrome because one gene from this chromosome 15 region (*UBE3A*) is normally paternally imprinted and is inactive in certain developmental stages. Because of the maternally derived deletion, these infants do not have the corresponding complementary active maternal genetic information.[9, 10, 33]

Interestingly, only about 70% of patients with either Angelman syndrome or Prader-Willi syndrome can be demonstrated by cytogenetic analysis to have this deletion. Furthermore, molecular analyses of the chromosomes of some individuals without cytologically detectable deletions have revealed submicroscopic deletions or mutations below the level of cytogenetic resolution. These molecular studies revealed that in the cells of approximately 5% of the individuals with these disorders, a portion of the imprinting center (within 15q11–q13) is either deleted or has a mutation responsible for the disorders. In addition, in 25% to 30% of the patients with Prader-Willi syndrome and in 3% of the patients with Angelman syndrome, *both* copies of chromosome 15 were either paternally or maternally derived and thus paternally or maternally imprinted. The critical region of corresponding active maternal or paternal genetic component is missing in these rare individuals because they have no maternally or paternally inherited chromosome 15.[9, 10, 23, 66]

It has now been recognized that uniparental inheritance of chromosomes, or *uniparental disomy* (UPD), can be the basis for syndromes demonstrating genomic imprinting in other genetic conditions. Two categories of UPD have been defined: *isodisomy*, which is the inheritance of two identical copies of a chromosome from the same parent; and *heterodisomy*, which is the inheritance of two different copies of the same chromosome from the same parent. This is not a trivial distinction if the parent contributing the chromosome is a carrier for a recessive disorder. An individual with uniparental isodisomy for a chromosome with a recessive disease gene would be affected with that disorder. Several cases of cystic fibrosis (CF) in children have been determined to be caused by isodisomy of chromosome 7 from a carrier parent.

The magnitude of genetic morbidity from UPD remains unknown, but its demonstration should not be surprising. As mentioned earlier, about 10% of all clinically recognized pregnancies that end in miscarriage are trisomies, which result from disomy in one gamete. Therefore, in meiosis, we would expect an approximately equal number of nullisomic gametes and disomic gametes to arise. An apparently "normal" conception could result from the rescue of a nullisomic gamete by fertilization of a gamete with

UPD for the missing chromosome.[9, 10, 66] Alternatively, fetuses with three of the same chromosomes could lose one chromosome, denoted as "trisomy rescue." If a fetus inherits two maternal chromosomes 15 and one paternal 15 and it loses the paternal chromosome, maternal UPD would result.

Not all chromosomes have been identified as having imprinted genes. For example, chromosomes 13 and 21 do not demonstrate any imprinting effects, and there are many chromosomes for which it is unknown whether an effect occurs. However, in addition to chromosome 15, UPD of several other chromosomes demonstrates an effect. A small number of cases of Beckwith-Wiedemann syndrome are due to the inheritance of both copies of the paternal chromosome 11. Some cases of Russell-Silver syndrome are due to UPD 7, and some cases of neonatal diabetes are due to UPD 6. Additionally, UPD 14 has been associated with developmental delay. In some of these syndromes, specific genes have been implicated as being imprinted, but in several cases, the causative genes are still not known.

Trinucleotide Repeat Expansions

A number of disorders, such as fragile X syndrome, Huntington disease, and myotonic dystrophy, have been characterized as having an underlying defect caused by expansion of a repeated trinucleotide sequence within the relevant gene. All these disorders have an unusual and nontraditional mendelian type of inheritance. For example, although myotonic dystrophy was known to be inherited as an autosomal dominant disorder, increasing severity could be seen in successive generations. The disorder could be "anticipated" in affected individuals. After analysis of the X-linked fragile X syndrome, Sherman and colleagues postulated several findings that appeared to be a paradox, given the standard X-linked recessive disorder.[60] These include:

1. The probability of offspring with mental retardation is increased by the number of generations through which the mutation has passed.
2. The probability of offspring with mental retardation is higher for both sons and daughters of affected women or women with affected sons.

The trinucleotide repeat expansion provides a rationale for this phenomenon and is discussed in greater detail later.

In addition, some of the genes involving mutations of trinucleotide repeats have been shown to be remarkably unstable as they are inherited from generation to generation. Although the inheritance pattern may be predictable, prediction of the phenotypic expression is extremely complex in such cases.[7] For example, there are documented cases of contraction of the CTG trinucleotide repeat numbers in myotonic dystrophy in transmission from affected parents to their children. In this particular disease, contraction is more likely to occur if the father is the affected parent.[1]

DNA DIAGNOSIS

Previously, many genetic diseases were diagnosed through an assay of the gene product (protein) or through detection of secondary effects or clinical symptoms (e.g., intestinal enzyme levels in CF or sonographic detection of polycystic kidneys). If the genetic locus involved in a single gene defect has been at least partially characterized, inheritance of the genetic defect can be followed at the DNA level. Because the genomic DNA is identical in every somatic cell, the diagnosis can be made using any available tissue, eliminating the need for active expression of the gene product in the sampled tissue or the onset of physiologic abnormalities.

DNA diagnosis relies on the detection of sequence variation among individuals. If the sequence of nucleotides from 10 unrelated individuals is analyzed, a variation in nucleotide sequence is encountered approximately once in every 200 base pairs of DNA. Most sequence variation is present within stretches of nonfunctional DNA that are interspersed with genes. (A gene is defined as a transcription unit capable of expression in the form of an RNA transcript.) Although this type of sequence variation is of no consequence to the individual, it has many uses in the identification of individuals and of the single gene defects individuals may carry. In DNA diagnosis, such DNA polymorphism can be used as a marker if it is known to be genetically linked to a disease locus.

Initially, the principle of linked markers was applied to disease diagnosis, using protein markers. An early example of this is the autosomal dominant disease myotonic dystrophy, which demonstrates genetic linkage to the blood group factor *secretor*. Although the two gene loci coding for these properties are completely unrelated functionally, allelic forms of the genes segregate together within a family, presumably as a result of physical linkage within the genome. More recently, these studies have used sequence variation of nonfunctional DNA.

The use of polymorphic DNA markers that are physically linked but functionally unrelated to a disease locus is called "linkage analysis" or "indirect diagnosis." This approach is versatile, because less knowledge of the disease gene is required, and the pool of potentially useful markers may be quite large. (Because the polymorphic variation is random, many markers are not informative in a given family.) However, it is inherently less accurate than a direct diagnosis, because the linkage pattern may be altered through genetic recombination. In addition, it is labor intensive, because the linkage pattern for each family must be ascertained independently.

It is important to note, however, that sequence variation (i.e., polymorphism) is still very valuable in genetics. In addition to linkage analysis, these polymorphic markers can be used for UPD studies, origin of nondisjunction analysis, identity analysis for both forensic and twin studies, chimerism analysis in bone marrow transplantation, and loss of heterozygosity in cancer studies.

With the proliferation of molecular genetic analysis and the completion of the sequencing of the human genome, the vast majority of genetic diagnosis is now done by direct diagnosis, or mutation analysis, of a given gene. Over 4000 genetic diseases have been postulated, but there are only a limited number in which the DNA sequence of at least part of a gene is available. Clinical or research DNA diagnosis is done on fewer than 100 genes, due to the frequency of disease and because all the specific mutations have not been identified for these genes.

The causes of the mutations that result in genetic diseases are sequence variations within functional genes. A mutation within a gene may be innocuous (in which case it is useful as a polymorphic marker), or, by having a detrimental effect on the function of the gene product, it may be the basis of genetic disease. When a deleterious mutation can be identified on the molecular level, genetic disease can be diagnosed directly. This approach requires knowledge of the nucleotide sequence of a disease gene. Mutations underlying genetic disease may be relatively disease specific, as in sickle cell anemia, in which most individuals with the disease have a single amino acid alteration (s single base change within codon 6 replaces glutamic acid with valine). This situation is more the exception than the rule, and in most genetic diseases, the mutations are heterogeneous and may be dispersed throughout the gene sequence. CF is a prime example of a genetic disease with marked heterogeneity. Since the identification of the CF gene in 1989, isolation and nucleotide sequencing of cystic fibrosis transmembrane conductance regulator (CFTR) genes from patients with CF have led to the delineation of more than 800 different mutations worldwide. Therefore, linkage analysis can be an approach in these CF families with rare and undefined mutations. Examples of prenatal diagnosis of CF using both direct mutation analysis and linkage analysis are shown in Figure 7–15.

Approach to Diagnosis

The primary methodologies used in DNA diagnosis are *Southern blot analysis* and the *polymerase chain reaction* (PCR) technique. PCR was introduced in 1986 and quickly became the state of the art of molecular diagnosis. Southern blot analysis and PCR are often used together for molecular diagnosis, but PCR has become the major diagnostic approach for most genetic disorders.

Southern blot analysis uses a class of bacterial enzymes called restriction endonucleases (Fig. 7–16). Each "restriction enzyme" has the ability to recognize a specific DNA sequence (four to eight nucleotides in length) and to cut double-stranded DNA at that position. Normally, the host organism uses this ability to protect itself from invasion by foreign organisms, but in the test tube, it is a powerful mechanism for

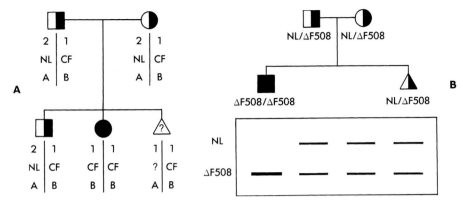

FIGURE 7–15. DNA diagnosis of cystic fibrosis. *A*, Linkage analysis using two flanking DNA probes "1,2" and "A,B." The first offspring (carrier) and the second offspring (affected) have inherited the parental haplotypes. In the current pregnancy, there has been a recombination between the two probes ("1" is no longer linked to "B"); therefore, this analysis is not useful in predicting the status of the fetus. *B*, Direct diagnosis using the ΔF508 mutation. Both parents are carriers of the ΔF508 mutation, and the affected offspring is homozygous for the mutation. The fetus also is a carrier. The results of polymerase chain reaction analysis are illustrated below the pedigree, where the three–base pair difference in size between the two alleles allows amplification products to be resolved by gel electrophoresis. ○, male; □, female; ●, ■, affected.

manipulating DNA from any source. Because digestion by restriction enzymes is sequence specific, DNA from any individual can be cut into a discrete series of fragments. The fragments produced are quite similar among individuals, but whenever sequence variation affects the recognition sequence of the enzyme in use, the size of one or more restriction fragments is altered. This is called restriction fragment length polymorphism (RFLP). An RFLP pattern that is useful in identifying an allele is one that is informative, and RFLP patterns demonstrated to be linked on a chromosome are called *haplotypes*.

Cloned DNA probes are used to analyze the large population of DNA fragments produced. A cloned probe is a specific, discrete fragment of DNA that has been isolated and propagated. The probe is used to visualize a small subset of the large number of fragments present in digested genomic DNA. Specifically, a probe anneals to those fragments that contain sequence homology to the probe. Artificially synthesized short segments of nucleic acids (oligonucleotides) also may be used as probes (see later).

In standard Southern blot analysis, gel electrophoresis is used to fractionate the DNA fragments through an electric field on the basis of size, thus dispersing the fragments in a predictable pattern. The DNA fragments are then immobilized on a firm support, a hybridization membrane. To detect the fragments of interest, a "tagged" DNA probe is applied to the membrane. Through complementary base pairing (hybridization), the probe adheres only to the homologous fragments in the genomic DNA. Because the DNA fragments are invisible to the naked eye, a "tag" is necessary to see where hybridization has occurred. Although the tag traditionally has been a radioactive compound, nonradioactive enzymatic tags are becoming increasingly useful.

The second major technologic advance in DNA diagnosis is PCR (Fig. 7–17). PCR allows physical amplification of a defined segment of DNA without having to isolate that segment from the remainder of the genomic DNA. This provides an efficient way of generating sufficient quantities of DNA from an individual for DNA diagnosis. Although this approach is extremely powerful, it requires at least partial determination of the nucleotide sequence of interest by DNA sequencing. Amplification is achieved through the use of two single-stranded oligonucleotide primers (20 to 30 nucleotides in length) that are homologous to the segment of interest and are of opposite polarity with respect to the target sequence. The primers thus define the boundaries of the segment of DNA to be amplified, because they direct DNA synthesis across the region of interest in opposite directions.

The basic steps in the PCR process are (1) *denaturation* of the DNA in the reaction, thus converting the DNA duplex to single strands; (2) *priming* by hybridization of the oligonucleotide primers to the target sequence; and (3) *strand synthesis* with DNA polymerase, beginning at each primer and using the denatured target DNA as a template. Amplification proceeds in a manner similar to DNA replication, except that only a discrete segment of genomic DNA is involved. The efficiency of this reaction allows routine amplification of fragments ranging from 50 to more than 2000 base pairs in length. The amplification products of a given target DNA are identical in length and sequence. Thus, PCR amplification of DNA from an individual who is heterozygous for a small deletion falling within the boundaries of the target yields two discrete amplification products that correspond to the normal and the deleted allele.

Repeated rounds of amplification result in the creation of more than 1 million copies of the target sequence. This process has been automated through the use of machines designed especially for this purpose and the availability of heat-stable DNA polymer-

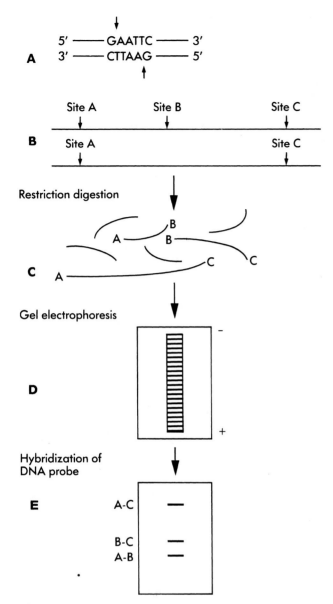

FIGURE 7–16. Restriction endonuclease digestion and Southern blot hybridization. *A,* Recognition sequence for the restriction endonuclease Eco RI. *B,* Illustration of restriction site polymorphism, where "Site B" is missing from the lower allele. *C,* DNA fragments generated by enzyme digestion of genomic DNA. *D,* Gel electrophoresis. *E,* Result of hybridization with a DNA probe homologous to region A–B–C.

ase that survives multiple rounds of temperature-driven DNA denaturation. PCR is not a method of DNA diagnosis in itself. It is an elegant, efficient way to obtain sufficient amounts of DNA for further analysis. The amplified DNA can be digested with restriction enzymes and used for Southern blot analysis (or a modification of that technique), or, in most applications, the amplification product can be visualized directly after gel electrophoresis, many times after cutting with an appropriate restriction enzyme.[37]

Presently, the vast majority of genetic diagnosis involves the use of PCR. This is true for a variety of reasons, including (1) only a small amount of tissue

(DNA) is needed, such as that obtained from a hair bulb or cheek swab; (2) PCR is especially effective for indirect analysis using polymorphic markers; and (3) although many initial studies used PCR to amplify probes for Southern blot analysis or to amplify segments for direct mutation analysis using restriction enzyme analysis, newer analyses use PCR to amplify segments for allele-specific oligonucleotides (ASOs) or for DNA sequencing.

With DNA sequencing for an increasing number of genes and specific mutations, many diagnostic analyses involve both ASO and direct DNA sequencing.[22, 61] ASO analysis involves the amplification of a DNA segment of the gene in question and hybridization (usually in a dot blot) with a specific oligonucleotide. This oligonucleotide may contain a normal (wild-type) sequence or a mutation. The hybridization is so precise that hybridization will not occur if there is one base change. Therefore, this can be used to detect whether an individual carries a normal and a mutant allele. Also, because of the proliferation of identified sequences, DNA sequencing is used more frequently for mutation analysis. These studies are used for many disorders, including *connexin 26* analysis for deafness, Rett syndrome, and prion disease.

Applications: Diagnosis of Fragile X Syndrome

The utility of DNA molecular technology in the diagnosis of genetic diseases is strikingly apparent when considering the advances made in the diagnosis of fragile X syndrome. Fragile X syndrome is the most common inherited cause of mental retardation, with an incidence of approximately 1 in 1200 among the male population and 1 in 2500 among the female population. In addition to mental retardation and behavioral problems, men affected with fragile X syndrome often have characteristic physical features, including a long face with prominent forehead and prognathia, large ears, and macro-orchidism. Affected women generally have a similar but milder phenotypic expression of facial characteristics and developmental handicap.[21] Before the underlying genetic defect leading to fragile X syndrome was elucidated, diagnosis depended on the expression of a fragile site on the long arm of the X chromosome at Xq27.3 in cells cultured under conditions of folate deprivation. However, diagnostic accuracy was limited by variable expression of the fragile site (generally less than 50% in affected individuals, and even more unpredictable in carrier individuals).

Localization and isolation of the gene causing fragile X syndrome dramatically reduced the issues related to diagnostic uncertainty. Fragile X syndrome is one of approximately eight recently characterized genetic diseases (along with Huntington disease and myotonic dystrophy) that have an underlying defect caused by expansion of a repeated trinucleotide sequence within the relevant gene (discussed previously). These disorders show expansions in the 5' untranslated region, in the 3' untranslated region, or within the gene itself. The expansion increases in

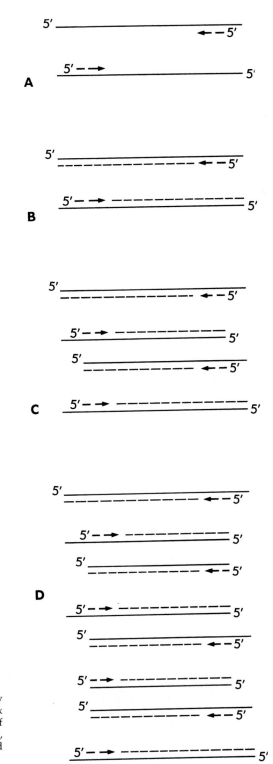

FIGURE 7–17. Polymerase chain reaction. In each round of amplification, newly synthesized strands are indicated by broken lines. *A,* Denatured DNA duplex showing hybridization of oligonucleotide primers. *B,* First-round synthesis of complementary strands, producing two DNA duplexes from the original one. *C,* Products of the second round of amplification. *D,* Products of the third round of amplification.

successive generations, leading to earlier detection and, in some cases, more severe phenotypic consequences. In the case of fragile X syndrome, the mutation involves expansion of the nucleotide sequence CGG, near the 5' untranslated end of the *FMR1* gene, to more than 200 repeats in affected individuals. Normal individuals carry approximately 6 to 50 CGG repeats, whereas the premutation state ranges from 50 to 200 repeats. The normal allele range and the premutation range overlap somewhat, but most normal alleles are less than 50 repeats, with an average of 29 to 30 repeats. Men and women carrying a premutation are unaffected, but there is a disparate risk to their offspring. A premutation can increase to a full expansion mutation *only* after transmission through a female meiosis. Therefore, a male premutation carrier can have only unaffected daughters with premutations, but they are at risk of transmitting an expanded mutation to their offspring. The larger the size of the premutation in a woman, the greater the risk of full mutation in her children.[67, 73]

Expansion to the full mutation of more than 200 CGG repeats is almost always associated with methylation of the promoter region of the gene and consequential gene inactivation. Although it is clear that gene inactivation by methylation is an important mechanism in the expression of the fragile X phenotype, the effects are not always predictable, especially in women. However, the methylation status and the size of the trinucleotide repeat of the *FMR1* gene form the basis for the accurate diagnosis of the genotype of individuals at risk of being carriers or being affected.

The techniques applicable to molecular diagnosis of fragile X syndrome are PCR analysis and Southern blot analysis. Each has intrinsic advantages and disadvantages. PCR analysis is used to amplify a fragment of DNA encompassing the repeat region. The size of the PCR-amplified DNA gives a close approximation of the number of CGG repeats in an allele of a given individual. PCR analysis is extremely accurate in sizing alleles in the normal, premutation, and borderline expansion ranges. Very large mutations involving high numbers of repeats are not as amenable to PCR amplification and may go undetected in PCR assays. In addition, rare cases of fragile X syndrome have been identified with a microdeletion in the Xq27.3 region, which precludes PCR amplification. Southern blot analysis is the tool of choice to demonstrate the presence of full mutations, and it also has the advantage of providing simultaneous assessment of methylation status. The size of the repeat and the methylation status of the *FMR1* allele can be determined by using a methylation-sensitive restriction endonuclease that is unable to cleave methylated sites. The disadvantages of Southern blot analysis include the need for larger quantities of genomic DNA, more labor-intensive procedures, and production of only an approximate, relative determination of allele size rather than a more precise estimate of the number of CGG repeats.[73] An example of *FMR1* diagnosis is shown in Figure 7–18. The American College of Medical Genetics has established guidelines for appropriate referrals for diagnostic testing of individuals and families that may be at risk for fragile X syndrome.[51]

The number of genetic diseases for which DNA diagnosis is feasible continues to grow. Early on, much of the effort in the development of these capabilities focused on severe diseases of childhood, such as CF and Tay-Sachs disease. There, the emphasis has been on prenatal testing for families wishing to avoid the birth of an affected child. DNA testing for many adult-onset diseases is either available or under development. Huntington disease is the prototype of an adult-onset disease for which presymptomatic DNA diagnosis is available, but the resulting information cannot be used to alter the course of the disease. In this situation, many at-risk individuals decline DNA testing. As DNA testing for more common conditions with genetic susceptibility factors becomes available, it is important to establish how the resulting information can be used and to involve the patient in the decision-making process.

MULTIFACTORIAL DISORDERS

Many of the more common birth defects, such as cleft lip and palate or spina bifida, cannot be explained on the basis of a mendelian pattern of inheritance, yet a

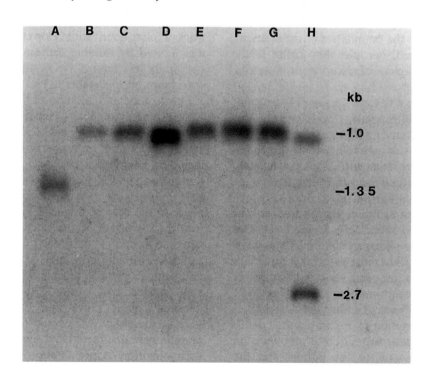

FIGURE 7–18. Molecular diagnosis of premutation carrier status in an affected female patient with fragile X syndrome, and Southern blot analysis of CGG repeats in genomic DNA digested by PST-1 and hybridized with probe PX6. Lanes B through G are results from normal men with unexpanded *FMR1* alleles about 1 kb in size. Lane A is DNA from a man with an *FMR1* premutation expanded to 1.35 kb with approximately 150 CGG repeats. Lane H is the DNA pattern from an affected woman with one normal allele of approximately 1 kb and a second allele of 2.7 kb, representing a full mutation with more than 600 CGG repeats.

familial tendency or liability has been recognized in their occurrence. Medical problems in adults, such as certain forms of cancer, hypertension, and diabetes mellitus, also fit into this category of increased familial risk. Although some specific forms of these disorders might be due to single gene defects (e.g., cancer), they are most often thought to result from a combination of additive genetic factors that lead to increased liability or threshold for expression plus environmental factors that trigger manifestations of the disorder in development. This combination of multiple gene liability and extrinsic environmental interaction is called *multifactorial inheritance*. Genetic traits that result from the additive effect of many genes are called *polygenic traits*. These terms often are used interchangeably in practice. Polygenic traits are generally quantitative rather than qualitative and follow a normal or gaussian distribution in the population. Common examples are height and blood pressure.

The evidence that genetic factors are important in common diseases and birth defects is derived from epidemiologic studies that compare the frequency of disease among related individuals with the frequency among the population at large. Some of the evidence for genetic influence can be summarized as follows:

1. Certain disorders occur more frequently among certain ethnic groups or those with particular racial backgrounds, such as neural tube defects in Ireland or northern India.
2. There is a higher frequency of specific birth defects among relatives of affected individuals, and this frequency is proportional to the degree of relatedness. For example, the percentage of siblings of an individual with cleft lip with or without cleft palate who are similarly affected is 4.1% (first-degree relative); of nieces and nephews, 0.8% (second-degree relative); and of first cousins, 0.3% (third-degree relative).[6]
3. The most convincing evidence of the genetic basis for multifactorial inheritance comes from twin studies. If a disorder is inherited in a mendelian fashion, there will be 100% concordance between monozygotic twins, who are genetically identical. Dizygotic twins, who share approximately half their genes, are expected to be 50% concordant. If a trait is multifactorial, with a significant genetic component, there is likely to be a high degree of concordance for identical twins (but less than 100%) and a much higher degree of concordance than for nonidentical twins. For example, the concordance for cleft lip and palate between monozygotic twins is 40%, whereas the concordance between dizygotic twins is only 4%—still significantly higher than in second- or third-degree relatives.

The observations with regard to multifactorial genetic traits have led to the threshold model of genetic liability. This model assumes that there is a continuous distribution of genetic risk for a specific disorder and that affected individuals fall to the extreme right of the genetic liability (Fig. 7–19). First-degree rela-

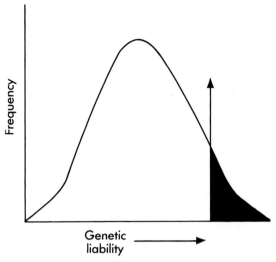

FIGURE 7–19. Model of genetic threshold for multifactorial disease. Liability for a particular trait follows a normal distribution, but abnormal classes or affected individuals exceed the threshold.

tives who share only half of their genes also have a genetic risk threshold that falls to the right of the general population, but not as extreme as the displacement in affected individuals. As the degree of relationship to the affected individual decreases, the genetic liability for the relative begins to approach the average liability for the general population.

Prediction of recurrence risks for multifactorial genetic disorders using the threshold model is based on empirical data and cannot be done specifically, as in mendelian disorders. There are, however, general guidelines with regard to these disorders and recurrence risks:

1. Recurrence risks represent average risks and vary among families. The exact risk cannot be given for any specific family member, but it decreases greatly with a decrease in the degree of relationship.
2. The risk within the family increases with the number of affected family members. For example, if one sibling has cleft lip with or without cleft palate, the risk of recurrence in another sibling is 4%; if two siblings are affected, the risk rises to 10%.
3. The risk increases with the severity of the malformation or the disease. The recurrence risk for unilateral cleft lip without cleft palate in a sibling is 2.5%, but it rises to 6% if the defect is bilateral with cleft palate.
4. When a multifactorial disorder is found more often in one sex than in the other, offspring of the lesser-affected sex are at higher risk. Congenital pyloric stenosis, for example, occurs five times more frequently in men than in women. The threshold of genetic liability for girls is therefore higher than for boys, and a girl who is affected is expected to have more genes or a larger genetic predilection to transmit to her offspring. Thus the risk for a son of an affected woman with pyloric

stenosis is 19.4%, and the risk for a daughter is 7.3%. Conversely, the risk for a son of an affected man is only 5.5%, and for a daughter is 2.4%.

One of the major difficulties in predicting and understanding recurrence risks for multifactoral genetic disorders is the role of environmental factors (see Chapter 12). The initial problem of identifying individuals with the genetic predilection is compounded by a lack of knowledge and understanding about the environmental components that trigger the developmental expression of birth defects or disease states. It seems likely that future research on genetic diseases will focus, first, on identification of genes that additively create threshold susceptibility and, second, on identification and alteration of environmental conditions that may lead to expression.[6, 40, 57]

A specialized type of multifactorial inheritance relates to the complex disorders. These disorders, such as asthma, hypertension, obesity, cancer, and heart disease, are still poorly understood, but because of their increased frequency, they are now being studied.[19, 55] It is hoped that future elucidation of the genes involved in these disorders will lead to new treatments.

ENVIRONMENTAL DISORDERS

Environmental causes of birth defects fall into three major categories: congenital infections, drug and chemical exposures, and physical agents, such as radiation exposure. Approximately 7% of congenital malformations are estimated to result from environmental factors. The degree to which an infant is affected by prenatal toxic exposure depends on two major factors: the stage in the embryo's or fetus's development at which the exposure occurs, and, as discussed previously, the genetic susceptibility of the mother and the fetus to the external toxic factor (see also Chapter 12).

During the period of gametogenesis, environmental exposure to toxic agents is probably lethal to these cells. There have been no studies in which preconceptual drug use has been shown to produce a statistically significant teratogenic effect on subsequent pregnancies. It is thought that the egg may be more vulnerable as a receptacle for toxic effects because of its extensive cytoplasmic, as well as nuclear, contribution to early embryonic development. In contrast, the contribution of sperm is limited to nuclear genetic information.

An "all or nothing" effect on cells resulting from potentially lethal environmental damage to the gamete probably extends from preconception throughout the postconceptual period to the time of primitive streak formation, about 3 weeks into human development. Exposure during this time most likely results in death of the embryo rather than survival of the fetus with major malformations.

Teratogenic effects of environmental agents are most severe during the subsequent period of develop-

ment, weeks 4 to 9 of gestation (see Chapter 12). Drugs for which a cause-and-effect relationship exists between exposure during this stage of gestation and major malformations include thalidomide, hydantoin, trimethadione, warfarin, amniopterin, ethanol, valproic acid, retinoic acid, and methyl mercury (resulting in Minamata disease) (see Chapter 10). Although high levels of androgens have been implicated as potentially masculinizing agents in the developing female embryo, only the effects of diethylstilbestrol (DES) on fetal development have been well documented. Birth control pills, in contrast, are thought to be unlikely teratogens. Infectious agents recognized as teratogens in the developing embryo include rubella, cytomegalovirus, herpes simplex types 1 and 2, toxoplasmosis, equine encephalitis virus, and syphilis. Varicella is considered a potential teratogen. Viral infections before the ninth week of gestation generally result in widespread damage to multiple organ systems (see Chapters 22 and 37). Extremely high levels of radiation exposure during this period appear to have a more limited effect, that of microcephaly. After the ninth week of gestation, the effects of teratogenic agents are more likely to be manifest as organ damage or growth disturbance rather than malformation. For each organ system, there is a critical period of development in which malformation may result from teratogenic interference. Table 7–1 lists the critical time frames for some of the more common congenital malformations.

Questions about teratogenic risks during pregnancy are always extremely difficult to answer. For most drugs, information about their safety or the possibility of low-level teratogenic effects has not been established in human beings, and extrapolation from animal studies may lead to erroneous conclusions. Mouse and rat embryos are relatively insensitive to thalidomide, but it is the most notorious of the recognized human teratogens and also severely affects monkey and rabbit embryos. Furthermore, case reports of exposure in humans are difficult to interpret because of the limited number of them and the wide variation in timing and amount of exposure. More information is available on the effect of radiation exposure in humans because of studies done on survivors of the atomic bomb explosions in Japan and their descendants and on survivors of the nuclear accident at Chernobyl. Radiation exposure of 10 rad or less to the mother is considered a reasonable upper limit for defining low risk to the fetus. Only under extremely unusual circumstances would diagnostic medical x-ray exposure exceed this limit. By comparison, the level of natural background radiation varies from 80 to 1000 mrad per year, depending on location, and a single chest x-ray would result in an exposure of approximately 100 to 200 mrad.

Counseling parents about birth defects with a suspected environmental cause must be a cautious undertaking. Parental guilt generated by such a suspected association can be overwhelming, and raising this issue may lead to questions of legal liability. If causality by an environmental agent can be estab-

TABLE 7–1   TIME FRAME FOR DEVELOPMENT OF COMMON CONGENITAL MALFORMATIONS

SITE OF MALFORMATION	MALFORMATION	TIME OF DEVELOPMENT
Face	Cleft lip	5–7 wks
	Posterior cleft palate	8–12 wks
Gastrointestinal tract	Esophageal atresia plus tracheoesophageal fistula	4 wks
	Rectal atresia (with fistula)	6 wks
	Malrotation	10 wks
	Omphalocele	10 wks
	Duodenal atresia	7–8 wks
Central nervous system	Anencephaly	3–4 wks
	Meningomyelocele	4 wks
Cardiovascular system	Transposition of great vessels	5 wks
	Ventricular septal defect	5–6 wks
Genitourinary system	Agenesis of the kidney	30 days
	Extroversion of the bladder	4 wks
	Bicornuate uterus	10 wks
	Retained testis (cryptorchidism)	36–40 wks
	Hypospadias	12 wks
Limb	Aplasia of the radius	38 days
	Syndactyly	6 wks

lished, however, parents may be reassured about future pregnancies, particularly if maternal immunity to a viral agent can be demonstrated or a certain drug can be avoided. Counseling parents about environmental toxic exposure during pregnancy should be done as neutrally as possible, presenting the most current information about the agent and all available options, including prenatal evaluation. The parents' decision to terminate a pregnancy must be reached on the basis of an honest presentation and interpretation of risk.[59]

GENETIC EVALUATION AND GENETIC COUNSELING

The evaluation plan to ascertain a possible genetic cause in an infant with congenital anomalies varies somewhat, depending on the child's age and condition. Obviously, evaluating a fetal death is more difficult than examining a living child. Nevertheless, vigorous efforts should be made to evaluate the fetus, particularly if it had suspected genetic abnormalities. One of the most frustrating problems for health care providers and families alike in attempting to assess the genetic risks for future pregnancies is the lack of information about the nature of abnormalities and the lack of etiologic evidence in a previous pregnancy loss. Couples coping with the death of a newborn with severe anomalies may refuse an autopsy and internal examination, only to find later that such information would have been helpful in defining genetic risks for future pregnancies and for other family members. One of the roles of the genetic counselor in this situation is to provide psychological support for the couple while explaining the need to obtain an-

swers that the couple will find valuable once their intense grief has subsided.

An organized plan for the evaluation of a fetus or child with suspected genetic disorders must always include a detailed family history, including pedigree and pregnancy history. This information provides important clues in separating genetic disorders from nongenetic causes. The minimal history should include the age, sex, and present health of all first-degree relatives (parents and siblings) and second-degree relatives (aunts, uncles, and grandparents). Questions about previous stillborns or spontaneous abortions should always be asked, because this valuable information is rarely volunteered. Ethnic background, as well as the possibility of consanguinity, should be elicited. The pregnancy history, including any maternal disease such as diabetes or epilepsy; maternal weight gain; fetal activity in utero; a detailed description of temporary maternal illness, particularly viral infections; and drug exposure, both over-the-counter and prescription, should be sought.

The physical examination of the fetus or child should be as extensive and detailed as possible, with particular attention paid to minor structural deviations (see also Chapter 26). Careful measurements of body proportions and facial features should be collected for comparison with standard measures for age and sex. Dermatoglyphic characteristics and ophthalmologic examinations may provide useful diagnostic clues. Radiologic studies, including bone films, computed tomography scans, and sonograms, should be used extensively for the examination of possible internal malformations. Laboratory tests are essential and should include cytogenetic studies, including FISH analysis; metabolic screening to rule out inborn errors of metabolism; and DNA studies, as appropriate. Last, photographs should be taken, as well as standard x-ray films, as part of a permanent file to provide a basis for comparison of progressive changes in the living child or to form the basis for re-evaluation of unknown disorders as new syndromes and diseases are delineated.

Although the foregoing aspects of genetic evaluation are generally attainable from a living child, it is often difficult to obtain similar evaluations of a fetus or stillborn. Unfortunately, such evaluations are not standard practice in many hospital pathology departments, and it is important to establish with the pathologist in advance the precise studies that may be informative for genetic assessment.

Counseling the parents of a child with a genetic disorder or birth defect should be tempered by recognition of the major emotional responses of the parents: anger, grief, and guilt. Because individual genetic diseases are so rare and because 95% occur with no family history, denial, frustration, and a sense of isolation are common reactions of parents and may impede their understanding of the nature of the disorder (see Chapter 32).

The course of genetic counseling after the birth of an affected child generally consists of two phases: first, an information-gathering stage focused on the nature of the problem and the prognosis for the child, and second, consideration of the genetic risks for future pregnancies or for other family members. If the couple anticipates future pregnancies, a major issue is whether prenatal diagnosis is possible and, if so, what diagnostic procedures are available and at what stage of the pregnancy. The time interval between the two phases of genetic counseling may be considerable for some couples, and emotional trauma may preclude their clear understanding of genetic issues, which is often difficult for even the most scientifically sophisticated parents. For these reasons, it is important that any counseling discussions be followed up by written explanations from the geneticist, reviewing and re-emphasizing the various points of concern.[26]

PRENATAL GENETIC DIAGNOSIS

Prenatal genetic evaluations fall into two general categories: generalized screening tests to identify pregnancies at risk, and specialized diagnostic tests to recognize a specific genetic risk to the fetus. Generalized screening can determine those couples with an increased risk for abnormality before the birth of an affected child. It is limited to a few genetic diseases associated with particular ethnic backgrounds, including screening for the carrier state for Tay-Sachs disease in individuals of Eastern European (Ashkenazi) Jewish heritage, for β-thalassemia in those of Mediterranean ancestry (Italians, Greeks, Sephardic Jews), for α-thalassemia in Chinese and Southeast Asian peoples, and for sickle cell trait and other hemoglobinopathies in blacks. As more information about the nature of common genetic diseases is learned, screening for the carrier state undoubtedly

will increase. The identification of the most common mutations in CF (see previous discussion) indicates that over 95% of the carriers for this disorder in those of Northern European ancestry and at least 90% in other populations can be identified. Although screening for CF is currently recommended only for those with a family history of the disorder, more widespread screening programs have been initiated at many genetics centers.

Another prenatal test that falls into the category of general screening is a maternal serum α-fetoprotein (AFP) determination performed at 15 to 20 weeks' gestation. This inexpensive test to measure the amount of AFP traversing from the fetal circulation into the maternal blood stream is unique in that both high and low levels of AFP correlate with increased risk for specific birth defects.

Elevations of maternal serum AFP identify nearly 100% of the fetuses with anencephaly, 70% to 85% with open spina bifida, and 70% with ventral wall defects, in addition to a diverse group of miscellaneous fetal anomalies (e.g., urogenital malformations) that affect amniotic fluid volume or fetal circulation and placental function. In addition to screening for fetal abnormalities, maternal serum AFP elevations are predictive for poor pregnancy outcome and complications in the third trimester, including increased risk for miscarriage, fetal death, stillbirth, prematurity, intrauterine growth retardation, and preeclampsia.[43]

Decreased levels of AFP interpreted in conjunction with maternal age were initially able to identify a cohort of pregnancies at increased risk for Down syndrome—a particularly valuable association, because 80% to 85% of babies with Down syndrome are born to women younger than age 35. Trisomy 13 and trisomy 18 fetuses also are found with reduced amounts of AFP.

Subsequent studies of maternal age and low maternal serum AFP in a prospective trial of women younger than 35 used a second-trimester Down syndrome risk of 1:270 (the specific risk for a woman who will be 35 at delivery) and a false positive rate of 5%. Initially, 4.7% screened positive for Down syndrome, 2% were reclassified as not at risk after sonographic dating correction, 2.7% were offered amniocentesis, and 2.1% chose the procedure. One case of Down syndrome was identified for every 90 amniocentesis procedures performed. When using maternal age and maternal serum AFP, the detection rate in women younger than 35 was approximately equal to that when using age alone in women older than 35.[43]

Two other maternal serum tests are used, in conjunction with AFP, for predictive Down syndrome screening. One, *unconjugated estriol* (uE$_3$), is a product of fetal adrenal gland and fetal liver biosynthesis, with placental modification before entering the maternal circulation. Levels of uE$_3$ that fall below the normal range suggest an increased risk for Down syndrome, as do low levels of AFP. However, higher than expected levels of β-*human chorionic gonadotropin* (β-hCG) in the second trimester of pregnancy correlate with Down syndrome in the fetus. AFP is the least sensitive discriminator in identifying Down syndrome pregnancies, with a sensitivity of about 15% to 20%, followed by uE_3, which detects about 25%. The most sensitive discriminator is β-hCG (40%).

Use of these three maternal serum tests in combination with maternal age has been adopted by centers throughout the United States and Europe. Triple screening has been tested prospectively in women younger than age 35, as well as in older women. Initially, 6.6% of younger women screened positive, with a risk of 1:270 or greater, but the true positive rate fell to 4.4% with sonographic correction of gestational dating. Of the remaining women who screened positive and who chose amniocentesis, one affected pregnancy was identified for every 36 amniocentesis procedures, for an overall Down syndrome detection rate of 58%.[46] When the triple screen was prospectively applied to a population of women age 35 or older, 89% of the cases of Down syndrome were identified, using a cutoff for amniocentesis of 1:200.[20] These results led to the suggestion that universal referral for amniocentesis because of maternal age can be modified by maternal serum triple-screen testing to reduce unnecessary amniocentesis procedures and to decrease the small risk of procedure-related pregnancy loss. This approach has been taken outside of the United States, but most referrals in the United States are still based on advanced maternal age.

New approaches for such screening have also been tested. Several laboratories are beginning to use a quadriplex marker screening, rather than just triple marker screening. The most recent addition to this testing is the substance inhibin. Inhibin is produced mainly from the placenta and is part of the transforming growth factor-β superfamily. Testing for serum inhibin A has been extremely promising, and it is estimated that its addition to triple screening will lead to positive screening of 7% to 8% of the population. Although β-hCG is the most sensitive discriminator for identifying Down syndrome pregnancies, inhibin is almost as effective, with a detection rate of 37%.[71]

Other testing, specifically in the first trimester, has been initiated. Three promising methodologies include PAPP-A, free β-hCG, and ultrasonographic detection of nuchal translucency. PAPP-A is a homodimer from the placenta whose function is unknown. In the first trimester, PAPP-A is decreased in Down syndrome, and free β-hCG is increased. When PAPP-A and β-hCG are combined with nuchal translucency detection, which measures skin thickness at the posterior neck, initial studies indicate that detection rates for Down syndrome are equal to those obtained with triple screening in the second trimester. Confirmatory studies of this methodology are still ongoing.

In pregnancies with this trisomy, serum levels of all three common second-trimester markers are greatly diminished, but the specificity for trisomy 18 detection is greatest with uE_3 measurement.[49] In addition to trisomy 18, 45,X pregnancies can be detected, but trisomy 13 pregnancies are not predictably screened

by triple-marker analysis of maternal serum. This is one reason why maternal serum screening has not been accepted as a standard of care in the genetics and obstetrics communities in the United States, particularly in women older than age 35.

Specialized prenatal diagnostic procedures are offered when there are known genetic risks. In contrast to the generalized screening tests, these procedures are individualized, require special techniques or training, and may involve procedure-related risk to the pregnancy. The generally accepted reasons for referral for genetic counseling and possible prenatal diagnosis include:

1. Advanced maternal age, usually 35 or older at delivery.
2. A previous fetus or child with a chromosomal abnormality or other major birth defect.
3. A family history of a specific genetic disorder.
4. One parent who is a known carrier for a chromosomal translocation or rearrangement with abnormal reproductive consequences.
5. A high or low maternal serum AFP level or abnormal triple screen.
6. A maternal disease associated with congenital malformations.
7. Parents who are known carriers of a specific genetic disorder.
8. Environmental exposure during pregnancy to drugs, medications, infections, or other recognized environmental hazards.
9. Known or suspected consanguinity.
10. Abnormal prenatal untrasonographic findings (see later).

ULTRASONOGRAPHIC DIAGNOSIS

The prenatal diagnostic procedure with the greatest potential for delineating abnormalities in a developing fetus is ultrasonography, which has come into widespread use as a safe, accurate method of defining fetal anatomy (see Chapter 8). It is estimated that approximately 80% of major fetal abnormalities can be diagnosed by this technology in the second trimester of pregnancy. Among the anomalies that can be diagnosed by the 16th week of pregnancy (or earlier, in many instances) by ultrasonographic examination are anencephaly, hydrocephalus, spina bifida, encephalocele, omphalocele, gastroschisis, renal agenesis, polycystic kidney disease, cystic hygroma, ascites, diaphragmatic hernia, and duodenal atresia.

Fetal echocardiography has been increasingly used to diagnose many congenital disorders of the heart and circulatory system. Disorders of the skeletal system, including those characterized by the absence of a bone, such as thrombocytopenia-absent radius syndrome, or by extra bone, such as polydactyly, also can be defined by ultrasonography. Skeletal dysplasias can be diagnosed by the characteristic shortening and bowing of the limbs compared with sonographic standards of limb length and appearance at comparable gestational ages. Defects in mineralization of bones found with disorders such as hypophospha-tasia or osteogenesis imperfecta also can be detected by ultrasonographic evaluation.[36]

The use of vaginal ultrasonographic probes and the improved resolution of modern ultrasonographic equipment have led to the diagnosis of many fetal anomalies, even in the first trimester, by experienced operators. The diagnostic limitation for first-trimester evaluations is manifestation of the anomaly in relation to the developmental sequence. For example, herniation of the bowel can occur until 13 weeks' gestation, so that a true diagnosis of omphalocele is precluded until the second trimester.

AMNIOCENTESIS

Amniocentesis has become widely accepted as the standard method for determining whether a fetus is affected by a wide variety of chromosomal disorders, metabolic diseases, or disorders detected by DNA analysis. The desquamated fetal cells and amniocytes from the amnion provide a source of mitotically active cells that can be used for cytogenetic evaluation or to establish cultures for enzymatic determinations or DNA analysis. Amniotic fluid itself can be used for AFP analysis, and acetylcholinesterase electrophoresis can be used to detect open neural tube defects in pregnant women with either a family history of such defects or elevations of maternal serum AFP. Enzyme analysis and metabolite measurements of amniotic fluid have provided diagnostic information in some genetic disorders, such as defects in the urea cycle, in which abnormal levels of metabolites may be found in the amniotic fluid. DNA analysis of amniotic fluid is possible for any disorder in which a PCR-based assay is used and only small amounts of DNA are needed.

Amniocentesis is traditionally performed at 16 to 18 weeks' gestation using ultrasonographic guidance. Approximately 20 to 30 mL of amniotic fluid is aspirated through a 20- to 22-gauge spinal needle into a sterile syringe. The first few milliliters of fluid are withdrawn in a separate syringe and discarded before aspiration of the sample for diagnosis. This is done to preclude contamination of the amniotic fluid cultures with maternal skin cells, which may lead to discrepant cytogenetic analysis. At this stage of pregnancy, the amniotic fluid volume of the uterus is rapidly replenished by the active urine output of the fetal kidneys. Amniocentesis is generally successful in greater than 95% of cases, with only one needle insertion necessary if performed by an experienced physician. Similarly, the success rate for establishing cell cultures from amniotic fluid cells is expected to be greater than 99%, although there may be wide variation in the rate of growth because of variation in the number of viable cells in the sample and the types of cells obtained. Cytogenetic analysis generally is completed within 7 to 12 days of the procedure.

The risk of pregnancy loss attributable to amniocentesis is low, probably less than 1 in 200, or 0.5% above pregnancy losses in control studies matched for maternal age. Chorioamnionitis after amniocentesis has been reported, but the actual frequency has not been documented. A reasonable estimate of risk for this particular complication is 1 in 1000 or less. Fetal injury during amniocentesis is unlikely because of the ultrasonic guidance for needle insertion and usually is limited to superficial scars or dimpling of the skin. Spotting or leakage of amniotic fluid for several days after the procedure has been reported, a complication that occurs in about 1 in 300 to 1 in 500 cases.[4, 42, 63]

The major drawback to midtrimester amniocentesis for prenatal genetic diagnosis is the late gestational age when fetal abnormalities are confirmed. The option for elective termination of an affected pregnancy is complicated by the extreme psychological trauma of loss of a fetus whose movements are already perceived and whose size makes the pregnancy loss public knowledge. In addition, there are the physical complications of undergoing induction of labor, followed by labor and delivery itself. For this reason, there has been a move toward earlier prenatal diagnosis by means of early amniocentesis or chorionic villus sampling (CVS).

Early amniocentesis usually is offered at 12 to 15 weeks' gestation and is performed in much the same manner as the standard amniocentesis procedure. Modifications of the technique include using only a 22-gauge spinal needle and removing 1 mL of amniotic fluid per week of gestation. Ultrasound guidance is essential for the earlier amniocentesis procedure. Despite the smaller volume of sample obtained at this stage of gestation compared with midtrimester amniocentesis, the diagnostic turn-around time for cytogenetic analysis is comparable. This may reflect a larger percentage of mitotically active cells per milliliter of amniotic fluid at earlier gestational ages. In general, the complication rate for pregnancy loss after early amniocentesis at 13 to 14 weeks is similar to the midtrimester risk. There is increased difficulty in obtaining fluid before 13 weeks' gestation and a greater chance of culture failure, as well as a slightly increased risk of procedure-related pregnancy loss. There have been some reports of increased risk for rupture of membranes if the procedure is performed before 13 weeks' gestation. At 12 weeks, the amnion and chorion may not be fused, requiring a more vigorous technique for inserting the needle to prevent membrane "tenting," which has been estimated to occur in 5% to 10% of these early amniocentesis procedures.[42]

CHORIONIC VILLUS SAMPLING

The earliest prenatal diagnostic procedure routinely offered is CVS, in which a biopsy of the villi of the developing placenta is obtained at 8 to 11 weeks' gestation (usually between 9 and 10 weeks) from the last menstrual period. CVS can be performed transcervically by inserting a fine plastic catheter through the vagina and cervical os and, under ultrasonographic guidance, advancing the catheter to the edge of the developing placenta, the chorion frondosum. After the catheter is in position within the placenta, the stylet is removed, and a 20-mL syringe containing a small amount of cell culture medium is attached to the catheter. The sampling is accomplished by moving the tip of the catheter back and forth while applying suction to the syringe. Samples of chorionic villi of approximately 10 to 50 mg wet weight are obtained, an amount more than adequate for cytogenetic, biochemical, or DNA diagnostic studies.

An alternative method for CVS is the transabdominal approach, which is particularly successful if the placenta is located in an anterofundal uterine position and inaccessible by the transcervical method. The transabdominal method involves placement of an 18- to 19-gauge spinal needle under ultrasonographic direction through the maternal abdominal and uterine wall into the body of the placenta, similar to amniocentesis. A syringe containing medium is attached to the needle, which is moved vertically as suction is applied to aspirate villi. Slightly smaller amounts and more fragmented villi are obtained by this method.[3, 29]

The diagnostic tests that can be performed on cultured amniotic fluid cells have been adapted for use with CVS. Cytogenetic analysis can be performed directly on the cytotrophoblastic layer of the villi, which contains many cells in active mitosis, as well as on cells cultured from the villus fragments. Cytogenetic analysis is never performed on the cytotrophoblastic cells alone, as these results are not always reflective of the fetus. Although the accuracy of CVS in predicting cytogenetically abnormal fetuses is roughly comparable to the accuracy of amniocentesis, there are some differences. The rate of maternal cell contamination in cultures obtained from CVS is greater than in cultures obtained from amniocentesis. Furthermore, the amount of chromosomal mosaicism and the type of cytogenetic mosaicism found in placental tissue are much greater than that observed in cells of fetal origin. For this reason, about 1% of patients undergoing CVS may be offered amniocentesis to obtain fetal cells for confirmation of a CVS cytogenetic diagnosis.

The background fetal loss rate after normal first-trimester ultrasonography is approximately 2.5% to 3%. Pregnancy losses attributable to CVS range from 0.5% to 2% above the background rate, with the lowest loss rates reported by centers with the most experience in CVS. Losses after transcervical CVS may be from three main mechanisms: infection, premature rupture of membranes, and placental disruption. Infection is less problematic with transabdominal CVS, a major advantage of this approach. An additional concern with CVS is possible limb abnormalities associated with the procedure. Limb reduction defects initially were reported out of London and Chicago after both transabdominal and transcervical CVS. An increased incidence of limb reduction defects after CVS was not found in the initial U.S. collaborative CVS report, and such defects have since been largely limited to CVS procedures performed earlier than 66 days' gestation, involving the use of a large catheter or the recovery of a large sample size of villi, and

perhaps in which the operator was inexperienced.[29, 52, 63] However, some studies suggest that limb reduction defects are increased in CVS procedures done after 11 weeks.

The risks associated with CVS, though small, are higher than those associated with amniocentesis. Patients must understand that the convenience of first-trimester termination of an abnormal fetus may be outweighed by an increased risk of losing a normal pregnancy. Patients with only a small risk for genetic abnormalities, such as those associated with maternal age of 35 or older, or with a history of infertility may be reluctant to consider CVS, whereas a couple with a 25% risk for a metabolic genetic disease in their offspring would most likely consider the pregnancy loss rate associated with CVS a minimal concern.

FETAL BLOOD SAMPLING

The final major category of specialized prenatal testing is fetal blood sampling, also known as *percutaneous umbilical blood sampling* or cordocentesis. Percutaneous umbilical blood sampling is basically a modification of the amniocentesis procedure and is generally limited to pregnancies of more than 19 weeks' gestation. Under ultrasonographic guidance, a 20- to 22-gauge spinal needle is directed to the umbilical vein at the level of cord insertion into the placenta (umbilical cord root). Small syringes are used to prevent excessive suction that could cause collapse of the vein. Once blood is obtained, it is important to ascertain that the sample is fetal and not maternal. The larger diameter of fetal cells compared with maternal blood cells is the basis for determining the purity of the sample. This is most effectively accomplished by a Coulter cell channelyzer, which determines the frequency distribution of fetal versus maternal cells based on erythrocyte volume. At later gestational ages, when the size discrepancy between fetal and maternal cells is less marked, the *Kleihauer-Betke test*, based on the tendency of adult cells to lyse in an acid solution, can be used to measure the purity of a fetal blood sample.

The major indication for fetal blood sampling is to obtain rapid cytogenetic analysis within 48 to 72 hours, usually in late gestations when a congenital anomaly is detected close to term or close to the legal time limit for elective termination. In cases of suspected cytogenetic mosaicism found in cells from amniotic fluid, in which the abnormal cell line may be derived from amnion rather than fetus, fetal blood sampling may provide reassurance about the cytogenetic status of the fetus. Factor VIII levels have been determined in fetal blood when the prenatal diagnosis of hemophilia A was inconclusive, and serum enzyme levels have been measured in cases of suspected inherited metabolic disease. Finally, fetal blood sampling has been used in cases of suspected congenital infection to measure immunoglobulin M levels and in instances of isoimmunization and suspected fetal anemia (see Chapter 44). Because production of immunoglobulin M antibodies depends on gestational age and may vary with the infectious agent involved, the development of PCR for quick, direct testing of microbial DNA to confirm a fetal infection (e.g., cytomegalovirus or toxoplasmosis) has meant a return to amniocentesis as the more common diagnostic approach (see Chapter 37). Currently, fetal blood sampling has a limited but specific application compared with amniocentesis, and experience tends to be restricted to major tertiary referral centers, where the procedure-related risks are generally quoted as 1% to 3%.[42, 63]

ASSISTED REPRODUCTION

The development of in vitro fertilization and other assisted reproduction techniques, as well as advances in molecular genetics, is changing the scope of obstetrics and prenatal diagnosis. Preimplantation genetic diagnosis separates conception from pregnancy, thus offering couples at risk an alternative to diagnosis of the fetus and possible late termination of a well-developed pregnancy. With preimplantation analysis of genetic status, the cessation of development in the affected embryo is easily managed. Preimplantation diagnosis also opens the possibility for the development and implementation of directed gene therapy to correct known genetic defects.

Assisted reproduction technologies were initially developed to treat women with obstructive tube disease but are much more broadly applied today. Hormonal manipulation produced superovulation, and the recovery of multiple follicles was made possible by ultrasonographic visualization of the stimulated ovaries. Access to ova and their polar bodies gave rise to a new source of tissue for genetic testing. With in vitro techniques and micromanipulation of embryos in culture, blastomere and trophectoderm can be isolated and analyzed, with only the unaffected embryos implanted into the uterus.

Single sperm analysis is not possible, because this reproductive cell would be destroyed in the process of genetic analysis. The first polar body, therefore, represents the best opportunity for preconception genetic diagnosis. It is accessible through the zona pellucida and can be removed without affecting conception or later development. Analysis of the DNA of the polar body is most appropriate for women who are carriers for autosomal recessive diseases, autosomal dominant diseases, or X-linked disorders. The chromosome in the polar body can be analyzed directly and identified as carrying the normal or mutant gene. By inference, the genetic status of the complementary chromosome status in the egg can be determined.

Two options are available for postconception preimplantation genetic diagnosis. Blastomere biopsy (of one to two cells) can be performed at the eight-cell stage of the embryo, or trophectoderm cells can be removed later from the blastocyst (blastocyst biopsy). The former is the preferred method and is most widely used. However, animal studies have shown that the blastocyst can be biopsied, or more than 100

cells of the trophectoderm removed, without loss of hCG function or risk of abnormal development. The latter technique has the advantage of removing greater numbers of cells from the embryo for genetic analysis. However, after this procedure, fewer embryos progress through the blastocyst stage, and pregnancy rates after transfer may decline. Because the trophoblast biopsy does not sample the embryonic disc directly, there is a risk of diagnostic error because of confined placental mosaicism, just as that found with CVS. Nevertheless, a very small number of successful pregnancies have been achieved in couples at risk for Lesch-Nyhan syndrome (X-linked), fragile X syndrome, Tay-Sachs disease, and CF with preimplantation diagnosis of blastocysts.[4, 45, 63, 70]

Technologic advances in both molecular genetics and molecular cytogenetics have revolutionized the field of preimplantation genetics. The development of PCR analysis has allowed DNA extracted from one to a few cells to be selectively expanded to an amount sufficient for genetic analysis. This DNA is amenable to most mutation detection methods, including heteroduplex analysis, single-strand confirmation polymorphism, fluorescent PCR, and restriction digestion. However, the power of PCR to amplify small amounts of DNA represents the greatest difficulty in the technology, because of several associated problems. Unintended replication of contaminating DNA, such as that of the sperm adherent to the zona pellucida, allele dropout, and reduced amplification efficiency can all be sources of diagnostic error. Advances in FISH have also been crucial in the advancement of preimplantation genetic diagnosis. Initially used for embryo sexing for the diagnosis of X-linked traits, these studies have been enhanced by probe and technologic developments. FISH is commonly done using multicolor analysis with nine probes (13, 14, 15, 16, 18, 21, 22, X, and Y) to diagnose the most frequent aneuploidies in both live births and spontaneous abortions. There is a 10% to 15% chance of a misdiagnosis, as testing of one cell has been shown to be problematic owing to mosaicism. Both chromosome paints and subtelomeric probes have been used to study the segregation of translocations.

CONCLUSION

The growing number of diagnostic procedures now available for prenatal genetic evaluation has given couples at high genetic risk, who otherwise might have forgone parenthood, the opportunity to have healthy children. Despite the criticism that prenatal genetic evaluations are nothing more than procedures to eliminate defective fetuses, studies based on interviews with couples who have high genetic reproductive risks have demonstrated a very positive effect. The availability of prenatal diagnosis has led to many more planned conceptions and births of normal children than terminations of fetuses diagnosed as genetically abnormal. As the technology improves, it is likely that prenatal diagnoses will have even more positive effects, allowing couples to have healthy children and reducing the burden of genetic disease.

■ REFERENCES

1. Ashizawa T, et al: Characteristics of intergenerational contractions of the CTG repeat in myotonic dystrophy. Am J Hum Genet 54:414, 1994.
2. Baird PA, et al: Genetic disorders in children and young adults: A population study. Am J Hum Genet 42:677, 1988.
3. Brambati B, et al: Transabdominal and transcervical chorionic villus sampling: Efficiency and risk evaluation of 2411 cases. Am J Med Genet 35:160, 1990.
4. Brock DJH, et al: Prenatal Diagnosis and Screening. Edinburgh, Churchill Livingstone, 1992.
5. Carrel L, et al: An assay for X inactivation based on differential methylation at the fragile X locus, FMR1. Am J Med Genet 64:27, 1996.
6. Carter CO: Genetics of common disorders. Br Med Bull 32:21, 1976.
7. Carter NP, et al: Reverse chromosome painting: A method for the rapid analysis of aberrant chromosomes in clinical cytogenetics. J Med Genet 5:299, 1992.
8. Caskey CT, et al: Triplet repeat mutations in human disease. Science 256:784, 1992.
9. Cassidy SB: Uniparental disomy and genomic imprinting as causes of human genetic disease. Environ Mol Mutagen 25(suppl 26):13, 1995.
10. Cassidy SB, et al: Prader-Willi and Angelman syndromes and disorders of genomic imprinting. Rev Mol Med 77:140, 1998.
11. Clark BA, et al: Molecular cytogenetics. In Reed G, et al (eds): Diseases of the Fetus and Newborn, 2nd ed, vol 2. London, Chapman & Hall, 1995.
12. Clarke LA: Mitochondrial disorders in pediatrics: Clinical, biomedical and genetic implications. Pediatr Clin North Am 39:2, 1992.
13. DeGrouchy J, et al: Clinical Atlas of Human Chromosomes, 2nd ed. New York, John Wiley & Sons, 1984.
14. Elias S, et al: Maternal Serum Screening for Fetal Genetic Disorders. New York, Churchill Livingstone, 1992.
15. Emery AEH, et al: Principles and Practice of Medical Genetics, 3rd ed, vols 1 and 2. New York, Churchill Livingstone, 1997.
16. Firth H: Chorion villus sampling and limb deficiency—cause or coincidence? Prenat Diagn 13:1313, 1997.
17. Gardner RJM, et al: Chromosome Abnormalities and Genetic Counseling, 2nd ed. New York, Oxford University Press, 1996.
18. Gelehrter TD, et al: Principles of Medical Genetics, 2nd ed. Baltimore, Williams & Wilkins, 1998.
19. Grundy SM: Multifactorial causation of obesity: Implications for prevention. Am J Clin Nutr 67:563S, 1998.
20. Haddow JE, et al: Prenatal screening for Down's syndrome with use of maternal serum markers. N Engl J Med 327:588, 1992.
21. Hagerman RJ, et al: Fragile X-Syndrome: Diagnosis, Treatment, and Research, 2nd ed. Baltimore, Johns Hopkins University Press, 1996.
22. Hahn M, et al: Hereditary colorectal cancer: Clinical consequences of predictive molecular testing. Int J Colorectal Dis 4:184, 1999.
23. Hall JG: Human diseases and genomic imprinting. Results Probl Cell Differ 25:119, 1999.
24. Hall JG: Medical genetics. Pediatr Clin North Am 39:1, 1992.
25. Han JY, et al: Molecular cytogenetic characterization of 17 rob(13q14) Robertsonian translocations by FISH, narrowing the region containing the breakpoints. Am J Hum Genet 55:960, 1994.
26. Harper PS: Practical Genetic Counseling, 5th ed. Oxford, Butterworth Heinemann, 1998.
27. Heard E, et al: X-chromosome inactivation in mammals. Annu Rev Genet 31:571, 1997.
28. Jacobs PA, et al: Estimates of the frequency of chromosome abnormalities detectable using moderate levels of banding. J Med Genet 29:103, 1992.
29. Jenkins TM, et al: First trimester prenatal diagnosis: Chorionic villus sampling. Semin Perinatol 5:403, 1999.
30. Jones KL: Smith's Recognizable Patterns of Human Malformation, 5th ed. Philadelphia, WB Saunders Co, 1997.
31. Kallioniemi OP, et al: Comparative genomic hybridization: A rapid new method for detecting and mapping DNA amplification in tumors. Semin Cancer Biol 1:41, 1993.
32. Kalousek DK: Current topic: Confined placental mosaicism and intrauterine fetal development. Placenta 15:219, 1994.
33. Knoll JHM, et al: Angelman and Prader-Willi syndromes share a common chromosome 15 deletion but differ in parental origin of deletion. Am J Med Genet 32:285, 1989.
34. Kumar A, et al: Molecular characterization and delineation of subtle deletions in de novo "balanced" chromosomal rearrangements. Hum Genet 2:173, 1998.
35. Kuwano A, et al: Detection of deletions and cryptic translocations in Miller-Dieker syndrome by in situ hybridization. Am J Hum Genet 49:707, 1991.
36. Lachman RS, et al: Fetal imaging in the skeletal dysplasias. Clin Perinatol 17:3, 1990.
37. Lewin B: Genes VII. New York, Oxford University Press, 2000.
38. Lyon MF: Imprinting and X-chromosome inactivation. Results Probl Cell Differ 25:73, 1999.
39. Lyon MF: X-chromosome inactivation. Curr Biol 9:R235, 1999.
40. Marx J: Dissecting the complex diseases. Science 247:1540, 1990.
41. McKusick VA: Mendelian Inheritance in Man, 12th ed. Baltimore, Johns Hopkins University Press, 1998. Available online at: http://www.ncbi.nlm.nih.gov/query.fcgi?db=OMIM
42. Milunsky A: Genetic Disorders and the Fetus: Diagnosis, Prevention and Treatment, 4th ed. Baltimore, Johns Hopkins University Press, 1998.
43. Milunsky A, et al: Predictive values, relative risks and overall benefits of high and low maternal serum α-fetoprotein screening in singleton pregnancies: New epidemiologic data. Am J Obstet Gynecol 161:291, 1989.
44. Mitelman F: An International System for Human Cytogenetic Nomenclature (ISCN, 1995). S. Karger, Basel, 1995.
45. Munne S, et al: Positive outcome after preimplantation diagnosis of aneuploidy in human embryos. Hum Reprod 9:2191, 1999.
46. New England Regional Genetics Group Prenatal Collaborative Study: Combining maternal serum α-fetoprotein measurements and age to screen Down's syndrome in pregnant women under age 35. Am J Obstet Gynecol 160:575, 1989.
47. NCI initiative: A resource of arrayed BAC clones for the identification of cancer chromosome aberrations. Available at: http://genomics.roswellpark.org/human/rfa_meeting.html/
48. Nielsen J, et al: Chromosome abnormalities found among 34,910 newborn children: Results from a 13-year incidence study in Arhus, Denmark. Hum Genet 87:81, 1991.
49. Palomaki GE, et al: Risk-based prenatal screening for trisomy 18 using alpha-fetoprotein, unconjugated estriol and human chorionic gonadotropin. Prenat Diagn 15:713, 1995.
50. Peterson MB, et al: Use of short sequence repeat DNA polymorphisms after PCR amplification to detect the parental origin of the additional chromosome 21 in Down syndrome. Am J Hum Genet 48:65, 1991.
51. Policy Statement, American College of Medical Genetics: Fragile X syndrome: Diagnostic and carrier testing. Am J Med Genet 53:380, 1994.
52. Report of NICHHD Workshop on Chorionic Villus Sampling and Limb and Other Defects, Oct 20, 1992. Teratology 48:7, 1993.
53. Robinson WP, et al: Molecular studies of chromosomal mosaicism: Relative frequency of chromosome gain or loss and possible role of cell selection. Am J Hum Genet 56:444, 1995.
54. Romero R, et al: Prenatal Diagnosis of Congenital Anomalies. Norwalk, Conn, Appleton & Lange, 1988.
55. Schmitz G, et al: Recent advances in molecular genetics of cardiovascular disorders: Implications for atherosclerosis and diseases of cellular lipid metabolism. Pathol Oncol Res 2:152, 1998.
56. Schrock, E, et al: Spectral karyotyping refines cytogenetic diagnostics of constitutional chromosomal abnormalities. Hum Genet 3:255, 1997.

57. Scott J: Molecular genetics of common diseases. BMJ 295:769, 1987.

58. Scriver CR, et al: The Metabolic and Molecular Bases of Inherited Disease, 7th ed. New York, McGraw-Hill, 1995.

59. Shepard TH: Catalog of Teratogenic Agents, 9th ed. Baltimore, Johns Hopkins University Press, 1998.

60. Sherman SL, et al: Trisomy 21: Association between reduced recombination and nondisjunction. Am J Hum Genet 49:608, 1991.

61. Shuber AP, et al: High throughput parallel analysis of hundreds of patient samples for more than 100 mutations in multiple disease genes. Hum Mol Genet 3:337, 1997.

62. Simon DK, et al: Mitochondrial disorders: Clinical and genetic features. Annu Rev Med 50:111, 1999.

63. Simpson JL, et al: Essentials of Prenatal Diagnosis. New York, Churchill Livingstone, 1993.

64. Sirko-Osadsa DA, et al: Molecular refinement of karyotype: Beyond the cytogenetic band. Genet Med 1:254, 1999.

65. Speicher MR, et al: Karyotyping human chromosomes by combinatorial multi-fluor FISH. Nat Genet 4:368, 1996.

66. Spence JE, et al: Uniparental disomy as a mechanism for human genetic disease. Am J Hum Genet 42:217, 1988.

67. Tarleton JC, et al: Molecular genetic advances in fragile X syndrome. J Pediatr 122:167, 1993.

68. Therman E: Human Chromosomes: Structure, Behavior, Effects, 3rd ed. New York, Springer-Verlag, 1993.

69. Thompson MW, et al: Genetics in Medicine, 5th ed. Philadelphia, WB Saunders Co, 1991.

70. Verlinsky Y, et al: Prepregnancy genetic testing for age-related aneuploidies by polar body analysis. Genet Test 4:231, 1997.

71. Wald NJ, et al: Antenatal screening for Down's syndrome. J Med Screen 4:181, 1997.

72. Warburton D: De novo balanced chromosome rearrangements and extra marker chromosomes identified at prenatal diagnosis: Clinical significance a distribution of breakpoints. Am J Hum Genet 5:995, 1991.

73. Warren ST, et al: Advances in molecular diagnosis of fragile X syndrome. JAMA 271:536, 1994.

8 Perinatal Ultrasound

Kevin Muise

Nancy E. Judge

Stuart C. Morrison

Ultrasound is the primary imaging modality used for obstetric evaluation. In addition to being accurate, ultrasound has the major advantage of being safe during pregnancy.

PRINCIPLES OF ULTRASOUND

Ultrasound is a form of high-frequency energy that is produced by applying an electric current across a piezoelectric crystal. The crystal converts voltage to vibration at frequencies above the 20,000-cycles-per-second (cps) threshold of human hearing. Beams of these longitudinal waves are pulsed from diagnostic ultrasound transducers at frequencies that range from 2 to 10 million cps (2 to 10 MHz).[19] The beams that return to the transducer after tissue contact are reconverted by the crystal array into electric impulses, which can be processed to generate images. The behavior of ultrasound waves is governed by both the velocity characteristics for sound traveling through a specific tissue and the tissue density. Acoustic impedance is the product of density and velocity. The lowest impedances occur in fluids with characteristics similar to water, and they result in nearly echo-free through penetration by the beam. Air and bone possess high acoustic impedances and produce extremely strong echoes. Ultrasound is reflected at the interfaces between tissues with different acoustic impedances. When the intersection of the surfaces is larger than the width of the ultrasound beam, as in borders between bone and fluid, virtually all of the signal is reflected back directly to the transducer and displayed as strong echoes. In contrast, the ultrasound beam is dispersed by smaller interfaces within tissue microarchitecture, resulting in weak, scattered echoes. Tiny structures scatter sound circumferentially (Raleigh scattering), an effect that is essential for the detection of red blood cells and for Doppler assessment of blood flow.[4] The combination of through transmission, strong specular echoes, and scattered echoes provides the information for the pixel displays that are characteristic of contemporary gray-scale ultrasound images.

An ultrasound transducer receives reflected echoes at a ratio of about 1000:1 compared with the transmitted pulses. The delay time, signal amplitude, and deflection of the returning echoes are used to construct a spatial map of the gray-scale interfaces. Images are assembled by the microprocessor of the ultrasound unit, and they are refreshed at a rate of 20 to 30 frames per second for video display. This approximates the flicker/fusion rate of the human eye and permits continuous, "real time" scanning. Current technical limits of ultrasound become apparent when imaging is performed at extreme sizes or in three dimensions.

Attenuation of ultrasound signals occurs in inverse proportion to wavelength, because longer wavelengths interact with fewer interfaces. At higher frequencies, more information (and potentially, undesirable "noise") is generated, because more interfaces are encountered and defined. Intracavity transducers that use very high frequency signals achieve excellent resolution because they bypass fat and soft tissue. The transvaginal approach is routinely used for studies of the uterus and ovaries, for ectopic pregnancy, and for evaluating embryonic and early fetal structures. Acoustic "windows" provided by a full maternal bladder or plentiful amniotic fluid enhance transabdominal ultrasound images. Conversely, visibility is severely restricted by obesity, scar tissue, bowel gas, calcifications, or oligohydramnios.

Refinements of the basic transducer during the past three decades have encompassed electronically focusing or steering the beam, incorporating arrays of crystals, and reshaping both beam paths and transducer "footprints" to improve imaging abilities. Improved processing of signals permits users to target portions of an image for enlargement, enhanced gain, contrast, position, and orientation. Additional capabilities have been provided by the incorporation of M-mode and Doppler ultrasound. M-mode imaging is used for cardiographic studies; Doppler ultrasound permits evaluation of velocity, direction, or presence of blood flow. Prenatal Doppler studies that attempt to quantitate velocity and flow are subject to inherent limitations that are secondary to the narrow and tortuous character of fetal vessels. Color enhancement of Doppler spectra has greatly facilitated cardiac examinations and review of small vessel, low-flow circulations, such as those of the uterus, placenta, fetal brain, and kidneys, and it has illuminated normal and pathologic conditions.

Three-dimensional ultrasound is one of the most recent developments in imaging. Advances in position sensor and computer processor sophistication permit the assignment of a precise spatial location in three orthogonal planes for each pixel. The resulting data can be used to generate volumetric images for display from various simulated viewpoints. Initial limitations of three-dimensional technology include nonuniform engineering, relatively long signal acquisition and processing intervals with consequent image degradation from movement artifacts, and a prerequisite for near-ideal two-dimensional views. To date, few centers have extensive experience with three-dimensional ultrasound, making it difficult to predict this application's eventual role.

BIOEFFECTS AND THE SAFETY OF ULTRASOUND

One reason for the popularity of prenatal ultrasound is its lack of ionizing radiation. The initial perception of safety has not significantly diminished in spite of significant potential bioeffects from high-frequency sound. The principal safety concern regarding diagnostic ultrasound is its conversion to thermal energy when the radiant energy is absorbed by human tissue. Thermal effects are greatest in and near bony structures in the human fetus. Current equipment design is controlled by both federal regulation and voluntary guidelines to minimize temperature changes over the full range of transducer types throughout gestation.[1, 34] Contemporary ultrasound machines display information about power, frequency, and duration of exposure, facilitating future studies. Ultrasound energy has also been associated with cell lysis, cavitation, intracellular shearing forces, alterations of cell permeability, and alterations in chromosomal function, usually under conditions substantially different from those encountered during diagnostic ultrasound.[8]

Prenatal exposure to ultrasound may first occur during embryogenesis as well as episodically during central nervous system differentiation and development. Study results generally have been negative with respect to detrimental outcomes in somatic, sensory, and neurobehavioral development. Teratogenic effects have not been confirmed, and currently there does not appear to be oncogenic potential inherent in fetal ultrasound exposure. The extraordinary prevalence of prenatal ultrasound in industrialized nations for imaging, office auscultation, and antepartum or intrapartum fetal monitoring seems likely to make studies of bioeffects increasingly difficult to perform and interpret.

DIAGNOSIS OF PREGNANCY AND FETAL LOSS

Pregnancy can be diagnosed sonographically by the fifth postmenstrual week. An embryo with cardiac activity is usually visualized during the sixth week of gestation by the vaginal approach.[42] Ultrasound combined with quantitative human chorionic gonadotropin (hCG) determinations has become the standard approach in evaluating ectopic and failed intrauterine pregnancies. Threshold values of serum hCG vary from institution to institution, but they are used to anticipate visualization of the gestational sac.[44] The persistent lack of embryonic components or the absence of embryonic cardiac activity at an appropriate gestational age as determined by sac size or crown-rump length is sufficient to diagnose an embryonic loss.[10] Serial scans at 5- to 7-day intervals may be helpful in questionable cases. Under most conditions, at later gestational ages, it is possible to confirm fetal death in utero by demonstration of the fetal heart in uninterrupted asystole. The complete, sustained absence of fetal umbilical flow, aortic pulsation, and fetal movement has been used to support a finding of recent intrauterine death. In more prolonged cases, typical findings may include overriding calvarial bones, scalp edema, hydropic changes, or distorted fetal postures. Ultrasound has become the standard method for detecting fetal death because of its accessibility and accuracy.

VAGINAL ULTRASOUND AND MORPHOLOGIC EVALUATION

A recent development in the evaluation of fetal anatomy is the use of high-frequency vaginal transducers (5 to 7 MHz) during the early fetal period. Because familiarity with the transvaginal appearance of normal embryonic development has improved, this technique is increasingly used for the early detection of anomalies and aneuploidy.[26, 41] In some cases, the premonitory findings are transient, as with nuchal cysts, and the first-trimester study may be the only indication for invasive karyotype testing.[15] The higher resolution permits detailed, accurate evaluation of many fetal anatomic sites several weeks before transabdominal study, as long as the examiner remains cognizant of normal developmental milestones (Fig. 8–1). The transvaginal approach has been especially effective in visualizing fetal structures deep in the maternal pelvis, in excluding placenta previa,[29] and in establishing chorionicity of early multiple gestations. In obese patients and in those with extensive abdominal scarring, endovaginal study may provide the only opportunity for morphologic evaluation.

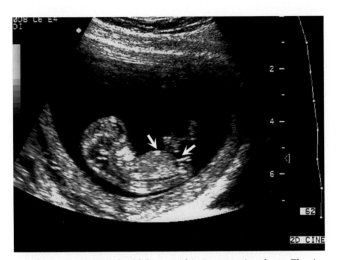

FIGURE 8–1. A 10-week-old fetus within its gestational sac. Physiologic midgut herniation is seen at this gestational age (arrows).

ESTIMATION OF GESTATIONAL AGE

CROWN-RUMP LENGTH

One of the most useful aspects of obstetric ultrasound is the ability to accurately assign gestational age throughout the majority of pregnancy. Only early hCG quantitation or known conception dating reliably exceeds the precision of an embryonic *crown-rump* measurement, which approximates gestational age to within plus or minus 3 to 5 days (Fig. 8–2).[16] Gestational sac measurements are also commonly used early in the first trimester, but they are less accurate because of variability in sac contours. The major disadvantage to these dating techniques is the early gestational age at which they must be performed. In many cases, the patient with poor dating information is also a late registrant for prenatal care. In other cases, the need for this level of dating accuracy is not recognized prospectively. A limitation of the crown-rump length is the reduced level of ana-

tomic detail that is provided by scans during the embryonic period. Morphology is often given precedence over chronology, with studies being postponed until the middle of the second trimester in an attempt to maximize the yield from a single scan.

CEPHALOMETRY

From the beginning of the second trimester, the most widely used method of estimating gestational age is the *biparietal diameter* (BPD). The measurement is taken at the level of the thalami, including the cavum septum pellucidum. The ovoid cross section of the skull is bisected at its widest point, measuring from the outer aspect of the superior table to the inner aspect of the inferior skull (Fig. 8–3). Through 34 weeks' gestation, the BPD is accurate to plus or minus 10 days. Thereafter, accuracy diminishes to plus or minus 3 weeks. The BPD may be compromised by molding and descent of the head into the maternal pelvis, and it is less reliable when the ratio between the BPD and the long axis of the skull is unusually large (brachycephaly) or small (dolichocephaly). *Head circumference* (HC) measurements may be more useful when the head assumes a less ovoid shape. The landmarks for the measurement of BPD and HC provide a useful starting point for a survey of the intracranial anatomy. The thalami and cerebral peduncles are hypoechoic sail-shaped and heart-shaped structures, respectively. The basilar artery can be seen pulsating on the anterior surface of the midbrain. The third ventricle is located between the anterior portions of the thalami and appears slitlike. The structures of the circle of Willis can be readily identified with color Doppler imaging. Using gray-scale ultrasound, pulsations of the internal carotid arteries may be seen in the region of the circle. Branches of the middle cerebral artery produce pulsations in the region of the sylvian fissures that appear as echogenic lines parallel to the lateral skull contour. Two echogenic lines parallel to the falx represent deep cerebral veins rather

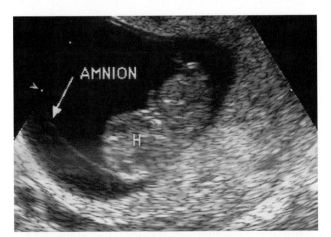

FIGURE 8–2. Transvaginal sonogram of a fetus at 8 weeks' gestation. Crown-rump length, which is the most accurate measurement for obstetric dating, is illustrated. Amnion (arrow) can be seen separate from the uterine wall. The head (H) can also be seen.

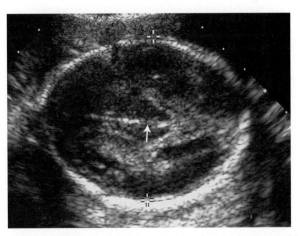

FIGURE 8–3. Biparietal diameter. Axial head scan shows suitable ovoid shape. Cursors measure a biparietal diameter at 22 weeks. The third ventricle is seen (arrow).

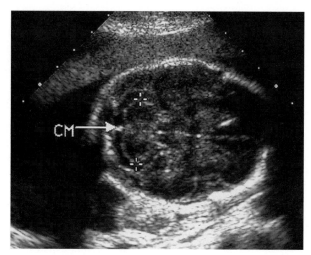

FIGURE 8–4. Axial view of the brain, demonstrating normal cerebellum and cisterna magna (CM). Edges of the cerebellar hemispheres are marked by cursors.

than the walls of the lateral ventricles, as once was thought.[7]

A strong midline echo represents the interhemispheric fissure and falx at superior levels and the septum pellucidum and third ventricle at more caudal levels. The choroid plexus is a strongly echogenic structure within the midportion of the lateral ventricles. The cerebellum and cisterna magna can be identified in the posterior fossa (Fig. 8–4). Imaging of these structures is frequently part of most basic and targeted ultrasounds.

ABDOMINAL CIRCUMFERENCE

The fetal abdomen is measured at the level of the liver, using the portal vein and the stomach as landmarks. Under ideal conditions, the abdominal cross section is nearly round (Fig. 8–5). The accuracy of the *abdominal circumference* (AC) is plus or minus 3 weeks at term. Measurement of the fetal abdomen is pivotal

for the estimation of fetal weight. The reliability of the AC in estimation of gestational age is dependent on fetal symmetry. Asymmetric intrauterine growth restriction (IUGR) initially results in a selective reduction of the AC and a corresponding decrease in the elapsed weeks assigned to this parameter. In contrast, macrosomia simulates a more advanced gestational age. Anomalies like diaphragmatic hernias, omphaloceles, masses, and cysts that alter or displace the abdominal contents may result in miscalculation of gestational age and estimated weight.

FEMUR LENGTH

The fetal femur is also used for estimating gestational age. The ideal *femur length* (FL) measurement captures the femoral shaft nearest the transducer in a perpendicular to the ultrasound beam (Fig. 8–6). Marked acoustic shadowing confirms that the appropriate angle has been obtained. Caliper placement is more critical for the femur than for the AC and cephalic evaluations, because the proportional error is greater in smaller structures. The measurement technique also is more demanding technically, because only the diaphysis should be included. The accuracy of FL in calculations of gestational age is plus or minus 3 weeks at term. In addition to technical considerations, the FL may be affected by abnormalities such as Down syndrome and skeletal dysplasias, severe IUGR or macrosomia, and in the third trimester, constitutional variation.

ESTIMATION OF FETAL WEIGHT

The fetal weight can be approximated on the basis of measurements of the major contributors to infant weight: head, trunk, soft tissue, and skeletal structures. Investigators have developed formulas that employ various combinations of AC or BPD, HC and FL, and other parameters.[20] A formula that reflects the birth weight distribution for a given demographic region is the most accurate. Most clinical facilities use calculations from one or more of the major investiga-

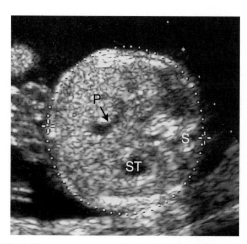

FIGURE 8–5. Transverse scan at the level of the abdominal circumference, which has been marked with dots. Fetal spine (S), portal vein (P), and stomach bubble (ST) are seen.

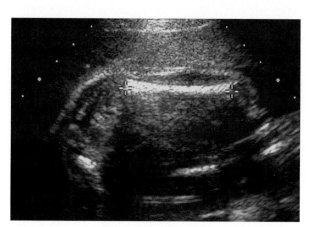

FIGURE 8–6. Femur length is demonstrated between cursors. Soft tissues and muscle of the thigh are anterior to the femur. Proximal femoral neck is to the left of image.

tors in the field, incorporated into the software of the ultrasound machines by the manufacturers. This approach is reasonable, as long as the results appear to be applicable to the local population. The reported accuracy of *estimated fetal weight* (EFW) is not usually approached in clinical settings, in part because the target population rarely mirrors the standard, and in part because subtle effects of technique in scanning and measurement are magnified across the two or three variables entered into EFW calculations. At the extremes of gestation, the error rate in calculating an EFW appears to exceed plus or minus 15%, with a potential for disastrous miscalculations if this limitation is not recognized. Even when accurate, the EFW of a previable fetus may overlap that of a potential survivor, rendering counseling more difficult. Equally frustrating is the difficulty in anticipating macrosomia at term, when weight estimates within the 15% range may differ by more than 500 gm from the actual birth weight.

OTHER FETAL MEASUREMENTS

A principal goal of fetal measurement is the assignment of gestational age when menstrual dating is inadequate. The chief limit of biometry in this pursuit is the interaction of aberrant growth with age-related findings. All of the standard measurements are affected, to varying degrees, by accelerated or reduced rates of intrauterine growth. Extremes of abnormal growth disrupt established relationships among the routine measurements, permitting identification of these conditions but compromising dating. Lesser, unrecognized degrees of macrosomia or growth lag are incorporated into faulty estimates of gestational age. The paucity of serious complications from these errors should be credited more to management that acknowledges the limitations of ultrasound than to intrinsic safety margins. Consequently, efforts have been made to identify structures reflecting gestational age that are unaffected by altered growth state. The transcerebellar diameter seemed to fulfill these requirements, but it was difficult to measure in the third trimester. Later studies suggested greater susceptibility to growth effects than originally anticipated.[23] Over the years, there have been more than 20 other fetal structures subjected to morphometric analysis. These data are expressed as regression equations against gestational age or in assorted ratios. These measurements are most helpful in cases in which the size of a particular anatomic feature is suspect, for example, when a structurally normal heart appears to occupy more of the chest cavity than anticipated, with skeletal dysplasias, or when intraocular distances seem abnormal.

FETAL ANOMALIES

(See also Chapter 28.)

Ultrasound reveals fetal malformations before birth. Many major fetal anomalies can be identified as early as 15 to 16 weeks of gestation. A few anoma-

---

■ **BOX 8–1**

INDICATIONS FOR ANTENATAL ULTRASOUND

A. Dating pregnancy
1. No accurate dates
2. Uterine size/dates discrepancy
   a. Suspected growth restriction
   b. Suspected large for dates; rule out
      (1) Multiple gestation
      (2) Polyhydramnios
      (3) Macrosomia
      (4) Uterine abnormality (e.g., fibroid tumor)
      (5) Molar pregnancy
B. Fetal/placental localization
1. Confirm pregnancy
2. Suspected missed abortion
3. Suspected ectopic pregnancy
4. Suspected placenta previa
5. Before amniocentesis
6. Before fetal transfusion/surgery
C. Survey of fetal anatomy; rule out congenital malformation, especially with/if
1. History of previous malformation
2. Maternal age more than 35 years
3. Diabetic pregnancy
4. Polyhydramnios/oligohydramnios
5. Abnormal presentation
6. Exposure to teratogens (e.g., alcohol, retinoic acid)
7. Suspicious maternal serum markers

---

lies do not become apparent until later in pregnancy. For example, the short femur of achondroplasia is not apparent until late in the second trimester. Indications for antenatal ultrasound examination are listed in Box 8–1.

CENTRAL NERVOUS SYSTEM

Fetal Ventriculomegaly

(See also Chapter 38.)

Strictly speaking, hydrocephalus and ventriculomegaly are not synonymous. *Hydrocephalus* implies raised intracranial pressure, and this functional observation cannot be made by ultrasound alone. The lateral ventricles may be enlarged because of a developmental abnormality, such as enlargement of the atrium and posterior horns of the lateral ventricles (colpocephaly), often in association with agenesis of the corpus callosum or type II Chiari malformation. The lateral ventricles may also be enlarged because of brain destruction from a variety of causes, including in utero infection with cytomegalovirus or ischemia.

A single measurement at the level of the atrium of the lateral ventricle has been proposed to define *ventriculomegaly*, with measurements greater than 10 mm considered to be abnormal.[13] The size of the

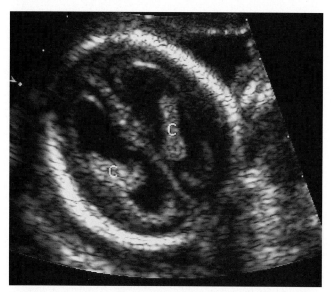

FIGURE 8–7. Ventriculomegaly. Dilated cerebral lateral ventricles with dangling choroid (C) can be seen.

lateral ventricular atrium is constant throughout pregnancy. The normal choroid plexus position depends on gravity, and in the standard axial view of the fetal brain, the dependent choroid plexus is attached at the level of the foramen of Monro and rests on the dependent wall of the lateral ventricle. Thus, the choroid plexus marks the position of the lateral ventricular wall even when the ventricular wall itself cannot be identified. A "dangling" choroid plexus can be used to gauge the extent and severity of ventricular enlargement (Fig. 8–7).

The clinical outcome with in utero diagnosis of large ventricles has been discouraging (Fig. 8–8).[24] Infants who survive are often mentally retarded and physically impaired. Unfortunately, it has proved impossible to define a group of fetuses with ventriculomegaly who would benefit from in utero shunting.

The finding of mild ventriculomegaly (atrial size between 10 and 12 mm) is associated with increased morbidity and mortality rates in some series and a good prognosis in others.[31]

Meningomyelocele and (Type II) Chiari Malformation

A *meningomyelocele* (Fig. 8–9) can occur in association with downward displacement of the hindbrain and with other associated anomalies of the brain. It may or may not include ventriculomegaly. Often hydrocephalus does not develop in these children until after birth. In cases of open neural tube defect, the α-fetoprotein level is elevated in both maternal serum and amniotic fluid (see Chapter 7).

A meningomyelocele is demonstrated by ultrasound as splaying or divergence of the posterior ossification centers, and it is best appreciated on the axial view of the spine. A fluid-filled sac may be seen, and the integrity of the overlying skin can be assessed. The diagnostic sensitivity of ultrasound for the detection of meningomyeloceles is 80% to 90%. Higher sensitivities have been described by experienced sonologists and with prior knowledge of an elevated serum α-fetoprotein. The level of meningomyelocele can also be ascertained by ultrasound examination. This information is helpful for predicting the outcome in affected children.

The following intracranial signs are associated with a meningomyelocele:

- small BPD or HC
- concave frontal bones (the "lemon" sign)
- distorted cerebellum (the "banana" sign)
- obliteration of the cisterna magna

Ventriculomegaly

The lemon sign refers to the appearance of the calvaria, which is similar in shape to a lemon, on axial

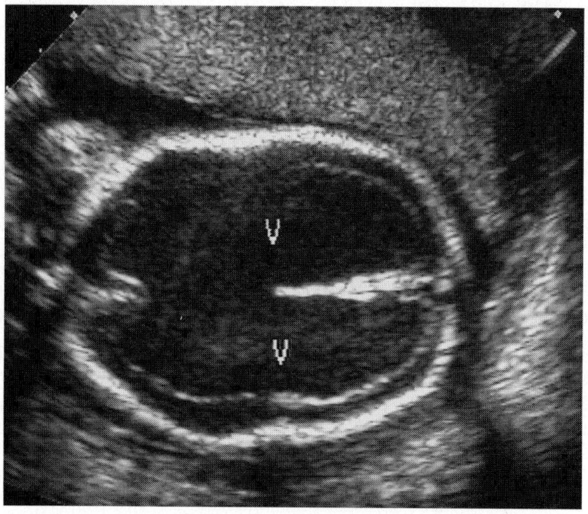

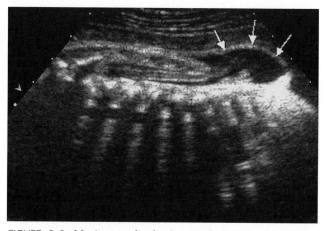

FIGURE 8–8. Severe ventriculomegaly. Dilated lateral cerebral ventricles (V) are surrounded by a small amount of brain parenchyma.

FIGURE 8–9. Meningomyelocele. Longitudinal view of a fetus, showing absence of posterior bony neural arch at the lower portion of the spine. The meningomyelocele sac is shown (*arrows*), and the spinal cord is seen in its normal position above this defect.

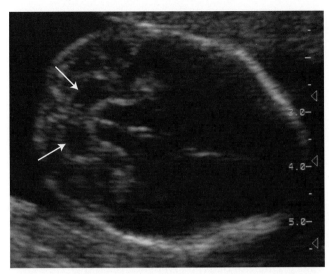

FIGURE 8–10. Lemon sign and banana sign. The concavity of the bony calvaria seen to the right of the image represents the lemon sign. Arrows mark the banana-shaped cerebellum.

scan (Fig. 8–10).[35] The biconcave frontal bones produce the distortion of the calvaria. This sign is age specific, demonstrated between 18 and 24 weeks. The sign is not totally diagnostic in that it is occasionally identified in otherwise normal children. The banana sign refers to the abnormal position of the cerebellum, which is wrapped in a crescent (banana-like) shape around the brain stem (see Fig. 8–10). Obliteration of the cisterna magna and distortion of the cerebellum are secondary to the downward displacement of the hindbrain associated with the type II Chiari malformation.

Anencephaly

Anencephaly, absence of the normal brain and calvaria superior to the orbits, can be detected by 14 to 15 weeks of gestation (Fig. 8–11). Usually, there is associated polyhydramnios (50%), but normally this does not appear until late in the second trimester. The maternal serum α-fetoprotein level is elevated in most cases. Approximately 50% have other associated anomalies, such as meningomyelocele, cleft palate, and clubfoot. Occasionally, the typical appearance is altered by the presence of echogenic material superior to the orbits. This material pathologically represents angiomatous stroma ("area cerebrovasculosa"). Anencephaly is incompatible with a meaningful postnatal survival beyond a few days.

Encephalocele

(See also Chapter 38.)

Protrusion of brain tissue within a meningeal sac is usually a straightforward obstetric ultrasound diagnosis. Most encephaloceles in the western world are occipital. Skin covers the encephalocele so that many are not associated with an elevated serum α-fetoprotein. Distinction should be made from soft tissue edema and a cystic hygroma of the neck. The identification of the bony calvarial defect allows a specific diagnosis (Fig. 8–12). Encephaloceles may occur as isolated anomalies, but they are also associated with the amniotic band syndrome (when the encephalocele is off midline) and a number of genetic syndromes, such as Meckel-Gruber syndrome.

Dandy-Walker Cyst

Dandy-Walker malformation is a fluid-filled cyst of the posterior fossa, with or without enlargement of the lateral ventricles (Fig. 8–13). Enlargement of the posterior fossa is always present with uplifting of the tentorium. Agenesis of the cerebellar vermis may also be recognized. The cerebellar hemispheres are rudimentary and are separated by the posterior fossa cyst.

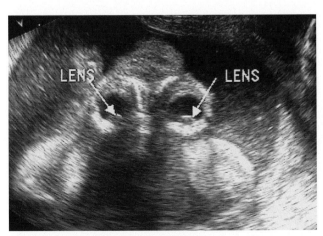

FIGURE 8–11. Anencephaly. Coronal image showing the orbits and eye lenses. Echogenic material superior to the orbits is angiomatous stroma.

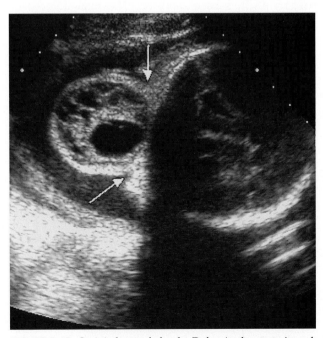

FIGURE 8–12. Occipital encephalocele. Defect in the posterior calvaria through which the brain has herniated *(arrows)* is seen.

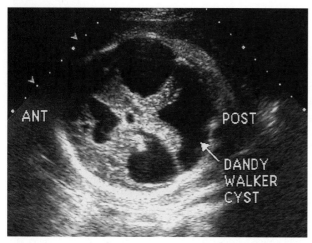

FIGURE 8–13. Dandy-Walker cyst. Transverse scan of the brain. Note the marked splaying of the cerebellar hemispheres. ANT, anterior; POST, posterior.

This diagnosis should not be made before 18 weeks because development of the cerebellar vermis may not be complete until this time.[9]

The Dandy-Walker variant shows direct communication between the fourth ventricle and the cisterna magna, but the posterior fossa is not enlarged.[18] Only mild hypoplasia of the inferior cerebellar vermis is present. An increased incidence of chromosomal abnormalities is reported.

Choroid Plexus Cyst

Choroid plexus cysts are identified in 1% to 2% of normal pregnancies during the second trimester, and they resolve by the early third trimester (Fig. 8–14). A slightly increased incidence of aneuploidy, especially trisomy 18, has been reported. The management of choroid plexus cysts is controversial. Amniocentesis

should probably not be offered solely from this finding, provided that a detailed ultrasound examination of the fetus is otherwise normal.

SPINE

Spinal anomalies that can be demonstrated on an ultrasound examination include congenital vertebral anomalies (Fig. 8–15) and diastematomyelia. *Diastematomyelia* is identified as an extra posterior echogenic focus between the fetal spinal laminae.[2] This is frequently associated with splaying of the posterior elements of the spine.

Sacrococcygeal teratoma is identified as a large mass arising posteriorly from the rump of the fetus. The posterior elements of the lumbosacral spine are intact. This tumor often is associated with polyhydramnios and premature delivery. Depending on the pathologic composition of the tumor, this mass may be cystic or solid. Extension into the fetal pelvis and abdomen can occur.

HEAD AND NECK

Normal anatomy is demonstrated after approximately 14 weeks, with visualization of the nose, orbits, forehead, lips, and ears. In the axial plane, the orbits are clearly seen, and measurements of the ocular diameter, interocular distance (which defines hypertelorism and hypotelorism), and binocular distance can be obtained. In the sagittal view, a profile of the face demonstrates the forehead, nose, and jaw (Fig. 8–16). The coronal view, the best view for the facial structures, demonstrates the orbits (including the lens), eyelids, nose, and lips. The coronal view is also the best plane for demonstrating facial clefting abnormalities, including cleft lip and cleft palate, which may be central or lateral (Fig. 8–17).[37] The complex anatomy of the fetal face is shown exquisitely by three-dimensional sonography.[22]

Cystic hygroma (lymphangioma) occurs in the region of the neck and in the occiput, and it may extend

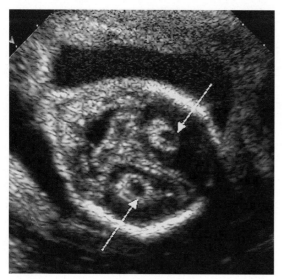

FIGURE 8–14. Choroid plexus cysts. Coronal view of the brain, showing bilateral choroid plexus cysts *(arrows)*.

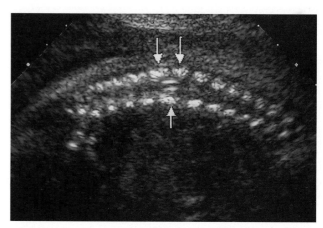

FIGURE 8–15. Coronal view through the fetal spine, showing a hemivertebra. The spinal ossification center *(upper left arrow)* has no mate.

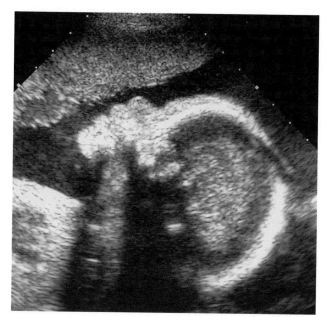

FIGURE 8–16. Sonogram demonstrates a normal forehead, nose, and jaw.

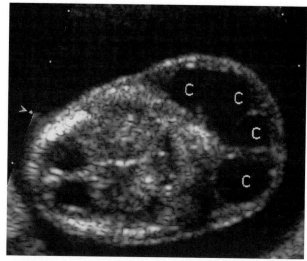

FIGURE 8–18. Transverse image through the head, showing cystic hygroma. C, septate cysts.

to involve the remainder of the trunk (Fig. 8–18). It is identified as a cystic mass that is septate. A posterior septum of the nuchal ligament helps define this lesion as a cystic hygroma. Testing for chromosomal abnormalities, including Turner syndrome, is mandatory. Increased nuchal translucency is now recognized with high frequency early in the pregnancy with trisomy 21. At the end of the first trimester, a nuchal lucency of 3 mm or greater has been shown to be a sensitive marker for this aneuploidy. Large-scale screening programs in low-risk populations have not yet validated this as a clinically appropriate screening study for the early detection of Down syndrome. The study also requires a level of technical expertise that will probably limit the value of this test.[43]

Other neck masses are rare, but they include anterior goiter and teratoma.

HEART

(See also Chapter 43.)

Fetal echocardiography has achieved prominence in perinatal ultrasound. The majority of fetal echocardiograms are obtained at 18 to 20 weeks of gestation; however, when using transvaginal ultrasound, the fetal heart may be evaluated as early as 12 weeks. The four-chamber view of the fetal heart should be part of all obstetric ultrasound examinations (Fig. 8–19). An abnormal four-chamber view has a 50% chance of signaling congenital heart disease in a non-selected population.[45] Fetal echocardiography includes assessment of the intracardiac structures and their relationships.

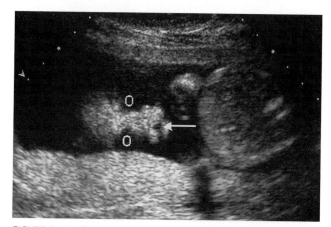

FIGURE 8–17. Coronal view of the face, showing right-sided cleft lip (arrow). Top of the head is to the left of the image. O, orbits.

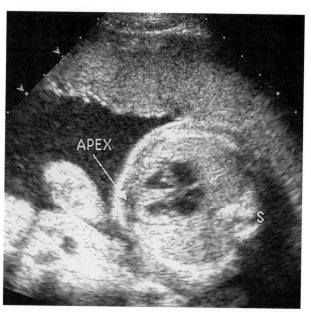

FIGURE 8–19. Four-chamber view of heart. The apex of the heart is to the left of the fetus. Right and left ventricles are approximately equal in size. S, spine.

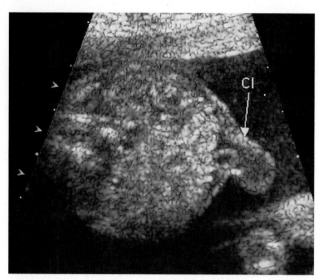

FIGURE 8–20. Cross section of the abdomen at the level of the umbilical vein, demonstrating fluid-filled loops of normal small bowel in the abdomen. CI, cord insertion.

GASTROINTESTINAL TRACT

(See also Chapter 45.)

Normal Bowel Appearance

The physiologic bowel migration that normally occurs into the proximal umbilical cord between 7 and 10 weeks of gestation can be identified on first-trimester scanning (see Fig. 8–1). It should never be mistaken for an anterior abdominal wall defect.[6] The normal fetal stomach is demonstrated between 13 and 15 weeks of gestation as a fluid-filled structure in the left upper quadrant of the abdomen. The normal stomach changes in size as it empties and fills. The fetal small bowel usually is not demonstrated early in gestation by ultrasound examination, but it may be seen as fluid-filled loops in the central region of the abdomen by the third trimester (Fig. 8–20). The large bowel is demonstrated from 22 weeks' gestation and is shown clearly in all fetuses by the third trimester. The large bowel normally is visible as a hypoechoic tubular structure in the periphery of the abdomen. Meconium in the large bowel is demonstrated in the third trimester. Occasionally, in the second trimester, meconium in the bowel results in increased echogenicity. This can be a normal finding that resolves toward the end of the second trimester. Echogenic fetal bowel may represent a nonspecific but abnormal finding that is a marker for a poor fetal outcome. The more echogenic the bowel, the worse the clinical outcome. Echogenic bowel has been associated with aneuploidy (trisomy 21), cystic fibrosis, bowel atresia, and IUGR.[36]

Obstruction at various levels of the gastrointestinal tract can be diagnosed by ultrasound. Obstruction of the proximal alimentary canal interferes with the normal process of amniotic fluid turnover, which involves swallowing and absorption of the amniotic fluid by the fetus. Thus, in proximal bowel obstruction, polyhydramnios is an invariable finding (see Chapter 21).

Esophageal Atresia and Tracheoesophageal Fistula

Nonvisualization of the fluid-filled stomach in association with polyhydramnios should alert the examiner to the diagnosis of *esophageal atresia*. Unfortunately, these two signs are not reliable, being identified in only 40% of cases. Nonvisualization of the stomach is not a specific sign of esophageal atresia. The proximal esophageal pouch is almost never visualized. Polyhydramnios is seen in two thirds of the cases, but commonly it does not develop until the third trimester. The VACTERL complex of congenital anomalies consists of *v*ertebral, *a*nal, *c*ardiovascular, *t*racheal, *e*sophageal, *r*enal, and *l*imb malformations. These systems should be investigated in the fetus with suspected *tracheoesophageal fistula*. Nonvisualization of the fluid-filled stomach also occurs with oligohydramnios when there is little fluid to swallow or with abnormalities of the central nervous system that interfere with swallowing.

Small Bowel Obstruction

With *duodenal atresia*, the presence of a distended stomach and proximal duodenum provides a double-bubble sign, likened to the x-ray appearance in the newborn period (Fig. 8–21). A close association (25%) with Down syndrome mandates a genetic amniocen-

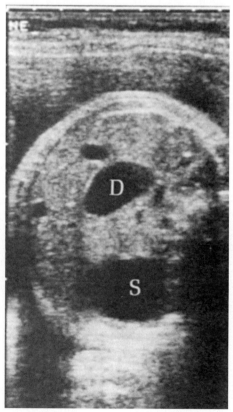

FIGURE 8–21. Duodenal atresia. Dilated stomach (S) and proximal duodenum (D) produce double-bubble sign. Duodenal obstruction can also be caused by annular pancreas or malrotation of the bowel.

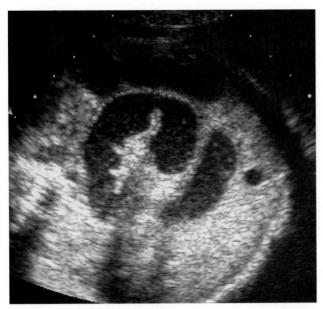

FIGURE 8–22. Ileal atresia. Transverse image of abdomen showing multiple dilated, fluid-filled loops of small bowel.

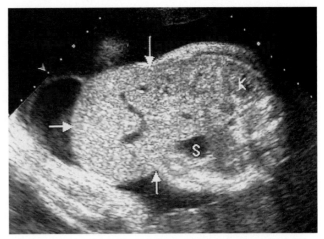

FIGURE 8–24. Omphalocele. Anterior abdominal wall defect (*arrows*) with surrounding membrane. The liver has herniated into this defect. S, stomach; K, kidney.

tesis when duodenal atresia is suspected. Other causes of a double bubble include annular pancreas, duodenal web, malrotation, and severe duodenal stenosis. Similarly, *ileal* and *jejunal atresia* can be diagnosed by the presence of multiple loops of bowel, which often exhibit peristalsis (Fig. 8–22).

A more distal bowel obstruction, as can be seen in meconium ileus, Hirschsprung disease, and anal atresia, will similarly produce dilated loops of bowel, but these are not usually apparent until the third trimester (Fig. 8–23). Meconium peritonitis is a chemical peritonitis that results from an intrauterine perforation from any cause. Peritoneal calcifications and free intraperitoneal fluid can be identified by ultrasound.

Anterior Abdominal Wall Defects

With an approximate incidence of omphalocele of 1 in 5000 births and of gastroschisis of 1 in 10,000 births, abdominal wall defects are among the more common abnormalities detected in the neonate. The presence of a midline abdominal wall defect into the base of the umbilical cord is an ultrasonic characteristic of an omphalocele (Fig. 8–24). A sac surrounds the herniated viscera and may include liver as well as bowel. Omphalocele is frequently associated with other congenital (e.g., Beckwith-Wiedemann syndrome) and chromosomal (trisomies 13 and 18) anomalies. With gastroschisis, herniated bowel loops are seen floating in the amniotic cavity, without covering membrane (Fig. 8–25). This defect is lateral to the umbilical cord insertion and is typically on the right side. Associated fetal abnormalities are rare.

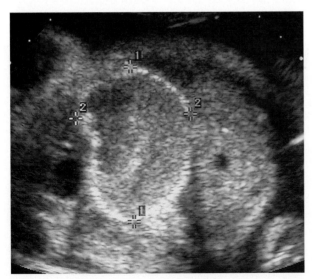

FIGURE 8–23. Transverse image of abdomen with meconium pseudocyst marked with cursors. This finding is associated with cystic fibrosis.

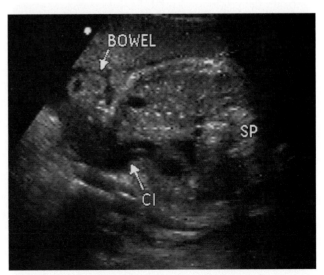

FIGURE 8–25. Gastroschisis. Transverse scan of the fetal abdomen, showing loops of bowel floating freely in the amniotic cavity to the right of the cord insertion (CI). SP, spine.

Diaphragmatic Hernia

The diagnosis of *congenital diaphragmatic hernia* is made when abdominal organs (usually stomach and loops of bowel) are seen in the thoracic cavity (Fig. 8–26). Fluid-filled loops of the bowel may show peristalsis in the thoracic cavity. Polyhydramnios, left-sided heart underdevelopment, and detection before 24 weeks' gestation are predictors of poor neonatal outcome.[32] (See Chapters 11, Part Two, 42, and 45.)

Diaphragmatic hernias show a mass effect with mediastinal shift and lung compression. Unfortunately, the extent of pulmonary hypoplasia as measured at the level of the four-chamber view of the heart cannot predict postnatal outcome. In utero surgical correction, hysterotomy with tracheal PLUG (*p*lug the *l*ung *u*ntil it *g*rows), remains experimental.

GALLBLADDER AND BILE DUCTS

(See also Chapter 46.)

Choledochal cyst is the localized dilation of the biliary system, and it most often involves the common bile duct. The lesion is recognized as a fluid-filled cyst in the right upper quadrant of the abdomen, separate from the gallbladder.

Echogenic material is rarely identified in the lumen of the fetal gallbladder during the third trimester (Fig. 8–27). It is suspected that this echogenic material is gallstones. Follow-up studies in neonates have shown resolution in the majority of cases. Children have been reported as asymptomatic.[11]

GENITOURINARY TRACT

(See also Chapter 49.)

The kidneys are identified as early as 12 to 14 weeks' gestation as circular structures lateral to the

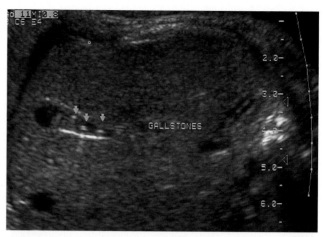

FIGURE 8–27. Transverse scan through abdomen, showing gallstones *(arrows)* in the fetal gallbladder.

fetal spine (Fig. 8–28). Normal fetal kidney size can be plotted against gestational age.[14] By the end of the third trimester, fat deposition results in an echogenic border and provides greater contrast for the demonstration of fetal kidneys. The bladder is seen as early as 13 weeks' gestation. Fetal adrenal glands are identified at the same time.

If a serious renal malfunction such as complete obstruction or bilateral renal agenesis is present, the absence of fetal urine production manifests as severe oligohydramnios. Oligohydramnios may not become apparent until 18 to 20 weeks' gestation. Infants born after prolonged oligohydramnios have a characteristic facial appearance with limb deformities and pulmonary hypoplasia, called Potter syndrome (or sequence). When oligohydramnios is encountered on an ultrasound examination, attention should be directed to the fetal urinary tract. The fetal bladder should be visualized after about 15 weeks. If the bladder is not seen at the first attempt, the patient should be rescanned at 30-minute intervals. Color

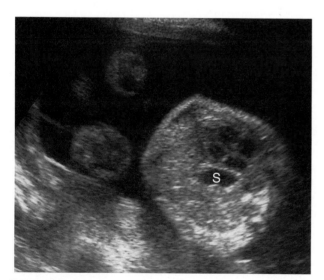

FIGURE 8–26. Diaphragmatic hernia. Transverse view of the fetal chest, showing the heart shifted to the right of the fetal chest by bowel. The stomach bubble (S) is to the left of the heart. There is polyhydramnios.

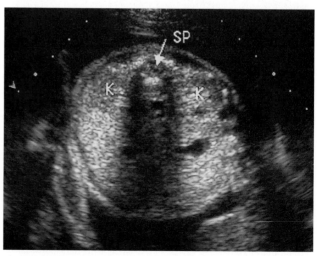

FIGURE 8–28. Transverse view of the abdomen, demonstrating two normal kidneys (K). SP, spine.

Doppler imaging clearly demonstrates the continuity with the two umbilical arteries on each side of the bladder (Fig. 8–29). Unfortunately, with oligohydramnios the lack of surrounding amniotic fluid makes it more difficult to see detailed fetal anatomy. Nevertheless, the inability to visualize the fetal bladder and kidneys in the presence of oligohydramnios is strongly suggestive of bilateral renal agenesis. The fetal adrenal glands are larger than in the neonate or infant, and they may be misinterpreted as kidneys in cases of renal agenesis. Care must be taken in diagnosing a unilateral absence of the kidney, because there may be a pelvic kidney.

Mild dilation of the renal pelvis is a common finding during pregnancy. Fetal renal pyelectasis is not related to maternal overhydration from drinking water to obtain a full maternal bladder. This is a normal finding that should not be misinterpreted as fetal hydronephrosis. Pyelectasis has been reported to be associated with Down syndrome. The identification of a single measurement to discriminate babies who will develop obstructive uropathy after birth has proved elusive. Pathologic dilation of the upper urinary tract was previously diagnosed when the renal pelvis measured 10 mm or greater in anteroposterior dimension (Fig. 8–30). This single measurement fails to identify hydronephrosis earlier than the third trimester. Measurements greater than 4 mm now have been proposed as being diagnostic earlier in pregnancy. Obstruction of the urinary tract produces a variable sonographic appearance, depending mainly on the time in gestation when this event occurs. Early in gestation, renal dysplasia, sometimes with cyst formation, is the consequence of obstruction. Later in gestation, dilation of the collecting system occurs.

Hydronephrosis may be unilateral because of obstruction of the ureteropelvic junction or bilateral because of obstruction of the lower urinary tract, such as obstruction caused by posterior urethral valves. In mild cases of hydronephrosis, only a dilated pelvis will be seen, and the renal parenchymal thickness will be normal. However, if hydronephrosis is severe, thinning of the renal parenchyma may be observed.

With posterior urethral valves, a distended and

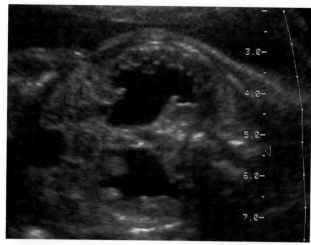

FIGURE 8–30. Coronal image showing bilateral ureteropelvic obstruction. Dilated renal pelvis with dilated calices is seen bilaterally.

often thick-walled bladder will be imaged in a male fetus. Hydronephrosis, usually bilateral, is also seen. There may be urinary ascites. Dilation of the posterior urethra helps distinguish this lesion from prune-belly syndrome (Fig. 8–31).

Multicystic dysplastic kidney appears as several noncommunicating cysts. The cysts vary in size and lack organization. This appearance is in contrast to the findings in severe hydronephrosis, in which there is an orderly arrangement of the enlarged renal pelvis surrounded by smaller calices. The size of these cysts can change. Bilateral renal anomalies (including bilateral multicystic renal dysplasia) are more common (40%) in the fetus (Fig. 8–32).

Dilated ureters may be secondary to obstruction at the ureterovesical junction (primary megaureter). Reflux has also been described in utero as producing dilated ureters. Autosomal recessive polycystic kidney disease produces bilateral enlargement of the kidneys, which retain their reniform shape. Polycystic

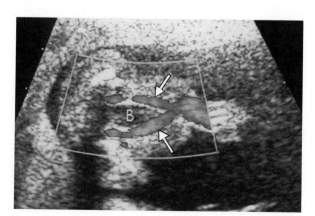

FIGURE 8–29. Fetal bladder. Cross section of pelvis. Bladder (B) is seen with two umbilical arteries running on each side (arrows).

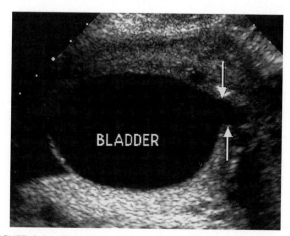

FIGURE 8–31. Posterior urethral valve. Coronal scan of the fetal pelvis, showing an enlarged bladder and dilated posterior urethra. Arrows are proximal to the posterior urethral valves. Note the oligohydramnios.

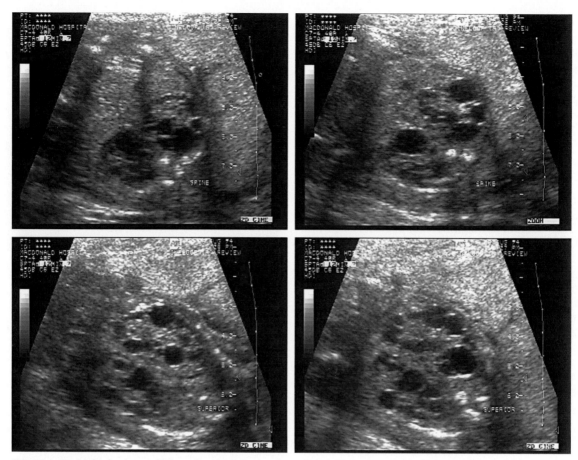

FIGURE 8–32. Multiple views of bilateral multicystic dysplastic kidneys. Note severe oligohydramnios.

kidneys are extremely echogenic (Fig. 8–33). Many other renal anomalies have been demonstrated in utero, including duplication of the kidney collecting system (Fig. 8–34) and extrophy of the bladder.

Distinction between the male and the female fetus by visualization of the external genitalia can be accomplished starting between 16 and 20 weeks' gestation (Figs. 8–35 and 8–36). Ovarian cysts can be demonstrated in utero. Often, ovarian cysts are abdominal in position and cannot be distinguished from other

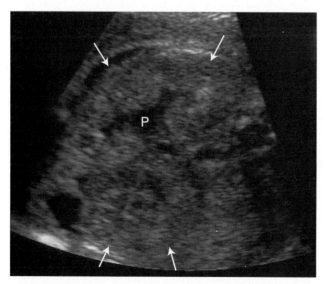

FIGURE 8–33. Polycystic kidneys. Transverse scan of the fetal abdomen, showing enlarged hyperechoic kidneys filling the fetal abdomen *(arrows)*. Oligohydramnios is present. P, renal pelvis.

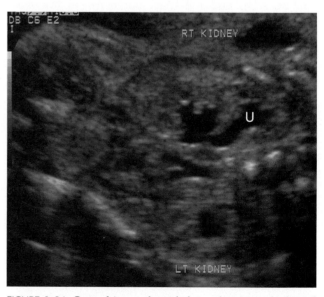

FIGURE 8–34. Coronal image through fetus, showing a duplicated renal collecting system in the right kidney. U, upper pole.

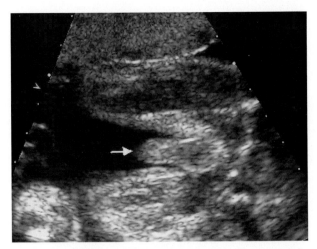

FIGURE 8–35. Male fetus. Arrow shows penis.

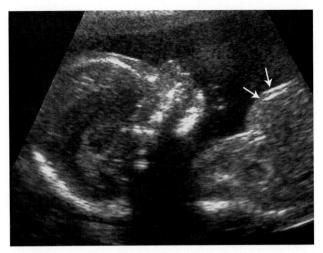

FIGURE 8–37. Thanatophoric dysplasia. Sagittal view of the fetus, revealing severe deformation of the rib cage with protrusion of the abdomen *(arrows)*.

abnormal cysts in the abdomen before delivery. These cysts may be fluid filled or septated with fluid levels. Hydrometrocolpos is another cause of a fluid-filled structure in the fetal pelvis.

MUSCULOSKELETAL SYSTEM

Examination of all four extremities and measurement of the FL should be included in an obstetric ultrasound examination. A previous history of a bony dysplasia makes this mandatory. Standardized tables list the lengths of all the limb bones in the second and third trimesters. Shortening of the limb bones to less than 3 standard deviations for gestational age on ultrasound examination is suggestive of a skeletal dysplasia. Because 5% of normal babies will be below the 5th percentile, it is reassuring that the majority of skeletal dysplasias show dramatic shortening at well below the 5th percentile. The gestational age of a fetus can then be ascertained by HC or BPD if the skull is not involved in the skeletal dysplasia.

Careful measurement of every bone in the peripheral skeleton is necessary, first to help define the category of bony dysplasia, and then, if possible, to give a specific diagnosis (see Chapters 28 and 52). Overall shortening of the limbs is called *micromelia*. Proximal shortening is called *rhizomelia* (femurs and humeri), *mesomelia* (forearms and legs), or *acromelia* (feet and hands). Fractures or curvatures of bones must be recorded, together with the bone density.

Pulmonary hypoplasia is a frequent cause of death in fetuses with lethal skeletal dysplasias. Lung volume can be assessed on the four-chamber view of the heart. Polyhydramnios may also be present with skeletal dysplasia.

Thanatophoric dysplasia is a uniformly lethal skeletal dysplasia that can be recognized in utero. There is severe micromelia, curvature of the femurs, and pulmonary hypoplasia (Fig. 8–37). One form of thanatophoric dysplasia shows a cloverleaf skull deformity. Achondrogenesis is a lethal skeletal dysplasia associated with severe micromelia. Lack of vertebral ossification helps define this skeletal dysplasia.

Lethal type II osteogenesis imperfecta demonstrates short fractured bones that are often bent or curved (Fig. 8–38). Bone density is decreased and is

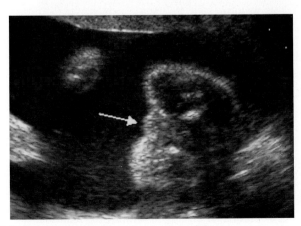

FIGURE 8–36. Female fetus. Arrow shows labia.

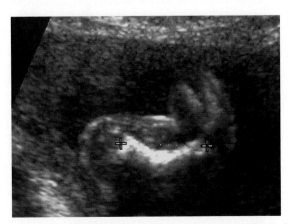

FIGURE 8–38. Osteogenesis imperfecta. Humerus with marked shortening and abnormal shape secondary to multiple fractures is indicated by cursors.

best appreciated in the calvaria.[33] The lethal neonatal form of hypophosphatasia may have a similar ultrasound appearance of severe demineralization.

Achondroplasia is the most common nonlethal skeletal dysplasia. Shortening of the femur defines this as a rhizomelic form of skeletal dysplasia. The retardation in the growth of the femur is not appreciated until the third trimester, limiting an early prenatal diagnosis.[27]

Other abnormalities of the musculoskeletal system include the malformation or absence (dysostosis) of various parts of the skeleton, for example, limb reduction anomalies such as radial clubhand or hemimelia (Fig. 8–39).

Pitfalls in the diagnosis of skeletal dysplasia should be appreciated. A phenocopy gives an infant the appearance of having a specific syndrome, but the cause may be some other factor, such as an infection, another genetic abnormality, or even medication taken during pregnancy. An example of a phenocopy is the occurrence of stippled epiphyses caused by the maternal ingestion of warfarin, which can produce a phenocopy of the skeletal dysplasia of stippled epiphyses.

TWO-VESSEL UMBILICAL CORD

A two-vessel umbilical cord or *single umbilical artery* (SUA) is identified on transverse section and may be

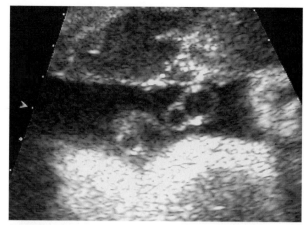

FIGURE 8–40. Two-vessel umbilical cord. A transverse scan of the umbilical cord, showing a single artery and vein.

confirmed by color Doppler imaging (Fig. 8–40). A color Doppler study of the fetal pelvis reveals absence of the umbilical artery as it courses around the bladder (Fig. 8–41). SUA is associated with other congenital anomalies, and its presence should prompt a careful anatomic survey. Unfortunately, the anomalies associated with SUA do not display a consistent pattern. It is unclear if isolated SUA is associated with aneuploidy, but discretion would suggest a discussion

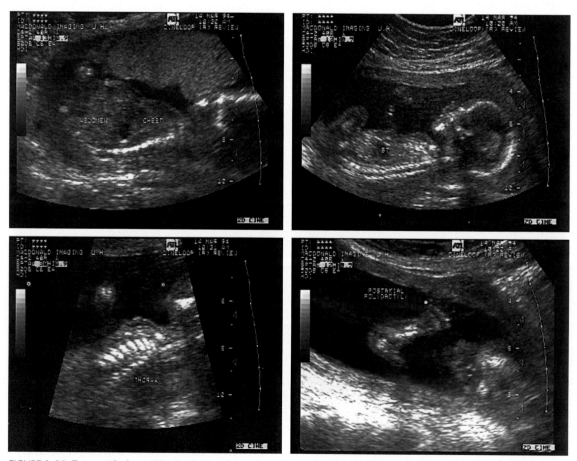

FIGURE 8–39. Fetus with short-ribbed polydactyly syndrome. Images show small chest with hypoechoic ribs, large amounts of amniotic fluid, and postaxial polydactyly.

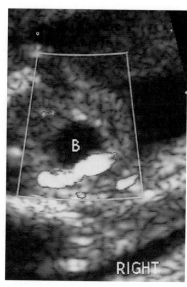

FIGURE 8–41. Transverse scan of the fetal pelvis at the level of the bladder (B), revealing absence of left umbilical artery.

and karyotyping if desired. Small size for gestational age is common in neonates with SUA and the fetus is at risk for IUGR. Serial third-trimester sonograms should be performed to assess fetal growth, and tests for fetal well-being may be indicated.[39]

AMNIOTIC FLUID VOLUME

(See also Chapter 21.)

The volume of amniotic fluid is an important indicator of development. Amniotic fluid volume above normal (polyhydramnios) or below normal (oligohydramnios) is associated with an increased risk of perinatal morbidity and death. Amniotic fluid volume increases through week 33 and then decreases. Ultrasound can be used to assess amniotic fluid volume. A common technique in this assessment is the *amniotic fluid index*.[40] This technique divides the maternal abdomen into four quadrants; the largest vertical pocket is measured in centimeters, and the total is calculated for the four quadrants. Tables of normal values are available. Abnormality of amniotic fluid volume requires additional investigation. (See Chapter 9.)

Causes of oligohydramnios include abnormalities in the production or maintenance of fluid. Renal agenesis and urinary tract obstructions are common causes of abnormalities of the production of amniotic fluid. The presence of amniotic fluid is associated with normal alveolar development. Absence of amniotic fluid is associated with pulmonary hypoplasia. Fetuses with rupture of membranes as the cause of oligohydramnios have a better prognosis than do those with renal abnormalities. The ultimate outcome of the pregnancy mirrors the gestational age at which the membranes ruptured. Oligohydramnios is also associated with IUGR. Uteroplacental insufficiency results in decreased perfusion of the fetal kidney with a subsequent decrease in urinary flow. A chronic hy-

poxic state leads to shunting of the fetal blood from the kidneys. Amniotic fluid may also be decreased in the post-term pregnancy because of placental aging. The finding of oligohydramnios in the post-term pregnancy is significant because it is associated with an increase in perinatal asphyxia. It is often the basis on which a decision to deliver the patient is made.

The diagnosis of polyhydramnios is made in approximately 1% of pregnancies, of which approximately two thirds are idiopathic. Other causes of polyhydramnios include maternal diabetes, multiple gestation, and fetal anomalies. Upper gastrointestinal tract obstructions have been associated with polyhydramnios, presumably because of the inability of the fetus to swallow amniotic fluid. Congenital diaphragmatic hernia, anencephaly, and dwarfism are also associated with polyhydramnios.

USE OF ULTRASOUND IN HIGH-RISK PREGNANCIES

INTRAUTERINE GROWTH RESTRICTION

Intrauterine growth restriction is associated with a significant perinatal mortality rate and long-term morbidity (see also Chapter 13). Our attempts to improve outcome rely on an ability to accurately identify the fetus at risk. Campbell[12] described two patterns of reduced fetal growth based on serial measurements of the fetal head and abdomen. *Asymmetric* growth restriction, the more common type, results in an accelerating discrepancy between the anticipated and observed values in the serial measurements of the fetal abdomen. Eventually, the growth of the BPD is affected. Uteroplacental insufficiency is the most common cause of asymmetric IUGR. *Symmetric* growth restriction usually begins earlier in the pregnancy, with concordant, steady growth of the head and abdomen along a growth curve appropriate for a fetus of much earlier gestational age. Symmetric IUGR is associated with chromosomal abnormalities and intrauterine infections. A single ultrasound study during the third trimester cannot distinguish between the last stage of asymmetric IUGR, in which the head measurements also lag, and symmetric IUGR. Dating errors can be difficult to distinguish from symmetric IUGR without independent data such as pregnancy test results.

Serial studies, although sensitive to IUGR, may not be available for many at-risk pregnancies. When the initial study occurs in the third trimester, ratios between the AC and the FL and between the AC and HC may be helpful in discriminating between errors in gestational age and asymmetric IUGR. When gestational age is known, the ultrasound EFW is one of the best predictors of IUGR. Unfortunately, studies have suggested that ultrasound identification of IUGR may be associated with increased interventions without demonstrable improvement in outcome.[28]

Once IUGR has been identified, additional testing is usually performed. Genetic and infectious disease testing should be considered with symmetric IUGR. In the latter portion of the third trimester, cordocentesis may be considered for obtaining karyotype and for excluding acidosis and hypoxia. Gravidas with asymmetric fetal IUGR should be evaluated for hypertension, connective tissue diseases, poor nutritional choices, cigarette smoking, and substance abuse. Cessation of maternal smoking and substance abuse, left-sided rest, and the use of nutritional and fluid supplements have been advocated in these cases, with amelioration noted only sporadically. Infants with asymmetric IUGR benefit from prompt delivery if pulmonary maturity is confirmed. In cases remote from term, however, serial tests of fetal well-being are mandated. Evidence of fetal compromise on antenatal testing may dictate the delivery of an infant of low birth weight, even when lung maturity is improbable.

ANEUPLOIDY

Fetal karyotyping is the only definitive method to diagnose or exclude chromosomal abnormalities. The techniques for obtaining cells with the fetal chromosomal complement remain invasive and carry a low but real risk of interruption or compromise of the pregnancy (see Chapter 7). Methods include chorionic villus sampling, amniocentesis, cordocentesis, placental biopsy, and rarely, fetal biopsy or aspiration. The risk of pregnancy loss ranges from a low of 1 in 400 (0.25%) to approximately 2% over background rates, depending on the technique and investigator. With a commonly accepted loss rate of 0.5%, midtrimester amniocentesis has been proposed as suitable for women older than 35 years of age at delivery. This belief exists because the empiric age-related risk of aneuploidy is greater than the procedure-related complication rate.[30]

Recent developments in noninvasive testing include the use of biochemical markers in combination with maternal age to assign a risk of trisomy 21 or 18 equivalent to that of a 35-year-old woman. With a similar aim, ultrasound markers for karyotypic abnormalities have been explored. The association of certain

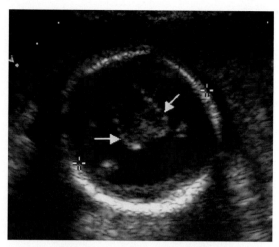

FIGURE 8–43. Coronal view through fetal brain with holoprosencephaly. Single cerebral ventricle can be seen with fused thalami *(arrows)*.

categories of physical anomalies with chromosomal defects is well accepted. The diagnosis of trisomy 18 must be considered likely in a fetus with an omphalocele, severe symmetric growth restriction, cardiac malformation, and overlapping digits (Fig. 8–42), as should the diagnosis of trisomy 13 in a fetus with holoprosencephaly (Fig. 8–43). Similarly, many of the serious structural defects identified by ultrasound have a prevalence of chromosomal abnormalities of more than 1 in 200. Chromosomal testing provides invaluable information for determining prognosis and shaping management decisions. Some structural variations have been evaluated separately as markers for chromosomal abnormalities, particularly for trisomy 21. Sonographic markers do not represent a significant risk to fetal well-being outside of their association with chromosomal abnormalities. Markers have included choroid plexus cysts, echogenic bowel, echogenic cardiac foci, reduced length of long bones relative to that expected from cephalic measurements, renal pyelectasis, and thickened nuchal folds (Fig. 8–44). The role of invasive testing in otherwise low-risk pregnancies that demonstrate one or more of these markers remains controversial, but it has gained increasing acceptance, particularly for nuchal thickening.[46] Conversely, the absence of ultrasound findings probably can be used to decrease the risk of abnormal outcomes assigned by empiric, genetic, or serologic testing. The appropriate sequence and role of current methods in a decision tree for invasive testing is the subject of ongoing investigation.

MULTIPLE GESTATION

(See also Chapters 18 and 23.)

The diagnosis of a multiple gestation is made reliably with ultrasound (Fig. 8–45). Visualization of multiple fetuses, gestational sacs, or both is diagnostic of multifetal pregnancy. Risks inherent in multiple gestation include IUGR and fetal death. Ultrasound examination can detect these abnormalities.

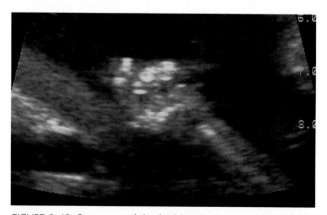

FIGURE 8–42. Sonogram of the fetal hand, showing the overlap of digits typical of a fetus with trisomy 18.

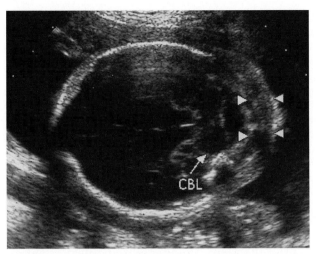

FIGURE 8–44. Transverse image of the fetal head, showing a thick nuchal fold *(arrowheads)*. CBL, cerebellum.

Structural defects are more common in twin pregnancies, and many anatomic abnormalities can be demonstrated by ultrasound. Polyhydramnios occurs in approximately 5% of twin gestations and may be monitored. A more severe form of IUGR is the placental transfusion syndrome, or twin-twin transfusion syndrome. This occurs in monozygotic twin pregnancies with a placental arteriovenous anastomosis and subsequent shunting. The typical prenatal ultrasound finding is that the donor twin is growth restricted with oligohydramnios and subcutaneous wasting. The recipient twin exhibits hydrops fetalis, congestive heart failure, and polyhydramnios.

RHESUS INCOMPATIBILITY AND HYDROPS FETALIS

(See also Chapters 20 and 21.)

With the introduction of rhesus immunoglobulin therapy, there has been a dramatic decline in the incidence of hydrops fetalis from isoimmunization and a small decrease in nonimmune hydrops. Ultrasound is useful for evaluating fetal compromise; excessive accumulation of amniotic fluid and the development of hydrops fetalis can be monitored.

ANTEPARTUM HEMORRHAGE

Third-trimester hemorrhage occurs during 3% of pregnancies. Placenta previa and abruptio placentae account for most antepartum hemorrhages, and ultrasound is instrumental in evaluating these conditions.

Placenta Previa

Placental localization through ultrasound is highly accurate. *Placenta previa* is a common finding in second-trimester ultrasound examinations, but its frequency is 0.3% to 0.5% at term. More than 90% of low placental implantations in second-trimester exams are shown to be in normal position at term. An early central placenta previa is more likely to be a placenta previa at term.[49] Sonographic detection of placenta previa depends on identification of the inferior margin of the placenta in relation to the internal os of the cervix (Fig. 8–46). For this reason, approaches other than transabdominal ones have been adopted. Transvaginal and transperineal ultrasonography have improved diagnostic accuracy without undue risk of hemorrhage in the patient with vaginal bleeding.[29] A placenta that is covering the internal os or is 2 cm or less away from the placental edge is believed to be clinically significant.[38] Partial placenta previa indicates that a portion of the internal os is covered. When the placenta approaches the edge of the internal os, the abnormality is called a marginal placenta previa. Anterior placenta previa is easier to visualize and diagnose than posterior. The accuracy of ultrasonography in diagnosing placenta previa is 90% to 97%, depending on experience. The cause of low placentation remains controversial. The major theories focus on endometrial damage that prevents effective pla-

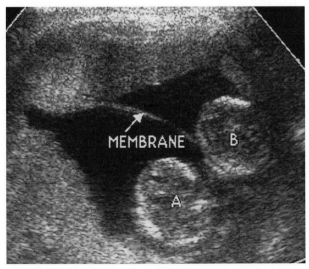

FIGURE 8–45. Twin pregnancy. Sonogram reveals a twin pregnancy with a cross section of the heads of fetuses A and B. Dividing membrane is seen.

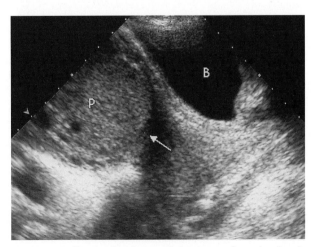

FIGURE 8–46. Transperineal scan of the maternal cervix, showing internal os *(arrow)* covered with placenta (P). B, maternal bladder.

centation. Prior cesarean section, therapeutic abortion, older age, and higher parity have been shown to increase the risk of placenta previa.

Abruptio Placentae

Abruptio placentae is the separation of the placenta with hemorrhage into the decidua basalis. The incidence varies from 0.2% to 2% of pregnancies. Conditions associated with abruptio placentae include a short umbilical cord, external trauma, sudden decompression of the uterus, maternal hypertension, folate deficiency, effects of cigarettes or cocaine, and uterine tumors. Bleeding from the abruption may appear through the vagina or remain retroplacental and concealed. Abruptio placentae is diagnosed clinically as an explanation for vaginal bleeding. Sonographically, a retroplacental hematoma may be visualized as an anechoic or complex fluid collection between the uterine wall and the placenta (Fig. 8–47). The sensitivity of the diagnostic ultrasound examination for abruptio placentae is unknown but is thought to be poor. A wide spectrum of sonographic findings, including hypoechoic and hyperechoic areas adjacent to the placenta, encompasses this entity.[21] It is known that in pregnancies in which abruption is seen, the outcome is poor.

ULTRASOUND PROCEDURES

(See also Chapter 7.)

Procedures performed during pregnancy involve removal of various fluids through needles placed into the uterus. Ultrasound is used to direct the operator's needle. Amniotic fluid can be removed, as can fetal blood and portions of the placenta or fetus. These tests are generally performed in concert with genetic counseling. By far the most common indication for invasive fetal testing is advanced maternal age. Advanced maternal age is currently defined as 35 years of age or older.

Amniocentesis for prenatal diagnosis is traditionally performed at about 16 weeks' gestation. Under direct ultrasound guidance, a spinal needle is placed into the amniotic cavity and fluid is aspirated. It is accepted that the fetal loss rate with amniocentesis is about 1 in 200.[30] When amniocentesis is performed at earlier gestational ages (i.e., 12 to 14 weeks), the pregnancy fetal loss rate appears to be equivalent.[3] Ultrasound-guided amniocentesis can be performed in multiple gestations, although there appears to be an increased loss rate.[25] Other uses for amniocentesis include evaluation of fetal lung maturity, measurement of bilirubin in isoimmunized patients, and examination of fluid for suspected viral or bacterial infection.

To obtain earlier prenatal diagnosis, *chorionic villus sampling* has been adopted. This procedure is performed from 10 to 12 weeks' gestation through two approaches, transcervical or transabdominal. The transcervical approach uses a polyethylene sampling catheter. Under ultrasound guidance, it is inserted into the uterus, and then the placental bed is sampled. In the transabdominal approach, a needle is used to sample the trophoblast. The transabdominal chorionic villus sampling technique may be used later in pregnancy, although it is then referred to as placental biopsy. Placental biopsy is often used in pregnancies with oligohydramnios. The risk of procedure-related loss after chorionic villus sampling is reported to be approximately the same as that for a mid-second-trimester amniocentesis.[48]

Fetal blood sampling is performed by directing the needle into the umbilical blood vessels. This procedure is commonly called *percutaneous umbilical blood sampling* (PUBS) or *cordocentesis*. The procedure allows the operator access to the fetal circulation for blood sampling and intravascular transfusion. Fetal blood is commonly obtained when a rapid karyotype would help in clinical decision making. Fetal blood may also be tested with a complete blood cell count in the fetus with suspected anemia or thrombocytopenia caused by isoimmunization (see Chapter 44). Blood products can be replaced in the fetus who requires this therapy. Hemoglobinopathies can be assessed through fetal blood. A blood gas measurement to determine pH and oxygen content can be performed in the fetus with suspected IUGR or distress. Additionally, blood can be cultured for viral organisms and tested for IgG and IgM in possibly affected pregnancies. Cordocentesis may be used for fetal drug therapy. Cordocentesis has been used to supply antiarrhythmic agents to fetuses with refractory arrhythmias.

Fetal liver, skin, and muscle tissues have been obtained through ultrasonographic biopsies.[17] Ultrasound is also used with selective reduction procedures.[47] Selective reduction is performed in the multifetal gestation, generally triplets or more, and the pregnancy is reduced to twins.[5] The technique

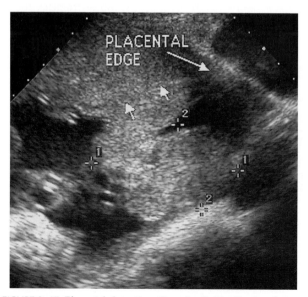

FIGURE 8–47. Placental abruption. Complex fluid collection *(between cursors)* and placental edge *(arrow)* are shown.

involves inserting a spinal needle into the fetal heart under ultrasound guidance and injecting potassium chloride, air, or digitalis, which results in fetal asystole. This procedure has also been used for reduction of twin pregnancies with an abnormal twin.

In summary, ultrasound is the most important modality for evaluating the pregnant uterus. Modern perinatal ultrasound has transformed the fetus from a static uterine passenger to a separate patient undergoing sophisticated diagnostic and therapeutic interventions.

■ REFERENCES

1. American Institute of Ultrasound in Medicine Bioeffects Committee: Bioeffects considerations for the safety of diagnostic ultrasound. J Ultrasound Med 7(Suppl):1, 1988.
2. Anderson NG, et al: Diastematomyelia: Diagnosis by prenatal sonography. Am J Roentgenol 163:911, 1994.
3. Assel BG, et al: Single-operator comparison of early and mid-second-trimester amniocentesis. Obstet Gynecol 79:940, 1992.
4. Blackwell RJ: The physics of ultrasound imaging. In Chervanak FA, et al (eds): Ultrasound in Obstetrics and Gynecology. Boston, Little, Brown, 1993.
5. Boulot P, et al: Effects of selective reduction in triplet gestation: A comparative study of 80 cases managed with or without this procedure. Fertil Steril 60:497, 1993.
6. Bowerman R: Sonography of fetal midgut herniation: Normal size criteria and correlation with crown-rump length. J Ultrasound Med 5:251, 1993.
7. Bowerman RA: Atlas of Normal Fetal Ultrasonographic Anatomy. Mosby-Year Book, 1992.
8. Brent RL, et al: Medical sonography: Reproductive effects and risks. In Chervanak FA, et al (eds): Ultrasound in Obstetrics and Gynecology. Boston, Little, Brown, 1993.
9. Bromley B, et al: Closure of the cerebellar vermis: Evaluation with second trimester US. Radiology 193:761, 1994.
10. Brown DL, et al: Diagnosis of early embryonic demise by endovaginal sonography. J Ultrasound Med 9:631, 1990.
11. Brown DL, et al: Echogenic material in the fetal gallbladder: Sonographic and clinical observations. Radiology 182:73, 1992.
12. Campbell S: Fetal growth. Clin Obstet Gynaecol 1:41, 1974.
13. Cardoza JD, et al: Exclusion of fetal ventriculomegaly with a single measurement: The width of the lateral ventricular atrium. Radiology 169:711, 1988.
14. Cohen HL, et al: Normal length of fetal kidneys: Sonographic study in 397 obstetric patients. AJR Am J Roentgenol 157:545, 1991.
15. Cullen MT, et al: Diagnosis and significance of cystic hygroma in the first trimester. Prenat Diagn 10:643, 1990.
16. Daya S: Accuracy of gestational age estimation by means of fetal crown-rump length measurement. Am J Obstet Gynecol 168:903, 1993.
17. Elias S, et al: Ultrasound-guided fetal skin sampling for prenatal diagnosis of genodermatoses. Obstet Gynecol 83:37, 1994.
18. Estroff JA, et al: Dandy-Walker variant: Prenatal sonographic features and clinical outcome. Radiology 185:755, 1992.
19. Fish P: Physics and Instrumentation of Diagnostic Medical Ultrasound. New York, John Wiley & Sons, 1990.
20. Hadlock FP: Sonographic estimation of fetal age and weight. Radiol Clin North Am 28:39, 1990.
21. Harris RD, et al: Sonography of the placenta with emphasis on pathological correlation. Semin Ultrasound CT MR 17:66, 1996.
22. Hata T, et al: Three dimensional sonographic visualization of the fetal face. AJR Am J Roentgenol 170:481, 1998.
23. Hill LM, et al: Ratios between the abdominal circumference, head circumference, or femur length and the transverse cerebellar diameter of the growth-retarded and macrosomic fetus. Am J Perinatol 11:144, 1994.
24. Hobbins J: Diagnosis and management of neural-tube defects today. N Engl J Med 324:690, 1991.
25. Jeanty P, et al: Single-needle insertion in twin amniocentesis. J Ultrasound Med 9:511, 1990.
26. Jurkovic D, et al: Ultrasound features of normal early pregnancy development. Curr Opin Obstet Gynecol 7:493, 1995.
27. Kurtz AB, et al: In utero analysis of heterozygous achondroplasia: Variable time of onset as detected by femur length measurements. J Ultrasound Med 5:137, 1986.
28. Larsen T, et al: Detection of small-for-gestational-age fetuses by ultrasound screening in a high-risk population: A randomized controlled study, Br J Obstet Gynaecol, 99:469, 1992.
29. Leerentveld RA, et al: Accuracy and safety of transvaginal sonographic placental localization. Obstet Gynecol 76:759, 1990.
30. Lowe CU, et al: The NICHD Amniocentesis Registry: The Safety and Accuracy of Midtrimester Amniocentesis. Washington DC, United States Department of Health, Education, and Welfare, 1978. DHEW Publication No (NIH) 78.
31. McGahan J: The fetal head: Borderlines. Semin Ultrasound CT MR 19:318, 1998.
32. Metkus AP, et al: Sonographic predictors of survival in fetal diaphragmatic hernia. J Pediatr Surg 31:148, 1996.
33. Munoz C, et al: Osteogenesis imperfecta type II: Prenatal sonographic diagnosis. Radiology 174:181, 1990.
34. National Council of Radiation Protection and Measurements: Exposure Criteria for Medical Diagnostic Ultrasound. I. Criteria Based on Thermal Mechanisms. Bethesda, Md, NCRP Publications, 1992. NCRP Report 113.
35. Nicolaides KH, et al: Ultrasound screening for spina bifida: Cranial and cerebellar signs. Lancet 2:72, 1986.
36. Nyberg DA, et al: Echogenic fetal bowel during the second trimester: Clinical importance. Radiology 188:527, 1993.
37. Nyberg DA, et al: Paranasal echogenic mass: Sonographic sign of bilateral complete cleft lip and palate before 20 menstrual weeks. Radiology 184:757, 1992.
38. Oppenheimer LW, et al: What is a low-lying placenta? Am J Obstet Gynecol 165:1036, 1991.
39. Persutte WH, Hobbins J: Single umbilical artery: A clinical enigma in modern prenatal diagnosis. Ultrasound Obstet Gynecol 6:216, 1995.
40. Phelan JP, et al: Amniotic fluid index measurements during pregnancy. J Reprod Med 32:601, 1987.
41. Rottem S, et al: Transvaginal sonographic diagnosis of congenital anomalies between 9 weeks' and 16 weeks' menstrual age. J Clin Ultrasound 17:307, 1990.
42. Schats R, et al: Embryonic heart activity: Appearance and development in early human pregnancy. Br J Obstet Gynaecol 97:989, 1990.
43. Seeds, JW: Ultrasonographic screening for fetal aneuploidy. N Engl J Med 337:1689, 1997.
44. Shapiro BS, et al: A model-based prediction for transvaginal ultrasonographic identification of early intrauterine pregnancy. Am J Obstet Gynecol 166:1495, 1992.
45. Tegnander E, et al: Prenatal detection of heart defects at the routine fetal examination at 18 weeks in a non-selected population. Ultrasound Obstet Gynecol 5:372, 1995.
46. Vintzileos AM, et al: The use of second-trimester genetic sonogram in guiding clinical management of patients at increased risk for fetal trisomy 21. Obstet Gynecol 87:948, 1996.
47. Wapner RJ, et al: Selective reduction of multifetal pregnancies. Lancet 225:90, 1990.
48. Young SR, et al: Single-center comparison of results of 1000 prenatal diagnoses with chorionic villus sampling and 1000 diagnoses with amniocentesis. Am J Obstet Gynecol 165:255, 1991.
49. Zelop CC, et al: Second trimester sonographically diagnosed placenta previa: Prediction of persistent previa at birth. Int J Gynaecol Obstet 44:207, 1994.

Estimation of Fetal Well-Being

9

part one
EVALUATION OF THE INTRAPARTUM FETUS

Barbara V. Parilla

Fetal heart rate (FHR) monitoring is currently the primary method used in the assessment of fetal well-being in the intrapartum period. Before the development of modern methods of assessment, *fetal distress* was usually diagnosed on the basis of criteria that are now considered to be faulty or erroneous. For example, meconium-stained amniotic fluid in the absence of an abnormal FHR pattern is an indication for aggressive airway management at delivery, but alone it is not diagnostic of fetal intolerance to labor. FHR monitoring involves evaluation of the pattern as well as the rate. It can help the physician identify and interpret changes in FHR patterns that may be associated with fetal conditions such as hypoxia, umbilical cord compression, tachycardia, and acidosis.

The ability to interpret FHR patterns and to understand their correlation with the condition of the fetus allows the physician to institute maneuvers such as maternal oxygen therapy, amnioinfusion, and tocolytic therapy to improve the abnormality. In addition, the antepartum history must be considered when evaluating the intrapartum fetus. Is it a normal-sized or growth-restricted fetus? Is there oligohydramnios or are there other complications that may affect the labor course? FHR monitoring alone should not be a substitute for informed clinical judgment.

A reassuring FHR monitoring strip is almost always associated with a nonacidotic fetus and a vigorous neonate at birth. However, nonreassuring pat-

terns are nonspecific and cannot reliably predict whether a fetus will be well oxygenated, depressed, or acidotic. Factors other than hypoxia may lead to a nonreassuring FHR, and an abnormal pattern may neither depict the severity of the hypoxia nor predict how it will progress if labor is allowed to continue. Nevertheless, because alterations in fetal oxygenation occur during labor and because many complications can occur during this critical period, some form of FHR evaluation should be provided to all patients.

For the purposes of this chapter, the following definitions are used:

Hypoxemia: Decreased oxygen content in the blood
Hypoxia: Decreased level of oxygen in tissue
Acidemia: Increased concentration of hydrogen ions in the blood
Acidosis: Increased concentration of hydrogen ions in tissue
Asphyxia: Hypoxia with metabolic acidosis

PHYSIOLOGY

The fetus is well adapted to extracting oxygen from the maternal circulation, even with the additional stress of normal labor and delivery. Transient and repetitive episodes of hypoxemia and hypoxia, even at the level of the central nervous system (CNS), are extremely common during normal labor, and they are generally well tolerated by the fetus. Furthermore, a progressive intrapartum decline in baseline fetal oxygenation and pH is virtually universal; levels of acidemia that would be ominous in an infant or adult are commonly seen in normal newborns. Only when hypoxia and resultant metabolic acidemia reach extreme levels is the fetus at risk for long-term neurologic impairment.[7] However, alterations in the fetoplacental unit resulting from labor or intrapartum complications may subject the fetus to decreased oxygenation, leading to potential damage to any susceptible organ system or even fetal death.

Oxygen delivery is critically dependent on uterine blood flow. Uterine contractions decrease placental blood flow and result in intermittent episodes of decreased oxygen delivery. Normally, the fetus tolerates contractions without difficulty, but if the frequency, duration, or strength of contractions become excessive, fetal hypoxemia may result. Maternal position and the use of conduction anesthesia can also alter uterine blood flow and oxygen delivery during labor. Finally, labor may be complicated by conditions such as preeclampsia, abruptio placentae, chorioamnionitis, and other pathologic situations that can further alter blood flow and oxygen exchange within the placenta.

Some fetuses are unusually susceptible to the effects of intrapartum hypoxemia, such as fetuses with growth restriction and those who are born prematurely. In these circumstances, hypoxia tends to progress more rapidly and is more likely to cause or aggravate metabolic acidemia, which, in extreme cases, correlates with poor long-term neurologic outcome. In severe cases, such hypoxia can lead to death.[1] (See Chapter 38, Parts Three and Four.)

The fetal CNS is susceptible to hypoxia. Experimentally induced hypoxia has been associated with consistent, predictable changes in the FHR.[2] Because the FHR and its alterations are under CNS control through sympathetic and parasympathetic reflexes, alterations in the FHR can be sensitive indicators of fetal hypoxia.

GUIDELINES FOR PERFORMING FETAL HEART RATE MONITORING

The FHR may be evaluated by intermittent auscultation with a DeLee-Hillis stethoscope or a Doppler ultrasound device or by electronic monitoring. Continuous FHR and contraction monitoring may be performed externally or internally. Most external monitors use a Doppler device with computerized logic to interpret and count the Doppler signals. Internal FHR monitoring is accomplished with a fetal electrode, which is a spiral wire placed directly on the fetal scalp or other presenting part. This method records the fetal electrocardiogram. In either case, the FHR is recorded continuously on the upper portion of a paper strip and every beat-to-beat interval is recorded as a rate. The lower portion of the strip records uterine contractions, which also may be monitored externally or internally.

Well-controlled studies have shown that intermittent auscultation of the FHR is equivalent to continuous electronic monitoring in assessing fetal condition when performed at specific intervals with a 1:1 nurse-to-patient ratio.[13] The intensity of FHR monitoring used during labor should be based on risk factors, and when they are present, the FHR should be assessed according to the following guidelines:

■ If auscultation is used during the active phase of the first stage of labor, the FHR should be evaluated and recorded at least every 15 minutes after a uterine contraction. If continuous electronic monitoring is used, the tracing should be reviewed at least every 15 minutes.

■ During the second stage of labor, if auscultation is being used, the FHR should be evaluated and recorded at least every 5 minutes. When electronic monitoring is used, the FHR strip should be reviewed every 5 minutes.

■ The optimal frequency at which intermittent auscultation should be performed in the absence of risk factors has not been established. One method is to evaluate the FHR at least every 30 minutes in the active phase of the first stage of labor and at least every 15 minutes in the second stage of labor.

RISKS AND BENEFITS

Currently, neither the most effective method of FHR monitoring nor the specific frequency or duration of monitoring to ensure optimal perinatal outcome has been identified by a significant body of scientific evidence.

Seven randomized, controlled trials have compared continuous electronic FHR monitoring with intermittent auscultation in patients at high risk and those at low risk, and no differences in intrapartum fetal death rates were found.[13] In contrast, a more recent randomized, controlled trial did show a significant reduction in perinatal deaths from asphyxia in the electronically monitored group.[17] It is not clear why this single study is so discordant with the others, but it does provide some promise that further studies may yet elucidate the real value of electronic FHR monitoring.

The primary risk of electronic FHR monitoring is a potential increase in the cesarean delivery rate. This effect has been observed in both retrospective trials and the majority of prospective, randomized trials. More accurate interpretation of FHR monitoring, fetal scalp blood pH determination, and the use of scalp stimulation to elicit FHR accelerations can lead to more precise interpretation of the fetal status, which may lead to a decrease in the cesarean delivery rate. Presently, direct fetal pulse oximeters are being studied, and may hold promise.

INTERPRETATION OF FETAL HEART RATE PATTERNS

The initial FHR pattern should be carefully evaluated for any abnormalities of the baseline and for the presence or absence of accelerations and decelerations. In one study, the first 30 minutes of electronic FHR monitoring identified about 50% of all fetuses that underwent cesarean delivery for a nonreassuring FHR pattern or fetal distress. Although the progression of decelerations usually explains changes in the baseline later in labor, abnormalities of the baseline on admission, such as fetal tachycardia or loss of variability,

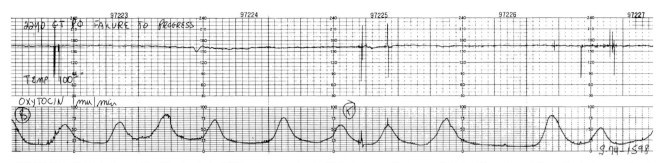

FIGURE 9–1. Fetal tachycardia. Heart rate is 165 beats per minute. This tachycardia is associated with maternal fever (note temperature). Also note the associated loss of variability. Because of the absence of associated decelerations and the presence of an explanation (fever), hypoxia is an unlikely cause. (From Freeman R, Garite T: Fetal heart rate monitoring. Baltimore, Williams & Wilkins, 1981, p 70.)

may be difficult to interpret because data regarding previous changes are lacking.

BASELINE FETAL HEART RATE

Rate and variability are two specific and important parameters of the baseline FHR. The baseline heart rate at term usually ranges from 120 to 160 beats per minute. The initial response of the FHR to intermittent hypoxia is deceleration, but baseline tachycardia may develop if the hypoxia is prolonged and severe. Tachycardia may also be associated with conditions other than hypoxia, such as maternal fever, intraamniotic infection, thyroid disease, presence of medication, and cardiac arrhythmia (Fig. 9–1). The presence of variability, or variation of successive beats in the heart rate, is a useful indicator of fetal CNS integrity. In the absence of maternal sedation, magnesium sulfate administration, or extreme prematurity, decreased variability, or flattening of the FHR baseline,

may serve as a barometer of the fetal response to hypoxia. Because decreased variability or flattening is presumed to be a CNS response, in most situations, decelerations of the FHR precede the loss of variability, indicating the cause (Fig. 9–2).

Periodic changes in the FHR are common in labor; they occur in response to contractions or fetal movement and include accelerations and decelerations.

ACCELERATIONS

Accelerations of the FHR seem to occur most commonly in the antepartum period, in early labor, and in association with variable decelerations. They are almost always associated with fetal movement. The presence of accelerations in the intrapartum period is always reassuring and reflects a normal fetal pH. The absence of accelerations in the intrapartum period is not alarming as long as the baseline FHR and variability are normal (Fig. 9–3).

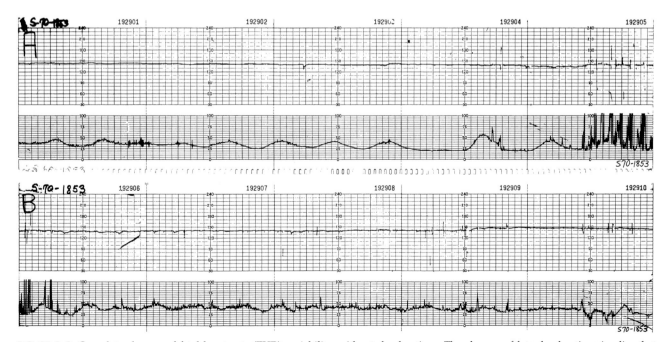

FIGURE 9–2. Complete absence of fetal heart rate (FHR) variability, without decelerations. The absence of late decelerations implies that fetal hypoxemia does not currently exist. However, the absence of FHR variability for this duration suggests fetal neurologic impairment antecedent to labor. (From Freeman R, Garite T: Fetal heart rate monitoring. Baltimore, Williams & Wilkins, 1981, p 138.)

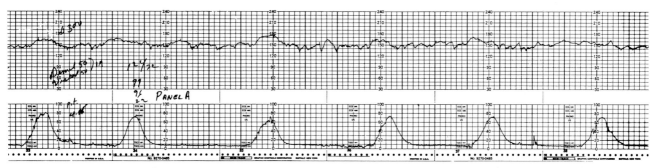

FIGURE 9–3. Normal, reassuring fetal heart rate (FHR) pattern. Note perturbations of FHR (small amplitude represents FHR variability; larger amplitude represents FHR reactivity). If seen during antepartum testing, this tracing would be interpreted as a reactive, negative contraction stress test. (From Freeman R, Garite T: Fetal heart rate monitoring. Baltimore, Williams & Wilkins, 1981, p 72.)

DECELERATIONS

In some instances of decreased oxygenation, the pattern of the FHR can identify the mechanism. For instance, umbilical cord compression coincides with variable decelerations.[3] Variable decelerations are the most common decelerations seen in labor, and they are generally associated with a favorable outcome. They are defined as slowing of the FHR with abrupt onset and return, and they are frequently preceded and followed by small accelerations of the FHR. These decelerations vary in depth, duration, and shape on the tracing, but they generally coincide with the timing of the uterine contractions (Fig. 9–4). Only when variable decelerations become persistent, progressively deeper, and longer lasting are they considered to be nonreassuring. Although progression is more important than absolute parameters, persistent variable decelerations to fewer than 70 beats per minute and lasting longer than 60 seconds are generally of concern, especially if they are accompanied by a change in baseline and decreased variability (Fig. 9–5). In addition, a slow return to baseline is worrisome because this reflects hypoxia persistent beyond the relaxation phase of the contraction.[8]

Late decelerations may be secondary to transient fetal hypoxia in response to the decreased placental perfusion associated with uterine contractions. Occasional or intermittent late decelerations are not uncommon during labor. These are U-shaped decelerations of gradual onset and gradual return that are usually shallow (10 to 30 beats per minute) and reach their nadir after the peak of the contraction (Fig. 9–6). When late decelerations become persistent, they are considered to be nonreassuring, regardless of the depth of the decelerations. Late decelerations caused by reflex and mediated by the CNS generally become deeper as the degree of hypoxia becomes more severe. However, as metabolic acidosis develops from tissue hypoxia, late decelerations are believed to be the result of direct myocardial depression, and they will not indicate the degree of hypoxia.[8]

Early decelerations are shallow and symmetric with a pattern similar to that of late decelerations, but they reach their nadir at the same time as the peak of the contraction and, therefore, look like mirror images of the contractions. They are infrequently seen and are thought to be caused by fetal head compression in the active phase of labor (Fig. 9–7).

A prolonged deceleration, often incorrectly referred to as bradycardia, is an isolated, abrupt decrease in the FHR to levels below the baseline that lasts at least 60 to 90 seconds. These changes are always of concern and may be caused by any mechanism that can lead to fetal hypoxia. The severity of the event causing the deceleration is usually reflected in the depth and duration of the deceleration, as well as by the degree to which variability is lost during the deceleration. When such a deceleration returns to the baseline, especially with more profound episodes, a transient fetal tachycardia and loss of variability may occur while the fetus is recovering from hypoxia (Fig. 9–8). The degree to which such decelerations are nonreassuring depends on their depth and duration,

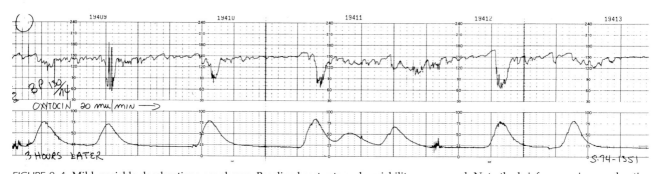

FIGURE 9–4. Mild, variable decelerations are shown. Baseline heart rate and variability are normal. Note the brief, reassuring acceleration preceding deceleration at panel 19412. (From Freeman R, Garite T: Fetal heart rate monitoring. Baltimore, Williams & Wilkins, 1981, p 78.)

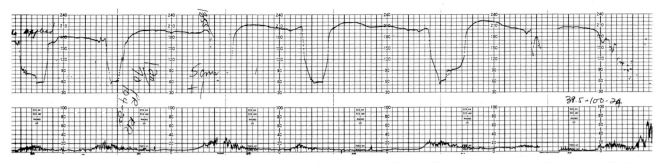

FIGURE 9–5. Severe, variable decelerations are shown, with baseline heart rate rising to 210 beats per minute and with virtually absent variability. Note the prolonged fetal heart rate "overshoot" in the midportion of the panel; it is an ominous tracing. This baby was premature, delivered by cesarean section, with Apgar scores of 1 at 1 minute and 2 at 5 minutes. (From Freeman R, Garite T: Fetal heart rate monitoring. Baltimore, Williams & Wilkins, 1981, p 80.)

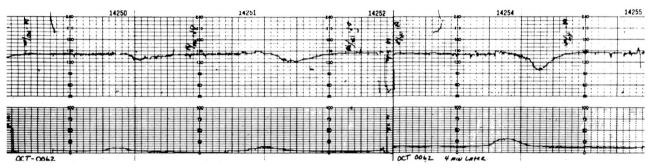

FIGURE 9–6. Late decelerations with absence of fetal heart rate (FHR) variability and reactivity. This is an ominous FHR pattern. (From Freeman R, Garite T: Fetal heart rate monitoring. Baltimore, Williams & Wilkins, 1981, p 201.)

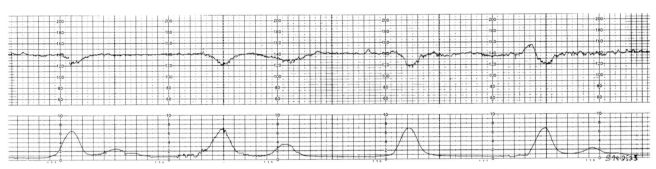

FIGURE 9–7. Early decelerations are shown with each contraction on this panel. They are uniform, mirror the contractions, and decelerate only 10 to 20 beats per minute. Fetal heart rate variability at the end of the panel is satisfactory, a reassuring sign. (From Freeman R, Garite T: Fetal heart rate monitoring. Baltimore, Williams & Wilkins, 1981, p 74.)

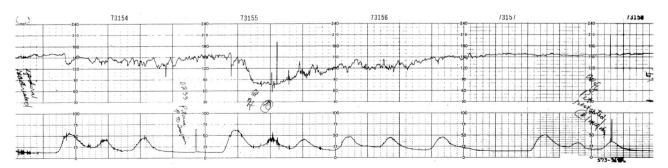

FIGURE 9–8. Prolonged deceleration associated with excessive uterine activity secondary to oxytocin hyperstimulation. A rebound tachycardia with decreased variability follows the prolonged deceleration. Oxytocin was stopped and restarted at a lower rate, and the heart rate subsequently returned to normal. (From Freeman R, Garite T: Fetal heart rate monitoring. Baltimore, Williams & Wilkins, 1981, p 85.)

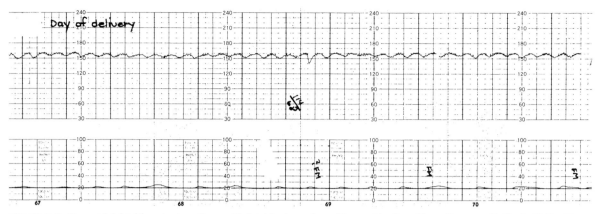

FIGURE 9–9. Sinusoidal fetal heart rate pattern with fetal hydrops from Rh sensitization. (From Freeman R, Garite T: Fetal heart rate monitoring. Baltimore, Williams & Wilkins, 1981, p 166.)

the loss of variability, the response of the fetus during the recovery period, and, most importantly, the frequency and progression of the recurrence.

A sinusoidal heart rate pattern consists of a regular oscillation of the baseline variability, resembling a sine wave. This smooth, undulating pattern, lasting at least 10 minutes, has a relatively fixed period of 3 to 5 cycles per minute and an amplitude of 5 to 15 beats per minute above and below the baseline (Fig. 9–9). This pattern may be associated with severe chronic, as opposed to acute, fetal anemia. It also has been described following the use of alphaprodine or other medications; in such circumstances, it may not represent fetal compromise. Additionally, severe hypoxia and acidosis occasionally manifest as a sinusoidal FHR; the reason for this is not understood. True sinusoidal patterns are quite rare. Unfortunately, small, frequent accelerations of low amplitude are easy to confuse with sinusoidal patterns. The former are benign and occur more frequently. A true sinusoidal FHR is always nonreassuring.

EVALUATION AND MANAGEMENT OF NONREASSURING PATTERNS

With a persistently nonreassuring FHR pattern in labor, the clinician should determine the etiology of the pattern, when possible, and attempt to correct it by specifically correcting the primary problem or by instituting general measures aimed at improving fetal oxygenation and placental perfusion. For example, it is not uncommon to see a prolonged deceleration or repetitive late decelerations following epidural placement secondary to splanchnic relaxation with resultant uterine hypoperfusion.[15] Measures such as ensuring that the woman is in the lateral recumbent position and administering an intravenous fluid bolus are helpful. If there is systemic hypotension, ephedrine administration should be considered. Excessive uterine contractions may also be responsible for decelerations (Fig. 9–10). Careful use of oxytocin is necessary to minimize uterine hyperstimulation. If nonreassuring FHR changes occur in patients receiving oxytocin, the infusion should be decreased or discontinued. Restarting the infusion at a lower rate and increasing it in smaller increments may be better tolerated. General measures that may improve fetal oxygenation and placental perfusion should also be used.

MATERNAL POSITION

Maternal position during labor can affect uterine blood flow and placental perfusion. In the supine position, the vena cava and aortoiliac vessels are compressed by the gravid uterus. This results in decreased return of blood to the maternal heart, leading to a reduction in cardiac output, blood pressure, and, therefore, uterine blood flow. In the supine position, aortic compression may result in an increase in the incidence of late decelerations and a decrease in fetal

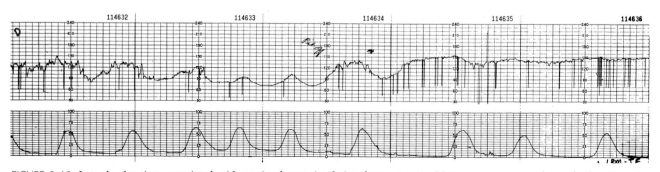

FIGURE 9–10. Late decelerations associated with uterine hyperstimulation from oxytocin. Note compensatory relative fetal tachycardia developing as recovery occurs. (From Freeman R, Garite T: Fetal heart rate monitoring. Baltimore, Williams & Wilkins, 1981, p 114.)

scalp pH. The lateral recumbent position (either side) is best for maximizing cardiac output and uterine blood flow. It is often associated with improvement in the FHR pattern.[6]

OXYGEN THERAPY

The arterial PO_2 in the fetus is normally about 25% of the arterial PO_2 in the mother. Despite this low PO_2, the fetal blood can carry a large amount of oxygen from the placenta because of the increased heart rate and the fetal hemoglobin's high affinity for oxygen. When there is evidence of a nonreassuring pattern, the administration of supplemental oxygen to the mother is thought to be useful. A significant increase in maternal oxygenation is accomplished with a tight-fitting face mask and an oxygen flow rate of 8 to 10 L per minute. Although such administration results in only a small increase in fetal PO_2, animal studies have suggested that a 30% to 40% increase in fetal oxygen content may occur.[11]

AMNIOINFUSION

For severe variable or prolonged decelerations, a pelvic exam should be performed to rule out umbilical cord prolapse or rapid descent of the fetal head (Fig. 9–11). If no cause for such decelerations is found, one can usually conclude that umbilical cord compression is responsible. In patients with decreased amniotic fluid volume, replacement of amniotic fluid with normal saline infused through a transcervical intrauterine pressure catheter has been reported to decrease both the frequency and severity of variable decelerations.[12] Investigators also have reported a decrease in newborn respiratory complications from meconium in patients who receive amnioinfusion. This result presumably is from the dilutional effect of amnioinfusion and possibly from prevention of in utero fetal gasping that may occur during episodes of hypoxia caused by umbilical cord compression.[9]

TOCOLYTIC AGENTS

Excessive uterine contractions accompanied by a nonreassuring FHR may require a tocolytic agent if general measures are not successful. Terbutaline and magnesium sulfate have been reported to be of value in rapidly improving fetal condition by promoting uterine relaxation during active labor. Even in the absence of uterine hypertonia, abnormal FHR patterns occurring in response to uterine contractions may be improved by the administration of tocolytic agents.[16] This approach is especially useful when unavoidable delays in effecting operative delivery are encountered.

EVALUATION AND MANAGEMENT OF PERSISTENT NONREASSURING FETAL HEART RATE PATTERNS

If the FHR pattern remains uncorrected, the decision to intervene depends on the clinician's assessment of the likelihood of severe hypoxia and the possibility of metabolic acidosis, as well as the estimated time to spontaneous delivery. For the fetus with persistent nonreassuring decelerations, normal FHR variability and the absence of tachycardia generally indicate the lack of acidosis. The presence of FHR variability should probably be confirmed with a fetal electrode in the presence of nonreassuring decelerations. Persistent late decelerations or severe variable decelerations associated with the absence of variability are always nonreassuring and generally require prompt intervention.

The presence of spontaneous accelerations of greater than 15 beats per minute and lasting at least 15 seconds almost always ensures the absence of fetal acidosis. Fetal scalp stimulation or vibroacoustic stimulation can be used to induce accelerations, which indicate the absence of acidosis.[4, 14] Conversely, there is about a 50% chance of acidosis in the fetus who fails to respond to stimulation in the presence of a nonreassuring pattern.[4, 14] In these fetuses, assessment of scalp blood pH should be considered to clarify the acid-base status. Surprisingly, this technique is underused in current obstetric practice.[5]

If the FHR pattern remains worrisome, either induced accelerations or repeat assessment of scalp blood pH is required every 20 to 30 minutes for continued reassurance. In cases in which the FHR pattern is persistently nonreassuring and acidosis is present or cannot be ruled out, the fetus should be promptly delivered by the most expeditious route, whether abdominal or vaginal.

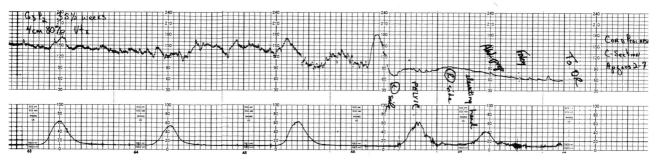

FIGURE 9–11. This patient showed a sudden, prolonged deceleration in the early active phase of labor. An immediate pelvic examination revealed cord prolapse, and a cesarean delivery was performed. (From Freeman R, Garite T: Fetal heart rate monitoring. Baltimore, Williams & Wilkins, 1981, p 83.)

PERINATAL ASPHYXIA AND CEREBRAL PALSY

With the advent and liberal use of electronic FHR monitoring in the 1970s, there was great hope that intrapartum fetal death and morbidity associated with intrapartum asphyxia could be virtually eliminated. This has not been proved in several prospective, randomized, controlled trials and retrospective, controlled studies.[2, 10]

In western industrialized countries, the rate of cerebral palsy in term infants (1–2:1000) has not changed in the past 20 years, despite new neonatal and obstetric technologies. However, a continuing misperception that birth asphyxia accounts for a significant portion of infants with cerebral palsy continues to exist, despite the lack of evidence to support this impression. Several clinical and experimental reports confirm that only severe and prolonged asphyxia is associated with an increased risk of subsequent neurologic dysfunction. In assessing a possible relationship between perinatal asphyxia and neurologic deficit in an individual patient, all of the following criteria must be present before a plausible link can be made[1]:

■ Profound umbilical artery metabolic or mixed acidemia (pH < 7.00)
■ Persistence of an Apgar score of 0 to 3 for longer than 5 minutes
■ Neonatal neurologic sequelae (e.g., seizures, coma, or hypotonia)
■ Multiorgan system dysfunction (e.g., cardiovascular, gastrointestinal, hematologic, pulmonary, or renal) (See also Chapter 38.)

When prolonged and severe asphyxia does occur, it is often followed by death. Most infants who survive severe birth asphyxia are clinically normal later.[1]

SUMMARY

Because alterations in fetal oxygenation occur during labor and because many complications can occur during this critical period, some form of FHR evaluation should be provided for all patients. By understanding the physiologic and pathophysiologic basis of FHR monitoring, as well as its capabilities and limitations, the clinician can reduce the need for interventions.

part two

ANTEPARTUM FETAL SURVEILLANCE

Susan E. Gerber

The primary goal of antenatal fetal surveillance is the avoidance of intrauterine fetal death. Pregnant women are counseled on the importance of fetal movement, and routine prenatal care provides for routine fetal surveillance. However, in certain populations with an increased risk of fetal demise, a greater degree of fetal surveillance may be warranted. This section addresses the methods used to perform such surveillance and the evidence for its use.

RATIONALE FOR SURVEILLANCE

The incidence of intrauterine fetal death at 20 weeks' gestation or later was 6.8 per 1000 births in the United States in 1997.[25] Intrauterine fetal death may result from a variety of causes, such as congenital malformations, fetal-maternal hemorrhage, congenital infection, isoimmunization, and antiphospholipid antibody syndrome. In many circumstances fetal deaths are precipitated by sudden catastrophic events, such as an abruptio placentae or cord prolapse. These events are often unpredictable and are not preventable by any form of antepartum surveillance; therefore, women at risk for such events may not benefit from increased surveillance. For example, maternal cocaine use may increase the risk of abruptio placentae and intrauterine fetal death, but without underlying uteroplacental insufficiency or growth restriction, such an event would not be predictable.

The methods commonly used for antenatal fetal surveillance rely on fetal biophysical parameters that are sensitive to hypoxemia and acidemia, such as heart rate and movement. These surveillance tools are useful in a fetus who is at risk for hypoxemia because of chronic uteroplacental insufficiency. It is hoped that if fetal surveillance identifies a fetus in jeopardy, the physician will have an opportunity to intervene before progressive fetal hypoxemia and acidosis lead to fetal death.

INDICATIONS FOR SURVEILLANCE

Pregnancies at increased risk for intrauterine fetal demise fall into two categories: those with maternal conditions and those with pregnancy-associated conditions. Table 9–1 lists some of the conditions in which antenatal surveillance should be considered. There are a number of situations in which a population is known to have an increased risk of fetal death, but the etiology is unclear. One such population is the 1% of all pregnant women that is found to have an unexplained elevated maternal serum α-fetoprotein. Although numerous studies have confirmed the elevated risk of fetal death in this population,[47] there is no consensus on whether antenatal surveillance reduces this risk.[49] Antenatal testing in such a population is commonly performed, but it remains controversial.

PHYSIOLOGIC BASIS FOR ANTENATAL SURVEILLANCE

In experiments involving animal and human fetuses, hypoxemia and acidosis have been shown to consis-

TABLE 9–1 INDICATIONS FOR ANTENATAL SURVEILLANCE

MATERNAL CONDITIONS	PREGNANCY-RELATED CONDITIONS
Antiphospholipid antibody syndrome	Pregnancy-induced hypertension
Hyperthyroidism (poorly controlled)	Decreased fetal movement
	Oligohydramnios
Hemoglobinopathies (hemoglobin SS, SC, or S-thalassemia)	Polyhydramnios
	Intrauterine growth restriction
	Multiple gestation
Cyanotic heart disease	Post-term pregnancy
Systemic lupus erythematosus	Isoimmunization (moderate to severe)
Hypertensive disorders	Previous fetal demise (unexplained or recurrent risk)
Chronic renal disease	Preterm, premature rupture of membranes
Diabetes mellitus	Unexplained third trimester bleeding

Data from American College of Obstetricians and Gynecologists: Antepartum fetal surveillance. Washington DC, American College of Obstetricians and Gynecologists, 1999. ACOG Practice Bulletin 9.

tently alter fetal biophysical parameters such as heart rate, movement, breathing, and tone.[22, 37, 42] The fetal heart rate (FHR) is normally controlled by the fetal central nervous system (CNS) and mediated by sympathetic or parasympathetic nerve impulses originating in the fetal brainstem. The presence of intermittent FHR accelerations associated with fetal movement, therefore, is believed to be an indicator of an intact fetal autonomic nervous system. In a study of fetal blood sampling in pregnancies resulting in healthy neonates, Weiner and colleagues established a range of normal fetal venous pH measurements. In this population, the lower 2.5th percentile of fetal venous pH was 7.37.[48] Manning and associates demonstrated that fetuses without heart rate accelerations had a mean umbilical vein pH of 7.28 ($\pm$ 0.11) and that those with abnormal movement had a mean pH of 7.16 ($\pm$ 0.08).[35] These and similar observations were the basis for the development of antenatal fetal testing modalities that are currently in use.

NONSTRESS TEST

In most institutions, the first-line assessment tool for fetal surveillance is the nonstress test (NST). Lee and coworkers first described the association between FHR accelerations and fetal movements in 1975.[32] Monitoring for the presence or absence of both elements was proposed as a method of evaluation of fetal well-being. The NST is performed in a nonlaboring patient (as opposed to the contraction stress test [CST], in which the patient has regular uterine contractions, either spontaneously or induced). At times, a woman undergoing an NST is found to have spontaneous contractions, thereby adding the reassurance of a negative CST.

With the patient in a recumbent, tilted position, the FHR is monitored with an external transducer for up to 40 minutes. The FHR tracing is observed for the presence of accelerations above the baseline. A reactive test is one in which there are at least two accelerations that peak 15 beats per minute above the baseline and last (not necessarily at the peak) for at least 15 seconds before returning to baseline (Fig. 9–12). The majority of NSTs are reactive within the first 20 minutes. For those that are not, possibly because of a fetal sleep cycle, an additional 20 minutes of monitoring may be needed. A nonreactive NST is one in which two such accelerations do not occur within 40 minutes, or if the acceleration peaks are fewer than 15 beats per minute.

Although it is noninvasive and easy to perform, the NST is limited by a high rate of false positive results. Normal fetuses often have periods of nonreactivity owing to benign variations such as sleep cycles. Vibroacoustic stimulation may be used safely in the setting of a nonreactive NST in order to elicit FHR accelerations without compromising the sensitivity of the NST.[50] In this situation, the operator places an artificial larynx on the maternal abdomen and activates the device for 1 to 3 seconds. This technique is often useful in situations in which the FHR has normal beat-to-beat variability and no decelerations but does not demonstrate any accelerations on an NST. If the test remains nonreactive, further evaluation with a biophysical profile or CST is warranted.

CONTRACTION STRESS TEST

The CST is designed to evaluate the FHR response to maternal uterine contractions. The principles that are applied to the evaluation of intrapartum FHR moni-

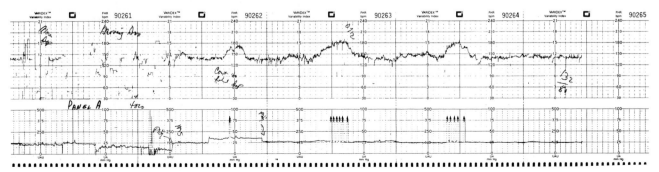

FIGURE 9–12. Reactive nonstress test, demonstrating accelerations occurring with fetal movement. (From Freeman R, Garite T: Fetal heart rate monitoring. Baltimore, Williams & Wilkins, 1981, p 163.)

toring (see Part One) are used here. In response to the stress of the contraction, a hypoxemic fetus demonstrates FHR patterns of concern, such as late decelerations, indicating worsening hypoxemia or fetal compromise.

Similar to the NST, for the CST the patient is placed in a recumbent tilted position and the FHR is monitored with an external fetal monitor. The FHR pattern is then evaluated while the patient experiences at least three contractions lasting 40 seconds within a 10-minute period. If the patient is not contracting spontaneously, contractions may be induced with either nipple stimulation or intravenous oxytocin. If no late or significant variable decelerations are noted on the FHR tracing, the CST is considered to be negative. If there are late decelerations following at least 50% of the contractions, the CST is positive. If late decelerations are present less than 50% of the time or if significant variable decelerations are present, the test is considered to be equivocal. Contraindications to the performance of this test include those clinical situations in which labor would be undesirable (e.g., placenta previa or prior classical cesarean section).

BIOPHYSICAL PROFILE

The biophysical profile (BPP) was developed by Manning and associates as an alternative tool to other methods of antenatal surveillance to evaluate fetal well-being.[38] As originally described, it combines the NST with four components evaluated by ultrasonography. In a 30-minute time period, the following observations are sought:

- Fetal breathing movements (one or more episode[s] lasting at least 30 seconds)
- Fetal movement (three or more discrete body or limb movements)
- Fetal tone (one or more episode[s] of active extension with return to flexion of a limb or trunk; or the opening and closing of a fetal hand; Fig. 9–13)
- Amniotic fluid volume (single vertical pocket of greater than 2 cm; Fig. 9–14)
- Reactive NST

Each component is assigned a score of 2 if present or 0 if absent. A combined score of 8 or 10 is considered to be indicative of fetal well-being. A score of 6 is considered to be equivocal, and it usually merits scheduled delivery at term or repeat testing in 24 hours in the preterm pregnancy. A score of 4 or lower is considered to be abnormal, and delivery is warranted except under extenuating circumstances. The BPP also has been analyzed with the four ultrasonographic parameters alone, and when all are present, it has been shown to have a false negative rate similar to the full BPP.[33]

AMNIOTIC FLUID VOLUME ASSESSMENT

Amniotic fluid volume is commonly estimated using ultrasonography. Decreased amniotic fluid volume, or

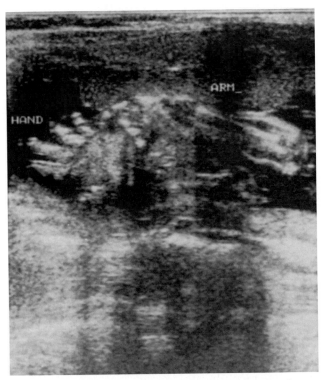

FIGURE 9–13. Ultrasound photograph of a fetal hand with poor tone (as reflected by extension), during biophysical profile. Fetal tone is generally the last biophysical parameter to be lost with deterioration of fetal state.

oligohydramnios, is typically defined in one of two ways: (1) no measurable vertical pocket of fluid greater than 2 cm, or (2) an amniotic fluid index of 5 cm or less.

The amniotic fluid index is calculated by measuring the maximal vertical pockets of fluid (without

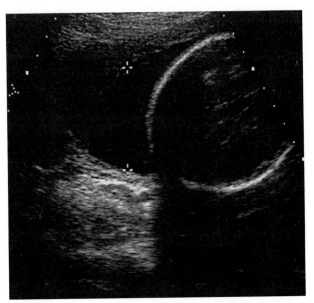

FIGURE 9–14. Ultrasound photograph of a maximum vertical pocket measured as part of either a biophysical profile or an amniotic fluid index. Note the absence of umbilical cord in the pocket measured.

loops of umbilical cord) in each of the four quadrants of the maternal abdomen (see Fig. 9–14).

Oligohydramnios, in most circumstances, is thought to be a reflection of fetal compromise. A decrease in placental perfusion results in decreased blood flow and, therefore, decreased oxygen delivery to the fetus. There is also decreased renal perfusion by the preferential shunting of blood to the fetal brain. Decreased renal perfusion results in decreased fetal urine output, which leads to a decreased amniotic fluid volume.

Oligohydramnios is commonly associated with post-term pregnancy, fetal growth restriction, maternal hypertension, and preeclampsia. In various clinical scenarios, oligohydramnios has been found to be associated with an increased risk of preterm delivery, low or very low birth weight, low Apgar scores, intrauterine fetal death, meconium-stained amniotic fluid, admissions to a neonatal intensive care unit, and cesarean delivery for nonreassuring fetal status.[20, 31, 44] In the term pregnancy, oligohydramnios is considered to be an indication for delivery. In the preterm pregnancy, immediate delivery may not be desirable, and in such cases, increased surveillance is warranted. However, in the preterm pregnancy with oligohydramnios, delivery is indicated for nonreassuring or abnormal fetal surveillance, or if there is no interval growth on ultrasound. (See also Chapter 21.)

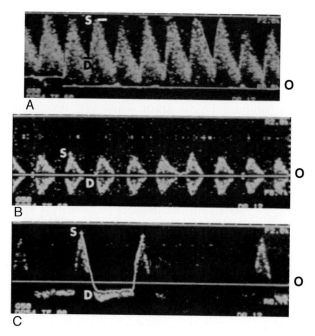

FIGURE 9–15. Composite photographs of three studies of fetal umbilical arterial velocimetry, ranging from normal to markedly abnormal. A, Normal velocimetry pattern. B, Absent diastolic flow, indicating increased placental resistance. C, Reversal of diastolic flow, indicating worsening placental function. S, systolic velocity; D, diastolic velocity.

MODIFIED BIOPHYSICAL PROFILE

Although the NST reflects the present fetal neurologic status and oxygenation, the amniotic fluid volume is a better measure of chronic placental function. Therefore, some authors have favored the use of the modified BPP, which consists of the combination of the NST and the amniotic fluid index. In a study of 15,482 women undergoing antenatal testing, Miller and colleagues found the modified BPP to have a lower false negative rate than the NST.[39] An abnormal result may be followed by the performance of a full BPP or a CST.

DOPPLER FLOW VELOCIMETRY

Ultrasonography of fetal blood flow is also used to evaluate fetal well-being antenatally. Doppler measurements of the pulsatile blood flow in the umbilical arteries directly reflect the status of the fetomaternal circulation (Fig. 9–15). A progressive decrease in placental function or blood flow is thought to manifest itself with an increased resistance to flow as evidenced by a diminution in the diastolic flow and eventual absence or reversal of flow during diastole in the fetal vessels. In clinical practice, commonly measured indices include the following:

- Systolic/diastolic ratio (S/D)
- Resistance index (S−D/S)
- Pulsatility index (S−D/A)

Doppler flow velocimetry of the fetal umbilical artery has been studied in a number of at-risk populations. Pregnancies with suspected intrauterine growth restriction have been extensively studied, and there is evidence that the use of umbilical artery Doppler flow velocimetry as a primary testing method results in fewer antenatal tests and less intervention with similar neonatal outcome when compared with pregnancies monitored by the NST.[30] However, Doppler flow velocimetry has not been found to convey any benefit in a low-risk population, or in high-risk populations other than those with suspected intrauterine growth restriction.[18] Selective use of Doppler velocimetry for traditional indications within a general population also has not been shown to result in decreased maternal hospitalization or improved neonatal outcome.[43] At our institution, pregnancies with suspected intrauterine growth restriction and absent or reversed end-diastolic flow undergo increased antenatal surveillance, with delivery if the NST or BPP is abnormal.

INTERPRETATION OF TEST RESULTS

The realistic goal of antepartum testing is to decrease the risk of intrauterine fetal demise or perinatal mortality in the tested population so that it approaches the rate for a low-risk population, without an excessive or unacceptable false positive rate that may result in unnecessary intervention. When corrected for congenital anomalies and unpredictable causes of intrauterine death, the rate of stillbirth in the tested population (after antepartum testing with normal results) has been reported to be approximately 1.9 per 1000 for the NST, 0.3 per 1000 for the CST, 0.8 per 1000 for the BPP, and 0.8 per 1000 for the modified BPP.[18] These rates are comparable to the risk of fetal death in a low-risk population.

The false positive rate is more difficult to ascertain because positive test results usually result in obstetric intervention, thereby significantly decreasing the likelihood of intrauterine death. However, one study demonstrated that 90% of nonreactive NSTs are followed by a negative CST result, consistent with a high false positive rate of the NST.[26] A study of CSTs in which physicians were blinded to the results found that in 61% of patients with positive tests there were no fetal late decelerations in labor, no low Apgar scores, and no significant neonatal morbidity.[46] Manning and associates reported on a cohort of 913 infants delivered following a BPP score of 6 or less. Nearly 40% of those with scores of 6 demonstrated no markers of fetal compromise at delivery, as defined by fetal distress in labor, NICU admission, 5-minute Apgar score of 7 or less, or umbilical cord pH less than or equal to 7.20. However, there was a significant inverse linear association between BPP score and these markers, and all fetuses with scores of 0 had at least one of these markers at delivery.[34]

In a clinically stable situation, reassuring tests (reactive NST, negative CST, and BPP of 8 or 10) are considered to be reliable for 1 week; therefore, testing is usually performed on a weekly basis. Labile conditions may merit more frequent testing, and the frequency is left to the discretion of the physician. If the indication for testing is not a persistent one (e.g., maternal perception of decreased fetal movement), there is no evidence to support the continuation of antenatal testing. In certain high-risk populations, the false negative rate of NST may be unacceptably high. The stillbirth rate within 1 week of a reactive NST is markedly higher for patients with diabetes mellitus (14 per 1000) and fetal growth restriction (20 per 1000).[21] Similarly elevated results have been reported for patients with prolonged gestations.[40] Boehm and coworkers found that the stillbirth rate decreased from 6.1 per 1000 to 1.9 per 1000 in their high-risk population when the frequency of testing was changed from once weekly to twice weekly.[23] For this reason, twice-weekly testing may be appropriate in select populations, such as those described.

FETAL GESTATIONAL AGE AND ANTENATAL SURVEILLANCE

FHR variability and reactivity vary with gestational age. Prior to 28 weeks' gestation, up to 50% of all NSTs may not be reactive. From 28 to 32 weeks' gestation, approximately 15% of normal fetuses have nonreactive NSTs.[18] Whereas fetal breathing movements and body movements are noted to decrease before the onset of spontaneous labor,[24] the biophysical parameters that compose the BPP score are present at early gestational ages and are therefore useful in the evaluation of a very premature fetus.

The optimal gestational age at which to begin ante-

natal surveillance depends on the clinical condition. In making this decision, the physician must weigh the risk of intervention at a premature gestational age against the risk of intrauterine fetal death. The American College of Obstetricians and Gynecologists recommends initiating testing at 32 to 34 weeks' gestation for most at-risk patients, with the acknowledgment that some situations may merit testing as early as 26 to 28 weeks' gestation.[18]

CLINICAL CONSIDERATIONS

It is important to remember that a large number of clinical situations not related to fetal well-being will temporarily affect the interpretation of antenatal surveillance techniques. Maternal cigarette smoking and alcohol ingestion decrease fetal movement, breathing, and heart rate reactivity.[28, 29, 36] Such commonly used maternal medications such as opioids and corticosteroids significantly decrease various fetal biophysical parameters, including movement, breathing, and heart rate reactivity, without compromising neonatal outcome.[19, 27, 41, 45] Maternal medical conditions such as an acute asthma exacerbation or diabetic ketoacidosis may result in nonreassuring fetal surveillance, including worrisome BPP scores. Delivery of the fetus in a mother in such an unstable condition is dangerous and undesirable. Fortunately, the improvement or elimination of such conditions usually results in an improvement in fetal status. This is accompanied by an improvement in antenatal testing results, and it negates the need for a premature delivery.

SUMMARY

In high-risk populations at increased risk of perinatal mortality, antenatal fetal surveillance plays a large role in prenatal care. Those pregnancies at risk for progressive deterioration of placental function leading to fetal hypoxemia and acidosis are most likely to benefit from the methods currently in use. The various modalities, including NST, CST, BPP, and umbilical artery Doppler velocimetry, rely on fetal biophysical parameters that are significantly associated with the presence or absence of fetal hypoxemia. As all tests are associated with a rate of false positive results, each test result should be interpreted within the clinical context presented by the patient.

■ REFERENCES

Part One: Evaluation of the Intrapartum Fetus

1. American College of Obstetricians and Gynecologists: Fetal and Neonatal Neurologic Injury. Washington DC, American College of Obstetricians and Gynecologists, 1992. ACOG Technical Bulletin 163.
2. American College of Obstetricians and Gynecologists: Fetal Heart Rate Patterns: Monitoring, Interpretation, and Manage-

ment. Washington DC, American College of Obstetricians and Gynecologists, 1995. ACOG Technical Bulletin 207.

3. Ball RH, Parer JT: The physiologic mechanisms of variable decelerations. Am J Obstet Gynecol 166:1683, 1992.

4. Clark SL, et al: The scalp stimulation test: A clinical alternative to fetal scalp blood sampling. Am J Obstet Gynecol 148:274, 1984.

5. Clark SL, Paul RH: Intrapartum fetal surveillance: The role of fetal scalp blood sampling. Am J Obstet Gynecol 153:717, 1985.

6. Clark SL, et al: Position change and central hemodynamic profile during normal third-trimester pregnancy and post partum. Am J Obstet Gynecol 164:883, 1991.

7. Fee S, et al: Severe acidosis and subsequent neurologic status. Am J Obstet Gynecol 162:802, 1990.

8. Freeman RK, et al: Fetal Heart Rate Monitoring, 2nd ed. Baltimore, Williams & Wilkins, 1991.

9. Macri CJ, et al: Prophylactic amnioinfusion improves outcome of pregnancy complicated by thick meconium and oligohydramnios. Am J Obstet Gynecol 167:117, 1992.

10. Melone PJ, et al: Appropriateness of intrapartum fetal heart rate management and risk of cerebral palsy. Am J Obstet Gynecol 165:272, 1991.

11. Meschia G: Placental respiratory exchange and fetal oxygenation. In Creasy RK, Resnik R, (eds): Maternal-fetal Medicine: Principles and Practice. Philadelphia, WB Saunders Co, 1999.

12. Nageotte MP, et al: Prophylactic amnioinfusion in pregnancies complicated by oligohydramnios: A prospective study. Obstet Gynecol 77:677, 1991.

13. Shy KK, et al: Effects of electronic fetal-heart-rate monitoring, as compared with periodic auscultation, on the neurologic development of premature infants. N Engl J Med 322:588, 1990.

14. Smith CV, et al: Intrapartum assessment of fetal well-being: A comparison of fetal acoustic stimulation with acid-base determinations. Am J Obstet Gynecol 155:726, 1986.

15. Steiger RM, Nageotte MP: Effect of uterine contractility and maternal hypotension on prolonged decelerations after bupivacaine epidural anesthesia. Am J Obstet Gynecol 163:808, 1990.

16. Tejani NA, et al: Terbutaline in the management of acute intrapartum acidosis. J Reprod Med 28:857, 1983.

17. Vintzileos AM, et al: A randomized trial of intrapartum electronic fetal heart rate monitoring versus intermittent auscultation. Obstet Gynecol 81:899,1993.

Part Two: Antepartum Fetal Surveillance

18. American College of Obstetricians and Gynecologists: Antepartum Fetal Surveillance. Washington DC, American College of Obstetricians and Gynecologists, 1999. ACOG Practice Bulletin 9.

19. Anyaegbunam A, et al: Assessment of fetal well-being in methadone-maintained pregnancies: Abnormal nonstress tests. Gynecol Obstet Invest 43:25, 1997.

20. Baron C, et al: The impact of amniotic fluid volume assessed intrapartum on perinatal outcome. Am J Obstet Gynecol 173:167, 1995.

21. Barrett J, et al: The nonstress test: An evaluation of 1,000 patients. Am J Obstet Gynecol 141:153, 1981.

22. Boddy K, et al: Foetal respiratory movements, electrocortical and cardiovascular responses to hypoxaemia and hypercapnia in sheep. J Physiol 243:599, 1974.

23. Boehm FH, et al: Improved outcome of twice weekly nonstress testing. Obstet Gynecol 67:566, 1986.

24. Carmichael L, et al: Fetal breathing, gross fetal body movements and maternal and fetal heart rates before spontaneous labour at term. Am J Obstet Gynecol 148:675, 1984.

25. Centers for Disease Control and Prevention, National Center for Health Statistics: Vital Statistics for the United States, vol II, Mortality, pt A. Hyattsville, Md, National Center for Health Statistics, 1999.

26. Evertson LR, et al: Antepartum fetal heart rate testing. I. Evolution of the non-stress test. Am J Obstet Gynecol 133:29, 1979.

27. Farrell T, et al: Fetal movements following intrapartum maternal opiate administration. Clin Exp Obstet Gynecol 23:144, 1996.

28. Fox HE, et al: Maternal ethanol ingestion and the occurrence of fetal breathing movements. Am J Obstet Gynecol 132:34, 1978.

29. Graca LM, et al: Acute effects of maternal cigarette smoking on fetal heart rate and fetal body movements felt by the mother. J Perinat Med 19:385, 1991.

30. Haley J, et al: Randomised controlled trial of cardiotocography versus umbilical artery Doppler in the management of small for gestational age fetuses. Br J Obstet Gynaecol. 104:431, 1997.

31. Hsieh TT, et al: Perinatal outcome of oligohydramnios without associated premature rupture of membranes and fetal anomalies. Gynecol Obstet Invest 45:232, 1998.

32. Lee CY, et al: A study of fetal heart rate acceleration patterns. Obstet Gynecol 45:142, 1975.

33. Manning FA, et al: Fetal biophysical profile scoring: Selective use of the non-stress test. Am J Obstet Gynecol 156:709, 1987.

34. Manning FA, et al: Fetal assessment based on fetal biophysical profile scoring. IV. An analysis of perinatal morbidity and mortality. Am J Obstet Gynecol 162:703, 1990.

35. Manning FA, et al: Fetal biophysical profile score. VI. Correlation with antepartum umbilical venous fetal pH. Am J Obstet Gynecol 169:755, 1993.

36. Manning FA, Feyerbend C: Cigarette smoking and fetal breathing movements. Br J Obstet Gynaecol 83:262, 1976.

37. Manning FA, Platt LD: Maternal hypoxemia and fetal breathing movements. Obstet Gynecol 53:758, 1979.

38. Manning FA, et al: Antepartum fetal evaluation: Development of a fetal biophysical profile score. Am J Obstet Gynecol 136:787, 1980.

39. Miller DA, et al: The modified biophysical profile: Antepartum testing in the 1990s. Am J Obstet Gynecol 174:812, 1996.

40. Miyazaki F, Miyazaki B: False reactive nonstress tests in post-term pregnancies. Am J Obstet Gynecol 140:269, 1981.

41. Mulder EJ, et al: Antenatal corticosteroid therapy and fetal behaviour: a randomised study of the effects of betamethasone and dexamethasone. Br J Obstet Gynaecol 104:1239, 1997.

42. Murata Y, et al: Fetal heart rate accelerations and late decelerations during the course of intrauterine death in chronically catheterized rhesus monkeys. Am J Obstet Gynecol 144:218, 1982.

43. Omtzigt AM, et al: A randomized controlled trial on the clinical value of umbilical Doppler velocimetry in antenatal care. Am J Obstet Gynecol 170:624, 1994.

44. Roberts D, et al: The fetal outcome in pregnancies with isolated reduced amniotic fluid volume in the third trimester. J Perinat Med 26:390, 1998.

45. Smith CV, et al: Influence of intravenous fentanyl on fetal biophysical parameters during labor. J Matern Fetal Med 5:89, 1996.

46. Staisch KJ, et al: Blind oxytocin challenge test and perinatal outcome. Am J Obstet Gynecol 138:399, 1980.

47. Waller DK, et al: Alpha-fetoprotein: A biomarker for pregnancy outcome. Epidemiology 4:471, 1993.

48. Weiner CP, et al: The effect of fetal age upon normal fetal laboratory values and venous pressure. Obstet Gynecol 79:713, 1992.

49. Wilkins-Haug L: Unexplained elevated maternal serum alpha-fetoprotein: What is the appropriate follow-up? Curr Opin Obstet Gynecol 10:469, 1998.

50. Zimmer EZ, Divon MY: Fetal vibroacoustic stimulation. Obstet Gynecol 81:451, 1993.

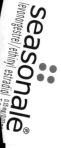

Jacob V. Aranda

David J. Edwards

Barbara F. Hales

Michael J. Rieder

DRUGS AND THE FETUS

EXPOSURE OF THE FETUS TO DRUGS

Although advances in prenatal diagnosis may soon permit physicians to consider the fetus the primary patient, the fetus is generally the passive recipient of drugs. Consequently, any drug effects on the fetus are usually undesirable. Such effects may vary from transient behavioral changes to irreversible structural defects. Concern has increased over the potentially harmful effects of drugs taken during pregnancy since the catastrophic teratogenic effects of thalidomide were discovered in the early 1960s.[100, 108] This drug, thought to be harmless, illustrated the totally unpredictable nature of drug toxicity in the fetus during the first trimester; thalidomide doses that induced analgesia in the mother with no demonstrable undesirable side effects produced major structural defects in the fetus.[108]

Although a number of drugs are possible teratogens in human beings, at present, only a few have been positively identified as such.[87, 172, 180] In the case of abnormalities that occur quite often in the population, physicians may not be alerted to the direct causal relationship between exposure of the fetus to the drug and the adverse effect. It has been estimated that to establish that a given drug changes the naturally occurring frequency of a congenital deformity by 1%, a sequential trial involving approximately 35,000 patients would be required.[39] The discovery that thalidomide caused congenital malformations was possible because this drug was widely used, induced dramatic and rare congenital defects, and had a high probability (estimated at 20% to 35%) of producing a teratogenic effect after exposure between the third and eighth week after conception.[108] Unfortunately, these three criteria are rarely met when one is attempting to assess the teratogenicity of other drugs. Thus, many of the data in the biomedical literature concern-

ing adverse effects of drugs on the fetus are circumstantial.

Maternal Consumption of Drugs

Drugs are usually administered for symptomatic relief of benign problems in the mother, with little or no consideration given to the unintended recipient, the fetus. The magnitude of the problem can be appreciated by considering that in several studies the average number of drugs prescribed during pregnancy was about four.[16, 35, 72] When self-prescribed drugs were included in these studies, the average number of drugs taken during pregnancy increased to between 8.7 and 11. Among obstetric patients, 92% to 100% took at least one physician-prescribed drug, and 65% to 80% also took self-prescribed drugs. Compounding this problem for women of childbearing age is additional occupational or environmental exposure to potential teratogens (see Chapter 12). In one controlled study, a significant association was found between fetal loss and the occupational exposure of nurses to antineoplastic drugs.[176]

From 1959 to 1965, a large-scale epidemiologic study investigated the possible teratogenic role of drugs, using a cohort of more than 50,000 mother-child pairs recruited in 12 centers in the United States.[72] The rates of exposure of these mother-child pairs to different drug groups are presented in Table 10–1. The highest rate of exposure was to analgesic and antipyretic drugs (about 32% of patients in the first trimester). On the basis of other studies, exposure to alcohol and cigarette smoke would also be expected to be high. Most studies of drug use during pregnancy performed since 1965 have found that the number of drugs consumed has stayed constant.[35] As average maternal age increases, and as more women with chronic diseases are able to complete pregnancy successfully, the rate of drugs used in pregnancy is likely to increase.

Placental Transfer of Drugs

(See also Chapter 11, Part One.)

The physiochemical properties that allow most drugs to cross cell membranes also permit their passive transport across the placenta into the fetus. The factors involved in placental transfer of drugs include lipid solubility and degree of ionization, molecular weight, protein binding, placental circulation, fetal circulation, and placental maturation and metabolism of drugs. Most drugs administered to the mother will reach the fetus; the extent of fetal exposure to a drug administered to the mother depends on its physiochemical properties, on the dose and duration of maternal treatment, and on the rate of maternal drug elimination. If the drug is readily diffused, it will equilibrate between maternal and fetal compartments very rapidly (Fig. 10–1). With fast transplacental equilibration and slow maternal elimination, the fetal pharmacokinetic profile will mimic the maternal pattern after either single or multiple drug doses. A drug that is polar or protein bound diffuses more slowly

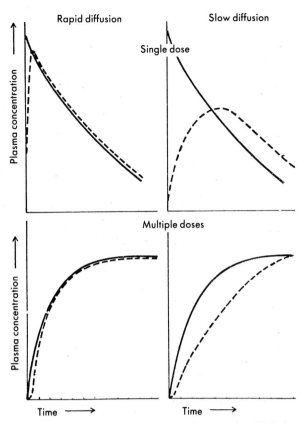

FIGURE 10–1. Schematic representation of maternal (*solid line*) and fetal (*dotted line*) plasma concentrations of drug with time after single or multiple IV doses. Simple transplacental diffusion rates that are rapid (*left*) or slow (*right*) are hypothesized; it is assumed that the half-lives of the drugs diffusing rapidly or slowly are the same. (From Neims AH, et al: Principles of neonatal pharmacology. In Schaffer AJ, et al [eds]: Diseases of the Newborn, 4th ed. Philadelphia, WB Saunders Co, 1977.)

	MOTHER-CHILD PAIRS EXPOSED (*n* = 50,282)	
DRUG GROUP	**Lunar Months 1–4**	**Any Time During Pregnancy**
Analgesics and antipyretic drugs	31.6	67.3
Immunizing agents	18.3	45.2
Antimicrobial and antiparasitic agents	16.1	34.9
Antinauseants, antihistamines, and phenothiazines	12.0	28.6
Caffeine and other xanthine derivatives	11.5	26.9
Drugs affecting the autonomic nervous system	9.3	24.9
Sedatives, tranquilizers, and antidepressants	6.2	28.4
Anesthetics, anticonvulsants, muscle relaxants, and stimulants	5.3	13.9
Inorganic compounds and certain vitamins	5.1	20.1
Hormones, hormone antagonists, and contraceptives	4.6	7.0
Cough medicines	1.9	15.8
Diuretics and drugs taken for vascular disorders	0.8	31.6

TABLE 10–1 PERCENTAGES OF DRUG EXPOSURE IN MOTHER-CHILD PAIRS FROM THE FIRST DAY OF THE LAST MENSTRUAL PERIOD TO 48 HOURS BEFORE DELIVERY

From Heinonen OP, et al: Birth defects and Drugs in Pregnancy. Littleton, Mass, Publishing Sciences Group, 1977.

into the fetus. However, high concentrations of a drug may still accumulate in the fetal compartment if multiple doses are administered to the mother (see Fig. 10–1).

Drug Ingestion by the Father

Although concern about the potential teratogenic effects of maternally ingested substances has grown in the past 30 years, the possibility that paternal drug exposure may have adverse effects on the progeny has not been of such widespread concern.[164] In animals, there is experimental evidence of adverse effects occurring in the progeny of males that ingest certain chemicals before mating; these include decreased litter size and birth weights, malformations, and increased neonatal mortality.* It is difficult to elucidate the mechanisms underlying this phenomenon. The drug itself may be present in semen and may cause alterations in development after fertilization; alternatively, drug exposure may directly alter the genetic material or its packaging in spermatozoa and conse-

* References 49, 79, 138, 164, 191, 198.

quently alter the developmental program of the zygote.

In human beings, a variety of paternal occupational exposures has been associated with adverse outcomes in progeny. These include exposure to wood, metals, solvents, pesticides, and hydrocarbons.[138] Further research is needed to investigate the relationship between paternal drug ingestion and perinatal outcome in human beings.

EFFECT OF DRUGS ON THE FETUS

The adverse effects of in utero exposure to drugs can vary from reversible effects such as transient changes in clotting time or fetal breathing movements to irreversible effects such as fetal death, intrauterine growth retardation, structural malformations, or mental retardation.[172, 180] The specific drug, the dosage, the route of administration, the timing of treatment, and the genotype of the mother or the fetus may be critical determinants of the effect of a drug on the fetus. The disease being treated may also be an important consideration. The factors that combine to influence the outcome of drug administration include diet and coadministration of other drugs. It is difficult to control these parameters in human beings. Thus, the incontrovertible establishment of a drug as a teratogen in human beings requires the combination of extreme situations such as those previously outlined for thalidomide. Consequently, it has been necessary to rely heavily on animal studies to assess the teratogenic potential of drugs.

The *timing* of drug exposure is frequently a critical determinant of the effect of a drug on the fetus (Fig. 10–2). The first week after fertilization is the "period of the zygote" (cleavage and gastrulation). During this time, the most common adverse effect of drugs is termination of pregnancy, which may occur before the woman even knows that she is pregnant. Exposure of the preimplantation embryo to embryotoxic drugs may retard development, perhaps by decreasing cell numbers in the blastocyst, or it may even produce malformations. The second to the eighth weeks of gestation are the "period of the embryo." It is mainly during this period of organogenesis that drugs produce dramatic and catastrophic structural malformations. Other adverse effects during this phase may include fetal wastage, transplacental carcinogenesis (e.g., diethylstilbestrol), and intrauterine growth retardation. From the third to ninth months of gestation, the "period of the fetus," differentiation of the central nervous system and the reproductive system continues. Certain drugs given during this period have been implicated as behavioral teratogens. Some drugs may cause disproportionate growth retardation (in infants whose head growth has been spared, after 30 or more weeks) or may alter the differentiation of the reproductive system or external genitalia.

Consideration of the irreversible adverse effects of drugs on development usually stops with birth. However, it is well known that sensory and other higher nervous system functions are not fully developed until well after birth. Thus birth is not really a termination point but only another milestone in development. Little is known about the long-term or delayed adverse effects of drugs administered to the mother during labor and delivery or drugs given directly to the neonate. When administered postnatally, antitumor agents such as cyclophosphamide can have long-term effects on the histogenesis of the cerebellum, on growth and development, and on reproductive function.

The effects on the fetus are highly dependent on the specific drug involved. There is no infallible means of predicting which drug will be "selectively toxic" to the fetus. Within some groups of drugs, each individual drug can cause the same type of

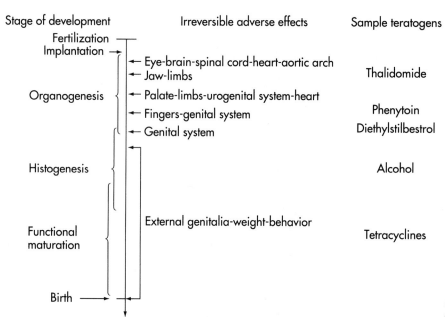

FIGURE 10–2. Critical periods in human embryogenesis.

malformation. The anticonvulsants, for example, are a family of drugs in which the core structure necessary for activity as an anticonvulsant appears to fulfill the requirements for inducing characteristic malformations.[119] In other families of drugs, such as the sedative-hypnotics, individual drugs with common therapeutic effects differ greatly with respect to their teratogenic potential. Thalidomide was withdrawn from the market because of its marked effect on the fetus. However, glutethimide, which has the same dioxopiperidine ring as thalidomide, is not teratogenic. It is obvious that more information on how drugs induce malformations is needed before knowledge of their molecular structure or pharmacologic action permits the prediction of teratogenicity.

The decision whether to give a drug during pregnancy is difficult. Some of the information available on the potential adverse effects of pharmacologic classes of drugs is summarized in Table 10–2. Table 10–3 summarizes the results of studies on the effects of in utero exposure to frequently used therapeutic agents.

Self-Administered Nontherapeutic Agents

Chronic ethanol intake during pregnancy is associated with a readily identifiable *fetal alcohol syndrome* (see Chapters 12 and 36) and has been cited as the most frequently documented cause of mental deficiency in the western world. Prenatal and postnatal growth retardation, mental deficiency, persistent microcephaly, and minor anomalies of the face, eyes, heart, joints, and genitalia have been identified.[26, 69, 80] The Collaborative Perinatal Study reported a mortality rate of 17% and mental retardation in 44% of infants of alcoholic mothers.[72]

A dose-response relationship may exist between the severity of fetal alcohol syndrome and alcohol consumption by the mother. Among women who have infrequent social exposure to alcohol in the first trimester, no increase in risk has been demonstrated. However, among babies born to mothers who drank 1.5 ounces or more of absolute alcohol daily (equivalent to about four or five drinks), 63% demonstrated neurologic impairment, 16% were born prematurely, and 28% were small for gestational age; 32% of the infants born to heavy drinkers had congenital malformations, and 16% had major malformations.[69] Binge drinking may be more harmful than if the same amount were consumed over a longer period. The mechanisms whereby alcohol produces teratogenic effects on the fetus are likely to include a direct toxic effect on the developing brain and impairment of placental-fetal blood flow.

It is now well established that *maternal smoking* substantially reduces the birth weight of offspring (see Chapters 12 and 13).[94, 127] There is a significant dose-response relationship, and early cessation of smoking can result in birth weights similar to those of offspring of nonsmoking mothers.[23] The largest studies also document a 30% to 35% increase in mortality rates resulting from abruptio placentae, placenta previa, prematurity, and respiratory disease. Some studies also report an increased incidence of spontaneous abortion in smoking mothers.[86]

Data concerning an association between smoking during pregnancy and congenital defects in the infant are conflicting.[42, 47, 123] There may be important functional consequences of exposure to cigarette smoke, such as decreased fetal breathing movements and increased fetal heart rate.[105, 146] Several studies have reported a significant relationship between maternal smoking during pregnancy and low achievement, increased hyperactivity, and "minimal cerebral dysfunction" in the offspring.[22, 37, 105]

Exactly which ingredients in cigarette smoke cause the effects is not known; nicotine, carbon dioxide, and thiocyanate have all been implicated. There does not seem to be a significant beneficial effect on birth weight or perinatal mortality rates from reducing the nicotine and tar content or smoking filtered cigarettes. Apparently, preventing the harmful effects of tobacco on the fetus can be achieved only from the cessation of smoking.[127]

Although caffeine has been found to be teratogenic in high doses in animal experiments, reports suggest little teratogenic danger to human beings.[121, 131] Administration of caffeine does alter ovine fetal respiratory activity,[148] however, and the presence of caffeine in most cord plasma samples suggests that it may alter human fetal respiratory activity or even neonatal breathing patterns.

Cocaine or "crack" use during pregnancy has been associated with reduced birth weight, premature labor, and abruptio placentae.[134] As many as one third of cocaine-exposed babies have neurologic problems that include depression of interactive behavior and poor organizational responses to environmental stimuli.[158] Smoking and consumption of alcohol, caffeine, and cocaine are highly correlated. The potential interaction of these influences, plus other drug and environmental factors, is presently being systematically considered.

Environmental Chemicals

(See also Chapter 12.)

Many chemicals are present in the environment; however, few have been shown to have teratogenic potential in animals or human beings.[211] In Ireland, the prevalence of anencephaly and spina bifida was related to heavy dietary consumption of blighted potatoes.[160, 192] Intrauterine methyl mercury poisoning (Minamata disease) was characterized by severe neurologic symptoms and convulsions.[70]

It has been suggested that deliberate inhalation of gasoline can cause congenital malformations characterized by profound retardation, initial hypotonia progressing to hypertonia, scaphocephaly, a prominent occiput, poor postnatal head growth, and additional minor abnormalities.[76] A syndrome of neurologic delay, craniofacial anomalies, and poor motor development has been described in infants of women who abuse solvents such as toluene. Polycyclic aro-

Text continued on page 151

TABLE 10–2 DRUGS ASSOCIATED WITH GROWTH AND CONGENITAL MALFORMATIONS

DRUGS	FETAL GROWTH	GROWTH RETARDATION	MENTAL RETARDATION	CENTRAL NERVOUS SYSTEM	CARDIOVASCULAR	MUSCULOSKELETAL	UROGENITAL	EYE AND EAR	THYROID
Antimicrobials									
Tetracycline						X			
Streptomycin								X	
Quinine								X	
Antineoplastics									
Methotrexate	X	X		X		X			
Busulfan, chlorambucil, cyclophosphamide	X	X		X		X	X	X	
Central nervous system drugs									
Cocaine				X	X				
Lithium					X				
Thalidomide						X		X	
Anticonvulsants									
Phenytoin		X	X			X			
Barbiturates			X		X	X			
Trimethadione			X		X	X	X	X	
Valproic acid		X		X		X			
Carbamazepine				X					
Steroid hormones									
Androgens							X		
Diethylstilbestrol							X		
Estrogen, progestins					X		X		
Iodine, propylthiouracil									X
Warfarin		X	X			X		X	
Alcohol		X				X		X	
Tobacco smoking	X	X	X						
Isotretinoin, vitamin A				X		X		X	

TABLE 10–3   EFFECTS ON THE FETUS OF IN UTERO EXPOSURE TO PHYSICIAN- OR
SELF-ADMINISTERED THERAPEUTIC AGENTS

SPECIFIC AGENT	STUDIES REPORTED	RESULTS AND RECOMMENDATIONS
Antineoplastic Agents (e.g., antimetabolites, alkylating agents, antitumor antibiotics)	Sieber et al, 1975[183]	As a group, these are the most potent teratogens known. It is difficult to delineate one agent because of frequent combined uses in addition to irradiation.
Antimetabolites (purine analogues, pyrimidine analogues, folic acid antagonists)	Milunsky et al, 1976,[114] Nicholson, 1968[128]	Potent teratogens; they are associated with skeletal defects.
Alkylating agents (busulfan, chlorambucil, cyclophosphamide, nitrogen mustard)	Diamond et al, 1960,[33] Garrett, 1974,[52] Greenberg et al, 1964,[57] Schardein, 1993,[172] Selevan et al, 1985,[176] Shotton et al, 1963,[182] Sieber et al, 1975[183]	Some reports have described drug-related defects; others have reported cases with no drug-related defects.
Antimicrobial Agents Sulfonamides	Richards, 1972,[163] Schardein, 1993[172]	Conflicting reports on teratogenicity; avoid use in third trimester because of theoretical risk of kernicterus.
Tetracyclines	Cohlan, 1977[27]	Results in staining of dentition; avoid use in second and third trimesters and early childhood.
Penicillins Cephalosporins	Nelson et al, 1971[126]	These appear to be safe when administered at any phase of pregnancy.

Aminoglycosides
  Streptomycin,
  dihydrostreptomycin
	Scheinhorn et al, 1977,[174] Warkany, 1979[206]	Auditory nerve defects and ocular nerve damage may occur in infants after prenatal exposure.

Antitubercular agents Isoniazid (INH)	Monnet et al, 1967[117]	Five children with severe encephalopathies were reported after prenatal exposure; prophylactic administration of vitamin B_6 to pregnant women receiving INH is often recommended.
Ethionamide, ethambutol, rifampin	Schardein, 1993[172]	No clear relationship with abnormal fetal development has been noted.
Antiparasitic agents	Schardein, 1993[172]	Quinidine has caused deafness; others, no definite teratogenicity.
Anticonvulsant Agents	Smith, 1977[186]	Women requiring anticonvulsant therapy should be counseled before becoming pregnant as to the nature and magnitude of risk to the fetus; overall risk of having a malformed child is about 1 in 10.
Hydantoins Phenytoin	Hanson, 1976,[68] Hanson et al, 1976[67]	Typical fetal hydantoin syndrome with mild to moderate growth and mental deficiencies, limb anomalies, and dysmorphic facies (low nasal bridge, short nose, mild ocular hypertelorism) has been reported.

Barbiturates, deoxybarbiturates
  Primidone, phenobarbital,
  secobarbital, amobarbital
	Bethenod et al, 1975,[15] Heinonen et al, 1977[72]	Postnatal effects are similar to those in fetal hydantoin syndrome; associated cardiovascular malformations also may occur.

Oxazoladinediones Trimethadione	Goldman et al, 1978[56]	Fetal trimethadione syndrome has been reported, with developmental delay, speech difficulty, V-shaped eyebrows, epicanthus, low-set ears, palatal anomaly, and irregular teeth.
Valproic acid	Jager-Roman et al, 1986[78]	Neural tube defects have been found.
Carbamazepine	Rosa, 1991[166]	Increased neural tube defects have been found.
Psychotropic Agents		The teratogenicity of most psychotropics is not established; caution is necessary in administering them during pregnancy; neonatal withdrawal syndrome can occur when drug is taken late in pregnancy.
Thalidomide	Schardein, 1993[172]	Teratogenic to human beings when administered in the first to eighth weeks of pregnancy; limb reduction anomalies.

Table continued on following page

TABLE 10–3 EFFECTS ON THE FETUS OF IN UTERO EXPOSURE TO PHYSICIAN- OR SELF-ADMINISTERED THERAPEUTIC AGENTS *Continued*

SPECIFIC AGENT	STUDIES REPORTED	RESULTS AND RECOMMENDATIONS
Psychotropic Agents *Continued*		
Benzodiazepines Diazepam, chlordiazepoxide	Heinonen et al, 1977,[72] Milkovich et al, 1976,[113] Rosenberg et al, 1983,[167]	Ingestion before parturition may cause hypotonia, apnea, and hypothermia.
Tricyclic antidepressants	Schardein, 1993[172]	Some evidence of increased malformations has been reported.
Monoamine oxidase inhibitors	Samojlik, 1965[170]	Few data are available on human beings; only phenelzine is reported as embryotoxic in rats.
Lithium	Jacobson, 1992,[77] Nora et al, 1974[133]	May induce malformations such as Ebstein anomaly. The increased risk is probably small.
Antinauseants; Antihistamines	Heinonen et al, 1977,[72] Paterson, 1977,[145] Shapiro et al, 1976,[179] Smithells et al, 1978[187]	No evidence of association with malformation in human beings.
Non-narcotic Analgesics; Anti-inflammatory, antipyretic Agents	Eriksson et al, 1973[43]	Little evidence exists to associate these with malformations (see specific exceptions following). As a group, considering their wide usage, they are not considered to be teratogenic in human beings.
Salicylates	Shapiro et al, 1976,[179] Turner et al, 1975[201]	Concern exists regarding effects on platelet function that could cause hemorrhagic complications in a traumatic birth; possible intrauterine closure of patent ductus arteriosus, pulmonary hypertension.
p-Aminophenols Acetaminophen	Schardein, 1993[172]	No evidence of toxicity or association with malformations after therapeutic doses.
Narcotic Analgesics	Rothstein et al, 1974,[169] Smith et al, 1975[185]	These appear to be nonteratogenic in human beings; withdrawal symptoms may occur in infants of narcotic-addicted women.
Hormones and Hormone Antagonists		
Androgens	Forsberg et al, 1969[49]	Increased risk of masculinization or pseudohermaphroditism in human beings has been reported.
Antiandrogens Cyproterone acetate	Forsberg et al, 1969[49]	These are associated with abnormal sexual development in male laboratory animals; effects in human beings are unknown.
Progestins Ethisterone, norethindrone	Wilkins, 1960[210]	Depending on the treatment period during pregnancy, association with equivocal or frankly masculinized external genitalia of varying degrees has been described.
Estrogens Diethylstilbestrol	Barnes et al, 1980,[11] Henderson et al, 1976,[73] Herbst et al, 1975,[74] Metzler et al, 1978[112]	These are associated with vaginal adenosis and adenocarcinoma in young women exposed in utero; in exposed men there was increased evidence of genitourinary tract disturbances but no increase in cancer incidence.
Antiestrogens Clomiphene		Multiple pregnancy has been reported.
Oral contraceptive agents	Levy et al, 1973,[101], Nora et al, 1973,[132] Ortiz-Perez et al, 1979,[140] Rothman et al, 1978[168]	No association between first-trimester exposure and malformations.
Corticosteroids (natural and synthetic mineralocorticoids and glucocorticoids)	Greenberger et al, 1985,[58] Heinonen et al, 1977,[72] Schardein, 1993[172]	All are teratogens in animals, producing cleft lip and palate. Large human studies have failed to demonstrate that these agents are major teratogens.
Antithyroid agents (iodides and propylthiouracil)		These may produce neonatal goiter and tracheal obstruction; also may be associated with hypospadias, aortic atresia, and developmental retardation.
Hypoglycemic Drugs (tolbutamide, chlorpropamide)	Landauer, 1972[92]	Neonatal hypoglycemia.
Insulin	Schardein, 1993[172]	Insulin is teratogenic to mice and rabbits but not to human beings

TABLE 10–3   EFFECTS ON THE FETUS OF IN UTERO EXPOSURE TO PHYSICIAN- OR SELF-ADMINISTERED THERAPEUTIC AGENTS *Continued*

SPECIFIC AGENT	STUDIES REPORTED	RESULTS AND RECOMMENDATIONS
Vitamins and Iron		These are used almost universally by pregnant women, with only rare reports of associated malformations (see following).
Vitamin A	Bernhardt et al, 1974,[14] Pilotti et al, 1965,[149] Schardein, 1993[172]	Hypervitaminosis A appears to be teratogenic in animals, and cases of related urinary malformations have been reported in human beings.
Isotretinoin	Lammer et al, 1985[91]	Characteristic pattern of malformations involving craniofacial, cardiac, thymic, and central nervous system structures has been found.
Iron-containing drugs	McBride, 1963,[109] Nelson et al, 1971[126]	Association with congenital malformations appears unlikely.
Diuretics		In general, these are not associated with congenital malformations.
Benzothiadiazides	Rodriguez et al, 1964,[165] Terrila et al, 1971[196]	Thrombocytopenia, altered carbohydrate metabolism, and hyperbilirubinemia have been reported in infants exposed late in gestation.
Cardiovascular Drugs (antiarrhythmics, digitalis, glycosides)		Very few reports relate these to malformations in human beings.
Antihypertensives Angiotensin-converting enzyme (ACE) inhibitors	Barr et al, 1994[12]	Hypoplasia of the skull calvaria, oligohydramnios, renal failure, death, and neonatal anemia have been reported.
Propranolol	Oakes et al, 1976,[135] Pruyn et al, 1979[153]	Associations with decreased uterine blood flow and intrauterine growth retardation have been reported; bradycardia and hypoglycemia may occur in the newborn infant.
Anticoagulants Warfarin	Schardein, 1993,[172] Warkany, 1976[205]	Only warfarin has shown teratogenicity in human beings. Exposure during the first trimester has been related to chondrodysplasia punctata and nasal hypoplasia associated with radiographic stippling of the epiphyses (Conradi disease). Exposure in the third trimester is known to cause fetal or placental hemorrhage; thus it is recommended that patients requiring anticoagulant therapy be treated with an agent that will not cross the placenta.
Cough and Cold Medicines Bronchodilators, centrally acting antitussive agents, decongestants, expectorants	Schardein, 1993[172]	Of these, only the iodide expectorants have been associated with adverse effects (fetal hypothyroidism and goiter).
Sympathomimetic amines (phenylephrine, phenylpropanolamine, ephedrine, dextroamphetamine)	Heinonen et al, 1977[72]	These have been associated with little risk to the developing fetus.

matic hydrocarbons and halogenated aromatic hydrocarbons (insecticides) are embryotoxic in animals[90, 211]; future studies may demonstrate that these environmental chemicals are also fetotoxic in human beings.[151]

Factors Modifying the Fetal Response to Drugs

GENETIC BACKGROUND. In addition to the drug itself, the dosage, timing during gestation, and genetic background of the individual fetus and mother may play an important role in determining susceptibility to the teratogenic effects of a drug.[50]

Experiments in mice differing at one allele demonstrated the importance of both the maternal and the fetal genotype in determining the outcome of exposure to a toxic drug.[90, 151] Fraser[50] demonstrated genetic (strain) differences in the susceptibility of inbred mice to the development of a cortisone-induced cleft palate. A recent study with mice deficient in glucose-6-phosphate dehydrogenase (G6PD) concluded that this enzyme was important in protecting the fetus against oxidative stress; after exposure to a teratogen, the incidence of fetal death and malformations was higher in G6PD-deficient mice than in controls.[129] In addition, a genetic defect in arene oxide detoxification may increase the risk that women with epilepsy who are treated with phenytoin may have babies with major birth defects.[193] Thus, congenital malformations may be under multifactorial control.

DRUG-DRUG INTERACTIONS. Individuals taking drugs rarely consume a single drug; rather, they use various combinations. Animal experiments have provided evidence that the administration of one drug can modify the teratogenicity of another. For example, treatment of rats with phenobarbital increased the teratogenicity of the antitumor drug cyclophosphamide.[64, 106] It is thought that phenobarbital pretreatment induced maternal hepatic cytochrome P-450, increasing the activation of cyclophosphamide to mutagenic or teratogenic metabolites. It has been suggested that the teratogenic effects of anticonvulsants are more common in women on multiple anticonvulsant therapy.

MECHANISMS OF DRUG TOXICITY IN THE FETUS. Various mechanisms have been postulated for the adverse effects of drugs on the fetus. Drugs may interact with a receptor, inhibit an enzyme, degrade a membrane, or chemically damage macromolecules, including nucleic acids, proteins, or lipids. The consequences of such actions may include mutations, altered differentiation, inhibition of the biosynthesis of structural proteins (e.g., collagen), inhibition of tissue interactions, and altered morphogenetic movements caused by selective cell death (Fig. 10–3).

We now know that many chemical carcinogens (or mutagens) are *precarcinogens* (or premutagens) and must be metabolically activated to reactive electrophilic metabolites, or "ultimate" carcinogens, to initiate the cell damage leading to cancer. Experiments

with limb bud and whole embryo culture techniques suggest that at least one teratogen, cyclophosphamide, requires activation to its ultimate teratogen.[45, 64, 106] There is also evidence that thalidomide, phenytoin, chlorcyclizine, and diethylstilbestrol require metabolic activation to be teratogenic.[19, 108, 112, 152] The ultimate teratogen may be a reactive intermediate of the drug or a reactive species of oxygen.[144] The mechanisms whereby active metabolites produce their effects are thought to involve reactions with DNA (leading to covalent modification of DNA, causing base substitution or frame shift mutations), with proteins (blocking crucial steps in cell metabolism), or with structural lipids (promoting lipid peroxidation).[90] We know that many active metabolites, because of their instability, react with any available cell nucleophile. Thus, a combination of these mechanisms may be involved.

Such reactive electrophilic metabolites can be detoxified by conjugation with nucleophiles such as glutathione, catalyzed by the glutathione S-transferases.[65] Animal experiments have revealed the presence of enzymes during development that may result in other deactivation processes, including hydration, glucuronidation, acetylation, or sulfation.

Determination of Adverse Drug Effects in the Fetus

Human studies of the effects of drugs during pregnancy are often retrospective. Amniocentesis and ultrasonography can be used to screen for some birth defects, but pregnancy is already well advanced by the time these can be used. An alternative, *chorionic villus sampling*, permits detection of genetic abnormalities in the first trimester. (See also Chapter 7.)

Epidemiologic studies can, after the fact, correlate a drug with a defect and thus prevent exposure of future fetuses.[39] However, to delineate the effects of drugs, taken either alone or in combination, on unidentified multiple factors in development is difficult in human beings, even in large epidemiologic studies. The fact that preclinical testing is often done in relatively small numbers of patients suggests the importance of careful postmarketing surveillance to detect an increase in uncommon problems and specific birth defects. The international availability of teratology information services provides a new source of data for prospective epidemiologic studies with a large sample size.

Data using animal models provide the initial information on the effects of drugs on the fetus. Such data permit the definition of drug dosage and timing of drug exposure during gestation under conditions in which the environment and genotype are controlled. This control of genotype and environment has increased our understanding of the mechanisms of drug-induced teratogenicity. Rodents, specifically mice and rats, are frequently chosen as animal models because they are easy to breed, are inexpensive, and have short gestational periods. Thalidomide is an unfortunate example of a human teratogen that is not

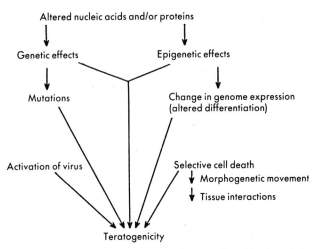

FIGURE 10–3. Potential mechanisms of drug-induced teratogenicity.

very teratogenic in rodents, but almost every drug that has since been found to be teratogenic in humans has been shown to cause similar teratogenic effects in animals.

Further study of the mechanisms of drug-induced teratogenicity may permit the development of anti-teratogens to prevent the fetotoxic effects of drugs essential for the mother during pregnancy. A number of such compounds (e.g., nicotinamide, ascorbate, cysteine, vitamins such as folic acid) have been studied in laboratory experiments.[93] Some of these approaches may be useful in decreasing the incidence of adverse pregnancy outcomes in humans; there is now strong evidence that adequate periconceptional maternal folic acid supplementation is associated with a reduction in the occurrence and recurrence of neural tube defects.

New, quick, inexpensive screening tests for teratogens need to be developed. Preferably, such tests should include metabolic routes of the drug similar to those in human beings. Whole embryo or organ culture techniques (limb bud, palate) are increasingly being accepted as screening systems to test for teratogens in vitro. Such systems can have drug-metabolizing enzymes incorporated (in liposomes or intact liver parenchymal cells) to activate any preteratogen such as thalidomide or cyclophosphamide. Other studies have suggested that the inhibition of tumor cell attachment may be useful in the prediction of drug teratogenicity in vitro.[19]

DRUG USE, DISPOSITION, AND METABOLISM IN THE NEWBORN INFANT

(See also Chapter 11, Part One.)

At birth, a term infant in North America receives at least three types of drugs: an ophthalmic antimicrobial agent, vitamin K, and an antibacterial agent for the cord. Low birth weight and sick infants in a neonatal intensive care unit additionally receive an increasing number of drugs, with the constant introduction of new drugs or old drugs with new indications in the neonatal therapeutic armamentarium. Thus the overall xenobiotic exposure of the fetus and newborn exceeds current estimates, particularly when environmental agents (e.g., lead, methyl mercury, volatile hydrocarbons) and drugs of habit (e.g., caffeine, alcohol) are taken into consideration.[58] Because many of these agents are pharmacologically active, their effects may be significant if sufficient amounts reach the fetus or newborn. Besides the usual oral or parenteral routes, unintentional portals of drug entry include the transplacental route; inadvertent direct fetal injection; pulmonary, skin, or conjunctival entry; or ingestion of breast milk.[156] Lack of awareness or underestimation of the degree of drug entry through these routes and of altered drug disposition and metabolism in the perinatal period has led to well-recognized therapeutic misadventures in neonatology. Prevention of toxic reactions to drugs and their rational and safe use require a thorough understanding of the

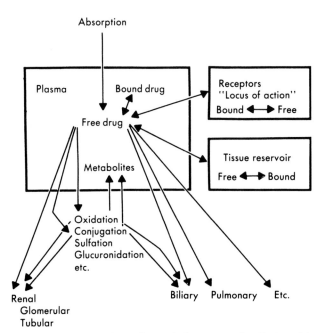

FIGURE 10–4. Interrelationships of absorption, distribution, biotransformation, and excretion of a drug and its concentration at the receptor site.

various pharmacologic profiles of each drug used in the treatment of the neonate.

Figure 10–4 illustrates many of the interrelationships of the absorption, distribution, binding, biotransformation, and excretion of a drug and its concentration at the locus of action.[177] To produce its characteristic effect, a drug must be present in appropriate concentrations at its sites of action or receptor sites. The concentration of drug at the receptor site depends not only on the amount of drug administered but also on the interrelationships listed. Those factors that have been evaluated in the newborn infant differ substantially from those in the adult and even in the young infant beyond the neonatal period.

ABSORPTION OF DRUGS IN THE NEONATE

Drug absorption is the passage of a drug from its site of administration into the circulation. In a sick neonate, the IV route is preferred because of ease of delivery, accuracy of dosage, possible poor peripheral perfusion, and poor gastrointestinal function. In neonates who can tolerate gastric feedings, the oral route of drug administration is the most convenient and probably the safest. Absorption of a drug or substance through the gastrointestinal system may be comprehensively defined as the net movement of a drug from the gastrointestinal lumen into the systemic circulation draining this organ. This process entails the movement of drugs across the gastrointestinal epithelium, which behaves like a semipermeable lipid membrane and constitutes the main barrier to absorption. The various processes operating to induce transepithelial membrane movement of drug molecules include (1) simple diffusion through lipid membranes or through aqueous pores of the membrane, (2) filtration through aqueous channels or membrane pores, and (3) carrier-mediated transport, such as active transport or facilitated diffusion and vesicular transport such as pinocytosis.[46] Of these, the most important is the process of simple diffusion, because most drugs administered orally are absorbed via this route. This is evident from the direct proportionality between the concentration of drug in the intestine and the amount of drug absorbed over a wide range of concentrations. Moreover, one drug does not compete with another for transfer, indicating that the process of absorption is a simple, nonsaturable one.

The rate and extent of drug absorption are partly determined by the physical and chemical characteristics of the drug.[171] Polarity, nonlipid solubility, and large molecular size tend to decrease absorption. In contrast, nonpolarity, lipid solubility, and small molecular size increase absorption. The degree of ionization, determined by the pK_a of the drug and the pH of the solution in which it exists, is an important determinant in drug absorption. The gastrointestinal epithelium is more permeable to the nonionized form because this portion is usually lipid soluble and favors absorption. The degree of drug ionization changes as the pH increases from the stomach through the distal portion of the gut. The slow gastric emptying time in the newborn may retard drug absorption and can be rate limiting. This is because the major absorption occurs in the proximal bowel, which has the greatest absorptive surface area. Conversely, a slow transit time or slow intestinal motility may facilitate the absorption of some drugs.[173]

These physiologic processes undergo substantial changes during the neonatal period.[71] Gastric acid production is generally low at birth, and the gastric pH is usually 6 to 8, decreasing within a few hours to pH values of 3 to 1.[1] Acid secretion is low in the first 10 days of life; it tends to rise thereafter and approaches adult values around 6 to 8 months of age. Intestinal motility is slow in the newborn, and transit time from the stomach to the cecum is generally prolonged relative to that in the adult. The gastric emptying time after milk feeding is considerably prolonged in the neonate and approaches adult values at age 6 to 8 months. The precise influence of milk feeding on neonatal drug bioavailability requires further evaluation.

Drug absorption requires an intact splanchnic vascular circulation. In sick neonates, especially those with hypotension, perfusion of the gut may decrease to maintain adequate perfusion of vital organs, resulting in decreased drug absorption.

Current evidence indicates that the amount of absorption of most drugs is independent of age, although the rate of absorption of certain drugs shows a nonlinear correlation with age. Heimann[71] studied the enteral absorption of various drugs (i.e., sulfonamides, phenobarbital, digoxin, methyldigoxin, D-xylose, and L-arabinose) and found reduced absorption rates in neonates relative to older children. Specific information concerning other drugs is becoming

available. These data indicate that gastrointestinal absorption of drugs is relatively slow in the neonate and undergoes maturational changes similar to those found in drug distribution, metabolism, and disposition. Although the neonatal drug absorptive deficit may influence the achievement of a desired pharmacologic effect, it is likely that its significance is minor relative to the age-related alterations in drug distribution, metabolism, and disposition.

PROTEIN BINDING OF DRUGS IN THE NEONATE

The unbound drug in plasma is considered to be the pharmacologically active fraction of the drug.[208] For some drugs, including theophylline, phenytoin, phenobarbital, penicillin, and salicylates, the binding to plasma protein is decreased in the newborn compared with that in the nonpregnant adult.[38] This suggests that a more intense pharmacologic response may be obtained in the newborn infant than in the adult for the same total drug concentration. The developmental changes in protein-drug binding and the postnatal age at which adult-like binding is achieved have not been defined with confidence for all drugs used in the neonatal period. Some drugs, such as phenytoin, may exhibit adult-like binding before the infant reaches 3 months of age.[157]

The reasons underlying this deficient plasma protein binding of drugs at birth may include decreased plasma albumin concentrations, possible qualitative differences in neonatal plasma proteins, and competitive binding by many endogenous substrates, such as hormones. Hyperbilirubinemia may accentuate this competition by displacing a drug, such as phenytoin, from its albumin-binding site.[136] This contrasts with the well-known bilirubin drug-protein binding interaction, in which drugs such as sulfonamides may displace bilirubin from its binding site.

Deficient plasma protein binding is usually not considered in calculating neonatal drug dosages. This factor must be considered in the application of adult therapeutic plasma concentrations to the neonatal patient. Moreover, decreased protein binding influences calculations of apparent volumes of distribution based on plasma concentrations of total drug. In terms of therapeutic monitoring, drug concentrations obtained from saliva reflect the concentrations of the unbound fraction in plasma.

DRUG METABOLISM AND DISPOSITION IN THE NEONATE

Many drugs are lipophilic and require conversion to more water-soluble metabolites for efficient elimination from the body. These metabolic processes are traditionally categorized as either phase I or phase II reactions. In a phase I reaction, a more polar compound is formed through oxidation, reduction, or hydrolysis of the parent molecule. Although often thought of as a detoxification process, phase I metabolites may be more pharmacologically active than the parent compound. It is the reactive product of phase

I metabolism that accounts for the carcinogenic and teratogenic effect of many xenobiotics. Phase II metabolism involves conjugation with endogenous substrates such as sulfate, acetate, or glucuronic acid. Drugs may be conjugated directly or made more amenable to conjugation following the introduction of a functional group by phase I metabolism (e.g., hydroxylation). It is well recognized that the neonate is deficient in many of the enzymes responsible for phase I and phase II drug metabolism.*

Unfortunately, these deficiencies have led to a number of adverse reactions, such as the "gray baby" syndrome associated with chloramphenicol use. Recent advances in our understanding of the ontogeny of the enzymes responsible for drug metabolism can explain past cases of drug toxicity in the neonate and help prevent such events in future.

Phase I metabolism is mediated primarily by the cytochrome P-450 enzymes. These enzymes are present in several tissues throughout the body (intestine, lung, kidney, adrenals) but are most highly concentrated in the liver. Numerous isoforms have been identified, but the primary enzymes involved in drug metabolism are listed in Table 10–4. Considerable individuality is evident with respect to substrate specificity, polymorphic expression, and susceptibility to induction and inhibition. The general pattern of development of these enzymes is illustrated in Figure 10–5. In fetal liver, studies have shown that CYP3A7

---

* References 29, 32, 63, 99, 159, 162.

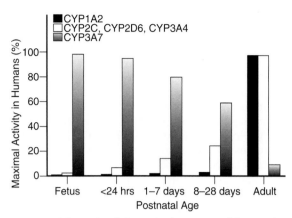

FIGURE 10–5. Maturational change in the activity of the cytochrome P-450 isoenzymes implicated in human drug metabolism. (See text for details.)

is by far the most significant P-450 enzyme in terms of protein expression and activity.*

CYP3A7 concentrations decline during the neonatal period, and in adults, the concentration is less than 20% that of CYP3A4.[89, 195] CYP3A4 is the most abundant P-450 enzyme in adults, accounting for 30% to 40% of hepatic P-450 and as much as 70% of the P-450 content of the intestine.[181, 207] The majority of other cytochrome P-450 enzymes develop rapidly in the neonatal period. Whether triggered by the loss of

---

* References 29, 63, 85, 89, 99, 159, 162.

TABLE 10–4 CHARACTERISTICS OF THE PRIMARY CYTOCHROME P-450 ENZYMES INVOLVED IN HUMAN DRUG METABOLISM

ENZYME	% OF TOTAL P-450 IN ADULT LIVER	POLYMORPHIC EXPRESSION	SELECTED SUBSTRATES	INHIBITORS
CYP1A2	15–20	No	Caffeine, theophylline, R-warfarin	Ciprofloxacin, erythromycin, amiodarone, fluvoxamine
CYP2C8/9	20–30 (includes CYP2C19)	<0.5% poor metabolizers (PMs)	Tolbutamide, phenytoin, S-warfarin, diclofenac, naproxen, ibuprofen	Sulphaphenazole, cimetidine, fluconazole, amiodarone
CYP2C19		Whites, blacks: 1–3% PMs Asians: 15–20% PMs	S-mephenytoin, omeprazole, diazepam, imipramine	
CYP2D6	1–5	Whites, blacks: 5–10% PMs Asians: 1–3% PMs	Debrisoquine, dextromethorphan, codeine, propafenone, amitriptyline, imipramine, fluoxetine, propranolol	Quinidine, haloperidol, fluoxetine
CYP3A4/5	30–40	No	Testosterone, ethinylestradiol, cyclosporine, carbamazepine, erythromycin, indinavir, saquinavir, ritonavir, lovastatin, midazolam, triazolam, quinidine, terfenadine, nifedipine, diltiazem, verapamil	Ketoconazole, itraconazole, erythromycin, verapamil, diltiazem, grapefruit juice, amiodarone, indinavir, ritonavir, clarithromycin

a maternal repressing factor or stimulated by transcription factors intrinsic to newborns, concentrations of CYP2D6 and CYP2E1 increase within hours of birth, followed closely by the CYP2C enzymes and CYP3A4.[89, 199, 200, 203] By 1 month of age, hepatic concentrations are approximately 25% to 30% of adult values. The notable exception is CYP1A2, which develops more slowly, reaching less than 5% of adult concentrations in the first month.[189] The total content of enzymes of the cytochrome P-450 3A subfamily remains relatively constant throughout the neonatal period and into adulthood, as declining concentrations of CYP3A7 are matched by increasing levels of CYP3A4.[89] It is generally assumed that premature babies exhibit greater impairment in drug metabolism than full-term infants, and this has been documented in several studies involving drugs metabolized by a wide range of cytochrome P-450 enzymes.[25, 96–98, 104, 124, 159] This may be due to a greater degree of immaturity in these enzymes at birth, a delay in the postnatal surge in P-450 concentration observed in full-term babies, or a combination of factors.

The pharmacokinetics of many drugs in neonates are consistent with the pattern of development of the P-450 enzymes shown in Figure 10–5. Caffeine, administered for the treatment of neonatal apnea, exhibits an extremely prolonged half-life of several days in neonates, compared with 4 to 6 hours in adults.[2, 6, 98] This is due to the delayed development of the CYP1A2 enzyme, which is responsible for demethylation of caffeine, the primary metabolic pathway.[23, 61, 62] The structurally related bronchodilator theophylline also exhibits reduced clearance and a prolonged half-life in neonates.[17, 36] However, the effect is not as dramatic as that observed with caffeine, because theophylline is partially oxidized by other cytochrome P-450 enzymes such as CYP2E1 in addition to CYP1A2.[62, 197] For drugs metabolized primarily by CYP2D6 or CYP2C, it seems reasonable to expect drug clearance to be low at birth but to increase rapidly during the first month of life. Data on tolbutamide and phenytoin, substrates for CYP2C9, support this view.[25] The half-life of tolbutamide was found to decrease from 46 hours to 6 hours within the first 2 days after birth in a neonate exposed to the drug by placental transfer from the mother.[25] The clearance of drugs metabolized by CYP3A4 may be reduced to a lesser extent in neonates than substrates for other P-450 enzymes if CYP3A7 is capable of contributing to the metabolic process. CYP3A4 and CYP3A7 show more than 85% amino acid sequence homology and have partially overlapping affinities for both endogenous and exogenous substrates.[55, 137] CYP3A7 appears to play an important role in the metabolism of steroids by the fetus and is 10- to 20-fold more active than CYP3A4 in catalyzing the 16α-hydroxylation of dehydroepiandrosterone. In addition, the ratio of 6β-hydroxycortisol to cortisol in urine declines in parallel with the decrease in CYP3A7 concentration in neonates, suggesting that CYP3A7 is involved in this reaction.[125] The catalytic activity of CYP3A4 toward drugs such as midazolam, carbamazepine, and nifedi-

pine is greater than that of CYP3A7, whereas the latter appears relatively active in metabolizing erythromycin.[55, 137] Even if catalytic activity is low, however, CYP3A7 may contribute to the overall clearance of a drug at birth owing to the high concentrations present. This may account for the observation that the elimination of CYP3A substrates such as carbamazepine[184] and the reverse transcriptase inhibitor nevirapine[122] in the first week of life is relatively similar to that observed in adults.

Phase II drug metabolism is mediated by a number of different enzymes, the most important of which are N-acetyltransferase (acetylation), sulfotransferase (sulfation), and uridine 5'-diphosphate glucuronosyltransferase (glucuronidation). Acetylation activity is polymorphically expressed in adults, with 10% to 20% of Asians and 40% to 60% of whites and African Americans being slow acetylators.[119] Delayed development in neonates is suggested by studies indicating that a much higher percentage (greater than 75%) of newborns and children younger than age 2 are phenotypic slow acetylators of caffeine and isoniazid compared with adults.[142, 143] Sulfation appears to be reasonably well developed at birth relative to other pathways of drug metabolism. The proportion of a dose of acetaminophen excreted as sulfate conjugate is higher in neonates than in older children or adults.[202] Increased sulfation compensates in part for reduced glucuronidation of acetaminophen and ritodrine in neonates.[18] Glucuronidation is an important route of metabolism for many drugs (acetaminophen, morphine, zidovudine) as well as endogenous compounds such as bilirubin.[32] Although glucuronosyltransferase (UGT) activity is generally presumed to be immature at birth, establishing a clear pattern for its development is complicated by the existence of numerous isoforms of the enzyme with broad and overlapping substrate specificity. UGT1A1, involved in the glucuronidation of bilirubin, is virtually absent in the fetus and develops slowly over several months after birth. A somewhat similar pattern of development exists for UGT1A6, responsible for glucuronidation of acetaminophen. UGT2B7 is expressed to a greater extent in the fetus and neonate (10% to 20% of adult values) and catalyzes the formation of morphine-3-glucuronide and morphine-6-glucuronide.[32] However, morphine clearance in neonates remains well below that of older children.[3] The UGT isoform involved in the metabolism of substrates such as zidovudine and chloramphenicol has not been clearly identified. Chloramphenicol is of particular interest, because impaired glucuronidation is the primary cause of the gray baby syndrome associated with use of this drug. Similar to observations with drugs metabolized by cytochrome P-450, glucuronidation in premature infants is impaired to a greater extent than in full-term infants.[115, 175]

Conclusions based on studies of drug metabolism in the neonate must be interpreted with caution, owing to the small numbers of subjects in many investigations and the potentially confounding effect of disease states on metabolism, as access to healthy babies during the first month of life is limited. Nonetheless, the available data suggest that:

1. The rate of drug metabolism is generally low at birth in full-term babies and even lower in premature infants, irrespective of the specific route of metabolism. Decreased clearance and a prolonged drug half-life require the administration of smaller doses at longer dosing intervals.
2. Many of the enzymes responsible for metabolism exhibit significant development during the first month of life. Dosing regimens appropriate during the first few days of postnatal life may be inappropriate 3 to 4 weeks after birth as dose requirements increase and dosing intervals decrease.
3. The development of individual drug-metabolizing enzymes varies widely between neonates and may be delayed in premature infants. Predicting clearance is difficult, and dosing regimens must be individualized for patients based on careful observation of response and monitoring of plasma concentrations whenever possible.

RENAL EXCRETION OF DRUGS

The kidneys are the most important organs for drug elimination in the newborn, because the most frequently used drugs, such as antimicrobial agents, are excreted via these organs.[110] Renal elimination of these drugs reflects and depends on neonatal renal function, characterized by low glomerular filtration rate, low effective renal blood flow, and low tubular function compared with that in the adult (see Chapter 49). Neonatal glomerular filtration rate is about 30% of the adult value and is greatly influenced by gestational age at birth.[59] The most rapid changes occur during the first week of life, and these events are reflected by the plasma disappearance rates of aminoglycosides, which are eliminated mainly by glomerular filtration.[178] These changes have been considered in the dosage regimen recommended for these drugs and other antibiotics.

Effective renal blood flow may influence the rate at which drugs are presented to and eliminated by the kidneys. Effective renal blood flow, as measured by para-aminohippurate (PAH) clearance, is substantially lower in infants relative to adult values, even when PAH extraction values are correlated (i.e., PAH extraction is 60% in infants, compared with greater than 92% in adults). Available data suggest that there is low effective renal blood flow during the first 2 days of life (34 to 99 mL/minute per 1.73 m²), which increases to 54 to 166 mL/minute per 1.73 m² by 14 to 21 days and further increases to adult values of about 600 mL/minute per 1.73 m² by age 1 to 2 years.[178] These data are probably not applicable to premature infants with very low birth weights, particularly those weighing less than 750 gm at birth. It is assumed, pending definitive data, that the glomerular filtration rate and renal blood flow in these micronates are substantially lower relative to bigger premature infants, such as those weighing more than 1000 gm at birth.

The pharmacokinetic behavior of drugs eliminated via the neonatal kidneys exhibits characteristics similar to those underlying hepatic biotransformation. For instance, the half-life of many antimicrobials, such as ampicillin (Fig. 10–6), shows marked interindividual variability at birth,[8] which narrows somewhat with advancing age. The plasma half-life also shortens progressively after birth, achieving adult rates of elimination within 1 month postnatally. The drug-dependent variability in the elimination process may reflect, in part, the major renal mechanism of drug excretion. Those drugs that undergo substantial elimination by glomerular filtration (e.g., aminoglycosides) may be excreted more rapidly than those requiring substantial tubular excretion (e.g., penicillins). These differences may reflect neonatal glomerular preponderance.

As with hepatic metabolism, renal excretion of certain drugs may be as efficient as in adults. For example, colistin, an antibiotic, is eliminated by neonates at rates similar to those in adults. However, as a rule, drug excretion via the neonatal kidneys is deficient relative to that in the adult. Pathophysiologic insults further compromise the inherent deficiency in drug

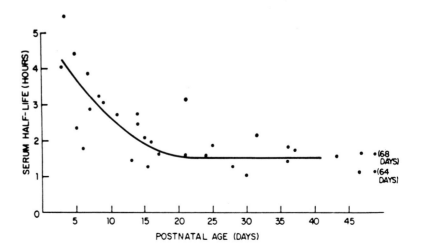

FIGURE 10–6. Postnatal changes in the serum half-life of ampicillin. (From Axline SG, et al: Clinical pharmacology of antimicrobials in premature infants. II. Ampicillin, methicillin, oxacillin, neomycin, and colistin. Pediatrics 39:97, 1967; copyright American Academy of Pediatrics, 1967.)

elimination, thus complicating individual drug dosage regimens.[30, 60] Moreover, very small infants, who receive the most drugs in the neonatal population, exhibit the worst functional deficiency in drug elimination. This can result in overdosage, as in the case of digoxin.[150] Neonates weighing less than 1000 gm achieved steady-state plasma concentrations of digoxin three times higher than did their counterparts born at term. Hypoxemia further decreases the slow glomerular and tubular function in neonates, thus leading to slower renal excretion of drugs, as has been shown with amikacin. A linear relationship between oxygen tension and hepatic oxidation has been reported, so drugs that require hepatic biotransformation or renal excretion may be excreted much more slowly in the face of hypoxemia. Determination of plasma concentration of drugs, coupled with appropriate caution and clinical awareness, helps ensure optimal and safe drug therapy in the neonate.

PHARMACOKINETIC CONSIDERATIONS, DOSAGE GUIDELINES, AND THERAPEUTIC MONITORING IN NEONATAL DRUG THERAPY

(See also Appendix A.)

Knowledge of the kinetic profile of a drug allows manipulation of the dosage to achieve and maintain a given plasma concentration. Many drugs administered in the newborn period exhibit a plasma disappearance curve (Fig. 10–7). In the example in the figure, the log of the plasma concentration decreases linearly as a function of time, with a brief but fast distribution (α) phase and a slower elimination (β) phase. This exemplifies a two-compartment model and first-order kinetics; that is, a certain fraction (not amount) of the drug remaining in the body is eliminated with time, and after the distribution phase, the plasma concentration reflects or is proportional to the

concentration of drug in other portions of the body. This model is applicable to a wide variety of drugs used in the neonatal period, although some drugs (e.g., gentamicin, diazepam, digoxin) fit a multicompartmental model. Others (e.g., ethanol) exhibit saturation kinetics; that is, a certain amount (not fraction) of the drug is eliminated per unit of time.[118] In newborn infants, in whom the elimination phase is extremely prolonged relative to the distribution phase, the relative contribution of the distribution phase to overall elimination and to dosage computations may not be significant. Thus, the entire body may behave kinetically as though it were a single compartment.

The administration of a loading dose (in milligrams per kilogram) to quickly achieve a given plasma drug concentration depends on the rapidity with which the onset of drug action is required. For many drugs used in neonates, loading doses are generally greater than for older children or adult subjects. The prolonged half-life warrants a substantially lower maintenance dosage given at longer intervals to prevent toxic effects or overdosage. The rapid postnatal changes in drug elimination require adjustment of maintenance dosage rates (in milligrams per kilogram per day) with advancing postnatal age; this adjustment may also be a function of the drug being used. Monitoring of drug concentrations is extremely useful if the desired pharmacologic effect is not attained or if adverse reactions occur. Moreover, therapeutic drug monitoring seems prudent, especially for drugs with a narrow therapeutic index used during a period in which there is rapid change in drug elimination.

In the clinical setting, therapeutic drug monitoring of anticonvulsants (phenytoin, phenobarbital, carbamazepine), antimicrobials (gentamicin, tobramycin, chloramphenicol, vancomycin), cardiac glycosides (digoxin),[209] and methylxanthines (caffeine, theophylline) is often useful in individualizing drug therapy.[4, 5, 9] Rapid microassay techniques such as enzyme multiplied immunoassay technique, high pressure liquid chromatography, and others require small volumes of blood samples and are well suited for neonates. Therapeutic drug monitoring to verify the appropriateness of the drug dosing schedule is useful when (1) dose adjustments are contemplated, (2) there is a lack of desired therapeutic effect, (3) there are adverse or toxic effects, and (4) factors modifying drug metabolism and elimination are present, such as abnormal renal and hepatic function. Because most drugs used in neonates exhibit first-order kinetics, the change in dose is proportional to the change in plasma drug concentration at steady state. Thus, a plasma phenobarbital concentration of 10 mg/L at a dose of 5 mg/kg per day would be expected to increase 100% to 20 mg/L if the dose were increased 100% to 10 mg/kg per day. Conversely, a plasma phenobarbital concentration of 10 mg/L would decrease to 5 mg/L if the phenobarbital dose were decreased 50% to 2.5 mg/kg per day. These predictions are expected to occur at steady state, where the fraction of the drug dose eliminated from the body is usually held constant.

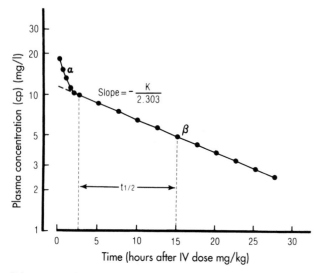

FIGURE 10–7. Representative plasma disappearance curve of a drug given intravenously, plotted semilogarithmically as a function of time. A fast distribution phase (α) is followed by a slower elimination phase (β).

TABLE 10–5   INFLUENCE OF FETAL MATURITY AND POSTCONCEPTIONAL AGE ON DRUG DOSE AND DOSE INTERVAL

DRUG	POSTCONCEPTIONAL AGE (WKS)	DOSE (MG/KG)	DOSE INTERVAL (HRS)
Gentamicin	<24	2.5	q36
	25–27	2.5	q24
	28–29	3.0	q24
	30–37	2.5	q18
	>37	2.5	q12
Vancomycin	<29	18	q24
	30–36	15	q12
	37–44	10	q8

Doses and intervals used at the McGill University Hospitals. Derived from published pharmacokinetic data and local therapeutic drug monitoring information compiled by I Alarcon, et al, McGill University–Jewish General Hospital, Montreal.

ROLE OF FETAL MATURITY AND ADVANCING POSTNATAL AGE ON NEONATAL DRUG DOSE AND DOSE INTERVAL

Infants with very low birth weights (500 to 750 gm) and those with low birth weights (751 to 1000 gm) are increasing in numbers in many neonatal intensive care units. This phenomenon is due to several factors, including attempts to decrease rates of perinatal death caused by fetal distress, fetal growth retardation, premature rupture of membranes, or simply inability to stop labor by existing tocolytic measures. The major organs for drug metabolism and drug excretion in these very small, premature neonates—namely, the liver and the kidneys—are substantially immature; therefore, the plasma clearance of drugs is exceptionally slow or diminished. This indicates that the total drug dose per day must be decreased and the intervals between drug doses must be much longer than in term newborns or more mature premature neonates (i.e., greater than 32 weeks' gestation). Drug doses, particularly for those agents excreted by the kidneys, are dynamically changing as functions of gestational age and postnatal age. These are exemplified by two commonly used agents, gentamicin and vancomycin (Table 10–5). In general, the total daily dose of the drug is directly related to gestational age. The lower the fetal or postconceptional age, the smaller the total daily drug dose. Moreover, fetal maturity is inversely related to dose interval. Thus, the younger the gestational age, the longer the dose interval. These dose adjustments reflect the relatively deficient drug elimination of very small premature infants.

DRUGS AND LACTATION

Until recently, investigations of drugs and other compounds in breast milk were hampered by the very small numbers of lactating women studied and the insensitivity of drug assay methods. Much of the early literature concerns isolated case reports and a small selection of drugs.[95] Several papers reviewed these data.[28] With today's higher incidence of breast feeding, there are more situations in which lactating women are exposed to various medications, and an increasing number of useful studies of drugs in breast milk can be expected. Currently, up to 80% of Canadian and American women breast-feed their infants. A comprehensive review of drugs in pregnancy and lactation can be found in the work by Briggs and colleagues.[20]

In addition to pharmaceuticals, environmental pollutants and nontherapeutic or "social" chemicals find their way into breast milk. Public awareness of these problems is high, and the physician is often called on for counseling.

PASSAGE OF EXOGENOUS COMPOUNDS FROM MATERNAL BLOOD TO MILK

The presence and concentration of compounds in breast milk depend on molecular weight, degree of ionization, protein binding in blood, lipid solubility, and specific uptake by mammary tissue.[102] Drugs that are not absorbed after oral ingestion do not appear in milk.

Small compounds with molecular weights of less than about 200 appear freely in breast milk and are presumed to have passed through pores in the mammary alveolar cell.[7] Large compounds such as insulin or heparin do not pass into milk. Intermediate-size compounds must penetrate the lipoprotein cell membrane by diffusion or active transport.

In general, drugs that are not ionized at blood pH traverse the alveolar cell membrane with greater ease than do highly ionized compounds. Because breast milk pH is 7 or slightly less, milk acts like a trap for weak bases.

Drugs pass the cell membrane only in their free form; thus, highly protein-bound drugs are less available for passage. Drugs or other chemicals that are very lipid soluble readily cross the alveolar cell, and because breast milk contains a considerable amount of lipid, these compounds are trapped in the milk. Drugs, for the most part, enter breast milk by passive diffusion. This is best described in pharmacokinetic terms as a three-compartment model, with the breast milk as a deep third compartment (Fig. 10–8). These principles also apply to drug metabolite transfer into breast milk.

Finally, certain compounds are actively taken up by mammary tissue and are found in breast milk in concentrations substantially higher than in blood.[34]

The amount of drug in breast milk can be calculated by the milk-plasma (M-P) ratio.[171] However, use of the M-P ratio is fraught with potential difficulties. It is better, if possible, to measure drug concentrations directly in breast milk.

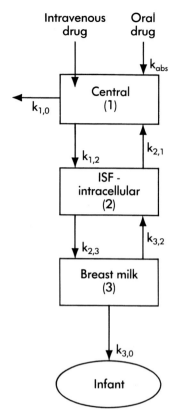

FIGURE 10–8. Three-compartment model for drug transfer into breast milk. ISF, interstitial fluid; k_{abs}, absorption rate constant; k_{xy}, rate constant for transfer from compartment x to compartment y. (Modified from Wilson JT: Determinants and consequences of drug excretion in breast milk. Drug Metab Rev 14:619, 1983.)

MODIFICATION OF PASSAGE OF COMPOUNDS INTO BREAST MILK

Drugs may be metabolized by the maternal body to active or inactive metabolites. These derivatives may be secreted into breast milk less readily than is the parent compound. The timing of maternal ingestion of a drug in relation to the time of milk synthesis may influence the concentration of drug in any particular breast milk feeding.

In animals, changes in mammary gland blood flow control the amount of drug presented to sites of uptake. Mammary tissue itself can metabolize certain compounds. Drugs already secreted into milk may be secreted back into the alveolar cell and then into blood. Moreover, the stage of lactation plays a role; drugs may be secreted more easily in the colostral phase. Finally, changes in milk composition during lactation or feeding may change the amount of drug in breast milk; for example, formula is more acidic than is milk expressed later in a feeding.[66, 194]

DELIVERY OF COMPOUNDS TO, AND DISPOSITION BY, THE INFANT

The total volume of milk consumed in a known period determines the dosage to the infant. Because daily volume intake of breast milk is exceedingly variable and impractical to measure routinely, one could assume a *high average* daily milk consumption to be about 1 L.

To produce an effect, the drug in the milk must either act locally in the gut or be absorbed. It is possible that the milk proteins will bind certain drugs and thereby impede absorption; it is also possible that the bowel of a very young infant may permit absorption of normally excluded large molecules.

The infant's disposition of the drug in milk changes with postnatal age. In addition, one must always be aware of the drug's potential for displacement of bilirubin from serum albumin.

COMPOUNDS IN BREAST MILK

Anticoagulants

Heparin does not enter breast milk. Newer synthetic heparin has a much lower molecular weight and thus has greater potential for passage into breast milk. Oral anticoagulants of the *inandione* group, as well as *bishydroxycoumarin* and *ethyl biscoumacetate,* are found in milk and have been associated with infant coagulopathies.[31] *Warfarin* must be considered the drug of choice; by virtue of its acidity and its high degree of protein binding, it is undetectable in breast milk.[139]

Anti-inflammatory and Analgesic Drugs

Acetylsalicylic acid (ASA) appears to pose no danger when used occasionally. Older infants have been found to receive about 0.2% to 0.3% of a single dose of ASA administered to the mother.[40] Although detailed studies do not exist, *acetaminophen* also seems to be safe.[7, 28]

Antimicrobial Drugs

Fortunately, most antimicrobial agents in breast milk appear to be safe for nursing infants. Drugs of the *penicillin* group may change the infant's intestinal flora and cause diarrhea and thrush; in theory, they could also incite hypersensitivity. The *cephalosporins* appear to be secreted in insignificant amounts in breast milk.[116, 212] The passage of the various *sulfonamide derivatives* is influenced by their differing degrees of ionization and protein binding; all have the potential to displace bilirubin from albumin. Thus, the sulfonamides should be avoided in a breast-feeding woman during the first week of the infant's life. Ingestion of *salicylazosulfapyridine* leads to the appearance of the metabolite sulfapyridine in breast milk; it has been estimated that the infant of a mother using this drug on a long-term basis will receive about 0.3% of the maternal dose per day.[13] *Erythromycin* is present in milk in a higher concentration than in maternal plasma, suggesting that the infant could receive a significant dose. The *tetracyclines* in breast milk have the potential to cause dental staining and should be avoided by women who are breast-feeding their infants. Most authors recommend that *chloramphenicol* not be taken by lactating women, even though the drug levels in milk would not produce a dose associated with gray baby syndrome. The *aminoglycosides* are poorly absorbed from the infant's gastrointestinal tract. *Isoniazid* and *PAS* have not been associated with ill effects in nursing infants. *Metronidazole* therapy in usual doses is not contraindicated for breast-feeding women.

Drugs Affecting the Cardiovascular System

The amount of *digoxin* present in milk depends on the maternal dose; infants whose mothers received 0.25 mg/day did not ingest enough digoxin in milk to have detectable blood levels.[24, 48, 103] Diuretics in general seem to be harmless, although if a nursing woman were to become dehydrated because of diuretic use, lactation would be greatly depressed. The effects of diuretics on milk composition are unclear. *Spironolactone* and its less active metabolite are secreted in breast milk, and an estimated 0.2% of the mother's daily dose is received by the infant.[82, 147] *Chlorthalidone* appears in small amounts in breast milk and could potentially accumulate in a young infant.[120] *Propranolol* seems to be safe. *Quinidine* is secreted in breast milk in a concentration about 60% that in maternal blood, but no ill effects have been observed.[75]

Drugs Affecting the Central Nervous System

Diazepam is converted in the body to an active metabolite, *desmethyldiazepam*, and both are excreted in breast milk. Both these compounds have a prolonged half-life in infants, and long-term use of diazepam by nursing women has been associated with lethargy and weight loss in their babies. The concentration of *barbiturates* in breast milk depends on their different degrees of ionization and lipid solubility. In anticonvulsant doses, they seem to be safe.[88, 130] *Chlordiazepoxide* in breast milk has been linked to depression in nursing infants. *Meprobamate* should probably be avoided because the drug achieves breast milk concentrations several times greater than maternal plasma levels.

Lithium is contraindicated during lactation because it has been found to cause significant cardiovascular and central nervous system signs in the infant. The *phenothiazines* and *tricyclic antidepressants* have been found in breast milk but appear to be safe in modest doses.[41, 53, 154, 190] The *amphetamines* also appear in breast milk and may cause jitteriness.

Phenytoin is found in breast milk in concentrations about one fifth those in maternal blood.[81] *Primidone* and *ethosuximide* both achieve breast milk levels near that of maternal blood, although significant symptoms in infants have not been noted.[81, 88]

Phenobarbital is metabolized much more slowly in neonates than in adults; it is possible that the drug may accumulate in breast-fed infants of phenobarbital-treated mothers. These infants should be monitored for lethargy and weight gain.[28]

Drugs Affecting the Endocrine System

Drugs of the *thiouracil* family, such as *methimazole, carbimazole,* and *iodides,* are contraindicated during breast feeding; they achieve a high breast milk concentration and can suppress the infant's thyroid function.[28] Revision of this dogma has been suggested, and *propylthiouracil* may be given to nursing mothers, provided the infant's thyroid function is monitored.

Thyroxine and other thyroid hormone preparations seem to be safe; endogenous thyroid hormone naturally secreted in breast milk may mask congenital cretinism during breast feeding.[28] The long-term effects of exogenous *glucocorticoids* and their derivatives in breast milk are not known. Women receiving *prednisone* and *prednisolone* excrete very small amounts of these compounds in breast milk.

A common problem is the use of *oral contraceptives* during lactation. Little is known about the effects of long-term exposure to small doses of these compounds in breast milk. Contraceptives with a high concentration of estrogen and progestin depress lactation, especially if they are begun soon after parturition. If their use is imperative, it is best to start treatment about 4 weeks after delivery, ensuring that lactation is already well established, and to use the lowest dosage possible. The infants should be followed with care, as there have been reports of gynecomastia and changes in vaginal epithelium. Study of late effects in exposed infants is urgently needed. The oral contraceptives in current clinical use are not contraindicated for mothers who are breast-feeding.[83, 188]

Other Drugs

Cimetidine, a histamine H_2-receptor antagonist, has been reported in breast milk in concentrations 3 to 12 times greater than in maternal blood; this drug may be actively transported into breast milk.[83, 188] Because cimetidine and ranitidine are known to be safe and effective when used for therapy in infants, they are not contraindicated during lactation. Omeprazole, a proton pump inhibitor, is extremely potent and should probably be avoided during lactation.

Theobromine from chocolate has been found in breast milk at a level of 80% of maternal serum.[161]

Theophylline ingestion by the mother has been associated with infant irritability. Extracts of *ergot* have been responsible for toxic reactions in nursing infants and should be avoided.[44] The use of *isotopes* for diagnosis or therapy should be avoided during lactation. An acceptable level of an isotope in breast milk is not known. It has been suggested that women not nurse for 10 days after exposure to ^{131}I, for 3 days after ^{99m}Tc exposure, and for 2 weeks after ^{67}Ga exposure. If radiopharmaceuticals are required during lactation, breast feeding should be avoided while the radioactive agent is present in breast milk. In cases of uncertainty, consultation should be obtained from a specialist in nuclear medicine.

The *quinolones* pass into breast milk. Given the

controversy over their potential effects on the developing musculoskeletal system, it is prudent to avoid using quinolones during lactation.

Nontherapeutic Agents in Breast Milk

(See also Chapter 12.)

CAFFEINE. One hour after the ingestion of an average cup of coffee, a peak breast milk caffeine level of about 1.5 gm/mL is obtained. Caffeine levels in breast milk are about half the corresponding maternal blood level. Although the daily amount of caffeine consumed by a nursing infant might be small, the long half-life of caffeine could cause symptoms such as wakefulness or jitteriness.

INGREDIENTS OF CIGARETTES. The *nicotine* content of breast milk from women smoking one pack per day has been found to be about 100 to 500 parts per billion. No symptoms have been ascribed to this degree of contamination. *Thiocyanate*, which is elevated in the blood of smoking women, does not appear in elevated amounts in their breast milk.[111]

ETHANOL. Ethanol, a small molecule, diffuses freely into breast milk and achieves levels equivalent to those in blood. The metabolite *acetaldehyde* does not appear in breast milk. Excessive ethanol intake by the mother may depress the nursing infant's central nervous system.

NARCOTICS. *Heroin, methadone, morphine,* and other *opiate derivatives* have been found in breast milk and may be responsible for both addiction and withdrawal symptoms in the nursing infant. Opiates used briefly appear to have little clinical effect. It has been suggested that women receiving methadone maintenance doses take their daily dose after the last breast feeding in the evening, as breast milk methadone levels peak about 4 hours after administration of the drug by mouth.

Environmental Pollutants in Breast Milk

(See also Chapter 12.)

LEAD. Lead has been found in both bovine and human milk, as well as in commercial infant formulas. The lead content of human milk has remained rather constant during the past four decades, in contrast to levels of some other pollutants. One study found the lead level in human milk in the United States to be about 0.03 gm/mL. There are no reports of signs and symptoms of lead toxicity from this source.

MERCURY. Metallic or inorganic mercury poisoning in adults is usually associated with occupational exposure. There are no reports of metallic mercury poisoning from consumption of breast milk. Organic mercury—more specifically, *methyl mercury*—has been used industrially in fungicides, in pulp and paper factories, and in chloralkali plants.[51] In the late 1950s, Minamata Bay, Japan, was contaminated with indus-

trial wastes containing methyl mercury; the compound found its way into human beings through contaminated fish. There was a high incidence of neurologic abnormalities in children born in this area, probably related to in utero exposure to the chemical rather than to exposure during lactation. Methyl mercury was found in breast milk in a concentration about 5% that in blood; the half-life for disappearance of mercury from breast milk was estimated to be about 70 days.

Several epidemics in Iraq in the last 15 years were traceable to contamination of grains with methyl mercury fungicides. A number of nursing infants ingested enough methyl mercury in breast milk to achieve blood levels above the toxic limit.

PESTICIDES. Organic pesticides are concentrated in body fat. Breast milk production, with its export of large quantities of lipid, is an efficient way for a woman to rid her body of these poisons.[204] The nursing human infant thus becomes the highest animal in the "food chain." *DDT* (dichlorodiphenyltrichloroethane) was first identified in breast milk in 1951, and levels have been falling slowly since its use was restricted in North America in the early 1970s. Current levels of DDT in breast milk vary geographically and are related to agricultural use of the compound. In Canada in 1979, average milk DDT was 44 ng/gm of breast milk. A 5-kg infant ingesting 1 kg of breast milk each day would thus take in about 0.009 mg/kg per day. The Food and Agriculture Organization and World Health Organization recommendation for the maximum allowable intake by an adult is about 0.005 mg/kg per day. Nonetheless, there are no known harmful effects to the infant from the ingestion of breast milk contaminated to this degree.

Many other pesticides have been found in breast milk, reflecting their commercial use in the particular region or country.[10] Concentrations of *dieldrin*, for instance, which was banned in the United States after 1974, are decreasing in breast milk.

INDUSTRIAL BY-PRODUCTS. The extremely toxic dioxin *TCDD* (2,3,7,8-tetrachlorodibenzo-*p*-dioxin) caused environmental contamination in Seveso, Italy, in 1976. Chloracne developed in children who were directly exposed; further effects remain to be determined. This toxin has been found in breast milk.

There has been great public interest in the *polychlorinated biphenyls* (PCBs).[54] This class of compounds has had 50 years of industrial use, primarily in the manufacture of electric apparatus (transformers, capacitors), although such use seems to be declining. Because of contamination of rivers and lakes by industrial effluent, PCBs are widely distributed in freshwater fish and in those animals that eat them. As with organic pesticides, PCBs remain in body fat stores and are excreted with the fat of breast milk. An epidemic of poisoning by PCBs (Yusho disease) occurred in 1968 in Japan, when a commercial rice oil product was inadvertently contaminated with PCBs. Fetuses exposed in utero suffered growth retardation both antenatally and postnatally. Several infants whose only exposure was via breast milk had weakness and apathy. It is of great concern that breast milk levels of PCBs in North America appear to be increasing. In Canada in 1979, the average PCB level in breast milk was 12 ng/gm, whereas women who are exposed occupationally to PCBs or who consume game fish from contaminated waters may have much higher levels in their breast milk.

The *polybrominated biphenyls (PBBs)* were brought to attention by an incident in Michigan in 1973 and 1974,[21] in which several hundred pounds of PBBs, normally used as fire retardants in the plastics industry, accidentally contaminated cattle feed; widespread intoxication of farm animals resulted. PBBs have the usual propensity to lodge in fat tissue and to persist in the body. To date, no ill effects have been noted in infants exposed to PBBs through their mothers' milk. In Michigan, breast milk PBB surveillance has provided an accurate picture of the contamination of the general population. This method of epidemiologic analysis of fat-soluble poisons has much to recommend it, because the collection of milk samples is far easier than the collection of adipose tissue specimens. Breast milk PBB levels in the contaminated areas of Michigan averaged 0.07 parts per million.

CONCLUSION

As with the helpless fetus in utero, the nursing infant is exposed to nearly everything entering the body of its mother.[141] The dangers, especially over the long term, are unclear. Environmental pollutants are almost impossible to avoid, and elimination of nontherapeutic (recreational) compounds involves changing lifestyles. Drug administration is the easiest to control, but often a difficult choice must be made between maternal therapy and potential infant harm. The following are some simple guidelines to be observed:

1. A lactating woman should not receive a drug that one would be reluctant to give directly to her infant at that particular postnatal or gestational age.
2. Drug secretion into milk is so variable that one should not attempt to *treat* an infant by administering the drug to the lactating mother.
3. Milk that is donated to milk banks must be free from contamination.
4. When maternal drug administration is necessary, one may attempt to minimize the dosage to the infant by withholding nursing at the time of maximum secretion of the drug into breast milk.
5. Signs and symptoms in a nursing child should be correlated with drug ingestion by the mother. In investigations it is most useful to measure levels of the drug and its metabolites in the infant's body fluids, rather than at isolated times in maternal blood or breast milk.
6. When therapy is necessary, it should be with single agents if possible. In the case of long-term therapy, consideration should be given to monitoring the infant's activity and growth.

■ REFERENCES

1. Agunod M, et al: Correlative study of hydrochloric acid, pepsin, and intrinsic secretion in newborns and infants. Am J Dig Dis 14:400, 1969.
2. Anderson BJ, et al: Caffeine overdose in a premature infant: Clinical course and pharmacokinetics. Anaesth Intensive Care 27:307, 1999.
3. Anderson BJ, et al: Size, myths and the clinical pharmacokinetics of analgesia in paediatric patients. Clin Pharmacokinet 33:313, 1997.
4. Aranda JV, et al: Pharmacokinetic aspects of theophylline in premature newborns. N Engl J Med 295:413, 1976.
5. Aranda JV, et al: Methylxanthines in apnea of prematurity. Clin Perinatol 6:87, 1979.
6. Aranda JV, et al: Pharmacokinetic profile of caffeine in the premature newborn with apnea. J Pediatr 94:663, 1979.
7. Atkinson HC, et al: Drugs in breast milk: Clinical pharmacokinetic considerations. Clin Pharmacokinet 14:217, 1988.
8. Axline SG, et al: Clinical pharmacology of antimicrobials in premature infants. II. Ampicillin, methicillin, oxacillin, neomycin, and colistin. Pediatrics 39:97, 1967.
9. Bada HS, et al: Interconversion of theophylline and caffeine in newborn infants. J Pediatr 94:993, 1979.
10. Bagnell PC, et al: Obstructive jaundice due to a chlorinated hydrocarbon in breast milk. Can Med Assoc J 117:1047, 1977.
11. Barnes AB, et al: Fertility and outcome of pregnancy in women exposed in utero to diethylstilbestrol. N Engl J Med 302:609, 1980.
12. Barr M Jr, et al: Teratogen update: Angiotensin-converting enzyme inhibitors. Teratology 50:399, 1994.
13. Berlin CM, et al: Disposition of salicylazosulfapyridine (Azulfidine) and metabolites in human breast milk. Dev Pharmacol Ther 1:31, 1980.
14. Bernhardt JB, et al: Hypervitaminosis A and congenital renal anomalies in a human infant. Obstet Gynecol 43:750, 1974.
15. Bethenod M, et al: Les enfants des antiepileptiques. Pediatrie 30:227, 1975.
16. Bologa M, et al: Drugs and chemicals most commonly used for pregnant women. In Koren G (ed): Maternal-Fetal Toxicology: A Clinician's Guide. New York, Marcel Dekker, 1994, p 89.
17. Bory C, et al: Metabolism of theophylline to caffeine in the premature newborn infant. J Pediatr 94:988, 1979.
18. Brashear WT, et al: Maternal and neonatal urinary excretion of sulfate and glucuronide ritodrine conjugates. Clin Pharmacol Ther 44:634, 1988.
19. Braun AG, et al: Teratogenic drugs inhibit tumour cell attachment to lectin-coated surfaces. Nature 282:507, 1979.
20. Briggs G, et al: A Reference Guide to Fetal and Neonatal Risk: Drugs in Pregnancy and Lactation, 5th ed. Baltimore, Williams & Wilkins, 1998.
21. Brilliant LB, et al: Breast-milk monitoring to measure Michigan's contamination with polybrominated biphenyls. Lancet 2:643, 1978.
22. Butler NR, et al: Smoking in pregnancy and subsequent child development. BMJ 4:573, 1973.
23. Cazeneuve C, et al: Biotransformation of caffeine in human liver microsomes from foetuses, neonates, infants and adults. Br J Clin Pharmacol 37:405, 1994.
24. Chan V, et al: Transfer of digoxin across the placenta and into breast milk. Br J Obstet Gynaecol 85:605, 1978.
25. Christesen HBT, Melander A: Prolonged elimination of tolbutamide in a premature newborn with hyperinsulinaemic hypoglycaemia. Eur J Endocrinol 138:698, 1998.
26. Clarren SK, et al: The fetal alcohol syndrome. N Engl J Med 298:1063, 1978.
27. Cohlan SQ: Tetracycline staining of teeth. Teratology 15:127, 1977.
28. Committee on Drugs, American Academy of Pediatrics: The

transfer of drugs and other chemicals into human milk. Pediatrics 93:137, 1994.

29. Cresteil T: Onset of xenobiotic metabolism in children: Toxicological implications. Food Addit Contam 15(suppl):45, 1998.
30. Dauber IM, et al: Renal failure following perinatal anoxia. J Pediatr 88:851, 1976.
31. DeSwiet M, et al: Excretion of anticoagulants in human milk. N Engl J Med 297:1471, 1977.
32. De Wildt SN, et al: Glucuronidation in humans: Pharmacogenetic and developmental aspects. Clin Pharmacokinet 36:439, 1999.
33. Diamond I, et al: Transplacental transmission of busulfan (Myleran) in a mother with leukemia: Production of fetal malformation and cytomegaly. Pediatrics 25:85, 1960.
34. Dickey RP: Drugs affecting lactation. Semin Perinatol 3:279, 1979.
35. Doering PL, et al: The extent and character of drug consumption during pregnancy. JAMA 239:843, 1978.
36. Dothey CI, et al: Maturational changes of theophylline pharmacokinetics in preterm infants. Clin Pharmacol Ther 45:461, 1989.
37. Dunn HG, et al: Maternal cigarette smoking during pregnancy and the child's subsequent development. II. Neurological and intellectual maturation to the age of 6½ years. Can J Public Health 68:43, 1977.
38. Ehrnebo M, et al: Age differences in drug binding by plasma proteins: Studies on human fetuses, neonates, and adults. Eur J Clin Pharmacol 3:189, 1971.
39. Ellenhorn MJ: The FDA and the prevention of drug embryopathy. J New Drugs 4:12, 1964.
40. Erickson SH, et al: Aspirin in breast milk. J Fam Pract 8:89, 1979.
41. Erickson SH, et al: Tricyclics and breast feeding. Am J Psychiatry 136:1483, 1979.
42. Ericson A, et al: Cigarette smoking as an etiologic factor in cleft lip and palate. Am J Obstet Gynecol 135:348, 1979.
43. Eriksson M, et al: Drugs and pregnancy. Clin Obstet Gynecol 16:199, 1973.
44. Erkkola R, et al: Excretion of methylergometrine (methylergonovine) into the human breast milk. Int J Clin Pharmacol 16:579, 1978.
45. Fantel AG, et al: Teratogenic bioactivation of cyclophosphamide in utero. Life Sci 25:67, 1979.
46. Faucett DW: Surface specialization of absorbing cells. J Histochem Cytochem 13:75, 1965.
47. Fedrick J, et al: Possible teratogenic effect of cigarette smoking. Nature 231:529, 1971.
48. Finely JP, et al: Digoxin excretion in human milk. J Pediatr 94:339, 1979.
49. Forsberg JG, et al: The reproductive tract of males delivered by rats given cyproterone acetate from days 7 to 21 of pregnancy. J Endocrinol 44:461, 1969.
50. Fraser FC: The multifactorial/threshold concept: Uses and misuses. Teratology 14:267, 1976.
51. Fumita M, et al: Mercury levels in human maternal and neonatal blood, hair and milk. Bull Environ Contam Toxicol 18:205, 1977.
52. Garrett MJ: Teratogenic effects of combination chemotherapy. Ann Intern Med 80:667, 1974.
53. Gelenberg AJ: Amoxapine, a new antidepressant, appears in human milk. J Nerv Ment Dis 167:635, 1979.
54. Giacoia GP, et al: Drugs and pollutants in breast milk. Clin Perinatol 6:181, 1979.
55. Gillam EMJ, et al: Expression of cytochrome P450 3A7 in *Escherichia coli*: Effects of 5' modification and catalytic characterization of recombinant enzyme expressed in bicistronic format with NADPH-cytochrome P450 reductase. Arch Biochem Biophys 346:81, 1997.
56. Goldman AS, et al: Fetal trimethadione syndrome. Teratology 17:103, 1978.
57. Greenberg LH, et al: Congenital anomalies probably induced by cyclophosphamide. JAMA 188:423, 1964.
58. Greenberger PA, et al: Management of asthma during pregnancy. N Engl J Med 312:897, 1985.
59. Guignard JP, et al: Glomerular filtration rate in the first three weeks of life. J Pediatr 87:268, 1975.
60. Guignard JP, et al: Renal function in respiratory distress syndrome. J Pediatr 88:845, 1976.
61. Ha HR, et al: Biotransformation of caffeine by cDNA-expressed human cytochromes P450. Eur J Clin Pharmacol 49:309, 1996.
62. Ha HR, et al: Metabolism of theophylline by cDNA-expressed human cytochromes P-450. Br J Clin Pharmacol 39:321, 1995.
63. Hakkola J, et al: Developmental expression of cytochrome P450 enzymes in human liver. Pharmacol Toxicol 82:209, 1998.
64. Hales BF: Modification of the mutagenicity and teratogenicity of cyclophosphamide in rats with inducers of the cytochromes P-450. Teratology 24:1, 1981.
65. Hales BF, et al: Developmental aspects of glutathione S transferase B (ligandin) in rat liver. Biochem J 160:231, 1976.
66. Hall B: Changing composition of human milk and early development of appetite control. Lancet 1:779, 1975.
67. Hanson JW: Fetal hydantoin syndrome. Teratology 13:185, 1976.
68. Hanson JW, et al: Risks to the offspring of women treated with hydantoin anticonvulsants, with emphasis on the fetal hydantoin syndrome. J Pediatr 89:662, 1976.
69. Hanson JW, et al: The effects of moderate alcohol consumption during pregnancy on fetal growth and morphogenesis. J Pediatr 92:457, 1978.
70. Harada M: Congenital Minamata disease: Intrauterine methylmercury poisoning. Teratology 18:285, 1978.
71. Heimann G: Enteral absorption and bioavailability in children in relation to age. Eur J Clin Pharmacol 18:43, 1980.
72. Heinonen OP, et al: Birth Defects and Drugs in Pregnancy. Littleton, Mass, Publishing Sciences Group, 1977.
73. Henderson BE, et al: Urogenital tract abnormalities in sons of women treated with diethylstilbestrol. Pediatrics 58:505, 1976.
74. Herbst AL, et al: Prenatal exposure to stilbestrol: A prospective comparison of exposed female offspring with unexposed controls. N Engl J Med 292:334, 1975.
75. Hill LM, et al: The use of quinidine sulfate throughout pregnancy. Obstet Gynecol 54:366, 1979.
76. Hunter AGW, et al: Is there a fetal gasoline syndrome? Teratology 20:75, 1979.
77. Jacobson S: Prospective multicentre study of pregnancy outcome after lithium exposure during first trimester of pregnancy. Lancet 339:530, 1992.
78. Jager-Roman E, et al: Fetal growth, major malformations, and minor anomalies in infants born to women receiving valproic acid. J Pediatr 108:997, 1986.
79. Joffe JM: Influence of drug exposure of the father on perinatal outcome. Clin Perinatol 6:21, 1979.
80. Jones KL, et al: Pattern of malformation in offspring of chronic alcoholic mothers. Lancet 1:7815, 1973.
81. Kaneko S, et al: The levels of anticonvulsants in breast milk. Br J Clin Pharmacol 7:624, 1979.
82. Karim A: Spironolactone: Disposition, metabolism, pharmacodynamics, and bioavailability. Drug Metab Rev 8:151, 1978.
83. Karpow S, et al: Cimetidine. JAMA 239:402, 1978.
84. Kaufman RE: Drug and therapeutics in infant and child. In Yaffe SJ, et al (eds): Pediatric Pharmacology. Philadelphia, WB Saunders Co, 1992, p 212.
85. Kitada M, Kamataki T: Cytochrome P450 in human fetal liver: Significance and fetal specific expression. Drug Metab Rev 26:305, 1994.
86. Kline J, et al: Smoking: A risk factor for spontaneous abortion. N Engl J Med 297:793, 1977.
87. Koren G, et al: Drugs in pregnancy. N Engl J Med 338:1128, 1998.
88. Koup JR, et al: Ethosuximide pharmacokinetics in a pregnant patient and newborn. Epilepsia 19:535, 1978.
89. Lacroix D, et al: Expression of CYP3A in the human liver: Evidence that the shift between CYP3A7 and CYP3A4 occurs immediately after birth. Eur J Biochem 247:625, 1997.
90. Lambert GH, et al: Genetically mediated induction of drug-metabolizing enzymes associated with congenital defects in the mouse. Teratology 16:147, 1977.
91. Lammer EJ, et al: Retinoic acid embryopathy. N Engl J Med 313:837, 1985.
92. Landauer W: Is insulin a teratogen? Teratology 5:129, 1972.

93. Landauer W: Antiteratogens as analytical tools. In Persaud TVN (ed): Teratogenic Mechanisms: Advances in the Study of Birth Defects. Baltimore, University Park Press, 1979.

94. Landesman-Dwyer S, et al: Smoking during pregnancy. Teratology 19:119, 1979.

95. Lawrence RA: Breast-feeding: A Guide for the Medical Profession. St. Louis, Mosby, 1980.

96. Lee TC, et al: Theophylline population pharmacokinetics from routine monitoring data in very premature infants with apnoea. Br J Clin Pharmacol 41:191, 1996.

97. Lee TC, et al: Population pharmacokinetic modeling in very premature infants receiving midazolam during mechanical ventilation: Midazolam neonatal pharmacokinetics. Anesthesiology 90:451, 1999.

98. Lee TC, et al: Population pharmacokinetics of intravenous caffeine in neonates with apnea of prematurity. Clin Pharmacol Ther 61:628, 1997.

99. Leeder SJ, et al: Pharmacogenetics in pediatrics: Implications for practice. Pediatr Clin North Am 44:55, 1997.

100. Lenz W: Kindliche Missbildungen nach Medikamenteinnahme wahrend der graviditat? Dtsch Med Wochenschr 86:2555, 1961.

101. Levy EP, et al: Hormone treatment during pregnancy and congenital heart defects. Lancet 1:611, 1973.

102. Levy M, et al: Excretion of drugs in human milk. N Engl J Med 297:789, 1977.

103. Loughnan PM: Digoxin excreted in human breast milk. J Pediatr 22:1010, 1979.

104. Lugo RA, et al: Pharmacokinetics of dexamethasone in premature neonates. Eur J Clin Pharmacol 49:477, 1996.

105. Manning FA, et al: Cigarette smoking and fetal breathing movements. Br J Obstet Gynaecol 83:262, 1976.

106. Manson JM, et al: In vitro metabolism of cyclophosphamide in limb bud culture. Teratology 19:149, 1979.

107. Martz F, et al: Phenytoin teratogenesis: Correlation between embryopathic effect and covalent binding of putative arene oxide metabolite in gestational tissue. J Pharmacol Exp Ther 203:231, 1977.

108. McBride WG: Thalidomide and congenital abnormalities. Lancet 2:1358, 1961.

109. McBride WG: The teratogenic action of drugs. Med J Aust 2:689, 1963.

110. McCracken GH Jr, et al: Antimicrobial Therapy for Newborns, 2nd ed. New York, Grune & Stratton, 1983.

111. Meberg A, et al: Smoking during pregnancy: Effects on the fetus and on thiocyanate levels in mother and baby. Acta Paediatr Scand 68:547, 1979.

112. Metzler M, et al: Oxidative metabolites of diethylstilbestrol in the fetal, neonatal, and adult mouse. Biochem Pharmacol 27:1087, 1978.

113. Milkovich L, et al: An evaluation of the teratogenicity of certain antinauseant drugs. Am J Obstet Gynecol 125:244, 1976.

114. Milunsky A, et al: Methotrexate-induced congenital malformations. J Pediatr 72:790, 1968; 10:192A, 1976.

115. Mirochnick M, et al: Zidovudine pharmacokinetics in premature infants exposed to human immunodeficiency virus. Antimicrob Agents Chemother 42:808, 1998.

116. Mischler TW, et al: Cephradine and epicillin in body fluids of lactating and pregnant women. J Reprod Med 21:130, 1978.

117. Monnet P, et al: Doit on craindre une influence teratogene eventuelle de l'isoniazide? Rev Tuberc (Paris) 31:845 1967.

118. Morselli PL, et al: Placental transfer of pethidine and norpethidine and their pharmacokinetics in the newborn. Eur J Clin Pharmacol 18:25, 1980.

119. Mrozikiewicz PM, et al: Determination and allelic allocation of seven nucleotide transitions within the arylamine N-acetyltransferase gene in the Polish population. Clin Pharmacol Ther 59:376, 1996.

120. Mulley BA, et al: Placental transfer of chlorthalidone and its elimination in maternal milk. Eur J Clin Pharmacol 13:329, 1978.

121. Mulvihill JJ: Caffeine as teratogen and mutagen. Teratology 8:69, 1973.

122. Musoke P, et al: A phase I/II study of the safety and pharmacokinetics of nevirapine in HIV-1-infected pregnant Ugandan women and their neonates (HIVNET 006). AIDS 13:479, 1999.

123. Naeye RL: Relationship of cigarette smoking to congenital anomalies and perinatal death. Am J Pathol 90:289, 1978.

124. Nakamura H, et al: Changes in the urinary 6β-hydroxycortisol/cortisol ratio after birth in human neonates. Eur J Clin Pharmacol 53:343, 1998.

125. Neims AH, et al: Developmental aspects of the hepatic cytochrome P450 monooxygenase system. Annu Rev Pharmacol Toxicol 16:427, 1976.

126. Nelson MM, et al: Associations between drugs administered during pregnancy and congenital abnormalities of the fetus. BMJ 1:523, 1971.

127. Newcombe RG: Cigarette smoking in pregnancy [letter]. BMJ 2:755, 1976.

128. Nicholson HO: Cytotoxic drugs in pregnancy. J Obstet Gynecol Br Comm 75:307, 1968.

129. Nicol CJ, et al: An embryoprotective role for glucose-6-phosphate dehydrogenase in developmental oxidative stress and chemical teratogenesis. FASEB J 14:111, 2000.

130. Niebyl JR, et al: Carbamazepine levels in pregnancy and lactation. Obstet Gynecol 53:139, 1979.

131. Nishimura H, et al: Congenital malformations in offspring of mice treated with caffeine. Proc Soc Exp Biol Med 104:140, 1960.

132. Nora JJ, et al: Birth defects and oral contraceptives. Lancet 1:941, 1973.

133. Nora JJ, et al: Lithium, Ebstein's anomaly, and other congenital heart defects. Lancet 2:594, 1974.

134. Nulman I, et al: Neurodevelopment of adopted children exposed in utero to cocaine. Can Med Assoc J 151:159, 1994.

135. Oakes GK, et al: Effect of propranolol infusion in the umbilical and uterine circulations of pregnant sheep. Am J Obstet Gynecol 126:1038, 1976.

136. Odell GB: The dissociation of bilirubin from albumin and its clinical implications. J Pediatr 55:268, 1959.

137. Ohmori S, et al: Differential catalytic properties in metabolism of endogenous and exogenous substrates among CYP3A enzymes expressed in COS-7 cells. Biochim Biophys Acta 1380:297, 1998.

138. Olshan AF, et al: Male-Mediated Developmental Toxicity. New York, Plenum Press, 1995.

139. Orme ML, et al: May mothers given warfarin breast-feed their infants? BMJ 1:1564, 1977.

140. Ortiz-Perez HE, et al: Abnormalities among offspring of oral and non-oral contraceptive users. Am J Obstet Gynecol 134:512, 1979.

141. Pagliaro LA, et al (eds): Problems in Pediatric Drug Therapy. Hamilton, Ill, Drug Intelligence Publications, 1995.

142. Pariente-Khayat A, et al: Caffeine acetylator phenotyping during maturation in infants. Pediatr Res 29:492, 1991.

143. Pariente-Khayat A, et al: Isoniazid acetylation metabolic ratio during maturation in children. Clin Pharmacol Ther 62:377, 1997.

144. Parman T, et al: Free radical–mediated oxidative DNA damage in the mechanism of thalidomide teratogenicity. Nature Med 5:582, 1999.

145. Paterson DC: Congenital deformities associated with Bendectin. Can Med Assoc J 116:1348, 1977.

146. Phelan JP: Diminished fetal reactivity with smoking. Am J Obstet Gynecol 136:230, 1980.

147. Phelps DL, et al: Spironolactone: Relationship between concentrations of dithioacetylated metabolite in human serum and milk. J Pharm Sci 66:1203, 1977.

148. Piercy WN, et al: Alteration of ovine fetal respiratory-like activity by diazepam, caffeine and doxapram. Am J Obstet Gynecol 127:43, 1977.

149. Pilotti G, et al: Hypervitaminosis A during pregnancy and neonatal malformations of the urinary apparatus. Minerva Ginecol 17:1103, 1965.

150. Pinsky WW, et al: Serum digoxin levels in premature infants [abstract]. Pediatr Res 10:196A, 1976.

151. Poland A, et al: 2,3,7,8-Tetrachlordibenzo-p-dioxin: Segregation of toxicity with the Ah locus. Mol Pharmacol 17:86, 1980.

152. Posner HS, et al: Experimental alteration of the metabolism of chlorcyclizine and the incidence of cleft palate in rats. J Pharmacol Exp Ther 155:494, 1967.

153. Pruyn SC, et al: Long-term propranolol therapy in pregnancy: Maternal and fetal outcome. Am J Obstet Gynecol 135:485, 1979.

154. Pynnonen S, et al: Carbamazepine: Placental transport, tissue concentrations in fetus and newborn, and level in milk. Acta Pharmacol Toxicol 41:244, 1977.

155. Raman-Wilms L, et al: Fetal genital effects of first-trimester sex hormone exposure: A meta analysis. Obstet Gynecol 85:141, 1995.

156. Rane A, et al: Plasma protein binding of diphenylhydantoin in normal and hyperbilirubinemic infants. J Pediatr 78:877, 1971.

157. Rane A, et al: Plasma disappearance of transplacentally transferred diphenylhydantoin in the newborn studied by mass fragmentography. Clin Pharmacol Ther 15:39, 1974.

158. Reider MJ: How much fire under the smoke? The effects of exposure to cocaine on the fetus. Can Med Assoc J 151:1567, 1994.

159. Renwick AG: Toxicokinetics in infants and children in relation to the ADI and TDI. Food Addit Contam 15(suppl):17, 1998.

160. Renwick JH: Spina bifida, anencephaly, and potato blight. Lancet 2:967, 1972.

161. Resman BH, et al: Breast milk distribution of theobromine from chocolate. J Pediatr 91:477, 1977.

162. Rich KJ, Boobis AR: Expression and inducibility of P450 enzymes during liver ontogeny. Microsc Res Tech 39:424, 1997.

163. Richards IDG: A retrospective inquiry into possible teratogenic effects of drugs in pregnancy. In Klingberg MA, et al (eds): Drugs and Fetal Development. New York, Plenum Press, 1972.

164. Robaire B, Hales BF: Paternal exposure to chemicals before conception: Some children may be at risk. BMJ 307:341, 1993.

165. Rodriquez SO, et al: Neonatal thrombocytopenia associated with ante-partum administration of thiazide drugs. N Engl J Med 270:881, 1964.

166. Rosa FW: Spina bifida in infants of women treated with carbamazepine during pregnancy. N Engl J Med 324:674, 1991.

167. Rosenberg L, et al: Lack of relation of oral clefts to diazepam use during pregnancy. N Engl J Med 309:1282, 1983.

168. Rothman KJ, et al: Oral contraceptives and birth defects. N Engl J Med 299:522, 1978.

169. Rothstein P, et al: Born with a habit: Infants of drug-addicted mothers. Pediatr Clin North Am 21:307, 1974.

170. Samojlik E: Effect of monoamine oxidase inhibition on fertility, fetuses, and reproductive organs of rats. I. Effect of monoamine oxidase inhibition on fertility, fetuses and sexual cycle. Endokrynol Pol 16:69, 1965.

171. Schanker LS, et al: Absorption of drug from the rat small intestine. J Pharmacol Exp Ther 123:81, 1958.

172. Schardein JL: Chemically Induced Birth Defects, 2nd ed. New York and Basel, Marcel Dekker, 1993.

173. Schedl HD, et al: Small intestinal absorption of steroids. Gastroenterology 41:491, 1961.

174. Scheinhorn DJ, et al: Antituberculous therapy during pregnancy. West J Med 127:195, 1977.

175. Scott CS, et al: Morphine pharmacokinetics and pain assessment in premature newborns. J Pediatr 135:423, 1999.

176. Selevan SG, et al: A study of occupational exposure to antineoplastic drugs and fetal loss in nurses. N Engl J Med 313:1173, 1985.

177. Sereni F, et al: Developmental pharmacology. Annu Rev Pharmacol Toxicol 8:453, 1968.

178. Sertel H, Scopes J: Rates of creatinine clearance in babies less than one week of age. Arch Dis Child 48:717, 1973.

179. Shapiro S, et al: Perinatal mortality and birth weight in relation to aspirin taken during pregnancy. Lancet 1:375, 1976.

180. Shepard TH: Catalog of Teratogenic Agents. Baltimore and London, Johns Hopkins University Press, 1992.

181. Shimada T, et al: Interindividual variations in human liver cytochrome P450 enzymes involved in the oxidation of drugs, carcinogens and toxic chemicals. J Pharmacol Exp Ther 270:414, 1994.

182. Shotton D, et al: Possible teratogenic effect of chlorambucil on a human fetus. JAMA 186:74, 1963.

183. Sieber SM, et al: Toxicity of antineoplastic agents in man: Chromosomal aberrations, antifertility effects, congenital malformations, and carcinogenic potential. Adv Cancer Res 22:57, 1975.

184. Singh B, et al: Treatment of neonatal seizures with carbamazepine. J Child Neurol 11: 378, 1996.

185. Smith DJ, et al: Increased neonatal mortality in offspring of male rats treated with methadone or morphine before mating. Nature 253:202, 1975.

186. Smith DW: Teratogenicity of anticonvulsive mediations. Am J Dis Child 131:1337, 1977.

187. Smithells RW, et al: Teratogenicity testing in humans: A method demonstrating safety of Bendectin. Teratology 17:31, 1978.

188. Somogyi A, et al: Cimetidine excretion into breast milk. Br J Clin Pharmacol 7:627, 1979.

189. Sonnier M, et al: Delayed ontogenesis of CYP1A2 in the human liver. Eur J Biochem 251:893, 1998.

190. Sovner R, et al: Excretion of imipramine and desipramine in human breast milk. Am J Psychiatry 136:451, 1979.

191. Soyka LF, et al: Lethal and sublethal effects on the progeny of male rats treated with methadone. Toxicol Appl Pharmacol 45:797, 1978.

192. Spiers PS, et al: Human potato consumption and neural-tube malformation. Teratology 10:125, 1974.

193. Strickler SM, et al: Genetic predisposition to phenytoin-induced birth defects. Lancet 2:746, 1985.

194. Syverson GB, et al: Drug disposition within human milk phases. J Pharm Sci 74:1085, 1985.

195. Tateishi T, et al: No ethnic difference between Caucasian and Japanese hepatic samples in the expression frequency of CYP3A5 and CYP3A7 proteins. Biochem Pharmacol 57:935, 1999.

196. Terrila L, et al: The effects and side-effects of diuretics in the prophylaxis for toxaemia of pregnancy. Acta Obstet Gynecol Scand 50:351, 1971.

197. Tjia JF, et al: Theophylline metabolism in human liver microsomes: Inhibition studies. J Pharmacol Exp Ther 276:912, 1996.

198. Trasler J, et al: Paternal cyclophosphamide treatment of rats causes fetal loss and malformations without affecting male fertility. Nature 316:144, 1985.

199. Treluyer M, et al: Expression of CYP2D6 in developing human liver. Eur J Biochem 202:583, 1991.

200. Treluyer M, et al: Cytochrome P-450 expression in sudden infant death syndrome. Biochem Pharmacol 52:497, 1996.

201. Turner G, et al: Fetal effects of regular salicylate ingestion in pregnancy. Lancet 2:338, 1975.

202. van Lingen RA, et al: Pharmacokinetics and metabolism of rectally administered paracetamol in preterm neonates. Arch Dis Child Fetal Neonatal Ed 80:F59, 1999.

203. Viera I, et al: Developmental expression of CYP2E1 in the human liver: Hypermethylation control of gene expression during the neonatal period. Eur J Biochem 238:476, 1996.

204. Vuori E, et al: The occurrence and origin of DDT in human milk. Acta Paediatr Scand 66:761, 1977.

205. Warkany J: Warfarin embryopathy. Teratology 14:205, 1976.

206. Warkany J: Antituberculosis drugs. Teratology 20:133, 1979.

207. Watkins PB, et al: Identification of glucocorticoid-inducible cytochromes P-450 in the intestinal mucosa of rats and man. J Clin Invest 80:1029, 1987.

208. Welbrandt W, et al: The concept of carrier transport and its corollaries in pharmacology. Pharmacol Rev 13:109, 1961.

209. Wettrel G, Andersson KE: Clinical pharmacokinetics of digoxin in infants. Clin Pharmacokinet 2:17, 1977.

210. Wilkins L: Masculinization of female fetus due to use of orally given progestins. JAMA 172:1028, 1960.

211. Wilson JG: Teratogenic effects of environmental chemicals. Fed Proc 36:1698, 1977.

212. Yoshioka H, et al: Transfer of cefazolin into human milk. J Pediatr 94:151, 1979.

11

Fetal Therapy

part one

PHARMACOLOGIC TREATMENT OF THE FETUS

Michael D. Reed and Jeffrey L. Blumer

Advances in medical science and diagnostic technology have provided us with new and exciting information about the dynamic nature of life in utero (Box 11–1). We have gained insight and understanding into the structure and function of the placenta. At the same time, advances in neonatal care have led to increased survival rates of infants of low and very low birth weight. Nevertheless, the innovations in diagnostic technology are what have added most to our understanding of human development and simultaneously have created some of our greatest clinical, ethical, and moral challenges.

Our ability to assess fetal vitality and genetic, biochemical, and physical "normality" has been greatly enhanced through the development of amniocentesis, fetoscopy, chorionic villus sampling, fetal blood sampling (cordocentesis), and real-time ultrasonography. Of these techniques, ultrasonography is perhaps the most seductive (see Chapter 8).[74] Because it is noninvasive, is safe, can be used serially, and is relatively less expensive than some of the other procedures, it has evolved almost to the point of attaining the status of a screening procedure (Box 11–2). Of course, the problem with the widespread use of ultrasonography

---

BOX 11–1

CHANGES IN MEDICAL SCIENCE AND TECHNOLOGY LEADING TO FETAL THERAPEUTICS

- Recognition of the structure and function of the placenta
- Advances in neonatal care leading to increased survival rates of infants of low and very low birth weight
- Amniocentesis
- Fetoscopy
- Real-time fetal ultrasonography
- Chorionic villus sampling
- Fetal blood sampling
- Fetal surgery

BOX 11–2

INDICATIONS FOR ANTENATAL ULTRASONOGRAPHY

- Determination of fetal viability when abortion or intrauterine fetal death is suspected
- Dating pregnancy when there is a consistent discrepancy between clinical and historical data
- Placenta localization in patients with vaginal bleeding, or when the fetus is in an unstable position
- Evaluation of pregnancy when there is a consistent, clinically significant discrepancy between uterine size and dates at any time
- Immediately before any amniocentesis
- Evaluation of fetal growth
- Determination of fetal number
- Suspected fetal congenital malformations
- Evaluation of fetal size in breech presentation
- Evaluation of amniotic fluid quantity
- Postdates pregnancy evaluation
- Suspected hydatidiform mole and possible associated pelvic masses
- As adjunct to special procedures, such as fetoscopy and intrauterine transfusion
- Pelvic mass evaluation
- Assessment of fetal well-being by observation of fetal activity (e.g., the biophysical profile)

167

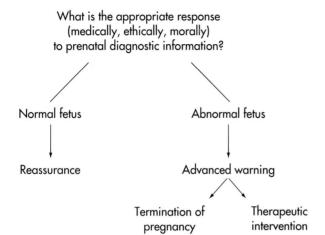

FIGURE 11–1. Dilemma confronted by parents and clinicians when presented with results of routine diagnostic evaluations of a fetus.

is that we find things. Most of the observations made are serendipitous; however, they may reflect grave or dire consequences for the outcome of the pregnancy.

Many clinicians believe that the use of ultrasound is both good and appropriate (Fig. 11–1). If the test reveals a normal fetus, both the parents and the physician are reassured. On the other hand, if it reveals fetal abnormalities, especially those that may be identified during the first trimester of pregnancy, decisions can be made regarding further (perhaps more invasive) evaluation, special medical needs required during delivery, special care needs required after birth, or, in extreme cases, whether to continue the pregnancy. However, these diagnostic advances have always been coupled with the idea that, as in other areas of medicine, the ability to make a diagnosis should be followed by the development of appropriate therapeutic interventions. This belief has led to an ever-expanding set of treatment options for recognized fetal disorders (Box 11–3).

From an intriguing concept several decades ago, fetal therapy has become a reality. There are now basically three approaches to treating fetal disease. The most common approach has been the use of drug therapy directed toward the recognized fetal disorder. In addition, several centers have begun to perform surgical procedures on fetuses with recognized malformations (see Part Two of this chapter). The third and most exciting of these approaches is the contemplation of fetal gene therapy to correct genetic defects ascertainable in utero.

This section of the chapter focuses primarily on the use of drug therapy to ameliorate or cure fetal disorders. It initially deals with the pharmacology of the maternal-fetal-placental unit. Then some of the more common fetal therapeutic interventions are discussed in more detail.

PHARMACOLOGY OF THE MATERNAL-FETAL-PLACENTAL UNIT

(See also Chapter 10.)

Three aspects of pharmacotherapy must be considered when one is treating patients (Fig. 11–2). In general, *pharmacokinetics* includes the processes of drug

---

■ **BOX 11–3**

APPROACH TO MANAGEMENT OF FETAL DISORDERS

- Selective abortion
  Anencephaly, hydranencephaly, and alobar holoprosencephaly
  Severe anomalies associated with chromosomal abnormalities (e.g., trisomy 13)
  Bilateral renal agenesis and infantile polycystic kidney disease
  Severe, untreatable, inherited metabolic disorders (e.g., Tay-Sachs disease)
  Lethal bone dysplasias (e.g., thanotophoric dysplasia, recessive osteogenesis imperfecta)
- Diagnosis in utero; treatment after delivery at term
  Esophageal, duodenal, jejunoileal, and anorectal atresias
  Meconium ileus (cystic fibrosis)
  Enteric cysts and duplications
  Small, intact omphalocele
  Small, intact meningocele, myelomeningocele, and spina bifida
  Unilateral, multicystic dysplastic kidney and hydronephrosis
  Craniofacial, extremity, and chest wall deformities
  Cystic hygroma, mesoblastic nephroma
  Small sacrococcygeal teratoma
  Benign cysts (e.g., ovarian, mesenteric, choledochal)
- May require premature delivery
- May require operative delivery
  Conjoined twins
  Giant omphalocele, ruptured omphalocele/gastroschisis
  Large sacrococcygeal teratoma or cystic hygroma
  Malformations requiring preterm delivery in the presence of inadequate labor or fetal distress
- May require treatment in utero

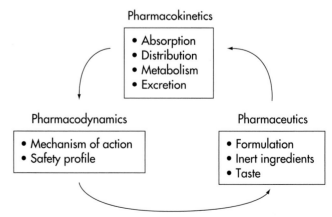

FIGURE 11–2. Determinants of effective drug therapy. Clinicians must account for all pharmacokinetic and pharmacodynamic characteristics of a drug when designing an optimal dose regimen.

absorption, distribution, metabolism, and excretion, whereas *pharmacodynamics* refers to the mechanisms of drug action and drug safety. The *pharmaceutic* aspects of drug therapy pertain to the actual formulation of the drug (e.g., tablet, liquid, suspension, capsule), including its inert ingredients. In therapeutics, if, for a given disorder and a given patient, a drug can be identified that has favorable characteristics in each of these three areas, therapy will be effective.

Identification of such a drug is usually a fairly complex problem that takes into account not only all the individual differences in physiology and biochemistry that determine individual differences in drug disposition but also any impact that the pathophysiologic state imposes on these processes. Moreover, differences in disease severity and expression must also be considered, along with any changes in the disease process during therapy. This complex set of issues must be considered each time a patient is treated.

In fetal therapy the situation is even more complex. In most instances the drug is administered to one individual, the mother, with the intent of its having a therapeutic effect in another, the fetus. Moreover, instead of dealing with the pharmacokinetic and pharmacodynamic processes in a single individual, one must consider three pharmacokinetically and pharmacodynamically distinct but intimately interconnected compartments—the mother, the fetus, and the placenta (Fig. 11–3).

MATERNAL DRUG DISPOSITION DURING PREGNANCY

Pregnancy is a period of change in female physiology.[91] A number of important changes directly influence drug disposition in both the maternal and the fetal environments (Table 11–1).

Drug Absorption

Among the changes seen during pregnancy that will potentially affect drug disposition, the decrease in intestinal motility is prominent. This decrease, in turn, may decrease the rate of absorption of orally administered medications. As a result, the observed peak maternal serum drug concentration will be blunted or delayed, or both. For the majority of clinical situations, these effects are of little clinical consequence in the treatment of maternal disorders and would appear to be of no clinical significance relative to fetal distribution. Alterations in the absolute peak serum drug concentration and time to peak will not influence the resultant fetal drug exposure, because it is the steady-state maternal drug concentration that appears to be the most important determinant of the extent of drug diffusion from the maternal to the fetal compartment, not the absolute peak serum drug concentration. For the relatively few drugs that are metabolized within the gastrointestinal tract (e.g., cyclosporine), this increased time within the gastrointestinal tract may lead to decreased maternal bioavailability.

Aerosolized (inhaled) medications may achieve greater absorption into the maternal systemic circulation after pulmonary exposure because of pregnancy-associated increases in minute ventilation. Similarly, maternal exposure to environmental toxins and pol-

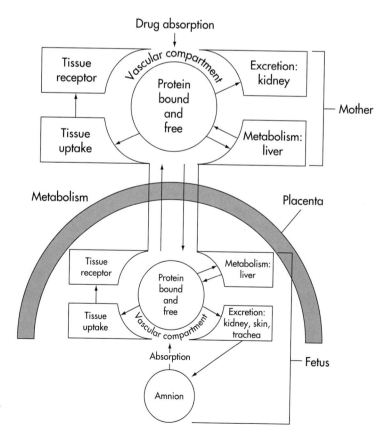

FIGURE 11–3. Drug disposition in the maternal-placental-fetal unit.

TABLE 11–1 INFLUENCE OF PREGNANCY ON PHYSIOLOGIC ASPECTS OF DRUG DISPOSITION

PHARMACOKINETIC PARAMETER BY SYSTEM	CHANGE
Absorption	
Gastric emptying	Increased
Intestinal motility	Decreased
Pulmonary function	Increased
Cardiac output	Increased
Blood flow to the skin	Increased
Distribution	
Plasma volume	Increased
Total body water	Increased
Plasma proteins	Decreased
Body fat	Increased
Metabolism	
Hepatic metabolism	±
Extrahepatic metabolism	±
Excretion	
Uterine blood flow	Increased
Renal blood flow	Increased
Glomerular filtration rate	Increased
Pulmonary function	Increased

Modified from Mattison DR, et al: Physiologic adaptations to pregnancy: Impact on pharmacokinetics. In Yaffe SJ, et al (eds): Pediatric Pharmacology: Therapeutic Principles in Practice. Philadelphia, WB Saunders, 1992, p 81.

lutants also increases during pregnancy. On average, maternal tidal volume increases approximately 39% with an accompanying average increase in minute ventilation of approximately 42% during pregnancy.[51] The primary determinant of drug exposure after aerosolized drug administration is minute ventilation, not the absolute dose of the medication per exposure. This fact is of greatest significance for medications that are characterized by excellent bioavailability after inhalation (e.g., adrenergic receptor agonists [epinephrine, albuterol], dexamethasone). It is unknown whether this enhanced pulmonary exposure during pregnancy poses any real threat to the mother or the fetus. Some investigators have attempted to extrapolate differences in exposure rates between men and women for certain environmental diseases (e.g., silicosis) based on enhanced exposure during pregnancy.[51] However, because this aspect of possibly enhanced drug exposure has not been specifically studied, its impact on fetal drug exposure remains unknown. Nevertheless, it seems prudent to monitor closely the therapeutic response and systemic effects of aerosolized medications, as well as the amount and types of environmental exposures encountered by pregnant patients.

With respect to percutaneous drug exposure or administration, the differences that occur in peripheral regional blood flow during pregnancy are of particular interest.[51, 52] During pregnancy, blood flow increases about sixfold in the human hand and about twofold in the human foot, with only small increases

observed in the human forearm and leg. These increases in perfusion take on added importance with the increasing number of medications administered topically as either patch formulations or ointments and creams. Although the primary determinant of dermal drug absorption is lipid solubility (stratum corneum and stratum lucidum) and water solubility (stratum granulosum, stratum spinosum, stratum basale, and the basement membrane), exposed surface area and blood flow to the skin are also important components. Although the increases in dermal blood flow are well documented, their impact on drug absorption has not been determined. Moreover, the specific regions that have been reported to receive greater blood flow do not represent the more common sites for application of patch drug formulations (e.g., chest, back). Thus, the possibility of enhanced systemic exposure from topically administered medications during pregnancy may be of limited clinical significance, with the exception of direct application of medications to the hand or foot.

The overall effects of changes in intestinal motility, minute ventilation, and regional blood flow during pregnancy remain largely unknown. It is the steady-state concentration of drug in the maternal circulation that will ultimately determine the amount of drug available for disposition to the fetal compartment. Because steady-state concentration is more a product of drug clearance than drug absorption, these changes in maternal physiology would be predicted to have little impact on fetal drug exposure. Nevertheless, data are lacking.

Drug Distribution

During pregnancy, several physiologic changes occur that may influence drug distribution (Tables 11–1 to 11–3). Maternal total body water, extracellular fluid, and plasma volumes all increase during gestation by about 32%, 36%, and 52%, respectively. These substantial changes in the sizes of various body fluid compartments occur gradually throughout pregnancy (see

TABLE 11–2 CHANGES IN MATERNAL BODY COMPOSITION THAT CAN INFLUENCE MATERNAL DRUG DISTRIBUTION CHARACTERISTICS

TIME OF GESTATION (wks)	BODY WEIGHT (kg)	BODY FAT	PLASMA VOLUME (L)	EXTRACELLULAR FLUID VOLUME (L)
0	50.0	16.5	2.50	11
10	50.6	16.8	2.75	12
20	54.0	18.6	3.00	13
30	58.5	20.0	3.60	14
40	62.5	19.8	3.75	15

Modified from Mattison DR, et al: Physiologic adaptations to pregnancy: Impact on pharmacokinetics. In Yaffe SJ, et al (eds): Pediatric Pharmacology: Therapeutic Principles in Practice. Philadelphia, WB Saunders, 1992, p 81.

TABLE 11–3   *HUMAN MATERNAL AND FETAL SERUM PROTEIN CONCENTRATIONS DURING PREGNANCY*

TIME OF GESTATION (wks)	SERUM ALBUMIN CONCENTRATION (mg/dL)		SERUM α_1-ACID GLYCOPROTEIN CONCENTRATION (mg/dL)	
	Maternal	**Fetal**	**Maternal**	**Fetal**
12–15	2.8	1.1	57	5
16–25	3.4	1.9	73	8
26–35	2.8	2.6	58	16
35–41	2.9	3.4	60	21

Modified from Hill MD, et al: The significance of plasma protein binding on the fetal/maternal distribution of drugs at steady-state. Clin Pharmacokinet 14:156, 1988.

Table 11–2). The increase in body water is the primary reason for the observed decreases in peak drug concentrations with standard dosing. When the drug dose is kept constant in the presence of increasing body water, the drug's apparent volume of distribution increases and steady-state drug concentrations decrease. Such a decrease in steady-state concentration will markedly influence the amount of drug available for diffusion across the placenta.

Maternal cardiac output also increases by about 40% to 50% by the middle of the second trimester, remaining elevated until delivery.[51] This increase in cardiac output is the result of increases in both heart rate (10 to 15 beats per minute) and stroke volume. More drug, therefore, will be presented for hepatic metabolism and renal elimination per unit time. The increase may also result in a decrease in the duration of time that drug resides in the villous space (see later) and is available for transfer to the fetal compartment. Furthermore, the volume of blood within the placenta increases with gestation, increasing from ~60 mL at 10 weeks to 950 mL at term.[91]

Coincident with the changes in body water distribution and cardiac output, the amount of maternal fat increases in a relatively constant proportion to the increase in body weight (see Table 11–1). In addition, concentrations of circulating serum proteins fluctuate during gestation (see Table 11–3), resulting in changes in the free fraction of various highly protein-bound drugs.[37] Unfortunately, the overall impact of changes in body composition and resulting changes in drug distribution on fetal drug exposure is largely unknown. Resulting interactions are complex, making predictions regarding their impact on fetal drug exposure speculative at best.

Drug Metabolism and Excretion

Few data exist to suggest any true change in the maternal rate of hepatic drug metabolism. In contrast, the renal plasma flow increases by about 30% and the glomerular filtration rate by about 50%. As a result, serum creatinine, urea, and uric acid concentrations are lower during pregnancy. These changes in renal function may also be expected to enhance the elimination of drugs primarily dependent on the kidneys for elimination from the body.

THE PLACENTA

(See also Chapter 23.)

After fertilization, the rapidly dividing conceptus travels down the fallopian tube toward the uterus. By day 3 the mulberry-appearing conceptus divides into approximately 16 cells and enters the uterus. This stage of embryo development, called the *morula*, consists of an inner cell mass and a surrounding layer, the outer cell mass. The inner cell mass gives rise to the *embryo*, whereas the outer cell mass forms the *trophoblast*, which helps to form the placenta. Once in the uterus, maternal fluids penetrate the zona pellucida and accumulate within the inner cell mass between the cells. This is the conceptus' first exposure to maternal fluids. Gradually, a cavity (the *blastocele*) forms, displacing the inner cell mass to one pole of the embryo. These changes signal the blastocyst stage of embryo development. The zona pellucida disappears, allowing implantation to take place. Around the sixth day after fertilization, the trophoblastic cells lining the inner cell mass begin to penetrate the uterine mucosa, attaching the conceptus to the myometrial epithelium. Proteolytic enzymes from the uterine mucosa and the trophoblast probably work in concert to allow implantation of the zygote. Thus, by the end of the first week after fertilization, the human zygote has passed through the morula and blastocyst stages of development and has begun implantation in the uterine mucosa. Up to this point, no interface for maternal-fetal exchange has been established.[19, 78]

By the second week of development, lacunae formed within the trophoblastic cell mass have fused to form interconnected lacunar networks. These lacunae function as early intervillous spaces of the placenta. Maternal blood seeps into and flows slowly throughout the lacunar system, establishing the uteroplacental circulation. Sometime around the end of the second week, primary chorionic villi form and begin to differentiate into the chorionic villi of the placenta. Early in the third week, mesenchyme grows into the primary chorionic villi, forming a placard of loose connective tissue. Mesenchymal cells in the villi differentiate into capillaries and form arteriovenous networks. Blood vessels from within these maturing villi become connected with the embryonic heart, later establishing the umbilical cord. By the end of the third week, blood of embryonic origin begins to circulate through the capillaries of the chorionic villi, and by the end of the fourth week the essential elements necessary for physiologic exchange between the mother and the embryo are well established.[19, 78]

From the fourth week of gestation until term, the surface area of the placenta increases dramatically to accommodate the increasing needs of the maturing fetus. In contrast, the thickness of the placental membrane decreases with advancing gestation. During late gestation, at about 32 weeks, fetal capillaries become oriented beneath the thin layers of syncytial trophoblast. In these areas the tissue barrier separating the maternal and fetal circulations may be less than 2 μm. This characteristic of the placenta, decreasing membrane thickness with advancing gestation, favors greater transfer of drugs during late gestation (from approximately 50 to 100 μm to 2 to 5 μm at term). These areas become specialized in the transport functions of the placenta (i.e., rapid diffusion of substances) rather than in the metabolic functions of the placenta. By term, the placenta has only a single cell layer of fetal chorionic tissue separating the fetal capillary endothelium and the maternal blood. This separation, with its loose intercellular connections, presents little hindrance to small molecule transfer.[19, 78]

Important Differences between Human and Animal Placentas

As described earlier, the human placenta is a network of specialized cells and tissues whose functional capacity evolves during gestation.[19, 78] These dynamic processes, which most likely vary with the time during gestation, influence the ability of drugs and other compounds to cross from the maternal compartment to the fetal compartment. Unfortunately, the many medical, ethical, and social barriers that limit our ability to study human placental development necessitate our reliance on studies of placental mechanics performed in various animal species to model the human system.

Although much has been learned about placental maturation and function from such studies, these data must be extrapolated to the human placenta with extreme caution. It is of utmost importance to recognize that the cellular arrangement of the human placenta differs markedly from that of many other mammals. The differences in placental structure between human beings and other mammals influence the rate at which a compound crosses in either direction and the extent to which it does so. Thus, the placental transfer for a particular drug or substrate defined in the rat or sheep may bear very little relationship to human placental function and substrate disposition.[19, 40, 78]

Studies that have compared the placental transport function and capacity for specific substrates between various animal species and human beings have revealed substantial differences.[9, 59, 78, 84] For this reason, one should rely solely on data derived in human systems to develop possible fetal treatment strategies. Some of these differences are most likely due to the anatomic differences between the placentas of various species. Some of the more important differences in placental structure in species commonly studied as potential models for human development are now discussed briefly. The reader who is interested in the embryology and structure of the placenta of various animal species in greater depth is referred to more detailed discussions of this topic.[19, 40, 78]

The placenta in most mammals is classified as *chorioallantoic*. It includes a chorion vascularized by blood vessels derived from the allantois. Once vascularized, the chorion gives rise to the placenta. In human beings, other primates, pigs, and ruminants, a chorioallantoic placenta persists throughout gestation. In contrast, many rodents and lagomorphs have two types of placentas that persist throughout gestation: the chorioallantoic placenta and the inverted yolk sac placenta. In these placentas, active transport mechanisms develop rapidly. In the human placenta, the transfer of most compounds, including drugs, appears to involve simple diffusion.[78] Thus, the drug transfer mechanics described in some animal placentas may bear no real relationship to drug transfer dynamics in human placentas.

The human placenta consists of three layers of fetal tissue: the trophoblastic epithelium covering the villi, the chorionic connective tissue, and the capillary endothelium. The surface area of the villi, which represent the real area for exchange, varies according to the time of gestation. At 28 weeks of gestation, the villous surface area is about 3.4 m², compared with about 12.6 m² at term.[59] Furthermore, the thickness of the placental membrane decreases with gestation, being thinnest, about 2 cm thick, in late gestation. These changes in placental surface area and thickness during gestation enhance the ability of most drugs to diffuse across the placenta.

Drug Transfer across the Placenta

(See also Chapter 10.)

Despite numerous studies and exhaustive reviews* that focus on the processes and extent of drug transfer across the placenta, very little specific information defines the mechanisms of drug transfer across the human placenta. This circumstance is a direct result of the difficulties inherent in studying the target population and of our reliance on data obtained from nonhuman model systems. It is difficult to obtain not only general information relative to drug disposition at the human maternal-placental-fetal interface (i.e., to what extent an administered dose of a drug crosses the placenta) but also information concerning the specific processes involved in drug disposition by the placenta. For example, very little is known regarding the rate at which the placenta metabolizes drugs or the extent to which it does so.[35]

A number of interdependent variables influence the rate and extent of drug transfer across the placenta from the maternal to the fetal compartment. It is believed by most investigators and clinicians that any compound found in the maternal circulation will cross the placenta into the fetal compartment.[29] The fundamental questions, therefore, are at what rate and to what extent. Unfortunately, even today, this information is only partially available for just a few chemical entities. Similarly, the mechanisms by which drugs are transferred across the placenta are known

---

*References 9, 19, 29, 59, 78, 84, 91.

only for a few select compounds; however, it is assumed that the majority of drugs cross the placenta via simple passive nonionic diffusion. An understanding of these transport mechanisms is important in the design of fetal drug therapy.

The physical variables that will influence drug transfer across the placenta include the surface area of the exchange membrane, the thickness of the endotheliosyncytial membrane, the integrity of the maternal blood flow and resultant hydrostatic pressure in the intervillous chambers, the blood pressure in fetal capillaries, and any differences between maternal and fetal osmotic pressures and pH. Maternal osmotic pressure is higher than that in the fetal compartment, whereas a pH difference between 0.1 and 0.15 units exists between the fetal and maternal blood (i.e., fetal umbilical blood is −0.1 pH unit lower than maternal blood).[19, 59] Further, the decreasing thickness of the placenta as term approaches facilitates further maternal-placental exchange during the later stages of gestation.

The possible modes of drug transfer across the placenta are listed in order of importance in Box 11–4. For the majority of drugs and other compounds, it is presumed that the primary mode of transfer is by simple passive nonionic diffusion. Simple diffusion does not require energy and is described by the Fick equation:

$$\text{Rate of diffusion} = K \cdot A \, (C_m - C_f) / d$$

where "K" is the diffusion constant of the drug, which is dependent on the drug's physiochemical characteristics; "A" is the surface area of the membrane to traverse; "C_m" and "C_f" are the concentrations of drug in maternal and fetal blood, respectively; and "d" is the thickness of the membrane to be traversed. Thus, "$C_m - C_f$" represents the concentration gradient across the placenta, which is primarily regulated by the surface area, A, and the thickness, d, of the placenta. In addition to the changes in surface area and membrane thickness described previously, one additional variable increases with increasing gestation and appears to be an important factor in placental drug transfer: uterine blood flow, which is a factor not considered in the Fick equation. At term, uterine blood flow is estimated to approach 150 mL/

minute per kg newborn body weight.[54] Depending on the physicochemical characteristics of the drug in this environment, blood flow has an important influence on the rate and amount of drug transfer.

Important physicochemical characteristics that influence drug transfer across membranes, including the placenta, are outlined in Box 11–5. Characteristics that facilitate placental transfer include high lipid solubility, un-ionized form under physiologic and pathophysiologic conditions, low molecular weight (<500 daltons), and low protein binding. Very few clinically important drugs meet all these "ideal" characteristics, which explains the high degree of variability reported in various studies of placental transfer. It appears that a classification system (based on these important physicochemical characteristics) for compounds and their ability to cross the placenta could be developed and used to guide fetal drug therapy. Unfortunately, this is not possible because of the tremendous interdependence of each of these physicochemical properties in determining the actual transfer across the placenta.

Further confusion regarding the extent to which a particular drug or compound may traverse the placenta is propagated by uncontrolled studies that compare a single maternal blood concentration to a (near) simultaneous concentration obtained from cord blood. Many published experiences have attempted to quantitate drug transfer as a ratio of fetal to maternal drug concentration using these single time point determinations. Unfortunately, the usefulness of such assessments is often limited and must be interpreted with extreme caution. This ratio is highly dependent on a number of very important variables, including the number of maternal doses administered (i.e., first dose administration versus steady-state) and the time

---

BOX 11–4

MECHANISMS OF DRUG TRANSFER ACROSS THE HUMAN PLACENTA*

Simple diffusion
Facilitated transport
Active transport
Pinocytosis (phagocytosis)

*Listed in order of importance.

BOX 11–5

PHYSICOCHEMICAL FACTORS THAT INFLUENCE THE TRANSFER OF COMPOUNDS ACROSS THE HUMAN PLACENTA

- Degree of lipid solubility
  Lipid soluble favored versus water soluble
- Molecular weight (mw)
  MW < 100 readily crosses the placenta
  MW 600–1000 variable placental transfer
  MW > 1000 impermeable
- Blood flow
  Drug (oxytoxics) can decrease or alter rate and extent of transfer
- pH
  Un-ionized form under physiologic or pathologic conditions favors transfer
- Protein binding
  Low protein binding favors transfer across the placenta

after the dose that the sample was obtained. The amniotic sac may be understood as an additional, separate anatomic compartment into which a drug must distribute. It is extremely unlikely that instantaneous distribution occurs for most drugs used clinically. Thus, lag time exists for drug distribution into the amniotic sac and to the fetus, markedly shifting the concentration time curve for the fetus, relative to the mother, to the right. Thus, the peak plasma concentration in the maternal circulation may occur at the trough in the fetus and conversely. It would appear that the determined absolute concentration and the interval relative to drug administration are much more important than a ratio of limited physiologic significance.

Metabolic Capability of the Human Placenta

The placenta performs many important functions that ensure homeostasis in the fetal environment. The placenta regulates the delivery of oxygen, nutrients, hormones, and other substrates from the maternal circulation to the fetus while removing metabolic end products from the fetal compartment. In addition, the human placenta is capable of synthesizing, metabolizing, and transferring a wide range of endogenous and exogenous substances. The degree to which the placenta metabolizes a drug, if at all, definitely influences the apparent amount that crosses the placenta and the amount of active drug that reaches the fetus.

Many cytochrome P-450, mixed-function oxidase enzymes have been isolated from the human placenta.[35, 63] Most of these enzymes appear to be located in the smooth endoplasmic reticulum and mitochondria of trophoblasts. Although each enzyme possesses its own substrate specificity, substantial overlap exists in the metabolizing capacity of these enzymes. Moreover, it is clear that a number of these enzymes are susceptible to modulation (i.e., induction or inhibition) by exogenous influences. In particular, some of the enzymes found in human placenta are inducible by cigarette smoking (e.g., CYP1A1).[35, 63] It is tempting to speculate that enhanced metabolism of important fetal substrates by the placentas of pregnant smokers is responsible for some of the known adverse fetal effects associated with smoking. However, no direct adverse fetal effects have been attributed to perturbation of placental enzyme activity.

Human placental microsomal enzymes are capable of biotransforming a wide variety of chemical species. A partial list of substrates shown to be metabolized by human placenta is outlined in Table 11–4. Although the number of different substrates biotransformed by enzymes located in human placenta is large, the actual content of cytochrome P-450 enzymes in placental tissue is low. Attempts to quantitate the functional drug-metabolizing enzyme capacity of the human placenta have led to disparate results, but the activity appears to be much lower than that determined in the fetal or adult liver.[35, 78] Thus, the actual contribution of placental enzyme activity to the biotransformation of administered drugs is believed to

TABLE 11–4 PARTIAL LISTING OF SUBSTRATES AND METABOLIC FUNCTIONS PERFORMED BY THE HUMAN PLACENTA

METABOLIC PATHWAY	SUBSTRATES
Hydroxylation	2-Acetylaminofluorene,* benzo[a]-pyrene,* chrysene,* warfarin,* phencyclidine, amphetamine, pentobarbital, aniline, biphenyl
N-Demethylation	Aminopyrine, diazepam, ethylmorphine, meperidine
O-Demethylation	Codeine, mescaline

*Increased rate of biotransformation in mothers who smoke cigarettes. Modified from Pasanen M, et al: Human placental xenobiotic and steroid biotransformation, catalyzed by cytochrome p450, epoxide hydrolase, and glutathione S-transferase activities and their relationships to maternal cigarette smoking. Drug Metab Rev 21:427, 1990.

be inconsequential and of limited clinical significance for most drugs administered either maternally or into the fetal compartment.[35, 78] Nevertheless, the differential placental metabolism of certain corticosteroids (e.g., prednisolone, in contrast to betamethasone) and the resultant poor clinical outcomes reported with prednisolone in enhancing fetal lung maturation[54, 97] suggest a potential effect of placental metabolism in certain fetal therapeutic endeavors (see "Augmentation of Fetal Lung Maturation"). In contrast, placental metabolism may be of greater importance relative to toxicology outcome than to the metabolism of therapeutically administered drugs.

In addition to mixed-function oxidase activity, the human placenta possesses some capacity to catalyze phase II reactions. Conjugation of substances to enhance water solubility and promote excretion is a primary mechanism of in vivo drug biotransformation. Similar to the low level of activity observed for the phase I enzymes, the enzymes catalyzing conjugation reactions are present in very limited quantities.[78] Thus, the overall activity of conjugation pathways by the human placenta is presumed to play only a minor role in fetal drug elimination.

Some important conjugating enzymes have been detected in human placenta.[10, 18, 34, 35, 63] Sulfotransferase, arylamine-N-transferase (i.e., N-acetyltransferase), and glutathione S-transferase activity have been detected in human placenta.[10, 18, 34, 35, 78] Of the three types of known glutathione S-transferase purified from human liver, only one isoenzyme has been identified in human placenta.[2] In contrast, glucuronidation by uridine diphosphate-glucuronosyltransferase activity has not been found in human placenta.[78] The importance of this lack of uridine diphosphate-glucuronosyltransferase activity in placenta relative to fetal drug disposition is unknown.

FETAL DRUG DISPOSITION

In contrast to our knowledge of drug disposition in the pregnant woman and in the placenta, our understanding of drug disposition in the fetus is inadequate. Contrary to the popular concept that the fetus resides in a privileged and protected environment, we now understand that the fetus is exposed to virtually every chemical entity to which the mother is exposed. Thus, the absorption of a drug into the fetal circulation is both rapid and complete. Most of it occurs through passive nonionic diffusion down concentration gradients between maternal and fetal blood that oppose each other in the placental villi, where they are separated by as little as a single layer of cells. In addition, the fetus may undergo continued drug exposure after drug elimination because of the recirculation of amniotic fluid via the fetal gastrointestinal tract.

Once a drug is within the fetal circulation, we have little knowledge of its fate or potential activity. Certainly, it will be distributed to fetal organs in a manner similar to that observed after birth. However, it is not known whether there are any unique fetal barriers to drug distribution analogous to the blood-brain barrier or the anterior chamber of the eye. In fact, it is not even known whether these barriers actually exist during fetal life.

Once a drug has reached various organs, it is not known whether it has any effect at all. It is clear that both receptor number and receptor affinity change during development. Likewise, receptor-effector coupling undergoes a programmed maturation. Thus, even though a drug may interact with specific receptors, it is possible that no pharmacologic effect will be discernible, because effector mechanisms have not yet developed.

There is no question that the mean residence time for drugs in the fetus is longer than that observed in older children and adults because of immaturity of drug clearance mechanisms. This is especially true for drugs that are cleared entirely by renal excretion. The ontogeny of glomerular filtration and tubular secretion has been well studied. In contrast, for those drugs undergoing significant metabolism, there are many unknown factors. Though most hepatic metabolism pathways are less active in the fetus than in the adult, this is not universally true. Moreover, in the fetus the adrenal gland has a significant complement of drug-metabolizing enzymes, which, although active during fetal and neonatal life, disappear by 6 months' postnatal age.[35] Thus, the true ability of the fetus to metabolize drugs is largely unknown, but it depends, in part, on the particular drug under consideration, the gestational age of the fetus, and its drug metabolism phenotype.

As noted earlier, multiple enzyme systems are involved in xenobiotic metabolism within the body.[35, 63] Of the phase I or oxidative enzymes, the oxidative cytochrome P-450 enzymes predominate. These CYP enzymes constitute a superfamily of heme-containing monooxygenases with 14 *CYP* gene families appearing to exist in mammals; the *CYP1*, *CYP2*, and *CYP3* families are the most important in human drug metabolism. Although the fetuses of many species appear to possess a very poor capacity to metabolize

TABLE 11–5   EXPRESSION OF CYTOCHROME P-450 FORMS IN THE FETAL LIVER AND THE ADRENAL GLAND

ORGAN/GLAND*	CYP FORM
Liver**	CYP1A, 3A, 3A7**
Adrenal**	CYP1A1, 2A5, 3A,** 3A7, CYPB1, CYP17

*Primary form/isoform expressed in specific site.
**Primary site for CYP expression in the human fetus (fetal adrenal > liver containing CYP protein).

xenobiotics, the liver of the human fetus is relatively well developed in its capacity to metabolize various compounds, and it appears to mirror those processes performed by the placenta (see Table 11–4). Nevertheless, the overall functional capacity of the fetal CYP activity is very low. Furthermore, human fetal liver metabolic capacity is qualitatively and quantitatively very different from activity observed in adult liver. The human fetal liver contains many different CYP forms (Table 11–5), though they are present in fewer number and in less density than in the adult liver. The total amount of CYP-450 in the fetal liver approximates 0.2 to 0.4 nmol/mg microsomal protein, which represents approximately 20% to 70% of that found in adult liver. Thus, the metabolic capacity of CYP-mediated reactions are less in the fetus than in adults.

The CYPs are found in many tissues in the extra-uterine organism, including liver, adrenal gland, lung, brain, kidney, and intestine (see Table 11–5). Of these CYP forms, minimal CYP3A7 is expressed in adult liver. Preliminary data suggest that fetal brain may express CYP2D6 and 2E1 and that several other embryonic and fetal tissues may be minimally involved in xenobiotic metabolism. Although our understanding of the expression of CYP forms by the fetus is growing exponentially, the extent of our understanding, unfortunately, remains limited. Nevertheless, available data are clear in that the overall functional capacity of the fetus to effectively metabolize xenobiotics is limited.

CLINICAL PHARMACOKINETICS AND THE MATERNAL-PLACENTAL-FETAL UNIT: CONCLUSIONS

Most of the pharmacologic agents present in the maternal circulation cross the placenta into the fetal circulation.[9, 35, 78, 84, 91] The false belief that the placenta is a "barrier" that maintains a secure, safe environment protected from the maternal environment has long been discounted. Thus, what is present in the maternal circulation should be considered to be present in the fetal circulation. The factors regulating drug transfer across the placenta (see Box 11–5) are the same as those that regulate drug transfer across biologic membranes in other parts of the body. Thus, the primary determinants of drug transfer across the placenta into the fetal compartment are the maternal steady-state drug concentration and the integrity of the maternal and fetal circulations.

The gross physiologic changes that occur during pregnancy (see Tables 11–1 to 11–3) influence both the ultimate steady-state drug concentration achieved and the time required to achieve it. The changes that occur in maternal fluid compartment volumes, renal function (see Tables 11–1 and 11–2), and protein binding (see Table 11–3) directly influence the maternal body stores of a drug and the amount of that drug in the maternal circulation. These factors then determine the concentration gradient achieved at the maternal-placental-fetal interface and, thus, the amount of drug available for fetal transfer.

For the majority of un-ionized, lipophilic compounds, the rate-controlling process in placental transfer is placental blood flow. Alterations in the hemodynamics of either the maternal or fetal circulation can markedly affect the placental transfer of most compounds. It seems obvious that alterations in total placental blood flow modulate the rate and extent of drug transfer from the mother to the fetus and, conversely, from the fetus to the mother. Numerous physiologic and therapeutic interventions can alter the hemodynamics of both circulations. For example, uterine contractions associated with labor, preeclampsia, hypertension, removal of amniotic fluid, and the administration of oxytocic drugs decrease placental blood flow.

Once a drug crosses the placenta, it enters the umbilical vein, flowing to the fetal liver via the portal circulation. Portions of this blood flow enter the fetal liver, and the remainder appears to bypass this route, flowing through the ductus venosus. Any drug present in the blood that flows through the fetal liver is available for metabolism. In contrast, compounds present in blood flowing through the ductus venosus bypass any initial metabolism, possibly allowing a greater amount of unmetabolized compound to be distributed to its receptors in the fetus. The clinical significance and ontogeny of this phenomenon are unknown.

Given the truly rudimentary nature of our understanding of drug disposition and action in the maternal-placental-fetal unit, it seems prudent to perform focused animal experiments and controlled clinical trials before embarking on generalized treatment of recognized fetal disorders. A number of influences result in marked variation in the amount of fetal drug exposure that occurs after maternal administration (Table 11–6). Most of our attempts at fetal therapy, however, have been much more empiric. The remainder of this chapter describes some of these attempts.

PHARMACOLOGIC TREATMENT OF SPECIFIC FETAL DISORDERS

The successful treatment of specific pathophysiologic disorders in the fetus by administering pharmacologic agents to the mother has permitted the development of therapeutic strategies to prevent or reverse a number of fetal abnormalities. Today, fetal therapy is com-

TABLE 11–6   LIMITATIONS TO ASSUMING A UNIFORM FETAL EXPOSURE FROM THE ADMINISTRATION OF A UNIFORM WEIGHT-ADJUSTED DOSE TO THE MOTHER

VARIATION EXISTS IN:	DUE TO DISPARITY IN:
Interindividual disposition	Maternal absorption Maternal distribution Maternal metabolism/ elimination
Placental transfer	Uterine blood flow Placental blood flow Placental thickness and surface area Placental metabolism
Fetal tissue exposure	Fetal position/site of placentation Fetal tissue distribution Fetal metabolism/ elimination

mon practice for a number of intrauterine disorders. Some relatively common disorders that have been successfully treated with fetal therapy are listed in Table 11–7. They represent only some neonatal diseases that occur and progress in utero, which underscores the present and future importance of fetal therapy to decreasing neonatal morbidity and mortality rates.

AUGMENTATION OF FETAL LUNG MATURATION

(See also Chapter 42, Part One.)

One of the earliest attempts to influence fetal development pharmacologically focused on lung matura-

TABLE 11–7   SOME DISORDERS IN WHICH FETAL THERAPY HAS BEEN ATTEMPTED

DISORDER	THERAPY
Mixed carboxylase deficiency	Biotin
Methylmalonic acidemia	Vitamin B_{12}
Neural tube defects	Folate
Hypothyroidism	Thyroid hormone
Adrenogenital syndrome	Steroids
Fetal arrhythmia	Digoxin
Fetal arrhythmia	Verapamil
Fetal arrhythmia	Procainamide
Fetal sedation	Valium
Fetal withdrawal (prevention)	Methadone
Pulmonary maturity	Steroids
Idiopathic thrombocytopenic purpura	Steroids
Fetal distress	Tocolysis
Toxoplasmosis	Spiramycin
Group B streptococcus	Ampicillin
Syphilis	Penicillin
Tuberculosis	Antitubercultotic agents

tion and the amelioration or prevention of neonatal respiratory distress syndrome (RDS).

The first description of pharmacologic acceleration of fetal lung development was reported in 1969.[47] This finding of corticosteroid-induced acceleration of the functional maturation of the lung was serendipitous because the primary purpose of this study was to compare the influence of mineralocorticoid and glucocorticoid effects on parturition. This early work was followed by a number of investigations involving a variety of animal models and clinical trials.[14, 46, 92] The exact mechanisms of corticosteroid enhancement of lung maturation are unknown, but they appear to be primarily a result of the drug's ability to augment structural changes in lung parenchyma through steroid-induced enzyme induction and stimulation of protein synthesis, as well as possible enhancement of surfactant synthesis.

The effects of corticosteroid administration on lung maturation are relatively rapid, occurring within 24 hours of maternal steroid therapy, and infants exposed for 24 hours or less are reported to have up to a 50% decrease in the incidence of RDS.[14, 92] The most dramatic effects on neonatal lung function are observed when maternally administered corticosteroid therapy is provided for somewhere between 1 and 7 days prior to delivery.[14, 92]

Controversy surrounding the effectiveness of corticosteroid therapy in reducing the incidence and severity of neonatal RDS has arisen from studies that have used various corticosteroid preparations. Investigators have used cortisone, prednisone, or prednisolone rather than betamethasone or dexamethasone, which have been associated with clinical success. The data from these studies show clearly that the specific corticosteroid preparation used was more important than the dose administered. Ward summarized corticosteroid dosing data from various clinical studies by normalizing the total amount of steroid administered per treatment course to "cortisol equivalents."[92] As shown in Table 11–8, it was not until the dose of hydrocortisone was raised to about 2000 cortisol equivalents that any positive effect on the incidence of RDS was observed. This dose is more than three times the effective dose in cortisol equivalents recommended for betamethasone. Furthermore, when as much as 250 mg of methylprednisolone was administered, equal to approximately 1000 cortisol equivalents, no decrease in the incidence of RDS was observed (see Table 11–8). It is very clear from these data that either betamethasone or dexamethasone is the corticosteroid analogue to be used to promote fetal lung maturation.

The studies using other corticosteroid analogues, including methylprednisolone,[75] prednisone, and prednisolone,[5] raise questions concerning the placenta, fetal metabolism, or drug disposition dynamics within the fetal compartment as important influences precluding therapeutic success. Beitins and colleagues,[5] in assessing the placental transfer of prednisone and prednisolone, clearly showed that substantial amounts of prednisolone were present in the maternal circulation, regardless of the formulation ad-

TABLE 11–8 ASSESSMENT OF SPECIFIC CORTICOSTEROID ANALOGUE AND MATERNAL DOSE USED TO ENHANCE FETAL LUNG MATURITY

CORTICOSTEROID	DOSAGE/TREATMENT COURSE (mg)*	
	No Decrease†	Decrease†
Cortisone	12 (9.6)	
Hydrocortisone	500 (500)	2000 (2000)
Methylprednisolone	250 (1000)	
Betamethasone		24 (600)

*Dose in parentheses represents milligrams of relative cortisol equivalent based on 1 mg cortisol (hydrocortisone), assigned a value of 1 mg cortisol equivalent.

†No decrease or a decrease in the incidence of severe hyaline membrane disease recorded after maternal administration of corticosteroid analogue.

Modified from Ward RM: Pharmacologic enhancement of fetal lung maturation. Clin Perinatol 21:523, 1994.

ministered (prednisone requires in vivo conversion to the active prednisolone moiety). In contrast, very little prednisolone was measured in cord blood. The study design of these investigators appears to be adequate for an accurate assessment of this observed discrepancy. An initial bolus dose was administered, followed by a 160-minute continuous IV infusion of the study drugs before paired blood sampling was performed, thus approximating steady-state conditions. Only 12% of the maternal prednisolone concentration was identified in the fetal circulation. These data strongly suggest prednisolone metabolism by the placenta as the most likely explanation for the lack of clinical benefit seen with methylprednisolone, even when it is given in very high doses.[75]

It is possible that the inactivation of prednisolone and other corticosteroid analogues (e.g., cortisone, hydrocortisone) is catalyzed by the 11β-hydroxysteroid dehydrogenase found in placental tissue.[57] Preparations of minced human placenta have been shown to metabolize cortisol and prednisolone to their inactive metabolites effectively, whereas only minimal metabolic activity was observed under identical laboratory conditions with dexamethasone (1.8% metabolized) and betamethasone (7.1% metabolized).[8] Another group of investigators,[45] using isolated, perfused placental cotyledons, observed more extensive metabolism of betamethasone (47%) and dexamethasone (54%), but the extent was still much lower than the 73% and 86% metabolism observed with cortisol and prednisolone, respectively. Extending these studies further, investigators have described efficient placental transfer that achieved equivalent maternal and cord blood concentrations with betamethasone[4] and dexamethasone.[56] Thus, the increased placental metabolism of nonhalogenated substituted corticosteroids (e.g., cortisone, prednisolone) and the attainment of high concentrations in the fetal circulation support the importance of using either betamethasone or dexamethasone as the corticosteroids of choice for fetal therapy to enhance the maturation of fetal lung function.

In conclusion, the majority of published studies using betamethasone or dexamethasone as their study compound have demonstrated a clear reduction in the incidence of neonatal RDS compared with its incidence in study infants who received placebo. The results of an exhaustive meta-analysis that included only published studies that involved randomized, blinded, placebo-controlled evaluations support this conclusion.[14] Complementing these impressive efficacy data are the long-term outcome data demonstrating no adverse delayed effects on infant growth or development.[14, 92] Studies tracking patients for up to 12 years after they received maternally administered corticosteroid in utero have not demonstrated any adverse effects on individual IQ scores, school performance, motor development, or overall growth. Recognizing that the effects of corticosteroid on the lungs are attenuated after 7 days, weekly courses have been advocated; however, the risks associated with repetitive antenatal dosing require critical evaluation.[39] Moreover, antenatally administered corticosteroids have been shown to have important extrapulmonary effects on other developing organs, including cardiovascular function, postnatal renal function, and adrenocortical function.[60]

IN UTERO PREVENTION OF INTRACRANIAL HEMORRHAGE

(See also Chapter 38, Part Five.)

Early brain injury in infants with very low birth weight remains an unfortunate and common clinical problem. The most common form of brain injury in these infants is periventricular-intraventricular hemorrhage (PIVH).[1, 62, 91] Advances in neonatal intensive care and the increasing use of prenatal corticosteroids to enhance fetal lung maturation[13, 92] have resulted in a lowering of the incidence to less than 20% in infants with very low birth weight.[68, 77] This positive corticosteroid effect may also be due to enhanced vascular integrity, decrease in RDS, or ability of these drugs to attenuate cytokine production.[85]

The importance of fetal treatment to prevent PIVH is underscored by the clear relationship between the incidence of PIVH and postnatal age. Nearly all of the PIVH observed in infants with very low birth weight is apparent within the first 4 days of life.[17, 22] These data clearly demonstrate the need for in utero measures to prevent PIVH rather than the use of focused therapy in early postnatal life.

Although numerous early studies, including a meta-analysis,[76, 86] suggested that antenatal phenobarbital is effective in decreasing the frequency and severity of intraventricular hemorrhage, more recent data strongly refute these earlier suggestions. In a well-designed, randomized, placebo-controlled study involving over 600 women whose fetuses were younger than 34 weeks' gestation (range, 24 to 33 weeks), the National Institute of Child Health and Human Development Neonatal Research Network[77] clearly demonstrated that properly dosed phenobarbital administered to the mother resulted in no greater benefit over placebo in these premature infants. Important to the findings of this study was that 59% and 58% of women receiving phenobarbital and placebo, respectively, received antenatal corticosteroids, which provide protection against intraventricular hemorrhage.[77]

FETAL THERAPY TO PREVENT MATERNAL-INFANT TRANSMISSION OF THE HUMAN IMMUNODEFICIENCY VIRUS

(See also Chapter 22 and Chapter 37, Part Four.)

Infection with the human immunodeficiency virus (HIV) (and the subsequent development of the acquired immunodeficiency syndrome [AIDS]) is one of the most important public health concerns of the 20th century. Because there is no known cure for this devastating disease, infants infected in utero are committed to a short, difficult, turbulent life. For this reason, aggressive attempts have been made to identify means to decrease the possibility of mother-to-child transmission of HIV.[13, 65, 99]

The risk of vertical transmission in the absence of maternal antiretroviral therapy is 25% to 30%. Unfortunately, the timing of vertical HIV transmission is not well established, complicating the institution of preventive therapies. Several factors increase the risk of maternal transmission to the fetus, including high viral load, rapidly replicating viruses, prolonged rupture of membranes, and conditions that may disrupt the integrity of the placenta, such as other active sexually transmitted diseases or chorioamnionitis.[71, 83, 89]

Strategies targeting prevention or decreasing the incidence of maternally transmitted HIV infection (vertical infection) have been developed, and they focus on the use of zidovudine (AZT).[71, 99] The effectiveness of perigestational therapy is unequivocal. Maternal AZT therapy clearly has been shown to reduce vertical transmission from 25.5% to 8.3%,[71, 83, 99] with evolving data suggesting that this transmission rate may be able to be reduced to less than 5% with more aggressive, multidrug therapy.

FETAL VACCINATION: PREVENTION OF CERTAIN FETAL INFECTIOUS DISEASES

It has been recognized for decades that active immunization of newborn infants is effective in preventing subsequent infection with certain pathogens, including diphtheria, pertussis, tetanus, and poliomyelitis. However, such a therapeutic strategy will not be effective in preventing the occurrence of these diseases immediately after birth,[49] because such disease implies infection in utero, for which fetal immunization would be needed for successful prevention. Direct immunization of the fetus is seldom contemplated because of its known and unknown risks, but passive immunization is possible through maternal immunization. This approach to protecting the infant from infection while in utero has been used successfully in the past for some infectious diseases (e.g., influenza, respiratory syncytial virus infection) and is a promising therapeutic strategy for others (Box 11–6).

The success of passive immunization of the fetus is dependent on the effectiveness of the transplacental transfer of immunoglobulins. In human beings, IgG is the only immunoglobulin that crosses the intact placenta. IgA, IgD, and IgM do not cross the human placenta.[32] Of primary importance to the passive immunization of the fetus, the IgG_1 subclass possesses the greatest affinity for the Fc receptor affording accumulation of this immunoglobulin in the fetus.[49]

The majority of this immunoglobulin crosses the placenta by simple passive diffusion, the mechanism by which nearly all compounds cross the placenta. The extent to which IgG crosses the placenta by passive diffusion is directly proportional to the maternal IgG concentration. In addition, Fc receptor–bound IgG located in the placental trophoblast membrane is actively transported across the placenta by endocytosis. This passage of IgG across the placenta occurs as early as 8 weeks of gestation and increases in quantity with advancing gestation. By 17 to 20 weeks, fetal IgG concentrations approach 100 mg/L.[24, 32] This transfer of maternal antibodies to the fetus protects the fetus from infection and transiently protects the neonate from a variety of infectious diseases.

On the basis of the data discussed earlier, investigators and clinicians have successfully provided passive immunization to the fetus. Some of the more important infectious diseases successfully prevented by in utero vaccination are listed in Box 11–6. This list should be considered only a temporary, partial list, because research and clinical experience with passive immunization by maternal vaccination is growing rapidly. Moreover, initial concerns regarding use of live virus vaccines during pregnancy are also under re-evaluation. The potential increased risk to the fetus of acquiring infection from maternally administered live virus vaccine has been a major concern to investigators and clinicians for decades. Nevertheless, available data do not support this concern and, in fact, have demonstrated the safe use of maternal vaccination with live virus preparations when needed.[49, 87]

Extensive experience with yellow fever vaccinations in pregnant women has yielded no evidence of an increased incidence of untoward fetal effects from the maternally administered vaccine.[49] Furthermore, current Centers for Disease Control and Prevention guidelines recognize the legitimate need for maternal administration of live virus vaccines if immediate protection is necessary because of imminent exposure to yellow fever or poliomyelitis. Despite these experiential data, it is clear that more detailed research is needed on the efficacy and maternal-fetal safety of live virus vaccinations during pregnancy.

Many of the available data describing the safety of in utero vaccination have been obtained under less than optimal conditions. Outbreaks of specific, serious infectious diseases in various parts of the world have required aggressive immunization programs that have included pregnant women. Reports of outbreaks involving pertussis,[41] tetanus,[31] and poliomyelitis[48] and a single case report of the use of human rabies vaccine[90] support the efficacy and safety of in utero vaccination with specific vaccine preparations. Similarly, outbreaks of meningococcal disease in Brazil, necessitating a mass public immunization campaign that included pregnant women, yielded the important information that antibodies effectively crossed the placenta and that the titers measured in the newborn infant and the mother were much higher than in control subjects.[11] These data suggest the efficacy of vaccination for the prevention of this epidemic-associated disease.

Additional investigations into the development of effective vaccines against other, more common infections that affect the fetus and neonate, including *Haemophilus influenzae* and the group B streptococci, continue. The role of these and other vaccines targeting protection of the fetus exposed to infectious diseases requires more specific study. Nevertheless, these data demonstrate the efficacy and overall safety of maternal immunization to protect mothers and their unborn children from certain infectious diseases.

CONGENITAL TOXOPLASMOSIS

(See also Chapter 22 and Chapter 37, Part Three.)

Toxoplasma gondii is an organism that is ubiquitous in nature and causes a variety of illnesses in human beings. Toxoplasmosis is one of the most common infections worldwide. The incidence varies with geographic region and an individual's level of immunocompetence. A recent resurgence in infections caused by *T. gondii* has been observed in patients with AIDS. The primary source of human infection is contact with soil or other objects contaminated with cat feces that contains sporulated cysts. A less common source of infection is the ingestion of poorly cooked meat contaminated with latent cysts. Estimates of the incidence of toxoplasmosis during pregnancy range from 3 to 6 cases per 1000 live births in "high-risk" countries and 1 to 2 cases per 1000 live births in "low-risk" countries.[43, 50]

Fetal infection with *T. gondii* is acquired from the mother. Organisms present in the maternal circulation infect the placenta first. After a lag period, organisms are released from the placenta and infect the fetus. The placenta serves as a reservoir for these parasites, continuously seeding the fetus throughout pregnancy.[28] The highest rate of maternal transmission to the fetus occurs when the mother acquires the disease late in gestation. In contrast, transplacental infection early in the first trimester is low, approximating 15%. This discrepancy in infection rates relative to trimester may reflect the differences in placental membrane thickness with gestation. Overall, the risk of fetal infection because of maternal toxoplasmosis approximates 40%. The risk of fetal infection depends on a number of variables, including the severity of maternal parasitemia, the maturity of the placenta, and the competency of the maternal immune system. It appears that clinically significant congenital toxoplasmosis involves transplacentally infected fetuses younger than 26 weeks' gestation.[50] Unfortunately, the risk or presence of fetal infection does not correlate with maternal symptoms, complicating the clinical approach to these patients.

Congenital toxoplasmosis is associated with a wide variety of serious sequelae. The so-called classic triad of hydrocephalus, chorioretinitis, and intracranial calcifications is rarely observed today. Greater than 90% of congenitally infected infants are free of symptoms at birth; if untreated, the infection will progress, resulting in serious sequelae such as intracranial calcifications, chorioretinitis, hearing impairment, and developmental delay. Common early and late manifestations of congenital toxoplasmosis are shown in Box 11–7. The clinical importance of these effects argues for rapid maternal and fetal diagnosis of the disease and prompt institution of appropriate therapy.

Complicating the decision to initiate therapy is the difficulty of making an accurate diagnosis. Maternal diagnosis is often based on evidence of recent primary infection assessed by the combination of seroconversion, a marked increased in antibody titers for several weeks, and the presence of IgM antibodies.

■ BOX 11–7

COMMON MANIFESTATIONS OF
CONGENITAL TOXOPLASMOSIS

Early*	Late†
Chorioretinitis	Mental retardation
Abnormal CSF (increased	Convulsions
protein level)	Spasticity and palsies
Anemia	Severely impaired vision
Convulsions	Hydrocephalus or
Intracranial calcifications	microcephaly
Jaundice	Deafness
Hydrocephalus	
Splenomegaly	
Lymphadenopathy	
Hepatomegaly	
Microcephaly	

---

*Occurring early after birth and within the first 3 months of life.

†Late in the course of disease; sequelae from no or inadequate treatment, severe disease, or both.

CSF, cerebrospinal fluid.

Although the findings may be positive, the exact timing of maternal infection often cannot be determined. In utero the diagnosis involves the identification of parasites in fetal blood or amniotic fluid. When the index of suspicion is high, attempts to isolate parasites from the placenta at birth should be performed. More recently, the use of a specific polymerase chain reaction has facilitated diagnostic determination.[28]

Therapy for toxoplasmosis during pregnancy is aimed at both preventing vertical transmission and treating the infected mother and the fetus. Because of the unpredictability and insensitivity of current diagnostic methods, it is not possible to assess the efficacy of fetal prevention methods accurately; thus, most clinicians who attempt therapy during pregnancy select drug regimens that may prevent or treat maternal disease.

One of the earlier drugs used for the treatment of toxoplasmosis was spiramycin. A macrolide antibiotic, spiramycin achieves high concentrations in the placenta and about 50% of maternal serum concentrations in the fetus.[50] The drug is primarily used in Europe, and few maternal or fetal side effects have been reported. Uncontrolled studies suggest a maternal benefit and a possible impact on vertical transmission, but they do not support any benefit of spiramycin in already infected fetuses. This differential effect of the drug relative to the fetus may merely reflect the very high concentrations achieved in the placenta compared with fetal tissue concentrations.

By far the most common drug regimen used to treat toxoplasmosis in newborns, pregnant women, and nonpregnant patients involves the combination of pyrimethamine and a sulfonamide (e.g., sulfadiazine). The combination of maternally administered spiramycin with pyrimethamine and sulfadiazine appears to provide the best treatment results in both mother and fetus. A large study involving the placentas obtained from 223 proven cases of toxoplasmosis supports this belief. Samples from these placentas were inoculated intraperitoneally into mice and revealed parasites in 76 of 85 mothers (89%) who were untreated or inadequately treated, in 89 of 118 placentas (75%) obtained from mothers who received 3 gm spiramycin for more than 15 days, and in only 10 of 20 placentas (50%) obtained from patients who received combined spiramycin, pyrimethamine, and sulfadiazine.[11, 28]

Daffos and associates in France demonstrated that in 15 spiramycin-treated women with documented toxoplasmosis who chose to continue their pregnancies to term, the addition of pyrimethamine plus sulfadoxine by 28 weeks of gestation resulted in 13 of 15 newborns' having no clinical evidence of disease at follow-up.[15] The two affected offspring had only mild chorioretinitis.

In conclusion, controlled data establishing treatment guidelines for toxoplasmosis infection during pregnancy are limited. If therapy is started early enough after maternal infection, spiramycin may reduce the incidence of fetal infection or possibly even prevent the transplacental transmission of parasite to the fetus. With active fetal infection, the addition of antiparasitic therapy beginning by the middle of the third trimester appears to provide effective therapy. The true efficacy of this regimen is unknown because of the large number of affected pregnancies that are electively terminated, but it appears to reduce the severity of neonatal infection and, thus, neonatal morbidity and mortality rates. To date, no published data have appeared describing teratogenic or adverse fetal effects of these drugs, which suggests their safety for use during pregnancy.

FETAL ENDOCRINE DISORDERS RESPONSIVE TO IN UTERO THERAPY: CONGENITAL ADRENAL HYPERPLASIA AND DISEASES OF THE THYROID GLAND

(See also Chapter 47, Parts Three and Four.)

Treatment of Congenital Adrenal Hyperplasia

Congenital adrenal hyperplasia (CAH) is an autosomal recessive disorder that results from a deficiency of one of many different enzymes required for the synthesis of cortisol from cholesterol within the adrenal cortex.[82] Deficiency of the 21-hydroxylase enzyme is the most common cause of CAH, occurring in approximately 1 in 140,000 live births. Another form of CAH, often referred to as virilizing CAH, is much less common and is the result of 11β-hydroxylase deficiency. Both of these deficiencies are responsive to prenatal therapy.[12, 61]

The normal synthetic pathway for cortisol synthesis from cholesterol is shown in Figure 11–4. Cortisol synthesis is stringently regulated by a negative feedback control loop involving the pituitary hormone adrenocorticotropic hormone (ACTH) and the hypothalamic hormone corticotropin-releasing hormone (CRH). With increasing cortisol secretion, glucocorticoid receptors in the higher centers bind to cortisol, signaling a diminished need for ACTH and CRH transcription. This action reduces the production of these hormones, which are responsible for stimulating cortisol secretion.[82] CAH is characterized by a reduction in cortisol synthesis caused by deficiency of 21-hydroxylase, leading to continuous overproduction of ACTH, adrenocortical hyperplasia, and the accumulation of 17α-hydroxyprogesterone and other precursors to 21-hydroxylase activity. These accumulated precursors are shunted into sex-steroid pathways, which promotes excessive production of virilizing

hormones such as testosterone and other potent androgens. The sex steroids are produced from 17-hydroxylated pregnenolone, progesterone, dehydroepiandrosterone, or androstenedione by the catalytic activity of 17,20-lyase.[61, 82] In addition, accumulation of products of 3β-hydroxysteroid dehydrogenase will affect aldosterone synthesis, with a resultant effect on fluid and electrolyte homeostasis.

Thus, the mechanisms of production of these important steroids are interrelated and will be perturbed by an early defect in 21-hydroxylase activity. Depending on the extent of enzyme deficiency and enhanced production of sex steroids, newborn infants with CAH may have varying anatomic anomalies. In a newborn female infant with severe virilizing CAH, it is not uncommon for the infant to have a single perineal orifice originating from a fused vagina and urethra. The clitoris is often very enlarged, with the appearance of a hypospadiac phallus. The labia majora are fused at the midline and rugose, empty of glans. 21-Hydroxylase deficiency is the most common recognized cause of ambiguous genitalia in the female newborn. The extent of the deformities varies with the variability in enzyme deficiency.[61, 82]

In contrast to female infants, newborn male infants with 21-hydroxylase or 11β-hydroxylase deficiency will have no apparent genital defects, with the exception of possibly an elongated penis.[82] Overall, the male fetus is at little risk of CAH-associated morbidity or death and responds well to corticosteroid replacement therapy after birth.

Intrauterine therapy is needed in fetuses known to have CAH because the resulting severe physical deformities in the female infant have an impact on the infant's parents, parent-infant bonding, family, friends, and the patient herself in later years.[61, 82] Fetal therapy should prevent the occurrence of associated structural genital anomalies, sparing the infant and family from surgical procedures and sequelae. For more than a decade,[16] in utero suppression of adrenal activity by maternal administration of dexamethasone has been employed for female fetuses identified to be deficient in 21-hydroxylase activity. More recently, Cerame and coworkers reported the successful treatment of a female fetus with 11β-hydroxylase deficiency with maternally administered dexamethasone (20 μg/kg per day divided in three equal doses).[12]

For the greatest possibility of completely preventing or minimizing the CAH-associated structural anomalies in susceptible female fetuses, dexametha-

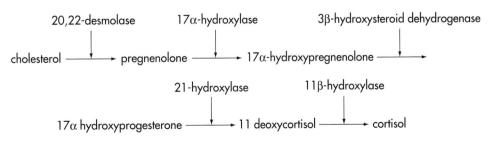

FIGURE 11–4. Normal synthetic pathway for cortisol production by the adrenal cortex.

sone therapy should be started as soon after conception as possible. The adrenal cortex is first detected by approximately 7 weeks' gestation, with fetal steroid production beginning in the latter half of the first trimester.[82] Complete prevention of genital virilization may require starting maternal dexamethasone before 6 weeks' gestation, when the affected adrenal gland appears to be capable of secreting androgens.[54] Obviously, the earliest suspicion that a fetus may be affected will come from genetic counseling of families with a history of an infant born with CAH. With parental consent, daily maternal dexamethasone therapy, 20 μg/kg per day in three equally divided doses, is started as soon after conception as possible. Further studies are then performed to assess the sex of the fetus and the presence of CAH. Chorionic villus sampling performed at approximately 9 to 10 weeks' gestation for first trimester diagnosis or by amniocentesis after 14 weeks of fetal age for second trimester diagnosis can be employed for the perinatal diagnosis of 21-OH deficiency (e.g., MLA-typing of cultured fetal cells or 21B gene analysis of extracted DNA).[61] After amniocentesis, if karyotype analysis (by 12 to 14 weeks' gestation) reveals a male fetus or DNA analysis reveals an unaffected infant, dexamethasone therapy may be discontinued. If the fetus is female and later DNA analysis reveals 21-hydroxylase or 11β-hydroxylase deficiency, dexamethasone therapy is continued to term. Unfortunately, the decision to treat must be made before a diagnosis is possible, exposing a fair number of fetuses to suprapharmacologic maternal doses of dexamethasone.

For infants born with classic 21-hydroxylase deficiency, sodium and mineralocorticoid replacement therapy is required. The most common approach to replacing mineralocorticoid activity is with the oral administration of 9α-fluorohydrocortisone, 50 to 100 μg per day, along with tailored sodium chloride supplementation.

The efficacy of maternal dexamethasone in preventing the anomalies associated with CAH is dependent on a number of factors including early institution and proper dosing of dexamethasone. The degree of structural deformity in the female infant will be directly related to the timing of the institution of therapy. Once the deformity has occurred, maternal dexamethasone therapy cannot reverse the deformity, but it may prevent its progression. A review of reported cases published between 1986 and 1993 revealed 9 of 11 affected female fetuses younger than 8 weeks' gestation treated without interruption had normal genitalia or only minor ambiguity, in comparison with 3 of 5 infants who started treatment at 8 to 10 weeks' gestation in whom much more severe ambiguity was displayed.[82] Pang reported her experience with prenatal dexamethasone administration in 54 fetuses (52 with classic 21-OH deficiency).[61] Of the newborns whose mothers received dexamethasone before 10 weeks of fetal age and continued therapy to birth, 34% had normal genitalia, 52% had mild virilized genitalia not requiring surgery, and 14% had significantly virilized genitalia requiring surgical re-

pair. Of the experience to date, maternally administered dexamethasone throughout gestation appears to be safe and without teratogenic effect (see later).[61] Moreover, before the advent of fetal therapy, all infants with profound enzyme deficiency were severely disfigured, whereas even delayed therapy was found to decrease the degree of deformity in affected offspring. Thus, early institution of dexamethasone therapy and strict maternal compliance are essential to a good outcome. However, initiation of maternal dexamethasone after 10 weeks of fetal age or discontinuation of dexamethasone treatment by the late second trimester is usually associated with severe virilization.[61]

Another important variable influencing the efficacy of maternal dexamethasone therapy is drug dose. The efficacy of maternal dosing on suppressing fetal adrenal activity can be assessed by monitoring the maternal blood or urine concentrations of the hormone estriol. This hormone accurately reflects the fetal synthesis of the precursor steroid 16α-hydroxydehydroepiandrosterone, an estriol precursor.[82] In mothers receiving adequate doses of dexamethasone, fetal adrenal activity is suppressed, and the maternal blood and urine concentrations of estriol will be zero.

As discussed earlier, when dexamethasone therapy is used to enhance fetal lung maturation, fetal exposure appears to be both safe and effective. Obviously, the duration of maternal dexamethasone therapy for CAH is substantially longer than that for the enhancement of fetal lung maturation, subjecting the fetus to a possibly greater risk of adverse effects. The published experience to date with long-term maternal dexamethasone therapy administered throughout gestation reveals no greater incidence of dexamethasone-associated fetal/neonatal adverse effects than what is seen with more limited use at the time of preterm delivery. Early suggestions that dexamethasone therapy may be associated with a higher incidence of cleft palate have been refuted in more recent, controlled evaluations.[27] Similarly, no influence of therapy has been observed in the subsequent mental and physical development of these infants.[27, 61, 82] Further, it is clear that female fetuses who do not receive effective prenatal therapy have marked differences in their social and behavioral development from unaffected controls.[7]

In contrast, clinically important dexamethasone-associated adverse effects have been observed in mothers taking the drug throughout pregnancy. All the known side effects associated with long-term corticosteroid therapy have been described in treated mothers, and they include Cushing syndrome, weight gain, edema, elevations in blood pressure or blood glucose concentrations, gastric distress, and irritability. Maternal side effects of chronic dexamethasone therapy are listed in Table 11–9. The incidence and severity of these effects appear directly related to the duration of therapy. Unfortunately, no known means of reducing the development or incidence of these side effects in the mother is available. Mothers receiving dexamethasone therapy should be monitored closely for the

TABLE 11–9 COMMON AND POTENTIAL MATERNAL ADVERSE EFFECTS ASSOCIATED WITH DEXAMETHASONE THERAPY* IN THE TREATMENT OF CONGENTIAL ADRENAL HYPERPLASIA

Excess weight gain (≥4.5–12 kg)
Cushingoid complications
   Moon face, increased facial hair
   Extreme striae causing permanent scarring (abdomen, hip, breasts, arms, thighs, shoulders)
Overt diabetes or diabetic OGTT
Hypertension
Extreme emotional lability
Epigastric pain
Fatigue, pedal edema
Potential risks not established
   Osteoporosis
   Aseptic necrosis of the hip
   Predisposition to cesarean section

*Chronic therapy, first trimester to term.
OGTT, oral glucose tolerance test.
Modified from Pang S: Congenital adrenal hyperplasia. End Metab Clin N Am 26:853, 1997.

occurrence of these and other dexamethasone-associated adverse effects, and the need to discontinue maternal dexamethasone therapy should be decided on a case-by-case basis. In addition, it may be possible to reduce the incidence and severity of dexamethasone-associated maternal adverse effects by determining the true maternal dose needed to suppress fetal adrenal activity. Lower maternal doses may decrease the severity of side effects, and the dose needed could be assessed by individual dose-response relationships focused on how much dexamethasone is needed daily to suppress maternal urinary estriol excretion, targeting a zero urinary concentration.

Treatment of Fetal Thyroid Disorders

(See also Chapter 47, Part Three.)

The fetus may demonstrate hypothyroidism, hyperthyroidism, or goiter associated with either hypothyroidism or hyperthyroidism. Concern over thyroid dysfunction in the fetus and the possibility of subsequent abnormal infant development has stimulated some investigators to consider in utero therapy as a way to avoid these potentially irreversible sequelae. Nevertheless, considerable controversy persists about whether fetal therapy is needed in the vast majority of cases of congenitally diagnosed thyroid disease.

The maturation and function of the thyroid gland represent a complex interplay among the thyroid, the pituitary, and the hypothalamus. By the 10th week of gestation, thyroid colloid, iodide uptake, and thyroid hormone synthesis have been demonstrated, and thyrotropin-releasing hormone has been identified in hypothalamic extracts.[25, 69] It is important to recognize that the normal ontogeny of fetal thyroid gland occurs relatively independent of the maternal environment.

The placenta appears to be freely permeable to iodide and thyrotropin-releasing hormone, only partially permeable to the iodothyronines, and impermeable to thyrotropin. Maturation of the gland continues throughout gestation and after birth. Thus, adequate maternal intake of iodine is important.

Of the congenital thyroid disorders, fetal hypothyroidism, as uncommon as it is, is the most frequently encountered congenital thyroid disease. The more frequent causes of fetal hypothyroidism are listed in Table 11–10.[25, 69] The majority of these cases are caused by abnormal thyroid, pituitary, or hypothalamic embryogenesis. Because of the infrequency of the disease and the cause of the dysgenesis, active diagnostic evaluation of the fetus to assess fetal thyroid status is unusual unless an abnormal thyroid gland is observed during an ultrasonographic evaluation performed for other reasons. In the remainder of patients with congenital hypothyroidism, abnormalities in thyroid hormone synthesis and disposition, abnormal gland function, and transient effects caused by maternal antibodies or maternal antithyroid drugs are generally implicated.[25, 69]

Considerable controversy surrounds the need to treat congenital hypothyroidism. Most infants born with thyroid gland dysgenesis or modest goiter have no symptoms and respond promptly to postnatal thyroid replacement therapy.[25, 69] Some investigators have suggested that untreated fetal hypothyroidism may be associated with mild IQ deficits and defects in bone maturation. Others believe sufficient thyroxine (T_4) from the euthyroid mother is usually adequate to

TABLE 11–10 CAUSES OF CONGENITAL HYPOTHYROIDISM WITH APPROXIMATE INCIDENCE

CAUSES	INCIDENCE
Thyroid dysgenesis	1:4000
Agenesis	
Dysgenesis	
Ectopia	
Thyroid dyshormonogenesis	1:30,000
TSH receptor defect	
Iodide trapping defect	
Organification defect	
Iodotyrosine deiodinase deficiency	
Thyroglobulin defect	
Transient hypothyroidism	1:40,000
Drug induced	
Maternal antibody induced	
Idiopathic	
Hypothalamic-pituitary hypothyroidism	1:70,000 to 1:100,000
Hypothalamic-pituitary anomaly	
Panhypopituitarism	
Isolated TSH deficiency	
TSH structural defect	

TSH, thyroid-stimulating hormone (thyrotropin).
Modified from Fisher DA: Fetal thyroid function: Diagnosis and management of fetal thyroid disorders. Clin Obstet Gynecol 40:16, 1997.

support normal fetal brain maturation.[25, 73] More data are needed from controlled longitudinal studies of infants with untreated congenital hypothyroidism to determine the true relationship, if any, between this fetal disorder and cognitive or developmental outcome. In contrast, fetal hypothyroidism resulting from maternal therapy with antithyroid medications (e.g., methimazole, propylthiouracil) requires diligent dosage adjustment to define the maternal requirement associated with the lowest dose to treat her hyperthyroidism. Other maternally consumed therapeutic agents with antithyroid activity on the fetus include lithium, amiodarone, and iodine.

Fetal hyperthyroidism with thyrotoxicosis is very uncommon, but when it occurs, it is nearly always associated with maternal Graves disease. Increased fetal thyroid function is due to the placental transfer of maternal thyroid-stimulating IgG antibody, which stimulates fetal T_4 secretion during the later stages of gestation. If T_4 stimulation is pronounced enough and expressed for a sufficient period, hyperthyroidism develops in the fetus, with classic symptoms including tachycardia, growth retardation, advanced bone maturation, and goiter.[25, 69, 70, 96] The most common initial manifestation of fetal hyperthyroidism is tachycardia.

Fetal goiter has been associated with tracheal compression and altered amniotic fluid volume.[96] In addition, fetal goiter may develop because of various abnormalities in thyroid function, including defects in thyroid hormone synthesis, maternal transfer of goitrogen, and, as described earlier, maternal autoimmune thyroid disease.[69] Goiter may be associated with either hypothyroidism or hyperthyroidism; therefore, if the diagnosis cannot be determined from the maternal history, further investigation may require direct determination of fetal thyroid function by performing hormone concentration studies of amniotic fluid or by using cordocentesis to obtain fetal blood samples.[19, 69, 70] Despite these advances in our ability to evaluate fetal thyroid status more critically, the risk to the infant of untreated congenital goiter in the euthyroid mother appears to be minimal. The success of postnatal therapy suggests that fetal therapy should be instituted only in cases of very large goiters, which may cause mechanical damage, or in situations associated with altered amniotic fluid volume.

Fetal hypothyroidism, with or without goiter, has been treated successfully with the intra-amniotic instillation of T_4. The optimal dose for intra-amniotic instillation of T_4 is not known; successful management of a small number of cases suggests a 250- to 500-μg dose of T_4, given intra-amniotically once weekly or semiweekly.[25, 69] Quantitation of trough hormone concentrations in the amniotic fluid may be useful in guiding the dosing interval for subsequent intra-amniotic dosing. In contrast, clinically important manifestations of fetal hyperthyroidism may best be treated with maternal administration of an antithyroid medication, either methimazole or propylthiouracil, with or without supportive therapy such as the use of propranolol. Methimazole is the preferred drug because a greater amount of this drug than of propyl-

thiouracil crosses the placenta. This increased transplacental transfer of methimazole is the primary reason that it is otherwise avoided during pregnancy. The use of propylthiouracil to treat maternal hyperthyroidism has less effect on the fetus. Monitoring of the fetal heart rate is usually sufficient to determine the success of therapy, with normalization of fetal heart rate occurring within 2 weeks. The maternal antithyroid drug dose is adjusted to maintain the fetal heart rate at approximately 140 beats per minute.

POLYHYDRAMNIOS

Amniotic fluid is the only environment of the fetus throughout gestation, and it supports and protects the fetus until the time of delivery. Controversy exists regarding the actual sources of amniotic fluid.[80] The volume of amniotic fluid increases with gestational age, reaching a plateau somewhere between 30 and 37 weeks (see also Chapter 21). The total volume of amniotic fluid is highly variable, but it usually ranges between 500 and 1100 mL. The actual amount produced is dependent on a number of variables controlled by the dynamic interactions among the maternal-placental-fetal compartments.[44] *Polyhydramnios* refers to an excess of amniotic fluid, usually more than 2000 mL.

The causes of polyhydramnios are many. The more important causes, listed in order of importance, are shown in Table 11–11.[6] The overall incidence of polyhydramnios appears to range between 0.13% and 3.5% of pregnancies. This rate remains relatively constant and independent of the method of diagnosing the disorder, although clinical assessment of amniotic fluid volume is not always reliable. Before ultrasonography became available, polyhydramnios was diagnosed on the basis of an abnormally large uterine size for gestational age and the inability to palpate aspects of the fetus.[44] Using ultrasound techniques, determination of the *amniotic fluid index* (AFI) is the most promising method for diagnosis. In 1987, Phelan and associates described a technique of dividing the uterus into quadrants and determining the vertical dimension of specific regions within each quadrant.[67] An AFI greater than 24 cm is considered to be diagnostic of polyhydramnios. Subsequent studies have

TABLE 11–11   CAUSES OF POLYHYDRAMNIOS

CAUSE*	% OF CASES
Idiopathic	~60
Fetal anomalies	~19
Gastrointestinal	
Central nervous system	
Cardiovascular	
Multiple gestation	~7.5
Maternal diabetes	~5
Other causes	~8.5

*Listed in order of importance.

verified the accuracy of the AFI in diagnosing polyhydramnios and its superiority to clinical assessment and other ultrasonographic methods.[21, 80] Using the AFI, Smith and coworkers diagnosed mild polyhydramnios in 97 of 1177 patients (8.2%).[80]

The need to treat polyhydramnios is dependent on maternal symptoms. Polyhydramnios per se causes no ill effects on the fetus; the mother alone is affected. Nevertheless, polyhydramnios may be a manifestation of many fetal disorders, necessitating close investigation of the fetus in identified cases. Indications for maternal treatment include maternal respiratory compromise, gastrointestinal difficulties or pain, or preterm labor. Available data suggest that indomethacin therapy, despite its risks, is most effective in cases of idiopathic polyhydramnios, maternal gastrointestinal obstruction or diabetes, or fetal nephrogenic diabetes insipidus (e.g., caused by maternal lithium therapy).[67]

Indomethacin is a propionic acid, nonsteroidal anti-inflammatory drug that competitively inhibits the activity of cyclooxygenase, which results in decreased prostaglandin synthesis. Its precise mechanism of action in decreasing amniotic fluid volume is unknown. Most investigators believe that indomethacin influences amniotic fluid production either by impairing fetal lung fluid production or enhancing its reabsorption, decreasing fetal urine production and/or increasing fluid movements across fetal membranes.[44] Preliminary data on sheep also suggest that maternal indomethacin administration may increase fetal respiratory movements, which, in combination with increased pulmonary fluid reabsorption, can lead to a decrease in amniotic fluid production. The overall effect of the drug is most likely due to a combination of these events.

Many different indomethacin dosage regimens have been used. An initial indomethacin regimen consisting of 25 mg PO administered every 6 hours (~1.4 to 1.5 mg/kg per day) may be effective. This dosage has been reported to decrease fetal urine production.[44] Maternal indomethacin doses greater than 2 mg/kg per day do not appear to afford any greater benefit, but they are clearly associated with increased maternal and fetal drug toxicity. These adverse effects may be dose limiting, especially when constriction of the ductus arteriosus occurs. The impact of this drug-induced effect on the fetus cannot be overemphasized. For this reason, maternal indomethacin probably should not be administered after 32 weeks of gestation, and it is contraindicated after 34 weeks of gestation.[23, 44]

With short-term indomethacin administration (i.e., ≤72 hours), the incidence of clinically important fetal adverse effects is small and necessitates no extraordinary patient monitoring. With longer courses of therapy, Kramer and colleagues recommend serial echocardiography to assess whether ductal constriction is present.[44] These authors obtain an initial fetal echocardiogram 24 hours after starting maternal indomethacin therapy and weekly during the treatment period. If ductal closure is noted, the maternal indomethacin

dose is reduced from 25 mg PO every 6 hours to 25 mg PO every 8 hours. Another fetal echocardiogram is obtained in 24 hours. If tricuspid regurgitation is noted with ductal constriction, indomethacin therapy is immediately discontinued. Fetal hydrops, postnatal persistence of the fetal circulation, and pulmonary hypertension may be manifestations of prolonged tricuspid regurgitation with severe ductal insufficiency. Indomethacin-induced constriction of fetal ductal tissue has been described as early as 24 weeks of gestation, and most authorities encourage close echocardiographic monitoring starting after 27 weeks.[44, 88]

In contrast to the serious indomethacin-associated adverse effects that can occur in the fetus, maternal tolerance of therapy is generally good, rarely requiring discontinuation of therapy. The most common maternal side effects of indomethacin therapy are gastric upset (e.g., heartburn), nausea, and headache. With long-term indomethacin administration, the incidence of headache, vertigo, or tinnitus appears to increase. When current indomethacin dosing recommendations have been followed, only rare instances of decreased maternal urine output and worsening maternal hypertension have been described. In addition, like all nonsteroidal anti-inflammatory drugs, indomethacin will interfere reversibly with platelet function and aggregation. Thus, patients with underlying coagulation disorders should not receive the drug.

FETAL ARRHYTHMIAS

(See also Chapter 43.)

For almost two decades, investigators and clinicians have successfully diagnosed and attempted to treat fetal cardiac dysrhythmias.[42] Today, antiarrhythmic therapy for fetuses with persistently abnormal cardiac rhythm is considered to be routine management.[79]

Abnormal cardiac rhythm occurs in approximately 1% to 3% of fetuses during the third trimester. It is presumed that the number is actually larger, considering the large number of fetuses that most likely have intermittent extrasystoles, which cause no symptoms and go undiagnosed. The most common means by which fetal cardiac dysrhythmias are diagnosed is through incidental observations obtained during regular clinic visits. Fetal echocardiography is the primary means by which the diagnosis of fetal dysrhythmia is confirmed and is used to assess whether other congenital cardiac abnormalities are present. Among fetuses who appear to have cardiac dysrhythmias on initial evaluation, approximately 80% are found to have extrasystoles, with the remaining 20% having some type of tachyarrhythmias or bradyarrhythmias.[42] Fortunately, most fetal cardiac dysrhythmias involve uncomplicated, nonsustained extrasystoles that do not require intervention. However, depending on severity, many sustained tachyarrhythmias do require therapeutic intervention.

Fetal tachycardia is most often defined as a fetal heart rate persistently more than 180 to 200 beats per minute, whereas *fetal bradycardia* is a persistent heart rate less than 100 beats per minute, regardless of gestational age.[81] The dysrhythmia should be categorized as either sustained or intermittent. *Sustained dysrhythmia* most often describes a duration of dysrhythmia for more than 50% of the time, whereas *intermittent dysrhythmia* is the occurrence of a dysrhythmia of shorter duration.[38] Recognizing the many difficulties in specifically assessing fetal cardiac rhythm with present technology, it is often difficult to delineate specifically the actual incidence of the specific type of dysrhythmia.

From available data, it appears that supraventricular tachycardia (SVT) is the most common form of tachyarrhythmia; the remaining tachyarrhythmias tend to involve atrial flutter (AF) and reciprocating or atypical SVTs[38] (see also Chapter 43). Although fetal dysrhythmias may be associated with any pathophysiologic perturbation of either the mother or fetus, tachyarrhythmias appear most often to represent primary abnormalities of the heart and/or conduction, with only a small percentage of cases caused by cardiac malformations, infection, or uterine contractions. Thus, when sustained fetal dysrhythmias are diagnosed and treatment is required, therapy usually involves the administration of an antiarrhythmic agent to the mother, with the goal of suppressing the abnormal fetal rhythm.

Untreated sustained fetal tachycardia or bradycardia can result in a terminal form of fetal heart failure culminating in fetal hydrops (see also Chapter 21). *Hydrops* refers to a group of physical findings, including anasarca, cardiac dilation, and hepatosplenomegaly. If fetal hydrops remains untreated, the perinatal mortality rate ranges from 50% to 98%. This staggering mortality rate and the recognition that a major cause is fetal dysrhythmia underscore the importance of prompt and successful treatment of sustained fetal dysrhythmias.[38, 79]

Extrasystoles rarely progress to tachyarrhythmia and, thus, rarely require therapeutic intervention. Nevertheless, patients should be monitored serially to ensure that the extrasystoles do not degenerate into more serious rhythm disturbances. Because there is no evidence that sustained fetal tachyarrhythmias resolve spontaneously and because the body of published experience describing successful resolution of the dysrhythmia with maternal antiarrhythmic drug therapy continues to grow, most authorities recommend a trial of antenatal antiarrhythmic therapy. Nevertheless, the decision is complex. The options include simple serial monitoring with repeated fetal echocardiograms and sonograms to assess disease progression, maternal antiarrhythmic drug therapy, direct fetal therapy, or premature delivery of the infant.[36, 79] Decisions must be made on a case-by-case basis. In contrast, fetal bradyarrhythmias do not respond to antiarrhythmic therapy. Thus, close monitoring is essential so that prompt delivery and postnatal therapy can be undertaken if fetal survival is jeopardized.[38, 58, 79]

The literature is replete with reports of successful management of fetal tachyarrhythmias with maternally administered antiarrhythmic drugs. The drugs most often used are listed in Box 11–8. Nevertheless,

---

> ■ **BOX 11–8**
>
> ### ANTIARRHYTHMIC MEDICATIONS USED TO TREAT FETAL TACHYARRHYTHMIAS
>
> Digoxin*   Verapamil*
> Procainamide   Amiodarone*
> Quinidine   Propafenone
> Propranolol   β-Methyldigoxin
> Flecainide*
>
> ---
>
> *Most frequently employed, either alone or in combination.

a review of the therapeutic outcome of 119 published cases of SVT or AF revealed that 50% of cases of SVT or AF failed to respond to maternally administered digoxin monotherapy.[38] Of the patients in whom therapy with digoxin initially failed, 80% of the patients with SVT and 60% of those with AF were treated successfully with the addition of a second maternally administered antiarrhythmic agent. The presence of fetal heart failure was associated with a poor response to digoxin monotherapy. This experience has been confirmed by the series of Simpson and associates, who have clearly shown the negative impact hydrops has on the fetal response to antiarrhythmic therapy (see later).[79]

Unfortunately, many clinically important variables influence maternal-fetal drug therapy and outcome, including differences in gestational age at the time of diagnosis, severity of underlying fetal cardiac dysrhythmia, presence of other maternal-fetal diseases, maternal digoxin dose, use of a maternal digoxin loading regimen on initiation of therapy, targeted or attained steady-state maternal serum digoxin concentrations, time of determining maternal-cord serum drug concentrations, and duration of monotherapy before the start of combination antiarrhythmic drug therapy. These variables preclude a detailed assessment of the true efficacy rate of digoxin monotherapy. Nevertheless, digoxin monotherapy appears to be efficacious in a large number of cases. In nonresponders, additional antiarrhythmic drugs are often therapeutic, most notably a calcium channel antagonist.[58, 79]

Appropriate dosing is one question that remains in treating fetal dysrhythmias through maternal drug administration. The answer to this important question must address the complex nature of the maternal-placental-fetal unit. Nevertheless, some general principles of drug therapy may be used to guide drug administration in this context (Box 11–9). The majority of the reported experience recommends targeting traditionally accepted therapeutic serum drug concentrations in the mother (Table 11–12), presumably to afford therapeutic concentrations in the fetus. These purported "therapeutic serum antiarrhythmic drug concentration ranges" are guidelines; they should not be interpreted as absolute. Furthermore, these concentration ranges have been assessed primarily in adult

GENERAL PRINCIPLES TO GUIDE MATERNAL
ANTIARRHYTHMIC DRUG THERAPY TO
TREAT FETAL DYSRHYTHMIAS

■ *Initiate maternal drug dosing aggressively.* Use loading
doses when appropriate. Repeatedly assess
maternal drug pharmacokinetics when possible to
account for pregnancy-associated differences in
drug disposition.
■ *Monitor mother closely for antiarrhythmic drug effects.*
Carefully assess mother for effects of
antiarrhythmic drug: presence, severity, and
tolerance. Carefully assess mother for any drug-
associated adverse effects.
■ *Monitor fetus closely for antiarrhythmic drug effects.*
Perform repeated assessment of fetal heart function
(e.g., echocardiography, continuous external fetal
heart rate monitoring). Target fetal monitoring to
coincide with expected or documented maternal
antiarrhythmic steady state.
■ *Aggressively adjust maternal antiarrhythmic drug
therapy as needed and tolerated.* Initial doses are
given to target upper limit of "usual" therapeutic
serum concentration range. Adjust doses upward
as needed for fetal heart effect and maternal
tolerance. Second antiarrhythmic agent indicated
only with maternal intolerance of maximal
antiarrhythmic monotherapy. Initiate
antiarrhythmic dosing of second agent as
aggressively as with first drug. Maintain dose of
first drug when adding second antiarrhythmic
drug.
■ *Unsuccessful maternal antiarrhythmic drug therapy
requires reassessment.* Reassess patient and cardiac
diagnosis. Ensure proper drug administration and
patient compliance. Consider direct fetal therapy
(e.g., intra-amniotic, intracord, fetal intramuscular).

than-usual doses to the mother to achieve serum drug
concentrations similar to those achieved in the non-
gravid state. If the desired therapeutic effect on the
fetal heart is not realized, the antiarrhythmic drug
dose should be increased, regardless of the maternal
serum concentration, until maternal intolerance limits
further dosage escalation or fetal therapeutic effect is
achieved. If maximally tolerated doses are administered without therapeutic success, the dose of the first
drug should be maintained constant and a second
drug should be added. Dosing with the second drug
should be initiated aggressively, again initially targeting the upper limit of the therapeutic serum concentration range. For antiarrhythmic drugs without
serum drug concentration monitoring parameters
(e.g., propranolol, propafenone), specific physiologic
parameters, such as maternal heart rate and blood
pressure, should be used to determine initial doses
and aggressive dose escalation (see Box 11-8).

Of the antiarrhythmic drugs available to treat fetal
arrhythmias, digoxin has been used most extensively.
It is the drug of choice for the treatment of fetal
tachyarrhythmias in the nonhydropic infant. Digoxin
is a positive inotrope, and it increases the refractory
period through the atrioventricular node. In the patient with a normal heart (e.g., the pregnant woman),
digoxin therapy may cause systemic hypertension as
a result of vasoconstriction, a decreased sinus rate,
and a slight decrease in cardiac output. Complicating
the routine monitoring of the serum digoxin concentration in both the fetus and the mother is the presence of endogenous digoxin-like immunoreactive
substances (EDLIS). These endogenous substances interact with current routinely employed immunoassay
laboratory methods used to quantitate digoxin concentrations in biologic fluids.[33, 38, 94] The presence of
EDLIS leads to a falsely elevated serum digoxin concentration. The physiologic role of these substances is
not understood, and maternal and fetal concentrations vary with time. Thus, an attempt to use a single,
baseline determination of the EDLIS concentration
before digoxin therapy to subtract from subsequent

patients with various underlying cardiac diseases.
Their relevance to the healthy mother and the fetus
with cardiac disease is unknown. Nevertheless, they
can be used as targets to guide initial maternal antiarrhythmic drug dosing, so that maternal serum drug
concentrations are balanced against maternal tolerance and fetal cardiac effects. From the limited published experience, it appears that a mother with
normal cardiovascular function is very tolerant to
the effects of maternally circulating antiarrhythmic
agents. A major challenge is clearly the mother whose
fetus (and who herself) has clinically significant cardiac disease.

Maternal drug dosing should be aggressive because of the many physiologic changes that occur
during pregnancy (see Tables 11-1 to 11-3) and influence maternal drug disposition. As discussed earlier,
most alterations necessitate administration of higher-

TABLE 11-12   THERAPEUTIC MATERNAL
SERUM ANTIARRHYTHMIC
DRUG CONCENTRATIONS

DRUG	INITIAL THERAPEUTIC MATERNAL SERUM CONCENTRATION*
Digoxin†	1–3 ng/mL
Procainamide	4–12 mg/L
N-Acetylprocainamide	10–30 mg/L
Quinidine	2–5 mg/L
Verapamil	100–120 ng/mL
Flecainide	0.4–1 mg/L
Amiodarone	0.5–2.5 mg/L

*Initial target maternal serum drug concentrations. Drug dose should
be adjusted as needed to treat fetal arrhythmia and as tolerated by the
mother.

†Must account for the presence of endogenous digoxin-like substances
(see text for details).

serum concentrations is inaccurate. Rather, to account accurately for the presence of these substances and to determine only the serum digoxin concentration derived from exogenous digoxin, one must send blood samples for specific analysis by high-performance liquid chromatography.

The overall modest success rate in treating fetal tachyarrhythmias with digoxin monotherapy (~50%) raises questions about the possible presence of factors that may decrease the efficacy of this drug in this setting. The presence of fetal hydrops decreases the likelihood of success with maternal digoxin monotherapy, but the reasons are unknown. It is possible that stress and other aspects of fetal hydrops may enhance digoxin binding to the placenta or to P-glycoprotein, an adenosine triphosphate–dependent drug-transporting protein.[20, 38] Digoxin binding to these components markedly reduces the concentration of pharmacologically active free digoxin, possibly reducing the efficacy of drug therapy. Moreover, the influence, if any, of fetal hydrops on the fetal distribution of digoxin is unknown. Thus, in fetuses with severe advanced cardiac disease, hydrops, or both, combination antiarrhythmic drug therapy should be employed to achieve and maintain control of the cardiac rhythm.[79]

Cardioactive drugs other than digoxin that have been used to treat fetal arrhythmias are listed in Box 11–8. In many cases, successful fetal therapy has been described in most digoxin nonresponders with the addition of one of these agents. Caution must be exercised when some of these medications are coadministered with digoxin because of known drug-drug interactions that lead to accumulation of digoxin. The possible impact of the coadministration of some of the more important antiarrhythmic medications with digoxin on resultant steady-state serum digoxin concentrations is shown in Table 11–13.

Procainamide appears to be the most common

drug coadministered with digoxin in digoxin-unresponsive patients. This drug combination has been reported to be well tolerated by the mother and fetus and to treat the fetal arrhythmia successfully in a number of cases.[38, 81] The frequent selection of procainamide most likely reflects the successful use of this drug combination in treating nonfetal tachyarrhythmias.

More recent data indicate the efficacy of the calcium-channel blocking drugs verapamil[38, 53] and flecainide[3, 38, 66] and suggest their possible superiority to procainamide as a second-line therapy alone or in combination with digoxin.[58, 79] These encouraging data on verapamil and, especially, flecainide suggest that diltiazem, a calcium-channel blocker with minimal cardiac depressant activity, might also be useful for the treatment of fetal tachyarrhythmias.

With advances in direct fetal administration of medications (e.g., cordocentesis, intra-amniotic drug injection, and direct fetal intramuscular or intraperitoneal injections),[30, 95] adenosine may be a reasonable drug for use in certain patients with complicated cases.[58] Adenosine slows the sinus rate and decreases (blocks) atrioventricular nodal conduction. After bolus administration, the drug's pharmacologic effect is observed within 20 to 30 seconds and is very short-lived. Adenosine's elimination half-life is approximately 10 seconds. Although the drug has been very effective in successfully terminating SVT in most patients receiving it, its effects are short-lived. SVT will recur in many patients, requiring additional maintenance antiarrhythmic therapy. Ito and coworkers described one 28-week fetus with hydrops and incessant SVT who, despite failure of maternal procainamide therapy, initially responded to direct fetal injections of adenosine on two occasions.[38] The SVT recurred until spontaneous delivery of the infant. Hansmann and colleagues have described success with the direct fetal administration of digoxin alone or in combination.[36] The potential need for repeated direct fetal injections of adenosine severely limits its clinical utility. In patients whose cases are difficult to manage, adenosine might be a useful adjunct for termination of SVT with longer-acting antiarrhythmics maternally administered to maintain the improved fetal cardiac rhythm.[58, 79]

DEFECTS IN NEURAL TUBE DEVELOPMENT AND FOLIC ACID

Of the congenital malformations diagnosed at birth, many involve the neural tube. Although these congenital malformations may be associated with other congenital anomalies, they are usually isolated defects.[55] Surviving infants with neural tube defects consume substantial medical resources throughout their lifetimes. For these reasons, efforts have focused on determining the factors that predispose the conceptus to the development of neural tube defects so that effective preventive therapy can be developed. Unfortunately, no specific inciting event can be identified in many infants born with a neural tube defect. Nev-

TABLE 11–13 PROBABLE INFLUENCE OF COMMONLY COADMINISTERED ANTIARRHYTHMIC MEDICATIONS ON THE STEADY-STATE SERUM DIGOXIN CONCENTRATION*

COADMINISTERED MEDICATION	INCREASE IN TROUGH SERUM DIGOXIN CONCENTRATION* (%)
Quinidine	100–200
Amiodarone	50–100
Verapamil	20–60
Flecainide	10–20

*Data are presented as possible percentage increases in the steady-state trough serum digoxin concentration. The actual effect on serum digoxin concentration from these digoxin drug-drug interactions is highly variable, necessitating close monitoring.

Modified from Ito S, et al: Drug therapy for fetal arrhythmias. Clin Perinatol 21:543, 1994.

ertheless, a considerable amount of data have been amassed and demonstrate the efficacy of folic acid supplementation in preventing neural tube defects in a large number of cases. Because of the timing of neural tube development, periconceptional folic acid supplementation appears to be of utmost importance.

The neural tube begins to form from the neural plate by the third week after fertilization (see also Chapter 38, Part Two).[64] The neural plate develops infolds that form the neural groove, with neural folds on both sides. During the middle of the fourth week after fertilization, the neural folds begin to fuse, forming the neural tube. By the end of the fourth week of gestation, closure of the neural tube is complete, with openings at the cranial (rostral neuropore) and caudal (caudal neuropore) ends. The cranial portion of the neural tube forms the brain, and the caudal end develops into the spinal cord.[72] Defects arise from failure of the neural tube to close anywhere along the tube but most commonly at the caudal or cranial portions. Spina bifida is caused by nonfusion of the embryonic halves of the vertebral arches, leading to a condition of diverse presentations and varying severity.

The cause of many neural tube defects is unknown. Some data suggest a possible association between maternal use of phenytoin, carbamazepine, or valproic acid and neural tube defects. A possible relationship between folate deficiency and the development of neural tube defects is suggested by the apparent association of poor diet, inadequate vitamin supplementation, and the use of folic acid antagonists during pregnancy with an increased risk of neural tube defects.[72] It is interesting that no apparent association exists between maternal folate-deficient megaloblastic anemia and an increased risk of having an infant with a neural tube abnormality.[72] The long period that often is necessary to manifest microscopic signs of megaloblastic anemia may reflect its absence in early gestation.

A number of studies have assessed the efficacy of folic acid supplementation in reducing the risk and incidence of congenital neural tube defects. Regardless of the finding, considerable controversy has surrounded these results. Valid concerns have been raised about the methods used, such as study sample size, use and types of appropriate controls, adequate data collection systems, retrospective versus prospective study design, and use of multivitamin preparations in contrast to folic acid alone. Nevertheless, the published experience strongly suggests that periconceptional administration of folic acid substantially reduces the risk of congenital neural tube abnormalities overall, as well as the risk of recurrence in a later pregnancy. Reduction in the risk of recurrence is important because the incidence of neural tube defects may be as high as 20-fold greater in women with a previous pregnancy resulting in the birth of an infant with a neural tube defect than in the general population (20 cases per 1000 live births versus an estimated prevalence rate in the general U.S. population of 1.3 cases per 1000 live births).[72] It is important to note that any effect of periconceptional folic acid

supplementation must be realized by the fourth week of gestation, at which time neural tube closure is complete. Folic acid supplementation after neural tube closure has no effect on the incidence or severity of congenital neural tube defects.

The maternal doses of folic acid that have been used to prevent the development of neural tube defects have varied. For the most part, folic acid doses have ranged from 0.4 to 4 mg daily. The evidence supports a dose between 0.4 and 0.8 mg per day to prevent folate-susceptible abnormalities. As stated earlier, folic acid therapy must be started as soon after conception as possible, if not before conception (e.g., planned pregnancy), and continued for at least 4 weeks of gestation. In late 1995, the U.S. Food and Drug Administration proposed folic acid enrichment of fortified grain products. The exact dose had not been determined, but the precise level of fortification was to exceed 140 µg per 100 gm of grain product, eliminating most neural tube defects.

ACCESS TO THE FETUS AND FETAL COMPARTMENT: DIRECT MANIPULATION

Advances in technology have greatly expanded opportunities to treat fetal disorders by guiding direct access to the fetus or the fetal compartment. Case reports have described successful in utero drug therapy by direct intraperitoneal injection into the amniotic fluid and by direct IM and IV drug administration to the fetus.[36] Weiner and coworkers described a fetus with SVT who did not respond to maternal digoxin administration but did respond to multiple IM injections of the drug.[95] Similarly, Gembruch and colleagues have successfully treated SVT with fetal IV digoxin administration.[30] Animal data assessing the clinical efficacy of intra-amniotic administration of surfactant to prevent RDS are encouraging. Nevertheless, these approaches to fetal drug therapy should be considered only when maternal therapy is not possible or is unsuccessful, because experience with the direct fetal administration of drugs is limited.

Questions remain regarding this approach to drug administration, including drug-dosing guidelines and associated risks such as in utero infection and the precipitation of premature labor. Assessment of drug dose is extremely difficult and, at present, empirical. Until more experience is acquired with this mode of fetal drug therapy, the dose for an IV, IM, or IP injection should be based on the weight of the fetus estimated with ultrasound and gestational age calculations. The drug dose administered would be the same dose per unit of body weight that is administered to infants of similar gestational ages.

Similarly, for intra-amniotic drug administration, the volume of amniotic fluid present could be estimated by ultrasound and used as a component of a fetal "volume of distribution" calculation, which, in turn, could be employed to calculate a dose required to achieve a target fetal drug concentration. Finally, once direct fetal drug therapy is instituted, elimination of the drug through the maternal circulation must also be taken into account. It may be necessary to provide some maternal drug dosing to retain an adequate drug concentration in the fetal compartment. Obviously, these approaches to fetal drug administration are only initial guidelines, and they require close fetal monitoring for efficacy and safety. The accuracy of achieving target drug concentrations in the fetus could be assessed by direct fetal blood sampling,[93] whereas overall efficacy is determined by critical clinical assessment for the desired pharmacologic effect.

THE FUTURE: FETAL GENE THERAPY

Most inherited disorders would benefit from therapeutic intervention as early as possible in life to prevent disease expression. Ideally, prevention could be achieved with gene therapy early in pregnancy. In theory, such therapy even during the last two trimesters of pregnancy could allow targeting of still-expanding stem cell populations that may no longer be accessible later in life.

To date, a limited number of studies have used viral vectors to direct fetal gene incorporation. All studies have been in animals, and the results are evolving.[98] Difficulties have been encountered in targeting specific genes to specific organs and determining the optimal time points for vector delivery. There is also concern that current strategies, which are aimed at somatic cells, provide insufficient safeguards against genelike transfection. Flake and associates described the successful treatment of a fetus with X-linked severe, combined immunodeficiency by in utero transplantation of paternal bone marrow.[26]

Thus, fetal gene therapy is an approach on the horizon. Though it appears to be poised for human trials, some important clinical and ethical issues remain to be resolved. When this technology is applied to human genetic disease, a vast new frontier in medicine will be opened.[98] It is hoped that our technologic capabilities will not exceed our ability to handle their consequences.

part two
SURGICAL TREATMENT OF THE FETUS

Timothy M. Crombleholme

As prenatal diagnosis has become increasingly sophisticated and as technologic advances have enhanced the range of diagnostic capabilities, invasive therapies have developed from our expanded under-

standing of the natural history and pathophysiology of structural anomalies.[102, 169] In the 1960s and 1970s, despite rapid progress in prenatal diagnosis, few invasive therapies were considered, much less employed.[100] Once a prenatal diagnosis was made, parents had only two choices: terminating pregnancy, if prior to 24 weeks, or continuing to term.[192] An additional option that was soon recognized was altering the delivery site so that appropriate pediatric specialists would be available immediately to treat the newborn with a congenital anomaly. As the natural history of many prenatally diagnosed anomalies became better understood, early delivery was recognized as an option to avoid ongoing damage caused by the anomaly in utero.[102] Fortunately, today there are more alternatives. In this chapter we present a comprehensive review of the treatment options currently available for the entire spectrum of fetal diagnoses that are potentially surgically correctable. The current indications, contraindications, and outcomes for shunting procedures, fetoscopic surgery, and open fetal surgery are reviewed.

FETAL SHUNTING PROCEDURES

A new era in invasive fetal therapy began in the early 1980s when several independent groups introduced shunting procedures for hydrocephalus and hydronephrosis.[135, 167, 175] These first few cases represented an extension of invasive fetal therapy from simple intrauterine blood transfusion for a medical illness to the first attempts at in utero treatment of structural anomalies.

During this period, hydronephrosis and hydrocephalus were recognized more frequently with ultrasound examination. The prenatal natural history of these lesions was established by serial sonographic observation of untreated cases.* Fetuses with high-grade obstructive uropathy followed to term were often born with advanced hydronephrosis, type IV cystic dysplasia, and pulmonary hypoplasia, conditions that were incompatible with life.[129, 145, 253] In the case of obstructive hydrocephalus, it was known that shunting in the newborn period improved neurologic outcome, and it was reasoned that decompression in utero might avert progressive brain damage.[218, 224, 292] At the time, the understanding of the natural history, pathophysiology, and patient selection criteria was rudimentary and incomplete at best. However, experimental work by numerous investigators, in appropriate animal models, helped to define the pathophysiology of these lesions and establish the theoretical basis for intervention.†

VENTRICULOAMNIOTIC SHUNTS

Among the most important lessons learned in invasive fetal therapy were the necessity to understand

---

*References 129, 131, 136, 143, 171, 245.
†References 107, 170, 172, 173, 187, 190, 236.

the natural history of the untreated condition and the ability to identify fetuses most likely to benefit from treatment. Based on the observation that postnatal shunting for hydrocephalus is beneficial, Birnholz and Frigoletto reported using serial percutaneous cephalocentesis to treat hydrocephalus in utero.[120] The results of their efforts were disappointing because the fetus had unrecognized intracranial abnormalities and Becker type muscular dystrophy. Shortly thereafter, ventriculoamniotic shunts were developed to provide consistent ventricular decompression.[135, 167] Although these procedures enjoyed a brief period of enthusiasm, results proved to be poor, often being related to undetected central nervous system (CNS) and non-CNS anomalies, and the shunts failed to provide consistent ventricular decompression because of obstruction or migration.[134, 228]

The fetus that is likely to benefit from ventriculoamniotic shunting is one with isolated progressive ventriculomegaly.* However, the incidence of associated CNS anomalies in reported series has varied from 70% to 84%, with many of these defects being undetected prenatally.† Previous studies list the incidence of isolated progressive ventriculomegaly from 0% to 56%, with most reports listing the incidence as only between 4% and 14%.‡ Even with improved diagnostic capabilities, identifying appropriate fetal intervention may be difficult.

If ventriculoamniotic shunting is to be reinstated, selection criteria must first be defined. These criteria would include fetuses with isolated progressive ventriculomegaly; accurate exclusion of other CNS and extra-CNS anomalies; and development of a valved shunt less likely to clog, become dislodged, or cause ventriculitis than previous versions.

THORACOAMNIOTIC SHUNTS

Thoracoamniotic shunting is the treatment of choice for management of the fetus with symptomatic fetal hydrothorax (FHT) before 32 weeks of gestation (Fig. 11–5). In contrast, thoracentesis is a diagnostic maneuver performed to obtain pleural fluid for differential cell count and culture and to establish whether the effusion is chylous. Even repeated thoracentesis provides inadequate decompression of the fetal chest. There have been several reports of thoracentesis for FHT performed with either complete resolution or a good outcome despite reaccumulation.[118, 214, 250] Others have had disappointing results with repeated thoracentesis for FHT, owing to rapid reaccumulation of the effusion and neonatal death from respiratory insufficiency.[223, 247] Spontaneous resolution of FHT may occur in as many as 10% of cases, and resolution following thoracentesis may or may not be related to the procedure. Thoracentesis alone cannot adequately decompress the fetal chest to allow pulmonary expansion and prevent pulmonary hypoplasia.[215]

---

*References 131, 134, 137, 205, 228, 254, 268, 276.
†References 131, 134, 137, 204, 205, 228, 254, 268, 276.
‡References 137, 204, 205, 219, 268, 276.

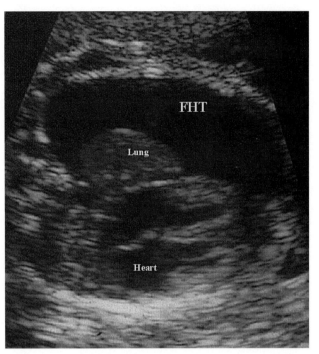

FIGURE 11–5. Fetal sonogram demonstrating larger tension fetal hydrothorax (FHT) compressing the adjacent lung and causing shift of the heart into the contralateral hemithorax. (From Shaaban AF, et al: The role of ultrasonography in fetal surgery and invasive fetal procedures. Semin Roentgen 34:62, 1999.)

Thoracoamniotic shunting for FHT, first reported by Rodeck and colleagues in 1988, provides continuous decompression of the fetal chest, allowing lung expansion.[265] If instituted early enough, this procedure allows compensatory lung growth and prevents neonatal death from pulmonary hypoplasia.

The indications for thoracoamniotic shunting are not well defined. Most authors consider the presence of FHT-induced hydrops or polyhydramnios as indications for shunting.[177, 223, 247, 265] In addition, we recommend thoracoamniotic shunting for primary FHT with evidence of effusion under tension even in the absence of hydrops (Fig. 11–6).[240] Because spontaneous resolution has been observed in even severe cases of FHT, we reserve thoracoamniotic shunting for cases in which tension hydrothorax recurs after two thoracenteses.

Thoracoamniotic shunts have also been used in the treatment of congenital cystic adenomatoid malformation (CCAM) of the lung with a dominant cyst (see also Chapter 42). Nicolaides and associates reported the first case of CCAM treated by shunt insertion in utero in 1987.[248] Decompression of a large type I CCAM in a fetus of 20 weeks' gestation by percutaneous placement of a thoracoamniotic shunt was subsequently reported by Clark in 1987.[133] This procedure resulted in resolution of both mediastinal shift and hydrops and successful delivery at 37 weeks of gestation. Postnatally, the infant underwent uneventful resection of the CCAM. Six subsequent cases of thoracoamniotic shunting in CCAM have been reported by Adzick and coworkers, with a good out-

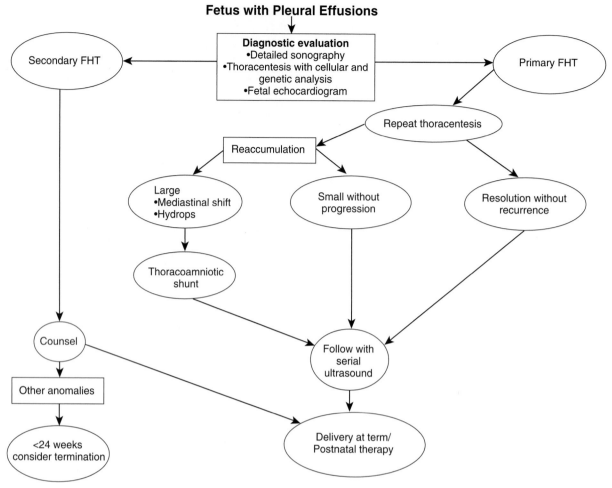

FIGURE 11–6. Proposed algorithm for the management of fetal hydrothorax.

come in five of the six fetuses treated.[101, 106] These cases are unusual for CCAM, because they were large cysts resulting in hydrops. More commonly, it is the type III CCAM, or microcystic lesions that become enlarged, resulting in hydrops and intrauterine fetal demise. In these later cases open fetal surgery and resection are indicated. However, in the rare instances in which there is a single large cyst in CCAM responsible for hydrops, thoracoamniotic shunting appears to be an appropriate treatment option.

VESICOAMNIOTIC SHUNTS

The first case of a fetus with obstructive uropathy treated in utero by vesicoamniotic shunting was reported by Golbus and associates in 1982.[174] Advances soon followed in diagnosis, technique, shunt design, and patient selection.* The procedure became widely implemented before stringent selection criteria for treatment were developed and therapeutic efficacy of the procedure was established. The widespread use of vesicoamniotic shunts also had the effect of shifting cases away from centers studying these questions and

*References 142–144, 157, 181, 188, 191, 202, 209, 245, 262, 267.

limiting attempts to better define the role of vesicoamniotic shunting in the management of fetal obstructive uropathy. A detailed discussion of vesicoamniotic shunting appears later (see "Prenatal Treatment" in the "Obstructive Uropathy" section).

OPEN FETAL SURGERY

Experience has demonstrated the usefulness of shunting procedures in some fetal conditions, but the limitations of these catheters have also become apparent. In addition to their problems with obstruction, dislodgment, and short functional life span, shunting procedures are not adequate for many conditions. The experience with open fetal surgery in the 1960s for the treatment of erythroblastosis fetalis was discouraging, and it was soon abandoned with the introduction of percutaneous techniques of fetal transfusion.[116, 165, 221] Harrison and colleagues introduced open fetal surgery for the treatment of obstructive uropathy in 1982.[189] Although the procedure (bilateral ureterostomy) was technically successful, the fetus made no urine, oligohydramnios persisted, and the infant died of pulmonary hypoplasia. Despite this initial unsuccessful result, a new era in fetal therapy was opened. Soon, successful open surgical procedures were reported in the treatment of obstructive uropathy,[143] congenital diaphragmatic hernia,[185, 194] cystic adenomatoid malformation,[106, 182] and sacrococcygeal teratoma (Table 11–14).[108] An appreciation of the fetal natural history of these conditions and the success of Harrison's group at the University of California at San Francisco encouraged groups in Philadelphia, Boston, Denver, Memphis, and Detroit in the United States as well as Seoul, Korea, Melbourne, Australia, and Paris, France, to undertake open fetal surgery.

Clinical experience is still quite limited, however, with just over 200 cases of open fetal surgery performed worldwide.

OBSTRUCTIVE UROPATHY

Posterior urethral valves (PUVs) are the leading cause of antenatally diagnosed lower urinary tract obstruction and are the structural genitourinary anomaly amenable to fetal therapy. PUVs are found only in the male population and have an incidence of 1 in 5000 births.[129] The mortality rate in these patients has been

TABLE 11–14 TREATABLE FETAL MALFORMATIONS

FETAL MALFORMATION	FETAL PRESENTATION	FETAL/NEONATAL CONSEQUENCE	FETAL TREATMENT OPTIONS
Amniotic band syndrome	Edematous limb from constricting band Umbilical cord constriction	Limb amputation Fetal death	Fetoscopic laser lysis of bands
Aqueductal stenosis	Rapidly progressive isolated hydrocephalus	Neurologic damage	Ventriculoamniotic shunt Ventriculoperitoneal shunt
Acardiac/acephalic twin (TRAP sequence)	Polyhydramnios	IUFD, hydrops, cardiac failure Multifocal leukoencephalomalacia	Fetoscopic cord ligation Fetoscopic cord coagulation
Complete heart block	Hydrops, slow heart rate	IUFD, neonatal death	Fetal epicardial pacemaker
Congenital diaphragmatic hernia (CDH)	Herniated viscera in chest	IUFD, pulmonary hypoplasia and respiratory insufficiency, neonatal death	Open fetal tracheal clip Fetoscopic tracheal clip Fetoscopic tracheal balloon
Cystic adenomatoid malformation of the lung (CCAM)	Chest mass, mediastinal shift Hydrops	Pulmonary hypoplasia, IUFD, neonatal death	Thoracoamniotic shunt (if there is dominant cyst) Fetal resection of CCAM (if it is solid tumor)
Fetal hydrothorax (FHT)	Mediastinal shift, hydrops, polyhydramnios	Pulmonary hypoplasia	Thoracoamniotic shunt
Myelomeningocele (MMC)	Neural tube defect, "lemon" sign, "banana" sign	Paralysis, hindbrain herniation Hydrocephalus	Open fetal MMC repair
Neck masses (cervical teratoma, lymphangioma)	Polyhydramnios, neck mass, absent stomach bubble	Inability to ventilate due to lack of airway Anoxic brain injury, neonatal death	EXIT procedure
Ovarian cyst	Wandering cystic abdominal mass	Ovarian torsion, polyhydramnios	Cyst aspiration
Posterior urethral valves	Hydronephrosis and oligohydramnios	Renal dysplasia and renal insufficiency Pulmonary hypoplasia and respiratory insufficiency	Vesicoamniotic shunt Cystoscopic laser ablation of valves Open vesicostomy
Sacrococcygeal teratoma (SCT)	High output failure Hydrops	IUFD, prematurity, tumor rupture, hydrops, hemorrhage	Open resection Radiofrequency coagulation
Twin-twin transfusion syndrome (TTTS)	Oligohydramnios and polyhydramnios, growth discordance	IUFD, heart failure Multifocal leukoencephalomalacia	Serial amnioreduction Microseptostomy Cord coagulation Selective laser photocoagulation

EXIT, ex utero intrapartum treatment; IUFD, intrauterine fetal death; TRAP, twin reversed arterial perfusion.

reported to be as high as 63%, especially when it is associated with severe oligohydramnios owing to pulmonary hypoplasia. (See also Chapter 49.)

The natural history and outcome of antenatally diagnosed obstructive uropathy differ significantly from those of postnatally diagnosed obstruction. Early reports of postnatally diagnosed obstructive uropathy did not appreciate the significance of respiratory difficulties in these patients. Subsequent reports of PUVs diagnosed at birth reveal a significant mortality associated with respiratory and renal insufficiency.[245] Oligohydramnios occurring before 24 weeks of gestation profoundly affects the fetal lung development during the critical transition from the canalicular to the alveolar phase of lung development. Profound oligohydramnios owing to PUV is also associated with clubfoot and Potter facies, and there is a 9% incidence of chromosomal anomalies in obstructive uropathy.[262]

Prenatal Diagnosis

The major diagnostic tool in obstructive uropathy remains antenatal ultrasonography.[129, 193, 203] With current techniques, fetal ultrasonography may detect urinary tract anomalies as early as 12 to 13 weeks of gestation.

The prenatal diagnosis of obstructive uropathy requires an understanding of physiologic and pathologic dilatation of the urinary tract. Hydronephrosis is the most common pathologic finding on prenatal ultrasonography in cases of fetal obstructive uropathy. The discovery of echogenic kidneys with pronounced cystic dysplasia is an ominous finding, universally associated with a poor overall prognosis. However, with less severe pathology, distinguishing pathologic dilatation of the renal pelvis (pelviectasis) from physiologic dilatation is difficult, especially early in pregnancy. Transient dilatation of the fetal urinary tract is a relatively common finding, occurring in 1 out of every 100 pregnancies. This frequency is far more common than that of pathologic obstruction, as found on postnatal evaluation and autopsies.

Measurements of the anteroposterior (AP) pelvic diameter and its ratio to the overall AP renal diameter have been proposed as criteria for discriminating between normal and abnormal pelvic dilatation.[114] In fetuses younger than 20 weeks' gestation, the parameters of abnormal pelvic distention have not been defined. A recent prospective study correlating screening ultrasonography in patients 16 to 23 weeks' gestation with postnatal outcome revealed that a pelvic diameter greater than 4 mm was 76% sensitive in identifying a pathologic obstruction.[113] Furthermore, fetuses with a urinary tract obstruction demonstrated a more rapid increase in this dilatation over the remainder of gestation than did fetuses without obstruction. For fetuses older than 23 weeks' gestation, threshold values associated with pathologic fetal hydronephrosis are an AP pelvic diameter greater than 10 mm and an AP pelvic–to–AP renal diameter ratio

greater than 0.5. The additional finding of caliectasis provides even stronger support to a pathologic etiology (Fig. 11–7A).[212] If any of these criteria are met, the patient should undergo further sonographic assessment and a full prognostic profile, including sequential taps of the fetal bladder for urinary electrolyte determination if oligohydramnios develops in a case of suspected bladder outlet obstruction.

Lower urinary tract obstruction must be distinguished from the other pathologic causes of fetal hydronephrosis. The presence of megacystis, thickened bladder wall, posterior urethral dilatation, bilateral hydronephrosis, and ureterectasis characterizes the changes associated with PUV (see Fig. 11–7B) and urethral atresia in contrast to the more common ureteropelvic junction obstruction, ureterovesical obstruction, and vesicoureteral reflux. These cases of lower urinary tract obstruction lead to oligohydramnios, as urinary output is the major component of amniotic fluid in the third trimester. In contrast, a unilateral obstruction, such as a ureteropelvic junction obstruction, does not lead to oligohydramnios, and it carries a universally favorable prognosis provided that the other kidney functions normally.[145]

Among cases of fetal urinary tract obstruction, a fetus with preserved renal function produces more hypotonic urine, whereas one with advanced renal dysfunction is a "salt waster," producing less hypotonic urine. The usefulness of assessing urine chemistry in fetal obstructive uropathy lies in the separation of fetuses into "good" or "poor" prognostic categories based on preservation of renal function reflected by the tonicity of the fetal urine.[144] In one study, urine samples taken from fetuses who subsequently had a good outcome revealed levels of Na^+ less than 100 mEq/L, Cl^- less than 90 mEq/L, and osmolarity less than 210 mOsm/L.[172] These values were chosen because they were two standard deviations from the mean values of fetuses with a good prognosis. Fetuses with urine chemistries beyond these values had irreversible renal damage and suffered from severe oligohydramnios and pulmonary insufficiency. The efficacy of these proposed criteria were subsequently confirmed to reflect postnatal outcome and appropriately select fetuses for intervention.[144] In a separate study, this approach was modified to include three sequential vesicocentesis at 24-hour intervals. This regimen permits a comparative analysis of stagnant urine (first sample) with fresh urine (third sample). Fresh urine samples more accurately reflect fetal renal function, and this approach increases the predictive value of fetal urinary electrolytes.[244]

Urinary β_2-microglobulin levels have become an important adjuvant in predicting the severity of renal damage. In one study, β_2-microglobulin levels below 2 mg/L were found to have as good a predictive value as urinary sodium levels below 70 mEq/L.[157] Furthermore, urinary β_2-microglobulin levels may have greater value in predicting the outcome of fetal obstructive uropathy in the absence of oligohydramnios. In one study, β_2-microglobulin levels from fetuses with evidence of obstructive uropathy but with-

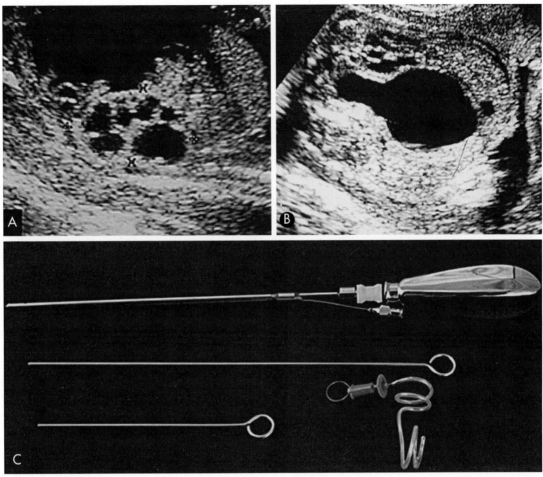

FIGURE 11–7. *A,* Fetal sonogram demonstrating hydronephrosis with caliceal dilatation owing to posterior urethral valves. *B,* Obstructed bladder outlet demonstrating the "keyhole" sign owing to posterior urethral valves. *C,* Standard trocar and Rocket catheter for fetal shunting procedures. (From Shaaban AF, et al: The role of ultrasonography in fetal surgery and invasive fetal procedures. Semin Roentgen 34:62, 1999.)

out oligohydramnios were significantly higher in those who eventually developed renal insufficiency at 1 year of age.[138] This distinguishing feature may enable the selective antenatal treatment of fetuses with a good prognostic profile who, despite normal amniotic fluid volume, are still at risk for ongoing renal damage.

Prenatal Treatment

The two goals of prenatal intervention in fetal obstructive uropathy are decompression of the obstructed fetal urinary bladder and restoration of amniotic fluid dynamics. Percutaneous vesicoamniotic shunting has been the most common technique used to accomplish these goals with minimal maternal morbidity in patients with isolated lower urinary tract obstruction and a good prognostic profile* (see Fig. 11–7C).

Because of the lack of a prospective, randomized trial, the most difficult question to address in the treatment of fetal obstructive uropathy is the efficacy

_____

*References 138, 144, 166, 172, 208, 228, 244.

of prenatal decompression. The only series that attempted to address this question, albeit in a retrospective analysis, was reported by Crombleholme and coworkers.[144] In fetuses predicted to have either good or poor prognoses by fetal urine electrolyte and ultrasound criteria, the survival rate was greater among those decompressed in utero, as opposed to those who were not decompressed. In the group of fetuses predicted to have a poor prognosis by selection criteria, 10 fetuses were treated. Three of those fetuses were electively terminated, four neonates died from pulmonary hypoplasia or renal dysplasia, and three neonates survived. All three survivors had restoration of normal amniotic fluid levels and no pulmonary complications, but two subsequently developed renal failure and underwent renal transplantation. Among the 14 patients with no intervention, there were no survivors (11 terminations and three neonatal deaths from pulmonary hypoplasia).

In the group of fetuses predicted to have a good prognosis by selection criteria, nine fetuses were treated, with one elective termination (after the development of procedure-related chorioamnionitis), no deaths, and eight neonatal survivors. Of the seven patients in the good prognosis group who were not treated, five survived and two died after birth. Two of the survivors later developed renal failure.

When oligohydramnios develops during the canalicular stage of lung development (16 to 24 weeks), the fetus usually has pulmonary hypoplasia that precludes survival.* When in utero intervention for obstructive uropathy associated with oligohydramnios restores amniotic fluid volume, neonatal demise from pulmonary hypoplasia is clearly averted.[144, 174] In the group of fetuses reported by Crombleholme and coworkers, there was a preponderance of oligohydramnios in the poor prognosis group (23 of 24) compared with the good prognosis group (7 of 16).[144] Despite this, fetuses from the good prognosis group seemed to survive as a direct result of fetal treatment. In the good prognosis group, six of the seven fetuses with oligohydramnios had intervention, and all six survived with normal renal function. However, the patient with oligohydramnios who was not treated died at birth of pulmonary hypoplasia. In the entire series, uncorrected oligohydramnios was associated with a 100% neonatal mortality rate. Normal or restored amniotic fluid volume was associated with a 94% survival rate.[144]

Although in utero decompression appears to prevent neonatal death from pulmonary hypoplasia, the effect of in utero decompression on renal function is less clear. The maternal morbidity of vesicoamniotic shunting has been reported to be minimal, but there has been a high incidence (14%) of associated chorioamnionitis.[144, 172] These cases of chorioamnionitis occurred before routine use of prophylactic antibiotics and during a period when long-term (4 to 16 hours) bladder catheterization, rather than aspiration, was used for fetal urine sampling. In addition, there have been reports of shunt-induced abdominal wall defects with herniation of bowel through trocar stab wounds and maternal ascites from leakage of amniotic fluid into the maternal peritoneal cavity.[228, 262, 267]

The usefulness of vesicoamniotic shunts is limited by brief duration of decompression, risk of infection, catheter obstruction or dislodgment, fetal injury during placement, and potentially inadequate decompression of the fetal urinary tract.[144, 145, 157, 172] These factors make vesicoamniotic shunts inappropriate for long-term decompression of the urinary tract early in gestation, and they are catalysts for development of open fetal surgical and fetoscopic techniques to treat obstructive uropathy in utero.[145, 157]

Dissatisfaction with catheter decompression led Harrison and colleagues to perform a small series of open fetal procedures for PUVs, initially bilateral ureterostomies, and, subsequently, open vesicostomy.[143, 189] Open vesicostomy is certainly the most definitive compression of the urinary tract. However, there are increased maternal risks with this approach. These issues have led some investigators to pursue percutaneous fetal cystoscopy and fulguration or la-

ser ablation of PUVs.[257, 258] Although this technique appears to be technically feasible, there have been no survivors in the initial experience.

Currently, once the diagnosis and favorable prognostic profile are confirmed, we recommend percutaneous vesicoamniotic shunting for fetal lower urinary tract obstruction. Fetoscopic cystoscopy is performed to assess the posterior urethra to determine if the fetus is a candidate for laser ablation of valves. Those who are not candidates for laser ablation have a vesicoamniotic shunt placed. Vesicostomy is reserved for cases in which vesicoamniotic shunting fails to decompress the bladder and restore amniotic fluid dynamics. Experienced ultrasound guidance is essential in vesicoamniotic shunt placement. Furthermore, serial sonography is critical to confirm sustained shunt function, good bladder drainage, decompression of the upper urinary tracts, and normalization of amniotic fluid volume.

CONGENITAL DIAPHRAGMATIC HERNIA

(See also Chapter 42, Parts Five and Eight.)

Congenital diaphragmatic hernia (CDH) is most often a posterolateral defect in the left hemidiaphragm (88%) on one side, which leads to herniation of the viscera into the thorax, resulting in pulmonary hypoplasia and respiratory embarrassment. CDH occurs in approximately 1 in 2500 to 5000 live births and as frequently as 1 in 2200 prenatal ultrasound studies.[103] This discrepancy between neonates who survive birth and transport to a tertiary newborn treatment center and fetuses diagnosed by prenatal ultrasonography supports the notion of a "hidden" mortality.[103, 104, 183] With inclusion of cases that never reach the treatment stage of disease, the mortality approaches 75%.[183] Although familial cases with an autosomal-dominant inheritance have been reported, most cases of CDH are sporadic.[141, 240]

Associated anomalies are seen in 25% to 57% of all cases of CDH and 95% of stillborns and include congenital heart defects, hydronephrosis, renal agenesis, intestinal atresia, extralobar sequestrations, and neurologic defects, including hydrocephalus, anencephaly, and spina bifida.[160, 255] Chromosomal anomalies, including trisomy 21, 18, and 13, occur in association with CDH in 10% to 20% of cases that are diagnosed prenatally.

Prenatal Diagnosis

The diagnosis of CDH is often an unexpected finding on routine prenatal ultrasound examination or a scan prompted by polyhydramnios. Critical ultrasound findings include the presence of viscera in the right or the left hemithorax above the level of the inferior margin of the scapula or at the level of the four-chamber view of the heart (Fig. 11–8A).[122, 232] The hypoechoic signal of the fluid-filled stomach, gallbladder, and bowel can be distinguished from the hyperechoic signal of the fetal lung. A small ipsilateral lung, a defect in the ipsilateral diaphragm, and a

---

*References 107, 187, 188, 191, 202, 245.

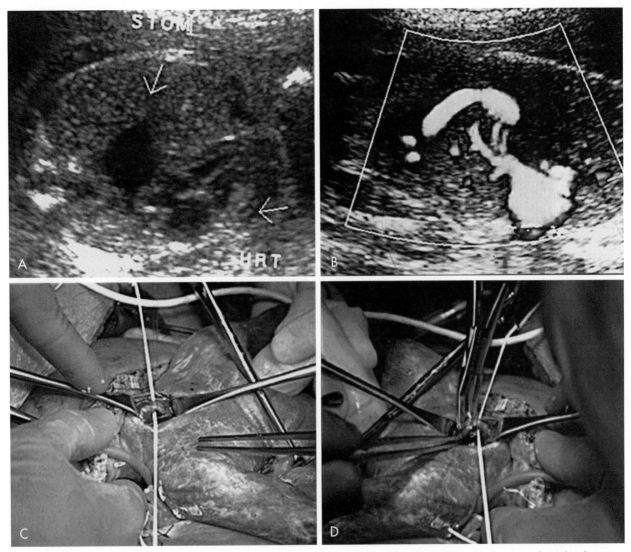

FIGURE 11–8. *A,* Fetal sonogram demonstrating a large congenital diaphragmatic hernia (CDH), with the stomach in the chest seen at the level of the four-chamber view of the heart. *B,* Power Doppler image demonstrating bowing of the sinus venosus toward the left in left CDH. *C,* Exposure of the fetal trachea during tracheal clip application. *D,* Application of fetal tracheal clip. (From Shaaban AF, et al: The role of ultrasonography in fetal surgery and invasive fetal procedures. Semin Roentgen 34:62, 1999.)

shift of the mediastinum away from the affected side are other common findings. In the case of a right-sided CDH, the liver is usually the only herniated organ, and it is difficult to distinguish it from the fetal lung because of their similar echodensities. Identification of the diaphragm does not exclude the possibility of CDH because some portion of the diaphragm is usually present in CDH.

The differential diagnosis includes type I CCAM, bronchogenic cysts, neurenteric cysts, and cystic mediastinal teratoma, which may mimic the appearance of a herniated bowel. Identification of abnormal upper abdominal anatomy and presence of peristalsis in herniated bowel loops helps distinguish CDH from other diagnoses. The location of the gallbladder in fetuses with CDH is helpful because it may be displaced to the midline or in the left upper quadrant or herniated into the right chest.[180]

In most severe cases, the liver and the stomach are present in the thorax. Bowing of the portal vein or sinus venosus to the left of the midline or coursing of the portal branches to the lateral segment of the left lobe of the liver above the diaphragm can be seen with color flow Doppler imaging and is the best sonographic predictor of liver herniation (see Fig. 11–8B).[122, 123, 184] In addition, the position of the stomach (easily seen in contrast to the more echogenic fetal lung) in a posterior or midthoracic location is also associated with liver herniation. Several sonographic features have been suggested as prognostic indications in CDH, including polyhydramnios, early gestation diagnosis (less than 24 weeks), stomach herniation, herniation of the left lobe of the liver, and evidence of fetal cardiac ventricular disproportion before 24 weeks of gestation.[163] However, no sonographic features of CDH have been uniformly helpful in predicting outcome. A more direct estimate of pulmonary hypoplasia is needed.

Currently, lung area–to–head circumference ratio (LHR) (two-dimensional area of right lung measured at the level of the four-chamber view of the heart), is being assessed prospectively to determine its value in predicting the postnatal outcome with conventional therapy. In the selection of fetuses with an LHR greater than 1.4, only 25% of fetuses in this group required extracorporeal membrane oxygenation (ECMO). However, no fetus with an LHR less than 1.0 survived, despite the use of ECMO. Fetuses with an LHR between 1.0 and 1.4 had a 38% rate of survival, with 75% requiring ECMO.[222] These findings suggest that an affected fetus with an LHR less than 1.4 has a poor chance for survival despite optimal postnatal management. Conversely, a fetus with an LHR greater than 1.4 would be expected to have a universally favorable outcome with conventional postnatal therapy. The current selection criteria for the fetal tracheal clip procedure in CDH at The Children's Hospital of Philadelphia are more stringent, including an isolated defect associated with liver herniation and an LHR of 1.0 (Fig. 11–9).

Prenatal Treatment

Despite the advances in neonatal care, such as high-frequency oscillatory ventilation, inhaled nitric oxide, and ECMO, the mortality rate of isolated CDH remains 60%. Out of frustration with these grim statistics, Harrison and colleagues pioneered fetal surgery for CDH.[184–186] Unfortunately, survival following complete in utero repair was poor. These failures were due to herniation of the left lobe of the liver. Reduction of the liver during repair inevitably resulted in kinking of the umbilical vein, leading to fetal bradycardia and cardiac arrest. Herniation of the left lobe of the liver became an exclusion criterion for complete in utero repair of CDH. However, even if cases with left lobe herniation are excluded, the survival rate in the series by Harrison and colleagues was only 41%, which is no better than with conventional postnatal therapy. A prospective trial sponsored by the National Institutes of Health confirmed these findings; thus, there is currently no indication for complete repair of CDH in utero. The shortcomings of in utero repair led to development of a new approach.

Known for decades, fetal tracheal occlusion results in accelerated fetal lung growth in animal models.[110] It was not until 1994, however, that tracheal occlusion was applied to the problem of CDH.[151] In the animal CDH models, tracheal occlusion can induce lung growth, increased alveolar surface area and alveolar number, as well as visceral reduction from the chest.[151, 195, 199, 280] The results of these experiments were so compelling that fetal tracheal occlusion was applied in human fetuses with severe CDH. Subsequently, a procedure was described using transuterine laparoscopy or *Fetendo*.[280, 285, 286] Definitive short- and long-term outcomes following these procedures are still pending. We are currently performing the fetal

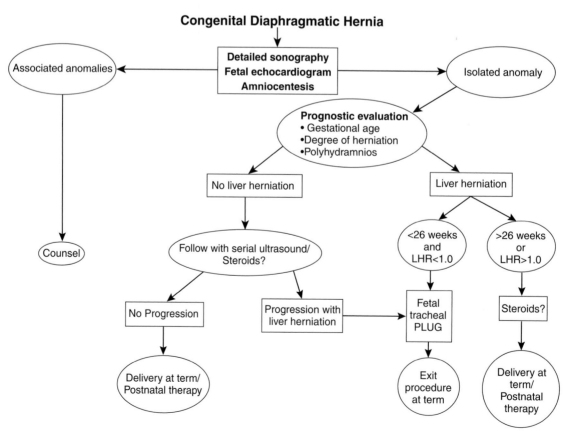

FIGURE 11–9. Proposed algorithm for the management of fetal congenital diaphragmatic hernia.

tracheal clip procedure in cases of isolated CDH before 26 weeks of gestation with liver herniation and an LHR less than 1.0. This procedure is performed through a small hysterotomy to expose the fetal neck and chest.

An incision is made just cephalic to the sternal notch to expose the trachea, which is meticulously dissected to avoid injury to the recurrent laryngeal nerves (see Fig. 11–8C, D). A hemoclip is then applied transversely across the trachea. The fetal neck incision and hysterotomy are then closed, and tocolytic agents are started.

Continuous tocolysis (with indomethacin or magnesium sulfate), aggressive pain control in the mother, daily ultrasonography, echocardiography, and maternal and fetal monitoring make up the foundation of the postoperative care plan. The most important modality to assess the fetus postoperatively is ultrasonography. The immediate postoperative concerns are the adequacy of amniotic fluid volume and the presence or absence of extra-amniotic clot at the site of hysterotomy closure. The patency of the ductus arteriosus is assessed daily by echocardiogram while the mother is on indomethacin therapy. During the maternal convalescence, fetal ultrasonography should be performed at least weekly to assess the physiologic effect of rising intrathoracic pressure resulting from growth of the pressurized lung. Serial LHR determinations reveal progressive rise in values as a result of tracheal occlusion. This effect can be quite dramatic in some patients, with increases in LHR from 0.6 to 5.5 over a period of 3 weeks. This situation can lead to cardiac compromise and fetal hydrops, mandating early delivery by ex utero intrapartum treatment (EXIT) procedure.[176] Otherwise, the fetus may be monitored until a planned EXIT procedure with removal of the tracheal clips can be performed near term.

CONGENITAL CYSTIC ADENOMATOID MALFORMATION

(See also Chapter 42, Part Five.)

CCAM is a rare pulmonary maldevelopment that is usually restricted to one lobe of the lung. Grossly, CCAM represents a multicystic mass of pulmonary tissue with proliferation of bronchial structures.[130, 281] These lesions may result from a failure of maturation of bronchiolar structures or focal pulmonary dysplasia arising in the fifth or sixth week of gestation. Histologic studies reveal rapid vascular and epithelial growth within the tumor.[130, 281] Recent findings of accelerated cellular proliferation and decreased apoptosis within resected CCAM specimens further suggest a benign neoplastic development.

CCAM is a rare anomaly that occurs slightly more often in the male population than in the female population. These lesions are almost always unilateral (85% to 95%), but occasionally they arise bilaterally (2%).[240] Associated anomalies include renal agenesis or dysgenesis, truncus arteriosus, tetralogy of Fallot, jejunal atresia, CDH, hydrocephalus, and skeletal anomalies. Approximately 6% of prenatally diagnosed CCAMs resolve spontaneously, but resolution does not correlate exactly with size.[226, 229]

Stocker and coworkers proposed a histologic classification of CCAMs as types I through III, according to cyst size and relative number.[281] A single cyst or a small number of large cysts between 3 and 10 cm is classified as a type I CCAM, which typifies 50% of postnatal cases. Multiple small cysts make up a type II lesion, occurring in approximately 40% of postnatal cases. Type III lesions are composed of relatively homogeneous microcystic tissue.

Prenatal Diagnosis

The prenatal diagnosis of CCAM can be difficult and relies on a number of sonographic features.[105, 229, 230, 240] Usually, a mass is identified in the fetal chest (Fig. 11–10A). This mass may be solid, cystic, or both, usually without evidence of systemic arterial blood flow by Doppler ultrasonography. If present, cysts may be solitary or multiple. With large CCAMs, mediastinal shift may occur away from the lesion, and polyhydramnios owing to esophageal compression may be present. In the worst cases, evidence of cardiac compression and fetal hydrops may be found. Fetal hydrops is universally associated with ensuing fetal demise and relates to cardiac or caval compression from tumor expansion within the thoracic cavity.

The differential diagnosis includes CDH; cystic hygroma; bronchogenic, enteric, or pericardial cysts; neuroblastoma; bronchopulmonary sequestration (BPS); and bronchial atresia or stenosis. Large microcystic CCAMs are highly echogenic and, thus, are distinguished easily from neuroblastoma. The absence of peristalsis helps distinguish CCAM from herniated bowel in a CDH. Using color and power Doppler imaging, the demonstration of a systemic blood supply emanating from the descending thoracic or abdominal aorta suggests the diagnosis of BPS or hybrid CCAM lesion.[241] A systemic arterial feeding vessel to an echogenic lung mass was previously considered pathognomonic of BPS; however, Cass and associates recently reported a series of "hybrid lesions," which histologically appear to be CCAMs but have a systemic arterial supply.[128] The natural history of hybrid lesions is uncertain because of the rarity of these lesions. The outcome for the fetus appears to be more favorable than with CCAM but less favorable than with BPS.

Sonographic criteria taken from studies correlating the Stocker classification, or microcystic versus macrocytic appearance, with fetal outcome have been unreliable in predicting the development of fetal hydrops. A more consistent correlation may exist between overall volume of the lesion at presentation and the likelihood of development of fetal hydrops. A detailed characterization of this relationship is currently under way in prospective studies at The Center for Fetal Diagnosis and Treatment. Our current management algorithm is shown in Figure 11–11.

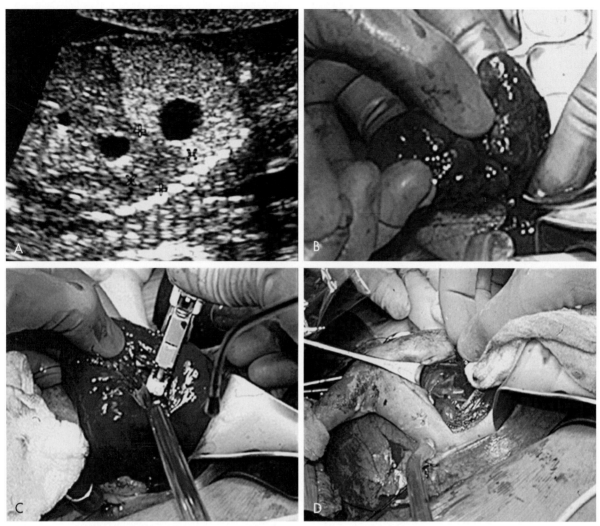

FIGURE 11–10. *A,* Fetal sonogram demonstrating an echogenic congenital cystic adenomatoid malformation of the lung (CCAM), with a single large cyst and compressed normal lung outlined by cursors posteriorly. *B,* Exposure of CCAM through fetal thoracotomy. *C,* Resection of CCAM from adjacent normal lung and hilum using surgical stapler. *D,* Fetal pleural cavity following resection of the CCAM. (From Shaaban AF, et al: The role of ultrasonography in fetal surgery and invasive fetal procedures. Semin Roentgen 34:62, 1999.)

Prenatal Treatment

A review of the first 13 fetuses treated by prenatal resection for life-threatening (hydropic) CCAM reveals an overall survival rate of 62% (8 of 13). This survival rate is remarkable, because untreated CCAM associated with hydrops is uniformly fatal. All of the surviving fetuses have had normal early neurologic development. The five fetuses that did not survive were massively hydropic and died either before (*n* = 1), during (*n* = 2), or shortly after (*n* = 2) the fetal operation. Maternal complications were minor. In addition, six fetuses with CCAM consisting of a dominant cyst and hydrops were treated by thoracoamniotic shunting, with four survivors.

Following maternal laparotomy and exposure of the uterus, the orientation of the fetus and the placenta is determined to plan the hysterotomy in the upper uterine segment overlying the fetal chest. The hysterotomy is made and the fetal arm and chest are exposed, leaving the head and remainder of the body within the amniotic sac. A fetal thoracotomy exposes the lobe containing the CCAM (see Fig. 11–10*B*). The mass is exteriorized, and any systemic feeding vessels and the pulmonary vein draining the CCAM are ligated. All normal adjacent lung is preserved and dissected from the CCAM using electrocautery. The lobar hilum is divided using a surgical stapler (see Fig. 11–10*C, D*). The thoracotomy is then closed. The fetus is returned to the amniotic cavity and the hysterotomy closed. Daily ultrasound examinations should be performed to confirm the resolution of placentomegaly and fetal hydrops, which usually takes 1 to 2 weeks. In addition, ultrasonography is helpful in assessing chorioamniotic separation or low amniotic fluid volume. Similarly, daily fetal echocardiography is needed to ensure resolution of pericardial effusions and to detect the presence of ductal constriction and tricuspid regurgitation while the patient is on postoperative indomethacin therapy. Later, weekly ultra-

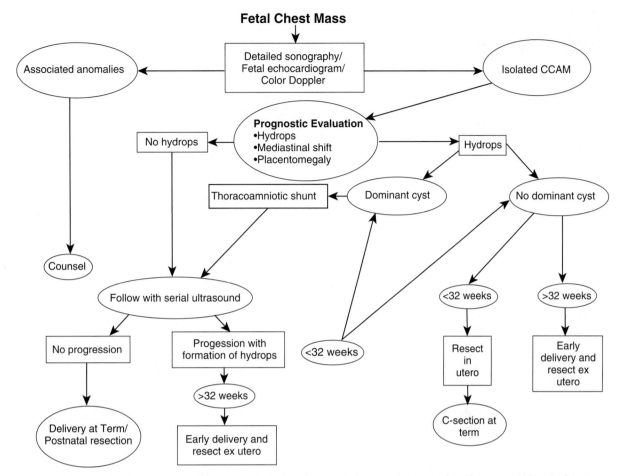

Fetal Chest Mass

FIGURE 11–11. Proposed algorithm for the management of fetal congenital cystic adenomatoid malformation (CCAM) of the lung.

sound studies should be performed to confirm compensatory fetal lung growth. Cesarean section is planned just before term or earlier for premature labor. In survivors of fetal surgery for CCAM the outcome has been excellent, with minimal or no need for postnatal ventilatory support.

SACROCOCCYGEAL TERATOMA

A sacrococcygeal teratoma (SCT) is formed from multiple neoplastic tissues that lack organ specificity, that are foreign to the sacrococcygeal region, and that are derived from all three germ layers.[162] SCT is thought to arise from totipotent somatic cells originating in the primitive knot (Hensen node) or caudal cell mass and, by an unknown mechanism, escape the normal inductive influences of the surrounding normal cells. SCT is the most common tumor of the newborn, occurring in 1 in 35,000 to 40,000 live births.[164, 227]

The American Academy of Pediatrics Surgical Section (AAPSS) classification system groups these tumors according to the relative amount of pelvic or external tumor present.[112] The importance of this classification system relates to the ease of detection and resection and, consequently, survival. Type I tumors are completely external and easily identified on prenatal ultrasound examination or at birth, leading to early referral and resection with less morbidity. In contrast, type IV tumors are completely internal and are usually recognized late, after they have undergone malignant transformation and become symptomatic. Type II has intrapelvic extension of SCT, and type III has intra-abdominal extension of SCT. Fortunately, most tumors are type I or II.

Although the postnatal mortality of SCT is quite low and relates to development of malignant transformation, prenatal mortality from SCT is over 50% as a consequence of associated physiologic derangement or mass effect of the tumor.[121, 140, 164, 216, 274] These effects are related to a vascular "steal" phenomenon, polyhydramnios-induced preterm labor, tumor rupture, or dystocia. Depending on tumor size, rate of growth, ratio of cyst to solid composition, and probably the tissue components of the tumor, the metabolic requirements of SCT vary dramatically. Furthermore, spontaneous internal or external hemorrhage of the SCT may result from necrotic or cystic degeneration of the tumor as it outgrows its blood supply or because of minor trauma in utero.[111] The resulting fetal anemia may initiate or exacerbate the effects of the vascular steal. Both mechanisms may indeed lead to high output failure, placentomegaly, and hydrops.

Prenatal Diagnosis

The diagnosis of SCT is usually made by obstetric ultrasonography performed as a screening procedure

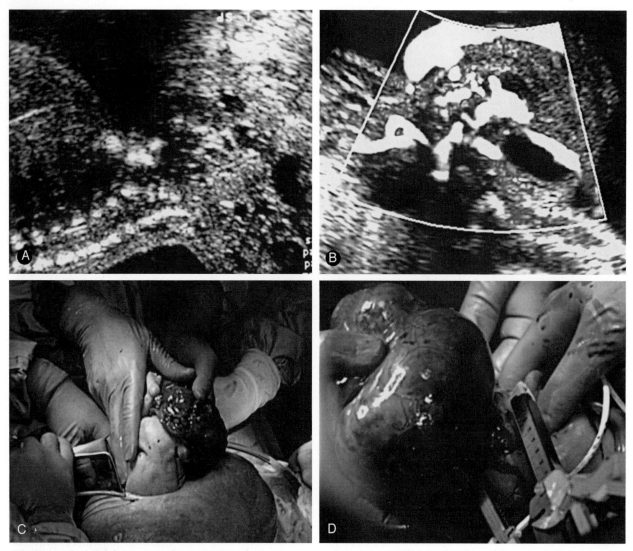

FIGURE 11–12. *A*, Fetal sonogram demonstrating a large sacrococcygeal teratoma (SCT) extending from the coccyx. *B*, Power Doppler image of a highly vascular SCT. *C*, Exposure of SCT during open fetal surgery for resection. *D*, Base of the SCT, including its vascular pedicle about to be divided using a surgical stapler. (From Shaaban AF, et al: The role of ultrasonography in fetal surgery and invasive fetal procedures. Semin Roentgen 34:62, 1999.)

or to assess uterine size too large for dates (polyhydramnios versus tumor enlargement).[213, 275] Characteristic findings are of a caudal or intrapelvic mass, which can be routinely identified during the second trimester (Fig. 11–12*A, B*). The sonographic appearance of a fetal SCT may be cystic, solid, or mixed, and it may demonstrate irregular echogenic patterns secondary to areas of tumor necrosis, cystic degeneration, internal hemorrhage, or calcification.[278] Other critical sonographic information includes the presence of abdominal or pelvic extension, evidence for bowel or urinary tract obstruction, assessment of the integrity of the fetal spine, and documentation of lower extremity function.[164, 242]

The major differential diagnosis includes myelomeningocele, meconium pseudocyst, and obstructive uropathy. Sonographically, detectable features that may exclude these other possibilities include the presence of normal kidneys, the absence of solid components and calcifications within the mass, the presence of spinal dysraphic features, and the lack of a meco-

nium appearance to the fluid contained within the cysts. Echocardiographic and Doppler ultrasound measurements are essential following the diagnosis of a large SCT. Echocardiographic features that should be monitored serially include inferior vena cava diameter, combined ventricular output, and descending aortic flow velocity. In addition, Doppler ultrasonography is useful to detect reversal of diastolic blood flow in the umbilical arteries, which is indicative of steal by the SCT. Most importantly, signs of fetal hydrops should be sought, including pleural or pericardial effusions, ascites, skin or scalp edema, cardiomegaly, or placentomegaly.[162] Follow-up examinations in fetuses with hemodynamically significant SCT demonstrate marked increases in combined ventricular output, descending aortic flow, and umbilical venous flow. Total placental flow increases dramatically. However, the portion of total descending aortic flow directed toward the placenta decreases as a result of steal of the descending aortic blood flow by the enlarging SCT. At least weekly, if not twice weekly, sonography and echocardiography should be performed in SCT to detect the development of high output failure as early as possible.

Prenatal Treatment

The published clinical experience with fetal surgery for SCT is a series of four patients treated at the University of California at San Francisco and The Children's Hospital of Philadelphia.[108, 162, 164] Review of the patients from these centers that were followed closely with serial ultrasonography and echocardiography reveals that the success of fetal intervention relies on early aggressive therapy before the onset of advanced physiologic or physical disturbance. If fetal intervention is to be successful, then candidates must be selected with the earliest signs of high cardiac output physiology before the development of frank hydrops and severe placentomegaly (Fig. 11–13). If lung maturity has been reached, treatment should be focused on cesarean section delivery for postnatal resection of the tumor. Before lung maturity, fetal surgery is an option as long as overt hydrops has not developed and there is no evidence of preterm labor.

The first successful in utero resection of a type II SCT was recently reported (see Fig. 11–12C, D).[108] The fetus had acute onset of placentomegaly and high output cardiac state. At 25 weeks of gestation, the exophytic portion of the tumor was successfully re-sected. The fetal anorectum was dissected off the tumor, and the division of the tumor was performed with a surgical stapler. The pregnancy proceeded uneventfully until premature rupture of membranes occurred at 30 weeks of gestation. The intrapelvic portion was resected postnatally without evidence of malignant transformation. In a situation similar to CCAM, close scrutiny must be given to the mother's postoperative fluid balance in SCT as the high output failure in the fetus resolves and placental flow improves. The situation is especially tenuous in cases of the maternal "mirror" syndrome. Routine postoperative echocardiographic assessment should include measurement of ventricular diameters, combined ventricular output, descending aortic flow, umbilical vein flow, and vena cava diameter. Consideration should be given to percutaneous umbilical blood sampling to check for fetal anemia and to perform fetal blood transfusion should evidence for high output failure persist. With resolution of high output failure, decreased or resolved polyhydramnios, and control of preterm labor, a cesarean delivery should be planned as close to term as possible.

MYELOMENINGOCELE

(See Chapter 38, Part Two.)

Myelomeningocele (MMC) is a protrusion of the meninges and spinal cord through a defect in the vertebral arches, muscle, and skin. Although a nonle-

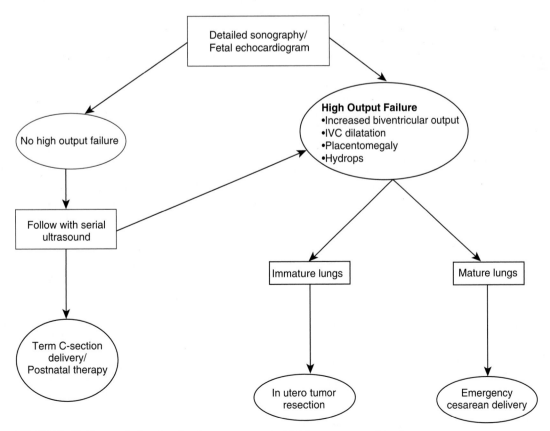

Fetal Sacrococcygeal Teratoma

FIGURE 11–13. Proposed algorthm for the management of fetal sacrococcygeal teratoma.

thal anomaly, MMC is associated with significant postnatal morbidity and lifelong disability.

MMC is a relatively common anomaly affecting 1 in 2000 live births.[153, 217, 277] The disabilities associated with MMC include paraplegia, hydrocephalus, sexual dysfunction, skeletal deformities, bowel and bladder incontinence, and cognitive impairment. Although most children with MMC have normal intelligence, 15% require some form of custodial care.

Dietary folate supplementation has been shown to prevent MMC in some cases.[243, 283] Folate must be supplemented soon after conception, but 50% of women of childbearing age do not take supplemental folate, and most pregnancies are unplanned. In addition, it is estimated that 30% of neural tube defects are refractory to folate supplementation. For these reasons, despite folate supplementation, MMC is an anomaly that likely will continue to affect children.

Traditionally, efforts to treat MMC have focused on postnatal surgical correction to prevent infection and to improve physical disabilities that cannot be corrected or reversed. The rationale for prenatal correction of MMC is to repair the defect before neurologic damage has occurred or when there is still potential for recovery.

The neurologic damage in MMC is hypothesized to result from the initial defective spinal cord development and the damage to the exposed spinal cord caused by failure of mesodermal migration. This has been referred to as the "two-hit hypothesis." Examination of the spinal cords of midgestation fetuses with MMC shows near-normal cord development in most cases.[139, 206, 235] In addition, leg movement in fetuses with MMC has been observed as early as 16 to 17 weeks of gestation. In contrast, most MMC fetuses exhibit severe neurologic impairment of the lower extremities by the time of birth, suggesting that the neurologic injury may occur later in gestation.[139, 235] This injury may occur during labor or as a result of passage through the birth canal.[225, 273] The neurologic injury may also occur by direct abrasion of the exposed cord against the uterine wall during gestation. An additional insult to the spinal cord may be a constituent of the amniotic fluid. However, amniotic fluid at 34 weeks of gestation was found to be more toxic to rat spinal cords in an in vitro organ culture model than was amniotic fluid from earlier in gestation.[152]

Animal models that mimic human MMC have been developed in primates,[237] rats,[201] pigs,[200] and sheep.[233, 234] Perhaps the model that comes closest to simulating human MMC is the ovine model. In this model, laminectomy is performed at 75 days of gestation and MMC repair is performed at 100 days of gestation. At birth, lambs that do not undergo repair have MMC-like lesions, flaccid paralysis, incontinence, and absent hind limb somatosensory-evoked potentials. In contrast, lambs that do undergo repair in utero are normal.[233, 234]

Prenatal Diagnosis

Elevation of maternal serum α-fetoprotein concentrations obtained in the first trimester of pregnancy identified 75% to 80% of pregnancies with MMC before 16 weeks of gestation.[211, 251] Amniocentesis is performed in at-risk cases identified by maternal serum α-fetoprotein concentration screening and amniotic fluid. α-Fetoprotein and acetylcholinesterase elevations confirm the presence of a neural tube defect. The structural defect can be readily identified by ultrasonography by 18 to 22 weeks' gestation.[211, 251] The presence of an MMC may also be suggested by the presence of a "lemon" sign, which is a scalloping of the frontal bones. A full anatomic survey should be performed to detect associated anomalies such as ventriculomegaly, Chiari malformation, and clubfoot. The presence or absence and quality of leg and foot movements should be performed, but it may be difficult to distinguish spontaneous from reflex fetal movement.[161] Ultrafast fetal magnetic resonance imaging (MRI) provides additional anatomic detail about the MMC and the brain.

Prenatal Treatment

The first attempted repair in utero of an MMC was reported in a letter by Bruner and colleagues in 1987, using a fetoscopic technique to apply a skin graft in two fetuses.[125] A full report of this experience revealed that four fetuses were operated on between 22 and 24 weeks' gestation.[126] There were two deaths: one from chorioamnionitis, requiring delivery 1 week postoperatively, and the second from placental abruption on the day of surgery. The two other fetuses delivered at 28 and 35 weeks' gestation. Both fetuses required ventriculoperitoneal shunting postnatally and surgery to close the defect, and it is not clear that there was any neurologic benefit. This fetoscopic approach has since been abandoned.

The first documented improvement from repair of MMC in utero was reported by Adzick and coworkers in 1998.[109] Open fetal surgical repair of a large T11 to S1 MMC was performed at 23 weeks of gestation. Postnatally, the infant had a right clubfoot with a neurologic L4 level and a left foot with an L5 level. Postnatal MRI demonstrated resolution of the hindbrain herniation, and there was no hydrocephalus. Almost all neonates with thoracolumbar MMC are paraplegic and require ventriculoperitoneal shunting for hydrocephalus. The outcome in this case suggested the potential neurologic benefit of in utero repair of MMC. Subsequent experience in 10 cases, between 22 and 25 weeks, by this same group demonstrated by pre- and postoperative fetal MRI that closure of the MMC in utero reverses the hindbrain herniation of the Chiari malformation. In addition, only 1 of the 10 required ventriculoperitoneal shunting.[282] Bruner and colleagues reported the Vanderbilt experience with 29 cases between 24 weeks and 30 weeks.[127] However, their series was marred by significant obstetric complications, including postoperative oligohydramnios in 48%, uterine dehiscence in 2 patients, and the need for postnatal ventriculoperitoneal shunting in 59%. There are differences in the approach between the groups in Philadelphia and Nashville; at The Children's Hospital of Philadelphia, researchers excluded from consideration fetuses of earlier gestation (before 24 weeks), fetuses with evidence of neurologic injury (manifested by clubbed feet), and fetuses with ventriculomegaly with lateral ventricles greater than 17 mm.

The results of fetal MMC repair are difficult to evaluate, especially given the limited duration of follow-up. Although hindbrain herniation definitely is reversed, ventriculoperitoneal shunting may still be needed. With longer follow-up time, both the Philadelphia and Nashville groups have observed a progressive rise in the number of patients requiring ventriculoperitoneal shunting. Whereas some patients in the Philadelphia series appear to have significantly improved neurologic level of function, most have not, and none of the patients in the Nashville group have shown improved neurologic function. These results will need to be evaluated in prospective trials with 4- to 5-year follow-up to determine if fetal MMC repair is truly beneficial. This is especially important, given the fetal deaths following fetal MMC repair for this nonlethal lesion.

FETAL AIRWAY OBSTRUCTION

Obstruction of the fetal airway presents a particularly difficult problem at delivery. A patent airway can be difficult to secure quickly, often necessitating emergent tracheostomy, which rarely can be performed in sufficient time to prevent anoxic brain injury or death. Cervical teratoma, lymphangioma, or intrinsic laryngeal or tracheal obstruction may compromise the fetal airway. Congenital high airway obstruction syndrome (CHAOS), resulting from tracheal or laryngeal occlusion, is relatively rare but almost always fatal.[198, 210] CHAOS most often involves occlusion at the level of the larynx by laryngeal atresia, with laryngeal webs or severe subglottic stenosis occurring less frequently. Similarly, cervical teratoma and lymphangioma may compromise the fetal airway by compression, resulting in complete occlusion of the fetal trachea.

Dilation of the airway distal to the obstruction results from impaired efflux of fetal lung fluid. Compensatory hypersecretion owing to stretch of the lung tissue accelerates this process.[179, 279, 289] Experimental models of CHAOS have confirmed this pathophysiology.[176] If left unchecked, the rising intrathoracic pressures eventually lead to placentomegaly and fetal hydrops as a result of compromised cardiac function. These conditions can be detected prenatally, thereby facilitating a planned and controlled delivery by EXIT procedure.

Prenatal Diagnosis

Giant fetal neck masses that occlude the airway are usually identified during routine ultrasonography. Most of these lesions are hypoechogenic cysts with a solid component present in teratomas. Intrinsic laryngeal obstructions are more difficult to diagnose.[210, 288] The trachea and lungs are dilated distal to the obstruction, and the diaphragms may be flattened or everted. The tense fluid accumulation gives the lungs an echogenic appearance. As CHAOS evolves, placentomegaly, fetal ascites, or generalized hydrops may develop. Absence of lung fluid efflux may be noted on color Doppler imaging of the dilated trachea during fetal breathing movements.

The frequency of associated CNS anomalies, renal anomalies, vascular anomalies, and esophageal atresia or fistula with laryngeal atresia may be as high as 50%. Fraser syndrome (cryptophthalmus, abnormal genitalia, syndactyly of the toes and fingers) has been described in association with laryngeal atresia.[272] With this association, there is an 85% incidence of major renal anomalies including unilateral or bilateral renal agenesis or multicystic renal dysplasia. Even if the kidneys are present, they are usually echogenic and poorly functioning, resulting in oligohydramnios. Therefore, the presence of fetal airway obstruction with oligohydramnios should raise the suspicion of Fraser syndrome and its poor prognosis.

Prenatal Treatment

Laryngeal obstruction from giant neck masses carries a good overall prognosis if the airway can be secured at delivery. Similarly, in the absence of associated anomalies, fetuses with laryngeal atresia may also do well. The EXIT procedure provides time with the fetus on placental support to secure the airway in these cases. Given proper anesthesia and uterine relaxation, sufficient uteroplacental gas exchange can be maintained for up to an hour. This time period permits either endoscopic or surgical control of the fetal airway without risk of fetal hypoxia.

The timing of the EXIT procedure relates to the well-being of the fetus. A fetus with airway obstruction from any cause may be followed to term (36 to 38 weeks) with serial ultrasonography, provided that there are no signs of hydrops. However, amnioreduction may be required in fetuses with neck masses associated with esophageal obstruction and severe polyhydramnios secondary to impaired swallowing. With the evolution of fetal hydrops or uncontrollable preterm labor, the EXIT procedure should be performed expeditiously.

In performing the EXIT procedure, the hysterotomy is created away from the placenta using a uterine stapling device to prevent hemorrhage. The fetal head and upper chest are delivered. If necessary, large cystic neck masses may be decompressed to permit delivery and to partially relieve the compression on the fetal airway. Fetal oxygenation is monitored with a pulse oximeter applied to the exposed fetal hand. Also, fetal cardiac function is assessed with continuous transthoracic fetal echocardiography. Deep anesthesia is maintained by maternal inhaled isoflurane in oxygen, providing uterine relaxation, fetal anesthesia, and preservation of uteroplacental gas exchange.

The EXIT procedure provides time for laryngoscopy and bronchoscopy if there is significant distortion of the airway (Fig. 11–14A). In addition, tracheostomy or even partial tumor resection may be

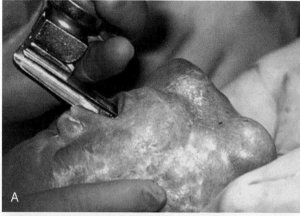

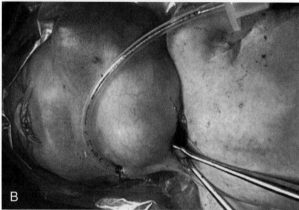

FIGURE 11–14. *A*, Direct laryngoscopy performed during ex utero intrapartum treatment (EXIT) procedure on a fetus with airway compromise owing to a giant cervical teratoma. *B*, Tracheostomy performed during the EXIT procedure, requiring tunneling of an endotracheal tube through the soft tissues of the neck because of the severe distortion of the fetal airway. (From Shaaban AF, et al: The role of ultrasonography in fetal surgery and invasive fetal procedures. Semin Roentgen 34:62, 1999.)

accomplished during placental support (see Fig. 11–14*B*). A recent report of five giant fetal neck masses confirmed the usefulness of this approach. Laryngoscopy was performed in all five cases, bronchoscopy in three, and tracheostomy in two. The mean time on placental support was 28 minutes (range, 8 to 54 minutes), with excellent uteroplacental gas exchange, as reflected by the results of cord blood gases.[220]

FETOSCOPIC SURGERY

Embryoscopy and fetoscopy have been used as diagnostic tools since the late 1960s. More recently, they have been used diagnostically to guide chorionic villus sampling and fetal skin and liver biopsies.[155, 178, 264] Fetoscopy also has been used therapeutically in the treatment of CDH for fetal tracheal clip application, in the release of amniotic bands, and in the treatment of twin reversed arterial perfusion sequence and twin-twin transfusion syndrome. The limitations of the initial fetoscopic procedures were largely related to the primitive optics and instrumentation available at

the time. The recent surge in operative laparoscopy has kindled rapid technical advances in optics and instrumentation.[271] These advances are illustrated by a recent report that details the usefulness of transabdominal fetoscopy in a case of Meckel-Gruber syndrome, in which a diagnosis could not be made by ultrasound examination.[260]

The same technologic advances that have made minimally invasive videoendoscopic surgery possible in children and adults offer the potential for minimally invasive fetal surgery[158, 159] (see Table 11–14). The small uterine puncture sites required for fetoscopic surgery, in theory, would prevent the morbidity of a large hysterotomy. Specifically, the fetoscopic approach could reduce the risks of preterm labor, hemorrhage, amniotic fluid leak, and uterine rupture and could eliminate the need for cesarean section delivery following fetal surgery.

TWIN REVERSED ARTERIAL PERFUSION SEQUENCE

Twin reversed arterial perfusion (TRAP) sequence occurs only in the setting of a monochorionic gestation and complicates approximately 1% of monochorionic twin gestations, with an incidence of 1 in 35,000 births.[207] In the TRAP sequence the acardiac/acephalic twin receives all of its blood supply from the normal "pump" twin. The term *reversed perfusion* is used to describe this scenario because blood enters the acardiac/acephalic twin through its umbilical artery and exits through the umbilical vein. Because of increased demand the abnormal circulation in TRAP sequence places on the heart of the pump twin, cardiac failure is the primary concern in TRAP sequence. If left untreated, the pump twin dies in 50% to 75% of cases. This is especially true when the acardiac/acephalic twin weighs more than 50% of the estimated weight of the pump twin.[239]

It is important to exclude a chromosomal abnormality before offering a fetoscopic procedure in TRAP sequence, because the incidence of chromosomal abnormality in the pump twin may be as high as 9%.[284] Fifty-one percent of TRAP sequence pregnancies are complicated by polyhydramnios, and 75% are complicated by preterm labor.[196] The difference in estimated fetal weight between the pump twin and the acardiac/acephalic twin is predictive of outcome. When the acardius–to–pump twin weight ratio exceeds 0.5, pump twin demise is predicted in 64% of cases.[239] If this weight ratio is greater than 0.7, the mortality rate of the pump twin is approximately 90%.

Techniques of sectio parva (selective removal of an anomalous twin)[263] and ultrasound-guided embolization[252] were used in an attempt to interrupt the vascular communication between the pump twin and the acardius. These procedures have been associated with substantial morbidity and unreliable outcomes, which led to the development of fetoscopic approaches to this problem. McCurdy and associates were the first to report a case of fetoscopic cord ligation in TRAP sequence.[231] The acardiac/acephalic twin's cord was successfully ligated, but only after the pump twin's cord was ligated and then released after the error was recognized. The pump twin developed persistent bradycardia and was noted to be dead on ultrasound examination on postoperative day 1.

Quintero and coworkers reported the first successful umbilical cord ligation for TRAP sequence.[256] The procedure was performed at 19 weeks of gestation, using two percutaneous trocars and a 1.9-mm endoscope. The cord was successfully ligated, and except for some mild postoperative uterine irritability, the patient responded well. Three weeks following the procedure the mother presented with leakage of amniotic fluid that subsequently resolved. The pregnancy continued until 36 weeks of gestation, when a healthy boy was delivered.

A total of 15 cases of fetoscopic umbilical cord ligation for TRAP sequence have now been reported.[231, 238, 256, 290] Ten of the 15 fetuses (67%) survived without neurologic deficit. The most common complication following fetoscopic cord ligation has been premature rupture of membranes. It is thought that this complication arises from the fixation of the amnion at the two trocar sites, causing tearing and leaking of the amnion with uterine enlargement during the pregnancy. Milner and Crombleholme have reported the evaluation and treatment of eight cases of TRAP sequence.[238] However, by size criteria of acardius–to–pump twin ratio greater than 0.7, only three cases required fetoscopic treatment. Two of these underwent fetoscopic cord ligation (Fig. 11–15), and the third case was treated by fetoscopic cord coagulation using a 3-mm bipolar coagulation grasper (Everest Medical, Minneapolis, Minn). Because this case of TRAP sequence occurred in a monoamniotic gestation, the umbilical cord of the acardius was coagulated in two spots and cut to prevent cord entanglement with the pump twin's cord. Two of the three

fetuses survived in small case series. We currently recommend fetoscopic bipolar cord coagulation for cases of TRAP sequence in which the acardius–to–pump twin weight ratio exceeds 0.7 or if any signs of cardiac decompensation are present in the pump twin. The fetoscopic cord coagulation technique is limited to earlier gestation pregnancies complicated by TRAP sequence. In later gestation fetuses, that is, after 22 weeks of gestation, the umbilical cord may be too large to safely coagulate with the bipolar cautery. In these cases, fetoscopic cord ligation is the preferred approach.

TWIN-TWIN TRANSFUSION SYNDROME

(See also Chapters 23 and 44.)

Twin-twin transfusion syndrome (TTTS), or oligohydramnios/polyhydramnios sequence, is a rare syndrome that occurs at an estimated rate of 0.1 to 0.9 per 1000 births.[115] This diagnosis carries an extremely poor prognosis, and it may be responsible for 15% to 17% of all perinatal deaths in twins. TTTS occurs only in the setting of monochorionic gestations.

It is estimated that 85% of monochorionic placentas have anomalous vascular connections; however, only 5% to 10% have sufficient imbalance to produce the TTTS.[246] It is also believed that the number of vascular anastomoses and types of anastomoses within a placenta determine if TTTS develops.

The natural history of TTTS is associated with a 60% to 100% mortality for both twins in the most severe cases.[117, 118, 132, 261] The most severely affected fetuses usually present with signs of TTTS before 20 weeks' gestation. Mothers commonly present clinically after 20 weeks' gestation with an acute increase in abdominal girth, discomfort, and occasionally respiratory compromise or preterm labor. Physical examination reveals tense polyhydramnios. However, pre-

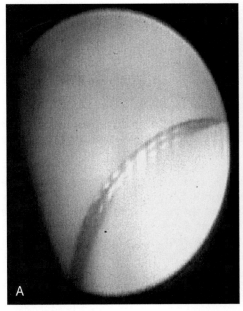 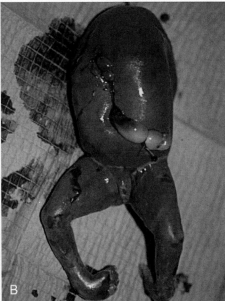

FIGURE 11–15. *A,* Fetoscopic view of cord ligation for twin reversed arterial perfusion (TRAP) sequence. *B,* Acardius/Acephalus following delivery that underwent cord ligation. (From Shaaban AF, et al: The role of ultrasonography in fetal surgery and invasive fetal procedures. Semin Roentgen 34:62, 1999.)

sentation before 20 weeks' gestation is usually asymptomatic, and diagnosis is usually a serendipitous finding on routine ultrasound.

Diagnostic criteria for TTTS include monochorionicity (chorionicity is best determined in the first trimester and is more difficult to determine in the second trimester), a marked discordance in amniotic fluid volume between the twins (thus the term *oligohydramnios/polyhydramnios sequence*), a size discordance with the larger twin in the polyhydramniotic sac (except in TTTS presenting before 20 weeks' gestation, in which size discordance may not be pronounced), same-sex twins, and a single placental mass.[124, 291] The most characteristic feature is the presence of a "stuck twin," in which the larger recipient twin has a large bladder and a polyhydramniotic sac and a smaller donor twin has a small bladder and is stuck against the uterine wall in an oligohydramniotic sac. A stuck twin can occur from causes other than TTTS, including premature rupture of membranes, placental insufficiency, urinary tract or other structural abnormalities, chromosomal anomalies, and infectious etiologies.

Initially, the twins present on ultrasound with a growth discrepancy between the larger recipient twin and the growth-restricted donor twin. It is not uncommon for the donor twin to have a velamentous umbilical cord insertion, which may exacerbate the growth discrepancy. The volume stress on the recipient heart in TTTS often leads to cardiac changes. The recipient may develop cardiomyopathy with ventricular dysfunction that culminates in fetal hydrops. These cardiac changes include ventricular hypertrophy, tricuspid valvular insufficiency, and, in advanced cases, an akinetic right ventricle and pulmonic valvular insufficiency.[293] Co-twin demise (usually the recipient) may occur as the fetal hydrops worsens. The surviving twin is at risk for severe neurologic injury caused by vascular resistance changes and consequent ischemic neurologic events. The surviving co-twin is also at risk for concomitant demise in 4% to 10% of cases.[154, 168]

Several treatment options exist for TTTS, including medical therapy, serial amnioreduction, amniotic septostomy, and fetoscopic approaches. Experience with medical therapy has been anecdotal, with case reports of resolution of TTTS with either digoxin or indomethacin therapy.[150, 266] These therapies have not been widely accepted or applied in patients diagnosed with TTTS.

Serial amnioreduction is one of the most commonly used and widely accepted therapies for TTTS. Its mechanism of action is unknown, but it appears to prolong gestation in addition to improving uteroplacental blood flow. Advocates of this therapy believe that amnioreduction increases the survival rate when compared with the natural history of TTTS and shows comparable survival to that observed with laser therapy.[156] The major criticism of amnioreduction is that it does not prevent the neurologic complications of TTTS.

Amniotic septostomy has been intentionally performed in a small number of cases.[269] Proponents of amniotic septostomy report equilibration of amniotic fluid volumes between the two fetuses that lasts for the duration of the pregnancy. Although the mechanism of amniotic septostomy is unclear, its success may be related to its effects on fetoplacental hemodynamics. I speculate that amniotic septostomy allows amniotic fluid to cross into the stuck twin's sac, resulting in a fluid bolus as the amniotic fluid is imbibed by the fetus. It is likely that restoration of amniotic fluid volume after just one or two amnioreductions is successful because of unintentional and unrecognized septostomy. An interesting observation is that TTTS does not seem to occur in monochorionic monoamniotic pregnancies, perhaps for the same reason that amniotic septostomy works. However, as with serial amnioreduction, amniotic septostomy would not be expected to prevent the neurologic sequelae in the event of either co-twin demise. In addition, if too large a septostomy is created, the twins are at risk for cord entanglement. Because of this risk, a microseptostomy is created, which is only a series of needle punctures of the intertwin membrane.

Fetoscopic laser as a treatment for TTTS was initially described by DeLia and colleagues in 1990.[147] Experimental work in both sheep and monkey models showed the efficacy of fetoscopic laser photocoagulation by using a neodymium:yttrium-aluminum-garnet laser before its use in the first three human cases was reported in 1990.[148, 149] The three women were treated at 18.5, 22, and 22.5 weeks of gestation after presenting with acute polyhydramnios. Two of the three procedures went uneventfully, but the third was complicated by a placental vessel perforation. The first two patients delivered at 27 and 34 weeks' gestation because of premature rupture of membranes. The third patient developed severe preeclampsia at 29 weeks' gestation, necessitating delivery. Four of the six infants survived.

A follow-up to these initial cases was published in 1995. DeLia and colleagues reported 26 patients treated by a fetoscopic laser.[146] The inclusion criteria were ultrasonographic findings consistent with TTTS, posterior placenta, gestational age younger than 25 weeks, and clinical polyhydramnios. The treated patients had a mean gestational age of 20.8 weeks (range, 18 to 24 weeks). One patient had surviving triplets, eight had surviving twins, nine had a single survivor (two neonatal and seven fetal deaths), and eight had no survivors (all had pregnancy loss within 3 weeks of the procedure). Surviving fetuses were delivered for obstetric reasons at a mean of 32.2 weeks (range, 26 to 37 weeks). Fifty-three percent (28 of 53) of fetuses survived, with 96% (27 of 28) showing normal development at a mean of 35.8 months of follow-up (range, 1 to 68 months).

A similar experience was reported by Ville and associates.[287] Forty-five women were treated at a median gestational age of 21 weeks (range, 15 to 28 weeks). The rate of fetuses surviving to delivery was also 53%. Among the survivors, the median gestational age at delivery was 35 weeks (range, 25 to 40 weeks), with a median interval between treatment and delivery of 14 weeks (range, 0 to 21 weeks). All of the survivors were developing normally at a median age of 12 months (range, 2 to 24 months).

A recent report from Germany compared outcomes of selective fetoscopic laser photocoagulation with those of serial amnioreduction for TTTS.[197] Unlike the technique described by DeLia, in which all vessels crossing the intertwin membrane are photocoagulated, the selective technique selects only those vessels for coagulation that appear to connect the circulations of the twins. These connections may be artery to vein, vein to vein, artery to artery, or connections within the placenta in which a cotyledon is perfused by an artery from one twin but drains by a vein returning to the other twin. Seventy-three women were treated between 1995 and 1997 in one center by fetoscopic laser photocoagulation, and 43 patients were treated at another center between 1992 and 1996 by serial amnioreduction. Women treated by fetoscopic laser instead of serial amnioreduction had a higher proportion of pregnancies with greater than one survivor (79% versus 60%), a lower number of spontaneous intrauterine fetal deaths (3% versus 19%), a lower incidence of abnormal ultrasonographic findings in the brains of surviving neonates (6% versus 18%), and an older gestational age at the time of delivery (33.7 versus 30.7 weeks). Based on this information, the authors concluded that fetoscopic laser photocoagulation is a more effective treatment for TTTS than serial amnioreduction.

Saade and coworkers argued that the vessels on the chorionic plate are only part of the chorioangiopagus and that more vascular connections occur deep within the cotyledons of the placenta.[270] Quintero and coworkers described the selective technique of fetoscopic laser photocoagulation for TTTS to address these deep communications.[259] The placental surface is fetoscopically inspected for what he terms *nonparticipating vessels* and *truly participating vessels* as well as the location of the intertwin membrane. Nonparticipating vessels occur in pairs with an artery entering a cotyledon and a vein returning to the same umbilical cord. In contrast, vessels truly participating in the TTTS are unpaired. An artery leaving the umbilical cord of the donor enters a cotyledon, but there is no vein returning to donor umbilical cord; rather, a vein draining this cotyledon can be seen on the other side of the vascular equator heading back to the umbilical cord of the recipient fetus. It is unlikely, however, that sufficient pressure changes could be transmitted across these deep communications within the cotyledons to account for the ischemic injury seen in surviving co-twins on fetal demise. Although these deep vessels may contribute to TTTS, they are unlikely to be responsible for all of its morbidity. It is for that reason that these unpaired vessels, along with any direct artery-to-vein, artery-to-artery, or vein-to-vein communications on the chorionic plate, are selectively laser photocoagulated.[259]

SUMMARY

Significant strides have been made in invasive fetal therapy. In recent years, progress seems to be accelerating, providing innovative treatment for fetuses with malformations that would otherwise be fatal. However, these pioneering efforts should not be mistaken for establishing invasive fetal therapy as the standard treatment for any condition. Although there is tremendous potential for fetal salvage in several highly lethal conditions, much experimental work remains to be done. Assessing the risk-to-benefit ratio for a mother with a fetus with a life-threatening malformation will evolve as technical advances diminish the potential risks of fetal surgery. Fetal surgery's contribution to advances in perinatal care and tocolytic management have implications far beyond the narrow sphere of fetal therapy. In the last analysis, the collateral advances that occur as a result of invasive fetal therapy may be the most important and lasting contributions of this experimental endeavor. The field of invasive fetal therapy is rapidly evolving and will undoubtedly provide new and exciting therapeutic options for the unborn patient.

■ REFERENCES

Part One: Pharmacologic Treatment of the Fetus

1. Abdel-Rahman AM, et al: Prevention of intraventricular hemorrhage in the premature infant. Clin Perinatol 21:505, 1994.
2. Ahmad H, et al: Primary and secondary structural analysis of glutathione S-transferase from human placenta. Arch Biochem Biophys 278:398, 1990.
3. Allan LD, et al: Flecainide in the treatment of fetal tachycardias. Br Heart J 65:468, 1991.
4. Anderson ABM, et al: Placental transfer and metabolism of betamethasone in human pregnancy. Obstet Gynecol 49:471, 1977.
5. Beitins IZ, et al: The transplacental passage of prednisone and prednisolone in pregnancy near term. J Pediatr 81:936, 1972.
6. Ben-Chetrit A, et al: Hydramnios in the third trimester of pregnancy: A change in distribution of accompanying fetal anomalies as a result of early ultrasonographic prenatal diagnosis. Am J Obstet Gynecol 162:1344, 1990.
7. Berenbaum SA, et al: Behavioral effects of prenatal versus postnatal androgen excess in children with 21-hydroxylase-deficient congenital adrenal hyperplasia. J Clin Endocrinol Met 85:727, 2000.
8. Blanford AT, et al: In vitro metabolism of prednisolone, dexamethasone, betamethasone and cortisol in the human placenta. Am J Obstet Gynecol 127:264, 1977.
9. Bounget P, et al: Models for placental transfer studies of drugs. Clin Pharmacokinet 28:161, 1995.
10. Cappillo M, et al: Sulphotransferase and its substrate: Adenosine-3'1-phosphate-5'-phosphosulphate in human fetal liver and placenta. Dev Pharmacol Ther 14:62, 1990.
11. Cavalho ADA, et al: Maternal and infant antibody response to meningococcal vaccination in pregnancy. Lancet 2:809, 1977.
12. Cerame BI, et al: Prenatal diagnosis and treatment of 11 β-hydroxylase deficiency. Congenital adrenal hyperplasia resulting in normal female genitalia. J Clin Endocrinol Metab 84:3129, 1999.
13. Clark CE, et al: Risk factor analysis of intraventricular hemorrhage in low-birth-weight infants. J Pediatr 99:625, 1981.
14. Crowley P: Antenatal corticosteroid therapy: A meta analysis of the randomized trials 1972–1994. Am J Obstet Gynecol 173: 322, 1995.
15. Daffos F, et al: Prenatal management of 746 pregnancies at risk for congenital toxoplasmosis. N Engl J Med 318:271, 1988.
16. David M, et al: Prenatal treatment of congenital adrenal hyperplasia resulting from 21-hydroxylase deficiency. J Pediatr 105:799, 1984.

17. DeCrespigny LC, et al: Timing of neonatal cerebroventricular hemorrhages with ultrasound. Arch Dis Child 57:231, 1982.

18. Derewlany LO, et al: Arylamine N-acetyltransferase activity of the human placenta. J Pharmacol Exp Ther 269:756, 1994.

19. Derewlany LO, et al: Role of the placenta in perinatal pharmacology and toxicology. In Radde IC, et al (eds): Pediatric Pharmacology and Therapeutics, 2nd ed, St Louis, Mosby, 1992, p 405.

20. Derewlany LO, et al: The transport of digoxin across the perfused human placental lobule. J Pharmacol Exp Ther 256:1107, 1991.

21. Didley GA, et al: Amniotic fluid assessment. I. Comparison of sonographic estimates versus direct measurements using a dye-dilution technique in human pregnancy. Am J Obstet Gynecol 167:986, 1992.

22. Dolfin T, et al: Incidence, severity and timing of subependymal and intraventricular hemorrhages in preterm infants born in a prenatal unit as detected by serial real-time ultrasound. Pediatrics 71:541, 1983.

23. Dudley DK, et al: Fetal and neonatal effects of indomethacin used as a tocolytic agent. Am J Obstet Gynecol 151:181, 1985.

24. Evans HE, et al: Serum immunoglobulin levels in premature and full-term infants. Am J Clin Pathol 56:416, 1971.

25. Fisher DA: Fetal thyroid function: Diagnosis and management of fetal thyroid disorders. Clin Obstet Gynecol 40:16, 1997.

26. Flake AW, et al: Treatment of x-linked severe combined immunodeficiency by in utero transplantation of paternal bone marrow. N Engl J Med 335:1806, 1996.

27. Forest MG, et al: Prenatal diagnosis and treatment of 21-hydroxylase deficiency. J Steroid Biochem Mol Biol 45:75, 1993.

28. Foulton W: Congenital toxoplasmosis: Is screening desirable? Scand J Infect Dis 84(Suppl):11, 1992.

29. Garland M: Pharmacology of drug transfer across the placenta. Obstet Gynecol Clin North Am 25: 21, 1998.

30. Gembruch U, et al: Direct intrauterine fetal treatment of fetal tachyarrhythmia with severe hydrops fetalis by antiarrhythmic drugs. Fetal Ther 3:210, 1988.

31. Gill TJ III, et al: Transplacental immunization of the human fetus to tetanus by immunization of the mother. J Clin Invest 72:987, 1983.

32. Gitlin D, et al: The selectivity of the human placenta in the transfer of plasma proteins from mother to fetus. J Clin Invest 43:1938, 1964.

33. Guedeney X, et al: Existence of a digitalis-like compound in the human fetus. Biol Neonate 59:133, 1991.

34. Guthenberg C, et al: Glutathione S-transferase from human placenta is identical or closely related to glutathione S-transferase from erythrocytes. Biochim Biophys Acta 661:255, 1981.

35. Hakkola J, et al: Xenobiotic-metabolizing cytochrome P450 enzymes in the human feto-placental unit: Role in intrauterine toxicity. Crit Rev Toxicol 28:35, 1998.

36. Hansmann M, et al: Fetal tachyarrhythmias: Transplacental and direct treatment of the fetus—a report of 60 cases. Ultrasound Obstet Gynecol 1:162, 1991.

37. Hill MD, et al: The significance of plasma protein binding on the fetal/maternal distribution of drugs at steady-state. Clin Pharmacokinet 14:156, 1988.

38. Ito S, et al: Drug therapy for fetal arrhythmias. Clin Perinatol 21:543, 1994.

39. Jobe AH, et al: Fetal versus maternal and gestational age effects of repetitive antenatal glucocorticoids. Pediatrics 102:1116, 1998.

40. Kaufman P: Functional anatomy of the nonprimate placenta. Placenta 1(Suppl):13, 1981.

41. Kendrick P, et al: Immunity response of mothers and babies to injections of pertussis vaccine during pregnancy. Am J Dis Child 70:25, 1945.

42. Kleinman CS, et al: In utero diagnosis and treatment of fetal supraventricular tachycardia. Semin Perinatol 9:113, 1985.

43. Koskiniemi J, et al: Toxoplasmosis needs evaluation: An overview and proposals. Am J Dis Child 143:724, 1989.

44. Kramer WB, et al: Treatment of polyhydramnios with indomethacin. Clin Perinatol 21:615, 1994.

45. Levitz M, et al: The transfer and metabolism of corticosteroids in the perfused human placenta. Am J Obstet Gynecol 132:363, 1978.

46. Liggins GC, et al: A controlled trial of antepartum glucocorticoid treatment for prevention of the respiratory distress syndrome in premature infants. Pediatrics 50:515, 1972.

47. Liggins GC: Premature delivery of foetal lambs infused with glucocorticoids. J Endocrinol 45:515, 1969.

48. Linder N, et al: Effect of third-trimester oral poliomyelitis vaccination (OPV) on newborn poliomyelitis antibody titers [abstract]. Pediatr Res 33:292A, 1993.

49. Linder N, et al: In utero vaccination. Clin Perinatol 21:663, 1994.

50. Matsui D: Prevention, diagnosis and treatment of fetal toxoplasmosis. Clin Perinatol 21:675, 1994.

51. Mattison DR, et al: Physiologic adaptations to pregnancy: Impact on pharmacokinetics. In Yaffe SJ, et al (eds): Pediatric pharmacology: Therapeutic principles in practice. Philadelphia, WB Saunders, 1992, p 81.

52. Mattison DR: Transdermal drug absorption during pregnancy. Clin Obstet Gynecol 33:718, 1990.

53. Maxwell DJ, et al: Obstetric importance, diagnosis and management of fetal tachycardias. BMJ 297:107, 1988.

54. Miller WL: Steroid hormone biosynthesis and actions in the maternal-fetal-placental unit. Clin Perinatol 25:799, 1998.

55. Myrianthopoulos NC, et al: Studies in neural tube defects. I. Epidemiologic and etiologic aspects. Am J Med Genet 26:783, 1987.

56. Osathanondh R, et al: Dexamethasone levels in treated pregnant women and newborn infants. J Pediatr 90:617, 1977.

57. Osinski PA: Steroid 11β-dehydrogenase in human placenta. Nature 187:777, 1960.

58. Owen P, et al: Fetal tachyarrhythmias. Br J Hosp Med 58:142, 1997.

59. Pacifici GM, et al: Placental transfer of drugs administered to the mother. Clin Pharmacokinet 28:235, 1995.

60. Padbury JF, et al: Extrapulmonary effects of antenatally administered steroids. J Pediatr 128:167, 1996.

61. Pang S: Congenital adrenal hyperplasia. End Metab Clin N Am 26:853, 1997.

62. Papile LA, et al: Incidence and evolution of subependymal and intraventricular hemorrhage: A study of infants with birth weights less than 1500 gm. J Pediatr 92:529, 1978.

63. Pasanen M, et al: Human placental xenobiotic and steroid biotransformations catalyzed by cytochrome P450, epoxide hydrolase, and glutathione S-transferase activities and their relationships to maternal cigarette smoking. Drug Metab Rev 21:427, 1990.

64. Pasternak JF, et al: Regional cerebral blood flow in the newborn beagle pup: The germinal matrix is a "low-flow" structure. Pediatr Res 16:499, 1982.

65. Peckham C, et al: Mother-to-child transmission of the human immunodeficiency virus. N Engl J Med 333:298, 1995.

66. Perry JC, et al: Fetal supraventricular tachycardia treated with flecainide acetate. J Pediatr 118:303, 1991.

67. Phelan JP, et al: Amniotic fluid volume assessment with four-quadrant technique at 36–42 weeks gestation. J Reprod Med 32:540, 1987.

68. Philip AGS, et al: Intraventricular hemorrhage in preterm infants: Declining incidence in the 1980s. Pediatrics 84:797, 1989.

69. Polk DH: Diagnosis and management of altered fetal thyroid status, Clin Perinatol 21:647, 1994.

70. Porreco RP, et al: Fetal blood sampling in the management of intrauterine thyrotoxicosis. Obstet Gynecol 76:509, 1990.

71. Public Health Service task force recommendations for the use of antiretroviral drugs in pregnant women infected with HIV-1 for maternal health and for reducing perinatal HIV-1 transmission in the United States. MMWR Morb Mortal Wkly Rep 47:1, 1998.

72. Rieder MJ: Prevention of neural tube defects with periconceptional folic acid. Clin Perinatol 21:483, 1994.

73. Rovert J, et al: Intellectual outcome in children with fetal hypothyroidism. J Pediatr 110:700, 1987.

74. Satoh S, et al: Clinical applications of the Doppler technique in monitoring the fetus. Clin Perinatol 26:853, 1999.

75. Schmidt PL, et al: Effect of antepartum glucocorticoid administration upon neonatal respiratory distress syndrome and perinatal infection. Am J Obstet Gynecol 148:178, 1984.

76. Shankaran S, et al: Antenatal phenobarbital therapy and neonatal outcome. I. Effect on intracranial hemorrhage. Pediatrics 97:644, 1996.

77. Shankaran S, et al: The effect of antenatal phenobarbital therapy on neonatal intracranial hemorrhage in preterm infants. N Engl J Med 337:466, 1997.

78. Simone C, et al: Drug transfer across the placenta: Considerations in treatment and research. Clin Perinatol 21:463, 1994.

79. Simpson JM, et al: Fetal tachycardias: Management and outcome of 127 consecutive cases. Heart 79:576, 1998.

80. Smith CV, et al: Relation of mild idiopathic polyhydramnios to prenatal outcome. Obstet Gynecol 79:387, 1992.

81. Southall DP, et al: Prospective study of fetal heart rate and rhythm patterns. Am J Dis Child 55:506, 1980.

82. Speiser PW, et al: Prenatal diagnosis and management of congenital adrenal hyperplasia. Clin Perinatol 21:631, 1994.

83. Sperling RS, et al: Maternal viral load, zidovudine treatment and the risk of transmission of human immunodeficiency virus type I from mother to infant. N Engl J Med 335:1621, 1996.

84. Szeto HH: Maternal-fetal pharmacokinetics and fetal dose-response relationships. Ann N Y Acad Sci 562:42, 1989.

85. The Developmental Epidemiology Network Investigators: The correlation between placental pathology and intraventricular hemorrhage in the preterm infant. Pediatr Res 43:15, 1998.

86. Thorp JA, et al: Antepartum vitamin K and phenobarbital for preventing intraventricular hemorrhage in the premature newborn: A randomized, double-blind, placebo-controlled trial. Obstet Gynecol 83:70, 1994.

87. Update on adult immunization: Recommendations of the Immunization Practices Advisory Committee (ACIP). MMWR Morb Mortal Wkly Rep 12:12, 1991.

88. Van DenVeyner I, et al: The effect of gestational age and fetal indomethacin levels on the incidence of constriction of the fetal ductus arteriosus. Obstet Gynecol 82:500, 1993.

89. Van Dyke RB, et al: The Ariel Project: A prospective cohort study of maternal-child transmission of human immunodeficiency virus type I in the era of maternal retroviral therapy. J Infect Dis 179:319, 1999.

90. Varner M, et al: Rabies vaccination in pregnancy. Am J Obstet Gynecol 143:717, 1982.

91. Ward RM: Pharmacological treatment of the fetus, clinical pharmacokinetic considerations. Clin Pharmacokinet 28:343, 1995.

92. Ward RM: Pharmacologic enhancement of fetal lung maturation. Clin Perinatol 21:523, 1994.

93. Wax JR, et al: Fetal blood sampling. Obstet Gynecol Clin N Am 20:533, 1993.

94. Weiner CP, et al: Digoxin-like immunoreactive substance in fetuses with and without cardiac pathology. Am J Obstet Gynecol 157:368, 1987.

95. Weiner CP, et al: Direct treatment of fetal supraventricular tachycardia after failed transplacental therapy. Am J Obstet Gynecol 158:570, 1988.

96. Weinstrom KD, et al: Prenatal diagnosis of fetal hyperthyroidism using funipuncture. Obstet Gynecol 76:513, 1990.

97. Yang K: Placental 11 beta-hydroxysteroid dehydrogenase: Barrier to maternal glucocorticoids. Rev Reprod 2:129, 1997.

98. Zanjani ED, et al: Prospects for in utero human gene therapy. Science 285:2084, 1999.

99. Zidovudine for the prevention of HIV transmission from mother to infant. MMWR Morb Mortal Wkly Rep 43:285, 1994.

Part Two: Surgical Treatment of the Fetus

100. Adamsons K Jr: Fetal surgery. N Engl J Med 275:204, 1966.

101. Adzick NS: Fetal thoracic lesions. Semin Pediatr Surg 2:103, 1993.

102. Adzick NS, Harrison MR: The unborn surgical patient. Curr Probl Surg 31:1, 1994.

103. Adzick NS, Harrison MR: The unborn surgical patient. Curr Prob Obstet Gynecol Fertil 18:173, 1995.

104. Adzick NS, et al: Diaphragmatic hernia in the fetus: Prenatal diagnosis and outcome in 94 cases. J Pediatr Surg 20:357, 1983.

105. Adzick NS, et al: Fetal cystic adenomatoid malformation: Prenatal diagnosis and natural history. J Pediatr Surg 20:483, 1985.

106. Adzick NS, et al: Fetal surgery for cystic adenomatoid malformation of the lung. J Pediatr Surg 28:806, 1993.

107. Adzick NS, et al: Pulmonary hypoplasia and renal dysplasia in a fetal urinary tract obstruction model. Surg Forum 38:666, 1970.

108. Adzick NS, et al: A rapidly growing fetal teratoma. Lancet 349:538, 1997.

109. Adzick NS, et al: Successful fetal surgery for spina bifida. Lancet 352:1675, 1998.

110. Alcorn D, et al: Morphological effects of chronic tracheal ligation and drainage in the fetal lamb lung. J Anat 123:649, 1977.

111. Alter DN, et al: Prenatal diagnosis of congestive heart failure in a fetus with a sacrococcygeal teratoma. Obstet Gynecol 71:978, 1988.

112. Altman RP, et al: Sacrococcygeal teratoma: American Academy of Pediatrics Surgical Section Survey—1973. J Pediatr Surg 9:389, 1974.

113. Anderson N, et al: Detection of obstructive uropathy in the fetus: Predictive value of sonographic measurements of renal pelvic diameter at various gestational ages. Am J Roentgenol 164: 719,1995.

114. Arger PH, et al: Routine fetal genitourinary tract screening. Radiology 156:485, 1985.

115. Arias F, et al: Treatment of acardiac twinning. Obstet Gynecol 91:818, 1998.

116. Asensio HS, et al: Intrauterine exchange transfusion. Am J Obstet Gynecol 95:1129, 1966.

117. Bebbington MW, et al: Selective feticide in twin transfusion syndrome using ultrasound guided insertion of thrombogenic coils. Fetal Diagn Ther 10:32, 1995.

118. Benacerraf BR, et al: Successful midtrimester thoracocentesis with analysis of lymphocyte population in the pleural fluid. Am J Obstet Gynecol 155:398, 1989.

119. Benirschke K, Kim CK: Multiple pregnancy. N Engl J Med 288:1276, 1973.

120. Birnholz JC, Frigoletto FD: Antenatal treatment of hydrocephalus. N Engl J Med 304:1021, 1981.

121. Bond SJ, et al: Death due to high-output cardiac failure in fetal sacrococcygeal teratoma. J Pediatr Surg 25:1287, 1990.

122. Bootstaylor BS, et al: Prenatal sonographic predictors of liver herniation in congenital diaphragmatic hernia. J Ultrasound Med 14:515, 1995.

123. Botash RJ, Spirt BA: Color Doppler imaging aids in the prenatal diagnosis of congenital diaphragmatic hernia. J Ultrasound Med 12:359, 1993.

124. Brennan JN, et al: Fetofetal transfusion syndrome: Prenatal ultrasonographic diagnosis. Radiology 143:535, 1982.

125. Bruner JP, et al: Endoscopic coverage of fetal open myelomeningocele in utero [letter]. Am J Obstet Gynecol 176:256, 1987.

126. Bruner JP, et al: Endoscopic coverage of myelomeningocele in utero. Am J Obstet Gynecol 180:153, 1999.

127. Bruner JP, et al: Fetal surgery for myelomeningocele and the incidence of shunt-dependent hydrocephalus. JAMA 282:1819, 1999.

128. Cass DL, et al: Cystic lung lesions with systemic arterial blood supply: A hybrid of congenital cystic adenomatoid malformation and bronchopulmonary sequestration. J Pediatr Surg 32:986, 1997.

129. Cendron M, et al: Prenatal diagnosis and management of the fetus with hydronephrosis. Semin Perinatol 18:163, 1994.

130. Cha I, et al: Fetal congenital cystic adenomatoid malformations of the lung: A clinicopathologic study of eleven cases. Am J Surg Pathol 21:537, 1997.

131. Chervenak FA, et al: The management of fetal hydrocephalus. Am J Obstet Gynecol 151:933, 1985.

132. Cheschier NC, Seeds JW: Polyhydramnios and oligohydramnios in twin gestations. Obstet Gynecol 71:882, 1988.

133. Clark SL, et al: Successful fetal therapy for cystic adenomatoid malformation associated with second trimester hydrops. Am J Obstet Gynecol 157:294, 1987.

134. Clewell WH: The fetus with ventriculomegaly: Selection and Treatment. In: Harrison MR, et al (eds): The Unborn Patient: Prenatal Diagnosis and Treatment, 2nd ed. Philadelphia, WB Saunders, 1991, p 444.

135. Clewell WH, et al: A surgical approach to the treatment of fetal hydrocephalus. N Engl J Med 306:1320, 1982.

136. Clewell WH, et al: Ventriculomegaly: Evaluation and management. Semin Perinatol 9:98, 1985.

137. Cochrane DD, et al: Intrauterine hydrocephalus and ventriculomegaly: Associated anomalies and fetal outcome. Can J Neurol Sci 12:51, 1984.

138. Coplen DE, et al: 10-year experience with prenatal intervention for hydronephrosis. J Urol 156:1142, 1996.

139. Copp AJ, et al: The embryonic development of mammalian neural tube defects. Prog Neurobiol 35:363, 1990.

140. Cousins L, et al: Placentomegaly due to fetal congestive failure in a pregnancy with a sacrococcygeal teratoma. J Reprod Med 25:142, 1980.

141. Crane JP: Familial congenital diaphragmatic hernia: Prenatal diagnostic approach and analysis of twelve families. Clin Genet 16:244, 1979.

142. Crombleholme TM: Invasive fetal therapy: Current status and future directions. Semin Perinatol 18:385, 1994.

143. Crombleholme TM, et al: Congenital hydronephrosis: Early experience with open fetal surgery. J Pediatr Surg 23:1114, 1988.

144. Crombleholme TM, et al: Fetal intervention in obstructive uropathy: Prognostic indicators and efficacy of intervention. Am J Obstet Gynecol 162:1239, 1991.

145. Crombleholme TM, et al: Prenatal diagnosis and management of bilateral hydronephrosis. Pediatr Nephrol 2:334, 1988.

146. DeLia JE, et al: Fetoscopic laser ablation of placental vessels in severe previable twin-twin transfusion syndrome. Am J Obstet Gynecol 172:1202, 1995.

147. DeLia JE, et al: Fetoscopic neodynium:YAG laser occlusion of placental vessels in severe twin-twin transfusion syndrome. Obstet Gynecol 75:1046, 1990.

148. DeLia JE, et al: Neodynium:YAG laser occlusion of ehesus placental vasculature via fetoscopy. Am J Obstet Gynecol 160:485, 1989.

149. DeLia JE, et al: Treatment of placental vasculature with a neodynium:YAG laser via fetoscopy. Am J Obstet Gynecol 151: 1126, 1985.

150. DeLia JE, et al: Twin transfusion syndrome: Successful in utero treatment with digoxin. Int J Gynecol Obstet 23:197, 1985.

151. DiFiore JW, et al: Experimental fetal tracheal ligation reverses the structural and physiological effects of pulmonary hypoplasia in congenital diaphragmatic hernia. J Pediatr Surg 29:248, 1994.

152. Drewek MJ, et al: Quantitative analysis of the toxicity of human amniotic fluid to cultured rat spinal cord. Pediatr Neurosurg 27:190, 1997.

153. Edmonds LD, James LM: Temporal trends in the prevalence of congenital malformations at birth based on the birth defects monitoring program, United States 1979–1987. MMWP Morb Mortal Wkly Rep 39:19, 1990.

154. Eglowstein M, D'Alton ME: Intrauterine demise in multiple gestation: Theory and management. J Maternal Fetal Med 2:272, 1993.

155. Elias S: Use of fetoscopy for the prenatal diagnosis of hereditary skin disorders. Corr Probl Prematol 16:1, 1987.

156. Elliott JP, et al: Aggressive therapeutic amniocentesis for treatment of twin-twin transfusion syndrome. Obstet Gynecol 77:537, 1991.

157. Estes JM, Harrison MR: Fetal obstructive uropathy. Sem Pediatr Surg 2:129, 1993.

158. Estes JM, et al: Endoscopic creation and repair of fetal cleft lip. Plast Reconstr Surg 90:743, 1992.

159. Estes JM, et al: Fetoscopic surgery for the treatment of congenital anomalies. J Pediatr Surg 27:950, 1992.

160. Fauza DO, Wilson JM: Congenital diaphragmatic hernia and associated anomalies: Their incidence, identification, and impact on prognosis. J Pediatr Surg 29:1113, 1994.

161. Filly RA: Ultrasound evaluation of the fetal neural axis. In Callen PW (ed): Ultrasonography in Obstetrics and Gynecology. Philadelphia, WB Saunders, 1994, p 189.

162. Flake AW: Fetal sacrococcygeal teratoma. Semin Pediatr Surg 2:113, 1993.

163. Flake AW: Fetal surgery for congenital diaphragmatic hernia. Semin Pediatr Surg 5:266, 1996.

164. Flake AW, et al: Fetal sacrococcygeal teratoma. J Pediatr Surg 21:563, 1986.

165. Freda VJ, Adamsons K Jr: Exchange transfusion in utero: Report of a case. Am J Obstet Gynecol 89:817, 1964.

166. Freedman AL, et al: Fetal therapy for obstructive uropathy: Specific outcomes diagnosis. J Urol 156:720, 1996.

167. Frigoletto FD Jr, et al: Antenatal treatment of hydrocephalus by ventriculoamniotic shunting. JAMA 248:2495, 1982.

168. Fusi L, Gordon H: Multiple pregnancy complicated by single intrauterine death: Problems and outcome with conservative management. Br J Obstet Gynaecol 97:511, 1990.

169. Garmel SH, D'Alton ME: Fetal ultrasonography. West J Med 159:273, 1993.

170. Glick PL, et al: Correction of congenital hydronephrosis in utero. III. Early mid-trimester ureteral obstruction produces renal dysplasia. J Pediatr Surg 98:681, 1983.

171. Glick PL, et al: Correction of congenital hydronephrosis in utero. IV. In utero decompression prevents renal dysplasia. J Pediatr Surg 19:649, 1984.

172. Glick PL, et al: Management of the fetus with congenital hydronephrosis. II. Prognostic criteria and selection for treatment. J Pediatr Surg 20:376, 1984.

173. Glick PL, et al: Management of ventriculomegaly in the fetus. J Pediatr 105:97, 1984.

174. Golbus MS, et al: In utero treatment of urinary tract obstruction. Am J Obstet Gynecol 142:383, 1982.

175. Golbus MS, et al: Prenatal diagnosis and treatment of fetal hydronephrosis. Semin Perinatol 7:102, 1983.

176. Graf JL, et al: Fetal hydrops after in utero tracheal occlusion. J Pediatr Surg 32:214, 1997.

177. Hagay Z, et al: Isolated fetal pleural effusion: A prenatal management dilemma. Obstet Gynecol 81:147, 1993.

178. Hahanemaamnn H, Mohr J: Antenatal fetal diagnosis in the embryo by means of biopsy from the extraembryonic membranes. Bull Eur Soc Hum Genet 2:23, 1968.

179. Harding R, et al: Upper airway resistance in fetal sheep: The influence of breathing activity. J Appl Physiol 60:160, 1986.

180. Harrison M: The fetus with a diaphragmatic hernia: Pathophysiology, natural history and surgical management. In Harrison M, et al (eds): The Unborn Surgical Patient: Prenatal Diagnosis and Treatment, 2nd ed. Philadelphia, WB Saunders, 1991, p 295.

181. Harrison MR, Filly RA: The fetus with obstructive uropathy: Pathophysiology, natural history, selection and treatment. In Harrison MR, et al (eds): The Unborn Patient: Prenatal Diagnosis and Treatment, 2nd ed. Philadelphia, WB Saunders, 1991, p 328.

182. Harrison MR, et al: Antenatal intervention for congenital cystic adenomatoid malformation. Lancet 336:965, 1990.

183. Harrison MR, et al: Congenital diaphragmatic hernia: The hidden mortality. J Pediatr Surg 13:227, 1978.

184. Harrison MR, et al: Correction of congenital diaphragmatic hernia in utero. V. Initial clinical experience. J Pediatr Surg 25:47, 1990.

185. Harrison MR, et al: Correction of congenital diaphragmatic hernia in utero. VI. Hard learned lessons. J Pediatr Surg 28:1411, 1993.

186. Harrison MR, et al: Correction of congenital diaphragmatic hernia in utero. VII: A prospective trial. J Pediatr Surg 32:1637, 1997.

187. Harrison MR, et al: Correction of congenital hydronephrosis in utero. I. The model: Fetal urethral obstruction produces hydronephrosis and pulmonary hypoplasia in fetal lambs. J Pediatr Surg 18:247, 1983.

188. Harrison MR, et al: Fetal hydronephrosis: Selection and surgical repair. J Pediatr Surg 22:556, 1987.

189. Harrison MR, et al: Fetal surgery for congenital hydronephrosis. N Engl J Med 306:591, 1982.

190. Harrison MR, et al: Fetal treatment 1982. N Engl J Med 307:1651, 1982.

191. Harrison MR, et al: Management of the fetus with congenital hydronephrosis. J Pediatr Surg 17:383, 1982.

192. Harrison MR, et al: Management of the fetus with a correctable congenital defect. JAMA 246:774, 1981.

193. Harrison MR, et al: Management of the fetus with a urinary tract malformation. JAMA 246:635, 1981.

194. Harrison MR, et al: Successful repair in utero of a fetal dia-

phragmatic hernia after removal of herniated viscera from the left thorax. N Engl J Med 322:1582, 1990.

195. Hashim E, et al: Reversible tracheal obstruction in the fetal sheep: Effects on tracheal fluid pressure and lung growth. J Pediatr Surg 30:1172, 1995.

196. Healey MG: Acardia: Predictive risk factors for the co-twins survival. Teratology 50:205, 1994.

197. Hecher K, et al: Endoscopic laser surgery versus serial amniocentesis in the treatment of severe twin-twin transfusion syndrome. Am J Obstet Gynecol 180:717, 1999.

198. Hedrick MH, et al: Congenital high airway obstruction syndrome (CHAOS): A potential for perinatal intervention. J Pediatr Surg 29:271, 1994.

199. Hedrick MH, et al: Plug the lung until it grows (PLUG): A new method to treat congenital diaphragmatic hernia in utero. J Pediatr Surg 29:612, 1994.

200. Heffez DS, et al: Intrauterine repair of experimental surgically created dysrhaphism. Neurosurgery 32:1005, 1993.

201. Heffez DS, et al: The paralysis associated with myelomeningocele: Clinical and experimental data implicating a preventable spinal cord injury. Neurosurgery 26:987, 1990.

202. Hislop A, et al: The lungs in congenital bilateral renal agenesis and dysplasia. Arch Dis Child 54:32, 1979.

203. Hobbins JC, et al: Antenatal diagnosis of renal anomalies with ultrasound. I. Obstructive uropathy. Am J Obstet Gynecol 148:868, 1984.

204. Holzgreve W, et al: Prenatal diagnosis and management of fetal hydrocephaly and lissencephaly. Childs Nervous System 9:408, 1993.

205. Hudgins RJ, et al: Natural history of fetal ventriculomegaly. Pediatrics 82:682, 1988.

206. Hutchins GM, et al: Acquired spinal cord injury in human fetuses with myelomeningocele. Pediatr Pathol Lab Med 16:701, 1996.

207. James WH: A note on the epidemiology of acardiac monsters. Teratology 16:211, 1977.

208. Johnson MP, et al: In utero surgical treatment of fetal obstructive uropathy: A new comprehensive approach to identify appropriate candidates for vesicoamniotic shunt therapy. Am J Obstet Gynecol 170:1770, 1994.

209. Johnson MP, et al: Sequential urinalysis improves evaluation of fetal renal function in obstructive uropathy. Am J Obstet Gynecol 173:59, 1995.

210. Kalache KD, et al: Prenatal diagnosis of laryngeal atresia in two cases of congenital high airway obstruction syndrome (CHAOS). Prenat Diagn 17:577, 1997.

211. Katz VL, et al: Role of ultrasound and informed consent in the evaluation of elevated maternal serum alpha-fetoprotein. Am J Perinatol 8:73, 1991.

212. Kleiner B, et al: Sonographic analysis of the fetus with ureteropelvic junction obstruction. Am J Roentgenol 148:359, 1987.

213. Kurjak A, et al: Ultrasound diagnosis and evaluation of fetal tumors. J Perinat Med 17:173, 1989.

214. Kurjak A, et al: Ultrasound diagnosis and fetal malformations of surgical interest. In Kurjak A (ed): The Fetus as Patient. Amsterdam, Excerpta Medica, 1985, p 243.

215. Laberge JM, et al: The fetus with pleural effusions. In Harrison MR (ed): The Unborn Patient, 2nd ed, Philadelphia, WB Saunders, 1991, p 314.

216. Langer JC, et al: Fetal hydrops and death from sacrococcygeal teratoma: Rationale for fetal surgery. Am J Obstet Gynecol 160:1145, 1989.

217. Lary JM, Edmonds LD: Prevalence of spina bifida at birth—United States, 1983–1990: A comparison of two surveillance systems. MMWP Morb Mortal Wkly Rep 45:15, 1996.

218. Lawrence KM, Coates S: The natural history of hydrocephalus: Detailed analysis of 182 unoperated cases. Arch Dis Child 37:345, 1962.

219. Levitsky DB, et al: Fetal aqueductal stenosis diagnosed sonographically: How grave is the prognosis. AJR 164:725, 1995.

220. Liechty KW, et al: Intrapartum airway management for giant fetal neck masses: The EXIT (ex utero intrapartum treatment) procedure. Am J Obstet Gynecol 177:870, 1997.

221. Liley AW: Intrauterine transfusion of foetus in haemolytic disease. Br Med J 2:1107, 1963.

222. Lipshutz GS, et al: Prospective analysis of lung-to-head ratio predicts survival for patients with prenatally diagnosed congenital diaphragmatic hernia. J Pediatr Surg 32:1634, 1997.

223. Longaker MT, et al: Primary fetal hydrothorax: Natural history and management. J Pediatr Surg 24:573, 1989.

224. Lorber J: Ventriculo-cardiac shunts in the first week of life: Results of a controlled trial in the treatment of hydrocephalus in infants born with spina bifida cystica or cranium bifidum. Dev Med Child Neurol (Suppl) 20:13, 1969.

225. Luthy DA, et al: Cesarean section before the onset of labor and subsequent motor function in infants with myelomeningocele diagnosed antenatally. N Engl J Med 324:662, 1991.

226. MacGillivray TE, et al: Disappearing fetal lung lesions. J Pediatr Surg 28:1321, 1993.

227. Mahour GH, et al: Sacrococcygeal teratoma: A 33-year experience. J Pediatr Surg 10:183, 1975.

228. Manning FA, et al: Catheter shunts for fetal hydronephrosis and hydrocephalus. Report of the International Fetal Surgery Registry. N Engl J Med 315:336, 1986.

229. Mashiach R, et al: Antenatal ultrasound diagnosis of congenital cystic adenomatoid malformation of the lung: Spontaneous resolution in utero. J Clin Ultrasound 21:453, 1993.

230. McCullagh M, et al: Accuracy of prenatal diagnosis of congenital cystic adenomatoid malformation. Arch Dis Child 71:F111, 1994.

231. McCurdy CM, et al: Ligation of the umbilical cord of an acardiac-acephalus twin with an endoscopic intrauterine technique. Obstet Gynecol 82:708, 1993.

232. Metkus AP, et al: Sonographic predictors of survival in fetal diaphragmatic hernia. J Pediatr Surg 31:148, 1996.

233. Meuli M, et al: Creation of myelomeningocele in utero: A model of functional damage from spinal cord exposure in fetal sheep. J Pediatr Surg 30:1028, 1995.

234. Meuli M, et al: In utero surgery rescues neurologic function at birth in sheep with spina bifida. Nat Med 1:342, 1995.

235. Meuli M, et al: The spinal cord lesion in human fetuses with myelomeningocele: Implications for fetal surgery. J Pediatr Surg 32:448, 1997.

236. Michejda M, Hodgen SD: In utero diagnosis and treatment of non-human primate fetal skeletal anomalies. I. Hydrocephalus. JAMA 246:1093, 1981.

237. Michejda M: Intrauterine treatment of spina bifida. Primate model. Z Kinderchir 39:259, 1984.

238. Milner R, Crombleholme TM: Troubles with twins: Fetoscopic therapy. Semin Perinatol 23:476, 1999.

239. Moore TR, et al: Perinatal outcome of forty-nine pregnancies complicated by acardiac twinning. Am J Obstet Gynecol 163:907, 1990.

240. Moran L, et al: Prenatal diagnosis and management of fetal thoracic lesions. Semin Perinatol 18:228, 1994.

241. Morin C, et al: Pulmonary sequestration with histologic changes of cystic adenomatoid malformation. Pediatr Radiol 19:130, 1989.

242. Morrow RJ, et al: Prenatal diagnosis of an intra-abdominal sacrococcygeal teratoma. Prenat Diagn 10:753, 1990.

243. MRC Vitamin Research Study Group: Prevention of neural tube defects: Results of the Medical Research Council Vitamin Study. Lancet 338:131, 1991.

244. Muller F, et al: Fetal urinary biochemistry predicts postnatal renal function in children with bilateral obstructive uropathies. Obstet Gynecol 82:813, 1993.

245. Nakayama DK, et al: Prognosis of posterior urethral valves presenting at birth. J Pediatr Surg 21:45, 1986.

246. Newton ER: Antepartum care in multiple gestation. Semin Perinat 10:19, 1986.

247. Nicolaides KH, Azar GB: Thoraco-amniotic shunting. Fetal Diagn Ther 5:164, 1990.

248. Nicolaides KH, et al: Chronic drainage of fetal pulmonary cysts. Lancet 2:618, 1987.

249. Patten BM: Embryological stages in the establishment of myeloschisis with spina bifida. Am J Anat 93:395, 1953.

250. Petres RE, et al: Congenital bilateral hydrothorax: Antepartum diagnosis and successful intrauterine surgical management. JAMA 248:1362, 1982.

251. Platt LD, et al: The California Maternal Serum alpha-Fetoprot-

ein Screening Program: The role of ultrasonography in the detection of spina bifida. Am J Obstet Gynecol 166:1328, 1992.

252. Porreco RP, et al: Occlusion of umbilical artery in acardiac-acephalic twin. Lancet 337:326, 1991.

253. Potter EL: Kidneys, ureters, urinary bladder, and urethra. In Potter EL, Craig JM (eds): Pathology of the Fetus and Neonate, 3rd ed. Chicago, Yearbook Medical, 1976, p 473.

254. Pretorius DH, et al: Clinical course of fetal hydrocephalus: 40 cases. Am J Radiol 144:827, 1985.

255. Puri P: Congenital diaphragmatic hernia. Curr Probl Surg 31:787, 1994.

256. Quintero RA, et al: Brief report: Umbilical-cord ligation to an acardiac twin by fetoscopy at 19 weeks of gestation. N Engl J Med 330:469, 1994.

257. Quintero RA, et al: In-utero percutaneous cystoscopy in the management of fetal lower obstructive uropathy. Lancet 346:537, 1995.

258. Quintero RA, et al: Percutaneous fetal cystoscopy and endoscopic fulguration of posterior urethral valves. Am J Obstet Gynecol 172:206, 1995.

259. Quintero RA, et al: Selective photocoagulation of placental vessels in twin-twin transfusion syndrome: Evaluation of a new technique. Obstet Gynecol Surv 53:S97, 1998.

260. Quintero RA, et al: Transabdominal thin-gauge embryo fetoscopy: A technique for early prenatal diagnosis and its use in the diagnosis of a case of Meckel-Gruber syndrome. Am J Obstet Gynecol 168:1552, 1993.

261. Rausen AR, et al: Twin transfusion syndrome. J Pediatr 66:613, 1965.

262. Robichaux AG III, et al: Fetal abdominal wall defect: A new complication of vesicoamniotic shunting. Fetal Diagn Ther 6:11, 1991.

263. Robie GF, et al: Selective delivery of an acardiac-acephalic twin. N Engl J Med 320:512, 1989.

264. Rodeck CH, et al: Fetal liver biopsy for prenatal diagnosis of ornithine carbamyl transferase deficiency. Lancet 2:297, 1982.

265. Rodeck CH, et al: Long-term in utero drainage of fetal hydrothorax. N Engl J Med 319:1135, 1988.

266. Roman JD, Hare AA: Digoxin and decompression amniocentesis for treatment of feto-fetal transfusion. Br J Obstet Gynecol 102:421, 1995.

267. Ronderos-Dumit D, et al: Uterine-peritoneal amniotic fluid leakage: An unusual complication of intrauterine shunting. Obstet Gynecol 78:913, 1991.

268. Rosseau GL, et al: Current prognosis in fetal ventriculomegaly. J Neurosurg 77:551, 1991.

269. Saade GR, et al: Amniotomy: A new approach to the 'stuck twin' syndrome. Am J Obstet Gynecol 172:429, 1995.

270. Saade GR, et al: Feto-fetal transfusion. In Fisk N, Moise KJ (eds): Transfusion in Fetal Therapy: Invasive and Transplacental. Melbourne, Australia, Cambridge University Press, 1997, p 227.

271. Sackier JM: Laparoscopy in pediatric surgery. J Pediatr Surg 26:1145, 1992.

272. Schauer GM, et al: Prenatal diagnosis of Fraser syndrome at 18.5 weeks gestation, with autopsy findings at 19 weeks. Am J Med Genet 37:583, 1990.

273. Scheller JM, Nelson KB: Does cesarean delivery prevent cerebral palsy or other neurologic problems of childhood? Obstet Gynecol 83:624, 1994.

274. Schmidt KG, et al: High-output cardiac failure in fetuses with large sacrococcygeal teratoma: Diagnosis by echocardiography and Doppler ultrasound. J Pediatr 114:1023, 1989.

275. Seeds JW, et al: Prenatal diagnosis of sacrococcygeal teratoma: An anechoic caudal mass. J Clin Ultrasound 10:193, 1982.

276. Serlo W, et al: Prognostic signs in fetal hydrocephalus. Childs Nerv Syst 2:93, 1986.

277. Shaw GM, et al: Epidemiologic characteristics of phenotypically distinct neural tube defects among 0.7 million California births, 1983–1987. Teratology 49:143, 1994.

278. Sheth S, et al: Prenatal diagnosis of sacrococcygeal teratoma: Sonographic-pathologic correlation. Radiology 169:131, 1988.

279. Silver MM, et al: Perinatal pulmonary hyperplasia due to laryngeal atresia. Hum Pathol 19:110, 1988.

280. Skarsgard ED, et al: Fetal endoscopic tracheal occlusion ('Fetendo-PLUG') for congenital diaphragmatic hernia. J Pediatr Surg 31:1335, 1996.

281. Stocker JT, et al: Congenital cystic adenomatoid malformation of the lung: Classification and morphologic spectrum. Hum Pathol 8:155, 1977.

282. Sutton LN, et al: Improvement in hindbrain herniation demonstrated by serial fetal magnetic resonance imaging following fetal surgery for myelomeningocele. JAMA 282:1826, 1999.

283. Use of folic acid for prevention of spina bifida and other neural tube defects—1983–1991. MMWR Morb Mortal Wkly Rep 40:513, 1991.

284. Van Allen MI, et al: Twin reversed arterial perfusion (TRAP) sequence: A study of 14 twin pregnancies with acardius. Semin Perinatol 7:285, 1983.

285. VanderWall KJ, et al: Fetal endoscopic ('Fetendo') tracheal clip. J Pediatr Surg 31:1101, 1996.

286. VanderWall KJ, et al: Fetendo-clip: A fetal endoscopic tracheal clip procedure in a human fetus. J Pediatr Surg 32:970, 1997.

287. Ville Y, et al: Preliminary experience with endoscopic laser surgery for severe twin-twin transfusion syndrome. N Engl J Med 332:224, 1995.

288. Watson WJ, et al: Prenatal diagnosis of laryngeal atresia. Am J Obstet Gynecol 163:1456, 1990.

289. Wigglesworth JS, et al: Fetal lung growth in congenital laryngeal atresia. Pediatr Pathol 7:515, 1987.

290. Willcourt RJ, et al: Laparoscopic ligation of the umbilical cord of an acardiac fetus. J Am Assoc Gynecol Laparosc 2:319, 1995.

291. Wittman BK, et al: Antenatal diagnosis of twin transfusion syndrome by ultrasound. Obstet Gynecol 58:123, 1981.

292. Young HF, et al: The relationship of intelligence and cerebral infantile hydrocephalus (IQ potential in hydrocephalic children). Pediatrics 52:38, 1973.

293. Zosmer N, et al: Clinical and echocardiographic features of in utero cardiac dysfunction in the recipient twin in twin-to-twin transfusion syndrome. Br Heart J 72:74, 1994.

12 Occupational and Environmental Risks to the Fetus

Cynthia F. Bearer

Occupational and environmental risks to the fetus are becoming increasingly important. In 1990, 58% of the U.S. work force consisted of women (approximately 49.3 million female workers).[69] Seventy-five percent of working women are of reproductive age.[77] It is estimated that up to 10% of employed women give birth in a given year.[77] In 1980, more than 1.25 million live births were to women who had worked at some time during the year before delivery.[77] Environmental exposures are increasing as both population and economic needs continue to expand. In 1900, there were 1.25 billion people on earth. This number doubled by 1950, then it doubled again to 5 billion by 1987. There are now more than 6 billion people on earth, and this number may double by the year 2050.[91] The pressures of population growth on the environment are reflected in increasing need for land, water, food, and fuels. With more people and increasing economic expansion come the problems of emissions and pollution from daily living, industry, commerce, and agriculture.[98] Land is overused; water, air, food, and soil are contaminated. Every human being on this planet is exposed to chemicals and other agents. This chapter describes the various types of exposures (nonconcurrent and concurrent with pregnancy), the unique pharmacokinetics of the fetus, and the spectrum of adverse outcomes known to be associated with occupational and environmental exposures (Fig. 12–1).

NONCONCURRENT EXPOSURES

Environmental exposures that affect newborns may occur before conception. The main effect of these exposures may be on the ovum or sperm, which then leads to the development of an abnormal fetus, but a woman's exposure may result in a delayed exposure to the developing fetus by the ongoing elimination of the chemical from the mother's body. Because the initial exposure is experienced by the mother before conception, these exposures are nonconcurrent with the pregnancy. For some chemicals, such as the organo-

halogens, the fetus can be affected by both nonconcurrent and concurrent maternal exposures.

PRECONCEPTUAL EFFECTS

Exposures Affecting the Ovum

The ova within women begin to develop in early fetal life. During female fetal development the oogonia are formed by meiotic division. Before birth, all oogonia have developed into primary oocytes and have completed the prophase of the first meiotic division (Fig. 12–2).[49] At the end of prophase, the chromosomes are condensed and spindle fibers connect them to the centrioles, which have reached the poles of the cell. The nuclear membrane has disappeared.[23] The oocyte remains in this state until puberty and perhaps for as long as 50 years. The oocyte may be vulnerable to environmental exposures. This hypothesis is supported by the increasing incidence of nondisjunctional events with increasing maternal age and, therefore, with prolonged environmental exposure. Environmental exposures to the oocyte have been shown in one study.[90] Xenobiotics (chemicals foreign to the metabolic network of the body) were measured in 18 samples of human follicular fluid collected during oocyte harvesting for in vitro fertilization. Concentrations of representative xenobiotics from this study are shown in Table 12–1. The significance of these concentrations is unknown.

Paternal Effects

Epidemiologic evidence suggests that preconceptual paternal exposures may constitute a risk to the fetus. Savitz and colleagues found associations between (1) stillbirth and paternal employment in the textile industry; (2) preterm delivery and paternal employment in the glass, clay, stone, textile, or mining industries; and (3) infants who are small for gestational age and paternal employment in the art or textile industries.[78] Paternal exposure to mercury vapor,[20] ethylene oxide, rubber chemicals, solvents used in

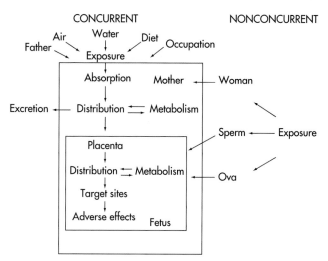

FIGURE 12–1. Maternal concurrent and nonconcurrent exposures and fetal exposure.

refineries, and solvents used in the manufacturing of rubber products[52] is associated with an increased relative risk of spontaneous abortion. Fathers employed in occupations associated with solvent exposure are at risk of having infants with anencephaly, with painters having the highest risk.[8] Male vehicle mechanics, automobile body repairmen, and welders have an increased risk of fathering a child with Wilms tumor.[66] The data on paternally mediated effects have been reviewed extensively.[54, 62]

One possible mechanism for paternally mediated

effects is the impairment of a paternal gene that is necessary for the normal growth and development of the fetus. In animals and human beings, the fetus requires genes derived from both the father and the mother, a phenomenon called *genetic imprinting.* Replacement of the father's genetic material with a second copy of the mother's genetic material (uniparental disomy), or vice versa, results in a nonviable conceptus.[34] One example of a defect in genetic imprinting is the Prader-Willi syndrome, caused by a functional mutation in paternal 15q, resulting in inactivation of the genes in that region of the chromosome. Angelman syndrome occurs if maternal 15q is affected. Environmental factors may play a role in functional uniparental disomy and lead to paternally mediated effects on the fetus. Two studies have shown an association between paternal exposure to hydrocarbons and Prader-Willi syndrome.[14, 88] In one study, approximately 50% of the fathers of patients with Prader-Willi syndrome were occupationally exposed to hydrocarbons.[14]

Certain birth defects are associated with older fathers, which provides additional evidence that paternal exposures may result in abnormalities of the fetus. These abnormalities include ventricular septal defects, atrial septal defects, and situs inversus.[50] The strongest association between advanced paternal age and birth defects is with achondroplasia.[76]

Another novel mechanism for preconceptual paternally mediated effects has been proposed by Yazigi and associates.[100] They found a high-affinity binding

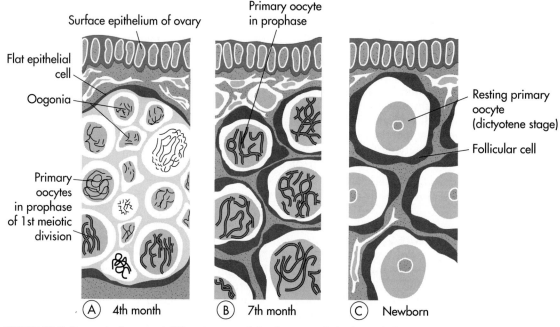

FIGURE 12–2. Segment of ovary at different stages of development. *A,* At 4 months' gestation; oogonia are grouped in clusters in the cortical part of the ovary. Some show mitosis, whereas others have already differentiated into primary oocytes and have entered prophase of first meiotic division. *B,* At 7 months' gestation; almost all oogonia are transformed into primary oocytes in prophase of first meiotic division. *C,* At birth; oogonia are absent. Each primary oocyte is surrounded by a single layer of follicular cells, forming primordial follicle. Oocytes have entered the dictyotene stage, in which they remain until just before ovulation, when they enter metaphase of first meiotic division. (From Langman J: Medical Embryology. Baltimore, Williams & Wilkins, 1975, p 11, with permission.)

TABLE 12–1   XENOBIOTICS IN HUMAN
FOLLICULAR FLUID

CONTAMINANT	MEAN CONCENTRATION (ppb)	SEM
Lindane	1.22	0.18
Total DDT	3.37	0.44
PCBs	8.03	0.88
Hexachlorobenzene	2.59	0.24
Dieldrin	0.13	0.03
Heptachlor epoxide	0.12	0.02

DDT, dichlorodiphenyltrichloroethane; PCBs, polychlorinated biphenyls; ppb, parts per billion; SEM, standard error of the mean.

From Trapp M, et al: Pollutants in human follicular fluid. Fertil Steril 42:146, 1984. Reproduced with permission of the publisher, the American Society for Reproductive Medicine (The American Fertility Society).

site for cocaine on sperm and postulated that sperm acted as a transporter of cocaine into the ovum.

SECONDARY FETAL EXPOSURE: MATERNAL BODY BURDEN

Nonconcurrent fetal exposure may result from either ongoing excretion of xenobiotics from maternal storage compartments or mobilization of contaminated compartments during pregnancy. Both adipose tissue and skeletal tissue are known storage sites for various chemicals.

Organohalogens are extremely stable chemicals both in the environment and in biologic systems. They bioaccumulate, becoming concentrated in tissues as they move up the food chain. Polychlorinated biphenyls (PCBs) are an example of this kind of chemical. They are ubiquitous in our environment because of their widespread use as liquid insulators for transformers and capacitors and because of their resistance to chemical and biologic breakdown. Their global distribution was first reported in 1966.[44] Their production peaked in 1970 and subsequently declined as more countries banned or limited their use.[41] Two major human poisonings have occurred through rice oil that was contaminated with PCBs, one in Japan in 1968 (called *Yusho*) and one in Taiwan in 1979 (called *Yu-Cheng*). In Taiwan, approximately 2000 adults had an illness characterized by hyperpigmentation, acne, and peripheral neuropathy. Of the first 39 hyperpigmented children born to poisoned women, 8 died.[40] In 1985, a cohort of 117 children born since the 1979 episode was found to have an excess of ectodermal defects and developmental delay.[73] Very few of these children were in utero during the actual poisoning episode. Their exposure to PCBs was from the elevated maternal body burden. In a more recent report,[15] Taiwanese children born up to 6 years after maternal exposure were as developmentally delayed as those children born within 1 year of maternal exposure (Fig. 12–3). The developmental delay persisted in these children at all times measured. Thus, these children had significant adverse effects from a mater-

nal exposure to PCBs that occurred up to 6 years before their birth.

The cognitive defects seen in the children with Yu-Cheng are comparable to those observed in American children exposed to higher levels of background PCBs. In North Carolina, small motor deficits were observed in children up to 2 years of age who had been prenatally exposed to PCBs through maternal body burden acquired through background exposure.[28] In Michigan, short-term memory deficits were measured in 4-year-old children with elevated cord blood levels of PCBs and whose mothers had regularly consumed sport fish contaminated with PCBs.[42] Further follow-up of these children at 11 years of age showed that those in the highest exposure group were three times more likely to have low-average IQ scores and twice as likely to be two years behind in reading comprehension.[43]

The major repository for lead is bone, where the turnover rate is approximately 25 to 30 years. Chronic lead exposure results in significant accumulation of lead in the skeleton. During pregnancy, calcium turnover is greatly increased,[46] which may increase mobilization of lead stores from bone. Lead mobilization was measured in one expectant couple by determining the isotopic ratio (IR) of lead, $^{206}Pb/^{207}Pb$ (Fig. 12–4).[57] The couple had initially lived in England, which has one IR for lead, and subsequently moved to Australia, which has a different IR for lead. If blood lead is primarily derived from air, then the IR of blood lead would parallel the IR prevalent in Australia. If blood lead is primarily derived from bone, then blood lead IR will not parallel that found in Australia; instead, it will be a reflection of the IR of lead absorbed in England during childhood. The man's blood lead IR paralleled that of Australia, whereas the woman's did not, indicating a significant source of lead for her other than an environmental one, probably from her skeletal stores. After delivery, her

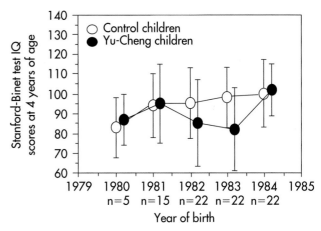

FIGURE 12–3. Stanford-Binet test IQ scores in 4-year-old children with Yu-Cheng and those in a control arm by year of birth. Error bars represent 1 standard deviation. Note that the contaminated rice was consumed in 1979. (From Chen Y-C, et al: Cognitive development of yu-cheng ["oil disease"] children prenatally exposed to heat degraded PCBs. JAMA 268:3216, 1992.)

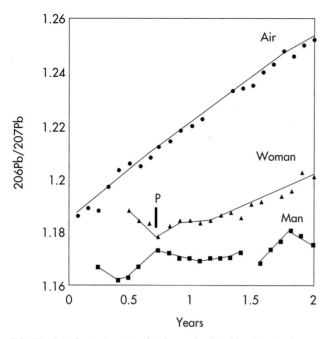

FIGURE 12–4. Isotopic ratio of airborne lead to blood lead of man and peripartum woman in 1974 and 1975. Declining isotopic ratio in the woman's blood before birth indicates a different source of lead from that of the man. Dietary sources of lead were the same. The only different source of lead for the woman is that coming from her skeleton during pregnancy. P, time of birth. (From Manton WI: Total contribution of airborne lead to blood lead. Br J Ind Med 42:168, 1985, p 169, with permission.)

blood lead IR also paralleled that prevalent in Australia. This hypothesis has been confirmed in two larger studies; one on pregnant Latin American women living in California,[75] the other on pregnant Eastern European women living in Australia.[32] Demonstration of significant fetal exposure because of an elevated maternal body burden of lead comes from two case reports of congenitally lead-poisoned children delivered to women inadequately treated for childhood plumbism.[83, 89]

CONCURRENT MATERNAL EXPOSURES

Exposures to the mother concurrent with pregnancy can come from many sources. Biologic markers of exposure to the fetus are being developed using meconium[3, 96] and hair.[72]

OCCUPATION

Several occupations have been shown to increase the risk of a poor outcome of pregnancy, and the studies showing that result have recently been reviewed.[69, 82, 95] Many studies are inconclusive or difficult to interpret. The strongest associations between workplace exposures and poor reproductive outcome have been found for lead, mercury, organic solvents, ethylene oxide, and ionizing radiation. Table 12–2 lists agents that are suspected to cause adverse pregnancy outcomes.[95]

PARAOCCUPATION

Other important sources of exposures to the mother occur through paraoccupational routes. These exposures occur when the father or others bring or track home occupational chemicals, when the home itself is in an occupational setting, or when industrial chemicals are brought home for home use.[55] Paraoccupational exposure occurred when a janitor in Alamogordo, New Mexico, brought home from a local seed company some grain that was intended for planting only. This grain had been treated with a fungicide containing organic mercury. The janitor used this grain to feed his hogs, one of which was subsequently slaughtered for consumption by the family. Three of nine children in the family became severely ill with organic mercury poisoning.[22, 70] The mother also ate the contaminated meat during the second trimester of her pregnancy. Both maternal serum and urine had elevated levels of mercury, as did the neonate's urine, indicating placental transfer of the mercury.[19] The newborn had gross tremulous movements of his extremities, which developed into myoclonic convulsions. At 1 year of age he could not sit up, and he was blind. The mother remained free of symptoms.

AIR

Air is an important source of exposure to the pregnant woman and fetus. For example, exposure of the mother to environmental tobacco smoke causes decreased birth weight,[33, 37, 59] an increased risk of sudden infant death syndrome (SIDS),[21, 63] and a predisposition to persistent pulmonary hypertension[2] (Fig. 12–5). In addition, exposure of the mother to fumes of naphthalene has resulted in severe fetal hemolysis in the absence of glucose-6-phosphate dehydrogenase deficiency.[25]

DIET

Diet may be an important vehicle for exposure. A tragic case occurred in Minamata Bay, Japan, where methyl mercury from an acetaldehyde-producing plant contaminated the food chain.[36] Pregnant women from a fishing village on the same bay gave birth to severely neurologically damaged infants, whereas they themselves had mild transient paresthesias or no symptoms at all.[58] The safe limit of both organic and inorganic mercury ingestion for pregnant women is the subject of much discussion and ongoing research.[56, 94]

PATHWAYS OF FETAL EXPOSURE

PLACENTA-DEPENDENT PATHWAYS

Two possible routes of fetal exposure to environmental hazards are placenta-dependent pathways and placenta-independent pathways (Box 12–1). For a placenta-dependent chemical to reach the fetus, it must

TABLE 12–2 AGENTS ASSOCIATED WITH ADVERSE FEMALE REPRODUCTIVE CAPACITY OR DEVELOPMENTAL EFFECTS IN HUMAN AND ANIMAL STUDIES*

AGENT	HUMAN OUTCOMES	STRENGTH OF ASSOCIATION IN HUMANS†	ANIMAL OUTCOMES	STRENGTH OF ASSOCIATION IN ANIMALS†
Anesthetic gases‡	Reduced fertility, spontaneous abortion	1, 3	Birth defects	1, 3
Arsenic	Spontaneous abortion, low birth weight	1	Birth defects, fetal loss	2
Benzo[a]pyrene	None	NA	Birth defects	1
Cadmium	None	NA	Fetal loss, birth defects	2
Carbon disulfide	Menstrual disorders, spontaneous abortion	1	Birth defects	1
Carbon monoxide	Low birth weight, fetal death (high doses)	1	Birth defects, neonatal death	2
Chlordecone	None	NA	Fetal loss	2, 3
Chloroform	None	NA	Fetal loss	1
Chloroprene	None	NA	Birth defects	2, 3
Ethylene glycol ethers	Spontaneous abortion	1	Birth defects	2
Ethylene oxide	Spontaneous abortion	1	Fetal loss	1
Formamides	None	NA	Fetal loss, birth defects	2
Inorganic mercury‡	Menstrual disorders, spontaneous abortion	1	Fetal loss, birth defects	1
Lead‡	Spontaneous abortion, prematurity, neurologic dysfunction in child	2	Birth defects, fetal loss	2
Organic mercury	CNS malformation, cerebral palsy	2	Birth defects, fetal loss	2
Physical stress	Prematurity	2	None	NA
Polybrominated biphenyls (PBBs)	None	NA	Fetal loss	2
Polychlorinated biphenyls (PCBs)	Neonatal PCB syndrome (low birth weight, hyperpigmentation, eye abnormalities)	2	Low birth weight, fetal loss	2
Radiation, ionizing	Menstrual disorders, CNS defects, skeletal and eye anomalies, mental retardation, childhood cancer	2	Fetal loss, birth defects	2
Selenium	Spontaneous abortion	3	Low birth weight, birth defects	2
Tellurium	None	NA	Birth defects	2
2,4-Dichlorophenoxyacetic acid (2,4-D)	Skeletal defects	4	Birth defects	1
2,4,5-Trichlorophenoxyacetic acid (2,4,5-T)	Skeletal defects	4	Birth defects	1
Video display terminals	Spontaneous abortion	4	Birth defects	1
Vinyl chloride‡	CNS defects	1	Birth defects	1, 4
Xylene	Menstrual disorders, fetal loss	1	Fetal loss, birth defects	1

*Major studies (Birnbaum LS, Tuomisto J: Non-carcinogenic effects of TCDD in animals. Food Additives and Contaminants 17:275, 2000) of the reproductive health effects of exposure to dioxin have shown that dioxin should be added to this list.
†1, limited positive data; 2, strong positive data; 3, limited negative data; 4, strong negative data.
‡Agent may have male-mediated effects.
CNS, central nervous system; NA, not applicable because no adverse outcomes were observed.
From Welch LS, et al (eds): Case studies in environmental medicine: Reproductive and developmental hazards. Washington, DC, 1993, Agency for Toxic Substances and Disease Registry, U.S. Department of Health and Human Services.

first enter the mother's blood stream and then cross the placenta in significant amounts. Not all environmental toxins meet these criteria; for example, asbestos and radon gas do not meet these criteria, unless they have been ingested. Three properties that enable chemicals to cross the placenta are low molecular weight, fat solubility, and resemblance to nutrients that are specifically transported. An example of a low-molecular-weight compound is carbon monoxide (CO), a constituent of environmental tobacco smoke. CO is an asphyxiant because it displaces oxygen from hemoglobin, forming carboxyhemoglobin (COHb). If enough COHb accumulates in the circulation, cellular metabolism is impaired by the inhibition of oxygen

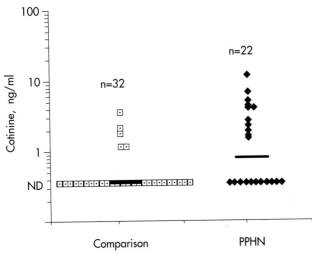

FIGURE 12–5. Distribution of cotinine concentrations of infants with persistent pulmonary hypertension of the newborn (PPHN) and a healthy comparison group after exclusion of mothers who smoke tobacco products. Mothers who smoke were identified by history of smoking or by umbilical cord cotinine concentrations greater than 13.7 ng/mL. Horizontal bars indicate medians of both groups. Medians were significantly different between the two groups (Mann-Whitney rank sum test: Z = 2.78941; P = .0053). (From Bearer CF, et al: Maternal tobacco smoke exposure and persistent pulmonary hypertension of the newborn. Environ Health Perspect 105:202, 1997, p 205.)

transport, delivery, and use. Fetal COHb accumulates more slowly than maternal COHb, but it increases to an equilibrium approximately 10% greater than in the maternal circulation.[38, 53] Thus, nonfatal CO poisoning of the mother may prove to be fatal to the fetus.[27]

Examples of fat-soluble chemicals that readily cross the placenta are ethanol and polycyclic hydrocarbons (benzo[a]pyrene, a carcinogen in environmental tobacco smoke, is a member of this class of compounds). Ethanol causes fetal alcohol syndrome (see Chapter 36). In pregnant ewes, IV infusion of ethanol results in identical maternal and fetal blood alcohol levels.[16] PCBs have been measured in equal concentrations in fetal and maternal blood.[11]

Calcium is a nutrient that is actively transported

BOX 12–1

PATHWAYS OF FETAL EXPOSURE

Placenta-dependent pathways
- Small molecular weight: carbon monoxide
- Lipophilic: benzo[a]pyrene, ethanol
- Specific transport mechanism: lead

Placenta-independent pathways
- Ionizing radiation
- Heat
- Noise
- Electromagnetic fields

---

across the placenta to provide the fetus with 100 to 140 mg/kg per day during the third trimester (see Chapter 47, Part Two).[86] It is believed that lead is transported by the calcium transporter. The fetal blood lead concentration is equivalent to the maternal blood lead concentration.[30] Recent animal studies have demonstrated that calcium supplementation may reduce the transfer of lead from prepregnancy maternal exposures to the fetus.[35]

PLACENTA-INDEPENDENT PATHWAYS

Placenta-independent hazards to the fetus include ionizing radiation, heat, noise, and, possibly, electromagnetic fields. Ionizing radiation is a well-characterized teratogen. Much of our knowledge comes from studies of the survivors of the atomic bombs in Hiroshima and Nagasaki. Children exposed in utero at younger than 18 weeks' gestation showed a dose response of increasing microcephaly with increasing dose of radiation. The lowest observable effect occurred at a dose of 1 to 9 rad (Fig. 12–6).[6] In comparison, the brain of a neonate undergoing cranial computed tomography with settings of 400 mA, 125 kV (peak), and a standard slice thickness of 4 mm receives a dose of 10.5 rad.[97] Because this level is close to that resulting in microcephaly, it has been recommended that computed tomography should be used sparingly for premature infants, particularly when other imaging techniques are available.[18] An excess of cancer among the Japanese exposed in utero has also been reported (Fig. 12–7).[101] Not all forms of radiation are hazardous to the fetus. Ultraviolet light does not penetrate to the fetus and does not constitute a future cancer risk.

Heat may directly penetrate to the fetus and cause birth defects. In a study of the effects of heat on the

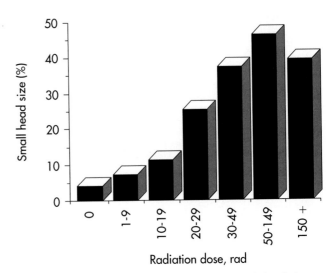

FIGURE 12–6. Percentage of Hiroshima children with head circumference 2 or more standard deviations below average, by fetal dose. Exposure occurred before 18 weeks of gestation. (From Blot WJ: Growth and development following prenatal and childhood exposure to atomic radiation. J Radiat Res [Tokyo] 16[Suppl]:82, 1975.)

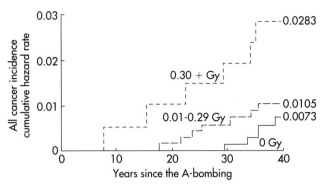

FIGURE 12–7. Cumulative hazard rate for cancer among survivors of intrauterine radiation in Hiroshima and Nagasaki, for three exposure groups through 1984. (From Yoshimoto Y, et al: Risk of cancer among children exposed in utero to A-bomb radiations, 1954. Lancet 2:667, 1988.)

outcome of pregnancy, 22,491 women undergoing α-fetoprotein screening were asked about their use of hot tubs, saunas, and electric blankets and whether they had experienced a fever during the first trimester.[60] The adjusted relative risk for neural tube defects with hot tub use was 2.8, with a 95% confidence interval of 1.2 to 6.5. With exposure to two of these heat sources, the relative risk increased to 6.5.

Noise has a waveform, which may be transmitted to the fetus (see Chapter 26, Part Two, and Chapter 29), and noise has been associated with certain birth defects, prematurity, and low birth weight.[19] In addition, noise-induced hearing loss may be evident following in utero exposure. In a study of 131 infants whose mothers worked in noisy conditions and received a noise dose of 65 to 95 LAeq.9m (dB) (a unit of noise dose calculated by an international standard and averaged over the 9 months of pregnancy), there was a threefold increase in the risk of a high-frequency hearing loss among infants whose mothers had received the highest doses of noise (Table 12–3).[48]

A unique source of exposure to the fetus occurs if

the fetus is born prematurely. Premature infants in the neonatal intensive care unit have several types of exposure in this highly artificial setting, including plasticizers,[71] noise,[5] electromagnetic fields,[1] and lead.[4] This subject has been discussed in several articles and is not reviewed here.[9]

FETAL PHARMACOKINETICS

FETAL DISTRIBUTION

The distribution of chemicals in the fetus differs from that in the adult (see Chapter 10 and Chapter 11, Part One). Because there is reduced protein binding in the fetus as a result of relative hypoproteinemia, chemicals can diffuse into tissues more readily. The blood-brain barrier is immature; therefore, chemicals can reach the brain easily. There is little or no body fat until approximately 29 weeks of gestation. Before that time, chemicals that normally accumulate in fat will accumulate in other fat-containing tissues, especially the brain. An example of this redistribution is shown in Figure 12–8.[26] DDT (an organochlorine pesticide, 1,1,1-trichloro-2,2-*bis*[*p*-chlorophenyl]ethane) was administered orally to mice at various ages that correspond to the human-brain growth spurt. The amount of radioactivity was measured in brain tissue after 24 hours and again after 7 days. There were striking differences in both the initial amount of DDT accumulated and the retention of DDT after 1 week. Twenty-day-old mice accumulated more DDT in their brains at 24 hours than mice at other ages. However, the DDT persisted longest in the animals given DDT at 10 days of age. In subsequent experiments, the mice treated at 10 days appeared to have more behavioral abnormalities than mice treated on either day 3 or day 19 of life, suggesting that the persistence of the pesticide was more important than the initial accumulation in regard to toxic effects. These results reflect the complexities of chemical distribution in the fetus

TABLE 12–3 COMPARISONS OF PERCENTAGES OF CHILDREN WITH HEARING LOSS AT 4000 Hz (>10 dB HL) BETWEEN CLASSES OF NOISE EXPOSURE DURING THEIR FETAL LIFE

| INDEPENDENT VARIABLE | CHILDREN WITH HEARING LOSS | | χ^2 (*p*) |
	No.	%	
LAeq.9m (dB)			
65–75	2	5.9	
75–85	3	7.0	8.3
85–95	13	24.1	(0.01)

From Lelande NM, et al: Is occupational noise exposure during pregnancy a risk factor of damage to the auditory system of the fetus? Am J Ind Med 10:427, 1986. Reprinted by permission of Wiley-Liss, Inc, a subsidiary of John Wiley & Sons, Inc.

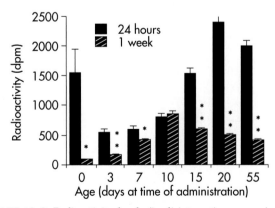

FIGURE 12–8. Radioactivity levels (in disintegrations per minute) in mouse brain 24 hours and 1 week after oral administration of 1.48 MBq [^{14}C]DDT per kg of body weight. Height of bars represents mean ± standard deviation; statistical difference between 24 hours and 1 week is indicated by $P < .01$ (*single asterisk*) and $P < .001$ (*double asterisk*). (From Eriksson P: Age-dependent retention of [^{14}C]DDT in the brain of the postnatal mouse. Toxicol Lett 22:326, 1984.)

as many organ systems continue to develop and mature.

FETAL METABOLISM

Chemicals are metabolized by a wide variety of enzymes, which differ among individuals both by genetic polymorphisms and by gestational age. *Ecogenetics* is the study of genetic predisposition to the toxic effects of chemicals.[37] An example of fetal ecogenetics is the susceptibility of some fetuses to the development of the fetal hydantoin syndrome with in utero exposure to phenytoin (see Chapter 10). Buehler and coworkers prospectively monitored 19 women receiving phenytoin during their pregnancy.[10] Epoxide hydrolase, an enzyme important in the metabolism of phenytoin, was measured in amniocytes from these pregnancies. Four of the samples had less than 30% of the standard activity (Fig. 12–9). All four infants corresponding to these samples had features of the fetal hydantoin syndrome; thus, their genetic background made them susceptible to an environmental exposure.

The expression of many proteins, including enzymes that metabolize xenobiotics, changes with gestational age. The developmental expression of alcohol dehydrogenase in the guinea pig is given in Figure 12–10.[13] Activity in the fetal liver is two orders of magnitude less than in the maternal liver. Even at 2 days of age, the difference in activity is still at one order of magnitude; therefore, environmental and occupational chemicals may not be cleared from the fetal compartment as rapidly as in the mother. On the other hand, the fetus may be protected against toxic effects if the active form of a chemical is its metabolite. An example of such a chemical is acetaminophen, the most common drug used in suicide attempts during pregnancy. Acetaminophen is metabolized by the P-450 cytochrome system to hepatotoxic and nontoxic

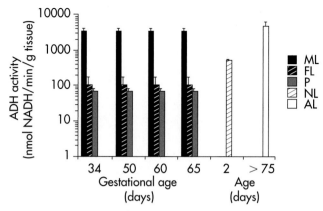

FIGURE 12–10. Activity of alcohol dehydrogenase (ADH) in guinea pig maternal liver (ML), fetal liver (FL), placenta (P), neonatal liver (NL), and adult liver (AL). Data are presented as mean ± SD ($n = 6$ at 34 days' gestation, $n = 5$ at 50 days' gestation, $n = 6$ at 60 days' gestation, $n = 6$ at 65 days' gestation, $n = 5$ at 2 postnatal days, and $n = 8$ at older than 75 postnatal days). (From Card SE, et al: Ontogeny of the activity of alcohol dehydrogenase and aldehyde dehydrogenase in the liver and placenta of the guinea pig. Biochem Pharm 38:2535, 1989. Used with permission from Elsevier Science Ltd., The Boulevard, Langford Lane, Kidlington OX5 1GB, United Kingdom.)

intermediates.[85] The expression of the P-450 enzymes is highly regulated both developmentally and by induction (see Chapter 11, Part One). Because many of these enzymes are poorly expressed in fetal tissues, the fetus may be protected from the effects of high doses of acetaminophen. In four case reports, the liver enzymes of neonates that were delivered on an emergency basis to overdosed women were normal or minimally elevated in the presence of severe maternal hepatotoxicity.[12, 47, 74, 87]

SPECTRUM OF OUTCOMES

Because of the complexity of development and of developmental processes from the fertilized egg to the newborn infant, sites of action of chemicals and radiation are numerous. An intrauterine exposure to radiation or chemicals may result in a broad array of phenotypic effects. Box 12–2 lists some of the phenotypes that may be seen.

Major malformations surpassed low birth weight and respiratory distress syndrome as the leading causes of infant death in 1990.[61] The rates for the top four causes of infant death per 100,000 live births were (1) major malformation, 198.1; (2) SIDS, 130.3; (3) disorders relating to short gestation and unspecified low birth weight, 96.5; and (4) respiratory distress syndrome, 7.4.[61] The environment has been linked to birth defects. A study of 371,933 women investigated the relative risk of a child being born with a birth defect similar to the birth defect affecting the preceding sibling (Table 12–4).[51] The relative risk of a similar birth defect was 11.6 (95% confidence interval, 9.3 to 14.0), and it dropped by more than 50% when the mother changed her living environment between the two pregnancies.

Reproductive dysfunction may also be a manifesta-

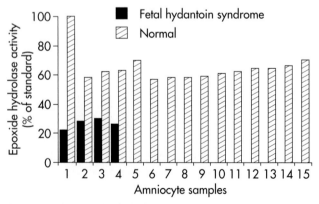

FIGURE 12–9. Epoxide hydrolase activity in amniocyte samples from 19 prospectively monitored fetuses. Samples from 4 fetuses subsequently given a diagnosis of fetal hydantoin syndrome are indicated by black bars. Samples from 15 fetuses subsequently confirmed not to have characteristic features of the syndrome are indicated by hatched bars. (From Beuhler BA, et al: Prenatal prediction of risk of the fetal hydantoin syndrome. N Engl J Med 322:1570, 1990, with permission. Copyright © 1990 Massachusetts Medical Society. All rights reserved.)

■ **BOX 12–2**

SPECTRUM OF PHENOTYPIC EFFECTS

- Preterm birth
- Growth retardation
- Microcephaly
- Major and minor malformations
- Deformations
- Metabolic dysfunction
- Cognitive dysfunction
- Behavioral dysfunction
- Malignancy

---

tion of occupational and environmental exposures. For example, when hamsters are exposed in utero to phenobarbital, they demonstrate altered neonatal behavior and reproductive maturation.[7] In studies of a cohort of adolescents exposed in utero to phenobarbital as part of a study to reduce postnatal hyperbilirubinemia, long-term effects, including lower testicular volume of exposed boys, were evident.[99] Dioxin and similar compounds have been shown to alter male reproductive function in wildlife.[17] Scientific debate continues over whether these observations in wildlife apply to human beings.

Permanent metabolic dysfunction has been associated with prenatal and neonatal exposure to monosodium glutamate (MSG) in animals. In female rats exposed neonatally to MSG, circulating growth hormone was reduced by 75% to 85%, and animals were mildly obese.[67] In addition, levels of a female-specific cytochrome P-450 were increased by almost 100%.[67] In male rats, neonatal exposure to MSG permanently blocked growth hormone secretion and resulted in stunted body growth, obesity, and impaired drug metabolism.[84] There was irreversible suppression of cytochrome P-450 2C11. These effects have now been linked to increased apoptosis in the developing brain of animals exposed to glutamate.[64] As a result of these observations in animals, MSG was removed from baby foods in 1969. The effects of both phenobarbital and MSG have been called delayed teratogenic expression because the effects of the exposure are not immediately apparent at birth.

Developmental neurotoxicity deserves special mention. The development of the central nervous system requires expression of unique proteins in specific cell populations within specific critical windows of time. Injury to these populations may result in neurodevelopmental disorders, such as mental retardation, autism, dyslexia, and attention-deficit/hyperactivity disorder. It is estimated that 3% to 8% of the 4 million children born each year in the United States are affected by a neurodevelopmental disability.[93] Some are caused by genetic aberrations (Down, fragile X), some by perinatal anoxia or meningitis, and some by exposure to drugs of abuse (ethanol, cocaine). However, the cause for most neurodevelopmental disabilities

is unknown. Environmental chemicals, such as lead, PCBs, and mercury, are known developmental neurotoxins. Alarmingly, of the 3000 chemicals produced or imported at over 1 million pounds a year, 43% have not received even minimal toxicologic assessment, and a mere 22% have been tested to determine whether they have the potential to cause developmental damage.[29] As of 1998, of all chemicals regulated by the U.S. Environmental Protection Agency, only 12 have had any developmental neurotoxicity testing.[92] Thus, it remains a real possibility that neurodevelopmental disabilities arising in the newborn period are a result of in utero chemical exposure.

CONCLUSION

In this chapter the many different sources of exposure and the timing of exposure to occupational and environmental chemicals have been described. The complexity of the maternal-fetal pharmacokinetics has been outlined, and many of the various types of outcomes have been discussed. The science of environmental medicine continues to evolve, elucidating sources of potential harm. What can one do now with the limited information available? First, women who work have a right by law to be informed about the chemicals with which they work,[68] and they have a right by law to be protected from harmful exposures. Materials safety data sheets are available to any employee who requests them. These sheets supply information of potential reproductive effects. Personal protective gear should be available, and increased monitoring of potential exposures should be instituted. In certain instances, temporary job shifting may prevent potential exposure. More insidious are the exposures that occur outside the workplace, which are often unknown to the person exposed. Sources of exposure include the chemicals and radiation in our environment—our water, our food, and our air. Current regulations rarely consider the unique susceptibilities and vulnerabilities of unborn children. Efforts should be made to inform the public and the legislature about these potential toxins so that safeguards to our children's health may be devised.

It is very challenging for the neonatologist confronted with a neonate with a problem resulting from an environmental exposure to determine the cause of that problem. Confirming the etiologic agent is almost impossible and requires several steps. First, a detailed exposure history is vital. Guidelines for taking this history can be found in a monograph from the U.S. Department of Health and Human Services, Agency for Toxic Substances and Disease Registry (ATSDR): *Case Studies in Environmental Medicine: Taking an Exposure History* (see "Additional Reading"). It is not enough to know the mother's occupation. One must ascertain exactly what she does at work, what the father does at work, what their hobbies are, what they do at home, what type of residence they have, and in what type of neighborhood they live. What is the composition of their diet? Do they smoke or use

TABLE 12–4 RISK OF SIMILAR AND DISSIMILAR BIRTH DEFECTS IN SECOND INFANTS OF MOTHERS WITH AN AFFECTED FIRST INFANT

DEFECT IN FIRST INFANT	NO. AT RISK	SECOND INFANT					
		Similar Defect			Dissimilar Defect		
		Observed	Expected	Relative Risk	Observed	Expected	Relative Risk
Clubfoot	2784	100	14.7	7.3 (5.9–9.1)*	59	42.0	1.4 (1.0–1.7)†
Genital defect	1447	25	5.1	4.9 (3.2–7.3)	35	24.2	1.5 (1.0–2.0)
Limb defect	957	25	2.2	11.3 (7.2–17)	41	17.1	2.4 (1.7–3.3)
Cardiac defect	567	6	1.0	6.0 (2.2–13)	11	10.5	1.1 (0.5–1.9)
Total cleft lip	436	18	0.6	31.4 (19–52)	10	8.2	1.2 (0.6–2.2)
Isolated cleft palate	144	3	0.1	44.5 (9.0–134)	2	2.9	0.7 (0.1–2.5)
All combined‡	9192	201	26.4	7.6 (6.5–8.8)†	249	164.6	1.5 (1.3–1.7)†

*Numbers in parentheses are 95% confidence intervals for the odds ratios.
†Asymptotic confidence interval (numbers are too large for exact calculation).
‡Includes all 23 categories of isolated defects and the category of multiple defects. In addition to those listed above, the categories were anencephaly; spina bifida; hydrocephalus; other; central nervous system defects; eye defects; ear, face, or neck defects; circulatory system defect; respiratory system defect; esophageal defect; abdominal wall defects; anal defect; renal defects, axial defects; skin, hair, or nail defect; or birth defect: Down syndrome and other chromosomal syndromes.

From Lie RT, et al: A population-based study of the risk of recurrence of birth defects. N Engl J Med 331:14, 1994. Reprinted by permission of The New England Journal of Medicine.

alcohol or other types of recreational drugs? Were medicines, both those prescribed and those available over the counter, used during the pregnancy? One must also be aware that taking this history has the potential for raising guilt feelings in the parents, and one must be prepared to address this issue.

Once the history of exposure has been taken, one must gauge the amount of exposure. An industrial hygienist may be able to make an estimate, but doing so is an expensive and time-consuming task. For certain types of exposure, biomarkers may be confirmatory. Examples are cord blood concentrations of cotinine for prenatal exposure to the products of tobacco smoke and urinary concentrations of mercury for mercury exposure.

Second, one must ascertain whether a neonate's particular problem is known to occur with a given type of exposure. Hotlines for teratology information are listed in the ATSDR monograph. Such hotlines operate much like poison control centers and have further information on associations between exposure and outcome.

Third, when an association is made between an exposure and an adverse outcome, one must determine the likelihood of that exposure having caused the adverse outcome. This assessment should be carried out with the help of the teratology hotline and any additional resources available (e.g., dysmorphologist, neuropsychologist). For example, methylethylketone (MEK), a commonly used solvent, has been shown to cause an increase in major malformations and intrauterine growth retardation in rats[24, 79] and mice.[80] In addition, human epidemiologic studies have shown an association between organic solvent exposure (in human studies rarely does one find exposure to only one organic solvent) and malformations.[39, 65, 45] Thus, it is reasonable to conclude that the microcephaly and mental retardation observed in a

child delivered to a woman exposed to MEK during her pregnancy are a result of this exposure. More formal criteria for assessing causation have been reviewed by Scialli.[81] What the mother should do to prevent a recurrence is a complicated issue. If the exposure is job related, job discrimination may result.[68] It may be necessary for both the patient and her doctor to work with the employer to find a suitable (and legal) alternative. Sometimes simple hygienic measures, such as changing contaminated clothing at work or frequent hand washing, are the only requirements. Additional interventions may be the use of personal protective devices and temporary job rotation to a position in which exposure does not occur.

The hotlines for teratology information are part of the Organization of Teratology Information Services (OTIS) and are listed in the ATSDR monograph *Case Studies in Environmental Medicine: Reproductive and Developmental Hazards*. This case study and others in the series can be obtained from the ATSDR, U.S. Department of Health and Human Services, Public Health Service, Centers for Disease Control and Prevention, Atlanta, GA 30333. To receive the complete series or any single monograph, call (404) 639-6204.

■ ADDITIONAL READING

Isaacson RL, et al (eds): The Vulnerable Brain and Environmental Risks, vols 1–3. New York, Plenum Press, 1992.

Paul M, (ed): Occupational and Environmental Reproductive Hazards: A Guide for Clinicians. Baltimore, Williams & Wilkins, 1993.

Persaud TVN: Environmental Causes of Human Birth Defects. Springfield, Ill, Charles C. Thomas, 1990.

Scarpelli DG, et al: Transplacental Effects on Fetal Health, vol 281. New York, Alan R. Liss, Inc, 1988.

Scialli AR: A Clinical Guide to Reproductive and Developmental Toxicology. Boca Raton, Fla, CRC Press, 1992.

Welch LS, et al, (eds): Case Studies in Environmental Medicine: Reproductive and Developmental Hazards. Atlanta, Agency for Toxic Substances and Disease Registry, U.S. Department of Health and Human Services, 1993.

Frank AL, et al, (eds): Case Studies in Environmental Medicine: Taking an Exposure History. Atlanta, Agency for Toxic Substances and Disease Registry, U.S. Department of Health and Human Services, 1992.

ACKNOWLEDGMENTS

The author gratefully acknowledges the editorial comments by Dr. Susan Cummins, Dr. Sophie Balk, and Dr. Robert Karp.

■ REFERENCES

1. Bearer CF: Electromagnetic fields and infant incubators. Arch Environ Health 49:352, 1994.
2. Bearer CF, et al: Maternal tobacco smoke exposure and persistent pulmonary hypertension of the newborn. Environ Health Perspect 105:202, 1997.
3. Bearer CF, et al: Ethyl linoleate in meconium: A biomarker for prenatal ethanol exposure. Alcohol Clin Exp Res 23:487, 1999.
4. Bearer CF, et al: Lead exposure from blood transfusion to premature infants. J Pediatr 137:549, 2000.
5. Bess FH, et al: Further observations on noise levels in infant incubators. Pediatrics 63:100, 1979.
6. Blot WJ: Growth and development following prenatal and childhood exposure to atomic radiation. J Radiat Res (Tokyo) 16(Suppl):82, 1975.
7. Bonner MJ: Prenatal and neonatal pharmacologic stress on early behavior and sexual maturation in the hamster. J Clin Pharmacol 34:713, 1994.
8. Brender JD, et al: Paternal occupation and anencephaly. Am J Epidemiol 131:517, 1990.
9. Brown AK, et al: Environmental hazards in the newborn nursery. Pediatr Ann 8:698, 1979.
10. Buehler BA, et al: Prenatal prediction of risk of the fetal hydantoin syndrome. N Engl J Med 322:1567, 1990.
11. Bush B, et al: Polychlorobiphenyl (PCB) congeners, p,p'-DDE, and hexachlorobenzene in maternal and fetal cord blood from mothers in upstate New York. Arch Environ Contam Toxicol 13:517, 1984.
12. Byer A, et al: Acetaminophen overdose in the third trimester of pregnancy. JAMA 247:3114, 1982.
13. Card SE, et al: Ontogeny of the activity of alcohol dehydrogenase and aldehyde dehydrogenase in the liver and placenta of the guinea pig. Biochem Pharmacol 38:2535, 1989.
14. Cassidy SB, et al: Occupational hydrocarbon exposure among fathers of Prader-Willi syndrome patients with and without deletions of 15q. Am J Hum Genet 44:806, 1989.
15. Chen Y-C, et al: Cognitive development of yu-cheng ("oil disease") children prenatally exposed to heat-degraded PCBs. JAMA 268:3213, 1992.
16. Clarke DW, et al: Activity of alcohol dehydrogenase and aldehyde dehydrogenase in maternal liver, fetal liver and placenta of the near-term pregnant ewe. Dev Pharmacol Ther 12:35, 1989.
17. Colborn T, et al (eds): Chemically Induced Alterations in Sexual and Functional Development: The Wildlife/Human Connection. Princeton, NJ, Princeton Scientific Publishing, 1992.
18. Committee on Environmental Health: Risk of ionizing radiation exposure to children: A subject review. Pediatrics 101:717, 1998.
19. Committee on Environmental Health: Noise: A hazard for the fetus and newborn. Pediatrics 100:724, 1997.
20. Cordier S, et al: Paternal exposure to mercury and spontaneous abortions. Br J Ind Med 48:375, 1991.
21. Council on Scientific Affairs, American Medical Association: Environmental tobacco smoke: Health effects and prevention policies. Arch Fam Med 3:865, 1994.
22. Curley A, et al: Organic mercury identified as the cause of poisoning in humans and hogs. Science 172:65, 1971.
23. Darnell J, et al: Molecular cell biology. New York, Scientific American Books, 1986, p 149.
24. Deacon MM, et al: Embryo- and fetotoxicity of inhaled methyl ethyl ketone in rats. Toxicol Appl Pharmacol 59:620, 1981.
25. Doctor B, Walsh-Sukys M: Severe fetal hemolysis secondary to maternal exposure to naphthalene fumes. J Pediatr 2000 (in review).
26. Eriksson P: Age-dependent retention of [14C]DDT in the brain of the postnatal mouse. Toxicol Lett 22:323, 1984.
27. Farrow JR, et al: Fetal death due to nonlethal maternal carbon monoxide poisoning. J Forensic Sci 35:1448, 1990.
28. Gladen BC, et al: Effects of perinatal polychlorinated biphenyls and dichlorodiphenyl dichloroethene on later development. J Pediatr 119:58, 1991.
29. Goldman LR, Koduru S: Chemicals in the environment and developmental toxicity to children: A public health and policy perspective. Environ Health Perspect 108:443, 2000.
30. Goyer RA: Transplacental transport of lead. Environ Health Perspect 89:101, 1990.
31. Grandjean P (ed): Ecogenetics. New York, Chapman & Hall, 1991.
32. Gulson BL, et al: Pregnancy increases mobilization of lead from maternal skeleton. J Lab Clin Med 130:51, 1997.
33. Haddow JE, et al: Second-trimester serum cotinine levels in nonsmokers in relation to birth weight. Am J Obstet Gynecol 159:481, 1988.
34. Hall J: Genomic imprinting: Review and relevance to human diseases. Am J Hum Genet 46:857, 1990.
35. Han S, et al: Effects of lead exposure before pregnancy and dietary calcium during pregnancy on fetal development and lead accumulation. Environ Health Perspect 108:527, 2000.
36. Harada M: Methyl mercury poisoning due to environmental contamination ("Minamata disease"). In Oehme FW (ed): Toxicity of Heavy Metals in the Environment. New York, Marcel Dekker, 1978, p 261.
37. Hauth JC, et al: Passive smoking and thiocyanate concentrations in pregnant women and children. Obstet Gynecol 63:519, 1984.
38. Hill EP, et al: Carbon monoxide exchanges between the human fetus and mother: A mathematical model. Am J Physiol 232:H311, 1977.
39. Holmberg PC, et al: Congenital defects of the central nervous system and occupational factors during pregnancy: Case referent study. Am J Ind Med 1:167, 1980.
40. Hsu S-T, et al: Discovery and epidemiology of PCB poisoning in Taiwan: A four-year follow-up. Environ Health Perspect 59:5, 1985.
41. International Agency for Research on Cancer (IARC): IARC Monographs on the Evaluation of the Carcinogenic Risk of Chemicals to Humans, Polychlorinated Biphenyls and Polybrominated Biphenyls, vol 18. Lyon, France, IARC, 1978.
42. Jacobson JL, et al: Effects of in utero exposure to polychlorinated biphenyls and related contaminants on cognitive functioning in young children. J Pediatr 116:38, 1990.
43. Jacobson JL, Jacobson SW: Intellectual impairment in children exposed to polychlorinated biphenyls in utero. N Engl J Med 335:783, 1996.
44. Jensen S: A new chemical hazard. New Sci 32:612, 1966.
45. Khattak S, et al: Pregnancy outcome following gestational exposure to organic solvents: A prospective controlled study. JAMA 281:1106, 1999.
46. Kumar R, et al: Vitamin D and calcium hormones in pregnancy. N Engl J Med 142:40, 1980.
47. Kurzel RB: Can acetaminophen excess result in maternal and fetal toxicity? South Med J 83:953, 1990.
48. Lalande NM, et al: Is occupational noise exposure during pregnancy a risk factor of damage to the auditory system of the fetus? Am J Ind Med 10:427, 1986.
49. Langman J: Medical Embryology. Baltimore, Williams & Wilkins, 1975, p 11.
50. Lian ZH, et al: Paternal age and the occurrence of birth defects. Am J Hum Genet 39:648, 1986.
51. Lie RT, et al: A population-based study of the risk of recurrence of birth defects. N Engl J Med 331:1, 1994.

52. Lindbohm M-L, et al: Effects of paternal occupational exposure on spontaneous abortions. Am J Public Health 81:1029, 1991.

53. Longo LD: Carbon monoxide in the pregnant mother and fetus and its exchange across the placenta. Ann N Y Acad Sci 174:313, 1970.

54. Lowery MC, et al: Male-mediated behavioral abnormalities. Mutat Res 229:213, 1990.

55. McDiarmid MA, et al: Fouling one's own nest revisited. Am J Ind Med 24:1, 1993.

56. Mahaffey KR: Methylmercury: A new look at the risks. Public Health Rep 114:396, 1999.

57. Manton WI: Total contribution of airborne lead to blood lead. Br J Ind Med 42:168, 1985.

58. Marsh DO: Dose response relationships in humans: Methyl mercury epidemics in Japan and Iraq. In Eccles CU (ed): The toxicity of methyl mercury. Baltimore, Johns Hopkins University Press, 1987, p 45.

59. Mathai M, et al: Passive maternal smoking and birthweight in a South Indian population. Br J Obstet Gynecol 99:342, 1992.

60. Milunsky A, et al: Maternal heat exposure and neural tube defects. JAMA 268:882, 1992.

61. MMWR: Infant mortality—United States, 1990. MMWR Morb Mortal Wkly Rep 42:161, 1993.

62. Narod SA, et al: Human mutagens: Evidence from paternal exposure? Environ Mol Mutagen 11:401, 1988.

63. Nicholl JP, et al: Epidemiology of babies dying at different ages from the sudden infant death syndrome. J Epidemiol Community Health 43:133, 1989.

64. Olney JW, et al: Environmental agents that have the potential to trigger massive apoptotic neurodegeneration in the developing brain. Environ Health Perspect 108 (Suppl 3):383, 2000.

65. Olsen J: Risk of exposure to teratogens amongst laboratory staff and painters. Dan Med Bull 30:24, 1983.

66. Olshan AF, et al: Wilms' tumor and paternal occupation. Cancer Res 50:3212, 1990.

67. Pampori NA, et al: Subnormal concentrations in the feminine profile of circulating growth hormone enhance expression of female-specific CYP2C12. Biochem Pharmacol 47:1999, 1994.

68. Paul M: Occupational and Environmental Reproductive Hazards: A Guide for Clinicians. Baltimore, Williams & Wilkins, 1993, p viii.

69. Persaud TVN: Environmental Causes of Human Birth Defects. Springfield, Ill, Charles C. Thomas, 1990, p 73.

70. Pierce PE, et al: Alkyl mercury poisoning in humans. JAMA 220:1439, 1972.

71. Ploniart SL, et al: Exposure of newborn infants to di-(2-ethylhexyl)-phthalate and 2-ethylhexanoic acid following exchange transfusion with polyvinylchloride catheters. Transfusion 33:598, 1993.

72. Pragst F, et al: Illegal and therapeutic drug concentrations in hair segments—a timetable of drug exposure? Forensic Sci Rev 10:81, 1998.

73. Rogan WJ, et al: Congenital poisoning by polychlorinated biphenyls and their contaminants in Taiwan. Science 241:334, 1988.

74. Rosevear SK, et al: Favourable neonatal outcome following maternal paracetamol overdose and severe fetal distress: Case report. Br J Obstet Gynecol 96:491, 1989.

75. Rothenberg SJ, et al: Maternal bone lead contribution to blood lead during and after pregnancy. Environ Res 82:81, 2000.

76. Rousseau F, et al: Mutations in the gene encoding fibroblast growth factor receptor-3 in achondroplasia. Nature 371:252, 1994.

77. Rudolph L, et al: Female reproductive toxicology. In LaDou J (ed): Occupational Medicine, vol 23, East Norwalk, Conn, Appleton & Lange, 1990, p 275.

78. Savitz DA, et al: Effect of parents' occupational exposures on risk of stillbirth, preterm delivery, and small-for-gestational age infants. Am J Epidemiol 129:1201, 1989.

79. Schwetz BA: Embryo- and fetotoxicity of inhaled carbon tetrachloride, 1,1-dicloroethane and methyl ethyl ketone in rats. Toxicol Appl Pharmacol 28:452, 1974.

80. Schwetz BA, et al: Developmental toxicity of inhaled methyl ethyl ketone in Swiss mice. Fundam Appl Toxicol 16:742, 1991.

81. Scialli A: A Clinical Guide to Reproductive and Developmental Toxicology. Boca Raton, Fla, CRC Press, 1992, p 257.

82. Scialli A: A Clinical Guide to Reproductive and Developmental Toxicology. Boca Raton, Fla, CRC Press, 1992, p 209.

83. Shannon M, et al: Lead intoxication in infancy. Pediatrics 89:87, 1992.

84. Shapiro BH, et al: Irreversible suppression of growth hormone dependent cytochrome P450 2C11 in adult rats neonatally treated with monosodium glutamate. J Pharmacol Exp Ther 265:979, 1993.

85. Snawder JE, et al: Loss of CYP2E1 and CYP1A2 activity as a function of acetaminophen dose: Relation to toxicity. Biophys Res Commun 203:532, 1995.

86. Steichen JJ, et al: Osteopenia and rickets of prematurity. In Polin RA, et al (eds): Fetal and Neonatal Physiology, vol 2, Philadelphia, WB Saunders, 1991.

87. Stokes IM: Paracetamol overdose in the second trimester of pregnancy: Case report. Br J Obstet Gynecol 91:286, 1984.

88. Strakowski SM, et al: Paternal hydrocarbon exposure in Prader-Willi syndrome [letter]. Lancet 2:1458, 1987.

89. Thompson GN, et al: Lead mobilization during pregnancy [letter]. Med J Australia 143:131, 1985.

90. Trapp M, et al: Pollutants in human follicular fluid. Fertil Steril 42:146, 1984.

91. United Nations. Available at http://www.zpg.org/Reports_Publications/Population_Facts/popfact82.html

92. United States Environmental Protection Agency: A Retrospective Analysis of Developmental Neurotoxicity Studies, 1999. SAP Report No 99-01B.

93. Weiss B, Landrigan PJ: The developing brain and the environment: An introduction. Environ Health Perspect 108:373, 2000.

94. Weiss J, et al: Human exposures to inorganic mercury. Public Health Rep 114:400, 1999.

95. Welch LS, et al (eds): Case Studies in Environmental Medicine: Reproductive and Developmental Hazards. Washington DC, 1993, Agency for Toxic Substances and Disease Registry, U.S. Department of Health and Human Services.

96. Whitehall JS, et al: Fetal exposure to pollutants in Townsville, Australia, detected in meconium. Pediatr Res 47:299A, 2000.

97. Wilson-Costello D, et al: Radiation exposure from diagnostic radiographs in extremely low birth weight infants. Pediatrics 97:369, 1996.

98. World Resources Institute, UN Environment Programme, and UN Development Programme: Population and health. In World Resources 1988–89. New York, Oxford University Press, 1988, p 33.

99. Yaffe SJ, et al: Effects of prenatal treatment with phenobarbital. Dev Pharmacol Ther 15:215, 1990.

100. Yazigi RA, et al: Demonstration of specific binding of cocaine to human spermatozoa. JAMA 266:1956, 1991.

101. Yoshimoto Y, et al: Risk of cancer among children exposed *in utero* to A-bomb radiations, 1954–1980. Lancet 2:665, 1988.

III Pregnancy Disorders and Their Impact on the Fetus

Intrauterine Growth Retardation

13

Robert M. Kliegman

Utpala (Shonu) G. Das

Fetal development is characterized by sequential patterns of tissue and organ growth, differentiation, and maturation that are determined by the maternal environment, uteroplacental function, and the inherent genetic growth potential of the fetus.[142] When circumstances are optimal, none of these factors has a rate-limiting effect on fetal growth and development. Thus, the healthy fetus should achieve complete functional maturity and genetically determined somatic growth, with the anticipation of an uncomplicated intrapartum course and a smooth neonatal cardiopulmonary and metabolic adaptation to extrauterine life.

However, fetal growth and development do not always occur under optimal intrauterine conditions.[69, 101] Those neonates subjected to aberrant maternal, placental, or fetal circumstances that restrain growth are a high-risk group and are traditionally categorized as having intrauterine growth retardation (IUGR). The cumulative effects of adverse environmental conditions and aberrant fetal growth threaten continued intrauterine survival; labor, delivery, and neonatal adaptation become increasingly hazardous. Similarly, postneonatal growth and development may be impaired as a result of IUGR and the subsequent problems encountered during the neonatal period. Neonates who have IUGR are a heterogenous group. Many with IUGR may in fact have intrauterine growth restriction as an adaptation to a suboptimal uterine environment. As we become more aware of the multiple etiologies producing IUGR, we must avoid generalizations about immediate and long-term consequences of IUGR. This chapter discusses normal and aberrant fetal growth and its sequelae.

Following is a list of synonyms for IUGR:

- Small for dates
- Small for gestational age
- Light for dates
- Chronic fetal distress
- Hypotrophic fetus
- Intrauterine growth stunting
- Intrauterine malnutrition
- Dysmature

- Clifford syndrome
- Postdates
- Postmaturity
- Failure to thrive in utero
- Fetal deprivation syndrome
- Pseudoprematurity

The terms *IUGR* and *small for gestational age* (SGA), although related, are not synonymous.[37, 121, 141] IUGR is a deviation from, or a reduction in, an expected fetal growth pattern and is caused by multiple adverse effects on the fetus. IUGR is due to processes that inhibit the normal growth potential of the fetus. Fetal growth at term may be predicted by anthropomorphic analysis of fetal dimensions with second-trimester ultrasonography. Deviations from the predicted weight at term may result in an infant with IUGR but may not result in an infant who is SGA. The term SGA describes an infant whose weight is lower than population norms or lower than a predetermined cutoff weight (-2 SD, 5%, 10%); the cause may be pathologic, as in an infant with IUGR, or nonpathologic, as in an infant who is small but healthy. All infants who are IUGR may not be SGA, because their weight may be above an arbitrary normative population growth percentile standard, but in comparison with siblings, ethnically derived fetal growth curves, or their own growth potential, their birth weight is less than expected. (See growth curves in Appendix B.)

Low birth weight as a classification includes premature infants (younger than 37 weeks), preterm infants who are SGA (younger than 37 weeks), and term (37 weeks or older) infants who are SGA.

FETAL GROWTH AND BODY COMPOSITION

Through anthropomorphic measurements that include fetal weight, length (crown-heel), abdominal circumference, and head circumference, fetal growth standards have been determined for various reference populations from various locations.[14, 37, 121] Although the range of birth weight at each gestational age in

TABLE 13–1 BIRTH WEIGHTS FROM SIX SOURCES

Nearest Week of Gestation	MEAN BIRTH WEIGHT (gm) ± 1 SD					
	Denver	**Baltimore**	**Montreal**	**Portland**	**Chapel Hill**	**12 U.S. Cities (Cluster Method)**
28	1150 ± 259	1050 ± 310	1113 ± 150	1172 ± 344	1150 ± 272	1165 ± 109
29	1270 ± 294	1200 ± 350	1228 ± 165	1322 ± 339	1310 ± 299	1295 ± 94
30	1395 ± 341	1380 ± 370	1373 ± 175	1529 ± 474	1460 ± 340	1440 ± 115
31	1540 ± 375	1560 ± 400	1540 ± 200	1757 ± 495	1630 ± 340	1601 ± 117
32	1715 ± 416	1750 ± 410	1727 ± 225	1881 ± 437	1810 ± 381	1760 ± 128
33	1920 ± 505	1950 ± 420	1900 ± 250	2158 ± 511	2010 ± 367	1955 ± 138
34	2200 ± 539	2170 ± 430	2113 ± 280	2340 ± 552	2220 ± 395	2160 ± 202
35	2485 ± 526	2390 ± 440	2347 ± 315	2518 ± 468	2430 ± 408	2387 ± 208
36	2710 ± 519	2610 ± 440	2589 ± 350	2749 ± 490	2650 ± 408	2621 ± 274
37	2900 ± 451	2830 ± 440	2868 ± 385	2989 ± 466	2870 ± 395	2878 ± 288
38	3030 ± 451	3050 ± 450	3133 ± 400	3185 ± 450	3030 ± 395	3119 ± 302
39	3140 ± 403	3210 ± 450	3360 ± 430	3333 ± 444	3170 ± 408	3210 ± 434
40	3230 ± 396	3280 ± 450	3480 ± 460	3462 ± 456	3280 ± 422	3351 ± 448
41	3290 ± 396	3350 ± 450	3567 ± 475	3569 ± 468	3360 ± 435	3444 ± 456
42	3300 ± 423	3400 ± 460	3513 ± 480	3637 ± 482	3410 ± 449	3486 ± 463
43		3410 ± 490	3416 ± 465	3660 ± 502	3420 ± 463	3473 ± 502

From Naeye RL, Dixon JB: Distortions in fetal growth standards. Pediatr Res 12:987, 1978, with permission.

these populations may vary (Table 13–1), the overall pattern of fetal growth (Fig. 13–1) is representative of these and subsequent groups. Both early and late fetal growth patterns appear to be linear, beginning at approximately 20 weeks' gestation and lasting until 38 weeks; thereafter the rate of weight gain begins to decline.

However, fetal growth curves based on prematurely born infants may result in inaccurate assessment of continued fetal growth. Premature infants often have had some degree of IUGR and thus skew the fetal growth curve to standards lower than those that would have been obtained if the fetus had not been born early. (See growth curves in Appendix B.)

Figure 13–2 demonstrates a similar linear relationship between fetal weight and gestational age. Near term, the fetal weight gain appears to decelerate; after birth, it again assumes the intrauterine rate. Fetal weight gain (grams per day) is constant during the second trimester, then accelerates during most of the third trimester, but declines near term. During the neonatal period the rate of gain accelerates again. This relative slowing of growth as the normal fetus approaches term is thought to be caused by some mild restraint of fetal growth. These restraining factors may be related to uterine size or placental function. Some fetuses, however, continue to grow in utero after week 40. During the neonatal period,

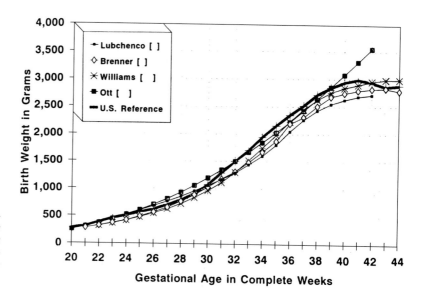

FIGURE 13–1. Fetal weight as a function of gestational age by selected references. (From Alexander GR, et al: A United States national reference for fetal growth. Obstet Gynecol 87:163, 1996. Reprinted with permission from the American College of Obstetricians and Gynecologists.)

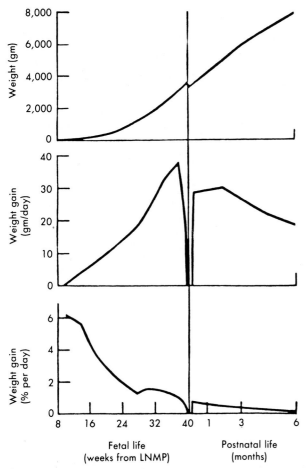

FIGURE 13–2. Smoothed curves for fetal and postnatal growth in grams and grams gained per day and expressed as percent increment of body weight (From Usher R, et al: In Davis J, et al (eds): Scientific Foundations of Pediatrics. Philadelphia, WB Saunders, 1974.)

growth resumes and approaches the in utero rate once this restraint has been eliminated.

Although weight gain per day is maximal before term, when growth is expressed as percent increment per day, it is greatest during embryonic and early fetal development (see Fig. 13–2). In the last half of pregnancy, the fetus gains 85% of its birth weight. However, the nature of fetal growth differs between early and later fetal life. During the embryonic and early fetal growth period, tissues and organs increase in cell number rather than cell size (the hyperplastic phase of cell growth, when total DNA content increases in new tissues). Later phases of growth include a period when cell size also increases (protein and RNA content), along with continued enhancement of cell number (mixed hyperplastic and hypertrophic phase). In muscle and brain (especially the cerebellum), this phase of growth may continue through adolescence and the second year of life, respectively. The final stage of growth is a purely hypertrophic phase, when only cell size increases.

The contribution of each tissue to body weight changes during fetal and postnatal development is depicted in Table 13–2. Muscle represents only 25% of fetal and neonatal body weight; once full adult maturity has been achieved, it accounts for 40% of the body's mass.[148] Fetal muscle growth, as well as all protein synthesis in the fetus, depends on active transport of essential amino acids across the placenta. Once provided with these precursors, fetal protein synthesis is autonomous and results in the net synthesis of proteins that have amino acid patterns equivalent to those in the adult. Although the building blocks may be the same, developmentally the fetal muscle has a lower fibrillar protein content, whereas the sarcoplasmic protein concentration remains unchanged as maturation proceeds. Besides those immunoglobulins (Ig), such as IgG, that cross the placenta, all protein present in the fetus has been synthesized de novo within fetal tissue.

Paralleling the patterns of fetal growth, the macromolecular composition of the body also undergoes sequential patterns of change. One general trend includes a decrease of total body and extracellular water content as the fetus and infant mature (Fig. 13–3; Table 13–3). Simultaneously, there is an increment of body protein and fat content (Fig. 13–4). Whereas the increase of tissue protein is gradual during development, the increment of fetal body fat is delayed until the third trimester. Once initiated, the deposition of subcutaneous and deep body adipose tissue accelerates more rapidly than the rate of protein accumulation.

Coinciding with the changes in the extracellular fluid space, the sodium and chloride concentrations in the fetus decline, whereas the expansion of the intracellular fluid space results in an increase in potassium concentration. (See also Chapter 34, Part One.) The decline in total body sodium is less than that for chloride, because sodium is also a component of fetal bone. Calcium, phosphorus, and magnesium are nevertheless the major minerals in bone. By term, the total body calcium/phosphorus ratio is 1.7:1.8, with 98% of calcium, 80% of phosphorus, and 60% of magnesium deposited within the bone.

TABLE 13–2   CONTRIBUTION OF ORGANS TO BODY MASS DURING DEVELOPMENT

TISSUE	FETUS 20–24 WEEKS (%)	TERM BABY (%)	ADULT (%)
Skeletal muscle	25	25	43
Skin	13	15	7
Skeleton	22	18	18
Heart	0.6	0.5	0.4
Liver	4	5	2
Kidneys	0.7	1	0.5
Brain	13	13	2

From Widdowson E: In Assali N (ed): Biology of Gestation, vol 2. New York, Academic Press, 1968, with permission.

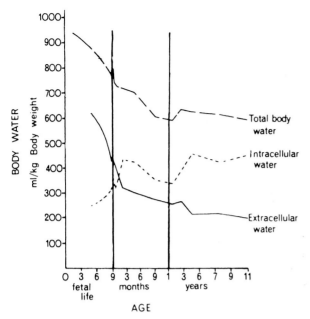

FIGURE 13-3. Developmental alterations of fluid space distribution. (From Uttley W, et al: Clin Endocrinol Metabol 5:3, 1976.)

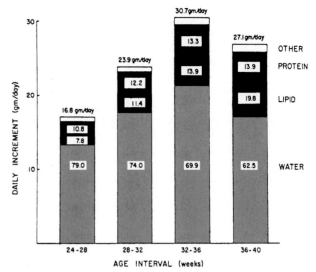

FIGURE 13-4. Composition of fetal weight gain. (From Ziegler E, et al: Body composition of the reference fetus. Growth 40:329, 1976.)

FETAL METABOLISM

Although the fetus is described as the perfect parasite, maternal and fetal nutritional deprivations can adversely affect fetal growth.[79] The fetus depends on maternal nutrient intake and maternal endogenous substrate stores as precursors for fetal tissue synthesis and as fuel for fetal oxidative metabolism. The oxygen consumed by the fetus in turn provides energy to support essential fetal "work," such as maintenance of transmembrane potentials and replacement of tis-

sue components that are continuously being renewed. In addition, fetal oxygen consumption is required for net synthesis of complex macromolecules such as DNA, RNA, protein, and lipid. Each gram of protein synthesized requires the expenditure of 7.5 cal, whereas a gram of triglycerides requires 11.6 cal. Because 4.85 cal use 1 L of oxygen, net tissue synthesis represents a substantial proportion of fetal oxygen consumption, which is approximately 4 to 6 mL/kg per minute. The energy cost of neonatal growth among premature infants constitutes the energy stored in tissue plus that expended for the synthesis of that tissue. Total energy cost per gram of new tissue is approximately 5.7 cal, whereas that remaining in

TABLE 13-3   BODY COMPOSITION OF THE REFERENCE FETUS

Gestational Age (Weeks)	Body Weight (gm)	PER 100 GM BODY WEIGHT				PER 100 GM FAT-FREE WEIGHT							
		Water (gm)	Protein (gm)	Lipid (gm)	Other (gm)	Water (gm)	Protein (gm)	Ca (mg)	P (mg)	Mg (mg)	Na (mEq)	K (mEq)	Cl (mEq)
24	690	88.6	8.8	0.1	2.5	88.6	8.8	621	387	17.8	9.9	4.0	7.0
25	770	87.8	9.0	0.7	2.5	88.4	9.1	615	385	17.6	9.8	4.0	7.0
26	880	86.8	9.2	1.5	2.5	88.1	9.4	611	384	17.5	9.7	4.1	7.0
27	1010	85.7	9.4	2.4	2.5	87.8	9.7	609	383	17.4	9.5	4.1	6.9
28	1160	84.6	9.6	3.3	2.4	87.5	10.0	610	385	17.4	9.4	4.2	6.9
29	1318	83.6	9.9	4.1	2.4	87.2	10.3	613	387	17.4	9.3	4.2	6.8
30	1480	82.6	10.1	4.9	2.4	86.8	10.6	619	392	17.4	9.2	4.3	6.8
31	1650	81.7	10.3	5.6	2.4	86.5	10.9	628	398	17.6	9.1	4.3	6.7
32	1830	80.7	10.6	6.3	2.4	86.1	11.3	640	406	17.8	9.1	4.3	6.6
33	2020	79.8	10.8	6.9	2.5	85.8	11.6	656	416	18.0	9.0	4.4	6.5
34	2230	79.0	11.0	7.5	2.5	85.4	11.9	675	428	18.3	8.9	4.4	6.4
35	2450	78.1	11.2	8.1	2.6	85.0	12.2	699	443	18.6	8.9	4.5	6.3
36	2690	77.3	11.4	8.7	2.6	84.6	12.5	726	460	19.0	8.8	4.5	6.1
37	2940	76.4	11.6	9.3	2.7	84.3	12.8	758	479	19.5	8.8	4.5	6.0
38	3160	75.6	11.8	9.9	2.7	83.9	13.1	795	501	20.0	8.8	4.5	5.9
39	3330	74.8	11.9	10.5	2.8	83.6	13.3	836	525	20.5	8.7	4.6	5.8
40	3450	74.0	12.0	11.2	2.8	83.3	13.5	882	551	21.1	8.7	4.6	5.7

From Ziegler E, et al: Body composition of the reference fetus. Growth 40:329, 1976, with permission.

structural or depot macromolecules represents 4.0 cal. Therefore, 1.7 cal are expended to produce 1 g of new tissue.[15] A similar relationship should occur in the third-trimester fetus, because energy requirements for growth should not change after birth.

Maternal metabolic adjustments during pregnancy are characterized by fuel and hormonal alterations that attempt to secure a continuous provision of substrates for use by the fetus.[4] During periods of alimentation, sufficient substrates are presented to the uteroplacental circulation while maternal fuel stores are simultaneously enriched. During the third trimester, maternal insulin resistance may partition ingested fuels toward the fetus. When fasting occurs during pregnancy, fuel mobilization is accelerated, as is evident by the rapid rise of maternal free fatty acids and ketone bodies. This accelerated mobilization of maternal adipose tissue stores is facilitated by a rapid decline of maternal insulin levels and an enhanced secretion of human placental somatomammotropin. This latter placental hormone has lipolytic activity and may also directly diminish maternal glucose oxidation. In addition, maternal glucose use is attenuated because free fatty acids and ketones replace glucose as a fuel in maternal tissues, whereas hypoinsulinemia reduces glucose uptake in the insulin-dependent tissue of the mother. Thus, fetal glucose provision may be continued. In addition, alternate substrates mobilized during maternal fasting, such as ketones, cross the placenta and may attempt to maintain fetal growth and development. Ketones may be oxidized or serve as precursors for fetal lipid or protein synthesis. This accelerated mobilization of fuels can ensure fetal growth during short periods of maternal fasting; however, prolonged periods of starvation adversely affect fetal outcome.

The substrates used to maintain fetal oxygen consumption have been most accurately determined in the ovine fetus (Table 13–4).[4, 36, 51, 92, 95] Glucose accounts for approximately 50% of fetal energy production in sheep when the mother is maintained in a high nutritional plane. Amino acids, in addition to

functioning as precursors for fetal protein synthesis, serve as an oxidizable fuel; they may contribute to 25% of ovine fetal oxygen uptake. Taken together, lactate and acetate may supply an additional 25%. Data from human pregnancies suggest that glucose oxidation may contribute a greater proportion of fetal energy production than in the ovine fetus.

Similarly, the fetal respiratory quotient has been estimated to be close to 1.0 in other mammalian species, which suggests that carbohydrate oxidation is the predominant source for fetal oxidative metabolism. As discussed previously, fasting during human pregnancy may result in an alteration of substrates presented to the fetus when maternal and subsequently fetal ketone bodies increase. Ketones may then serve as fuels for energy production and also as precursors for amino acids, proteins, and lipids.[103] Although free fatty acids, especially the essential fatty acids, must cross the placenta, their role in fetal energy production is limited because they are probably deposited in structural or depot tissues (Fig. 13–5).[66, 144]

In addition to the provision of substrates for fetal oxygen consumption and growth, tissue growth also depends on an appropriate fetal endocrine milieu (Table 13–5). Among the hormones, insulin has been implicated as a possible "growth hormone" of the fetus.[49] Because insulin does not usually cross the placenta, this growth-enhancing hormone must be of fetal origin. Insulin promotes fetal deposition of adipose and glycogen stores while potentially stimulating amino acid uptake and protein synthesis in muscle. In the absence of fetal insulin production, as in conditions such as pancreatic aplasia, transient neonatal diabetes mellitus, or congenital absence of the islets of Langerhans, fetal growth is severely impaired.[49] Moreover, when the peripheral action of insulin is attenuated by diminished receptor or postreceptor events, as in leprechaunism, fetal growth may be impaired.

There are at least five fetal monogenic disorders that effect fetal insulin secretion or action and subsequent fetal weight.[49, 50, 81, 146] Alterations of the fetal glucokinase gene, which causes insulin release after it senses ambient glucose concentrations in the pancreas, results in IUGR when the mutation produces reduced enzyme function. Fetal weight reduction due to a loss of function mutation may be as great as 500 gm. If the mother also has this mutation, she probably has maturity onset diabetes of youth and will be hyperglycemic, which may attenuate the fetal growth retardation. In contrast, gain of function mutations of this pancreatic glucose–sensing enzyme enhances fetal insulin secretion and may increase fetal weight. Another genetic cause of fetal hyperinsulinism is the mutation of the sulfonylurea receptor of the potassium inward rectifier channel. Persistent activation of this channel causes fetal hyperinsulinism and enhanced fetal weight.

Pancreatic agenesis (homozygous mutation of insulin promoter factor 1) and transient neonatal diabetes (commonly, paternal isodisomy or duplication of

TABLE 13–4 OXIDIZABLE SUBSTRATES IN THE OVINE FETUS*

SUBSTRATE	TOTAL OXYGEN CONSUMPTION ACCOUNTED FOR (%)
Glucose	50
Amino acids	25
Lactate	20
Acetate	5–10
Free fatty acids	Not significant
Fructose	Not significant
Glycerol	Not significant
Keto acids	Not significant

*Sheep placenta is impermeable to free fatty acids and ketones, in contrast to that of other mammals, which may be permeable to these substrates.

From Milley J, et al: Metabolic requirements for fetal growth. Clin Perinatol 6:365, 1979, with permission.

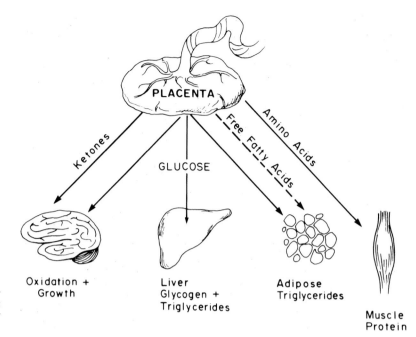

FIGURE 13–5. Placental nutrient support and disposition of substrates. (Modified from Adam PAJ: In Falner F, et al: Human Growth, vol 1. New York, Plenum Press, 1978.)

TABLE 13–5 HORMONAL EFFECT ON FETAL GROWTH

HORMONE	CONCENTRATION*	GROWTH EFFECT	COMMENT
Growth hormone (GH)	High	None? Length?	Absent tissue GH receptor (appears late in gestation)
Thyroid	Low	None on growth ↑ Epiphyseal maturation	Fetus inactivates thyroxine (T_4) to reverse triiodothyronine (T_3) Postreceptor defect Stimulates epidermal growth factor
Androgens	High	Minimal	Specific receptors on gonadal tissue

Insulin	Normal	Major	Action by:
			  ↑ Nutrient uptake
			  ↑ Binding to type I insulin-like growth factor (IGF) receptor
			  ↑ Release of IGFI

Vitamin D			
24,25-D$_3$	High	Anabolic for bone	Receptors on cartilage
1,25-D$_3$	Low		
Insulin-like growth†:			
Factor I (IGFI)	Low	Purported growth factor	Levels ↑ with gestational age
Factor II (IGFII)	Low	Purported growth factor	Levels ↑ before term but low at term
Epidermal growth factor (urogastrone)	Absent	Mitogen for epidermal cells and fibroblasts	Affects eye opening and tooth eruption in mice
Nerve growth factor	High	Mitosis of ganglion and glial cells	Maturation of adrenergic neurons and sympathetic nervous system
Platelet-derived growth factor	Unknown	Mitogenic for connective tissue	Related to tumor growth factors

*Compared with postnatal values.

†IGFI is identical to somatomedin C. IGFI and IGFII bind to specific receptors, stimulate mitosis, and are the mediators of growth hormone's effect on postnatal growth. These growth factors may function at the site of origin (paracrine) or through an endocrine mechanism by circulating on specific bindings proteins. Type I IGF receptors are structurally similar to the insulin receptor and have high affinity for IGFI and IGFII and low affinity for insulin. Type II IGF receptors have less affinity for insulin. In utero growth hormone exerts little or no regulation of somatomedins or IGF, whereas other hormones (fetal insulin or placental lactogen) or substrates (glucose) may regulate somatomedin secretion. Placental lactogen stimulates IGFII but not IGFI production by fetal fibroblasts. These hormones do not cross the placenta and are released by many cells, especially fibroblasts and hepataocytes.

chromosome 6q22–q33) are also associated with IUGR. The leprechaun syndrome (homozygous or compound heterozygous insulin receptor mutation) produces IUGR due to insulin resistance.

On the other hand, those neonates having prolonged periods of hyperinsulinism in utero, such as infants of diabetic mothers or infants with Beckwith-Wiedemann syndrome or hyperinsulinemic hypoglycemia (nesidioblastosis), demonstrate enhanced adipose and muscle tissue mass, resulting in excessive birth weight. (See also Chapter 47, Part One.) Amniotic fluid levels of C-peptide, a cleavage protein of proinsulin, vary directly with fetal growth status: C-peptide is reduced with IUGR and increased with fetal macrosomia.[73, 136]

Fetal growth hormone probably does not influence fetal growth, because there are few growth hormone receptors on fetal liver.[85] The birth weight of a panhypopituitary fetus is not very different from that of a normal fetus. Maternal levels of placental-derived growth hormone are low in cases of IUGR.[24] Placental growth hormone increases maternal nutrient provision to the fetus and is thought to enhance mobilization of maternal substrates for fetal growth.

The final common pathway of growth hormone action is mediated by the generation of insulin-like growth regulatory factors, the somatomedins (see Table 13–5). Insulin-like growth factor (IGF) type I is a single polypeptide encoded on chromosome 12. IGFI messenger RNA (mRNA) and its receptor are present in many fetal cells and are not regulated by growth hormone.[108, 136] IGFII is also a single polypeptide and is encoded on chromosome 11. Its mRNA is much more abundant (200-fold to 600-fold) in most fetal tissues than that for IGFI. IGFI and IGFII are 60% homologous to each other and 40% homologous to insulin. IGFI may be regulated by substrate availability. Its level declines in fetal models of IUGR but increases in infants who are large for gestational age. Fetal levels of IGFI correlate best with fetal weight. IGFI and IGFII receptor binding initiates transmembrane signaling, which activates cell metabolism and DNA synthesis.

IGFI and IGFII are present in fetal plasma as early as 15 weeks of gestation. Nonetheless, plasma levels may not reflect tissue-specific action because these proteins act as competence factors for the cell division cycle in a paracrine or autocrine, rather than an endocrine, manner. Knockout gene models deleting IGFI or IGFII genes or both demonstrate an additive reduction of fetal growth with both gene deletions.[36] Deletion of the paternal IGFII gene with genomic imprinting also produces IUGR.

IGFs are modulated by six IGF-binding proteins (IGFBP), which usually attenuate or occasionally enhance IGF bioavailability and are subject to regulatory signals similar to those that regulate IGF protein synthesis.[47, 59, 136, 137] Fetal IGFBP-1 serum levels are inversely related to birth weight and may restrict the availability of IGFI to fetal tissues.[136] In animals, overexpression of IGFBP-I produces IUGR. Acute fetal hypoxia and possibly fetal catecholamine release re-

duce IGFI levels but increase IGFBP-1 levels in the ovine fetus.[60, 62] Reduced nutrient availability and lower insulin levels associated with some models of IUGR reduce fetal IGFI levels while they increase IGFBP-1 levels. Fetal IGFBP-3 serum levels usually parallel those of IGFI and are thus increased in fetuses who are LGA but reduced in fetuses with IUGR. In the second trimester, amniotic fluid levels of IGFI, IGFII, and IGFBPI do not predict birth weight.[137]

Maternal nutrient availability is also regulated by IGFI. IUGR is associated with reduced maternal IGFI levels or when IGFBP-I is increased. In mice, increasing maternal IGFI levels result in heavier fetal weight; in sheep, maternal IGFI infusions result in increased fetal glucose levels and enhanced placental amino acid uptake.

Epidermal growth factor (EGF) in the neonate mediates mitosis and development of ectodermal and mesodermal structures; in rodents, EGF mediates eye opening and tooth eruption. EGF is a single 53-amino-acid polypeptide chain derived from the prepro-EGF peptide and may play a minor role in fetal growth and development; there is no fetal EGF RNA expression. Nonetheless, EGF receptors are abundant in the fetus, autophosphorylate themselves, and phosphorylate cytoplasmic proteins. EGF receptor phosphorylation is attenuated in the placenta of women who smoke and who deliver IUGR infants.[40, 42] Transforming growth factor–α, which is 40% homologous to EGF, binds to the EGF receptor, is involved in angiogenesis, and may be the fetal ligand for this receptor, which is similar to the c-erb B proto-oncogene. Fetal growth is regulated by growth factors and growth factor receptors that are similar to products of nuclear proto-oncogenes. Uncontrolled or constitutive (loss of regulated inhibition) activity of oncogenes is characteristic of malignant transformation, in contrast to the controlled and regulated activity of these proto-oncogene products (growth factors or receptors) during growth. Leprechaunism, an IUGR syndrome, in addition to having insulin resistance, also demonstrates EGF resistance because of an abnormal EGF receptor.

Leptin (from Greek leptos, thin) is a 16 kDa 167 amino acid discovered in 1994 as the product of the obese (ob) gene. The human leptin gene is on chromosome 7q31, consisting of more than 15,000 base pairs and 3 exon sites. Leptin is primarily produced in white adipose tissue but has recently been shown to be produced in the human placenta and gastric epithelium. Leptin has been shown to regulate body weight through a negative feedback loop between adipose tissue and the hypothalamic satiety centers.

Studies have shown that in children and adults, serum leptin concentrations correlate with body fat mass as well as body weight. There is also a gender difference that persists into adulthood; namely, girls have higher serum leptin levels than do boys. This gender difference has not been proven conclusively in the fetus and neonate.

Leptin has been detected in amniotic fluid and cord blood of the newborn and can be seen as early as 29 weeks of gestational age.[5] Amniotic fluid leptin is derived from the mother, whereas cord blood leptin is derived from the placenta and fetal tissues.[87] While cord blood leptin levels appear to correlate with birth weight, maternal leptin concentration is not an accurate indicator of fetal growth.* There is also a correlation between cord blood leptin level and fetal fat mass. This relationship suggests that leptin may have a role in fetal growth, but this role still needs to be defined. Cord blood leptin levels have shown to be significantly decreased in newborns with IUGR. This logically follows, given that increases in cord blood leptin correlate with the exponential increase in fat mass that occurs during the last trimester and that this fat mass is greatly reduced in fetuses or newborns with IUGR. Further, in the newborn group with IUGR, there is a positive correlation between cord blood leptin levels and body mass index (which indicates fat mass) and not with body weight. The relationship between leptin and fetal growth needs to be more clearly defined.

The role of other hormones, notably corticosteroids and thyroid hormone, has not been well defined for fetal growth. Nonetheless, repeated doses of dexamethasone to the mother may reduce birth weight and possibly brain growth. With thyroid hormone deficiency in the human athyrotic cretin, birth weight is not altered. These hormones, however, probably have a more significant role as regulatory signals for the initiation of maturation and differentiation in fetal tissues. (See also Chapter 47, Part Three.)

FETAL ORIGIN OF ADULT DISEASES: METABOLIC IMPRINTING/PROGRAMMING

Reduced birth weight has been associated with certain adult morbidities that would not be obvious based on our understanding of IUGR and its immediate neonatal sequelae.† Low birth weight in the fetus has been related to the subsequent risk of adult onset hypertension, non–insulin-dependent diabetes, stroke, obesity, and coronary artery disease. Four potential fetal phenotypes may predict adult morbidities: thin babies may have insulin resistance in utero, and this continues after birth; short babies with reduced abdominal circumference may have raised LDL cholesterol; short and fat babies may develop non–insulin-dependent diabetes; and those with a large placenta are at risk for hypertension.[8] One recognized risk for adult coronary artery disease is those infants born thin who in later life become obese.

The fetal organ hypothesis states that poor maternal nutrition programs the fetus and produces reduced birth weight and subsequent adult onset diseases.[18, 27, 49, 143] This suggests that such programming occurs during a critical or sensitive period in early fetal life. Studies have confirmed a relationship between poor maternal diet and blood pressure in offspring. Potential programming or imprinting mechanisms include changes in cell-cell interaction, alterations in fetal angiogenesis or innervation, reduction in cell number, clonal selection of cell types (cells with poor availability of nutrients such as lipids may be selected to produce more endogenous lipids), metabolic differentiation (enzymes, transporters, transcription factors, gene expression), and hepatocyte polyploidization (extra chromosome copies can enhance gene expression and alter metabolism). These adaptive fetal processes may be beneficial to the fetus but may permanently alter metabolism and result in adverse metabolic diseases as adults.[143]

Although genetic influences may have a role in postnatal and adult metabolic disorders, the fetal origin hypothesis has been demonstrated in the smaller or discordant fetus of identical twins. In addition, babies after ovum donation tend to have birth weight that correlates to the recipient mother. Furthermore, thin mothers who have poor weight gain in pregnancy have offspring with higher blood pressures than offspring of thin mothers with adequate weight gain during pregnancy. Although postnatal influences such as smoking and socioeconomic status have additional effects, the fetal origin hypothesis remains relevant.

Various monogeneic disorders also affect birth weight (see above).[49, 50, 124, 146] Fetal insulin resistance or poor production may be one primary overriding problem and not just the poor maternal nutrition found in some offspring with postnatal insulin resistance. The opposing hypotheses are noted in Figure 13–6.[49]

EPIDEMIOLOGY OF LOW BIRTH WEIGHT

(See also Chapter 2.)

The term *low birth weight* refers to infants born weighing less than 2500 gm. The neonatal mortality rate is directly related to the low birth weight rate in a given population. These high-risk infants are a heterogeneous group consisting of infants born preterm (less than 37 weeks) and those born at term but of reduced weight.[37, 121, 141]

IUGR is the predominant cause of low birth weight in developing areas and nations with low birth weight rates greater than 10%. Socioeconomic improvement decreases the proportion of IUGR. Between 20% and 30% of preterm infants also have obviously decreased growth for gestational age. Although there appear to be differences in the relative incidence of IUGR and premature birth in different countries, risk factors associated with birth of an infant with low birth weight are similar (Box 13–1).

The rate of reduced weight at term gestation is probably twice as great among black infants as white. This may be partially independent of socioeconomic variables (which are of paramount importance), because black infants often have lower birth weight than infants of Hispanic or Asian parents of similar socioeconomic status. The risk of low birth weight is

---

*References 26, 45, 64, 84, 88, 131

†References 8, 18, 49, 75, 78, 81, 106, 143, 146

Intrauterine Environment   **Fetal Genetics**

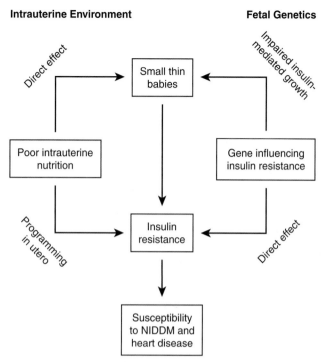

FIGURE 13–6. Two alternative explanations for association of small, thin babies with later onset of insulin resistance, NIDDM, and ischemic heart disease: intrauterine environment and fetal genetics. (From Hattersley AT, et al: The fetal insulin hypothesis: An alternative explanation of the association of low birthweight with diabetes and vascular disease. Lancet 353:1789, 1999. Copyright © 1999 by The Lancet Ltd.)

related to the occupation not only of the child's parents but also of the grandparents. There is a strong familial aggregation of births of low birth weight in both white and black families. Provision of adequate nutrition to the future mother and other environmental factors may alter that future mother's growth and future reproductive capability. This intergenerational effect explains in part the observation that mothers of infants of low birth weight were themselves neonates of low birth weight (see the preceding section "Fetal Origin of Adult Diseases"). Although medical complications of pregnancy occur equally in all socioeconomic groups, many adverse behavioral attitudes or practices contribute to the greater low birth weight rate among women of low socioeconomic status.

MATERNAL CONTRIBUTIONS TO ABERRANT FETAL GROWTH

PHYSICAL ENVIRONMENT

Certain otherwise normal mothers are prone to repeated delivery of infants who are SGA; the recurrence rate may be 25% to 50%.[71, 102] Many of these women themselves were born SGA, raising the possibility of intergenerational transmission of a physical regulator of fetal growth. A proportion of these women also remains small throughout life and are

identifiable by low prepregnancy weight and stature. These women may exert a restraint on fetal growth by some unknown regulator, possibly related to their own stature, previous nutritional status, or uterine capacity. In breeding experiments using Shetland ponies and Shire horses, the offspring resulting from breeding a male Shire to a female Shetland was similar in birth weight to a Shetland pony, whereas the birth weight of offspring born to a male Shetland and a female Shire approached that of a Shire. The smaller Shetland female apparently exerts a growth restraint on the genetic potential derived from the larger Shire

---

■ **BOX 13–1**

OVERVIEW OF RISK FACTORS* FOR LOW BIRTH WEIGHT

Demographic
Race (black)
Present low
    socioeconomic status
Socioeconomic status of
    infant's grandparents

Pregnancy
Multiple gestation
Birth order
Anemia
Elevated hemoglobin
    concentration
    (inadequate plasma
    volume expansion?)
Fetal disease
Preeclampsia and
    hypertension
Infections
Placental problems
Premature rupture of
    membranes
Heavy physical work
Altitude

Prepregnancy
Low weight for height
Short stature
Chronic medical illness
Poor nutrition
Low maternal weight at
    mother's birth
Previous infant of low
    birth weight
Uterine or cervical
    anomalies
Parity (none or more
    than five)

Behavioral
Low educational status
Smoking
No care or inadequate
    prenatal care
Poor weight gain
    during pregnancy
Alcohol abuse
Illicit and prescription
    drugs
Short interpregnancy
    interval (less than 6
    months)
Age (less than 16 or
    over 35 years)
Unmarried
Stress (physical and
    psychological)

*Many of these variables are risk factors for both IUGR and prematurity. These variables are not necessarily univariant risk factors but rather interact in a complex relationship. Only a few factors exert an independent effect. The relationship between black race and low birth weight remains a significant factor, with a twofold increase in the incidence of prematurity and IUGR when controlled for other risks.

Modified from Committee to Study the Prevention of Low Birthweight: Prevention of Low Birthweight. Washington, DC, Institute of Medicine, National Academy Press, 1985.

male. Similar observations are noted in humans. When ova are donated to a recipient mother, the fetal weight correlates best with that of the recipient mother.[143]

Another risk for IUGR is maternal failure to expand plasma volume during pregnancy. Such women have reduced placental weights and a hematocrit level that does not reflect an expanded plasma volume.[113]

Maternal genetic factors have a major direct effect on fetal growth. This influence depends on a transfer of maternal genes but also on the other, unexplained maternal genetic factors related in part to uteroplacental function. The observation that sisters of mothers with infants who are SGA are at higher risk of having infants who are SGA than their sisters-in-law gives further evidence of maternal genetic influences on fetal growth. The mother's genetic component to fetal growth is less than 25%.

Paternal factors have less effect on fetal growth. Paternal genes affect fetal growth directly by transfer of genetic material, which may be modified (accelerated or inhibited) by maternal factors. Paternal genotypic potential is best expressed as a function of postnatal growth.

Other constraints on fetal growth may be exerted during *multiple gestations*, because fetal growth declines when the number of fetuses increases. The onset of growth retardation in multiple gestations is also related to the number of fetuses: growth restraint begins sooner with triplets than twins (Fig. 13–7). In multiple gestations, the uterine constraint appears to occur when combined fetal size approaches 3 kg. Placental implantation site, uterine anomalies, vascular anastomoses, and nutritional factors may also interfere with growth in these pregnancies. The uterine capacity itself may also place a constraint on optimal fetal growth.

MATERNAL NUTRITION

Prepregnancy weight and pregnancy weight gain are two important independent variables that affect fetal growth.[1, 56, 99, 115, 125] Underweight mothers and those affected with malnutrition deliver infants with diminished birth weight. Weight gain during pregnancy in nonobese patients correlates significantly with fetal birth weight. Poor weight gain as early as 16 weeks' gestation may predict low birth weight. The effect of prepregnancy weight in obese women is independent of pregnancy weight gain and offsets the frequently observed poor weight gain of these overweight women (Fig. 13–8). Infants who are SGA are unusual for obese women, whereas macrosomia is common. This may be related to large maternal nutrient stores. Calculating the pregravid body mass index (BMI)

$$BMI = Prepregnancy\ weight\ (kg)/Height^2\ (m) \times 100$$

helps the clinician determine the target for pregnancy weight gain, which may reduce the risk of IUGR. A low BMI (<19.8) may require a pregnancy weight gain of 12.5 to 18 kg; a normal BMI (19.8 to 26) may require a weight gain of 11.5 to 16 kg; and a high BMI (>26 to 29) may require a weight gain of 7 to 11.5 kg, whereas obese women (BMI > 29) may need a weight gain of only 6 kg. Appropriate weight gain during pregnancy based on BMI may mitigate the risk of IUGR.[56]

The effects of maternal nutritional status on fetal growth are minimal during the first trimester of pregnancy. This is related to the large surfeit of nutrients presented to the relatively small, undemanding embryo and early fetus. As fetal growth accelerates, the requirements for fetal growth increase and may not be sufficiently provided by an inadequate maternal diet. Earlier attempts to limit weight gain in preg-

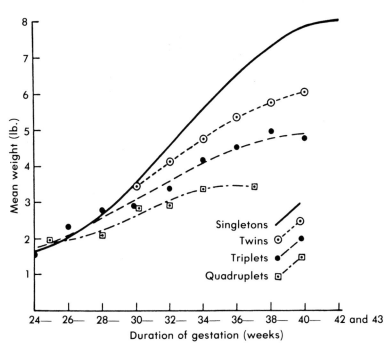

FIGURE 13–7. Birth weight–gestational age relationships in multiple gestation, denoting origin of aberrant fetal growth. (From McKeown T, et al: Endocrinology 8:386, 1952.)

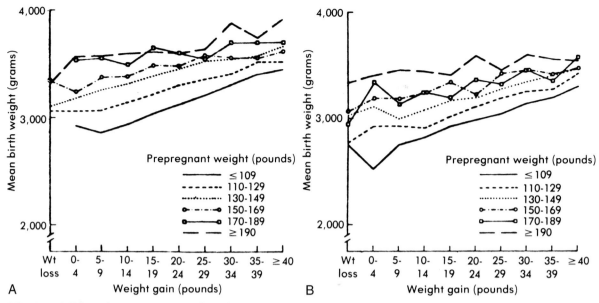

FIGURE 13–8. Effect of prepregnancy weight and weight gain during pregnancy among white women *(A)* and black women *(B)*. Note the reduced birth weight at term at all levels of maternal weight variables among black women. Also note that weight gain during pregnancy has its most positive effect on birth weight among lean women. Nonetheless, prepregnancy weight among obese, usually nondiabetic, women has the greatest effect on birth weight. (From Niswander K, et al: Weight gain during pregnancy and prepregnancy weight. Obstet Gynecol 33:482, 1969. Reprinted with permission from the American College of Obstetricians and Gynecologists.)

nancy with a 1200-kcal diet to prevent preeclampsia resulted in a 10-fold increase in growth retardation. In an otherwise healthy population of Dutch women experiencing a short period of famine during the Hunger Winter of 1944–1945, fetal growth was most severely affected when deprivation occurred in the third trimester.[125] Substrate deficiency during this period resulted in an overall reduction in birth weight of 300 gm. Maternal weight gain and placental weight were even more drastically reduced, demonstrating preferential use of nutrients for the fetus. Poor nutrition may also reduce uterine blood flow, placental transport, and villous surface area (Fig. 13–9). Observations similar to those of the Dutch experience occurred during a more severe and prolonged famine in wartime Leningrad, where birth weight was reduced by 500 gm at term.

There may even be an intergenerational effect of being in utero during maternal starvation. The daughters of women who experienced starvation during the Dutch famine of 1944–1945 have an increased risk of delivering infants of low birth weight if the daughters were exposed to starvation in utero during the first or second trimester. The reduction in the next generation's birth weight is approximately 200 to 300 gm.[82]

As illustrated in Figure 13–9, decreased caloric uptake below critical caloric needs may result in diminished fetal growth. Increased maternal caloric expenditure may occur two ways: excessive physical activity and greater waste of calories. The nutritional aspects of cigarette smoking may be an example of the second way. Furthermore, the diminished heat expenditure that occurs among obese women may result in caloric storage and explain in part their excessively large babies. Increased maternal storage of calories may be exemplified by the "selfish mother" hypothesis. These women may not develop the usual insulin resistance during pregnancy and may direct ingested calories toward their own tissue stores. These women have fasting hypoglycemia and/or ac-

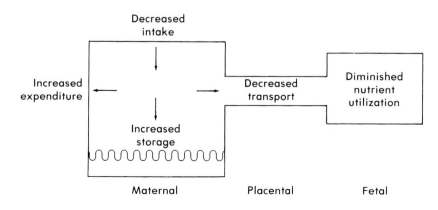

FIGURE 13–9. Interrelationship of caloric intake and expenditure and fetal nutrient availability. Multiple mechanisms can reduce nutrient availability or utilization (even in the presence of adequate fuel availability).

celerated disappearance of glucose after intravenous glucose tolerance testing. The opposite occurs among women of low socioeconomic status who receive food supplementation; their skinfold thickness decreases as fetal weight increases. Decreased transport may reflect placental defects in function, nutrient supply, or blood flow. Decreased blood flow may be caused by peripheral vascular disease or failure to expand blood volume and cardiac output, as in normal pregnancy. Fetuses with insulin resistance or decreased numbers of cells may not be able to grow despite adequate nutrient supply. Examples of fetuses with diminished cell numbers include fetuses affected by rubella embryopathy, autosomal trisomies, and other genetic causes of IUGR.

Attempts at improving the low birth weight outcome in high-risk populations (characterized by having poor nutritional histories) have demonstrated a positive effect of nutritional supplementation. Additional calories, rather than protein supplementation, correlate best with enhanced fetal weight. Caloric supplements greater than 20,000 cal per pregnancy reduced the number of infants with low birth weight; every 10,000 cal supplemented above the standard diet improved fetal weight by an average of 29 gm. In Gambia, supplementation during seasonal periods of food shortage resulted in a net positive caloric intake of more than 400 kcal/day. This increased fetal weight 224 gm and reduced the low birth weight rate from 28% to less than 5%. A threshold of 1500 kcal/day was observed, which augmented fetal weight when the mother was in positive caloric balance.[107] In the United States, WIC program participation has reduced the number of births that are SGA.[2]

Protein supplementation may even have adverse neurodevelopmental effects on the fetus. Aside from periods of famine and geographic areas where malnutrition is endemic, other conditions associated with poor maternal nutrition and suboptimal fetal growth are included in Box 13–2. Adolescent women, in particular, are at risk because of their own growth requirements in addition to those of the fetus.[118]

Certain maternal metabolic aberrations are associated with suboptimal fetal growth. Mothers who demonstrate excessively low fasting blood glucose values and those whose blood glucose levels are not sufficiently elevated after an oral glucose tolerance test are at risk of delivering an infant who is SGA. A "selfish mother" hypothesis has been proposed to explain the poor growth of these infants (see Fig. 13–9).

CHRONIC DISEASE

Of all disease mechanisms that interfere with fetal growth, those resulting in uterine ischemia, hypoxia, or both have the most extreme effect. Chronic maternal hypertension caused by either primary renal parenchymal disease, such as nephritis, or those conditions extrinsic to parenchymal disorders, such as essential hypertension, significantly alters fetal growth and well-being.[119] This effect is related to the

---

■ BOX 13–2

WOMEN WITH POOR NUTRITION AND RISK OF SUBOPTIMAL FETAL GROWTH

- Adolescent women, especially those who are not married
- Women with low prepregnancy weights
- Women with inadequate weight gain during pregnancy
- Women who have low income or problems in purchasing food
- Women with a history of frequent conception, especially with short interpregnancy intervals
- Women with a history of giving birth to infants with low birth weight
- Women with diseases that influence nutritional status: diabetes, tuberculosis, anemia, drug addiction, alcoholism, or mental depression
- Women known to be dietary faddists or with frank pica
- Women who do heavy physical work during pregnancy

From Christaksis G: Am Public Health 63(suppl):57, 1973.

---

duration of hypertension and to the absolute elevation of the diastolic pressure and is most severe in the presence of end-organ disorders, such as retinopathy. Well-controlled hypertension, without the development of preeclampsia, may not affect fetal growth.

Pregnancy-induced hypertension is of paramount importance to perinatologists in relation to its effect on fetal growth and well-being. (See also Chapter 14.) This disease, which may affect uteroplacental perfusion and fetal growth long before clinical signs of edema, proteinuria, and hypertension develop, reduces uterine blood flow, as determined by Doppler flow velocity waveforms of the uterine artery. Preeclampsia is characterized by retention of the spiral arteries muscle layer, reduced perfusion of the intervillous space, necrotizing atherosis, and decreased trophoblastic invasion of the decidual spiral arteries. Such trophoblastic invasion depends on decidual laminin, fibronectin, maternal cytokines, and trophoblastic integrins and proteases. Similar arterial pathologic changes may be present in idiopathic IUGR. In pregnancies complicated by eclampsia, fetal growth deviates from the expected norm from 32 weeks onward (Fig. 13–10). Treatment of hypertension in pregnancy with antihypertensive drugs may further contribute to IUGR. This is independent of the medication; with a 10–mm Hg decline, fetal weight may be reduced 145 gm.[140] Vascular insufficiency resulting from advanced maternal diabetes mellitus, especially in the presence of end-organ disease in the kidney or retina, also produces IUGR despite the presence of maternal hyperglycemia. (See also Chapter 15.) Women with serious autoimmune disease associated with the lupus

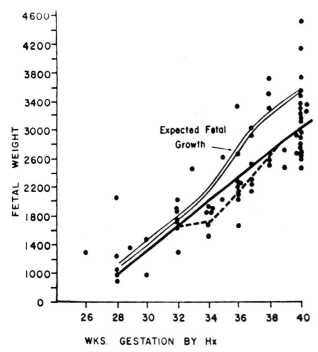

FIGURE 13–10. Fetal weight after eclampsia. Broken line demonstrates mean weight alteration. (From Zuspan F: Clin Obstet Gynecol 9:954, 1966.)

anticoagulant are also a high-risk population for preeclampsia and IUGR. (See also Chapter 17.)

Another major category associated with diminished fetal weight gain is that resulting from maternal hypoxemia. Severe cyanotic congenital heart disease, such as tetralogy of Fallot or Eisenmenger complex, is the best example of this mechanism, whereas sickle cell anemia is representative of diseases that can produce local uterine hypoxia and ischemia. The maternal morbidity rate is high with cyanotic heart disease. Nutritional anemias are not usually associated with aberrant fetal growth. In sickle cell anemia, the abnormal cells may interfere with local uterine perfusion during episodes of sickling, and growth retardation is observed.[16]

A common and nonpathologic factor related to maternal hypoxia is the diminished environmental oxygen saturation that is present at high altitudes. Infants born in the mountains of Peru demonstrate lower birth weights than do Peruvian infants born at sea level. Placental mass has hypertrophied in these newborns in an attempt to compensate for the lower circulating maternal oxygen concentration. These neonates are not born with polycythemia as a response to fetal hypoxia, as proposed for other infants who are SGA. The decline in body weight becomes manifest at an altitude of 2000 m, which corresponds to a barometric pressure of 590 mm Hg.[98]

DRUGS

(See also Chapters 10, 12, 28, and 36.)

The effects of maternal drug administration on the fetus are usually considered primarily in terms of teratogenicity.[31] However, a continuum of fetal compromise may be present because many malformation syndromes are associated with diminished birth weight, whereas other agents may interfere only with fetal growth. Some drugs associated with IUGR are included in the following list*:

- Amphetamines
- Antimetabolites (e.g., aminopterin, busulfan, methotrexate)
- Bromides
- Cigarettes (possibly carbon monoxide, thiocyanate, nicotine)
- Cocaine
- Ethanol (acetaldehyde)
- Heroin
- Hydantoin
- Isotretinoin
- Methadone
- Methylmercury
- Phencyclidine
- Polychlorinated biphenyls
- Propranolol
- Steroids (prednisone)
- Toluene
- Trimethadione (Tridione)
- Warfarin

Many of the typically abused drugs have been implicated as agents producing fetal growth retardation by reducing maternal appetite and by being associated with lower socioeconomic groups. However, at least for heroin, methadone, and ethanol, a cellular toxic effect acting directly on cell replication and growth appears to be involved. This is most evident in fetal alcohol syndrome: the prenatal onset of growth retardation persists during postnatal periods despite adequate food intake. A placental transfer block for specific amino acids has been observed in fetal alcohol syndrome.

The effects of cocaine on fetal growth may be multifactorial and include uterine artery vasospasm, reduced maternal prepregnancy weight, reduced weight gain during pregnancy, and, possibly, direct fetal endocrine effects. Multidrug use, poor nutrition, and poor prenatal care are common among many drug-dependent women.

Cigarette smoking during pregnancy reduces eventual fetal birth weight, which is directly related to the number of cigarettes smoked.[80] Birth weight at term is reduced an average of 170 gm if more than 10 cigarettes per day are used; smoking more than 15 per day may reduce weight by 300 gm. The mechanism of fetal growth retardation is uncertain, but nicotine and subsequent catecholamine release may produce uterine vasoconstriction and fetal hypoxia. Carbon monoxide and cyanide may cause a more direct effect: after binding to hemoglobin, carbon monoxide and cyanide may diminish oxygen unloading from the mother to the fetus and from the fetus to its tissues. Nutritional supplementation does not completely

---

*References 28, 55, 74, 80, 86, 116

eliminate the reduced fetal weight. Moreover, the effects of cigarettes may be greatest at advanced maternal age.

Drugs such as propranolol and other beta-blocking agents and corticosteroids probably have a direct effect on the fetus, although the confounding influence of the chronic maternal illnesses for which these agents are prescribed may also contribute to IUGR.

SOCIOECONOMIC STATUS

Poor environmental conditions related to lower socioeconomic status have been associated with infant malnutrition of both prenatal and postnatal onset. With improvement of these conditions, birth weight is enhanced. This was extensively studied after living conditions improved in postwar Japan. The improvement in birth weight during this era occurred only in infants born during the latter part of the third trimester; nutritional and environmental effects seem greatest during this period of fetal growth.[48, 130]

Many maternal factors, such as drug abuse, poor nutritional habits, and cigarette smoking, are interrelated and are covariables associated with poor socioeconomic status.[11, 145] Factors such as adverse environmental living conditions and low levels of education are more prevalent among reproductive-age women of lower socioeconomic status. Adolescent and single-parent families and the failure to seek adequate prenatal advice are also more common. Many investigations have demonstrated that such women are at risk of having babies with IUGR. It has been suggested that if chronic maternal illness and certain behavioral characteristics are eliminated and prenatal care is available, the remaining women of lower socioeconomic status do not have a higher incidence rate of infants who are SGA. The specific behavioral characteristics more common among poor women are noted in Box 13–1.[48, 118]

These behavioral variables may be related to an attitude difference among these women, who choose a different lifestyle and constitute a subgroup, and may not specifically represent the entire population. Thus, these behaviors may be based on choice and not necessarily on environment.

PLACENTAL DETERMINANTS

Optimal fetal growth depends on efficient function of the placenta as both a nutrient supply line and an organ of gaseous exchange. Placental functional integrity requires additional energy production because placental oxidative metabolism may equal that of the fetus. This large energy requirement is essential for maintaining fetal growth-promoting roles, which include active transport of amino acids, synthesis of protein and steroid hormones, and support of placental maturation and growth. Placental growth parallels that of the fetus; however, toward term there is a greater decline in the rate of placental weight gain than in the rate of weight gain by the fetus. During

this decline of placental weight, the fetus also exhibits a decrease in the rate of weight change, which suggests that placental function and weight gain have declined and led to reduced fetal growth. However, despite the change in the rate of placental weight gain, the placenta continues to mature. The placental villous surface area continues to increase with advancing gestational age (Fig. 13–11); simultaneously, the syncytial trophoblast layer continues to thin, and vascularization of the terminal villi continues to improve.[77] Functionally, urea clearance is enhanced toward term in the ovine placenta (Fig. 13–12), suggesting that permeability and diffusing distance improve as the placenta approaches term. Birth weight has been correlated with placental weight (Fig. 13–13) and villous surface area (see Fig. 13–11), suggesting that macroscopic and microscopic events are related to optimal placental function. Uterine blood flow, and thus placental oxygen or nutrient transfer, may be reduced if maternal blood volume contracts. Failure to expand plasma volume, which normally occurs in the last half of gestation, has been associated with IUGR. These high-risk women may be identified by an elevated hemoglobin level.

When placental insufficiency occurs, there may be a functional failure of the placenta as a respiratory or nutritive organ or both. Placental insufficiency associated with maternal nutritional deficiency has more than one effect on fetal growth. In addition to diminished fetal substrate provision, placental metabolism is altered directly, as proposed in Figure 13–9. Diminished placental growth adversely affects total nutrient transfer, whereas reduced placental production of

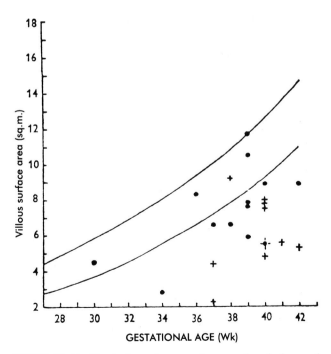

FIGURE 13–11. Chorionic surface area in normal and abnormal pregnancies. ●, Maternal hypertension; +, normotensive IUGR. (From Aherne W, et al: Quantitative aspects of placental structure. J Pathol Bacteriol 91:132, 1966.)

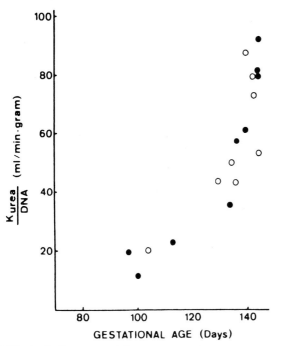

FIGURE 13–12. Urea permeability per gram of the ovine placenta. ●, Singletons; ○, twins. (From Kulhanek J, et al: Changes in DNA content and urea permeability of the sheep placenta. Am J Physiol 226:1257, 1974.)

- Fetal vessel thrombosis
- Circumvallate placenta
- Reduced capillarization
- Reduced terminal villus branching
- Elevated vascular tone
- Increased glucose utilization
- Confined chromosomal mosaicism (trisomy of 2, 3, 7, 8, 9, 13, 14, 15, 16, 18, 22, or X)
- Reduced spiral artery recruitment

Multiple gestations may produce significant placental disorders in suboptimal sites of implantation or, more often, related to abnormal vascular anastomoses in diamniotic monochorionic twinning (Fig. 13–14). As a result of arteriovenous interconnections, one twin serves as the donor and develops IUGR, losing nutrient supplies, whereas the other is the recipient and has satisfactory growth. These anastomoses may be detectable on careful gross examination of the placenta.[111] Ablation of vascular communications in the second trimester, by fetoscopic neodymium:yttrium-aluminum-garnet laser photocoagulation, may reduce the morbidity of the twin-twin transfusion syndrome, which develops in 5% to 17% of monozygotic twins.[33] (See also Chapters 18 and 23.)

Other detectable potential causes related to aber-

chorionic somatomammotropin attenuates maternal mobilization of fuels to the fetus. Reduced placental energy production and protein synthesis limits active transport of amino acids and facilitates transport of glucose.

When placental insufficiency complicates maternal vascular disease such as preeclampsia, placental weight and volume also diminish.[65] In addition, a decline in villous surface area (see Fig. 13–11) and a relative increase in nonexchanging tissue occur. At the same time, these placentas demonstrate thickening of the capillary basement membrane.

Following is a list of additional findings in placental disorders associated with diminished birth weight[20, 38, 109]:

- Twins (implantation site)
- Twins (vascular anastomoses)
- Chorioangioma
- Villitis (caused by *t*oxoplasmosis, *o*ther [congenital syphilis and viruses], *r*ubella, *c*ytomegalovirus, and *h*erpes simplex virus [TORCH])
- Villitis (unknown cause)
- Avascular villi
- Ischemic villous necrosis
- Vasculitis (decidual arteritis)
- Multiple infarcts
- Syncytial knots
- Chronic separation (abruptio placentae)
- Diffuse fibrinosis
- Hydatidiform change
- Abnormal insertion
- Single umbilical artery (?)

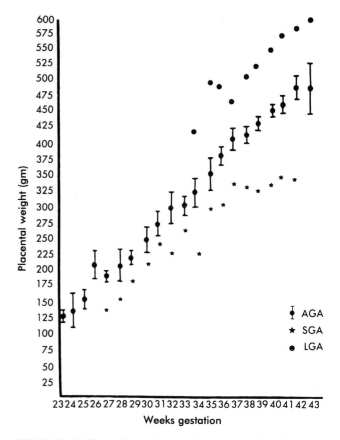

FIGURE 13–13. Placental weight-gestational age relationship in appropriate for gestational age (I, *AGA*), small for gestational age (*, *SGA*), and large for gestational age (●, *LGA*) neonates. Mean placental weight ±SEM. (From Molteni R, et al: Relationship of fetal and placental weight in human beings. J Reprod Med 21:327, 1978.)

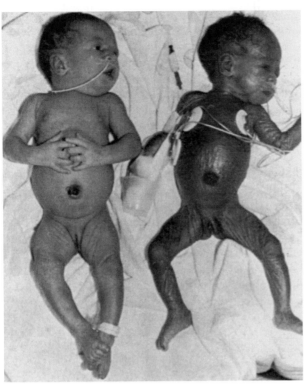

FIGURE 13–14. Diamniotic monochorionic twins, 36 weeks' gestational age, with birth weights of 1.3 and 2.0 kg.

major determinants of early fetal growth; nutritional and environmental problems should not affect the fetus until the requirements for tissue growth increase during the third trimester. Indeed, reduced first trimester growth as determined by crown-rump length is a risk factor for IUGR. This risk is even stronger in the presence of raised maternal α-fetoprotein levels.

Approximately 20% of birth weight variability in a given population is determined by the fetal genotype; maternal hereditary and environmental factors contribute an additional 65%; the remaining contributing factors are unknown. Birth order affects fetal size: infants born to primiparous women weigh less than subsequent siblings. The second child and each additional child weigh an average of 180 gm more than the firstborn. This relationship is not true for multiparous adolescent pregnancies in which subsequent births during adolescence produce neonates with lower term weights than that of the firstborn. Male sex of the fetus is associated with greater birth weight, beginning to become predominant after 28 weeks' gestation. At term, boys weigh approximately 150 gm more than girls. A male twin, in addition to affecting its own somatic growth, can also enhance the growth of its female twin. Androgenic hormonal stimulation of fetal growth may contribute to these observed differences. Also, a theory states that maternal-fetal antigenic (HLA, ABO) differences are responsible for this effect.[58] These antigenic differences result in enhanced

rant fetal growth include chorioangiomas, large retroplacental infarcts and hemorrhages, abnormal cord insertion patterns, and (questionably) single umbilical artery. Combined reductions of uterine and umbilical blood flow have also been detected in IUGR.[63] Furthermore, increased vascular resistance has been demonstrated in these circulations (Table 13–6). In addition, reduced placental prostacyclin (a potent vasodilator) production may be present in IUGR.[65] Increased placental vascular tone may be fixed or dynamic. The latter may be due to reduced activity of placental nitric oxide synthase or increased circulating fetal levels of angiotensin II or endothelium.

FETAL DETERMINANTS

Optimal fetal growth depends on adequate provision of substrates, their effective placental transfer, and the inherited regulatory factors within the fetal genotype that affect nutrient utilization. In addition to substrates, oxygen must be transferred, and an appropriate hormonal milieu must be present. There must also be sufficient room within the uterus. In the absence of adverse environmental effects, the inherent growth potential of the fetus may be achieved.

Genetic determinants of fetal growth are inherited from both parents, and population norms must be established to detect aberrant fetal growth. For example, the average birth weight of Cheyenne Indians is 3800 gm at term, whereas that of the New Guinea Luni tribe is 2400 gm. Such genetic potentials are the

TABLE 13–6 ABNORMALITIES OF UTEROPLACENTAL AND FETAL BLOOD FLOW IN IUGR PREGNANCIES

OBSERVATION	COMMENT
50% ↓ Uteroplacental flow	^{113}InCl to mother
↓ Uterine flow in malnutrition	Failure to increase cardiac output with pregnancy
↓ Placental nutrient transfer	
↑ Uterine artery systolic/ diastolic waveform ratio	Suggests increased uterine artery resistance
↑ Umbilical artery velocity waveform	
↑ Fetal descending aortic pulsatile index*	Suggests increased peripheral vascular resistance
↓ Fetal descending aortic end-diastolic velocity	
↑ Fetal descending aortic resistance index	Suggests decreased cardiac output, shunting away from descending aorta to brain, and fetal distress
↓ Fetal descending aortic peak velocity	
Reversed diastolic flow	Suggests severe reduction in flow and fetal compromise
↓ Umbilical venous flow	Associated with impending fetal distress
↓ Placental prostacyclin production	May promote platelet aggregation or diminish uterine vessel dilation

$$*\text{Pulsatile index} = \frac{\text{Peak velocity} - \text{End-diastolic velocity}}{\text{Mean blood flow velocity}}$$

placental trophoblastic invasion of the decidua, improving placental and subsequent fetal growth. As a corollary, interference with maternal immunologic function may inhibit this antigenic growth advantage and explain in part the diminished birth weights after maternal immunosuppressive therapy.

Alternately, chromosomes may carry growth-determining genes; genetic material on the Y chromosome may enhance the growth of the male fetus. Similarly, chromosomal deletions or imbalances result in diminished fetal growth. For example, Turner syndrome (XO) is associated with diminished birth weight. The converse is not true: additional X chromosomes beyond the norm are associated with reduced fetal growth. For each additional X chromosome (in excess of XX), birth weight may be reduced 300 gm. Similarly, autosomal trisomies, such as Down syndrome, are also associated with abnormal fetal growth. Chromosomal aberrations often result in diminished fetal growth by interfering with cell division. An intrinsic defect in cultured fibroblasts from patients with trisomy 21 has been observed in tissue culture. Single-gene defects may also reduce fetal growth. The inborn errors most notably associated with diminished fetal weight are included in the following outline. Many syndromes with autosomal-recessive, autosomal-dominant, polygenetic, or unknown inheritance are also associated with poor fetal growth and occasionally may produce marked IUGR. (See also Chapter 28.)

Monogenic disorders that affect fetal growth often impair insulin secretion or insulin action. These include reduced fetal insulin secretion by an attenuated insulin-sensing mechanism from a loss of function mutation in the pancreatic glucose-sensing enzyme glucokinase. Reduced insulin action is noted in leprechaun syndrome, a mutation in the insulin receptor. IUGR has also been reported with deletion of the IGFI gene. More complicated genetic mechanisms associated with IUGR include maternal uniparental disomy for chromosome 6, which probably unmasks an autosomal-recessive gene mutation. Parental uniparental disomy of chromosome 6 is associated with transient neonatal diabetes and IUGR.

Infectious agents are typically sought as being responsible for early onset of IUGR.[12] Of these, cytomegalovirus and rubella virus are the most important identifiable agents associated with marked fetal growth retardation. After maternal viremia, both agents invade the placenta, producing varying degrees of villitis, and subsequently gain access to fetal tissues. The effects of placentitis itself on fetal growth are unknown, but once congenital fetal infection has occurred, these viral agents have direct adverse effects on fetal development. Intracellular rubella virus inhibits cellular mitotic activity in addition to producing chromosomal breaks and subsequently cytolysis. In addition, this virus produces an obliterative angiopathy that further compromises cell viability. Cytomegalovirus also causes cytolysis, resulting in areas of focal tissue necrosis. These viral agents therefore reduce cell number and subsequent birth weight by simultaneously inhibiting cell division and producing cell death. (See also Chapters 22 and 37.)

Following are examples of factors affecting fetal growth.[138]

A. Chromosome disorders associated with IUGR
    1. Trisomies 8, 13, 18, 21
    2. 4p syndrome
    3. 5p syndrome
    4. 13q, 18p, 18q syndromes
    5. Triploidy
    6. XO
    7. XXY, XXXY, XXXXY
    8. XXXXX
B. Metabolic disorders associated with diminished birth weight
    1. Agenesis of pancreas
    2. Congenital absence of islets of Langerhans
    3. Congenital lipodystrophy
    4. Galactosemia (?)
    5. Generalized gangliosidosis type I
    6. Hypophosphatasia
    7. I-cell disease
    8. Leprechaunism
    9. Maternal and fetal phenylketonuria
    10. Maternal renal insufficiency
    11. Maternal Gaucher disease
    12. Menkes syndrome
    13. Transient neonatal diabetes mellitus
C. Syndromes associated with diminished birth weight
    1. Aarskog-Scott syndrome
    2. Anencephaly
    3. Bloom syndrome
    4. Cornelia de Lange syndrome
    5. Dubovitz syndrome
    6. Dwarfism (e.g., achondrogenesis, achondroplasia)
    7. Ellis–van Creveld syndrome
    8. Familial dysautonomia
    9. Fanconi pancytopenia
    10. Hallermann-Streiff syndrome
    11. Meckel-Gruber syndrome
    12. Microcephaly
    13. Möbius syndrome
    14. Multiple congenital anomalads
    15. Osteogenesis imperfecta
    16. Potter syndrome
    17. Prader-Willi syndrome
    18. Progeria
    19. Prune-belly syndrome
    20. Radial aplasia; thrombocytopenia
    21. Robert syndrome
    22. Robinow syndrome
    23. Rubinstein-Taybi syndrome
    24. Seckel syndrome
    25. Silver syndrome
    26. Smith-Lemli-Opitz syndrome
    27. VATER (*v*ertebral defects, imperforate *a*nus, *t*racheoesophageal fistula, and *r*adial and *r*enal dysplasia) and VACTERL (*v*ertebral abnormalities, *a*nal atresia, *c*ardiac abnormalities, *tra*-

cheoesophageal fistula, and/or *e*sophageal atresia, *r*enal agenesis and dysplasia, and *l*imb defects) syndromes
   28. Williams syndrome
D. Congenital infections associated with IUGR
   1. Rubella
   2. Cytomegalovirus
   3. Toxoplasmosis
   4. Malaria
   5. Syphilis
   6. Varicella
   7. Chagas disease

THE INFANT WITH IUGR/SGA

DEFINITION

Since the introduction of gestational age assessment and further subdivision of each neonatal period into categories of large, appropriate, and small for gestational age, it has become increasingly apparent that the infant of low birth weight (less than 2500 gm) is not always premature (earlier than 37 weeks). Worldwide, more than 20 million infants are born weighing less than 2500 gm. Between 30% and 40% of these infants are born at term gestation and are therefore undergrown (SGA status). As discussed previously, population norms need to be determined for each specific genetic group, especially those characterized by unusual inherited patterns of fetal growth. In general, these population norms established in various North American and European cities describe the usual fetal growth pattern for industrial societies and may be used as the reference norms for similar ethnic groups (see Fig. 13–1; see Table 13–1). Each curve defines either standard deviations or percentile units that include the normal variability or distribution of birth weights at each gestational age. By definition, infants less than two standard deviations or those at less than the third percentile (10th for Denver curves because of the lower birth weight at higher altitudes) are classified as SGA. Therefore, between 2.5% and 10% of each population has SGA status. The use of population means, however, is at times misleading. Within a sibship, fetal birth weight is less variable and more consistent than that for an entire population. Compared with family members, 80% of infants with congenital rubella infection were classified as SGA, whereas only 40% were SGA when population standards were used. Fetal growth assessment must therefore be considered in the context of prior reproductive history and clinical examination of the newborn.

Infants with IUGR may or may not be SGA. Alternately, infants who are SGA may not have been affected by growth-restricting processes that produce IUGR. Weight parameters at birth may be insensitive in determining IUGR. The ponderal index (wt/l³) or other body proportion ratios (head circumference to weight or length, femur length to abdominal circumference, head circumference to abdominal circumference) may be useful in detecting additional cases

of IUGR during the fetal or neonatal period. IUGR resulting from placental insufficiency usually reduces birth weight more than length and to a greater degree than head circumference and would be evident by a reduced ponderal index with a smaller, albeit relatively large (spared), head circumference. The greater the severity of IUGR, the greater is the deviation of weight, length, and (less so) head circumference from gestational age norms. Alterations of body proportion ratios may create a continuum rather than a dichotomous classification of birth weight status (appropriate for gestational age [AGA] versus SGA).

Deviations of fetal weight from a predetermined genetic potential produce IUGR with or without SGA status. Second-trimester fetal anthropomorphic and biometric ultrasonography can be used to predict an ideal weight, which may be modified by intrinsic and extrinsic growth-limiting factors. Any variation from the predicted weight would be considered IUGR. The growth potential realization index assesses deviations from norms of weight and of head, abdominal, and thigh circumferences. This index is applied to the infant after birth by calculating a neonatal growth assessment score that includes the deviation of each growth parameter from its related normative value for that gestational age. A neonatal growth assessment score of zero indicates ideal growth, and scores greater than 20 indicate IUGR but not necessarily SGA.

ABERRANT FETAL GROWTH PATTERNS

Fetal growth retardation may have its origins early or late during fetal development. Infants who demonstrate reduced fetal growth early in gestation constitute approximately 20% of all infants who are SGA. They are symmetrically growth-retarded: head circumference, weight, and length are proportionately affected to equivalent degrees. These fetuses and infants continue to grow, albeit with reduced net effect (Fig. 13–15A). In addition to inherent genetic growth constraint, other factors may produce diminished growth potential in these neonates. Congenital viral infections usually have their worst effect if infection occurs during the first trimester, when they have a significant effect on cell replication and subsequently birth weight. Similarly, abnormal genetic factors, such as single gene deletions and chromosomal disorders, also reduce the intrauterine growth rate at an early stage of development. Very early onset of growth delay has been reported in anomalous infants of diabetic mothers. Box 13–3 lists characteristics and examples of IUGR.

Growth retardation of a later onset is usually associated with impaired uteroplacental function or nutritional deficiency during the third trimester (see Fig. 13–15B). Nutrient supplies, oxygen, and uteroplacental perfusion are in excess of their requirements during early fetal development and should not interfere with fetal growth until the growth rate exceeds the provision of substrates or oxygen or both. During the last trimester, the fetal growth rate and net tissue

BOX 13–3

CHARACTERISTICS AND EXAMPLES OF IUGR

Symmetric

Early onset
Constitutional or "normal" small
Low profile biparietal diameter
↓ Growth potential
Normal ponderal index
Low risk for perinatal asphyxia
Brain symmetry to body size, short femur
Normal blood flow in internal carotid artery
Proportionate abdominal circumference
Normal maternal and fetal arterial waveform velocity
Glycogen and fat content relative
Low risk for hypoglycemia

Examples

Genetic
TORCH
Chromosomal
Anomalad syndromes

Asymmetric

Late onset
Environmental
Late flattening biparietal diameter
Growth arrest
Low ponderal index
↑ Risk for asphyxia
Brain sparing, normal femur length
Redistribution to internal carotid artery bloodflow
Decreased abdominal circumference
↓ Maternal and fetal arterial waveform velocity
↓ Glycogen and fat content
↑ Risk for hypoglycemia

Examples

Chronic fetal distress (hypoxia)
Preeclampsia
Chronic hypertension
Diabetes classes D to F
Poor caloric intake

accretion increase markedly; if the uteroplacental supply line is compromised, IUGR will develop. The anthropomorphic findings among these infants demonstrate a relative sparing of head growth, whereas body weight and somatic organ growth are more seriously altered. Spleen, liver, adrenal, thymus, and adipose tissue growth is affected to the greatest extent in these newborns who are late-onset SGA (Figs. 13–16 and 13–17). The relative sparing of fetal head (brain) growth is caused by preferential perfusion of the brain with well-oxygenated blood containing adequate substrates after redistribution of the cardiac output during periods of fetal distress. Infants with IUGR resulting from unknown or nutritional causes may have successfully adapted to a "hostile" in utero environment with reduced growth. After birth, in a more favorable environment, catch-up growth ensues.

ANTENATAL CARE

Diagnosis

Antenatal diagnosis of IUGR has proved difficult. Many of these infants deliver at or beyond term with-

out prior antenatal detection. At best, when sought with careful maternal physical examination, accurate dating, and risk assessment analysis, only 50% of these infants may be identified before birth. Antenatal detection is an essential component of care for these infants because they require intensive obstetric and neonatal management to reduce their excessive perinatal morbidity and mortality rates. This poor outcome is associated with unexplained antepartum or intrapartum fetal death, neonatal asphyxia, and major neonatal adaptive problems. Neonatal risks are increased at each respective gestational age (Fig. 13–18).[91] Antenatal identification and intensive perinatal care of mother, fetus, and, later, the neonate are imperative components that result in improved outcome for these infants.

Currently, careful measurement and recording of fundal height at each antenatal visit are a reasonable clinical screening aid in the diagnosis of IUGR. When dates are confirmed by onset of quickening, audible heart tones and accurate menstrual history, size-date discrepancy (i.e., fundal height less than or lagging behind the norm for gestational age) is suggestive of IUGR. History findings that may be components of a risk assessment score for IUGR include a history of a previous infant who was SGA, vaginal bleeding, multiple gestation, low prepregnancy weight, and poor pregnancy weight gain, as noted earlier. Chronic maternal illness and preeclampsia are also high-risk situations indicating possible IUGR.

Laboratory tests, including determination of maternal serum estriol level, placental lactogen, and various pregnancy-associated proteins, have been unreliable markers for IUGR. The diagnosis of chronic fetal distress in the absence of obvious alterations of fetal heart rate patterns is now possible with cordocentesis (*percutaneous umbilical blood sampling*). Although not indicated for all patients with IUGR, fetal blood sampling may demonstrate hypoxia, lactic acidosis, hypoglycemia, and normoblastemia caused by chronic fetal distress. Hypoxia may precede fetal acidosis. Fetal blood sampling may also permit rapid karyotyping of the fetus with IUGR with malformations and the identification of TORCH infections through the assessment of antibody titers, culture, or DNA diagnosis of TORCH agents.

Ultrasonographic assessment of the fetus can help detect the presence of IUGR. Either used as a routine two-step process (dating/sizing in mid–second trimester; follow-up assessment at 32 to 34 weeks) or based on risk analysis, fetal ultrasonography is the primary method for identifying fetuses with IUGR.[9, 17, 46, 135] Ultrasonography includes real-time biometric and anthropomorphic analysis of fetal growth parameters (head circumference, biparietal diameter, abdominal circumference, femur length), detection of anomalies, and identification of *oligohydramnios*.[30, 89, 110] The latter is a risk factor for congenital anomalies, severe IUGR with reduced urine production, pulmonary hypoplasia, variable decelerations from cord compression, and intrauterine fetal death in as many as 5% to 10% of affected fetuses. The risk of congenital

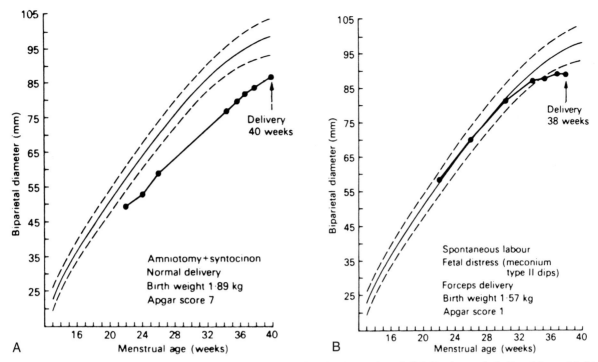

FIGURE 13–15. Low-profile *(A)* and late-flattening *(B)* patterns of IUGR. (From Campbell S: Fetal growth. In Beard R, et al (eds): Fetal Physiology and Medicine. Philadelphia, WB Saunders, 1976, p 271.)

anomalies with oligohydramnios increases from 1% to 9% with mild-to-severe amniotic fluid deficits; at the same time, the risk of IUGR increases from 5% to 40%. Second-trimester oligohydramnios, with elevated α-fetoprotein levels, has a particularly poor prognosis. (See also Chapter 21.)

The degree of oligohydramnios can be determined ultrasonographically and quantitated by means of the four-quadrant *amniotic fluid index* (AFI). The vertical

diameters of four pockets of amniotic fluid are added to determine the amniotic fluid index. Between 26 and 38 weeks of gestation, the amniotic fluid index is 12.9 ± 4.6 cm; an index of less than 5 cm signifies severe oligohydramnios.[89]

Morphometric analysis of fetal growth parameters includes determination of serial biparietal diameters as analyzed by absolute number and rate of change (see Fig. 13–15; Figs. 13–19 and 13–20). Head sparing

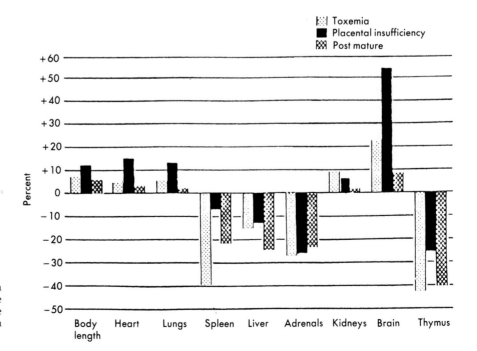

FIGURE 13–16. Deviation of organ weights following IUGR. (From Naeye R, et al: Judgment of fetal age. 3. The pathologist's evaluation. Pediatr Clin North Am 13:849, 1966.)

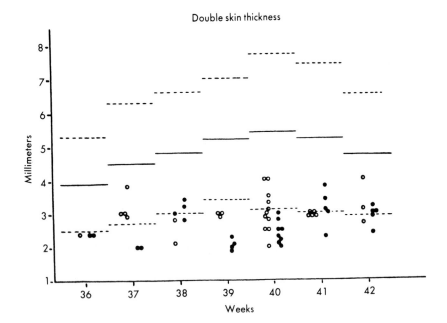

FIGURE 13–17. Skinfold thickness is a major determinant of neonatal subcutaneous fat deposits. Fetal malnutrition with (●) and without (○) severe clinical signs of wasting. (From Usher R: Clinical and therapeutic aspects of fetal malnutrition. Pediatr Clin North Am 17:169, 1970.)

in asymmetric IUGR may make fetal measurements of the biparietal diameter less sensitive; however, truncometry, by measuring the fetal abdominal circumference (in part, liver size) at the level of the umbilical vein, may add accuracy (Fig. 13–21). Using ratios of fetal growth parameters (Fig. 13–22) and adding the use of femur length and the fetal ponderal index may increase the sensitivity of fetal biometry.[30, 110]

Doppler flow velocity waveforms, assessed in the maternal and fetal circulations, may detect increased maternal and fetal vascular resistance before the onset of IUGR.[57, 67, 100, 134, 135] Maternal arcuate arterial flow may reflect trophoblastic invasion of the myometrium because increased flow may be associated with increased vascular invasion and better placental perfusion. Alternately, decreased maternal arcuate arterial waveform velocity may demonstrate increased maternal vascular resistance and decreased uteroplacental perfusion. Uterine vessel velocimetry is less accurate than waveforms in fetal vessels in predicting IUGR and fetal hypoxia.

Chronic fetal distress with hypoxia (with or without acidosis) is associated with fetal Doppler arterial waveform velocities that indicate reduced systemic (descending aorta, umbilical artery) flow and usually increased cerebral (internal carotid artery) flow (head sparing).[100] The greatest risk is associated with absent or even more seriously with reversed diastolic flow in systemic fetal arteries.[67] Various ratios of systolic-to-diastolic flow velocity waveforms have been used and include the systolic-to-diastolic ratio, systolic-diastolic/systolic (resistance index) or systolic-diastolic/mean (pulsatility index). Ratios or indexes greater than two standard deviations from the mean are associated with IUGR, whereas reversed or absent diastolic waveforms represent severe fetal hypoxia and increase the risks of intrauterine fetal death. In addition, umbilical venous pulsation and reversed flow in the vena cava suggest serious cardiac compromise from hypoxia or anemia. These Doppler waveform abnormalities may precede classic signs of fetal distress such as abnormal results on an oxytocin challenge test.

Antenatal Management

(See also Chapter 9.)

Once the diagnosis of IUGR is suspected and strengthened by ultrasonography, it is essential to institute appropriate maternal fetal care and closely monitor the well-being of the fetus. With severe IUGR, maternal activity should be limited and bed rest initiated, with the mother assuming a left lateral recumbent position to ensure optimal uterine blood

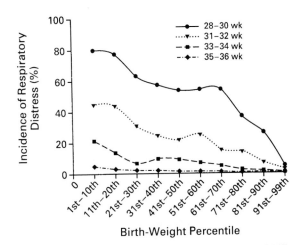

FIGURE 13–18. Incidence of respiratory distress among 12,317 preterm infants, according to birth weight percentile after stratification according to gestational age (28 to 30 weeks, 31 or 32 weeks, 33 or 34 weeks, and 35 or 36 weeks). (From McIntire DD, et al: Birth weight in relation to morbidity and mortality among newborn infants. N Engl J Med 340:1234, 1999. Copyright © 1999 Massachusetts Medical Society.)

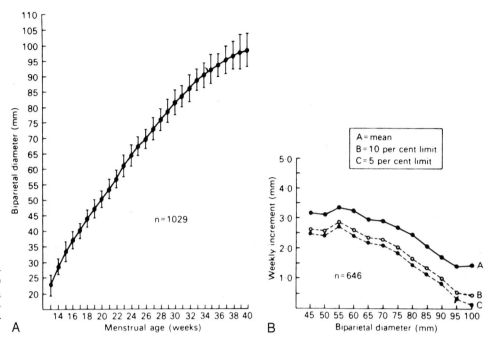

FIGURE 13–19. Absolute measurement *(A)*, and rate of change *(B)* of fetal biparietal diameter. (From Campbell S: Size at Birth. Amsterdam, Elsevier Scientific Publications, 1974.)

flow. Administration of oxygen (55% O_2 at 8 L/min) to the mother has resulted in improved fetal oxygenation, some growth, and normalization of fetal aortic blood flow velocity in some IUGR fetuses with chronic fetal distress.[10]

Assessment of fetal well-being should begin once the diagnosis is suspected and the fetus has approached a gestational age compatible with extrauterine survival. An inexpensive screening tool is a log of fetal activity recorded by the mother; normal activity is a reasonable sign of well-being. A specific period should be monitored, such as after a meal, and fetal activity should be recorded each day. In addition to this maternal record, a systematic approach to fetal evaluation should be performed routinely and frequently. Classically, the *oxytocin challenge test* (OCT)

has been used to predict the potential for fetal demise or acute intrapartum death in a marginally oxygenated, compromised fetus. This test requires the intravenous administration of oxytocin, which must result in three uterine contractions within 10 minutes. Late decelerations denote relative uteroplacental insufficiency and suggest that the oxygenation of the fetus may be impaired. A positive OCT result (three late decelerations with three contractions) also suggests that the fetus may not tolerate the contractions that occur during labor. This is not a universal observation; a significant percentage of these infants may be able to withstand spontaneous or oxytocin-induced labor without the development of fetal acidosis. Fewer decelerations than those for a positive OCT result should be considered suspect, and the test

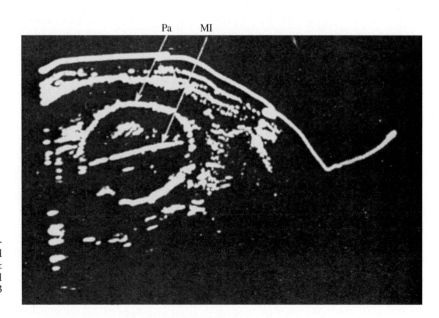

FIGURE 13–20. Sonogram demonstrating determination of the biparietal diameter. Pa, parietal bone; MI, midline echo. (From Campbell S: In Beard R, et al (eds): Fetal growth. Fetal Physiology and Medicine. Philadelphia, WB Saunders, 1976, p 271.)

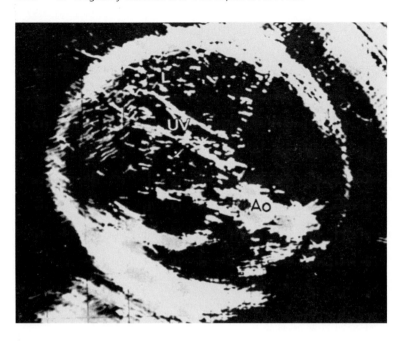

FIGURE 13–21. Truncometry at the level of fetal liver (L), umbilical vein (UV), and aorta (Ao). (From Campbell S: Size at Birth. Amsterdam, Elsevier Scientific Publications, 1974.)

should be repeated (along with technically unsatisfactory tracings) within the next 24 to 48 hours.

Because technical and time difficulties are related to the OCT and because contraindications exist for its use, such as a previous classic cesarean section, placenta previa, and concern about inducing premature labor, the *nonstress test* (NST) has been employed. This test examines fetal well-being by determining the acceleration of the fetal heart rate after spontaneous fetal movement. A healthy fetus (nonhypoxic) will respond to its own body movements with a mean acceleration of 15 beats per minute above the baseline heart rate. In addition, the frequency of fetal movements should be ascertained; at the same time, examination of beat-to-beat and long-term variability can offer additional useful information. The NST can also supplement the OCT, because fetuses with a positive OCT result but a reactive NST result and normal beat-to-beat variability are more likely to tolerate labor without untoward problems. Under stable maternal conditions and with signs of fetal well-being (negative OCT result and [or] reactive NST result), these tests may be repeated weekly.

The false-positive rate for OCT (25%) and NST

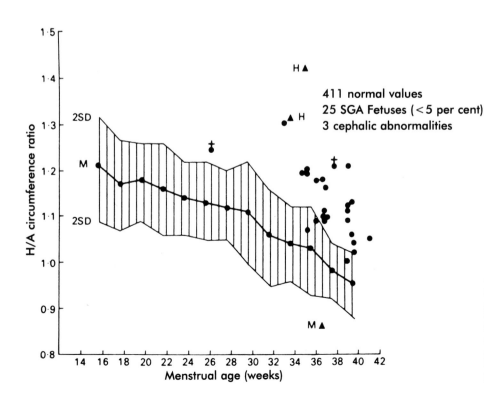

FIGURE 13–22. Assessment of aberrant fetal growth by the head-abdomen circumference ratio. H, hydrocephalus; M, microcephalus; +, fetal demise; ●, SGA; ▲H, hydrocephaly; ▲M, microcephaly. (From Campbell S: Fetal growth. In Beard R, et al (eds): Fetal Physiology and Medicine. Philadelphia, WB Saunders, 1976, p 271.)

(20%) is high compared with the false-negative rate for OCT (0.4 in 1000) and NST (6.8 in 1000). The rate of intrauterine fetal death is high after a positive OCT result (32%) but lower with a nonreactive NST result (12%). Therefore, the contraction stress test is more predictive of fetal death and has fewer false-negative results. However, more false-positive results are obtained than with the NST.

Biophysical determinants have been used successfully to assess fetal well-being.[83] The combined analyses of fetal breathing movements, gross body movements, fetal tone, fetal heart reactivity to movement, and qualitative amniotic fluid volume have improved the antenatal management of IUGR (Table 13–7). This *biophysical profile* provides a nonweighted score that can identify the fetus at risk. A biophysical profile score of 8 to 10 carries a 0.8% chance of fetal death, whereas a score of 0 predicts a fetal mortality rate of 40%. This analysis takes approximately 30 minutes and should be repeated weekly with scores of 8 to 10. If the score is less than 8, the biophysical profile should be repeated that afternoon. If the score is again less than 8, an OCT should be performed and a decision made to deliver the infant, regardless of gestational age, unless severe anomalies are determined. A low biophysical profile correlates with fetal hypoxia determined by cordocentesis. Assessment of fetal aortic flow with the pulsatile index (see Table 13–7) may also help determine optimal timing for delivery. If fetal lung maturity is present and aortic blood flow is reduced with other evidence of fetal distress, the fetus may need to be delivered before term.

With continued careful fetal surveillance and a stable maternal-fetal environment, a course of nonintervention is indicated.

The mode of delivery is not necessarily dictated by the abnormalities recorded by biophysical or electrophysiologic surveillance of the fetus. Some patients can tolerate labor after a positive OCT result, with oxygen administration and a left lateral recumbent position. However, it would be judicious to avoid labor in those situations complicated by a nonreactive NST result, a flat baseline, absent or reversed diastolic flow, and a positive OCT result. Similarly, premature infants who are SGA, in particular those with a breech presentation and those whose mothers have a completely unfavorable cervix, should be delivered by the abdominal route. Particular attention should be given to the asymmetrically (late-flattening) growth-retarded fetus with chronic fetal distress who tolerates labor poorly and readily develops signs of acute fetal distress, compared with the symmetrically undergrown fetus and the normal fetus.[43, 44] Whether labor is induced or spontaneous, continuous intrapartum fetal heart rate monitoring combined with appropriate use of fetal scalp pH determinations must be employed. (See also Chapter 9.) If late decelerations become evident, scalp blood pH might be evaluated, and if fetal acidosis has developed, delivery should be expedited.

During labor, uterine contractions may further compromise marginal placental perfusion and fetal gas exchange. The myocardium of these fetuses may have diminished glycogen stores, a key energy source partially responsible for the fetal ability to withstand asphyxia. Because there is a high incidence of intrapartum birth asphyxia, it is essential that the delivery be coordinated with the neonatal team, which should be prepared to resuscitate a depressed or asphyxiated neonate. In addition, combined obstetric-pediatric management is indicated if meconium is present in

---

TABLE 13–7 BIOPHYSICAL PROFILE SCORING: TECHNIQUE AND INTERPRETATION*

BIOPHYSICAL VARIABLE	NORMAL (SCORE = 2)	ABNORMAL (SCORE = 0)
Fetal breathing movements	≥ 1 episode of ≥ 30 sec in 30 min	Absent or no episode of ≥ 30 sec in 30 min
Gross body movements	≥ 3 Discrete body or limb movements in 30 min (episodes of active continuous movement considered as single movement)	≤ 2 Episodes of body or limb movements in 30 min
Fetal tone	≥ 1 Episode of active extension with return to flexion of fetal limb(s) or trunk (opening and closing of hand considered normal tone)	Slow extension with return to partial flexion or movement of limb in full extension or absent fetal movement
Reactive fetal heart rate	≥ 2 Episodes of acceleration of ≥ 15 beats/min and of ≥ 15 sec associated with fetal movement in 20 minutes	< 2 Episodes of acceleration of fetal heart rate or acceleration of < 15 beats/min in 20 min
Qualitative amniotic fluid volume	≥ 1 Pocket of fluid measuring ≥ 1 cm in two perpendicular planes	Either no pockets or a pocket < 1 cm in two perpendicular planes

*See Manning FA, et al: Antepartum fetal evaluation: Development of a biophysical profile. Am J Obstet Gynecol 136:787, 1980.
Modified from Manning FA, et al: Fetal assessment based on fetal biophysical profile scoring. Am J Obstet Gynecol 151:343, 1985.

the amniotic fluid. This event often follows periods of fetal hypoxia and stress, occurring with greatest frequency in the term or post-term neonate who is SGA. Obstetric management should include oropharyngeal suctioning immediately after delivery of the head. Immediately after birth, the neonatal team should further clear the oropharynx, and possibly also the trachea, of additional meconium. (See also Chapter 42, Part Five.)

Saline *amnioinfusion* may be beneficial in the presence of oligohydramnios and an amnionic fluid index of less than 5 cm.[128] Titration to an index of greater than 8 cm may lower the incidence of meconium-stained fluid, variable decelerations, end-stage bradycardia, fetal distress, and acute fetal acidosis.

One problem in managing these pregnancies is determining the course of action when the fetus stops growing. Unfortunately, under stable maternal conditions and if no other signs of compromise are detected in the fetus, the best alternative is to leave the fetus in utero, provide good nutrition, and continue fetal surveillance. The question of whether to deliver these fetuses should be tempered by the accuracy of the diagnosis and the ability to manage all potential neonatal problems efficiently, including appropriate alimentation. Although lung maturity may be present, the many other problems associated with prematurity should temper a decision for delivery before 30 weeks. These additional risks of prematurity must be balanced against the risk of fetal death in an adverse environment.

Approach to the Infant Who Is SGA

After birth, the infant who is SGA may develop significant neonatal problems (Table 13–8). In the delivery room it is essential to ensure optimal neonatal cardiopulmonary physiologic adaptation while ensuring minimal heat loss in a warm environment. Once stabilization has been established, a careful physical examination should be performed.[114]

When infants with obvious anomalies and syndromes and those born to mothers with severe illness or malnutrition are excluded, there still remains a heterogeneous population of infants who are SGA.[97, 147] These infants have a characteristic physical appearance; the heads look relatively large for their undergrown trunks and extremities, which seem wasted. The abdomen is scaphoid, misleading one to suspect a diaphragmatic hernia. The extremities have little subcutaneous tissue or fat, which is best exemplified by a reduced skinfold thickness (see Fig. 13–17). In addition, the skin appears to hang; it is rough, dry, and parchment-like; and it desquamates easily. Fingernails may be long, and the hands and feet of these infants tend to look too large for the rest of the body. The facial appearance suggests the look of a "wise old person," especially compared with that of premature infants (Fig. 13–23). Cranial sutures may be widened or overriding; the anterior fontanel is larger than expected, representing diminished membranous bone formation. Similarly, epiphyseal ossification at the

knee (chondral bone) is also retarded. Decreased bone mineralization may also be present.[25, 96] When meconium is passed in utero, there is often yellow-green staining of the nails, skin, and umbilical cord, which may also appear thinner than usual. Many of these infants have subclinical chronic fetal hypoxia, which is detectable by cordocentesis or Doppler waveform velocimetry.

Gestational age assessment of the infant who is SGA may result in misleading data when based on physical criteria alone. Vernix caseosa is frequently reduced or absent as a result of diminished skin perfusion during periods of fetal distress or because of depressed synthesis of estriol, which enhances vernix production. In the absence of this protective covering, the skin is continuously exposed to amniotic fluid and begins to desquamate after birth. Sole creases are determined in part by exposure to amniotic fluid and therefore appear more mature. Breast tissue formation also depends on peripheral blood flow and estriol levels and become markedly reduced in infants who are SGA. In addition, the female external genitalia appear less mature because of the absence of the perineal adipose tissue covering the labia. Ear cartilage, as noted in bone ossification, may also be diminished.

Neurologic examination for gestational age assessment may be affected less by IUGR than the physical criteria. Infants with IUGR achieve appropriate neurologic maturity functionally. Peripheral nerve conduction velocity and visual- or auditory-evoked responses correlate well with gestational age in normal neonates and are not impaired after IUGR. These aspects of neurologic maturity are not sensitive to deprivation, and occasionally maturity may even become accelerated. Determinants of active or passive tone and posture may be reliable in infants who are SGA, assuming that infants with significant central nervous system and metabolic disorders are excluded.

Specific organ maturity occurs despite diminished somatic growth. Cerebral cortical convolutions, renal glomeruli, and alveolar maturation all relate to gestational age and are not retarded with IUGR. As a result of stress in utero, these infants may occasionally accelerate the maturity of specific organ systems, such as the lung, thus explaining the low incidence of respiratory distress syndrome in preterm neonates who are SGA.

When examined in closer detail, infants who are SGA demonstrate specific behavioral characteristics that suggest, despite electric neurologic maturity, that functional central nervous system maturity may be impaired.[6, 7] In the absence of significant central nervous system disease, these neonates demonstrate abnormal sleep cycles and diminished muscle tone, reflexes, activity, and excitability. This hypoexcitability suggests an adverse effect on polysynaptic reflex propagation and implies that central nervous system functional maturity does not necessarily proceed independently of the intrauterine events that result in IUGR.

Once stabilized and assigned a gestational age, the

TABLE 13-8   PERINATAL PROBLEMS OF THE NEONATE WHO IS SGA

PROBLEM	PATHOGENESIS	ASSESSMENT/PREVENTION/ TREATMENT
Fetal death	Placental insufficiency, chronic fetal hypoxia	Biophysical profile Vessel velocimetry Cordocentesis Maternal O_2 Early delivery
Asphyxia	Acute fetal hypoxia superimposed on chronic fetal hypoxia, acidosis Placental insufficiency ↓ Cardiac glycogen stores	Antepartum and intrapartum monitoring Efficient neonatal resuscitation
Meconium aspiration pneumonia	Hypoxic stress	Pharyngeal-tracheal aspiration
Fasting hypoglycemia	↓ Hepatic glycogen ↓ Gluconeogenesis ↓ Counterregulatory hormones Cold stress Asphyxia-hypoxia	Early oral or intravenous alimentation or both
Alimented hyperglycemia	"Starvation diabetes"	Glucose infusion not to exceed 8 mg/kg per min except with hypoglycemia
Polycythemia/hyperviscosity	Placental transfusion Fetal hypoxia ↑ Erythropoietin	Neonatal partial exchange transfusion
Temperature instability	Cold stress Poor fat stores Catecholamine depletion Hypoxia, hypoglycemia Reduced fasting oxygen consumption	Neutral thermal environment Early alimentation
Dysmorphology	TORCH Syndrome complexes Chromosome disorders Teratogen exposure	Disease-specific therapy or prevention
Pulmonary hemorrhage (rare)	Hypothermia, polycythemia ↓ O_2/DIC	Avoid cold stress, hypoxia Endotracheal administration of epinephrine PEEP
Immunodeficiency	"Malnutrition" effect TORCH	Unknown Specific therapy if available
Decreased bone mineral density	Possible substrate deficiency or altered vitamin D metabolism	Appropriate postnatal oral calcium and vitamin D intake

DIC, disseminated intravascular coagulation; PEEP, positive end-expiratory pressure.

neonate who is SGA should be examined in more detail to direct the diagnostic work-up as detailed in the following outline:

A. History and physical examination.[34, 114, 122]
B. Accurate growth parameters
C. Findings:
   1. Dysmorphic features suggesting:
      a. Chromosome abnormality
      b. Syndrome
      c. Drugs (fetal exposure)
   2. Blueberry-muffin rash, petechiae, hepato-splenomegaly, and ocular pathologic changes suggesting:
      a. Rubella
      b. Cytomegalovirus
      c. Other infection
   3. Neither 1 nor 2 suggests:
      a. Chronic fetal hypoxia
      b. Constitutional factors
      c. Genetic factors
      d. Nutritional factors
      e. Toxins.
      f. Placenta (e.g., twins)
      g. Unknown

Dysmorphic features, "funny-looking facies," and abnormal hands, feet, and palmar creases, in addition to gross anomalies, suggest congenital malformation syndromes, chromosomal defects, or teratogens. Ocular disorders, such as chorioretinitis, cataracts, glaucoma, and cloudy cornea, in addition to hepato-splenomegaly, jaundice, and a blueberry-muffin rash, suggest a congenital infection. (See also Chapters 22 and 37.) The remaining infants constitute a heterogeneous group that represents most neonates who are SGA. Multiple gestations are the most recognizable cause in this category. TORCH infections resulting in extremely low birth weight are unusual in the absence of other clinical signs of congenital infection; how-

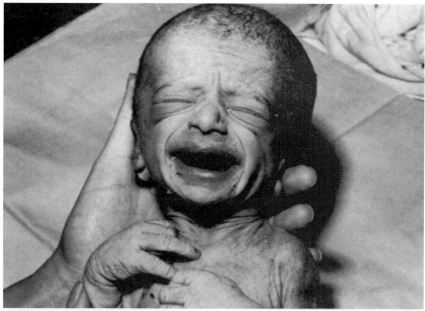

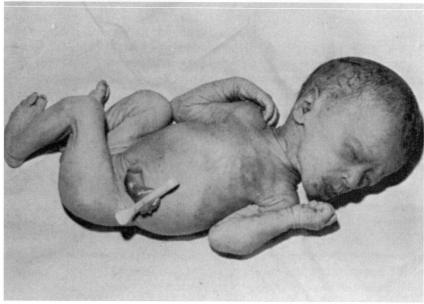

FIGURE 13–23. Term infant who is SGA demonstrating wizened facies and dry, desquamating, hanging skin. Birth weight: 1500 gm.

ever, a screening determination on cord blood for IgM values and a urine culture for cytomegalovirus may be indicated.[12] Radiographic examination of the long bones together with ultrasonography of the head are diagnostically useful. Careful data related to the present and past reproductive history of the mother, in addition to ongoing neonatal management and close observation, are indicated in the remaining large number of neonates who are SGA whose underlying disorders may never be determined.

Neonatal Problems

The perinatal mortality rate among infants who have IUGR is 10 to 20 times that among infants who are AGA. Intrauterine fetal death from chronic fetal hypoxia, immediate birth asphyxia, the multisystem disorders associated with asphyxia (hypoxic-ischemic encephalopathy, persistent fetal circulation, cardiomyopathy), and lethal congenital anomalies are the main contributing factors to the high mortality rate for fetuses and neonates who have IUGR. Problems due to prematurity such as respiratory distress syndrome are also more common with IUGR (see Fig. 13–18). Neurologic and other morbidities are also more frequent in infants who have IUGR; they have a rate 5 to 10 times that of infants who are AGA. Most intrauterine fetal deaths occur between 38 and 42 weeks' gestation and can be potentially avoided by careful assessment and intervention as noted in Table 13–8.

Asphyxia

Perinatal asphyxia and its sequelae constitute the most significant immediate problem of infants who have IUGR. As discussed, uterine contractions may add an additional hypoxic stress on the chronically hypoxic fetus with a marginally functioning placenta. The ensuing acute fetal hypoxia, acidosis, and cerebral depression may result in fetal death or neonatal asphyxia. IUGR accounts for a large proportion of stillborn infants with hypoxia in utero. Myocardial infarction, amniotic fluid aspiration, and signs of cerebral hypoxia are noted in the stillborn infants with IUGR. With repeated episodes of fetal asphyxia or persistent hypoxemia, myocardial glycogen reserves are depleted, further limiting the fetal cardiopulmonary adaptation to hypoxia. If inadequate resuscitation occurs at birth and Apgar scores are low, the combination of intrapartum and neonatal asphyxia places the infant in double jeopardy for a continuum of central nervous system insult. The sequelae of perinatal asphyxia include multiple organ system dysfunction potentially characterized by hypoxic ischemic encephalopathy, ischemic heart failure, meconium aspiration pneumonia, persistent fetal circulation, gastrointestinal perforation, and acute tubular necrosis. Concomitant with these sequelae, there may be metabolic derangements such as hypoglycemia. Hypocalcemia is partly caused by excessive phosphate release from damaged cells or acidosis; it is exacerbated by sodium bicarbonate and diminished calcium intake. Hypocalcemia does not occur more often with IUGR unless these problems are present. Meconium aspiration syndrome may complicate the clinical picture and further compromise respiratory function and oxygenation with the development of pneumonitis and pneumothorax.

Neonatal Metabolism

Fasting hypoglycemia develops in infants who are SGA more than in any other neonatal subgroup or category.[23] The propensity for hypoglycemia is greatest during the first 3 days of life; however, some of these infants have ketotic hypoglycemia months later. Key to the occurrence of hypoglycemia are the diminished hepatic glycogen stores (Fig. 13–24). Glycogenolysis constitutes the predominant source of glucose for the neonate during the immediate hours after birth.[72, 117] Later in the day, when glycogen stores become depleted, fasting glucose production results from the incorporation of lactate and gluconeogenic amino acid precursors into glucose. Infants who are SGA demonstrate an inability to increase blood glucose concentration after oral or intravenous administration of alanine, the key gluconeogenic amino acid.[52, 76] Hypoglycemic infants who are SGA have elevated alanine and lactate levels, suggesting that substrate availability is not rate-limiting for gluconeogenesis and that the enzymes or cofactors are not active. Hypoglycemic infants probably have reduced hepatic glucose production. Nonhypoglycemic infants who are SGA do demonstrate equivalent rates of gluconeogenesis from alanine as compared with nonhypoglycemic neonates who are AGA.[41]

Immediately after birth, fasting infants who are SGA may have lower plasma-free fatty acid levels than normally grown infants. Fasting blood glucose levels in infants who are SGA directly correlate with plasma-free fatty acid and ketone body levels. In addition, once fed, infants who are SGA have deficient use of intravenous triglycerides. After the intravenous administration of triglyceride emulsion, infants who are SGA have high free fatty acid and triglyceride levels, but ketone body formation is attenuated.[112] This suggests that use and oxidation of free fatty acids and triglycerides are diminished in neonates who are SGA. Free fatty acid oxidation is important because it spares peripheral tissue use of glucose, whereas hepatic oxidation of free fatty acids may contribute the reducing equivalents and energy re-

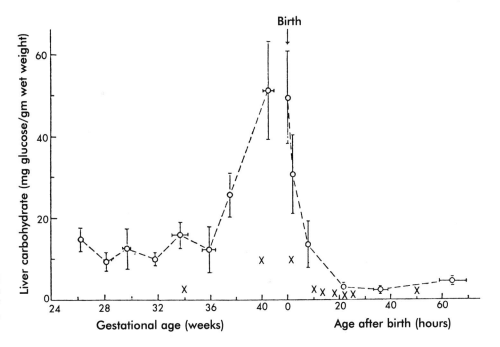

FIGURE 13–24. Fetal and neonatal hepatic glycogen content (X) in patients with IUGR. (From Shelly H, et al: Neonatal hypoglycemia. Br Med Bull 22:34, 1966.)

quired for hepatic gluconeogenesis. Deficient provision or oxidation of fatty acids may be partly responsible for the development of fasting hypoglycemia in these infants (Fig. 13–25).

Endocrine alterations have also been implicated in the pathogenesis of hypoglycemia in infants who are SGA. Hyperinsulinemia or excessive sensitivity to insulin may be one factor.[3, 29] Catecholamine release is deficient in these neonates during periods of hypoglycemia. Although basal glucagon levels may be elevated, exogenous administration of glucagon fails to enhance glycemia. These data suggest an abnormality of counter-regulatory hormonal mechanisms during periods of neonatal hypoglycemia in infants who are SGA.

With improved standards of care and attempts at early enteral feeding or intravenous alimentation, fasting hypoglycemia in the neonate who is SGA is a less common event. Before the start of alimentation, careful monitoring with Dextrostix reagent strips for determining blood glucose values identifies infants with asymptomatic hypoglycemia. If whole blood glucose concentrations decline to less than 45 mg/dL during the first 3 days in term infants or preterm infants and no untoward symptoms have occurred, early feeding or glucose infusion at 4 to 8 mg/kg per minute should begin. After this initial rate, the infusion should be titrated until blood glucose values achieve normal levels. If the hypoglycemia is symptomatic, particularly when seizure activity intervenes, an intravenous mini-bolus of 10% dextrose in water at 200 mg/kg should be given, followed by an infusion as just described. Infants at greatest risk of having hypoglycemia are those who have been asphyxiated and those who appear most undergrown

according to the ponderal index (Fig. 13–26). Similarly, breast-fed twins who are not supplemented with a carbohydrate source are at risk, particularly the smaller twin, and should be monitored carefully. (See also Chapter 47, Part One.)

TEMPERATURE REGULATION

(See also Chapter 29.)

After the birth of an infant whose gestation was complicated by uteroplacental insufficiency, the neonate's initial body temperature may be elevated. When placental function fails, the neonate's heat-eliminating capacity also becomes deficient, resulting in fetal hyperthermia. On exposure to the cold environment of the delivery room, infants who are SGA can increase their heat production (oxygen consumption) appropriately because brown adipose tissue stores are not necessarily depleted as a result of IUGR.[70, 120] However, the infants' core temperature drops if the cold stress continues, implying that heat loss has exceeded heat production. Heat loss in these infants is partly caused by the large body surface area exposed to cold and the deficiency of an insulating layer of subcutaneous adipose tissue stores. Indeed, magnetic resonance imaging detection of reduced fetal fat stores is highly suggestive of IUGR that may result in fetal distress. Infants who are SGA therefore have a narrower neutral thermal environment than term infants but a broader one than premature neonates. In infants who are SGA, hypoglycemia or hypoxia, or both, interferes with heat production and may contribute to thermal instability. In all infants, particularly those who are SGA, a neutral thermal environment should be sought to prevent excessive

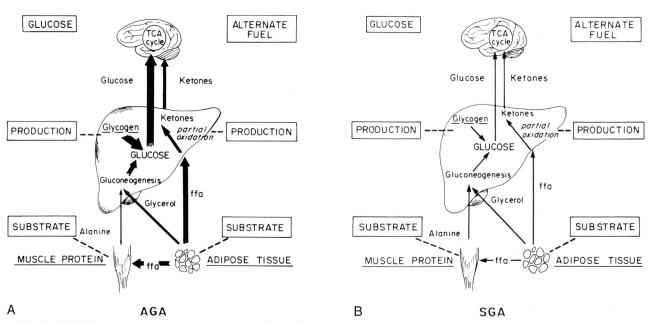

FIGURE 13–25. Postnatal glucose and fatty acid metabolic relationships in neonates who are AGA *(A)* and SGA *(B)*. *Arrows* depict magnitude of flux. Infants who are SGA demonstrate both diminished glycogen stores and gluconeogenesis. In addition, they may have attenuated fatty acid oxidation. (Modified from Adam PAJ: In Falkner F, et al (eds): Human Growth, vol 1. New York, Plenum Press, 1978.)

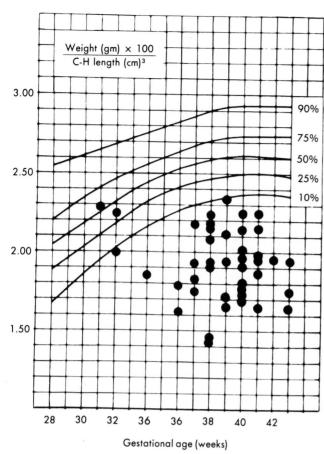

FIGURE 13–26. Relationship between ponderal index and neonatal hypoglycemia in IUGR. ● Hypoglycemic infants. (From Jarai I, et al: Body size and neonatal hypoglycemia in intrauterine growth retardation. Early Hum Dev 1:25, 1977.)

heat loss and to promote appropriate postnatal weight gain.

When nursed in a neutral thermal environment, infants who are SGA demonstrate the usual decline of the respiratory quotient after birth, representing a shift toward free fatty acid oxidation. During the first 12 hours after birth, basal oxygen consumption may be diminished in neonates who are SGA. Similar observations have been recorded in utero among fetal lambs that are spontaneously SGA, suggesting in both situations that there is a deficiency of potentially oxidizable substrates. Supporting this hypothesis is the marked increment of oxygen consumption that occurs in well-alimented infants who are SGA. This latter observation is also analogous to the rise of energy production after the nutritional rehabilitation of infants with marasmic-kwashiorkor. The increment of oxygen consumption after fetal or infantile malnutrition represents the energy cost of growth. Infants who are SGA usually have a significantly smaller postnatal weight loss because they are maturationally capable of achieving an adequate caloric intake earlier than premature neonates. Because of this enhanced caloric intake, infants who are SGA have a higher oxygen consumption than less mature neonates. Nutritional balance studies of premature infants who are SGA

demonstrated an increase of fecal fat and protein loss, despite faster rates of growth compared with premature infants who are AGA. Energy storage was lower with IUGR, suggesting less fat deposition.

A subgroup of neonates who are SGA does not demonstrate an elevation of oxygen consumption after appropriate caloric intake. These infants have had low-profile intrauterine growth and may be considered to have had "primordial fetal growth retardation." Their growth is set and fixed at a slower rate, and their eventual growth potential is reduced. The diminished body cell number in congenitally infected infants and in those with chromosomal disorders exemplifies primordial growth retardation in these neonates.

HYPERVISCOSITY-POLYCYTHEMIA SYNDROME

(See also Chapter 44.)

The plasma volume immediately after birth of infants who are SGA averages 52 mL/kg, as compared with 43 mL/kg in infants who are AGA. Once equilibrated at 12 hours of life, the plasma volume becomes equivalent in the two groups. In addition to an enhanced plasma space, the circulating red blood cell mass is expanded. Fetal hypoxia and subsequent erythropoietin synthesis induce excessive red blood cell production.[123] Alternately, a placental-fetal transfusion during labor or periods of fetal asphyxia may result in a shift of placental blood to the fetus. Nonetheless, the elevation of the hematocrit level potentially increases blood viscosity, which interferes with vital tissue perfusion. The altered viscosity adversely affects neonatal hemodynamics and results in an abnormal cardiopulmonary and metabolic postnatal adaptation, producing hypoxia and hypoglycemia. These infants are at increased risk of having necrotizing enterocolitis. In the event that polycythemia is present (central hematocrit level greater than 65%) with such symptoms, appropriate therapy is directed at correcting hypoxia and hypoglycemia, and a partial exchange transfusion to reduce blood viscosity and to improve tissue perfusion should be considered. (See also Chapter 44.)

OTHER PROBLEMS

Immunologic function of infants who are SGA may be depressed, as are older infants with the postnatal onset of malnutrition.[21, 39] Neonates with congenital rubella syndrome have functional deficiency of both T and B lymphocytes. This may, however, be related to continued intracellular viral infection. Other infants who are SGA may also manifest varying degrees of immunologic dysfunction that persist into childhood. Deficiencies have been demonstrated in lymphocyte number and function, which include decreased spontaneous mitogenesis and reduced response to phytohemagglutinin. Similarly, these infants tend to have lower immunoglobulin levels during infancy and to demonstrate an attenuated antibody response to oral polio vaccine. (See also Chapter 37, Part One.) IUGR is associated with a slower than normal production of long-chain polyunsaturated fatty acids.[133] Intestinal absorption of xylose is also attenuated. At birth, cord prealbumin and bone mineral content are low in term infants who are SGA. Thrombocytopenia, neutropenia, prolonged thrombin and partial thromboplastin times, and elevated fibrin degradation products are also problems among infants who are SGA.[93, 94, 105] Sudden infant death syndrome may be more common after IUGR. Inguinal hernias also typically follow preterm IUGR. Additional problems and their management are noted in Table 13–8.[6, 132]

FOLLOW-UP

Excluding the infants who are SGA who are severely affected with serious congenital malformations and viral infections, the remaining neonates should benefit from optimal antenatal detection, very careful management of pregnancy, and avoidance of hypoxic fetal distress. In addition, with ideal neonatal intensive care, the morbidity and mortality rates for infants who are SGA should be reduced to a minimum, and postnatal developmental handicaps should be diminished. Nonetheless, these infants continue to contribute to the excessive fetal and neonatal morbidity and mortality rates. The neonatal mortality rate is much greater than that for term neonates but only slightly increased for age-matched premature neonates. The incidence of fetal death remains higher for infants who are SGA. In addition to the etiologic events that lead to the development of IUGR, these infants have additional multisystem problems that further compromise survival and future growth or development. Among these fetuses, the perinatal mortality rate is 10 times that of infants who are AGA. The incidence of intrauterine fetal death is greatest among the most severely undergrown infants. Both antepartum and intrapartum events contribute to fetal death. Lethal congenital malformations and birth asphyxia are the two leading causes of death among neonates who are SGA. Infants with very low birth weight who are SGA (less than 1500 gm) are at significant risk of reduced postnatal growth and development in addition to chronic neonatal sequelae such as BPD or ROP.

DEVELOPMENTAL OUTCOME

When infants with congenital infections and severe malformations are excluded, there remains a heterogenous group of undergrown neonates. Intellectual and neurologic functions in these remaining infants depend heavily on the presence or absence of adverse perinatal events, in addition to the specific cause of IUGR.[13] Cerebral morbidity will be worsened by the significant alterations in fetal blood flow, as determined by reversed diastole umbilical artery blood flow, by hypoxic-ischemic encephalopathy subsequent to birth asphyxia, and by the postnatal problems of hypoxia and hypoglycemia.[90] Therefore, the prognosis must consider all the potentially adverse

perinatal circumstances in addition to IUGR.[6, 61, 126, 127] When these perinatal problems are minimal or are avoided, the neonate who is SGA may still demonstrate cerebral developmental handicaps, especially in the presence of relative head growth retardation.[104, 129, 139] If term neonates who are AGA are used as a standard, term infants who are SGA demonstrate developmental problems when they are examined at follow-up at age 2 years, 5 years, and older. Even when compared with premature neonates, term infants who are SGA continue to have developmental disadvantages. Follow-up of these infants reveals little difference in intelligence quotient or neurologic sequelae; however, their school performance is poor, partly because of behavioral and learning disorders. Preterm infants who are SGA may have an even greater percentage of abnormal neurodevelopmental outcomes than term neonates who are SGA. Those early-onset infants who are SGA, demonstrating decreased growth of the biparietal diameter before 26 weeks' gestation, and those with symmetric growth retardation have diminished developmental quotients in infancy. However, some follow-up observations in both term and preterm neonates who are SGA are favorable: these neonates compare well with their counterparts who are AGA. Cerebral palsy is uncommon following uncomplicated IUGR. Infants who are SGA are a heterogeneous group, and the populations investigated may vary in the severity of neurodevelopmental handicap; similarly, antenatal detection and perinatal management varies among high-risk centers. It therefore appears that these latter favorable reports may represent the outcome after optimal obstetric management and neonatal care. Adults who were SGA tend to have a normal IQ, but they demonstrate school difficulties, and fewer become professionals. Despite this, they report to be well-adjusted and socially satisfied with their lives.[126]

Another major determining influence on neonatal neurodevelopmental outcome in infants who are SGA is the family's socioeconomic status. Parent educational background, place of rearing, and environmental conditions all have a strong effect on outcome. Infants who are SGA born to families of higher socioeconomic status demonstrated little developmental difference on follow-up, whereas those born to poorer families had significant developmental handicaps. (See also Chapter 39.)

GROWTH

Postnatal growth after IUGR depends in part on the cause of the growth retardation, the postnatal nutritional intake, and the social environment.[32, 53, 54] Although birth weight correlates best to maternal weight, postnatal growth is related to both maternal and paternal growth characteristics. Neonates who are SGA who have primordial growth retardation related to congenital viral, chromosomal, or constitutional syndromes remain small throughout life. Those infants whose intrauterine growth was inhibited late in gestation because of uterine constraint, placental

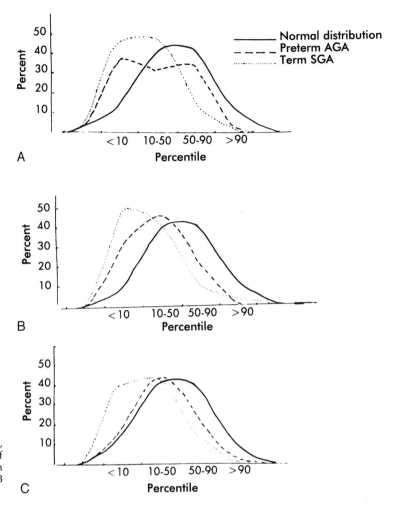

FIGURE 13–27. Eventual physical growth of SGA term, AGA premature, and AGA term neonates at 4 years of age. *A*, Height; *B*, weight; *C*, head circumference. (From Lubchenco L: The High-Risk Infant. Philadelphia, WB Saunders, 1976.)

insufficiency, or nutritional deficits will have catch-up growth after birth and approach their inherited growth potential when provided with an optimal environment.[68] Those infants with a low ponderal index or asymmetric growth retardation have an accelerated growth phase once adequate postnatal caloric intake has been established, which suggests release of an in utero constraining factor after birth. This postpartum acceleration of growth occurs within the first 6 months of life, placing the infant on a new percentile growth tract. Catch-up growth may be enhanced by nucleotide supplementation of formula in term infants who are SGA. Despite the catch-up period, some of these infants remain smaller than appropriately grown neonates (Fig. 13–27), especially those who had the onset of growth retardation before 26 weeks. Growth hormone therapy for primordial IUGR and for IUGR of unknown cause has produced growth acceleration in a small number of patients.[22, 35] Some infants with IUGR demonstrate abnormal postnatal growth hormone physiology, suggestive of growth hormone resistance.

The goal of future management plans for the improvement of growth and developmental outcome in neonates who are SGA must have its origins close to the onset of IUGR. Once growth retardation has developed, early identification and careful avoidance of undue hypoxic stress and nutritional deficits should enhance the survival and quality of life of these high-risk neonates.[19]

■ REFERENCES

1. Abrams B, et al: Maternal weight gain in women with good pregnancy outcome. Obstet Gynecol 76:1, 1990.
2. Ahluwalia IB, et al: The effect of WIC participation on small-for-gestational-age births: Michigan, 1992. Am J Pub Health 88:1374, 1998.
3. Antunes JD, et al: Childhood hypoglycemia: Differentiating hyperinsulinemic from nonhyperinsulinemic causes. J Pediatr 116:105, 1990.
4. Ashmead GG, et al: Maternal-fetal substrate relationship in the third trimester in human pregnancy. Gynecol Obstet Invest 35:18, 1993.
5. Auwerx J, et al: Leptin. Lancet 351:737, 1998.
6. Azzopardi D, et al: Phosphorus metabolites and intracellular pH in the brains of normal and small for gestational age infants investigated by magnetic resonance spectroscopy. Pediatr Res 25:440, 1989.
7. Bardin C, et al: Outcome of small-for-gestational age and appropriate-for-gestational age infants born before 27 weeks of gestation. Pediatrics 100:E4, 1997.
8. Barker DJP: Early growth and cardiovascular disease. Arch Dis Child 80:305, 1999.
9. Bastide A, et al: Ultrasound evaluation of amniotic fluid:

Outcome of pregnancies with severe oligohydramnios. Am J Obstet Gynecol 154:895, 1986.

10. Battaglia C, et al: Maternal hyperoxygenation in the treatment of intrauterine growth retardation. Am J Obstet Gynecol 167:430, 1992.

11. Berg CJ, et al: Gestational age and intrauterine growth retardation among white and black very low birthweight infants: A population-based cohort study. Paediatr Perinat Epidemiol 8:53, 1994.

12. Berge P, et al: Impact of asymptomatic congenital cytomegalovirus infection on size at birth and gestational duration. Pediatr Infect Dis 9:170, 1990.

13. Besson-Duvanel C, et al: Long-term effects of neonatal hypoglycemia on brain growth and psychomotor development in small-for-gestational-age preterm infants. J Pediatr 134:492, 1999.

14. Brenner W, et al: A standard of fetal growth for the United States of America. Am J Obstet Gynecol 126:555, 1976.

15. Brooke O, et al: Energy retention, energy expenditure, and growth in healthy immature infants. Pediatr Res 13:215, 1979.

16. Brown AK, et al: The influence of infant and maternal sickle cell disease on birth outcome and neonatal course. Arch Pediatr Adolesc Med 148:1156, 1994.

17. Burke G, et al: Is intrauterine growth retardation with normal umbilical artery blood flow a benign condition? BMJ 300:1044, 1990.

18. Campbell DM, et al: Diet in pregnancy and the offspring's blood pressure 40 years later. Br J Obstet Gynaecol 103:273, 1996.

19. Cance-Rouzaud A, et al: Growth hormone, insulin-like growth factor-I and insulin-like growth factor binding protein-3 are regulated differently in small-for-gestational-age and appropriate-for-gestational-age neonates. Biol Neonate 73:347, 1998.

20. Challis DE, et al: Glucose metabolism is elevated and vascular resistance and maternofetal transfer is normal in perfused placental cotyledons from severely growth-restricted fetuses. Pediatr Res 47:309, 2000.

21. Chandra R: Serum thymic hormone activity and cell-mediated immunity in healthy neonates, preterm infants, and small-for-gestational-age infants. Pediatrics 67:407, 1981.

22. Chatelain P, et al: Dose-dependent catch-up growth after 2 years of growth hormone treatment in intrauterine growth-retarded children, J Clin Endocrinol Metabol 78:1454, 1994.

23. Chessex P, et al: Metabolic consequences of intrauterine growth retardation in very low birthweight infants. Pediatr Res 18:709, 1984.

24. Chowen JA, et al: Decreased expression of placental growth hormone in intrauterine growth retardation. Pediatr Res 39:736, 1996.

25. Chunga Vega F, et al: Low bone mineral density in small for gestational age infants: Correlation with cord blood zinc concentrations. Arch Dis Child 75:F126, 1996.

26. Cinax P, et al: Plasma leptin levels of large for gestational age and small for gestational age infants. Acta Paediatr 88:753, 1999.

27. Clark PM, et al: Weight gain in pregnancy, triceps skinfold thickness, and blood pressure in offspring. Obstet Gynecol 91:103, 1998.

28. Clarren S, et al: The fetal alcohol syndrome. N Engl J Med 298:1063, 1978.

29. Collins J, et al: Hyperinsulinism in asphyxiated and small for dates infants with hypoglycemia. Lancet 2:311, 1984.

30. Combs CA, et al: Sonographic estimation of fetal weight based on a model of fetal volume. Obstet Gynecol 82:365, 1993.

31. Cordero JF: Effect of environmental agents on pregnancy outcomes: Disturbances of prenatal growth and development. Med Clin North Am 74:279, 1990.

32. Cosgrove M, et al: Nucleotide supplementation and the growth of term small for gestational age infants. Arch Dis Child 74:F122, 1996.

33. DeLia JE, et al: Fetoscopic neodymium:yag laser occlusion of placental vessels in severe twin-twin transfusion syndrome. Obstet Gynecol 75:1046, 1990.

34. Deter RL, et al: Neonatal growth assessment score: A new approach to the detection of intrauterine growth retardation in the newborn. Am J Obstet Gynecol 162:1030, 1990.

35. De Zegher F, et al: Early, discontinuous, high dose growth hormone treatment to normalize height and weight of short children born small for gestational age: Results over 6 years. J Clin Endocrin Metabol 84:1558, 1999.

36. DiGiacomo JE, et al: Placental-fetal glucose exchange and placental glucose consumption in pregnant sheep. Am J Physiol 258:E360, 1990.

37. Draper ES, et al: Prediction of survival for preterm births by weight and gestational age: Retrospective population-based study. BMJ 319:1093, 1999.

38. Edwards A, et al: Sexual origins of placental dysfunction. Lancet 355:203, 2000.

39. Ferguson S: Prolonged impairment of cellular immunity in children with intrauterine growth retardation. J Pediatr 93:52, 1978.

40. Fondacci C, et al: Alterations of human placental epidermal growth factor receptor in intrauterine growth retardation. J Clin Invest 93:1149, 1994.

41. Frazer T, et al: Direct measurement of gluconeogenesis from $[2,3^{13}C_2]$ alanine in the human neonate. Am J Physiol 240:615, 1981.

42. Gabriel R, et al: Alteration of epidermal growth factor receptor in placental membranes of smokers: Relationship with intrauterine growth retardation. Am J Obstet Gynecol 170:1238, 1994.

43. Gaziano EP, et al: Is it time to reassess the risk for the growth-retarded fetus with normal Doppler velocimetry of the umbilical artery? Am J Obstet Gynecol 170:1734, 1994.

44. Gazzolo D, et al: Predictors of perinatal outcome in intrauterine growth retardation: A long-term study. J Perinat Med 22:71, 1994.

45. Gomez L, et al: Leptin values in placental cord blood of human newborns with normal intrauterine growth after 30–42 weeks of gestation. Horm Res 51:10, 1999.

46. Hadlock F, et al: Estimation of fetal weight with the use of head, body, and femur measurements: A prospective study. Am J Obstet Gynecol 151:333, 1985.

47. Hakala-Ala-Pietilia TH, et al: Elevated second-trimester amniotic fluid concentration of insulin-like growth factor binding protein-1 in fetal growth retardation. Am J Obstet Gynecol 169:35, 1993.

48. Hanke W, et al: Heavy physical work during pregnancy: A risk factor for small-gestational-age babies in Poland. Am J Ind Med 36:200, 1999.

49. Hattersley AT, et al: The fetal insulin hypothesis: An alternative explanation of the association of low birthweight with diabetes and vascular disease. Lancet 353:1789, 1999.

50. Hattersley AT, et al: Mutations in the glucokinase gene of the fetus result in reduced birth weight. Nat Genet 19:268, 1998.

51. Hay WW, et al: Effects of glucose and insulin on fetal glucose oxidation and oxygen consumption. Am J Physiol 256:E704, 1989.

52. Haymond M, et al: Increased gluconeogenic substrates in the small for gestational age infant. N Engl J Med 291:322, 1974.

53. Hediger ML, et al: Growth and fatness at three to six years of age of children born small- or large-for-gestational-age. Pediatrics 104:E33, 1999.

54. Hediger ML, et al: Growth of infants and young children born small or large for gestational age. Arch Pediatr Adolesc Med 152:1225, 1998.

55. Hersh J, et al: Toluene embryopathy. J Pediatr 106:922, 1985.

56. Hickey CA, et al: Prenatal weight gain, term birth weight, and fetal growth retardation among high-risk multiparous black and white women. Obstet Gynecol 81:529, 1993.

57. Hitschold T, et al: Low target birth weight or growth retardation? Umbilical Doppler flow velocity waveforms and histometric analysis of fetoplacental vascular tree. Am J Obstet Gynecol 168:1260, 1993.

58. Hoff C, et al: Maternal-fetal ABO/Rh antigenic relationships and human fetal development. Am J Obstet Gynecol 154:126, 1986.

59. Holmes RP, et al: Maternal insulin-like growth factor binding protein-1, body mass index, and fetal growth. Arch Dis Child Fetal Neonatal Ed 82:F113, 2000.

60. Hooper SB, et al: Catecholamines stimulate the synthesis and

release of insulin-like growth factor binding protein-1 (IGFBP-1) by fetal sheep liver in vivo. Endocrinology 134:1104, 1994.

61. Hutton JL, et al: Differential effects of preterm birth and small gestational age on cognitive and motor development. Arch Dis Child 76:F75, 1997.

62. Iwamoto HS, et al: Effects of acute hypoxemia on insulin-like growth factors and their binding proteins in fetal sheep. Am J Physiol 263:E1151, 1992.

63. Iwata M, et al: Prenatal detection of ischemic changes in the placenta of the growth-retarded fetus by Doppler flow velocimetry of the maternal uterine artery. Obstet Gynecol 82:494, 1993.

64. Jacquet D, et al: Ontogeny of leptin in human fetuses and newborns: Effect of intrauterine growth retardation on serum leptin concentrations. J Clin Endocrin Metab 83:1243, 1998.

65. Jogee M, et al: Decreased prostacyclin production by placental cells in culture from pregnancies complicated by fetal growth retardation. Br J Obstet Gynaecol 90:247, 1983.

66. Jones JN, et al: Altered cord serum lipid levels associated with small for gestational age infants. Obstet Gynecol 93:527, 1999.

67. Karsdorp VHM, et al: Clinical significance of absent or reversed end-diastolic velocity waveforms in umbilical artery. Lancet 344:1664, 1994.

68. Keet M, et al: Follow-up study of physical growth of monozygous twins with discordant within-pair birth weights. Pediatrics 77:336, 1986.

69. King A, et al: Unexplained fetal growth retardation: What is the cause? Arch Dis Child 70:F225, 1994.

70. Kinnala A, et al: Differences in respiratory metabolism during treatment of hypoglycemia in infants of diabetic mothers and small-for-gestational-age infants. Am J Perinatol 15:363, 1998.

71. Klebanoff MA, et al: Second-generation consequences of small-for-dates birth. Pediatrics 84:343, 1989.

72. Kliegman RM: Alterations of fasting glucose and fat metabolism in intrauterine growth-retarded newborn dogs. Am J Physiol 256:E380, 1989.

73. Krew MA, et al: Relation of amniotic fluid C-peptide levels to neonatal body composition. Obstet Gynecol 84:96, 1994.

74. Kuzma J, et al: Maternal drinking behavior and decreased intrauterine growth: Alcoholism. Clin Exp Res 6:396, 1982.

75. Lamont D, et al: Risk of cardiovascular disease measured by carotid intima-media thickness at age 49–51: Lifecourse study. BMJ 320:273, 2000.

76. LeDune M: Response to glucagon in small for dates hypoglycemic and nonhypoglycemic newborn infants. Arch Dis Child 47:754, 1972.

77. Lee M, et al: Fetal microcirculation of abnormal human placenta: Scanning electron microscopy of placental vascular casts from small for gestational age fetus. Am J Obstet Gynecol 154:1133, 1986.

78. Leon DA: Twins and fetal programming of blood pressure. BMJ 319:1313, 1999.

79. Leturque A, et al: Fetal glucose utilization in response to maternal starvation and acute hyperketonemia. Am J Physiol 256:E699, 1989.

80. Lieberman E, et al: Low birthweight at term and the timing of fetal exposure to maternal smoking. Am J Public Health 84:1127, 1994.

81. Lucas A, et al: Fetal origins of adult disease: The hypothesis revisited. BMJ 319:245, 1999.

82. Lumey LH: Decreased birthweights in infants after maternal in utero exposure to the Dutch famine of 1944–1945. Paediatr Perinat Epidemiol 6:240, 1992.

83. Manning FA, et al: Fetal biophysical profile score VI: Correlation with antepartum umbilical venous fetal pH. Am J Obstet Gynecol 169: 755, 1993.

84. Marchini G, et al: Plasma leptin in infants: Relations to birth weight and weight loss. Pediatrics 101:429, 1998.

85. Massa G, et al: Serum growth hormone binding proteins in the human fetus and infant. Pediatr Res 32:69, 1992.

86. Mastrogiannis DS, et al: Perinatal outcome after recent cocaine usage. Obstet Gynecol 76:8, 1990.

87. Masuzaki H, et al: Nonadipose tissue production of leptin: Leptin as a novel placental-derived hormone in humans. Nature Med 3:1029, 1997.

88. Matsuda J, et al: Serum leptin concentration in cord blood: Relationship to birth weight and gender. J Clin Endocrin Metab 82:1642, 1997.

89. McCurdy CM, et al: Oligohydramnios: Problems and treatment. Semin Perinatol 17:183, 1993.

90. McDonnell M, et al: Neonatal outcome after pregnancy complicated by abnormal velocity waveforms in the umbilical artery. Arch Dis Child 70:F84, 1994.

91. McIntire DD, et al: Birth weight in relation to morbidity and mortality among newborn infants. N Engl J Med 340:1234, 1999.

92. Marconi AM, et al: Steady state maternal-fetal leucine enrichments in normal and intrauterine growth-restricted pregnancies. Pediatr Res 46:114, 1999.

93. Meberg A: Hematologic syndrome of growth-retarded infants. Am J Dis Child 143:1260, 1989.

94. Mehta P, et al: Thrombocytopenia in the high-risk infant. J Pediatr 97:791, 1980.

95. Milley J, et al: Metabolic requirements for fetal growth. Clin Perinatol 6:365, 1979.

96. Minton S, et al: Decreased bone mineral content in small for gestational age infants compared with appropriate for gestational age infants: Normal serum 25-hydroxyvitamin D and decreasing parathyroid hormone. Pediatrics 71:383, 1983.

97. Morrison L, et al: Weight-specific stillbirths and associated causes of death: An analysis of 765 stillbirths. Am J Obstet Gynecol 152:975, 1985.

98. Mortola JP, et al: Birth weight and altitude: A study in Peruvian communities. J Pediatr 136:324, 2000.

99. Niswander K, et al: Weight gain during pregnancy and prepregnancy weight. Obstet Gynecol 33:482, 1969.

100. Noordam MJ, et al: Doppler colour flow imaging of fetal intracerebral arteries and umbilical artery in the small for gestational age fetus. Br J Obstet Gynaecol 101:504, 1994.

101. Ott WJ: Intrauterine growth retardation and preterm delivery. Am J Obstet Gynecol 168:1710, 1993.

102. Ounsted M, et al: Maternal regulation of intrauterine growth. Nature 220:995, 1966.

103. Paton JB, et al: Placental transfer and fetal effects of maternal sodium β-hydroxybutyrate infusion in the baboon. Pediatr Res 25:435, 1989.

104. Pena IC, et al: The premature small-for-gestational-age infant during the first year of life: Comparison by birth weight and gestational age. J Pediatr 113:1066, 1988.

105. Perlman M, et al: Blood coagulation status of small for dates and postmature infants. Arch Dis Child 50:424, 1975.

106. Poulson P, et al: Low birth weight is associated with NIDDM in discordant monozygotic and dizygotic twin pairs. Diebetologia 40:439, 1997.

107. Prentice A, et al: Prenatal dietary supplementation of African women and birthweight. Lancet 1:489, 1983.

108. Reece EA, et al: The relation between human fetal growth and fetal blood levels of insulin-like growth factors I and II: Their binding proteins and receptors. Obstet Gynecol 84:88, 1994.

109. Robinson J, et al: Placental control of fetal growth. Reprod Fertil Dev 7:333, 1995.

110. Robson SC, et al: Ultrasonic estimation of fetal weight: Use of targeted formulas in small for gestational age fetuses. Obstet Gynecol 82:359, 1993.

111. Rodis JF, et al: Intrauterine fetal growth in concordant twin gestations. Am J Obstet Gynecol 162:1025, 1990.

112. Sabel K, et al: Interrelation between fatty acid oxidation and control of gluconeogenic substrates in small for gestational age (SGA) infants with hypoglycemia and with normoglycemia. Acta Paediatr Scand 71:53, 1982.

113. Salas SP, et al: Maternal plasma volume expansion and hormonal changes in women with idiopathic fetal growth retardation. Obstet Gynecol 81:1029, 1993.

114. Sanderson DA, et al: The individualised birthweight ratio: A new method of identifying intrauterine growth retardation. Br J Obstet Gynaecol 101:310, 1994.

115. Scholl TO, et al: Weight gain during pregnancy in adolescence: Predictive ability of early weight gain. Obstet Gynecol 75:948, 1990.

116. Seidler A, et al: Maternal occupational exposure to chemical

substances and the risk of infants small-for-gestational-age. Am J Ind Med 36:213, 1999.

117. Shelly H, et al: Neonatal hypoglycemia. Br Med Bull 22:34, 1966.

118. Shults RA, et al: Effects of short interpregnancy intervals on small-for-gestational age and preterm births. Epidemiology 10:250, 1999.

119. Sibai B, et al: Pregnancy outcome of intensive therapy in severe hypertension in first trimester. Obstet Gynecol 67:517, 1986.

120. Sinclair J: Heat production and thermoregulation in the small for date infant. Pediatr Clin North Am 17:147, 1970.

121. Smith GCS, et al: First-trimester growth and the risk of low birth weight. N Engl J Med 339:1817, 1998.

122. Snijders RJM, et al: Fetal growth retardation: Associated malformations and chromosomal abnormalities. Am J Obstet Gynecol 168:547, 1993.

123. Snijders RJM, et al: Fetal plasma erythropoietin concentration in severe growth retardation. Am J Obstet Gynecol 168:615, 1993.

124. Spiro RP, et al: Intrauterine growth retardation associated with maternal uniparental disomy for chromosome 6 unmasked by congenital adrenal hyperplasia. Pediatr Res 46:510, 1999.

125. Stein Z, et al: Prenatal nutrition and birth weight: Experiments and quasi-experiments in the past decade. J Reprod Med 21:287, 1978.

126. Strauss RS: Adult functional outcome of those born small for gestational age. JAMA 283:625, 2000.

127. Strauss RS, et al: Growth and development of term children born with low birth weight: Effects of genetic and environmental factors. J Pediatr 133:67, 1998.

128. Strong TH, et al: Prophylactic intrapartum amnioinfusion: A randomized clinical trial. Am J Obstet Gynecol 162:1370, 1990.

129. Sung I-K, et al: Growth and neurodevelopmental outcome of very low birth weight infants with intrauterine growth retardation: Comparison with control subjects matched by birth weight and gestational age. J Pediatr 123:618, 1993.

130. Tafari N, et al: Effects of maternal undernutrition and heavy physical work during pregnancy on birth weight. Br J Obstet Gynaecol 87:222, 1980.

131. Tamura T, et al: Serum leptin concentrations during pregnancy and their relationship to fetal growth. Obstet Gynecol 91:389, 1998.

132. Tsang R, et al: Studies in calcium metabolism in infants with intrauterine growth retardation. J Pediatr 86:936, 1975.

133. Uauy R, et al: Long chain polyunsaturated fatty acid forma-tion in neonates: Effect of gestational age in intrauterine growth. Pediatr Res 47:127, 2000.

134. Valcamonico A, et al: Absent end-diastolic velocity in umbilical artery: Risk of neonatal morbidity and brain damage. Am J Obstet Gynecol 170:796, 1994.

135. Van Splunder P, et al: Fetal atrioventricular, venous, and arterial flow velocity waveforms in the small for gestational age fetus. Pediatr Res 42:765, 1997.

136. Verhaeghe J, et al: C-peptide, insulin-like growth factors I and II and insulin-like growth factor binding protein-1 in umbilical cord serum: Correlations with birth weight. Am J Obstet Gynecol 169:89, 1993.

137. Verhaehge J, et al: IGF-I, IGF-II, IGF binding protein-1, and C-peptide in second trimester amniotic fluid are dependent on gestational age but do not predict weight as birth. Pediatr Res 46:101, 1999.

138. Verkerk PH, et al: Impaired prenatal and postnatal growth in Dutch patients with phenylketonuria. Arch Dis Child 71:114, 1994.

139. Villar J, et al: Heterogeneous growth and mental development of intrauterine growth-retarded infants during the first 3 years of life. Pediatrics 74:783, 1984.

140. Von Dadelszen P, et al: Fall in mean arterial pressure and fetal growth restriction in pregnancy hypertension: A meta-analysis. Lancet 355:87, 2000.

141. Wang X, et al: Familial aggregation of low birth weight among whites and blacks in the United States. N Engl J Med 333:1744, 1995.

142. Warshaw J: Intrauterine growth retardation: Adaptation or pathology? Pediatrics 76:998, 1985.

143. Waterland RA, et al: Potential mechanisms of metabolic imprinting that lead to chronic disease. Am J Clin Nutr 69:179, 1999.

144. Werner JC, et al: Palmitate oxidation by isolated working fetal and newborn pig hearts. Am J Physiol 256:E315, 1989.

145. Wilcox A, et al: Why small black infants have a lower mortality rate than small white infants: The case for population-specific standards for birth weight. J Pediatr 116:7, 1990.

146. Woods KA, et al: Intrauterine growth retardation and postnatal growth failure associated with deletion of the insulin-like growth factor I gene. N Engl J Med 335:1363, 1996.

147. Yogman MW, et al: Identification of intrauterine growth retardation among low birth weight preterm infants. J Pediatr 115:799, 1989.

148. Ziegler E, et al: Body composition of the reference fetus. Growth 40:329, 1976.

14 Hypertensive Disorders of Pregnancy

Dinesh M. Shah

Hypertensive disorders of pregnancy are one of the most serious complications in pregnancy because of their potential to cause serious maternal and perinatal morbidity and mortality. Although a substantial number of these patients have relatively good outcome, difficulty in differentiating among various hypertensive conditions, inability to predict which patients are at highest risk, and variability in the progression of preeclampsia make these disorders the greatest challenge of clinical medicine in obstetrics.

CLASSIFICATION

Various systems of classification of these disorders have been used. Some of the terminology, like pregnancy-induced hypertension, have misleading connotations about the underlying mechanism. This is a result of lack of clear understanding about the etiologic factors and lack of a gold standard diagnostic test. The classification originally prepared by the Committee on Terminology of the American College of Obstetrics and Gynecology[33] was revised by the National Institutes of Health Working Group on Hypertension in Pregnancy.[55] This revised classification proposes that hypertensive disorders of pregnancy be divided into four categories: (1) preeclampsia-eclampsia, (2) transient hypertension, (3) chronic hypertension, and (4) preeclampsia superimposed on chronic hypertension.

PREECLAMPSIA-ECLAMPSIA

Preeclampsia is new-onset hypertension with proteinuria with or without edema. Edema alone with hypertension is not reliable for diagnosis of preeclampsia because edema occurs frequently, even in normal pregnancy, and it is difficult to distinguish physiologic collection of fluid from pathologic edema. However, edema occurring in nondependent sites, rapidly increasing edema (as evidenced by rapid weight gain of more than or equal to 2.27 kg or 5 lb/week), or persisting facial edema after upright posture is assumed for several hours should be suspected as pathologic edema. Hypertension is defined as blood pressure greater than 140/90 mm Hg or mean arterial pressure (MAP) greater than 105 mm Hg. Proteinuria is defined as protein excretion of 30 mg/dL in a random specimen (equal to 1+ on urine strips) or 300 mg in a 24-hour urine specimen.

Eclampsia is the development of convulsions or coma or both in the clinical setting of preeclampsia.

TRANSIENT HYPERTENSION

Transient hypertension is hypertension as previously defined after the 20th week of pregnancy or during the first 24 hours postpartum without evidence of proteinuria or other signs of preeclampsia and in the absence of evidence of preexisting hypertension.

CHRONIC HYPERTENSION

Chronic hypertension is hypertension diagnosed before pregnancy or before the 20th week of pregnancy. Hypertension is defined as blood pressure greater than 140/90 mm Hg. This definition may overlook isolated systolic or diastolic hypertension. Some investigators have therefore suggested use of MAP greater than 105 mm Hg as the alternate diagnostic criterion. MAP is calculated as diastolic pressure plus one-third pulse pressure[63] (pulse pressure = systolic pressure minus diastolic pressure). Hypertension diagnosed any time during pregnancy but persisting beyond the 42nd postpartum day is also classified as chronic hypertension.

SUPERIMPOSED PREECLAMPSIA

Superimposed preeclampsia is either aggravation of hypertension or onset or increase in degree of proteinuria in a patient with a chronic hypertensive disorder. Aggravation of hypertension is an increase in systolic pressure by 30 mm Hg or diastolic pressure by 15 mm Hg.

COMMENTARY ON CLASSIFICATION

Increases of 30 mm Hg in systolic and of 15 mm Hg in diastolic blood pressure have been shown to be unreliable criteria for diagnosis of preeclampsia. The

263

majority of patients with an increase of this magnitude do not have a hypertensive disorder.[110]

One of the difficulties of diagnosing hypertension before the 20th week of gestation is that a patient's blood pressure is generally lower in the first half of pregnancy compared with the nonpregnant state. The lowering of blood pressure is a result of the vasorelaxant effect of gestation, thereby masking the diagnosis of hypertension in some patients before the 20th week of pregnancy. Patients with chronic hypertension have been shown to have a greater decline in their blood pressure than normal patients.[6, 93] Diagnosis of chronic hypertension as persisting after the 42nd postpartum day is useful only for classifying patients retrospectively, e.g., for grouping patients in a study, but not useful for clinicians in managing the index pregnancy.

PREECLAMPSIA-ECLAMPSIA

PATHOPHYSIOLOGY

One of the most fundamental abnormalities recognized in preeclampsia-eclampsia is uteroplacental ischemia.[45, 60] This is based on (1) histopathologic examination of placenta revealing ischemic lesions,[3] (2) study of the uterine vascular bed revealing vascular lesions called acute atherosis,[92, 117] (3) restriction of fetal growth secondary to reduced uteroplacental blood flow,[44, 62] and (4) radionuclide studies of uteroplacental perfusion demonstrating reduced clearance of radionuclide.[46, 49] Therefore, understanding the pathogenic mechanism requires understanding uterine vascular modeling in implantation and placentation and understanding the mechanisms of regulation of blood flow in the maternal uteroplacental vasculature.

Uterine Vascular Modeling

Terminal uterine vessels are known as spiral arteries. In the process of gestational development, under the influence of sex steroids, these vessels grow in length and to some degree in diameter.[30, 72] Trophoblastic invasion of these vessels occurs in the process of implantation and development of the placenta. Trophoblastic invasion results in complete replacement of endothelium by a layer of trophoblastic cells. Furthermore, the medial coat of the vessel, which consists of smooth muscle cells and connective tissue, is completely replaced by the invading trophoblasts.[66] At the end of this remodeling, the spiral artery is made of a thin adventitial layer internally lined by trophoblasts considerably dilated in diameter and is known as the uteroplacental vessel.[11]

It has been suggested that this trophoblastic invasion occurs in two phases. The first phase extends from the time of implantation until the 10th to 12th week of gestation[66]; invasive growth progresses to two-thirds depth in the decidua. The second phase extends from the 12th to the 16th to 18th week of gestation. The vessels are remodeled up to the termi-

nal resistance portion of the vessel into the myometrial layer. This results in a marked decrease in the resistance of the blood flowing into the uteroplacental vessels and thence into the intervillous space. Furthermore, as placentation progresses, trophoblastic invasion incorporates greater numbers of vessels, until an average of 100 decidual arteries are tapped for intervillous circulation.[11]

In patients who eventually develop preeclampsia, the second-phase trophoblastic invasion has been suggested to be deficient in the depth of the invasion[65, 92] but not limited to the placental bed site.[90] This deficiency allows greater numbers of decidual spiral arteries to maintain intact the resistance portion of the vessel with inadequate dilation of these vessels. More important, the contractile portion of these vessels remains intact. This has profound implications for the effect of vasomotor regulators of circulation.

Vasomotor Regulation of Uteroplacental Circulation

REGULATION OF UTERINE BLOOD FLOW. It is now well recognized that many organs have mechanisms for regional regulation of blood flow. The uterus is similar to the kidney in its embryologic origin, anatomic vascular arrangement, and mechanisms for regulation of blood flow. Like the kidney, uteroplacental circulation produces various vasodilators and vasoconstrictors including eicosanoids,[108] endothelin,[39] nitric oxide,[47] renin,[51, 86, 105] and angiotensinogen.[52, 86]

Various aberrations have been described to occur in these vasomotor regulators in preeclampsia. Prostaglandin production has been shown to be decreased in preeclampsia; however, such deficiency accounts for only a small degree of change in blood pressure[24, 28] (3 to 5 mm Hg). Thromboxane is considered a counter-regulatory vasoconstrictor eicosanoid to prostacyclin, and its production has been shown to be increased.[23] Viewing these two facts together, it has been suggested that the balance of eicosanoids is disturbed in preeclampsia.[24, 112] Some investigators have suggested that endothelin levels may be increased in preeclampsia.[107] Others have shown this not to be the case.[85]

In experimental gravid animal models, pharmacologic interventions to decrease nitric oxide production are associated with development of systemic hypertension.[119] However, nitric oxide production by measurements of urinary metabolite has been shown not to be deficient in human preeclampsia.[15]

ROLE OF THE RENIN-ANGIOTENSIN SYSTEM. The renin-angiotensin system has been suggested to be involved in the pathogenesis of preeclampsia.[103] The role of angiotensin II in the regulation of uterine blood flow directly or through alterations of eicosanoids has been suggested in experimental settings. Uterine venous angiotensin II levels have been shown to be higher in the hypertensive human pregnancy.[68] More important, systemic vasculature has been shown to become more responsive to angiotensin II in preeclampsia.[26] In view of evidence for uteroplacental ischemia and evidence for local renin and angiotensinogen production in the uterus, it is reasonable to assume that uterine vasculature is also modified to become more sensitive to angiotensin II in human preeclampsia. This vascular maladaptation, i.e., increased responsiveness to angiotensin II and development of hypertension, was first described by Goldblatt and recently confirmed in renin gene overexpression models with development of hypertension.[53] This emphasizes the role of renin in the evolution of vascular maladaptation. The change in the vasculature in renin-mediated hypertension is primarily driven by functional changes in the vasculature. Such functional changes in vasculature in renin-mediated hypertension are biochemically mediated by (1) alterations in the cyclooxygenase pathway of arachidonic acid metabolism and increased thromboxane production,[44a, 45a, 115] (2) protein kinase C–mediated mechanism and its effect on calcium handling by the vascular smooth muscle,[57, 58] (3) alterations in Na$^+$-K$^+$ pump and co-transport,[59] and (4) change in endothelin expression and release.[8] Initial change in vasculature in renin-mediated vasoconstriction appears to be mediated through increased sympathoadrenal activity. Many of these alterations have been described in human preeclampsia,[23, 24, 28] including increased sympathoadrenal activity.[83]

Takimoto and colleagues[106] reported the development of preeclampsia-eclampsia syndrome by crossbreeding transgenic mice, with the introduction of human renin (*REN*) and human angiotensinogen (*ANG*) in the mouse genome. Specifically, when male mice carrying human *REN* were mated with female mice carrying human *ANG*, preeclamptic syndrome developed, and REN overexpression was demonstrated on the fetal side of the placenta. One unique aspect of the mouse model of preeclampsia is that fetal renin from the placenta appeared to transfer to maternal circulation much more readily than that reported in humans.[42] In human preeclampsia, it has been demonstrated that renin gene expression is increased in the decidua vera on the maternal side.[88] Circulating levels of renin have been shown to peak earlier in women who develop superimposed preeclampsia, as compared with women with chronic hypertension who do not.[1] Increased renin production from the uterus has been shown to occur in response to decreased blood flow to the uterus in experimental settings.[118] Collectively, these data demonstrate a role of increased renin production in the uteroplacental interphase in the pathogenic mechanism of preeclampsia. Angiotensinogen mutation with increased angiotensin II production and susceptibility to development of preeclampsia has been shown in some populations but not in others.[113] Because other biochemical aberrations that mediate vascular maladaptation are renin-mediated, the proximate role for renin from uteroplacental interphase in initiating the pathogenesis of preeclampsia may be proposed (Fig. 14–1).

In addition to development of systemic hypertension, alterations in regional organ circulation occur in

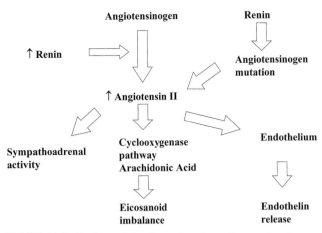

FIGURE 14–1. Renin-angiotensin system in pathogenesis of preeclampsia.

sites that are normally renin-angiotensin–dependent. This reduction in local blood flow may then explain the spectrum of clinical manifestations of preeclampsia.

VASOMOTOR IMPLICATIONS OF VASCULAR MODELING. The intactness of the resistance portion of the uteroplacental vessels with preserved ability for vasoconstriction should have profound implications for uteroplacental ischemia. These vessels should also become increasingly responsive to angiotensin II that is produced locally. Thus, the local renin-angiotensin system may initiate vasoconstriction-mediated ischemia and cellular injury in the uteroplacental vascular bed.

Pathophysiologic Basis of Clinical Manifestation

The renin-angiotensin system is involved in physiologic regulation of blood flow in various organs. These sites include the heart and systemic vasculature and the uterus, kidney, liver, and brain (Table 14–1). These are, therefore, also the sites for major clinical manifestations of preeclampsia-eclampsia, which emphasizes the role of *RAS* in the pathogenesis of this disorder. Clinical manifestations are described here according to the systemic or regional circulations involved. The primary mechanism at all sites is increased responsiveness to angiotensin II, leading to increased vascular resistance initially and vasoconstriction later with attendant hypoxemia and cellular damage. Furthermore, when vasoconstriction and hypoxemia occur, endothelial dysfunction sets in, and free radical formation and lipid peroxidation may further accelerate the process.[80] Endothelial dysfunction may occur earlier in individuals with susceptibility for such endothelial damage (e.g., thrombophilic conditions).[40] Other studies suggest such individuals may not be at an increased risk.[91]

CARDIOVASCULAR MANIFESTATIONS. Increased sympathoadrenal activity may mediate increases in car-

TABLE 14–1   FINDINGS AND CLINICAL MANIFESTATIONS OF PREECLAMPSIA

VASCULATURE OR SYSTEM	FINDINGS	CLINICAL MANIFESTATIONS
Cardiovascular	Increased cardiac output (CO) and systemic vasoconstriction	Systemic hypertension (HTN)
	Increased hydrostatic pressure	Generalized edema
	High CO and HTN	Intravascular hemolysis
Uteroplacental	Uteroplacental insufficiency	Fetal somatic growth deficiency; fetal hypoxemia and distress
	Decidual ischemia	Abruptio placentae; placental infarcts
	Decidual thrombosis	Thrombocytopenia
Renal	Decreased renal blood flow and glomerular filtration rate; endothelial damage	Proteinuria; elevated creatinine and decreased creatinine clearance; oliguria
	High AII responsiveness of tubular vasculature	Elevated uric acid
	All of the above	Renal tubular necrosis and renal failure
Cerebrovascular	Cerebral motor ischemia	Generalized grand mal seizures, i.e., eclampsia
	High cerebral perfusion pressure with regional ischemia	Cerebral hemorrhage
	Cerebral edema	Coma
	Regional ischemia	Central blindness; loss of speech
Hepatic	Ischemia→hepatic cellular injury	Elevated liver enzymes
	Mitochondrial injury	Intracellular fatty deposit
Hematologic	Intravascular hemolysis	Schistocyte burr cells; elevated free hemoglobin and iron; decreased haptoglobin levels
	Decidual thrombosis, release of FDP	Thrombocytopenia; antiplatelet antibodies

diac output. Increase in cardiac work demanded by increased cardiac output is generally well tolerated by young patients, but it may occasionally precipitate left ventricular failure. Decreased renal perfusion, high hydrostatic pressure due to the cardiovascular changes, and decrease in oncotic pressure due to proteinuria compounded by fluid overload may result in development of pulmonary edema.

Systemic vasculature is most frequently and fairly consistently involved with vasoconstriction, the primary manifestation being development of hypertension. Usually, both systolic and diastolic blood pressures are elevated, and hypertension has proportionality to renal manifestations, especially proteinuria, at least in uncomplicated cases. Hypertension to some degree depends on increased sympathoadrenal activity, which explains the fluctuations in blood pressure and accelerations related to anxiety.

High cardiac output, in the face of markedly increased peripheral vascular resistance, results in traumatic intravascular hemolysis. This may result in a decreased haptoglobin level, increased free hemoglobin level, increased bilirubin levels, burr cells and schistocytes in the peripheral blood, and an increased free serum iron level.

UTERINE VASCULATURE. Initially, the presence of high cardiac output and increased vascular resistance without change in vessel diameter results in increased uteroplacental perfusion.[18] Later, with a marked increase in local vasoconstriction, regional blood flow decreases.

Uteroplacental ischemia and placental infarcts are well-recognized pathologic findings of preeclampsia-eclampsia syndrome.[60, 61] Decreased uteroplacental blood flow explains increased frequency of somatic growth deficiency in this condition.[44, 116] (See also Chapter 13.) Severe reductions in uteroplacental blood flow may result in fetal hypoxemia, clinically manifested as fetal distress, hypoxemic multiorgan failure, or death. Uteroplacental interphase hypoxemia can also result in cellular injury to the decidua and injury to the vascular wall itself, with resultant small hemorrhages. These two processes—hypoxemic cell injury and hemorrhage—may result in small disruptions of placental attachment, which in turn may cause further disruption of the vascular wall as a result of mechanics of physical separation, resulting in bleeding in the uteroplacental interphase. This explains development of abruptio placentae. Uteroplacental interphase vessels normally have fibrin deposition, a process that can be aggravated by vasoconstriction, and further decreases in the blood flow in these vessels, explaining decidual thrombosis and initiation of thrombocytopenia with local platelet consumption.[75] Dissemination of small fibrin degradation products from these vessels and release of tissue thromboplastin from decidual and trophoblast cell injury may result in disseminated intravascular coagulopathy.[70]

RENAL VASCULATURE. Decreased renal blood flow and high renal perfusion pressure and associated hypoxemia may result in glomerular injury, in turn resulting in proteinuria. Glomerular injury may be associated with fibrin deposits in the basal layer and swelling of endothelial cells, resulting in glomerular endotheliosis seen in renal histology.[22] A severe decrease in renal blood flow may result in oliguria, and severe vasoconstriction and hypoxemia with cellular injury may explain renal tubular necrosis seen occasionally in preeclampsia. Decreased renal tubular blood flow (this vasculature is sensitive to angiotensin II) results in proximal tubular exchange of urate in favor of plasma, which explains frequent association of elevated serum uric acid as a manifestation of preeclampsia. Elevated uric acid is thus more accurately reflective of angiotensin II responsiveness,[19, 21] thereby explaining the ability of elevated uric acid to predict fetal death better than by systemic hypertension.[77]

Decreased glomerular filtration rate, combined with proteinuria-induced decrease in oncotic pressure and high hydrostatic pressure due to increased cardiac output, increased vascular resistance, and sodium and obligatory water retention (aldosterone effect), causes increased dependent and even generalized edema of preeclampsia.

Rare cases of diabetes insipidus of nephrogenic origin occur, and measurements of arginine vasopressin levels are generally normal, with placental aminopeptidase being responsible for rapid degradation of arginine vasopressin, resulting in functional deficit.

HEPATIC VASCULAR CHANGES. Angiotensin II responsiveness of hepatic vasculature is well recognized; it has been used for selective chemotherapy for tumors by angiotensin II infusion–induced vasoconstriction of normal vasculature to protect normal liver tissue. In later phases of disease, hepatic vasoconstriction-mediated hypoxemia and cellular injury are expected to result in release of hepatic enzymes into the circulation, with elevation of liver enzymes in blood.[38] Hepatic vasculature in the subcapsular region appears particularly susceptible to injury, resulting in small hemorrhages. In combination with disseminated intravascular coagulopathy, these hemorrhages may become larger and cause major subcapsular hematomas of the liver. Tissue injury with edema of liver parenchyma and capsule and stretching of the capsule may explain the hepatic origin of epigastric pain.

HELLP syndrome[114] is an acronym applied to preeclamptic women with a combination of intravascular hemolysis (H), elevated liver enzymes (EL), and thrombocytopenia or low platelets (LP).

Acute fatty liver of pregnancy (AFLP)[36, 52] is a condition with a predominantly hepatic manifestation frequently associated with thrombocytopenia and frequently occurring without cardiovascular manifestations of preeclampsia. Cellular hypoxemic injury explains mitochondrial damage, disruption of fatty acid metabolism, and deposition of microvesicular fat in hepatic cells. Susceptible individuals (those with a carrier state of deficiency of enzymes of fatty acid metabolism and short- and long-chain fatty acid dehydrogenase) may develop AFLP.[35, 109] AFLP occurs, in most cases, independent of preeclampsia. There appears to be some overlap in the pathophysiology of AFLP and preeclampsia with AFLP, with hepatic manifestations being predominant in individuals with such susceptibility. Mitochondrial enzyme defects may thus present as gene defects or be acquired through free radical–mediated cellular injury.

CENTRAL NERVOUS SYSTEM. High cardiac output and increased vascular resistance may be associated with greater regional circulation in the brain at higher perfusion pressure.[2] However, some regions of the brain, especially in advanced stages of the disease, may have locally decreased perfusion.

Vasoconstriction and hypoxemia in the microvasculature of the brain result in cellular injury with extracellular release of intracellular sodium, which provides the means for aberrant electrical impulse generation. The motor cortex appears to be particularly susceptible to such cellular injury, with resultant convulsions and eclampsia.[71] Vasoconstriction of different regions of the brain gives varied manifestations such as (1) frontal cortex: frontal headache, (2) occipital cortex: visual disturbances and central blindness, and (3) Broca's area: loss of speech. Blindness may also develop as a result of retinal detachment. Most patients who develop blindness recover completely without medical intervention. In cases of cerebral edema, coma and loss of recent memory of specific convulsive episodes occur.

Cerebrovascular accidents occur as a result of cerebral vasospasm, hypoxemia-induced vascular damage, and systolic hypertension causing mechanical rupture/disruption of vessel wall. Current data in developed countries suggest that almost 70% of hypertension-related maternal mortality is due to cerebrovascular accidents.[74]

Hyperreflexia has been recognized as a sign of neurologic irritability in epilepsy and is also seen prior to eclamptic seizures, but many women have normally active deep tendon reflexes without neurologic irritability.

CLINICAL CONSIDERATIONS

Predisposing Factors

There are several factors associated with or suggested to be associated with an increased risk of preeclampsia-eclampsia:

1. Parity: Both eclampsia and preeclampsia are recognized to occur more frequently in the first pregnancy.[7]
2. Age: Relationship is described as a J-shaped curve with slightly increased incidence in young primigravidae and a more pronounced increased incidence in older primigravidae.[7]
3. Race: Incidence of hypertension is not increased in African Americans, contrary to a commonly held belief, although a higher incidence of proteinuria is observed.[96]
4. Familial factors: In a study of women with eclampsia, their daughters had an incidence of preeclampsia of 26%; their sisters had an

incidence of 37%, and daughters-in-law had an incidence of 8%.[4]

5. Genetic: Genetic predisposition has been suspected on the basis of increased familial incidence,[4] suggesting a recessive trait possibly of maternal origin.

6. Diet: Most studies suggest that protein, carbohydrate, or total calorie intake does not influence the incidence of preeclampsia.

7. Social status: There have been several reports that suggest that lower socioeconomic populations have higher incidence of preeclampsia and severe preeclampsia.

8. Twin pregnancies: Twinning is associated with a higher incidence of preeclampsia compared with singleton gestation. Furthermore, severe preeclampsia occurs more frequently in monozygotic twinning, especially in multiparous women.

9. Diabetes: The incidence of preeclampsia is generally thought to be increased in diabetic pregnancies.[12, 81]

10. Hydatidiform mole: The higher incidence and early onset of preeclampsia are well recognized in molar gestation[61]; these features are also observed in triploidy gestations, which usually have partial mole.[100]

11. Hydrops fetalis: The incidence of preeclampsia appears to be increased only in nonimmune hydrops fetalis.[84]

12. Polyhydramnios: Increased incidence of preeclampsia observed in association with polyhydramnios is related to causes of polyhydramnios—multiple gestation, diabetes, and hydrops fetalis.[84]

13. Climate and season: Despite considerable interest and analysis, climatic and seasonal factors do not seem to contribute to the incidence of preeclampsia.

14. Cigarette smoking: The incidence of preeclampsia is lower in smokers compared with nonsmokers.[101] However, if preeclampsia does occur, fetal risks are greater in smokers compared with nonsmokers.

Differential Diagnosis

One of the most fundamental issues faced by clinicians is differentiation of a preexisting hypertensive disorder from the development of preeclampsia. This is because preeclampsia is a progressive disorder of increasing severity, which demands intervention in the form of delivery to halt the progression of the disease. This contrasts with preexisting hypertensive disorders, which exhibit stable manifestations, allowing clinicians to prolong gestation. This difference in clinical course of action has profound implications for prevention of interventional prematurity. Because preeclampsia is a progressive disease, observation of the patient may reveal progression of the disorder. However, this approach is fraught with the risk of the patient developing serious complications

of preeclampsia. Therefore, such an approach is valid when the severity of suspected "preeclampsia" is judged to be mild or moderate and gestational age is preterm enough to justify prolongation of gestation and postponement of delivery. This philosophy should maximize perinatal outcome within the bounds of maternal safety.[16, 89]

Preexisting essential hypertension should be suspected in the absence of proteinuria and other laboratory findings, especially if there is a family history of hypertension, and in the presence of maternal obesity. Corroborative information on "mild" elevations in blood pressure prior to pregnancy may be obtained by careful inquiry into all previous health care encounters by the patient, including visits for contraceptive advice.

Preexisting chronic hypertension secondary to renal disease may be readily diagnosed in cases with type I diabetes mellitus or known systemic lupus erythematosus. In other patients, preexisting renal disease should be suspected when proteinuria is in marked disproportion to the degree of hypertension, especially in multiparous patients[49] and whenever a patient presents with clinical manifestations of preeclampsia at preterm gestation. This is supported by renal biopsy data showing that 43% of multiparae presenting with preeclampsia had evidence of preexisting renal parenchymal/vascular disease.[22] It is further supported by follow-up data on patients presenting with preeclampsia prior to 34 weeks' gestation, of whom almost 70% had laboratory or renal biopsy evidence of preexisting renal disease.[34] Because most patients with chronic hypertension have essential hypertension, new-onset proteinuria in patients with essential hypertension makes the diagnosis of superimposed preeclampsia easier to make. However, this requires that an estimation of proteinuria be obtained earlier in pregnancy by quantitative laboratory analysis (e.g., from a 24-hour urine collection). In the presence of preexisting proteinuria in chronic hypertensive disorders of renal cause, a physiologic increase in proteinuria early in the third trimester is difficult to distinguish from pathologic proteinuria due to superimposed preeclampsia. Under these circumstances, development of other laboratory abnormalities, e.g., thrombocytopenia, may assist the diagnosis. Generally, proteinuria in the severe range—5 gm/24 hours or greater—should be regarded as superimposed preeclampsia in patients with preexisting proteinuria.

Development of convulsions or coma not related to a hypertensive disorder may occur as a result of neurologic causes; therefore, presence of hypertension, proteinuria, or edema provides corroborating background. In a small number of patients, the disease process may progress so rapidly that manifestation of convulsions might occur without or prior to development of proteinuria.

Variability in Progression of Preeclampsia

A characteristic of preeclampsia that is well recognized by clinicians is the variability in progression of

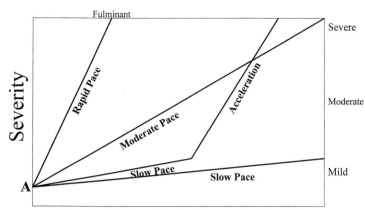

FIGURE 14–2. Four representative samples of rate of progression of the preeclamptic process, starting at point A and ending in mild, moderate, severe, or fulminant disease over a variable course of time.

the disease (Fig. 14–2). Therefore, it is necessary to establish an algorithm for each individual case in order to monitor progression.

Figure 14–2 graphically depicts various scenarios of the progression of preeclampsia, indicating that the clinician may encounter these patients at different stages of the disease process.

At point A, all patients may have similar degrees of severity, e.g., mild preeclampsia. If intervention in the form of delivery is not carried out because of prematurity, then the monitoring algorithm should initially consider the possibility of rapid progression. If rapid progression is not observed in 24 to 48 hours, then frequency of laboratory testing and monitoring of other parameters may be reduced in frequency until some clinical signs are detected that suggest acceleration of the disease process. Clinically, this may manifest as acceleration of hypertension or development of increasing facial edema along with glistening sheen described as toxemic facies. When such a change is observed clinically, additional testing of laboratory parameters may be necessary to reevaluate the patient.

Severity of Preeclampsia

Preeclampsia may be categorized for its severity, arbitrarily defined as mild or severe; in clinical settings it may also be reasonable to consider moderate severity. Severe preeclampsia is defined based on the following criteria[10]:

1. Systolic blood pressure greater than 160 mm Hg or diastolic blood pressure greater than 110 mm Hg.
2. Proteinuria of 5 gm or more per 24 hours (3+ or 4+ on urine dipping strip examination).
3. Oliguria defined as urine output of 500 mL or less in 24 hours.
4. Visual disturbances, i.e., scotomata (black spots or flashes).
5. Epigastric pain.
6. Cerebral symptoms, e.g., persistent frontal headache.
7. Pulmonary edema or cyanosis.

Mild preeclampsia should include hypertension, systolic blood pressure 140 to 150 mm Hg, diastolic blood pressure 90 to 100 mm Hg, and proteinuria 300 to 1000 mg per 24 hours (1+ on urine dip strip). Moderate preeclampsia may be defined as systolic blood pressure 150 to 160 mm Hg, diastolic blood pressure 100 to 110 mm Hg, and proteinuria more than 1 gm but less than 2.5 gm per 24 hours.

Principles of Management

The goals of management of women with preeclampsia-eclampsia include prevention of maternal morbidity and mortality and reduction of perinatal morbidity and mortality. Arrest of disease progression and recovery is most effectively achieved by delivery.[27] Many patients require hospitalization for evaluation and monitoring.[31]

Diagnostic parameters are standard hospitalization criteria, and they have contributed to prevention of eclampsia. Clinicians need to continue to pay close attention to the blood pressure profile because the mean duration from acceleration of hypertension to the time at which delivery is indicated is approximately 3 weeks.[89] Such acceleration of hypertension may herald the failure of uteroplacental circulation and activation of vasomotor mechanisms with progressive evolution of the disorder.

Assessment of fetal well-being by fetal heart rate monitoring, nonstress test, and ultrasonic biophysical profile is used for antepartum assessment. (See also Chapter 9.) Continuous electronic fetal heart rate monitoring of baseline rate, beat-to-beat variability, and presence of decelerations are used in the intrapartum period for detection of fetal distress. Fetal growth evaluation by ultrasound is indicated in antepartum inpatient monitoring of preeclampsia.

INDICATIONS FOR DELIVERY. The following are indications for delivery:

1. Preeclampsia of any severity at term.
2. Moderately severe preeclampsia near term, i.e., after 34 weeks' gestation.
3. Eclampsia at any gestational age.

4. Rapidly progressive preeclampsia with secondary system involvement, e.g., thrombocytopenia and elevated liver enzymes, at any gestational age.
5. Clinical unequivocal evidence of fetal compromise, e.g., persistent nonreactive nonstress test, poor biophysical profile score, or spontaneous repetitive deceleration in fetal heart rate monitoring, at any gestational age.
6. Established evidence of fetal pulmonary maturity.

INTRAPARTUM TREATMENT. *Antihypertensives*: As indicated previously, severe hypertension has serious cerebrovascular consequences in terms of parenchymal ischemia and hemorrhage. Decisive treatment of hypertension is generally indicated for hypertensive episodes. Blood pressure criteria used by the author are generally diastolic pressure of greater than 105 mm Hg or systolic pressure 160 mm Hg or greater. Sublingual nifedipine and an intravenous bolus of hydralazine as the primary antihypertensives are used. There is no evidence of inadvertent precipitation of angina and myocardial infarction with use of sublingual nifedipine in this generally healthy young population. However, caution is indicated in use of nifedipine for older mothers (age 40 and over), when there is a family history of coronary artery disease at young age, and especially in women who are heavy smokers. Labetalol and clonidine have also been used for the same purpose (Table 14–2).

Corticosteroids: There is evidence to support that glucocorticoids may be used safely in patients with preeclampsia for accelerating fetal pulmonary maturation.[79]

METHOD OF DELIVERY. Cesarean section is best reserved for specific obstetric clinical indications. Availability of cervical ripening agents containing prostaglandins makes the success of vaginal delivery more feasible. Vaginal delivery following induction of labor remains the mainstay method for patients with preeclampsia and most cases of eclampsia because induction of labor in patients with preeclampsia may be easier than predicted by cervical findings.[120]

SEIZURE PROPHYLAXIS AND TREATMENT OF ECLAMPSIA. Magnesium sulfate infusion for prevention of seizures is routinely recommended by most authorities in the United States. This is partly because the signs and symptoms of preeclampsia are not reliable predictors of eclampsia.[99] The secondary reason for this approach is the fact that magnesium sulfate infusion is remarkably safe prophylaxis.[69, 71] Several other agents have been used in the past for seizure prophylaxis, including phenytoin. However, an international randomized trial now supports use of magnesium sulfate as the agent of choice over phenytoin for such prophylaxis.[14]

Magnesium sulfate is well recognized as the treatment for prevention of further seizures in patients presenting with eclampsia.[69] Magnesium sulfate can be safely used even in patients on nifedipine (a calcium channel blocker), because there is no evidence of adverse consequences and there is no sound theoretical basis for avoiding such a combination.

The most commonly used regimen of magnesium sulfate is intravenous infusion[121] given as a 2- to 4-gm bolus over 5 to 30 minutes followed by continuous infusion starting at 1 gm/hr and increasing up to 2 gm/hr to maintain therapeutic levels of 4 to 6 mEq/L. Use of intramuscular injection of magnesium sulfate has fallen out of favor because of pain associated with the injections and lack of precision in maintaining therapeutic levels. Close supervision of the patient's deep tendon reflexes and urine output measurements is important.

Neonatal serum magnesium concentrations are very similar to those of the mother.[71] Stone and Pritchard[102] reported that Apgar scores do not correlate with magnesium levels. Clinical observations by neonatologists suggest higher frequency of neonatal hypotonia and decreased intestinal motility in infants exposed to magnesium sulfate. (See also Chapter 47, Part Two.)

Prevention of Preeclampsia

Until all aspects of the pathogenic mechanisms are well defined, prevention of preeclampsia remains an

---

TABLE 14–2 PHARMACOTHERAPY FOR MATERNAL HYPERTENSIVE EMERGENCIES

DRUG	INITIAL DOSE	REPEAT DOSES	COMMENTS/PRECAUTIONS
Hydralazine (bolus)	5 mg IV bolus; response time 10–15 minutes	5–10 mg every 20–30 minutes	If no response with total dose of 20 mg, consider alternatives.
Hydralazine (infusion)	40 mg in 500 mL D5/LR; begin at 15–25 mL/hour	Begin at 1 mL/min, titrate against blood pressure	
Nifedipine	10 mg sublingual, response time 10 minutes with maximum effect at 30 minutes	10 mg in 30 minutes	If no response after 20 mg, consider alternatives; avoid in elderly or with family history of coronary disease, especially if smokers.
Clonidine	0.1 mg PO	0.1 mg in 30 minutes, then 0.1 mg every hour	Patient must be placed on equivalent maintenance dose tid.
Labetalol	20-mg IV bolus, response time 5–10 minutes	20-mg dose or begin infusion of 1–2 mg/min	Check cardiac functional suppression.

unrealized goal. Studies of aspirin and calcium supplementation have not supported their use in either low-risk or high-risk populations.[43, 95] To some extent, this may be a result of the heterogeneity of the disorder.[56]

Outcome in Preeclampsia-Eclampsia

PERINATAL OUTCOME. Perinatal mortality is increased in women with preeclampsia-eclampsia.[54, 99] Fortunately, the fetal death rate has decreased in recent times,[20, 62] but perinatal morbidity due to clinically indicated interventional prematurity continues to be a major problem.[89] Major causes of perinatal morbidity and mortality are uteroplacental insufficiency, abruptio placentae,[54, 63] and interventional prematurity.[89] Fetal death rate correlates with clinical parameters that reflect the disease process. The fetal death rate has been shown to increase with increases in both hypertension and degree of proteinuria[25] and also with high uric acid levels.[77]

Perinatal morbidity is primarily a result of the need for delivery. Despite the fact that prematurity remains the single most important threat to the infants of hypertensive mothers, analysis suggests that these infants may have better outcomes than preterm infants delivered spontaneously.[87] Recent improvements in perinatal mortality appear to be due to reduction in fetal but predominantly neonatal death rates.

MATERNAL MORTALITY AND MORBIDITY. Maternal mortality is still a major risk from hypertensive disorders.[37, 41] Marked improvements in maternal morbidity and mortality have occurred in recent times. These improvements are attributable to improvements in medical care (e.g., blood transfusion, prevention of aspiration), in methods of stabilization (e.g., reduced use of sedation) of eclamptic and severe preeclamptic patients, and expedited delivery after stabilization. Maternal mortality rates close to zero have been achieved.[99] In areas of the world where good medical care is readily available, cerebrovascular accidents remain the single most common reason for maternal mortality, accounting for 60% to 70% of all deaths due to hypertensive disorders.[74] Therefore, future decrease in maternal mortality and morbidity rates in hypertensive disorders in developed parts of the world will come from assertive and decisive treatment of severe hypertension.

REMOTE PROGNOSIS. Long-term follow-up studies of eclampsia by Chesley and coworkers[5] revealed that in women with hypertension in the first pregnancy, 33% had a hypertensive disorder in any subsequent pregnancy, and 5% had a recurrence of eclampsia. Multiparous women with eclampsia had recurrence of hypertension in 50% of subsequent pregnancies.[5] Sibai and associates[97] reported a 45% recurrence of preeclampsia in women with severe preeclampsia, and they also showed that risk of such recurrence is higher in women who develop preeclampsia in the late second or early third trimester.[98] McGillvry[50]

showed that of the women with preeclampsia in their first pregnancy, 15% to 25% developed a hypertensive disorder in subsequent pregnancies. Renal biopsy data from the University of Chicago suggest that approximately 22% of primigravidae with preeclampsia have an underlying renal disorder.[22] Collectively, these data suggest that 15% to 45% of primigravid women who develop preeclampsia, severe preeclampsia, or eclampsia have essential hypertension or renal parenchymal disease, or both, as the primary cause.

Some investigators have suggested an increased risk of developing hypertension later in life in women who develop preeclampsia in their first pregnancy.[17] However, these studies are better explained as having erroneously included chronic hypertensive disorders in the patients being studied. Long-term follow-up studies of preeclampsia-eclampsia in first pregnancy by Chesley and coworkers[5] suggest there was no increase in the rate of hypertension. However, multiparous women do exhibit excess rates of hypertension and cardiovascular mortality, which are best explained by underlying hypertensive disorders.

OTHER HYPERTENSIVE DISORDERS

TRANSIENT HYPERTENSION

This transient disorder, previously referred to as gestational hypertension, typically occurs in the third trimester. Recurrence of nonproteinuric hypertension of this type in 15% to 25% of the patients with hypertensive disorders suggests an underlying hypertensive disorder, especially if there is a family history of essential hypertension. Under such circumstances, and in the absence of signs and symptoms of preeclampsia, antihypertensive treatment should be considered.[64] In the author's experience, such antihypertensive therapy reduces the need for hospitalization and makes outpatient monitoring and management easier. Patients managed as outpatients benefit from ambulatory blood pressure monitoring. Antihypertensive treatment is similar to that for patients with chronic hypertension. Acceleration of hypertension or need for progressively increasing antihypertensive therapy may indicate development of "superimposed preeclampsia" or misdiagnosis of the preeclamptic patient as having transient hypertension. Careful evaluation of signs and symptoms of preeclampsia before beginning antihypertensive therapy can minimize such difficulties. Patients with severe hypertension without evidence of preeclampsia may have severe hypertension due to cocaine abuse.[111] All patients with severe hypertension manifesting in an episodic manner should have a toxicology urine screen test performed for accurate diagnosis and appropriate treatment of hypertension and substance abuse.

CHRONIC HYPERTENSION

Chronic hypertension in pregnancy is hypertension (i.e., blood pressure greater than 140/90 mm Hg) diagnosed before the 20th week of gestation or hypertension before pregnancy. Overt hypertension is easily diagnosed, although latent hypertension does not become manifest until later in pregnancy. Latent hypertension is frequently diagnosed as transient hypertension as described previously.

Classification

A. Primary hypertension: essential or idiopathic—most common type observed.
B. Secondary hypertension (secondary to a known cause):
   1. Renal: parenchymal (glomerulonephritis, chronic pyelonephritis, interstitial nephritis, polycystic kidney) and renal vascular in origin. Renal parenchymal disease is the second most common cause of chronic hypertension, other causes being rare.
   2. Adrenal gland
      a. Cortical: Cushing syndrome and hyperaldosteronism.
      b. Medullary: pheochromocytoma.
   3. Other: coarctation of aorta and thyrotoxicosis.
C. Chronic hypertensive disease with superimposed preeclampsia.

A patient should be considered to be at risk of chronic hypertensive disease of pregnancy in the presence of one or more of the following:

1. A diastolic blood pressure in a nonpregnant state or before the 20th week of gestation that consistently exceeds 80 mm Hg.
2. A history of hypertension.
3. A history of secondary causes of hypertension (e.g., renal disease).
4. A family history of hypertension.
5. Hypertension in a previous pregnancy.
6. Hypertension with oral contraceptives.

Evaluation of the Pregnant Hypertensive Patient

1. A complete physical examination, including a funduscopic examination for severe hypertension.[13]
2. Evaluation of heart size if long-standing or significant hypertension is a factor.
3. Auscultation over the renal arteries to rule out a bruit consistent with renovascular hypertension; however, a bruit is rarely first detected by obstetricians.
4. Simultaneous palpation of the femoral and radial arteries to rule out coarctation of the aorta, again rarely first detected by obstetricians.

Screening Laboratory Data

A complete urinalysis for protein and for microscopic sediment should be done to diagnose renal disease. A 24-hour urinalysis for protein and determination of creatinine clearance should be performed to assess renal function. Serum electrolyte levels to rule out primary hyperaldosteronism may be sent only if the diagnosis is not obviously essential hypertension or renal disease.

If blood pressure elevation is episodic and reaches systolic pressures of 180 mm Hg and diastolic pressures above 110 mm Hg, measurement of urinary catecholamines to rule out pheochromocytoma should be done. These cases should also have a toxicology screen.[111]

Ultrasonography of the kidneys may be considered when clinically relevant (e.g., chronic pyelonephritis) to assess renal size and pelvic dilation if the patient did not have a diagnostic study before pregnancy. Electrocardiography and an echocardiogram may be considered depending on the severity of the hypertension.

Preconception Counseling

If possible, counseling should be provided before conception to the woman who has chronic hypertension. This is important in order to establish adequate control of hypertension and to make changes in the antihypertensive regimen. It is important to establish baseline data and to teach self-monitoring of blood pressure. If the patient is taking diuretic medication, she should be advised that she should discontinue use of this medication before conception. An appropriate diet that curtails heavy salt use is recommended. Patients on angiotensin-converting enzyme inhibitors should be advised to discontinue them because of serious risks of fetal defects and pregnancy loss.

Management During Pregnancy

Bed rest is suggested to increase uterine blood flow and promote nutrition to the fetus.[104] Uterine size and compression of the inferior vena cava and aorta are factors that alter blood pressure recordings in the supine position in the third trimester of gestation. The currently recommended position for outpatient blood pressure measurement, as advocated by the American Heart Association, is the sitting position. The brachial artery blood pressure is highest when sitting, lower when lying on the back, and lowest when lying on the side.

HOME BLOOD PRESSURE MONITORING. All patients with chronic hypertension benefit from self-monitoring of blood pressure. Not only do self-monitored blood pressure readings tend to be lower, but they also reflect patients' blood pressure readings in their environment more accurately. The author advises taking blood pressure measurements at least three times a day. If the patient works outside the home, blood pressures should be taken both during the workweek and weekend. This identifies the effects of the environment on blood pressure. Newer digital blood pressure monitors are easy to use and moderately inexpensive. For these reasons it is time to abandon the use of stethoscope for self-monitoring. It is important to check calibration of the patient's machine in the office. Self-monitoring reduces antihypertensive use and need for hospitalization.[73]

OTHER CONSIDERATIONS. Therapeutic abortion is generally not necessary or recommended, but the decision regarding whether to continue the pregnancy should be determined on an individual basis. It is essential to establish the estimated date of confinement. History, early pelvic examination, and early ultrasonography aid in this process. Ultrasonography is needed (at 3- to 6-week intervals from 24 to 28, 28 to 32, and 32 to 36 weeks) during pregnancy to detect intrauterine growth restriction, which is most likely to develop after the 30th week of gestation.

PHARMACOTHERAPY. There is no current proof that pharmacotherapy (Table 14–3) alters fetal salvage or prevents preeclampsia, but it controls major accelerations of maternal blood pressure during pregnancy. This may reduce the risk of complication of severe hypertension, especially of cerebrovascular accidents. Antihypertensive medication should be started when home diastolic blood pressure consistently exceeds 84 mm Hg or office blood pressure readings consistently exceed 90 mm Hg. The current drug of choice is methyldopa (Aldomet).[76] During the past decade, beta blockers such as propranolol or atenolol have been used.[82] However, these agents increase the risk of intrauterine growth retardation and may increase fetal morbidity. Alternative drugs now available include calcium channel blockers,[9] clonidine, and labetalol.[32, 93] All drugs may cross the placenta; however, these drugs have not been shown to cause any birth defects, except angiotensin-converting enzyme inhibitors.[29, 67] One should avoid using two antihypertensives of the same class whenever a patient needs more than one agent to control the hypertension. This is most likely to occur for agents acting on the adrenergic system; for example, avoid combining methyldopa with labetalol. It is better to use a vasodilator such as nifedipine as a second agent.

COMPLICATIONS. Chronic hypertension is associated with a fourfold to eightfold increase in the incidence of abruptio placentae. Planned delivery at or near term may be advisable. The patient should be observed for preeclampsia as indicated by an increase in blood pressure and development of proteinuria. The patient should be hospitalized if preeclampsia is suspected.

ANTEPARTUM FETAL EVALUATION

1. Serial ultrasound to diagnose intrauterine growth retardation.
2. Nonstress tests twice a week from 32 weeks of gestation.
3. Fetal movement activity count from 32 weeks; at least 4 movements per hour or 3 movements in 30 minutes, indicating fetal health.

LABOR AND DELIVERY. If a decision is made to proceed to delivery and the cervix is not favorable for induction of labor, vaginal administration of prostaglandin may be used. Continuous electronic fetal monitoring should be performed during labor. Regional analgesia with epidural administration is ideal, as is also the case for patients with preeclampsia. It is recommended that a pediatrician be available for evaluation of the newborn.

In summary, women who have chronic hypertension usually do well during pregnancy, although 5% to 10% have major catastrophic events. It is recommended that patients with chronic hypertension may take oral contraceptives postpartum; a barrier form of contraception is an alternative. For women who have completed their childbearing, a permanent form of contraception may be desirable.

SUPERIMPOSED PREECLAMPSIA-ECLAMPSIA

As previously described, this is a condition that supervenes on a preexisting hypertensive disorder of whatever cause. Clinically, this is the most severe form of disease; it is associated with the most severe degree of hypertension and proteinuria. When a diagnosis of superimposed preeclampsia is made, it generally indicates need for expedited delivery. Establishment of baseline data on renal and other functions during the prenatal course is helpful for comparison. Usually, liver function abnormality would indicate superimposed preeclampsia; however, association of

TABLE 14–3 COMMON ANTIHYPERTENSIVE AGENTS FOR CHRONIC HYPERTENSION IN PREGNANCY

AGENT	MECHANISM OF ACTION	DOSE
Methyldopa	Centrally acting alpha agonist	250 mg bid–500 mg qid
Clonidine	Centrally acting alpha agonist	0.1–0.6 mg tid, rarely exceeding 0.4 mg tid
Nifedipine (long acting) XL	Calcium channel blocker	30 mg XL qd to 60 mg XL bid; maximum dose 120 mg/day
Norvasc	Calcium channel blocker	5–10 mg qd
Labetalol	Beta blocker	Starting dose 100 mg bid; usual dose 200–400 mg bid; maximum dose 1600–2400 mg

methyldopa with elevation of liver enzymes without development of superimposed preeclampsia is known to occur. When such a diagnosis is entertained, hospitalization is essential for evaluation, close supervision, monitoring, and delivery.

■ REFERENCES

1. August P, et al: Longitudinal study of the renin-angiotensin-aldosterone system in hypertensive pregnant women: Deviations related to the development of superimposed preeclampsia. Am J Obstet Gynecol 163:1612, 1990.
2. Belfort MA, et al: Preeclampsia may cause both overperfusion and underperfusion of the brain: A cerebral perfusion based model. Acta Obstet Gynecol Scand 78:586, 1999.
3. Brosens I, Renaer M: On the pathogenesis of placental infarcts in pre-eclampsia. J Obstet Gynaecol Br 79:794, 1972.
4. Chesley LC, et al: The familial factor in toxaemia of pregnancy. Obstet Gynecol 32:303, 1968.
5. Chesley LC, et al: The remote prognosis of eclamptic women. Am J Obstet Gynecol 124:446, 1976.
6. Chesley LC, Annitto JE: Pregnancy in patients with hypertensive disease. Am J Obstet Gynecol 53:372, 1947.
7. Christianson RE: Studies on blood pressure during pregnancy. Am J Obstet Gynecol 125:509, 1976.
8. Chua BH, et al: Regulation of endothelin-1 mRNA by angiotensin II in rat heart endothelial cells. Biochem Biophys Acta 117:201, 1993.
9. Constantine G, et al: Nifedipine as a second line antihypertensive drug in pregnancy. Br J Obstet Gynaecol 94:1136, 1987.
10. Cunningham FG, Lindheimer MD: Hypertension in pregnancy. N Engl J Med 326:927, 1992.
11. DeWolf FD, et al: Ultrastructure of the spiral arteries in the human placental bed at the end of normal pregnancy. Am J Obstet Gynecol 117:833, 1973.
12. Diamond MP, et al: Complication of insulin-dependent diabetic pregnancies by preeclampsia and/or chronic hypertension: Analysis of outcome. Am J Perinatol 2:263, 1985.
13. Dimmitt SB, et al: Usefulness of ophthalmoscopy in mild to moderate hypertension. Lancet 20:1103, 1989.
14. Duley L, et al: Which anticonvulsant for women with eclampsia? Evidence from the collaborative eclampsia trial. Lancet 345:1455, 1995.
15. Egerman RS, et al: Neuropeptide Y and nitrite levels in pre-eclamptic and normotensive gravid women. Am J Obstet Gynecol 181:921, 1999.
16. Entman SS, Shah DM: Conservative therapy of toxemia of pregnancy: Standard, innovative and experimental approaches. Perinatol Neonatol 9:58, 1985.
17. Epstein FH: Late vascular effects of toxemia of pregnancy. N Engl J Med 271:391, 1964.
18. Everett RB, et al: Relationship of maternal placental blood flow to the placental clearance of maternal plasma dehydroisoandrosterone sulfate through placental estradiol formation. Am J Obstet Gynecol 136:435, 1980.
19. Fadel HE, et al: Hyperuricemia in pre-eclampsia. Am J Obstet Gynecol 125:640,1975.
20. Ferranzzani S, et al: Proteinuria and outcome of 444 pregnancies complicated by hypertension. Am J Obstet Gynecol 162:366, 1990.
21. Ferris TF, Gorden P: Effect of angiotensin and norepinephrine upon urate clearance in man. Am J Med 44:359, 1968.
22. Fisher KA, et al: Hypertension in pregnancy: Clinical-pathological correlations and remote prognosis. Medicine 60:267, 1981.
23. Fitzgerald DJ, et al: Thromboxane A_2 synthesis in pregnancy-induced hypertension. Lancet 335:751, 1990.
24. Fitzgerald DJ, FitzGerald GA: Eicosanoids in the pathogenesis of preeclampsia. In Laragh JH, Brenner BM (eds): Hypertension: Pathophysiology, Diagnosis and Management, vol. 2. New York, Raven Press, 1990, p 1789.
25. Friedman EA, Neff RK: Pregnancy outcome as related to hypertension, edema and proteinuria. In Lindheimer MD, Katz AI, Zuspan FP (eds): Hypertension in Pregnancy. New York, Wiley, 1976, p 13.
26. Gant NF, et al: A study of angiotensin II pressor response throughout primigravid pregnancy. J Clin Invest 51:2682, 1973.
27. Gilstrap LC, et al: Management of pregnancy-induced hypertension in the nulliparous patient remote from term. Semin Perinatol 2:73, 1978.
28. Goodman RP, et al: Prostacyclin production during pregnancy: Comparison of production during normal pregnancy and pregnancy complicated by hypertension. Am J Obstet Gynecol 142:817, 1982.
29. Hanssens M, et al: Fetal and neonatal effects of treatment with angiotensin-converting enzyme inhibitors in pregnancy. Obstet Gynecol 78:128, 1991.
30. Harris JWS, Ramsey EM: The morphology of human uteroplacental vasculature. Contrib Embryol 38:43, 1966.
31. Hauth JC, et al: Management of pregnancy-induced hypertension in the nullipara. Obstet Gynecol 48:253, 1976.
32. Horvath JS, et al: Clonidine hydrochloride: A safe and effective antihypertensive agent in pregnancy. Obstet Gynecol 66:634, 1985.
33. Huges EC (ed): Obstetric-Gynecologic Terminology. Philadelphia, FA Davis, 1972.
34. Ihle BU, et al: Early onset pre-eclampsia: Recognition of underlying renal disease. Br Med J 294:79, 1987.
35. Ibdah JA, et al: A fetal fatty-acid oxidation disorder as a cause of liver disease in pregnant women. N Engl J Med 340:1723, 1999.
36. Kaplan MM: Acute fatty liver of pregnancy. N Engl J Med 313:367, 1985.
37. Kaunitz AM, et al: Causes of maternal mortality in the United States. Obstet Gynecol 65(5):605, 1985.
38. Killam AP, et al: Pregnancy-induced hypertension complicated by acute liver disease and disseminated intravascular coagulation: Five case reports. Am J Obstet Gynecol 123:823, 1975.
39. Kubota T, et al: Synthesis and release of endothelin-1 by human decidual cells. J Clin Endocrinol Metab 75:1230, 1992.
40. Kupferminc MJ: Increased frequency of genetic thrombophilia in women with complications of pregnancy. N Engl J Med 340:9, 1999.
41. Lawson HW, et al: Maternal mortality related to preeclampsia and eclampsia in the United States 1979–1986. Morbid Mortal Wkly Rep CDC Surveill Summ 40:1, 1991.
42. Lentz T, et al: Prorenin secretion from human placenta perfused in vitro. Am J Physiol 260:E876, 1991.
43. Levine RJ, et al: Trial of calcium to prevent preeclampsia. N Engl J Med 337:69, 1997.
44. Lin CC, et al: Fetal outcome in hypertensive disorders of pregnancy. Am J Obstet Gynecol 142:255, 1982.
44a. Lin L, et al: The role of prostanoids in renin-dependent and renin-independent hypertension. Hypertension 17:517, 1991.
45. Lindheimer MK, Katz AI: Pathophysiology of preeclampsia. Annu Rev Med 32:273, 1981.
45a. Luft FC, et al: Angiotensin-induced hypertension in the rat: Sympathetic nerve activity and prostaglandins. Hypertension 14:396, 1989.
46. Lunell NO, et al: Uteroplacental blood flow in pregnancy-induced hypertension. Scand J Clin Lab Invest 169:28, 1984.
47. Matsumoto M, et al: Endothelium-derived relaxation of the pregnant and nonpregnant canine uterine artery. J Reprod Med 37:529, 1992.
48. McCartney CP, et al: Renal structure and function in pregnant patients with acute hypertension. Am J Obstet Gynecol 90:579, 1964.
49. McClure Browne JC, et al: The maternal placental blood flow in normotensive and hypertensive women. J Obstet Gynaecol 60:141, 1953.
50. McGillvry I: Some observations on the incidence of pre-eclampsia. J Obstet Gynecol 65:536, 1958.
51. Morgan T, et al: Human spiral artery renin-angiotensin system. Hypertension 32:683, 1998.
52. Muise KJ, Shah DM: Acute fatty liver of pregnancy: Etiology of fetal distress and fetal wastage. Obstet Gynecol 69:482, 1987.

53. Mullins JJ, et al: Fulminant hypertension in transgenic rats harbouring the mouse Ren-2 gene. Nature 344:541, 1990.

54. Naeye RL, Friedman EA: Causes of perinatal death associated with gestational hypertension and proteinuria. Am J Obstet Gynecol 133:8, 1979.

55. National High Blood Pressure Education Program Working Group: Report on high blood pressure during pregnancy. Am J Obstet Gynecol 163:1689, 1990.

56. Ness RB, Roberts JM: Heterogeneous causes constituting the single syndrome of preeclampsia: A hypothesis and its implications, Am J Obstet Gynecol 175:1365, 1996.

57. Ochsner M, et al: Protein kinase C inhibitors potentiate angiotensin II–induced phosphionositide hydrolysis and intracellular Ca2+ mobilization in renal mesangial cells. Eur J Pharmacol 245:15, 1993.

58. O'Donnell ME: Endothelial cell sodium-potassium-chloride co-transport: Evidence of regulation by Ca2+ and protein kinase C. J Biol Chem 266:11559, 1991.

59. Orlov SN, et al: Na(+)-K(+) pump and Na(+)-K(+) co-transport in cultured vascular smooth muscle cells from spontaneously hypertensive and normotensive rats: Baseline activity and regulation. J Hypertens 10:733, 1992.

60. Page EW: On the pathogenesis of pre-eclampsia and eclampsia [review]. J Obstet Gynaecol Br Commonw 79:883, 1972.

61. Page EW: The relation between hydatid moles, relative ischaemia of the gravid uterus and the placental origin of eclampsia. Am J Obstet Gynecol 37:291, 1939.

62. Page EW, Christianson R: Influence of blood pressure changes with and without proteinuria upon outcome of pregnancy. Am J Obstet Gynecol 126:821, 1976.

63. Page EW, Christianson R: The impact of mean arterial pressure in the middle trimester upon the outcome of pregnancy. Am J Obstet Gynecol 125:740, 1976.

64. Pickles CJ, et al: The fetal outcome in a randomized double-blind controlled trial of labetalol versus placebo in pregnancy-induced hypertension. Br J Obstet Gynaecol 96:38, 1989.

65. Pijnenborg R, et al: Placental bed spiral arteries in the hypertensive disorders of pregnancy. Br J Obstet Gynaecol 98:648, 1991.

66. Pijnenborg R, et al: Trophoblastic invasion of human decidua from 8 to 18 weeks of pregnancy. Placenta 1:3, 1980.

67. Piper JM, et al: Pregnancy outcome following exposure to angiotensin-converting enzyme inhibitors. Obstet Gynecol 80:429, 1992.

68. Pipkin FB, et al: The uteroplacental renin-angiotensin system in normal and hypertensive pregnancy. Contrib Nephrol 25:49, 1981.

69. Pritchard JA: The use of the magnesium ion in the management of eclamptogenic toxemias. Surgery Gynecol Obstet 100:13, 1955.

70. Pritchard JA, et al: Coagulation changes in eclampsia: Their frequency and pathogenesis. Am J Obstet Gynecol 124:855, 1976.

71. Pritchard JA, Pritchard SA: Standardized treatment of 154 consecutive cases of eclampsia. Am J Obstet Gynecol 123:543, 1975.

72. Ramsey EM, Harris JWS: Comparison of uteroplacental vasculature and circulation in the rhesus monkey and man. Contrib Embryol 381:59, 1966.

73. Rayburn WF: Self blood pressure monitoring during pregnancy. Am J Obstet Gynecol 148:159, 1984.

74. Redman CWG: The treatment of hypertension in pregnancy. Kidney Int 18:267, 1980.

75. Redman CWG, et al: Early platelet consumption in preeclampsia. Br Med J 1:467, 1978.

76. Redman CWG, et al: Fetal outcome in trial of antihypertensive treatment in pregnancy. Lancet 2:753, 1976.

77. Redman CWG, et al: Plasma-urate measurements in predicting fetal death in hypertensive pregnancy. Lancet 1:1370, 1976.

78. Redman CWG, et al: Treatment of hypertension in pregnancy with methyldopa: Blood pressure control and side effects. Br J Obstet Gynaecol 84:419, 1977.

79. Ricke PS, et al: Use of corticosteroids in pregnancy-induced hypertension. Obstet Gynecol 48:163, 1976.

80. Roberts JM, et al: Clinical and biochemical evidence of endothelial cell dysfunction in pregnancy syndrome preeclampsia. Am J Hypertens 4:700, 1991.

81. Roberts JM, Perloff DL: Hypertension and the obstetrician-gynecologist. Am J Obstet Gynecol 127:316, 1977.

82. Rubin PC, et al: Placebo-controlled trial of atenolol in treatment of pregnancy-associated hypertension. Lancet 1:431, 1983.

83. Schobel HP, et al: Preeclampsia: A state of sympathetic overactivity. N Engl J Med 335:1480, 1996.

84. Scott JS: Pregnancy toxaemia associated with hydrops fetalis, hydatidiform mole and hydramnios. J Obstet Gynaecol 65:689, 1958.

85. Shah DM, et al: Circulating endothelin-1 is not increased in severe preeclampsia. J Matern Fetal Med 1:177, 1992.

86. Shah DM, et al: Definitive molecular evidence of RAS in human uterine decidual cells. Hypertension 36:159, 2000.

87. Shah DM, et al: Neonatal outcome of premature infants of mothers with preeclampsia. J Perinatol 15:264, 1995.

88. Shah DM, et al: Reproductive tissue renin gene expression in preeclampsia. Hypertens Pregnancy 19:341, 2000.

89. Shah DM, Reed G: Parameters associated with adverse perinatal outcome in hypertensive pregnancies. J Hum Hypertens 10:511, 1996.

90. Shanklin DR, Sibai BM: Ultrastructural aspects of preeclampsia. Am J Obstet Gynecol 161:735, 1989.

91. O'Shaughnessy KM, et al: Factor V Leiden and thermolabile methylenetetrahydrofolate reductase gene variants in an East Anglian preeclampsia cohort. Hypertension 33:1338, 1999.

92. Sheppard BL, Bonnar J: An ultrastructural study of uteroplacental spiral arteries in hypertensive and normotensive pregnancy and fetal growth retardation. Br J Obstet Gynaecol 88:695, 1981.

93. Sibai BM, et al: A comparison of no medication versus methyldopa or labetalol in chronic hypertension during pregnancy. Am J Obstet Gynecol 162:960, 1990.

94. Sibai BM, et al: Pregnancy outcome in 303 cases with severe preeclampsia. Obstet Gynecol 64:319, 1984.

95. Sibai BM, et al: Prevention of preeclampsia with low-dose aspirin in healthy, nulliparous pregnant women. N Engl J Med 329:1213, 1993.

96. Sibai BM, et al: Risk factors for preeclampsia in healthy nulliparous women: A prospective multicenter study. Am J Obstet Gynecol 172:642, 1995.

97. Sibai BM, et al: Severe preeclampsia-eclampsia in young primigravid women: Subsequent pregnancy outcome and remote prognosis. Am J Obstet Gynecol 155:1011, 1986.

98. Sibai BM, et al: Severe preeclampsia in the second trimester: Recurrence risk and long-term prognosis. Am J Obstet Gynecol 165:1408, 1991.

99. Sibai BM, et al: The incidence of nonpreventable eclampsia. Am J Obstet Gynecol 154(3):581, 1986.

100. Sorem KA, Shah DM: Advanced triploid pregnancy and preeclampsia. South Med J 88:1144, 1995.

101. Spinillo A, et al: Cigarette smoking in pregnancy and risk of pre-eclampsia. J Hum Hypertens 8:771, 1994.

102. Stone SR, Pritchard JA: Effect of maternally administered magnesium sulfate on the neonate. Obstet Gynecol 35:574, 1970.

103. Symonds EM: Aetiology of preeclampsia: A review. J R Soc Med 73:871, 1980.

104. Symonds EM: Bed rest in pregnancy. Br J Obstet Gynaecol 89:593, 1982.

105. Symonds EM: Renin and reproduction. Am J Obstet Gynecol 158:754, 1988.

106. Takimoto E, et al: Hypertension induced in pregnant mice by placental renin and maternal angiotensinogen. Science 274:995, 1996.

107. Taylor RN, et al: Women with preeclampsia have higher plasma endothelin levels than women with normal pregnancies. J Clin Endocrinol Metab 71:1675, 1990.

108. Terragno NA, et al: Prostaglandins and the regulation of uterine blood flow in pregnancy. Nature 249:57, 1974.

109. Treem WR, et al: Acute fatty liver of pregnancy and long-chain 3-hydroxyacyl-coenzyme A dehydrogenase deficiency. Hepatology 19:339, 1994.

110. Villar MA, Sibai BM: Clinical significance of elevated mean arterial blood pressure in second trimester and threshold increase in systolic or diastolic blood pressure during third trimester. Am J Obstet Gynecol 160:419, 1989.

111. Volpe JJ: Effect of cocaine use on the fetus. N Engl J Med 327:399, 1992.

112. Walsh SW: Preeclampsia: An imbalance in placental prostacyclin and thromboxane production. Am J Obstet Gynecol 152:335, 1985.

113. Ward K, et al: A molecular variant of angiotensinogen associated with preeclampsia. Nat Genet 4:59, 1993.

114. Weinstein L: Syndrome of haemolysis, elevated liver enzymes, and low platelet count: A severe consequence of hypertension in pregnancy. Am J Obstet Gynecol 142:159, 1982.

115. Wilcox CS, et al: Thromboxane mediates renal hemodynamic response in infused angiotensin II. Kidney Int 40:1090, 1991.

116. Wildschut HIJ, et al: The effect of hypertension on fetal growth. Hypertens Pregnancy 2:437, 1983.

117. Wolf FD, et al: The ultrastructure of acute atherosis in hypertensive pregnancy. Am J Obstet Gynecol 123:164, 1975.

118. Woods LL: Role of renin-angiotensin system in hypertension during reduced uteroplacental perfusion pressure. Am J Physiol 257:204, 1989.

119. Yallampalli C, Garfield RE: Inhibition of nitric oxide synthesis in rats during pregnancy produces signs similar to those of preeclampsia. Am J Obstet Gynecol 169:1327, 1993.

120. Zuspan FP: Factors affecting delivery in preeclampsia: Condition of the cervix and uterine activity. Am J Obstet Gynecol 100:672, 1968.

121. Zuspan FP: Problems encountered in the treatment of pregnancy-induced hypertension: A point of view. Am J Obstet Gynecol 131:591, 1978.

15 Pregnancy Complicated by Diabetes Mellitus

Carol Andrea Lindsay

Diabetes mellitus is a group of metabolic diseases, all having hyperglycemia in common, that result from defects in insulin secretion, insulin action, or both.[29] Diabetes mellitus is classified in one of three ways: type I (insulin-dependent diabetes), type II (non–insulin-dependent diabetes), or gestational diabetes mellitus. Diabetes mellitus in pregnancy is further subdivided according to the classification of Priscilla White (Table 15–1). She reported that the prognosis for pregnancy is related to (1) control of maternal diabetes, (2) occurrence of congenital fetal defects, (3) degree of maternal vascular disease, (4) gestational age at delivery, (5) duration of diabetes, (6) age of onset of diabetes, and (7) balance of the sex hormones of pregnancy.[98]

Gestational diabetes mellitus is defined as carbohydrate intolerance of variable severity with onset or first recognition during pregnancy.[64] Of the 3% to 5% of pregnancies complicated by diabetes mellitus, 80% to 90% are gestational diabetes.[15, 16, 29] Risk factors for the development of gestational diabetes mellitus include age older than 25 years; obesity defined as pregravid body mass index (BMI) greater than 27.3 kg/m^2; family history of diabetes mellitus; persistent glucosuria; and history of prior pregnancies complicated by macrosomia, congenital malformation, or stillbirth.[45] Other risk factors include sedentary lifestyle, prior gestational diabetes, hypertension, or dyslipidemia.[29] Ethnicity also plays a role in the risk of development of diabetes mellitus, with people of color having a higher incidence.[45] However, more than 50% of all patients who exhibit abnormal glucose tolerance lack the risk factors mentioned.[54]

PATHOPHYSIOLOGY

The pathophysiology of diabetes mellitus is complex, with hyperglycemia being a common manifestation. Type I diabetes mellitus primarily represents insulin deficiency that results in chronic hyperglycemia and disturbances of protein and lipid metabolism.[35] People with type I diabetes require insulin for survival, and in the absence of insulin, they are at risk of developing diabetic ketoacidosis.[14] They are also at increased risk of developing microvascular and macrovascular complications.[29]

Type II diabetes mellitus results from an imbalance between insulin sensitivity and B cell function. This type of diabetes mellitus has an insidious onset and generally is seen in older and more obese patients,[14] although there is an alarming increase of incidence in obese adolescents. Decreased insulin sensitivity is manifested as increased hepatic glucose production and decreased peripheral use of glucose. In both type II diabetes and gestational diabetes there is decreased hepatic and peripheral insulin sensitivity and relatively decreased insulin response for the degree of hyperglycemia.[14]

B cell function is represented by insulin production.[14] The B cell response is abnormal, that is, there is an inadequate insulin response for a given degree of glycemia[23, 70]; however, because of the decrease in insulin sensitivity, insulin response may actually be greater than in women with normal glucose toler-

TABLE 15–1 MODIFIED WHITE'S CLASSIFICATION OF DIABETES MELLITUS IN PREGNANCY*

CLASS	DESCRIPTION
A1	Onset during pregnancy, treated with diet only
A2	Onset during pregnancy, requiring insulin therapy
B	Onset at ≥ 20 years old, < 10 years' duration
C	Onset 10–19 years old, 10–19 years' duration
D	Onset < 10 years old, ≥ 20 years' duration or background retinopathy
F	Any duration or age of onset with the presence of nephropathy
H	Any duration or age of onset with the presence of atherosclerotic heart disease
R	Any duration or age of onset with the presence of proliferative retinopathy
T	Any duration or age of onset with the presence of a renal transplant

*If a patient falls into two or more classes, she is assigned to the most severe class.

Adapted from White P: Pregnancy complicating diabetes. Am J Med 7:609, 1949, with permission from Excerpta Medica Inc.

ance.[14] As a consequence, women with type II diabetes may have normal or increased insulin levels.[29]

In women with normal glucose tolerance in pregnancy, more endogenous insulin is required to maintain normal glucose tolerance.[63] As a result, plasma insulin levels are greater in these women than in weight-matched nonpregnant women.[63] This extra insulin compensates for the 60% reduction in the response of the peripheral tissue to insulin.[63] In lean women, maternal metabolism is adapted to allow for increased maternal fat stores early in pregnancy and increased availability of carbohydrate and protein to the fetus in late pregnancy when increased fetal growth occurs.[14]

Gestational diabetes is characterized by a 60% decrease in peripheral insulin sensitivity and the inability of the pancreas to produce adequate insulin in response to a glucose load.[1] Several hormones produced by the placenta have antagonistic effects on insulin, leading to this decrease in insulin sensitivity.[1] These hormones may include human placental lactogen (human chorionic somatomammotropin) and progesterone,[1] although definitive proof is lacking and mechanisms are poorly understood. As a consequence of decreased insulin sensitivity, levels of plasma glucose, free fatty acids, branched chain amino acids, and ketone bodies are elevated.[1]

SIGNS AND SYMPTOMS

Many women with gestational diabetes and type II diabetes are asymptomatic; however, any signs and symptoms of hyperglycemia should be evaluated, including fatigue, polyuria, polydipsia, weight loss, polyphagia, and blurred vision.[29] In the first trimester, women with type I diabetes may experience periods of hypoglycemia.[54] In the presence of infection, these women are at increased risk for developing ketoacidosis.

DIAGNOSIS

Screening based on risk factors has recently been advocated by the American Diabetes Association.[29] Screening should be performed between 24 and 28 weeks of gestation. Some advocate earlier screening in women with significant risk factors. Factors that increase a woman's risk for gestational diabetes include age older than 25 years, obesity, having a first-degree relative with diabetes mellitus, being a member of an ethnic group at high risk (Hispanic, American Indian, Asian, African American), history of abnormal glucose metabolism, history of poor obstetric outcome, history of previous gestational diabetes mellitus, and concomitant glucocorticoid therapy.[29, 54, 62]

Screening is generally performed with a 50-gm, 1-hour oral glucose tolerance test. The cutoff for which further testing is indicated ranges from 130 to 140 mg/dL. At a cutoff of 140 mg/dL, the false negative rate is approximately 10%.[30] The sensitivity at this level is 75%, with 6% to 15% of the tests being abnormal.[1, 10, 14] Lowering the cutoff to 130 mg/dL enhances sensitivity but impairs specificity.[54] At 130 mg/dL the sensitivity increases to nearly 100%, but 15% to 25% of the population must undergo a diagnostic test as a result of an abnormal value.[10, 14]

An abnormal screening test is followed by a 100-gm, 3-hour oral glucose tolerance test. The criterion for diagnosis of gestational diabetes is at least two abnormal values on the 3-hour glucose tolerance test. This criterion was initially set forth by O'Sullivan and Mahan.[76] Abnormal values were set to reflect the risk for the woman subsequently developing glucose intolerance after delivery, not based on perinatal outcome. Abnormal values were defined as two or more values greater than 2 standard deviations above the mean.[76] In 1979, the National Diabetes Data Group revised the O'Sullivan criterion, which was based on whole blood to reflect plasma values.[73] Carpenter and Coustan further refined the National Diabetes Data Group criteria to reflect the glucose oxidase methods by which plasma glucose is currently obtained, rather than the former Smogyi method.[11, 73] These criteria are fasting blood glucose of 95 mg/dL or less, 1-hour blood glucose of 180 mg/dL or less, 2-hour blood glucose of 155 mg/dL or less, and 3-hour blood glucose of 140 mg/dL or less, with either a 75-gm or 100-gm glucose load. These criteria have been recommended by the American Diabetes Association and the 4th International Workshop Conference on Gestational Diabetes.[31, 62]

Glycosylated hemoglobin, although not useful for diagnosis, is useful for managing patients with type I or type II diabetes. Higher levels indicate poorer glycemic control. It should be noted that in pregnancy, erythropoiesis is increased, leading to younger red blood cells, which cause the red blood cells of pregnant women to be less glycated than those in nonpregnant women.[10]

Women who have one abnormal value on the oral glucose tolerance test are also at increased risk for fetal macrosomia.[55] Repeat testing at 32 to 34 weeks has been recommended in this group because 33% of these women will have a positive test at that time.[74]

Women who are diagnosed with gestational diabetes should undergo testing for glucose intolerance in the postpartum period because of their increased risk of developing diabetes mellitus.[76] The diabetes that occurs following gestational diabetes is primarily type II diabetes, but in 3% to 5% of these patients, type I diabetes is diagnosed; this is important because women with type II diabetes are at increased risk for the development of hyperlipidemia and increased risk of cardiovascular disease.[62] Fifty to sixty percent of women with prior gestational diabetes develop type II diabetes during their lifetime.[51] Diabetes mellitus in nonpregnant individuals is defined as a glucose level of 126 mg/dL or greater after an 8- to 14-hour fast or as a 2-hour postprandial glucose of 200 mg/dL or greater after a 75-gm oral glucose tolerance test.[31, 62, 86] The diagnosis should be confirmed on two separate occasions.[29] The diagnosis can also be made in the symptomatic patient with a random plasma glucose concentration greater than 200 mg/dL.[29]

Impaired glucose tolerance is diagnosed when the fasting plasma glucose level is 110 mg/dL or greater but less than 126 mg/dL or when the 2-hour value is 140 to 199 mg/dL. Impaired glucose tolerance is not a clinical diagnosis but rather a risk factor for future development of diabetes and cardiovascular disease.[29, 31] Finally, if the fasting plasma glucose is less than 110 mg/dL and the 2-hour value is less than 140 mg/dL, glucose tolerance is normal, but frequent testing is recommended.[31]

MANAGEMENT OF DIABETES MELLITUS IN PREGNANCY

Glucose control is the mainstay of the management of diabetes in pregnancy, whether the diabetes is pregestational or gestational. Women can monitor their own blood glucose, with the goal being maintenance of glucose levels between 60 and 120 mg/dL.[54] Recommended regimens for glucose evaluation for women with gestational diabetes mellitus vary widely from weekly office visits to eight daily checks. Euglycemia can be achieved with self-monitoring of blood glucose (SMBG).[42] In general, SMBG is thought to be superior to monitoring that is less frequent.[14, 35, 62, 85] One of the most frequently used protocols involves fasting blood sugar, which is checked before each meal, 2 hours after each meal, and at bedtime.[77] If nocturnal hypoglycemia is suspected, an additional capillary glucose level test at 3:00 AM can be added.[77]

Target levels of glucose in pregnancy are as follows: fasting, before meals and bedtime snack, 60 to 95 mg/dL; 1 hour after meals, 130 to 140 mg/dL; 2 hours after meals, 120 mg/dL or less; and 2:00 AM to 6:00 AM, 60 to 90 mg/dL.[14, 37, 54, 63, 77] When the mean plasma glucose values are maintained below 100 mg/dL during pregnancy, perinatal mortality is reduced to that of a control population with normal glucose tolerance.[21, 43] Maintaining euglycemia may also improve the rates of several fetal or neonatal complications such as macrosomia, hyperbilirubinemia, hypocalcemia, respiratory distress syndrome, and intrauterine fetal demise (see Chapter 47, Part One).[36, 54] A reduction in maternal complications may also be seen, for example, in the reduced need for cesarean delivery.[85]

In addition to SMBG, daily urine tests for ketones are advocated.[27] Ketonuria may be a result of accelerated fat catabolism.[62] Ketonuria has been associated with lower IQ scores than expected in the offspring of pregnancies complicated by diabetes.[17] Checking the first voided urine sample can determine if the patient has an adequate caloric intake and is taking adequate insulin.[14] Ketonuria can also be a sign that a woman with type I diabetes mellitus is developing diabetic ketoacidosis.

The amount of weight gain recommended in pregnancy is based on prepregnancy weight. In obese

patients, defined as BMI greater than 29 kg/m², a weight gain of approximately 7 kg is recommended during pregnancy[37]; in lean patients, with BMI less than 19.8 kg/m², a weight gain of up to 18 kg is recommended.[62] For women with a normal BMI that is between 19.8 and 26 kg/m², weight gain ranging from 11 to 16 kg is recommeded.[46] Most women with gestational diabetes are 50% to 70% overweight.[57] Caloric requirements are weight based. Obese patients can be managed on diets consisting of as few as 1600 kcal per day as long as ketonuria does not develop.[54] Women with normal weight require from 2200 to 2400 kcal per day[14]; approximately 30 to 35 kcal/kg ideal body weight is recommended.[16] The amount of calories is similar to that required by the pregnant woman with normal glucose tolerance and may be less[1]; however, attention must be paid to the composition and distribution. It is recommended that the patient eat three meals and one to three snacks each day.[54, 77] This approach requires consumption of 10% to 15% of calories at breakfast, up to 10% as a midmorning snack, 20% to 30% at lunch, up to 10% as a midafternoon snack, 30% to 40% at dinner, and up to 10% as a bedtime snack.[41] The composition of the diet is as follows: 50% to 60% complex carbohydrates, 12% to 20% protein, 20% to 30% fat.[4, 14, 16, 54, 63]

Exercise can be used as an adjunct to diet in the management of gestational diabetes. Regular aerobic exercise has been shown to lower fasting and postprandial glucose concentrations.[62] Non–weight-bearing exercise has shown similar results.[9] In some cases, exercise may prevent the need for insulin therapy in those women whose diabetes cannot be controlled by diet alone.[39]

If target glucose levels are not attained on a consistent basis, insulin may be required. Patients undergoing frequent SMBG are more likely to require insulin; however, there was a significant reduction in adverse pregnancy outcomes.[36] Insulin requirements may decrease between 10 and 16 weeks of gestation in women with pregestational diabetes.[97] In patients with type I diabetes, the dose of insulin required to maintain euglycemia frequently doubles by the third trimester.[77] After 36 weeks, however, insulin dose requirements may be reduced.[60]

The major maternal complication of insulin therapy is hypoglycemia. Maternal hypoglycemia most frequently occurs in the context of a missed meal, decreased carbohydrate content of meal, or increased physical activity.[3] Occasionally, in the woman with pregestational diabetes, the continuous subcutaneous insulin infusion pump is used. However, this method has never been demonstrated to be superior to multiple insulin injections for maintaining euglycemia.[22] The type of insulin therapy should be individualized based on a particular patient's needs. In general, oral hypoglycemic agents are not used during pregnancy because they may produce fetal hyperinsulinemia[1, 14] and neonatal hypoglycemia.

Antepartum testing is important in order to decrease the risk of intrauterine fetal demise and neonatal mortality, especially in patients with fasting and postprandial hyperglycemia.[5] There are four main components to antenatal testing: laboratory evaluation, ultrasound, fetal movement counts, and fetal heart rate testing. (See Chapter 9.)

Women with diabetes are at a 10-fold increased risk for neural tube defects. These women should be offered maternal serum α-fetoprotein screening at 16 to 18 weeks' gestation, followed by a detailed ultrasound examination.[54] Maternal serum α-fetoprotein levels are affected by maternal race and weight and are lower in pregnancies complicated by diabetes,[14] and the risk for neural tube defects in these women is elevated.

Ultrasound is useful for management of pregnancies complicated by diabetes. Because women with pregestational diabetes have an increased risk of congenital anomalies, level II ultrasound at 18 to 20 weeks' gestation can be used to detect fetal malformation. Echocardiography is usually performed at 20 to 22 weeks' gestation because there is a fivefold increase in the risk of cardiac malformations in the fetuses of women with diabetes mellitus.[54] In addition, in the third trimester, ultrasound can be used to estimate fetal weight and to detect polyhydramnios.[54] Women with diabetes are at risk for fetal growth disturbances, so serial ultrasound testing in the third trimester at 4- to 6-week intervals should be considered.[54] The mother should also monitor the activity of her fetus, starting at approximately 28 weeks' gestation, by counting fetal movements.

There is fairly universal agreement that women with pregestational diabetes and gestational diabetes requiring insulin should have antenatal testing. Whether women with uncomplicated gestational diabetes managed with diet alone require antenatal testing remains controversial. There are no prospective trials evaluating the appropriate use of antenatal testing in the woman with uncomplicated gestational diabetes. Antenatal testing or fetal heart rate monitoring commonly consists of nonstress testing. In women with pregestational diabetes or gestational diabetes requiring insulin twice weekly, nonstress testing is begun at 32 to 34 weeks of gestation, earlier if in the presence of vascular disease, poor diabetes control, hypertension, previous intrauterine fetal demise, or other pregnancy complications.[6, 54, 66, 77, 87] At 40 weeks, nonstress testing is considered in women with gestational diabetes managed on diet alone.[77] Some investigators recommend only the use of fetal movement assessment by the mother in the woman with well-controlled gestational diabetes, that is, in the absence of hypertension, adverse obstetric history, or other risk factors.[21] The rationale for this approach is that abnormal results are unusual in this group of women.[21] Other investigators recommend weekly nonstress testing beginning at 36 weeks.[1, 14]

The appropriate timing of delivery for the woman with gestational diabetes has not been clearly established. In the past, women with diabetes delivered between 35 and 36 weeks of gestation, but the current recommendation is to delay elective delivery until term, when lung maturity can be ensured. When considering the timing of delivery, one must be aware of certain goals in the management of the woman with diabetes. The main goal of management is to prevent fetal demise or fetal compromise, such as from a traumatic birth from the macrosomic fetus at the time of delivery, while ensuring fetal lung maturity.[34] The woman with uncomplicated gestational diabetes need not deliver before 40 weeks unless there is a specific maternal or fetal indication.[90] This approach gives women a better chance to enter labor spontaneously, resulting in a smaller number of inductions of labor and, consequently, fewer cesarean deliveries for failed induction.[27] This approach is especially successful if strict control of diabetes is maintained, which results in greater rates of spontaneous labor.[27]

After 38 weeks, delivery is considered if the patient has poor glycemic control, poor compliance, a fetus with macrosomia, vasculopathy, or history of prior fetal demise.[19] Early delivery reduced the rate of macrosomia, the incidence of traumatic births, and cesarean deliveries in the woman with gestational diabetes.[34]

Determination of lung maturity with lecithin-to-sphingomyelin ratios can be used when dates are uncertain or early delivery is considered. Before 38 or 39 weeks' gestation, an amniocentesis should be considered to document lung maturity.[54] The presence of phosphatidylglycerol is the marker for pulmonary maturation. Although its presence may be delayed in women with diabetes,[54] it is a reliable predictor of lung maturity. In the presence of a positive phosphatidylglycerol result, the risk of respiratory distress syndrome is 1%. Expectant management beyond 38 weeks increases the incidence of infants who are large for gestational age; however, if the cervix is unfavorable for delivery, expectant management may be considered.[77]

In general, vaginal delivery is advocated in the woman with diabetes in the absence of other obstetric indications for cesarean section. The cesarean delivery rate remains high in women with diabetes, however, ranging from 20% to 60%.[54] Elective cesarean delivery is advocated for the woman with diabetes who has a fetus with an estimated fetal weight greater than 4000 to 4500 gm.[34]

POSTPARTUM MANAGEMENT

Breast feeding should be encouraged in women with diabetes mellitus; it results in increased high-density lipoprotein and decreased blood glucose levels.[49] In addition, no adverse metabolic effects of breast feeding have been found.[1] Breast feeding also is associated with a lower long-term risk of obesity and diabetes in the offspring.[62]

At the postpartum visit, follow-up testing for overt diabetes is recommended in all women with gestational diabetes. Testing should be performed yearly thereafter because these women are at high risk for the subsequent development of diabetes. The risk of subsequent development of diabetes is determined by the severity of glucose intolerance during pregnancy; that is, diabetes mellitus develops in 29% of women who required insulin but in only 7% of women managed on diet alone.[50] Of those patients with abnormal glucose tolerance postpartum, 78% require insulin during pregnancy, whereas of patients with normal postpartum glucose tolerance, 40% require insulin during gestation.[16] Other predictors of abnormal glucose tolerance postpartum include gestational age at diagnosis of gestational diabetes and fasting glucose level at the time of the antepartum oral glucose tolerance test.[16] Increased maternal age and hyperglycemia at 2 hours during antenatal testing are also associated with an increased likelihood of abnormal glucose tolerance and overt diabetes postpartum.[1] Postpartum, the presence of impaired glucose tolerance results in an 80% risk of a woman developing diabetes within 5 years or a 16% annual incidence of diabetes.[51] Modifiable risk factors, which can be adjusted to decrease the risk of a woman developing diabetes postpartum, include diet, weight loss, exercise, smoking cessation, and medications that adversely affect glucose metabolism (corticosteroids, nicotinamide, high-dose thiazide diuretics).[1, 62] Each 10-pound gain of weight above the initial postpartum weight increases the risk for the development of diabetes twofold.[51] The recurrence rate for gestational diabetes ranges from 30% to 50%,[1, 71] with the risk increasing with age and postpartum weight gain.[32, 71] Subsequent pregnancy after a history of prior gestational diabetes is associated with a greater chance of the development of type II diabetes, with a relative risk of 3.34.[51]

COMPLICATIONS

Complications of pregestational diabetes that have an impact on pregnancy include hypertension, nephropathy, retinopathy, and urinary tract infections, such as pyelonephritis, neuropathy, and diabetic ketoacidosis.* Maternal complications of diabetes in pregnancy include hypoglycemia, pregnancy-induced hypertension, progression of diabetic retinopathy, cephalopelvic disproportion, malpresentation, cesarean section, and operative vaginal delivery.[1, 77] Adverse effects seen in the embryonic period from conception to 8 weeks include spontaneous abortions and congenital malformations.[77, 80] Beyond 8 weeks, particularly in late second and early third trimester, the pregnancy is at risk for fetal hyperinsulinism, macrosomia, polyhydramnios, cardiac septal hypertrophy, chronic hypoxia, fetal growth restriction in women with hypertension or vascular disease, intrauterine fetal death, and increased perinatal mortality.[14, 77, 80, 88, 96] In the intrapartum period, one must be concerned with shoulder dystocia and neonatal trauma.

HYPERTENSION IN PREGNANCY

One of the major risks of gestational diabetes mellitus is the development of hypertensive disorders. The risk is approximately two- to threefold higher in women with gestational diabetes mellitus than in

women with normal glucose tolerance.[58, 62, 75] The incidence rate of pregnancy-induced hypertension in women with diabetes is 11.7%, ranging from 10% in women with gestational diabetes to 15.7% in women with class D, F, or R diabetes mellitus[20] (see Table 15–1). Chronic hypertension is seen in 9.6% of all women with diabetes and up to 16.9% in women with class D, F, or R diabetes mellitus.[20] The incidence rate of hypertensive complications in all pregnant women with diabetes is 18%, ranging from 14.6% in women with gestational diabetes to 30.9% in women with class D, F, or R diabetes mellitus.[20] These complications are most frequent in women with class D, F, or R, followed by classes A, B, and C.[20]

NEPHROPATHY

Class F diabetes includes the 5% to 10% of patients with underlying renal disease.[54] *Nephropathy* is defined as reduced creatinine clearance or proteinuria of at least 400 mg in 24 hours, measured in the first trimester, in the absence of urinary tract infection.[54, 65] These patients are at increased risk for preeclampsia, intrauterine growth restriction, and premature delivery.[54] As gestation progresses, nephropathy may worsen, particularly in patients with a serum creatinine concentration greater than 1.5 mg/dL.[20]

Patients with nephropathy should be followed with serial 24-hour urine collections for total protein and creatinine clearance.[14] Fetal testing can begin at 28 weeks in patients with well-controlled diabetes with normal fetal growth and no vascular diseases.[14]

RETINOPATHY

The longer a woman has diabetes and the greater the degree of hyperglycemia, the more likely the woman is to develop proliferative diabetic retinopathy.[24, 25] Any woman who has had diabetes for more than 5 years requires a retinal examination.[61] Pregnancy increases the risk of progression of diabetic retinopathy twofold.[54] Progression to proliferative retinopathy from background retinopathy or no retinal disease is rare; however, untreated proliferative retinopathy may progress to vision loss.[52] Of patients with untreated proliferative retinopathy, 86% have progression of their disease during pregnancy, whereas only 16% of patients with background retinopathy have disease progression.[25] Photocoagulation before or during pregnancy may help prevent the progression of retinal disease.[25] The course of background retinopathy for the pregnant woman is not different than that for the nonpregnant woman.[25] Women who have severe florid disc neovascularization that is unresponsive to laser therapy may be at a significant risk for visual deterioration, and termination of pregnancy should be considered.[54]

DIABETIC KETOACIDOSIS

Diabetic ketoacidosis is a complication seen primarily in women with type I diabetes, but it can be seen in women with type II or gestational diabetes. A preg-

---

*References 1, 21, 29, 77, 78, 84.

nant woman can develop diabetic ketoacidosis at a much lower glucose concentration than can a nonpregnant woman. In this condition, dehydration leads to hypovolemia and hypotension, which can result in a reduction of blood flow to the placenta.[54] The fetal mortality rate in maternal diabetic ketoacidosis may exceed 50%.[21] Diabetic ketoacidosis is usually the result of inadequate circulating insulin.[21] It can occur at much lower circulating glucose levels in pregnant women than in nonpregnant women, with cases being reported with glucose levels as low as 150 to 200 mg/dL.[21] Normally, the accelerated starvation of pregnancy is characterized by increases in plasma free fatty acids, ketones, and glycerol and by decreases in maternal glucose concentrations and gluconeogenic amino acids.[14] There is an increase in plasma concentrations of glucose and insulin after a meal.[13] There is also an increased fetal-placental transfer of glucose,[54] contributing to lower fasting plasma glucose levels in late gestation. These normal physiologic changes contribute to the development of diabetic ketoacidosis at much lower glucose concentrations in the pregnant woman than in the nonpregnant woman.

HEART DISEASE

Class H diabetes is an infrequently seen class of diabetes in pregnancy, representing ischemic heart disease.[54] In women with a previous myocardial infarction or an infarction during pregnancy, the maternal mortality rate exceeds 50%.[54] These patients should be evaluated with an electrocardiogram. If any abnormalities are noted, an echocardiogram or a modified stress test to assess ventricular function should be performed prior to conception.[54]

CONGENITAL ANOMALIES

Women with diabetes are at risk for the development of fetal anomalies. The congenital anomaly most specific to pregnant women with diabetes mellitus is caudal dysplasia (sacral agenesis), which occurs 200 to 400 times more often in women with diabetes than in pregnant women without diabetes.[54] Although this lesion is most specific for diabetes, it is not the most frequently encountered anomaly in the pregnancies of women with diabetes mellitus, because it is so rare.[27] Neural tube defects and congenital heart defects are far more common.[21] Malformations of the central nervous system, such as anencephaly, open myelomeningocele, and holoprosencephaly, are increased 10-fold, whereas cardiac anomalies, such as transposition of the great vessels and ventricular septal defects, are increased fivefold.[54] Other anomalies commonly observed in women with pregestational diabetes are discussed in Chapter 47, Part One.

The congenital malformation rate in infants of women with diabetes is 5% to 10%.[27, 54, 65, 93] This rate represents a two- to fourfold higher rate of anomalies when compared with a control population.[53, 54, 63] The rate of malformation is related to glucose control during organogenesis. Congenital anomalies have be-

come the most common cause of perinatal loss in women with pregestational diabetes,[54] accounting for 30% to 50%.[92] The perinatal mortality rate in pregnancies complicated by diabetes is less than 4%, with approximately 50% of these being due to congenital anomalies,[21, 65] which makes congenital anomalies the leading cause of perinatal deaths in these pregnancies.[63]

Why women with diabetes are at such a high risk for congenital anomalies is uncertain. The high risk may be due to an increased supply of substrate leading to an oxidative stress on the developing fetus, which in turn generates excess free oxygen radical formation that may ultimately be teratogenic.[14, 80] Tight metabolic control during organogenesis reduces the rate of anomalies.[79]

MACROSOMIA

The rate of *macrosomia,* defined as an estimated fetal weight in the 90th percentile or higher for gestational age, is 8% to 14% in normal pregnancies and 25% to 45% in pregnancies complicated by diabetes.[8, 38, 48] The Pedersen hypothesis states that the increase in fetal growth is the result of increased concentrations of maternal glucose, which crosses the placenta and results in fetal hyperglycemia and subsequently hyperinsulinemia.[79] This hyperinsulinemia affects primarily insulin-sensitive tissues such as fat.[14, 33] In fetuses of women with diabetes, the internal organs are enlarged, specifically the liver, heart, adipose tissue, adrenal tissue, and pancreatic islet tissue.[54, 80] It is thought that the macrosomic infant of the woman with diabetes has excessive fat deposition on the shoulders and trunk. This excess fat increases the risk of shoulder dystocia when compared with infants of similar weight in women with normal glucose tolerance.[69] Increasing maternal glycemia is a risk factor for fetal macrosomia.* Normalizing glucose values decrease the risk of macrosomia but does not eliminate it.[96]

Abdominal circumference obtained from ultrasonography is useful in detecting macrosomia. Studies have shown that an abdominal circumference greater than the 90th percentile taken within 2 weeks of delivery identified 78% of macrosomic fetuses.[95] Maternal weight was positively correlated with birth weight as well.[44]

Fetuses of women with diabetes experienced shoulder dystocia five times more often than those of women with normal glucose tolerance, with a 23.1% incidence rate of shoulder dystocia in infants weighing 4000 to 4499 gm and a 50% rate in infants weighing 4500 gm or more.[2] Shoulder dystocia complicates 0.2% to 2% of deliveries in women with normal glucose tolerance,[2, 56] compared with 3% to 9% of pregnancies complicated by diabetes.[28] Most cases of shoulder dystocia in women with diabetes occur in the macrosomic infant.[19] In women without diabetes, approximately 60% of shoulder dystocia cases occur

---

*References 8, 36, 37, 40, 57, 62, 85, 88.

in infants weighing 4000 gm or more; the comparable rate in women with diabetes is 84%.[56] Therefore, induction of labor at term for diabetic mothers of infants who are large for gestational age has been advocated by some investigators.[18] Cesarean delivery has been recommended for women with diabetes with estimated fetal weight of 4000 to 4500 gm, although predictions of birth weight by antenatal ultrasound or clinical examination are poor.[2, 7]

Macrosomia also is associated with a number of maternal and neonatal complications. There is an increased risk of cephalopelvic disproportion and shoulder dystocia that leads to traumatic birth injury and asphyxia.[54] These risks are highest when birth weight is greater than 4 kg and is greater in infants of diabetic mothers than in infants of women without diabetes whose children have a similar birth weight.[2, 14] These infants are at risk for birth trauma such as Erb palsy and clavicular fracture (see Chapter 27).[96] Erb palsy has the potential for a long-term morbidity because the neurologic deficit may be permanent in approximately 5% to 15% of cases.[59] The rate of Erb palsy in macrosomic, vaginally delivered infants weighing 4500 gm or more is 5%, compared with 0.7% in those weighing less than 4500 gm.[80] Thirty percent of the infants of women with diabetes with birth weight greater than 4500 gm had shoulder dystocia.[2] Additional neonatal complications associated with shoulder dystocia include neonatal depression and a greater incidence of an Apgar score of less than 7. The combination of diabetes and fetal weight of more than 4000 gm is the best predictor of subsequent development of shoulder dystocia, accounting for 54.7%.[2]

POLYHYDRAMNIOS

(See also Chapter 21.)

Polyhydramnios is seen more frequently in pregnancies that are complicated by diabetes. The reported rate ranges from 15% to 18%.[20, 96] The etiology is unknown; however, possible mechanisms include fetal hyperinsulinemia or hyperglycemia, increasing the fetal osmotic load, leading to fetal polyuria.

HYPOXIA

Hyperinsulinemia has also been linked to hypoxemia in the fetus,[54] which leads to an increase in oxygen consumption and a decrease in arterial oxygen content.[12] When such a fetus becomes hypoxic, the maternal hyperglycemia accentuates the rise in lactate and the decline in pH in the fetus.[62] There is also increased erythropoietin-induced red blood cell production in response to fetal hyoxia,[89] resulting in polycythemia in the neonate.

INTRAUTERINE GROWTH RESTRICTION

(See also Chapter 13.)

Growth disturbances (i.e., fetuses who are too big or too small) can complicate pregnancies in women with diabetes. Women with class A, B, or C diabetes are more likely to have macrosomic infants, but in women whose pregnancies are complicated by diabetic vasculopathy, there is an increased incidence of intrauterine growth restriction, which is thought to be caused by reduced uterine blood flow.[54]

INTRAUTERINE FETAL DEMISE

Maternal and fetal hyperglycemia and hyperinsulinemia may lead to fetal acidemia and hypoxia[96]; therefore, the incidence of intrauterine fetal demise, which is related to glucose control, is increased in women with diabetes. In women with gestational diabetes, the stillbirth rate increases when the postprandial glucose level is greater than 120 mg/dL, which is similar to pregestational diabetes with glucose levels of 160 mg/dL or greater.[19] Patients who are poorly compliant with prenatal care are also at increased risk for demise, particularly if they also have poor glucose control.[19]

PERINATAL MORTALITY RATE

As the fasting glucose levels rise above 105 mg/dL, the likelihood of adverse perinatal outcomes increases.[30] In pregnancies complicated by diabetes, the perinatal mortality rate has been reported to be as high as 31 to 38 out of 1000.[27, 90] If gestational diabetes is undiagnosed or untreated, the risk of perinatal mortality increases.[87] Hyperglycemia, defined as fasting blood sugar greater than 105 mg/dL and 2-hour postprandial blood sugar greater than 120 mg/dL, is the greatest risk factor for intrauterine or neonatal death.[54] Perinatal mortality also is influenced by the age of onset of diabetes, the duration of disease, and the presence of vasculopathy.[54] Women with gestational diabetes who are normoglycemic have a lower perinatal mortality rate.[54] Similarly, those requiring insulin are at greater risk of prenatal mortality than those whose diabetes is controlled by diet alone.[54]

OFFSPRING

In addition to the mothers, children of women with gestational diabetes are at increased risk for the development of type II diabetes or impaired glucose tolerance.[26, 62, 91] Children of mothers whose pregnancies were complicated by diabetes are also at risk for becoming obese as adolescents and adults.[21, 62, 83, 94, 96] These facts may represent the influence of the metabolic abnormalities in the intrauterine environment, such as hyperglycemia rather than genetic influences alone.[81, 82]

PRECONCEPTUAL COUNSELING

Because women with diabetes are at significant risk for complications during pregnancy, preconceptual counseling is recommended. It is preferable for a woman to establish normal glucose levels at least 1 year before attempting conception.[51] The glycosylated hemoglobin should be within two standard deviations of the mean,[30] which may reduce the rate of spontaneous abortions and congenital anomalies to nearly normal.[14, 68]

Before conception, the patient should undergo evaluation of glucose control with management of hemoglobin A_{1c} (HbA$_{1c}$), renal function with serum creatinine, 24-hour urine for total protein and creatinine clearance, and a rubella titer.[77] Measurement of glycosylated HbA$_{1c}$ gives retrospective insight into glycemic control. Higher first-trimester glycosylated hemoglobin is associated with a greater likelihood of anomalies.[65] Therefore, the goal is to establish good control with normal levels of hemoglobin A_{1c} before conception. After conception these laboratory studies should be repeated each trimester.

In addition to laboratory studies, patients should be evaluated for the presence of proliferative retinopathy with a retinal examination; if present, therapy should be instituted before conception. Because women with diabetes are at increased risk for asymptomatic bacteriuria and pyelonephritis, periodic urine cultures are necessary, with aggressive treatment of any positive cultures. Some also advocate an electrocardiogram as a baseline study for women older than 30 years.[47, 54, 67] Because women with diabetes are at increased risk for neural tube defects, they should be started on folate supplementation 4 mg daily once they are trying to conceive, continuing through the first 12 weeks of gestation. This supplement may decrease the risk of neural tube defects.[72]

Because diabetes mellitus is a complex constellation of diseases with variable effects both on the mother and on her fetus, preconceptual counseling in order to achieve optimal maternal health prior to conception is highly recommended. In addition, maintenance of euglycemia prior to conception and throughout gestation is highly recommended to reduce the incidence of maternal, fetal, and neonatal complications.

■ REFERENCES

1. Abrams RS, Coustan DR: Gestational diabetes update. Clinical Diabetes 8:19, 1990.
2. Acker DB, et al: Risk factors for shoulder dystocia. Obstet Gynecol 66:762, 1985.
3. American Diabetes Association: Clinical practice recommendations: American Diabetes Association 1991–1992. Diabetes Care 15:30, 1992.
4. American Diabetes Association: Special report: Principles of nutrition and dietary recommendations for individuals with diabetes mellitus, 1979. Diabetes 28:1027, 1979.
5. American Diabetes Association: Summary and recommendations of the Second International Workshop-Conference on Gestational Diabetes Mellitus. Diabetes 34 (Suppl 2):123, 1985.
6. Barret JM, et al: The non-stress test: An evaluation of 1000 patients. Am J Obstet Gynecol 141:153, 1981.
7. Benedetti TJ, Gabbe SG: Shoulder dystocia: A complication of fetal macrosomia and prolonged second stage of labor with midpelvic delivery. Obstet Gynecol 165:837, 1991.
8. Buchanan TA, et al: Utility of fetal measurements in the

9. Bung P, et al: Exercise in gestational diabetes. An optional therapeutic approach? Diabetes 40(Suppl 2):182, 1991.
10. Carr SR: Screening for gestational diabetes mellitus: A perspective in 1998. Diabetes Care 21:B14, 1998.
11. Carpenter MW, Coustan DR: Criteria for screening tests for gestational diabetes. Am J Obstet Gynecol 144:768, 1982.
12. Carson BS, et al: Effects of a sustained insulin infusion upon glucose uptake and oxygenation of the ovine fetus. Pediatr Res 14;147, 1980.
13. Catalano PM: Carbohydrate metabolism and gestational diabetes. Clin Obstet Gynecol 37:25, 1994.
14. Catalano PM, et al: Diabetes Mellitus in Reproductive Endocrinology, Surgery, and Technology. Philadelphia, Lippincott-Raven, 1996.
15. Catalano PM, et al: Carbohydrate metabolism during pregnancy in control subjects and women with gestational diabetes. Am J Physiol 264:E60, 1993.
16. Catalano PM, et al: Incidence and risk factors associated with abnormal postpartum glucose tolerance in women with gestational diabetes. Am J Obstet Gynecol 165:914, 1991.
17. Churchill JA, et al: Neuropsychological deficits in children of diabetic mothers. A report from the Collaborative Study of Cerebral Palsy. Am J Obstet Gynecol 105:257, 1969.
18. Conway DL, Langer O: Elective delivery of infants with macrosomia in diabetic women: Reduced shoulder dystocia versus increased Cesarean deliveries. Am J Obstet Gynecol 178:922, 1998.
19. Conway DL, Langer O: Optimal timing and mode of delivery in the gestational diabetic pregnancy. Prenat Neonat Med 3:555, 1998.
20. Cousins L: Pregnancy complications among diabetic women: Review 1965–1985. Obstet Gynecol Surv 42:140, 1987.
21. Coustan DR: Diabetes in Pregnancy in Neonatal and Perinatal Medicine, St. Louis, Mosby, 1996.
22. Coustan DR, et al: A randomized clinical trial of the insulin pump versus intensive conventional therapy in diabetic pregnancies. JAMA 225:631, 1986.
23. DeFronzo RA: Lilly Lecture 1987. The triumvirate: Beta cell, muscle, liver: A collusion responsible for NIDDM. Diabetes 37:667, 1988.
24. The Diabetes Control and Complications Trial Group: The effect of intensive diabetes treatment on the progression of diabetic retinopathy in insulin-dependent diabetes mellitus. The Diabetes Control and Complications Trial. Arch Ophthalmol 113:36, 1995.
25. Dibble CM, et al: Effect of pregnancy on diabetic retinopathy. Obstet Gynecol 59:699, 1982.
26. Dornhorst A, Rossi M: Risk and prevention of type 2 diabetes in women with gestational diabetes. Diabetes Care 21:B43, 1998.
27. Drury MI, et al: Pregnancy in the diabetic patient: Timing and mode of delivery. Obstet Gynecol 62:279, 1983.
28. Elliot JP, et al: Ultrasonic prediction of fetal macrosomia in diabetic patients. Obstet Gynecol 60:159, 1982.
29. The Expert Committee on the Diagnosis and Classification of Diabetes Mellitus: Report of the Expert Committee on the Diagnosis and Classification of Diabetes Mellitus. Diabetes Care 20:1183, 1997.
30. Gabbe SG: The gestational diabetes mellitus conferences: Three are history: Focus on the fourth. Diabetes Care 21:B1, 1998.
31. Gabbe SG: Unresolved issues in screening and diagnosis of gestational diabetes mellitus. Prenat Neonat Med 3:523, 1998.
32. Henry OA, Bleisher NA: Long-term implication of gestational diabetes for the mother. Baillieres Clin Obstet Gynaecol 5:461, 1991.
33. Hill DJ, et al: Growth factors and the regulation of fetal growth. Diabetes Care 21:B60, 1998.
34. Hod M, et al: Antepartum management protocol: Timing and mode of delivery in gestational diabetes. Diabetes Care 21:B113, 1998.
35. Hollander P: Approaches to the treatment of type I diabetes. Laboratory Medicine 8:522, 1990.
36. Homko CJ, et al: Is self-monitoring of blood glucose necessary in the management of gestational diabetes mellitus? Diabetes Care 21:B118, 1998.

management of gestational diabetes mellitus. Diabetes Care 21:B99, 1998.

37. Jovanovic L: American Diabetes Association's Fourth International Workshop-Conference on Gestational Diabetes Mellitus: Summary and discussion. Therapeutic interventions. Diabetes Care 21:B131, 1998.
38. Jovanovic L, et al: Metabolic and immunologic effects of insulin lispro in gestational diabetes. Diabetes Care 22:1422, 1999.
39. Jovanovic-Peterson L, et al: Randomized trial of diet versus diet plus cardiovascular conditioning on glucose levels in gestational diabetes. Am J Obstet Gynecol 161:415, 1989.
40. Jovanovic-Peterson L, et al: Maternal postprandial glucose levels and infant birth weight: The diabetes in early pregnancy study. Am J Obstet Gynecol 164:103, 1991.
41. Jovanovic-Peterson L, ed: Medical Management of Pregnancy Complicated by Diabetes, 2nd ed. Alexandria, Va, American Diabetes Association, 1995.
42. Jovanovic L, et al: Feasibility of maintaining normal glucose profiles in insulin-dependent pregnant diabetic women. Am J Med 68:105, 1980.
43. Karlsson K, Kjellmer I: The outcome of diabetic pregnancies in relation to the mother's blood sugar level. Am J Obstet Gynecol 112:213, 1972.
44. Khojandi M, et al: Gestational diabetes: The dilemma of delivery. Obstet Gynecol 43:1, 1974.
45. King H: Epidemiology of glucose intolerance and gestational diabetes in women of childbearing age. Diabetes Care 21:B9, 1998.
46. King JC: New National Academy of Sciences guidelines for nutrition during pregnancy. Diabetes 40(Suppl 2):151, 1991.
47. Kitzmiller JL, et al: Preconception management of diabetes continued through early pregnancy prevents the excess frequency of major congenital anomalies in infants of diabetic mothers. JAMA 265:731, 1991.
48. Kitzmiller JL: Macrosomia in infants of diabetic mothers: Characteristics, causes, prevention. In Jovanovic L, et al (eds): Diabetes in Pregnancy: Teratology, Toxicology and Treatment. New York, Praeger, 1986.
49. Kjos SL, et al: The effect of lactation on glucose and lipid metabolism in women with recent gestational diabetes. Obstet Gynecol 82:451, 1993.
50. Kjos SL, et al: Hormonal choices after gestational diabetes: Subsequent pregnancy, contraception, and hormone replacement. Diabetes Care 21:B50, 1988.
51. Kjos SL, et al: Postpartum screening and contraceptive use in women with gestational diabetes. Prenat Neonat Med 3:563, 1998.
52. Klein BEK, et al: Effect of pregnancy on the progression of diabetic retinopathy. Diabetes Care 13:34, 1990.
53. Kucera J: Rate and type of congenital anomalies among offspring of diabetic women. J Reprod Med 7:73, 1971.
54. Landon MB, Gabbe SG: Diabetes mellitus and pregnancy. Obstet Gynecol Clin North Am 19:633, 1992.
55. Langer O, et al: Management of women with one abnormal oral glucose tolerance test value reduces adverse outcome in pregnancy. Am J Obstet Gynecol 161:593, 1989.
56. Langer O, et al: Shoulder dystocia: Should the fetus weighing >4000 grams be delivered by cesarean section? Am J Obstet Gynecol 165:831, 1991.
57. Langer O: Insulin and other treatment alternatives in gestational diabetes mellitus. Prenat Neonat Med 3:542, 1998.
58. Lavin J, et al: Clinical experience with 107 diabetic pregnancies. Am J Obstet Gynecol 147:742, 1983.
59. Levine MG, et al: Birth trauma: Incidence and predisposing factors. Obstet Gynecol 63:792, 1984.
60. McManus RM, Ryan EA: Insulin requirements in insulin-dependent and insulin-requiring GDM women during final month of pregnancy. Diabetes Care 15:1323, 1992.
61. Medical Management of Pregnancy Complicated by Diabetes. Alexandria, Va, American Diabetes Association, 1993.
62. Metzger BE, Coustan DR: Summary and Recommendations of the Fourth International Workshop-Conference on Gestational Diabetes Mellitus. The Organizing Committee. Diabetes Care 121:B161, 1998.
63. Metzger BE, Freinkel N: Diabetes and pregnancy: Metabolic changes and management. Clinical Diabetes 8, 1990.
64. Metzger BE: Summary and recommendations of the Third International Workshop Conference on Gestational Diabetes Mellitus. Diabetes 40(Suppl 2):197, 1991.
65. Miller E, et al: Elevated maternal hemoglobin A1c in early pregnancy and major congenital anomalies in infants of diabetic mothers. N Engl J Med 304:1331, 1981.
66. Miller JM, Horger EO: Antepartum heart rate testing in diabetic pregnancy. J Reprod Med 30:515, 1985.
67. Mills JL, et al: Lack of relations of increased malformation rates in infants of diabetic mothers to glycemic control during organogenesis. N Engl J Med 318:671, 1988.
68. Mills J, et al: Incidence of spontaneous abortion among normal and insulin-dependent diabetic women whose pregnancies were identified within 21 days of conception. N Engl J Med 319:1617, 1988.
69. Modanlou HD, et al: Large-for-gestational age neonates: Anthropometric reasons for shoulder dystocia. Obstet Gynecol 60:417, 1982.
70. Moller DE, Flier JS: Insulin resistance-mechanisms, syndromes and implications. N Engl J Med 325:938, 1991.
71. Moses RG: The recurrence rate of gestational diabetes in subsequent pregnancies. Diabetes Care 19:1349,1996.
72. MRC Vitamin Study Research Group: Prevention of neural tube defects: Results of the Medical Research Council Vitamin Study. Lancet 338:131, 1991.
73. National Diabetes Data Group: Classification and diagnosis of diabetes mellitus and other categories of glucose intolerance. Diabetes 28:1039, 1979.
74. Neiger R. Coustan DR: The role of repeat glucose tolerance tests in the diagnosis of gestational diabetes. Am J Obstet Gynecol 165:787, 1991.
75. Olofsson P, et al. Diabetes and pregnancy: A 21 year Swedish material. Acta Obstet Gynecol Scand (Suppl 122):3, 1984.
76. O'Sullivan JB, Mahan CM: Criteria for the oral glucose tolerance test in pregnancy. Diabetes 13:278, 1964.
77. Pasui D, McFarland KF: Management of diabetes in pregnancy. American Family Physician 55:2731, 1997.
78. Pedersen J, et al: Assessors of fetal perinatal mortality in diabetic pregnancy. Diabetes 23:302, 1974.
79. Pedersen J: The Pregnant Diabetic and Her Newborn: Problems and Management, 2nd ed. Baltimore, Williams & Wilkins, 1977.
80. Persson B, Hanson U. Neonatal morbidities in gestational diabetes mellitus. Diabetes Care 21:B79, 1998.
81. Pettitt DJ, et al: Abnormal glucose tolerance during pregnancy in Pima Indian women. Long-term effects on offspring. Diabetes 40(Suppl 2):126, 1991.
82. Pettitt DJ, Knowler WC: Long-term effects of the intrauterine environment, birth weight and breast-feeding in Pima Indians. Diabetes Care 21:B138, 1998.
83. Phillips DIW: Birth weight and the future development of diabetes: A review of the evidence. Diabetes Care 21:B150, 1998.
84. Pirart J: Diabetes mellitus and its degenerative complications: A prospective study of 4400 patients observed between 1947 and 1973. Diabetes Care 1:252, 1978.
85. Reece EA, Homko CJ: Optimal glycemic control, fetal morbidity and monitoring protocols in gestational diabetes mellitus. Prenat Neonat Med 3:526, 1998.
86. Report of the Expert Committee on the Diagnosis and Classification of Diabetes Mellitus. Diabetes Care 20:1183, 1997.
87. Rosenn BM, Miodovnik M: Antenatal fetal testing in pregnancies complicated by gestational diabetes mellitus: Why, who and how? Prenat Neonat Med 3:550, 1998.
88. Sermer M, et al: The Toronto tri-hospital gestational diabetes project. Diabetes Care 21:B33, 1998.
89. Shannon K, et al: Erythropoiesis in infants of diabetic mothers. Pediatr Res 20:161, 1986.
90. Shea MA, et al: Diabetes in pregnancy. Am J Obstet Gynecol 111:801, 1971.
91. Silverman BL, et al: Long-term effect of the intrauterine environment: The Northwestern University Diabetes in Pregnancy Center. Diabetes Care 21(Suppl 2):B142, 1998.
92. Simpson JL, et al: Diabetes in pregnancy, Northwestern University Series (1977–1981). I. Prospective study of anomalies in offspring of mothers with diabetes mellitus. Am J Obstet Gynecol 146:263, 1983.
93. Sinclair SH, et al: Macular edema and pregnancy in insulin dependent diabetes. Am J Opthalmol 97:154, 1984.

94. Slaine DR, et al: Long term outlook for the offspring of the diabetic woman. In Jovanovic L (ed): Controversies in Diabetes in Pregnancy. New York, Springer-Verlag, 1988.

95. Tamura RK, et al: Diabetic macrosomia: Accuracy of third trimester ultrasound. Obstet Gynecol 67:828, 1986.

96. Uvena J, Catalano PM: Short- and long-term effects of gestational diabetes mellitus on the neonate. Prenat Neonat Med 3:517, 1988.

97. Weiss PA, Hoffman H: Intensified conventional insulin therapy for the pregnant diabetic patient. Obstet Gynecol 64:629, 1984.

98. White P: Pregnancy complicating diabetes. Am J Med 7:609, 1949.

16 Obstetric Management of Prematurity

Patrick S. Ramsey

Robert L. Goldenberg

Preterm labor is defined as contractions with cervical change occurring at less than 37 gestational weeks. *Preterm delivery,* as defined by the World Health Organization, is delivery that occurs at more than 20 and less than 37 gestational weeks. In the United States, the prematurity rate is approximately 8% to 10%, whereas in Europe it varies between 5% and 7%. In spite of advances in obstetric care, the rate of prematurity has not changed substantially over the past 40 years and may actually have increased slightly in recent decades.[82] Prematurity remains a leading cause of neonatal morbidity and mortality worldwide, accounting for 60% to 80% of deaths of infants without congenital anomalies.[281] Recent advances have furthered understanding of the pathophysiology of preterm labor and may serve as a basis for novel approaches to address this important clinical problem. In this chapter, we review various issues related to preterm labor and delivery, including complications, pathophysiology, risk factors, preventive strategies, and treatment.

PREMATURITY

Spontaneous preterm labor accounts for 40% to 50% of all preterm deliveries, with the remainder resulting from preterm premature rupture of membranes (PPROM) (25% to 40%) and obstetrically indicated preterm delivery (20% to 25%).[294, 421] Because the risk of neonatal mortality and morbidity near term is low, great attention has been focused on early preterm birth (23 to 32 weeks' gestation).[5] Although preterm birth in this gestational age group represents less than 1% to 2% of all deliveries, this group contributes to nearly 50% of long-term neurologic morbidity and to about 60% of perinatal mortality.

Survival of preterm babies is highly dependent on the gestational age at the time of the preterm birth.[130] Neonatal mortality rates have declined over recent years largely because of improved neonatal intensive care.[143, 427] In general, for a given gestational age, female infants demonstrate a greater rate of survival than do male infants, and African American neonates tend to do better than white neonates (see Chapter 2).[72] Neonatal survival dramatically improves as gestational age progresses, with over 50% surviving at 25 weeks' gestation and over 90% surviving at 28 or 29 weeks' gestation.[72] The gestational age–specific neonatal mortality rates are listed in Table 16–1. Similarly, neonatal survival rates increase as infant birth weight increases: 501 to 750 gm, 49%; 751 to 1000 gm, 85%; 1001 to 1250 gm, 93%; and 1251 to 1500 gm, 96%.[406] In the United States, survival rates of 20% to 30% have been noted in neonates delivered at 22 to 23 weeks' gestation; however, these premature infants are often left with long-term neurologic impairment.[164, 166, 281]

Neonatal morbidity remains a significant clinical problem that may result from prematurity. Morbidities include respiratory distress syndrome, intraventricular hemorrhage, periventricular leukomalacia, necrotizing enterocolitis, bronchopulmonary dysplasia, sepsis, patent ductus arteriosus, cerebral palsy, mental retardation, and retinopathy of prematurity. The risk for these morbidities is directly related to gestational age at delivery and birth weight. The gestational age–specific neonatal morbidity rates are listed in Table 16–2.[372] Use of antenatal corticosteroids (betamethasone or dexamethasone) has been shown to reduce the incidence and severity of respiratory distress syndrome, intraventricular hemorrhage, and necrotizing enterocolitis.[83, 234, 326] In spite of these benefits, the use of antenatal corticosteroids has not been widespread until recently. (See Chapter 11, Part One, and Chapter 42.)

Cerebral palsy, defined as a nonprogressive motor dysfunction with origin around the time of birth, complicates approximately 2 per 1000 live births. Most cases of cerebral palsy do not have a specific identifiable cause. Although most cases of cerebral palsy occur in term infants, the relative risk for an early preterm infant developing cerebral palsy is nearly 40 times that of a term infant. Intrauterine infection recently has been shown to be associated with the subsequent development of periventricular leukomalacia, intraventricular hemorrhage, and cerebral palsy.[90, 106, 327, 415] Intrauterine infection and the

TABLE 16–1   NEONATAL SURVIVAL BY GESTATIONAL AGE AT DELIVERY

GESTATIONAL AGE (WKS)	SURVIVAL BY GESTATIONAL AGE (%)	WEEKLY IMPROVEMENT IN SURVIVAL (%)
22	0.0	0.0
23	1.8	1.8
24	9.9	8.1
25	15.5	5.6
26	54.7	39.2
27	67.0	12.3
28	77.4	10.4
29	85.2	7.8
30	90.6	5.4
31	94.2	3.6
32	96.5	2.3
33	97.9	1.4

Modified from Copper RL, et al: A multicenter study of preterm birth weight and gestational age specific mortality. Am J Obstet Gynecol 168:78, 1993.

various inflammatory cytokines appear to increase substantially the risk of cell death, resulting in leukomalacia, periventricular hemorrhage, and, ultimately, cerebral palsy.[246, 442] Infants born at the same gestational age but without evidence of infection appear to have a substantially lower risk for periventricular damage and cerebral palsy. Children with extremely low birth weight (less than 1000 gm) have substantially higher rates of mental retardation, cerebral palsy, and visual disabilities, as well as neurobehavioral dysfunction and poor school performance.[165, 166, 428] Approximately 10% of surviving newborns who weigh less than 1000 gm at birth develop cerebral palsy.[4] Although more infants with very low birth weight survive, the rate of cerebral palsy ranges from 13 to 90 per 1000 for survivors weighing 500 to 1500 gm.[386]

PATHOGENESIS

The pathogenesis of preterm labor is not well understood; it is unclear whether preterm labor represents an idiopathic activation of the normal labor process or whether it results from a different pathologic mechanism.[334] It is becoming clear that the factors that lead to the development of preterm labor are multifactorial and are distinct from those that occur with term labor, representing a pathologic rather than a physiologic process. Central to all pathophysiologic pathways leading to the onset of term or preterm labor are three main biologic events: cervical ripening, formation and expression of myometrial oxytocin receptors, and myometrial gap junction formation.[127, 369] Prostaglandins E_2 (PGE_2) and $F_{2\alpha}$ ($PGF_{2\alpha}$) are believed to be important factors involved in these events, based on several findings. First, increased prostaglandin levels are present in amniotic fluid, maternal plasma, and urine during labor.[96, 334] These prostaglandins have been shown to facilitate cervical ripening and to promote myometrial gap junction formation.[248, 264] Further support for the important role of prostaglandins in the process of parturition comes from the observation that exogenous prostaglandins administered by various routes are effective for facilitating cervical ripening and for inducing labor at any point in gestation. Finally, prostaglandin synthetase inhibitors are effective agents that can delay the onset of parturition, arrest preterm labor, and delay abortions.[56] From these data it is relatively clear that the prostaglandins are an important component of the parturition process. What is less clear, however, is the mechanism or mechanisms by which this cascade of events that culminates in parturition begins. Several theories exist regarding the initiation of parturition: (1) progesterone withdrawal, (2) oxytocin initiation, and (3) premature decidual activation.

The progesterone withdrawal theory stems from the large body of work previously done with sheep. Endogenous progesterone is known to inhibit decidual prostaglandin formation and release.[1] As parturition nears, the fetal adrenal axis becomes more sensitive to adrenocorticotropic hormone (ACTH), inciting the increased secretion of cortisol. Fetal cortisol then stimulates trophoblast 17α-hydroxylase activity, which decreases progesterone secretion and leads to a subsequent increase in estrogen production. This reversal in the estrogen-to-progesterone ratio results

TABLE 16–2   MAJOR NEONATAL MORBIDITIES BY GESTATIONAL AGE AT DELIVERY

MORBIDITY	GESTATIONAL AGE (WKS)																	
	23	24	25	26	27	28	29	30	31	32	33	34	35	36	37–38	39–40	41–42	43–44
RDS %	83.3	86.7	87.0	92.6	83.9	64.3	52.8	54.7	37.3	28.0	33.9	13.5	6.4	3.3	.4	.3	.5	1.6
IVH %	16.7	25.0	30.4	29.6	16.1	3.6	2.8	1.9	2.0	.0	.0	.0	.0	.0	.0	.0	.0	.0
Sepsis %	33.3	25.0	8.7	33.3	35.6	25.0	25.0	11.3	13.7	2.8	5.4	3.5	2.3	1.3	.3	.4	.4	.5
NEC %	16.7	8.3	17.4	11.1	9.7	25.0	13.9	15.1	7.8	5.6	1.8	3.1	.3	.9	.0	.1	.0	.0
PDA %	16.7	33.3	60.9	48.1	38.7	42.9	44.4	22.6	15.7	9.3	1.6	1.7	1.3	.4	.3	.2	.4	1.0
Admission to NICU %	100.0	100.0	100.0	100.0	100.0	100.0	100.0	94.3	96.1	98.1	83.9	70.3	41.5	24.1	10.2	9.6	12.6	16.9

IVH, intraventricular hemorrhage, grade III or IV; NEC, necrotizing enterocolitis; NICU, neonatal intensive care unit; PDA, patent ductus arteriosus; RDS, respiratory distress syndrome.

Modified from Robertson PA, et al: Neonatal morbidity according to gestational age and birth weight from five tertiary centers in the United States, 1983–1986. Am J Obstet Gynecol 166:1629, 1992.

in increased prostaglandin formation.[57] Although this mechanism is well established in sheep, it does not appear to be the primary initiator of parturition in humans. First, there is a minimal decrease of progesterone levels in pregnant women prior to the onset of labor. Moreover, administration of progesterone to women in labor or preterm labor has no inhibitory effect.[124] Withdrawal of progesterone at the cellular level as a result of the presence of binding proteins has been proposed.[226, 396] Changes in the binding of progesterone to plasma proteins or changes in the metabolism of progesterone have also been implicated.[249, 297] To date, these proposed mechanisms are not well supported in the literature.

The second parturition theory involves oxytocin as an initiator of labor. As term approaches, the number of myometrial oxytocin receptors increases substantially. Because oxytocin is intimately related to the initiation of uterine contraction and has been shown to promote the release of prostaglandins, it is logical to suggest that oxytocin plays an important role in the initiation of labor.[125, 126, 371] Accepting oxytocin as the initiating agent for the onset of labor, however, is difficult for two reasons: blood levels of oxytocin do not rise before labor and the rate of clearance of oxytocin remains constant during pregnancy.[242] It is important to note that the prostaglandin levels in amniotic fluid are lower with oxytocin-induced labor than with spontaneous labor.[343] Oxytocin probably ensures uterine contractions, prevents blood loss after labor, and plays a crucial role in lactation. The involvement of oxytocin in parturition likely represents a final common pathway.[126]

The final and most likely theory regarding preterm labor involves premature decidual activation.[58] Whereas decidual activation may in part be mediated by the fetal-decidual paracrine system, in many cases, especially those involving early preterm labor, this activation occurs in the context of an occult upper genital tract infection (Fig. 16–1).[59, 13, 129, 350] Indeed, there is a growing body of evidence that has established a strong link between upper genital tract infection and spontaneous preterm delivery.[13, 41, 129, 146, 344, 378, 383] Colonization or infection of the upper genital tract results in inflammation and disruption of the choriodecidual interface, initiating a cascade of events that ultimately result in spontaneous labor.[129] These events are well supported by the biochemical changes that have been observed within the amniotic fluid, trophoblast, and decidua of patients with spontaneous preterm labor. Further support for this hypothesis comes from studies of midtrimester amniotic fluid, obtained at the time of genetic amniocentesis, which demonstrate that elevated interleukin-6 (IL-6) levels are often associated with subsequent spontaneous abortion, fetal death, or preterm labor.[384, 437, 438] Elevated IL-6 levels likely result from a subclinical upper genital tract infection that is often present many weeks before the eventual onset of preterm delivery or adverse pregnancy outcome. In addition to IL-6, amniotic fluid levels of the proinflammatory cytokines interleukin-1 (IL-1) and tumor necrosis factor–α

(TNF_α) have been associated with intrauterine infection and preterm labor.[14, 193, 207, 256]

IL-1 and TNF_α are known to be present in amniotic fluid during labor and are produced by the decidua and fetal membranes in vitro.[28, 79, 80, 331] These cytokines have been shown to induce production of other cytokines in vitro, including IL-6 by the decidua and chorion and interleukin-8 (IL-8) by the decidua, amnion, and chorion.[97, 98, 218, 417] IL-1, IL-6, and TNF_α result in stimulation of prostaglandin synthesis by amnionic, chorionic, and decidual cells in vitro.[260, 302, 303] Concentrations of PGE_2 and $PGF_{2\alpha}$ and their metabolites increase dramatically during labor.[96] The sources of these prostaglandins are the amnion, chorion laeve, and decidua parietalis. The amnion and the chorion are the sources of PGE_2.[301, 338] The decidua also is capable of producing PGE_2, but it is the only source of $PGF_{2\alpha}$.[338, 400] IL-8 is a granulocyte chemotactant and activator that, in turn, releases specific collagenases and elastases. These substances cause the breakdown of the cervical-chorionic-decidual extracellular matrix, leading to cervical ripening, separation of the chorion from the decidua, and, possibly, membrane rupture.

It appears that most cases of spontaneous preterm labor and delivery, especially those occurring early in gestation, are the result of occult upper genital tract infection with coincident activation of the decidua.[146] Interestingly, an inverse relationship exists between bacterial colonization of the chorioamnion and amniotic fluid and gestational age at delivery in women with spontaneous preterm labor.[62, 63, 177] Chorioamnion colonization is associated with nearly 80% of the very early spontaneous preterm births. In contrast, microbial colonization of the upper genital tract appears to play a much less important role in the initiation of parturition at or near term.[62, 177] The strong association between microbial chorioamnion colonization and preterm birth is an important advance in our understanding of the mechanisms involved in spontaneous preterm delivery and represents a potential target for therapeutic intervention.[177]

RISK FACTORS

The identification and management of preterm labor have been directed at defining various epidemiologic, clinical, and environmental risk factors that are related to preterm labor and delivery.[142] Early identification of these risk factors may allow modification of the traditional approaches to prenatal care and ultimately may reduce the rate of preterm delivery. In this section we review the major risk factors that are associated with preterm delivery (Table 16–3).

DEMOGRAPHICS

In the United States, race is a significant risk factor for preterm delivery. African American women have a prematurity rate of about 16% to 18%, whereas the prematurity rate for white women is 7% to 9%. Neonates of very low birth weight (less than 1500

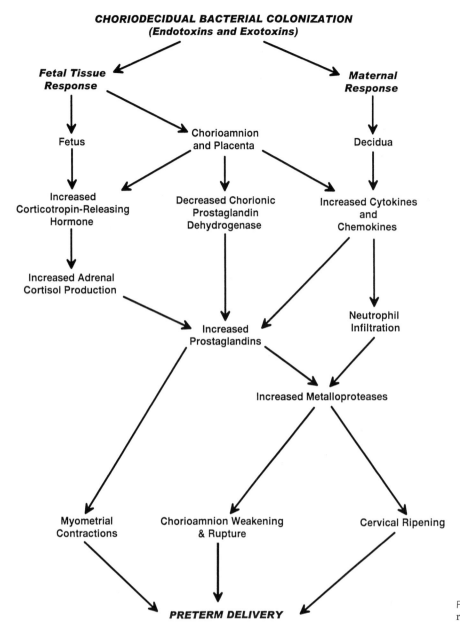

FIGURE 16–1. Pathogenesis of infection-related preterm labor and delivery.

gm) demonstrate the greatest risk of neonatal morbidity and death, and they are disproportionately represented by African American neonates.[2] Various other factors have been implicated, including maternal age. Women younger than 17 years and older than 35 years carry a higher risk of preterm delivery.[298] When similar age groups are compared by race, African American women still have a higher rate of preterm deliveries.[2] Less education and lower socioeconomic status also have been shown to be risk factors, although probably they are not independent of each other.[115] When these factors are controlled, African American women continue to have a higher rate of preterm delivery than other ethnic groups. The cause of preterm birth also appears to differ ethnically: preterm labor is more common in white women; PPROM is more common in African American women.[289] (See Chapter 2.)

Various behavioral factors increase the risks. Nutritional status, either poor or excessive weight gain, seems to have an adverse affect.[435] Women with a low body mass index (less than 19.8 kg/m²) are at higher risk than other women for preterm delivery. Smoking plays a more significant role in growth retardation than it does in preterm delivery; however, women who smoke have about a 20% to 30% increase in preterm births, compared with nonsmokers.[361, 398] In the United States, where an estimated 20% to 30% of pregnant women smoke, 10% to 20% of all preterm births can be attributed to maternal smoking.[267] The increasing use of cocaine during pregnancy is another important behavioral factor.[263] The pathophysiology may be similar to that of smoking, in which there is vasoconstriction that leads to an increased rate of abruption.[441] (See Chapters 12 and 36.)

Other behavioral factors are the degree of physical

TABLE 16–3 RISK FACTORS ASSOCIATED WITH PRETERM DELIVERY

Demographic Factors
- Age
- Race
- Socioeconomic status

Behavioral Factors
- Smoking
- Substance abuse
- Poor nutrition
- Absent or inadequate prenatal care

Maternal Medical Conditions
- Poor obstetric history
- Uterine/cervical malformations
- Myomata
- DES exposure
- Hypertension
- Diabetes
- Other medical conditions

Current Pregnancy Complications
- Multiple gestation
- Excess or decreased amniotic fluid
- Vaginal bleeding
- Low body mass index (< 19.8 kg/m²)
- Fetal anomalies
- Abdominal surgery
- Infection (systemic or local)

DES, diethylstilbestrol.

activity and stress during pregnancy. Several studies have evaluated the effects of employment on preterm delivery, with results including an increase in the rate of preterm deliveries, no difference in the rate of preterm deliveries, or an actual decrease in premature deliveries in the working group.[271, 285, 321] Unfortunately, none of these studies addresses the physical activity of domestic labor. Activity in the standing position does increase uterine irritability, which is probably caused by uterine compression of pelvic vessels, resulting in a decreased venous return to the heart. Contractions of the uterus may relieve this compression. A Swiss study demonstrated increased uterine activity in 66% of singleton pregnancies in relation to standing, and in all cases of twins studied.[393] Maternal stress also appears to be associated with an increased risk for preterm birth. Copper and coworkers, in a study of 2593 women assessed between 25 and 29 weeks of gestation, showed that maternal stress was significantly associated with spontaneous preterm birth.[74] What seems reasonably clear is that women who work hard physically for long hours and are under increased stress do have an increased risk of preterm birth.

OBSTETRIC HISTORY

Obstetric history plays an important role in the occurrence of preterm labor. Prior preterm delivery is one of the most significant risk factors. The risk of recurrent preterm birth in women with a history of preterm delivery ranges from 17% to 40%, and it appears to be dependent on the number of prior preterm deliveries. Carr-Hill and Hall, in a study of 6572 Scottish women, demonstrated a threefold increased risk for preterm delivery in women with one prior preterm delivery (15%) compared with women with no previous preterm delivery (5%) (Table 16–4).[55] For women who had two previous preterm births, a sixfold increase in the risk for recurrent preterm delivery was noted (30%). Similarly, Bakketeig and associates demonstrated that for every preterm birth, the risk in the subsequent pregnancy increased, whereas for every term delivery, the risk decreased.[20] Mercer and coworkers recently reported on 1711 women who had a prior preterm delivery, noting a 2.5-fold increased risk of spontaneous preterm delivery in the subsequent pregnancy.[294] Interestingly, the younger the gestational age of the prior preterm delivery, the greater the risk for a subsequent spontaneous preterm delivery.

Prior second-trimester abortions, whether single or multiple, also increase the risk of preterm delivery. However, the picture is not as clear for prior first-trimester abortions, either spontaneous or induced. Several studies evaluating one first-trimester abortion reported no increased risk, and data regarding multiple first-trimester abortions are inconsistent.[66, 251]

UTERINE AND CERVICAL ABNORMALITIES

Congenital müllerian anomalies are associated with a higher risk of preterm delivery.[183] Approximately 3% to 16% of all preterm births are associated with a uterine malformation. Heinonen and colleagues evaluated 126 patients with known uterine anomalies involving 256 pregnancies.[183] Overall, the incidence of preterm labor varied greatly depending on the type of uterine anomaly. Unicornuate, didelphic, and bicornuate abnormalities had preterm labor rates ranging from 18% to 80%, whereas the rates for a septate uterus varied from 4% to 17%, depending on whether the division was incomplete or complete.

Uterine leiomyomata also have been associated with an increased risk of preterm delivery because of an increased incidence of antepartum bleeding and PPROM. Of the various types of myoma, submuco-

TABLE 16–4 RECURRENCE RATES FOR SPONTANEOUS PRETERM DELIVERY ACCORDING TO PRIOR PREGNANCY OUTCOME

FIRST BIRTH	SECOND BIRTH	NEXT PREGNANCY (%)
Term	—	5
Preterm	—	15
Term	Preterm	24
Preterm	Preterm	32

From Carr-Hill RA, Hall MH: The repetition of spontaneous preterm labour. Br J Obstet Gynecol 92:921, 1985.

sal and subplacental myomata appear to be most strongly associated with preterm delivery.[320]

Cervical incompetence is another important risk factor that can lead to preterm delivery. The classic clinical description of cervical incompetence includes a history of painless cervical dilatation occurring between 12 and 20 weeks that leads to either preterm labor or PPROM. A history of a second-trimester pregnancy loss has been the cornerstone of the diagnosis of cervical incompetence. Various etiologic factors, such as cone biopsies of the cervix and traumatic forceps deliveries have been identified as potential causes of cervical incompetence.

A significant factor associated with congenital causes of cervical incompetence is intrauterine exposure to diethylstilbestrol (DES). It has been estimated that between 1 and 1.5 million female fetuses were exposed to DES between the late 1940s and 1971. These women have an increased risk of preterm delivery that ranges from 15% to 28% and an increased risk of spontaneous abortion that ranges from 20% to 40%.[216, 407] Women exposed to DES who have associated anomalies, such as T-shaped uterus, cervical incompetence, or vaginal structural anomalies, have a greater risk of preterm delivery than those who do not demonstrate changes. Because most women exposed to DES in utero are now older than 30 years of age, this risk factor is now seen only rarely and is expected to disappear in the next few years.

Upper and lower genital tract structural abnormalities range from 33% to 66% in women exposed to DES.[215] Visible cervical and vaginal abnormalities occur in about 25% to 50% of these patients. Changes include transverse septa, cervical collars, hoods, cockscombs, abnormal mucus, and cervical incompetence.[407] The upper genital tract also has associated abnormalities, such as the T-shaped uterus, synechiae and diverticula, and structural alteration of the fallopian tubes.[216] Women exposed to DES have an increased incidence of preterm labor and delivery in comparison with control subjects, and those with visible cervicovaginal abnormalities tend to have worse outcomes.[78] Normal cervicovaginal anatomy in women exposed to DES does not rule out the possibility of cervical incompetence, as documented by Ludmir and associates.[258]

Trauma during various obstetric or gynecologic procedures can cause cervical incompetence. Cervical conization, performed for the diagnosis and treatment of cervical intraepithelial neoplasia by cold knife, laser, or loop electrosurgical excision procedure (LEEP), has also been associated with cervical incompetence in subsequent pregnancies.[208] An extensive review of the literature by Harger showed a minimal role for these procedures in relation to cervical incompetence, with only the depth of the biopsy determining the subsequent risk.[172] First-trimester dilatation and curettage, if performed by an experienced operator with the preoperative use of *Laminaria digitata*, appears to confer minimal risk for subsequent cervical incompetence.[395]

Distinguishing between cervical incompetence and preterm labor can at times be difficult. Several techniques have been used to diagnose cervical incompetence in nonpregnant women. These techniques include passage of a number 8 Hegar dilator with ease through the internal os, measurement of the pressure necessary to pull a Foley balloon catheter inflated with 1 mL of water through the internal os, and identification of an abnormal cervical canal and isthmic funnel angle by either hysterosalpingography or hysteroscopy. All these methods evaluate cervical incompetence in the nonpregnant state, making the results at best suggestive in relation to cervical function or to anatomy in the pregnant woman.[347]

MULTIPLE GESTATION

Multiple gestation carries one of the highest risks of preterm delivery. Approximately 50% of twin and nearly 100% of multiple gestations of a higher order end before 37 completed weeks. A British study reported that as the number of fetuses increases, the average duration of gestation decreases.[61] Whereas the average length of gestation for singleton pregnancies is 39 weeks, the average length of gestation is significantly shorter for twins (35 weeks), triplets (33 weeks), and quadruplets (29 weeks).[61] In a recent report evaluating the clinical predictors of preterm labor, multiple gestation resulted in a greater than 40-fold increase in the rate of preterm delivery, compared with control subjects with a singleton pregnancy.[182] (See Chapter 18.)

BLEEDING

Vaginal bleeding caused by placenta previa or abruption is associated with almost as high a risk of preterm delivery as is multiple gestation.[182] In a study by Heffner and associates, bleeding in the first or second trimester was associated with an increased risk of preterm delivery.[182] A retrospective study of 341 patients with PPROM documented a relative risk of 7.4 when antepartum bleeding occurred in more than one trimester.[174] Additionally, second-trimester bleeding not associated with either placenta previa or abruption has also been significantly associated with preterm birth. Ekwo and coworkers observed a strong association between bleeding in the second trimester and PPROM (relative risk, 15.1; 95% confidence interval, 2.8 to 81) and preterm labor (relative risk, 19.7; 95% confidence interval, 2.1 to 186).[104] The mechanism responsible for the development of preterm labor in the setting of vaginal bleeding appears to be related to thrombin deposition with subsequent production of prostaglandins and plasminogen activators that stimulate an array of degradative enzymes, leading to destruction of the extracellular matrix.

INFECTION

Infections of the decidua, fetal membranes, and amniotic fluid have been associated with preterm delivery (see Fig. 16–1).* Intra-amniotic infection or chorioamnionitis complicates 1% to 5% of term pregnancies and nearly 25% of preterm pregnancies.[17] Heffner and associates demonstrated that clinical chorioamnionitis had a relative risk for preterm delivery of 48 over control subjects, representing the strongest correlation among all risk factors examined.[182] Romero and colleagues demonstrated that intra-amniotic infection was present in 16.1% of 367 patients.[377] Most women initially did not manifest overt signs and symptoms of chorioamnionitis, but approximately 60% had clinical signs at some point during their pregnancies. Sixty-five percent of cases with positive amniotic fluid cultures were refractory to tocolysis treatment versus 16% with negative culture results, and PPROM was more likely to occur (40% versus 3.8%).

There is a growing body of evidence that establishes a strong link between occult upper genital tract infection and spontaneous preterm delivery.† Histologic chorioamnionitis has been strongly associated with prematurity and extremely low birth weight (less than 1000 gm).[163, 191, 319] Guzick and coworkers prospectively evaluated placentas from 2774 women with preterm delivery.[163] Histologic chorioamnionitis was more common in preterm deliveries than in term deliveries (32.8% versus 10%). In women with PPROM, 48.6% had histologic evidence of chorioamnionitis. (See Chapter 22.)

Watts and colleagues investigated a series of patients with preterm labor, demonstrating that positive amniotic fluid cultures were present in 19% of women with spontaneous preterm labor and intact membranes with no clinical evidence of intrauterine infection.[433] In addition, the likelihood of a positive amniotic fluid culture in this investigation was inversely proportional to gestational age.[433] An association between histologic chorioamnionitis and preterm delivery has also been established.‡ Hillier and coworkers evaluated placental microbiology and histology in women who delivered prematurely compared with those who delivered at term.[191] Isolation of microorganisms from the chorioamnion of women who delivered preterm was strongly associated with histologic chorioamnionitis (odds ratio, 7.2; 95% confidence interval, 2.7 to 19.5).[191] Organisms that have been associated with histologic chorioamnionitis include species of the genera *Ureaplasma, Mycoplasma, Gardnerella, Bacteroides,* and *Mobiluncus.*[62, 192, 433] Further support for this hypothesis is derived from data-linking the presence of pathogenic organisms in both the amniotic fluid and chorioamnion with spontaneous labor in otherwise asymptomatic women with intact membranes.§ Cassell and coworkers demonstrated the poor sensitivity of amniotic fluid cultures in identifying upper genital tract microbial colonization, noting that women were twice as likely to have microbial

colonization of the chorioamnion than of the amniotic fluid.[63] Interestingly, an inverse relationship exists between colonization of the chorioamnion and amniotic fluid and gestational age at delivery in women with spontaneous preterm labor.[62, 63, 177] Chorioamnion colonization is associated with nearly 80% of the very early spontaneous preterm births. In contrast, microbial colonization of the upper genital tract appears to play a much less important role in the initiation of parturition at or near term.[62, 177]

Numerous theories exist regarding the underlying pathogenesis of intra-amniotic infection: (1) ascending infection from the vagina and cervix, (2) transplacental passage through hematogenous dissemination, (3) retrograde seeding from the peritoneal cavity through the fallopian tubes, and (4) iatrogenic means as a result of intrauterine procedures such as amniocentesis and chorionic villous sampling. There is some evidence to support each of these theories, but evidence from several sources supports ascending infection. Histologic chorioamnionitis is more common and severe at the site of membrane rupture than at other locations.[113] In cases of congenital pneumonia, inflammation of the chorioamniotic membrane is present and the bacteria identified are similar to those found in the genital tract.[31]

The mechanism may start with excessive overgrowth of certain organisms within the vagina and cervical canal. These microorganisms gain access to the intrauterine cavity by infecting the decidua, the chorion, and, finally, the amnion, leading to the amniotic cavity itself. Therefore, bacteria are able to cross intact membranes. The fetus then becomes infected by aspiration or swallowing of infected amniotic fluid or by direct contact, which may result in localized infection such as pneumonitis, otitis, or conjunctivitis. Seeding of these areas can lead to generalized fetal sepsis. Sepsis may also result from maternal bacteremia, leading to a placental infection that is passed to the fetus through the umbilical cord.[377]

Prostaglandins play a crucial role in the mechanism of both preterm and term labor. Stimulation of these prostaglandins because of intra-amniotic infection may be mediated by bacterial endotoxins. $PGF_{2\alpha}$ and PGE_2 and their metabolites are in increased concentrations in patients with preterm labor and intra-amniotic infection.[381] Bacterial products are sources of phospholipase A_2 and C, and they can stimulate prostaglandin production by the human amnion. Lipopolysaccharide, which is a known endotoxin in gram-negative organisms, is present in the amniotic fluid of patients with gram-negative infections and can stimulate the amnion and decidua to make prostaglandins.[375, 379] However, the quantities of endotoxin required to stimulate prostaglandin production by the amnion are generally not found in the amniotic fluid of women with preterm labor and intra-amniotic infection. These endotoxins stimulate the production of various cytokines by the host, which, in turn, stimulate prostaglandin production.

There is an increased presence of PGE_2 and $PGF_{2\alpha}$ in the amniotic fluid of women with intra-amniotic

---

*References 41, 42, 146, 155, 228, 278, 299, 344, 378, 383, 430.
†References 13, 41, 129, 146, 278, 344, 378, 383.
‡References 163, 191, 192, 278, 319, 344, 378.
§References 42, 62, 63, 177, 228, 434.

infection and PPROM.[376] Amniotic fluid concentrations of endotoxins are higher in women with preterm labor and PPROM than in those without preterm labor and PPROM.[380] Twenty-eight percent of patients with PPROM have positive results on amniotic fluid cultures without labor, which suggests that it takes more than the presence of bacteria to stimulate prostaglandin production and labor.

Various organisms have been implicated as causal agents for preterm labor and PPROM. Asymptomatic bacteriuria occurs in 2% to 10% of all pregnant women, and 30% to 50% develop pyelonephritis if the infection is left untreated.[211] In a recent meta-analysis by Romero and colleagues, asymptomatic bacteriuria carried a higher relative risk of subsequent premature birth than was found in control subjects (odds ratio, 1.9). Treatment of these patients lowered the risk of prematurity.[382]

Neisseria gonorrhoeae infection is associated with prematurity. Amstey and coworkers collected culture specimens from 5065 women at their initial prenatal visit and at 36 weeks of gestation, reporting an infection rate of 4.4%.[9] Preterm delivery was more common in patients with positive culture results (25.2% versus 12.5%). The rate of premature rupture of membranes that occurred anytime before labor was higher in the positive culture group than in the group of control subjects (26% versus 19%).[9]

Group B streptococci (GBS) plays a major role in neonatal morbidity and death, especially in premature infants. Reporting on genital colonization, Regan and associates cultured cervical specimens from 6706 pregnant women on admission to the hospital and found a prevalence of 13.4%.[363] The incidence rate of preterm delivery at less than 32 weeks of gestation was higher in colonized than noncolonized women (5.4% versus 1.26%). The rate of PPROM that occurred 1 hour before the onset of contractions also was greater in the colonized group (15.3% versus 7%). Bobitt and colleagues obtained vaginal cultures monthly, beginning at 24 weeks of gestation and at the time of admission.[42] Positive culture results were obtained in 11.3% of the patients. A higher rate of low birth weight was noted in the colonized group than in the noncolonized group (8.4% versus 3.4%), and the rate of PPROM also was higher (5.6% versus 1.7%). Moller and colleagues collected urine culture specimens between 12 and 38 weeks of gestation, reporting an overall positive culture rate (regardless of the colony count) of 2.5%.[307] Prematurity was more frequent in the positive culture group (20% versus 8.5%), as was PPROM (35% versus 15%).

In a randomized, controlled, double-blind trial of women with a urine culture who tested positive for GBS and who were treated with antibiotics, Thomsen and coworkers reported that the treated group had a lower rate of premature delivery than the nontreated group (37.5% versus 5.4%).[413] The rate of occurrence of PPROM was statistically significant between the two groups (53% versus 11%). These studies demonstrate that asymptomatic bacteriuria with GBS is a risk factor for preterm delivery and that eradication

with antibiotics decreases the risk. However, no study to date has shown that treatment of GBS genital tract colonization decreases the risk of PPROM. In the Thomsen study, all patients with urinary colonization also had positive results on cervical and vaginal cultures, possibly indicating that the presence of GBS in the urine may be a marker of more severe forms of genital tract colonization.[413]

In 1996, the Centers for Disease Control and Prevention in conjunction the American College of Obstetricians and Gynecologists and the American Academy of Pediatrics set forth recommendations regarding different approaches to the prevention of GBS disease.[64] Two prevention strategies were recommended. In the first strategy, intrapartum antibiotic prophylaxis is offered to women who are identified as GBS carriers through prenatal screening cultures collected at 35 to 37 weeks' gestation and to women who develop premature onset of labor or rupture of membranes prior to 37 weeks' gestation. In the second strategy, which does not use cultures, intrapartum antibiotic prophylaxis is provided to women who develop one or more risk conditions at the time of labor or membrane rupture. For intrapartum chemoprophylaxis, IV penicillin G (5 mU initially, followed by 2.5 mU every 4 hours) until delivery is recommended. IV ampicillin (2 gm initially, followed by 1 gm every 4 hours until delivery) is an acceptable alternative to penicillin G. Clindamycin or erythromycin may be used for women who are allergic to penicillin, although the efficacy of these drugs for GBS disease prevention has not been measured in controlled trials.

Another infection reported to be associated with prematurity is *Chlamydia trachomatis*. Harrison and associates screened 1365 women, noting an 8% incidence rate of cultures that tested positive for infection.[175] Although no differences were documented in the prematurity rate, PPROM was more common in women with positive IgM titers than in those without (41.1% versus 7.5%). Gravett and colleagues showed that a positive culture result had a significant association with preterm delivery before 34 and 37 weeks, with odds ratios of 4.0 and 4.7, respectively.[154] A chlamydial infection also had an elevated odds ratio (2.7) for PPROM. Similarly, Andrews and coworkers reported that patients with chlamydia noted during pregnancy have an odds ratio of 2.0 for spontaneous preterm birth.[15] These studies demonstrate a correlation between *C. trachomatis* infection and prematurity, especially related to PPROM as the event leading to preterm birth.

Bacterial vaginosis is a common lower genital tract infection found in approximately 20% to 40% of African-American women and 10% to 15% of white women.[111, 134, 291] Bacterial vaginosis is a clinical syndrome characterized by a decrease in the normal vaginal lactobacilli-dominant microflora, resulting in a predominance of bacteria such as *Gardnerella vaginalis*, *Prevotella* organisms, *Bacteroides* organisms, *Peptostreptococcus* organisms, *Mobiluncus* organisms, *Mycoplasma hominis*, and *Ureaplasma urealyticum*.[189] Characteristically, patients with symptomatic bacterial vaginosis complain of a watery, homogeneous grayish discharge with a fishy amine odor.

Bacterial vaginosis has been associated with an increased risk for preterm labor and delivery.* Gravett and colleagues previously showed a relative risk of 2.7 and 2.0 for PPROM and preterm delivery, respectively, at less than 37 weeks' gestation.[154] Presently, there are more than 15 studies showing an association between bacterial vaginosis and spontaneous preterm birth. Nearly 40% of early spontaneous preterm births, especially in African American women, may be attributable to bacterial vaginosis.[118, 119] Bacterial vaginosis seems to be associated more with early preterm birth than with late preterm birth. Additionally, two randomized clinical trials have demonstrated that treatment of bacterial vaginosis in patients at high risk for preterm delivery resulted in substantial reductions in the preterm birth rates.[178, 310] Based on the present data available, treatment of bacterial vaginosis appears to be effective in preventing preterm birth only in high-risk populations. Data from a study of low-risk women with bacterial vaginosis in Australia and a recently completed study in the United States by the National Institute of Child Health and Human Development Network of Maternal-Fetal Medicine Units (NICHD/MFMU), evaluating and treating asymptomatic women with bacterial vaginosis, failed to demonstrate a reduction in preterm delivery.[51, 284]

Most women with bacterial vaginosis never manifest any signs or adverse outcomes related to colonization, and it is likely that bacterial vaginosis is only a surrogate marker for a more important, presently unrecognized condition that may cause preterm birth.[377] One compelling theory is that bacterial vaginosis is a marker for occult upper genital tract infection†; therefore, premature births, attributed to bacterial vaginosis or prevented by its treatment, may instead be related to an associated upper genital tract infection.

Many other maternal infections and colonizations are associated with preterm birth.‡ One of the difficult questions to answer is whether these relationships are causal or merely associations. Gonorrhea, chlamydia, *Trichomonas*, syphilis, and other genital pathogens and infections are more frequently found in women who have a spontaneous preterm birth. However, the population of women affected by these infections often has other risk factors for preterm birth (low socioeconomic status, malnutrition, smoking, substance abuse, bacterial vaginosis, and others). These confounding variables make it difficult to establish causality because most studies have not controlled for these variables. In general, gonorrhea and chlamydia have been associated with a twofold increased risk for preterm delivery.[353, 409] Similarly, trichomoniasis appears to be associated with a 1.3-fold increased risk for preterm

delivery.[75, 387] GBS has been associated with prematurity in some studies; however, most studies demonstrate no association.[176, 307, 363, 413, 439] Many of the other sexually transmitted diseases, such as human immunodeficiency virus, hepatitis B, and genital herpes simplex virus, have been associated with an increased risk for spontaneous preterm birth in some but not most studies. Syphilis is widely reported to be associated with a twofold increased risk of preterm birth, and this relationship is relatively consistent among most studies.

OTHER RISK FACTORS

In addition to the risk factors already discussed, various other factors have been associated with an increased risk for preterm labor (see Table 16–3). Extremes in the volume of amniotic fluid, such as polyhydramnios or oligohydramnios, have been associated with an increased risk for preterm labor (see Chapter 21). Similarly, fetal anomalies, especially those involving multiple organ system and central nervous system abnormalities, carry a higher risk. Maternal abdominal surgery in the late second and third trimesters causes an increase in uterine activity, leading to preterm delivery.[195] Maternal medical conditions, such as gestational or pre-existing diabetes and hypertension (essential or pregnancy induced), are associated with a higher rate of preterm delivery; however, these preterm births are often classified as indicated preterm deliveries due to maternal complications rather than as the result of spontaneous preterm labor.[182] Asymptomatic bacteriuria is associated with an increased rate of prematurity.[382] Systemic infections, such as bacterial pneumonia, pyelonephritis, and acute appendicitis, often lead to increased uterine activity, potentially leading to premature delivery. Periodontal disease has also been shown to be associated with an increased risk of spontaneous preterm delivery.[192]

PREDICTION

Achieving the ultimate goal of reducing the incidence of preterm labor and delivery has been complicated because preterm deliveries have multiple causes. Deliveries indicated for maternal or fetal reasons account for approximately 20% to 25% of preterm births. PPROM is associated with another 25% to 40%, and under these conditions prevention with tocolysis is generally contraindicated. Of the 40% to 50% of idiopathic cases, nearly half occur beyond 34 weeks of gestation, when the use of tocolysis would be of questionable benefit. Consequently, only about 15% to 20% of patients in preterm labor are candidates for treatment.[188, 420] This frustrating statistic has led to various attempts to identify risk factors that may predict preterm labor. Three main areas of prediction are explored in this section: classic, biochemical, and ultrasound.

---

*References 111, 154, 194, 228, 230, 277, 282, 283, 368.

†References 13, 156, 169, 191, 225, 229.

‡References 34, 108, 137, 154, 180, 236, 237, 274, 277, 359.

CLASSIC PREDICTORS

Cervical change is the first of the classic clinical predictors. In one of the largest studies to date, Papiernik and associates evaluated 8303 pregnancies followed with weekly cervical examinations to determine whether precocious cervical change was associated with preterm birth.[346] These investigators noted that regardless of gestational age at delivery, cervical changes occurred approximately 3 to 4 weeks before delivery. After controlling for other risk factors in their study, they found that cervical dilatation of more than 1 cm carried a twofold to threefold increased relative risk for preterm delivery. Unfortunately, no sensitivity or positive predictive value was reported, although the authors claimed a reduction in the preterm birth rate from about 7% to 5% during an 8-year period while using this screening strategy.

Mortensen and colleagues evaluated cervical changes in 1300 pregnancies with examinations performed at 24, 28, and 32 weeks.[316] They divided their population into high- and low-risk groups on the basis of various factors. Cervical changes in the low-risk group were extremely poor predictors of preterm delivery, with a positive predictive value of 4%. In the high-risk group, however, the predictive value was 25% to 30%, with a sensitivity of 65%.[316]

Another potentially important clinical factor is the presence of uterine contractions. In a study involving approximately 2500 patients, excluding those with multiple gestation, vaginal bleeding, PPROM, and polyhydramnios, Nageotte and associates evaluated uterine activity differences in patients with preterm, term, and post-term deliveries.[324] The authors demonstrated an increase in uterine activity beginning 6 weeks before delivery, regardless of gestational age at birth, and a surge in uterine activity occurring within 72 hours of delivery in all three groups.[324] Unfortunately, these patients depended on tocodynamometry to determine this increase in frequency. When patients are instructed to self-detect an increase in uterine activity, they can identify only 15% of the contractions noted by tocodynamometry.[329] In another study, which used contractions as a screening tool, Main and coworkers evaluated intermittent uterine monitoring in an office setting.[268] One hundred thirty-nine patients were screened for 1 hour on at least three occasions between 28 and 32 weeks of gestation; a minimum of six contractions per hour during at least one occasion was used as a minimum. The test had a sensitivity of 75% and a positive predictive value of 32%.[268] The preterm delivery rate was 11.5%, which is higher than would be expected. Copper and coworkers evaluated the use of tocodynamometry and cervical examination at 28 weeks of gestation in 589 nulliparous women to determine whether patients at risk for preterm delivery could be identified.[73] The investigators noted that the best predictors of spontaneous preterm birth were the presence of a soft- or medium-consistency cervix and two or more contractions in 30 minutes. The risk for spontaneous preterm delivery increased from 4.2% for those patients with no con-

tractions detected to 18.2% for those patients having four or more contractions in 30 minutes.

In a study from the NICHD/MFMU network, Iams and associates again found that although an association was noted between the reported presence of contractions and preterm delivery, monitoring contractions was not useful clinically in defining a population at especially high risk for spontaneous preterm birth.[204, 205] Uterine activity does appear to play a role in preterm delivery; however, the use of home uterine monitoring as a screening tool in most, it not all, populations is not justified because of problems in identifying patients at risk and cost.

Attempts were made beginning in the early 1980s to combine these various classic factors into a risk scoring system to determine which patients were in jeopardy for preterm delivery. Creasy and colleagues combined socioeconomic factors (age, height, weight, previous medical history, smoking, work habits) and aspects of the current pregnancy into a risk scoring system.[81] A total of 10 points or more indicated a high risk of preterm delivery (Table 16–5). The initial study was promising, with a positive predictive value of 38%. Subsequent studies of various populations had much lower positive predictive values, in the range of 18% to 22%.[187, 266, 318, 341] One of the problems with the Creasy risk scoring system is the emphasis placed on a previous preterm delivery, which by itself elevates a patient into a high-risk category. Unfortunately, 50% of preterm deliveries happen in primigravidae, whose obstetric histories lower the predictive value even further.[188] Overall, classic predictors have had limited success in predicting preterm delivery, and no well-done study has demonstrated a reduction in preterm birth with their use.

BIOCHEMICAL PREDICTORS

The biochemical process leading to the initiation of either term or preterm labor has not been well established in humans. Recently, however, important insights into the pathophysiology of spontaneous preterm labor have helped to identify various biochemical markers that may predict preterm delivery (see Fig. 16–1).

Perhaps one of the most important and powerful biochemical markers identified to date is fetal fibronectin.[255] A glycoprotein found in the extracellular matrix surrounding the extravillous trophoblast at the uteroplacental junction, fetal fibronectin is a prototypical example of a marker of choriodecidual disruption.[116] Typically, fetal fibronectin is absent from cervicovaginal secretions from around the 20th week of gestation until near term.[18] Detection of elevated cervicovaginal levels of fetal fibronectin has been shown to be strongly associated with an increased risk for preterm delivery in patients at high risk for preterm delivery.* Lockwood and associates examined the concentrations of fetal fibronectin in amniotic fluid, cervical and vaginal secretions, and maternal serum

---

*References 18, 134, 136, 138, 202, 253, 349.

TABLE 16-5   SYSTEM FOR DETERMINING RISK OF SPONTANEOUS PRETERM DELIVERY*

POINTS ASSIGNED	SOCIOECONOMIC FACTORS	MEDICAL HISTORY	DAILY HABITS	ASPECTS OF CURRENT PREGNANCY
1	Two children at home Low socioeconomic status	Abortion × 1 Less than 1 yr since last birth	Works outside home	Unusual fatigue
2	Maternal age < 20 yrs or > 40 yrs Single parent	Abortion × 2	Smokes > 10 cigarettes per day	Gain of < 5 kg by 32 wks
3	Very low socioeconomic status Height < 150 cm Weight < 45 kg	Abortion × 3	Engages in heavy work or stressful work that is long and tiring	Breech at 32 wks Weight loss of 2 kg Head engaged at 32 wks Febrile illness
4	Maternal age < 18 yrs	Pyelonephritis		Bleeding after 12 wks Effacement Dilatation Uterine irritability
5		Uterine anomaly Second-trimester abortion DES exposure Cone biopsy		Placenta previa Polyhydramnios
10		Preterm delivery Repeated second-trimester abortion		Twins Abdominal surgical procedure

*Score is computed by adding the number of points given to any item. The score is computed at the first visit and again at 22 to 26 weeks' gestation. A total score of > 10 places the patient at high risk of spontaneous preterm delivery.
DES, diethylstilbestrol.
Modified from Creasy RK, et al: System for predicting spontaneous preterm birth. Obstet Gynecol 55:692, 1980.

from 163 uncomplicated pregnancies that resulted in delivery at term.[253] Fetal fibronectin was detected in only 4% of cervical and 3% of vaginal secretions between 21 and 37 weeks. In 65 patients with PPROM, 93% had fetal fibronectin in amniotic fluid and in vaginal or cervical secretions. In the preterm labor group, the presence of fetal fibronectin had a sensitivity of 81% and a specificity of 82% in predicting preterm labor.[253] Three subsequent studies of symptomatic women[255, 315] and asymptomatic women[254, 255, 324] have reported sensitivities in the 80% to 90% range and positive predictive values of 30% to 60%.

Goldenberg and coworkers demonstrated that detection of elevated cervicovaginal fetal fibronectin levels (greater than 50 ng/mL) at 24 weeks of gestation in asymptomatic women was strongly associated with subsequent spontaneous preterm delivery, with odds ratios of 59.2 (95% confidence interval, 35.9 to 97.8) for preterm delivery before 28 weeks of gestation, 39.9 (25.6 to 62.1) for preterm delivery before 30 weeks of gestation, and 21.2 (14.3 to 62.1) for preterm delivery before 32 weeks of gestation.[136] Additionally, fetal fibronectin levels have been correlated with cervical length, bacterial vaginosis, IL-6, and peripartum infection.[132, 134] These data clearly suggest that fetal fibronectin is one of the most potent markers identified to date for spontaneous preterm delivery. It is clear that infection of the upper genital tract with disruption of the choriodecidual interface is a feature common to many cases of preterm birth.

Measurement of estriol has recently been promoted as a potential biochemical marker that may be of use to predict preterm delivery. Estriol is a unique hormone of pregnancy that is produced almost entirely by the trophoblast from precursors derived from the fetal adrenal gland and liver. Initial investigations with urinary and plasma estriol attempted to use this assay to measure fetal well-being in utero.[25, 26, 27, 168] Subsequent investigations, however, failed to demonstrate a significant difference in perinatal outcome based on estriol-based management.[94, 100, 392]

Levels of estriol have been shown to rise throughout pregnancy, with a characteristic exponential increase 2 to 4 weeks before the spontaneous onset of labor at term.[91, 286] Interestingly, patients induced at term in the absence of spontaneous labor fail to demonstrate this increase in estriol.[311] Several investigations have assessed the use of salivary estriol levels to identify patients at risk for preterm delivery,[92, 288] suggesting that detection of an early estriol surge may identify patients at risk for preterm labor and delivery. Estriol appears to be a better marker for late rather than early spontaneous preterm birth; hence, the clinical utility of this biochemical marker is unclear. As with many other markers, estriol measurement has not demonstrated a reduction in the preterm birth rate.

Various other serologic, cervical, and amniotic fluid markers have been evaluated as predictors for preterm delivery, including α-fetoprotein (AFP), human chorionic gonadotropin (hCG), human placental lactogen (hPL), corticotropin-releasing hormone, C-reactive protein, alkaline phosphatase, ferritin, placental iso-ferritin, progesterone, estradiol, matrix metalloproteinase, IL-6, TNFα, and granulocyte colony-stimulating factor.* Each of these markers has been shown to have modest correlation with spontaneous preterm delivery.

Progesterone and estradiol are potentially interesting markers, based on the theory that progesterone withdrawal may be the initiating event. An early study noted a fall in progesterone levels before the onset of term labor and abortion.[422] Subsequent investigations have measured total or free progesterone, estradiol, or the estradiol-to-progesterone ratio during term or preterm labor.[10, 170] One prospective study examined both progesterone and estradiol concentrations weekly with no correlation.[39]

Corticotropin-releasing hormone (CRH), a placental peptide produced during the second and third trimesters that may play a role in the initiation of parturition, also is elevated weeks before the onset of preterm labor.[114, 354, 364, 432, 440] Wolfe and associates prospectively followed 168 patients with serial plasma CRH levels from 24 weeks of gestation and found that plasma levels rose at a 25% faster rate in the preterm group than in the term labor group, although this factor did not achieve statistical significance.[440] Tropper and colleagues demonstrated that CRH levels were significantly higher in maternal serum and umbilical cord serum in patients who delivered preterm as compared with control group patients who were matched for gestational age and who delivered at term.[418] Berkowitz and coworkers, however, observed that CRH levels were not predictive of preterm birth or PPROM. They did note that CRH binding protein levels decreased as term neared, suggesting that the bioavailability of CRH may increase coincident with the onset of parturition.[33] Leung and associates furthered these observations through an evaluation of 1047 women at low risk between 15 and 20 weeks of gestation.[245] Elevated midtrimester serum CRH levels were significantly associated with preterm delivery before 34 weeks. Using an arbitrary cutoff of 1.9 multiples of the median to predict preterm birth, elevated CRH had a sensitivity of 72.9%, a specificity 78.4%, a positive predictive value of 3.6%, and a negative predictive value of 99.6%. The use of CRH as a marker for preterm delivery holds promise because results are elevated not only in preterm labor but also with PPROM and intrauterine infection.[65, 99]

Various degradative enzymes have been characterized in relation to the prediction of women at risk for preterm delivery. Serum collagenases are one group of these potential markers. IL-1 stimulates cervical, decidual, and other cells to produce various collagenases, resulting in breakdown of the collagen matrix of the cervix. Rajabi and colleagues measured serum levels of collagenase at various gestational ages.[356]

They found that the levels remained relatively constant until the onset of labor, when an increase of 66% occurred over control values. In preterm deliveries this rise was eightfold greater than in control values.

Increasing interest also has focused on the metalloproteinases and their inhibitors in relation to preterm labor. Metalloproteinases-2 (MMP-2) and metalloproteinases-9 (MMP-9) have been associated with preterm labor, PPROM in particular.[19, 121] Fortunato and coworkers demonstrated that elevated amniotic fluid levels of MMP-2 and MMP-9 were associated with PPROM, suggesting that the metalloproteinases may play a role in degradation of the chorioamnion basement membrane, resulting in membrane weakening and rupture.[121] Athayde and associates further explored the association of amniotic fluid MMP-9 levels and preterm delivery, noting that MMP-9 levels were increased in patients who had preterm labor and who delivered prematurely as compared with patients with preterm contractions who delivered at term and with a control group without complications.[19] Tu and colleagues evaluated plasma MMP-9 levels to determine whether they predict subsequent spontaneous preterm birth.[419] Serum MMP-9 levels appeared to remain unchanged throughout pregnancy until the spontaneous onset of labor, at which time MMP-9 levels significantly increased. MMP-9 levels, however, did not increase before the onset of labor. Although MMP-9 levels may be a useful marker for true labor, their elevated levels do not seem to be useful to predict which patients may be at risk for developing preterm labor.

Cervical granulocyte elastase activity also has been the subject of several studies.[209, 210] Granulocytes are stimulated by IL-8, which is elevated in amniotic fluid of labor patients. Granulocyte elastase is one specific granulocyte degradative enzyme that may play a role in parturition. This elastase activity is increased in both term and preterm labor, which suggests that it may be involved in cervical ripening and in degradation of fetal membranes, leading to PPROM.[209, 210]

Given the association of occult upper genital tract infection with early spontaneous preterm birth, certain serum, amniotic fluid, and cervicovaginal inflammatory markers have also been evaluated as potential markers for the prediction of spontaneous preterm delivery. Both serum and cervical IL-6 levels have been found to be significantly elevated at 24 weeks of gestation in women with subsequent spontaneous preterm birth before 35 weeks.[132, 322] Elevated cervical IL-6 levels also are strongly associated with elevated fetal fibronectin levels.[132] Rizzo and associates characterized cervical and amniotic fluid levels of several inflammatory cytokines (IL-1, IL-6, TNFα) in a series of patients with preterm labor and intact membranes.[370] Elevated concentrations of these cytokines in cervical fluid were significantly associated with the presence of intra-amniotic infection. Cervical IL-6 appears to have the strongest association, with high levels (greater than 410 pg/mL) having a relative risk of 7.7 (95% confidence interval, 3.5 to 17.8) for intra-amniotic infection.[370] Serum granulocyte colony-

---

*References 35, 47, 48, 77, 93, 122, 131, 135, 139–141, 144–146, 185, 257, 279, 296, 313, 358, 373, 394, 399, 411, 412, 424, 436, 438, 439.

stimulating hormone and ferritin levels have been shown to be significantly elevated in asymptomatic women who subsequently have a spontaneous preterm birth before 35 weeks.[140, 145] Additionally, elevated levels of cervical ferritin and lactoferrin in asymptomatic women also have been shown to be significantly associated with subsequent spontaneous preterm birth.[144, 358]

Clearly, additional biochemical markers with improved sensitivity and specificity are needed. Use of these biochemical markers, alone or in combination, may improve our ability to predict which patients are at greatest risk for spontaneous preterm delivery. Of particular interest is the potential for a cervicovaginal multiple marker test. Recently, Goldenberg and co-workers demonstrated that the use of a serum multiple marker test may enhance the predictive value of the presently available serologic markers for spontaneous preterm birth.[147] Further studies are needed to address these issues.

ULTRASOUND PREDICTORS

Cervical changes occur approximately 3 to 4 weeks before delivery regardless of gestational age. Detection is dependent on digital examination, which presents problems such as introduction of infection and interobserver differences. If the external portion of the cervix is closed, it is impossible to evaluate the internal os by digital examination. Detection of these changes may be possible only late in the process, limiting our ability to affect treatment. Ultrasonography provides a more objective approach to examination of the cervix. Various cervical changes described by ultrasound studies may have predictive value, including cervical length, dilatation of the internal os, dynamic changes that occur in the cervix with time, and cervical funneling or wedging.

Several studies have compared digital examination with ultrasound. Sonek and coworkers assessed 83 patients at risk for preterm labor, reporting that a digital examination tended to underestimate cervical length by about 1 to 1.5 cm.[402] In 45% of patients, ultrasound detected changes before digital examination. Subsequent reports documented that ultrasound changes are more predictive than digital examination.[148, 339] Okitsu and colleagues noted that alterations in length and internal os dilatation occurred approximately 10 weeks before delivery, whereas the more dynamic changes occurred 4 weeks before delivery.[339] Digital examination changes, however, occurred only 3 to 4 weeks before delivery.[346]

Transvaginal ultrasound is far superior to transabdominal ultrasound. Transabdominal ultrasound is more difficult technically because the distance between the transducer and the cervix is relatively long. Cervical length and internal os dilatation, when measured transabdominally, are affected by bladder filling and emptying. Finally, fetal parts can cause acoustic shadowing of the cervix. Transperineal ultrasonography is also an effective modality to access cervical length. Transperineal cervical length assessment appears to correlate well with findings from digital cervical examination and from transvaginal sonographic assessment.[232, 366]

In a study by Smith and associates, patients at low risk were observed serially by means of transvaginal ultrasonography.[401] The average cervical length (37 mm) did not change significantly between 10 and 30 weeks and decreased slightly after week 32. Most additional studies have reported lengths of more than 30 mm as normal. Anderson and colleagues evaluated 113 patients with no history of preterm labor or cervical incompetence with transvaginal ultrasound and digital examination before 30 weeks of gestation.[11] A cervical length of less than 39 mm (50th percentile) had a sensitivity of 76% and a specificity of 59% in predicting preterm labor.[11] Other studies using various cutoff points for cervical length, ranging from 17.6 to 30 mm, demonstrated sensitivities of 72% to 100% and positive predictive values of 55% to 76%.[148, 201]

In a large multicenter trial, Iams and associates provided the clearest insights into the relationship between cervical length and spontaneous preterm delivery.[203] In this prospective study of 2915 women with a singleton pregnancy at 24 weeks' gestation, transvaginal sonographic determination of cervical length was made at 24 weeks and again at 28 weeks. Cervical length shorter than 26 mm (10th percentile) at 24 weeks was significantly associated with spontaneous preterm birth before 35 weeks (relative risk, 6.19; 95% confidence interval, 3.84 to 9.97; $P < .001$). The investigators concluded that an inverse relationship exists between cervical length and the frequency of preterm delivery.[203] The risk of spontaneous preterm birth is increased in women who have a short cervix demonstrated by transvaginal ultrasonography during pregnancy. Andrews and coworkers evaluated the use of cervical length determination before 20 weeks of gestation in women with a history of previous spontaneous preterm delivery to determine whether early cervical changes predict spontaneous preterm delivery.[16] In this study of 69 women, the presence of either a short cervical length (the 10th percentile for the study population [22 mm]) or cervical funneling was significantly associated with an increased risk for spontaneous preterm delivery, defined as earlier than 35 weeks of gestation. Owen and colleagues furthered these insights, evaluating the use of cervical length in a cohort of women at high risk screened between 16 and 18 weeks of gestation, and they demonstrated that a cervical length of 25 mm or shorter is significantly associated with increased risk for spontaneous preterm delivery before 35 weeks (relative risk, 3.4; 95% confidence interval, 2.2 to 5.4; $P < 0.0001$).[342] In contrast to cervical length in singleton pregnancies, cervical length in multiple gestations is significantly different, likely reflecting a greater risk for subsequent preterm delivery.[233, 357]

Another important factor is dilatation of the internal os. In a study by Okitsu and colleagues, dilatation of the internal os of greater than 5 mm carried a sensitivity of approximately 70% and a positive predictive value of 33.3%.[339] Gomez and associates found similar results using dilatation of greater than 7 mm as an indicator.[148]

Parulekar and coworkers studied 56 patients with a history compatible with cervical incompetence and found that 15 patients demonstrated dynamic findings in which the internal os changed from closed to 42 mm dilatated, with no alteration of cervical length.[348] These changes occurred in 1- to 3-minute intervals. Fifty percent of these patients delivered at less than 37 weeks. Okitsu and colleagues found that these changes had a positive predictive value of 22%.[339] The findings can be influenced by the patient's respiration, Valsalva maneuver, fundal pressure, and changes in amniotic fluid levels.

Ultrasound assessment of the cervix is a novel approach identifying patients who may be at higher risk for spontaneous preterm delivery, one that has only begun to be explored. As with the other modalities, data have not shown that ultrasound cervical screening results in a reduction in preterm births.

PREVENTION

Programs that attempt to decrease the rate of preterm delivery have traditionally focused on two main approaches to define high-risk status: (1) education and surveillance programs and (2) uterine activity monitoring.[70]

Education and surveillance programs train women to recognize the symptoms of preterm labor. In addition, weekly vaginal examinations may detect early cervical changes before the onset of true labor. One of the largest intervention studies was conducted by Papiernik and associates in France from 1971 to 1982.[345] Over the study interval, the preterm birth rate in the region studied decreased from 5.4% to 3.7% as the apparent result of a proactive educational program for the prevention of preterm birth. This investigation, however, was uncontrolled, and changes in antenatal care provided to the women make it difficult to assume that the improvement was due solely to the educational program. In two subsequent studies modeled after the Papiernik design, no statistically significant differences were observed.[290, 443]

Several theories may explain why these studies have failed to demonstrate significant improvements. For example, the level of education and supervision may not have been adequate for the patient population under evaluation. The highest incidence of preterm delivery tends to be in the indigent population, in which education and surveillance are more difficult to achieve. One of the most significant reasons, however, may be that early symptoms of premature labor are often subtle and varied, with diagnostic sensitivity of less than 50%.[71, 214] Women often do not perceive contractions until labor is relatively advanced. In a study by Newman and coworkers, women who had been trained in self-palpation of uterine activity identified only 15% of the contractions detected by a monitor, and as few as 11% could identify 50% of their contractions.[329]

Home monitoring of uterine activity was proposed as a potential solution to this problem. Katz and associates were the first to study home uterine monitoring performed intermittently (1 to 2 hours per day), with the data transmitted by telephone to a medical center for interpretation.[212] Retrospective analysis showed that more than four contractions per hour carried a higher risk of preterm labor, with a sensitivity of 80%. The greatest uterine activity occurred 24 to 48 hours before preterm labor. In a subsequent report, Katz and associates, using greater than four contractions per hour as an indicator of risk of preterm labor, obtained a somewhat lower sensitivity at 57%, with a positive predictive value of 72%.[213]

Because home monitoring may result in early recognition of preterm labor, the question arises of whether home monitoring and early treatment if needed lead to a delay in delivery. Morrison and colleagues conducted a prospective randomized trial in 67 women at high risk for preterm delivery.[314] Women were randomized to either home uterine monitoring or to self–uterine palpation. Results from this small study demonstrated significantly increased delay in delivery and a greater percentage of patients who reached term in those who were monitored with home uterine monitoring. Katz and associates conducted a prospective randomized study of home uterine activity monitoring to address the same issue.[213] The treatment group underwent home monitoring beginning at 24 weeks and continuing through 36 weeks of gestation, with preterm labor education and daily nursing support given by telephone. If preterm contractions occurred more often than four times an hour, the patients were admitted to the hospital for monitoring and examination. If cervical change was noted, the women received tocolytic therapy. The control group received standard antenatal care. Women in the home uterine monitoring group had a significant increase in the duration of pregnancy compared with those in the control group. Criticism of these data includes the possible overdiagnosis of preterm labor and the role played by nursing support. It is possible that nursing calls rather than uterine monitoring resulted in early diagnosis.

Only one study has completely separated the issue of home monitoring from nursing support. Mou and coworkers randomly assigned 377 high-risk patients to monitoring or no monitoring groups.[317] The monitored group phoned in their data but received no medical advice. The diagnosis of preterm labor was clearly defined by the investigators. There was a statistically significant difference in outcome, with the monitored patients demonstrating differences in mean cervical dilatation, older gestational age at birth, higher birth weight, and less neonatal intensive care.

Several studies have evaluated the use of nursing support with and without home uterine monitoring. All patients received home nursing support and were subsequently randomized to home monitoring or no monitoring groups. Unfortunately, there was no control group receiving only standard antenatal care without monitoring. In a study by Iams and associates, no difference was demonstrated between the monitored and unmonitored groups.[200] A study by Dyson and colleagues concluded that daily nursing support was more effective than home monitoring, although only in a twin subgroup.[102] A critical review of these data by McClean and coworkers suggests that this conclusion may be invalid because the same nursing team was involved in both groups.[280] One of the largest and most recent studies was conducted by Dyson and colleagues.[103] These investigators enrolled 2422 women at high risk, including 844 with twins, into a three-armed trial to receive weekly contact with a nurse, daily contact with a nurse, or a uterine contraction monitor and daily contact with a nurse. No significant differences were noted among the three treatment arms with respect to the rate of preterm delivery before 35 weeks, mean cervical dilatation at the time of preterm labor diagnosis, or neonatal outcomes. Women who received daily nurse contact and monitoring had more visits and were more frequently treated with prophylactic medications than women who received weekly nurse contact.

Whereas some of the earlier and smaller trials with home uterine activity monitoring demonstrated a significant decrease in preterm births among enrolled subjects,[213, 314] subsequent studies have not.[40, 69, 102, 103, 205] Therefore, it appears that home uterine activity monitoring is of no benefit in reducing the frequency of preterm birth.

TREATMENT

One of the main problems encountered when deciding on the optimal therapeutic intervention to prevent spontaneous preterm labor is the ability to accurately distinguish between preterm labor and preterm contractions. Traditionally, this distinction is made by the combination of persistent uterine contractions with change in the dilatation or effacement of the cervix by digital examination. Another dilemma is with regard to the aggressiveness with which we desire to treat preterm labor. Clearly, gestational age plays an important role in this decision. Before 32 weeks' gestation, an aggressive approach seems reasonable because of the neonatal consequences of early preterm birth; however, beyond this gestational age, when neonatal morbidity and mortality rates approach those of term infants, maternal treatment becomes more controversial. Many of the therapies that are discussed in this section have the potential for significant maternal and fetal side effects, and the risks of these adverse events may outweigh the benefits of treatment.

The therapeutic interventions implemented in the setting of preterm labor have the following purposes: (1) to prevent premature onset of contractions and labor, (2) to control contractions when they do occur and delay the time from onset of contractions to the actual time to delivery, and (3) to optimize fetal status and maturation before preterm delivery.[143] In this section we review many of the contemporary obstetric therapeutic strategies proposed to achieve the above-mentioned goals. As our clinical strategies have evolved with time, some therapies have been relinquished to the history books (e.g., ethanol tocolysis), and they are not discussed here.

BED REST

Bed rest represents one of the most common interventions implemented for the prevention or treatment of threatened preterm labor, but limited data exist that demonstrate a significant benefit. Goldenberg and coworkers reviewed the use of bed rest for the treatment of a variety of pregnancy complications.[133] In spite of bed rest having been prescribed for over 20% of pregnancies for a wide range of conditions, there is little evidence of its effectiveness. Unfortunately, well-done, prospective randomized studies that independently evaluate bed rest's potential effects for the treatment or prevention of preterm labor in singletons have not been performed. No benefit to reducing preterm birth has been found when bed rest was used in treating women pregnant with twins.

HYDRATION AND SEDATION

One of the mainstays in the initial treatment of preterm labor is the use of PO or IV hydration to differentiate true preterm labor from preterm contractions before cervical change. Several theories suggest why hydration may be effective in treating preterm contractions. Hydration inhibits the release of antidiuretic hormone through the Henry-Gauer reflex. This reflex, however, has been demonstrated only in animals.[38] A second theory is based on the fact that patients with preterm labor may have hypovolemia, with plasma volumes below normal. Significant delays in delivery have been reported to occur in patients with preterm contractions whose plasma volumes are expanded with albumin.[149] Few studies have evaluated the use of hydration in a prospective manner. Pircon and colleagues conducted a prospective randomized study of 48 women with preterm contractions.[352] Twenty-eight women were randomly assigned to a hydration and bed rest group and the remaining 20 women were assigned to a control bed rest alone group. No differences were found in the percentage of patients whose contractions stopped with hydration and bed rest compared to those being treated with bed rest alone. In addition, patients whose contractions were stopped by either treatment remained at an increased risk of preterm delivery.[352] Guinn and associates reported similar findings in a prospective randomized study of 179 women with preterm contractions.[161] Patients in this investigation were randomized to observation alone, IV hydration, or a single dose of subcutaneous terbutaline. No significant differences were noted among the three groups with regard to mean days to delivery or the incidence of preterm delivery; hence, IV hydration appears to offer no clinical benefit.

Sedation is also a common strategy used to differentiate between preterm labor and preterm contractions. Similar to studies of hydration, there are limited data documenting the efficacy of sedation in this clinical setting. Helfgott and coworkers performed a prospective comparative study of 119 women with preterm labor who were randomly assigned to treatment with hydration and sedation or to the control group receiving treatment with bed rest alone.[184] Women randomized to the hydration and sedation group received 500 mL of IV lactated Ringer's irrigation over 30 minutes and 8 to 12 mg of IM morphine sulfate. The results from this investigation demonstrated no significant difference between the hydration/sedation group and the bed rest group with regard to contraction cessation and preterm delivery.

Overall, the literature does not support the use of hydration, sedation, or both in the initial treatment of preterm labor. In many cases, initial hydration with IV infusion of fluid occurs before the start of IV infusion of a tocolytic agent. Rehydration with a large fluid bolus may increase the risk of fluid overload and subsequent development of pulmonary edema when used in the setting of tocolytic therapy, especially the β-sympathomimetic agents.

PROGESTERONE

Based on the progesterone withdrawal hypothesis of parturition initiation, interest has been placed on the potential use of progesterone or similar progestins for the treatment or prevention of preterm labor and delivery. Although progesterone or 6α-methyl-17α-hydroxyprogesterone (medroxyprogesterone) has been shown to have no inhibiting effect on acute preterm labor,[124, 340] a meta-analysis of six randomized controlled trials of 17α-hydroxyprogesterone caproate to prevent preterm labor and delivery revealed a significant decrease in preterm birth (odds ratio, 0.5; 95% confidence interval, 0.3 to 0.85).[217] Further studies evaluating this therapy are warranted.

CERCLAGE

Use of cerclage is generally limited to a patient with a history consistent with incompetent cervix. A cerclage is basically a suture placed circumferentially around the internal cervical os to strengthen the cervix. The cerclage can be placed either vaginally (McDonald cerclage, Shirodkar cerclage) or abdominally, depending on the cervical anatomy and obstetric history. The timing of cerclage placement is important; elective placement has a much higher success rate and a much lower complication rate than placement after cervical changes have begun to occur.[45] Generally, the optimal time for placement of a cerclage is early in the second trimester (12 to 14 weeks). By 12 weeks, the risk of spontaneous miscarriage in the first trimester is reduced, and major anatomic fetal abnormalities, such as anencephaly, can be detected by ultrasound before cerclage placement. In patients at high risk of aneuploidy or metabolic abnormalities, chorionic villus sampling can be performed before cerclage placement. There is no consensus on the gestational age beyond which cerclage placement is contraindicated; however, with fetal viability beginning around the 24th week of gestation, the risk of complications related to cerclage placement may outweigh the potential benefit after this time in pregnancy.

Initial studies evaluating the efficacy of a cerclage claimed success rates of 75% to 90%.[151] The primary limitation of these early studies was that the women involved served as their own control subjects in a comparison of pregnancy outcome with those of previous pregnancies. This is an important confounding variable because data support the occurrence of a successful pregnancy after repeated midtrimester losses.[173] Subsequently, several randomized, controlled studies have attempted to evaluate the efficacy of cerclage in patients without a classic history of cervical incompetence. Dor and associates examined twin pregnancies in which 50 patients were randomly assigned to cerclage or no cerclage groups.[95] No statistical difference was found in gestational age at delivery or in incidence of PPROM. Rush and colleagues[388] and Lazar and coworkers,[241] using similar study designs, evaluated 700 patients, finding no statistical difference in gestational age at delivery or perinatal mortality rate between the cerclage and control groups. In both reports there was a higher incidence of hospitalization and treatment with tocolytic agents for patients in the cerclage group. In a meta-analysis of all three studies, Grant again showed no statistically significant differences in outcomes between the cerclage and control groups.[151] There was, however, a nonsignificant increase in preterm delivery noted in the cerclage placement group.

One of the largest studies to date was conducted by the Royal College of Obstetricians and Gynaecologists, in which 1292 patients with histories of early deliveries or prior cervical surgery were randomly assigned to cerclage or no cerclage groups.[152, 153] Significantly fewer deliveries occurred before 33 weeks in the cerclage group (13% versus 17%). There was, however, a higher incidence of puerperal pyrexia in the cerclage group.[152] Limitations of the above-mentioned studies include ill-defined subjective enrollment criteria and lack of statistical power to adequately address neonatal morbidity outcomes. The advent of transvaginal cervical sonography may provide a way to objectively enroll patients for future cerclage intervention trials. Several prospective, randomized, multicenter clinical trials are ongoing to further elucidate the role of cerclage for the prevention of preterm birth. At the present time, cerclage is indicated only for patients with a classic history of cervical incompetence, and even in these women, the intervention is not supported by data from randomized clinical trials.

Contraindications to cerclage placement include prior rupture of membranes, evidence of intrauterine infection, major fetal anomalies, active vaginal bleeding of unknown cause, and active labor. Potential morbidities associated with cerclage placement include the risk of anesthesia, bleeding, infection, rupture of membranes, maternal soft tissue injury, and spontaneous suture displacement. Cerclage placement does not appear to incite prostaglandin release or initiate labor.[335] Complications associated with delivery include cervical laceration, which ranges in incidence from 1% to 13%.[172] Rare cases of uterine rupture have been reported in patients in whom labor occurred before suture removal. The increased incidence of cesarean delivery may be due to scarring of the cervix from the procedure.

Removal of the cerclage is normally accomplished at about 36 to 37 weeks of gestation unless labor ensues before that time. The cerclage should be removed promptly in the setting of PPROM to reduce the risk of infection because the suture left in situ may act as a wick for ascending infections.[259]

TOCOLYTICS

β-Sympathomimetic Agents

Three types of β-sympathomimetic receptors exist in humans: β_1, receptors that occur primarily in the heart, small intestine, and adipose tissue; β_2, receptors that are found in the uterus, blood vessels, bronchioles, and liver; and β_3, receptors that are found predominantly on white and brown adipocytes.[240] Stimulation of the β_2 receptors results in uterine smooth muscle relaxation. These β-sympathomimetic agents are structurally related to catecholamine, and when administered in vivo, they stimulate all β-receptors throughout the body. Although some β-sympathomimetic agents have been proposed as β_2 selective agents, at the dosages used pharmacologically, stimulation of all receptor types often occurs.[252] Such stimulation results in many of the side effects associated with the β-sympathomimetic agents. Of the β-sympathomimetic agents, the β_2 selective agents (e.g., ritodrine, terbutaline) have been the primary drugs used for the treatment of preterm labor.

RITODRINE. Ritodrine is the only medication approved by the U.S. Food and Drug Administration for the treatment of preterm labor. This approval resulted largely from studies performed by Barden and associates[24] and by Merkatz and colleagues,[295] in which ritodrine demonstrated efficacy similar to that of other tocolytic agents but with fewer side effects. In addition, pregnancy prolongation was statistically significant, with a reduction in neonatal morbidity and mortality. Subsequent reports have not been as positive regarding neonatal morbidity and mortality. The Canadian Preterm Labor Investigators Group conducted a prospective, randomized, placebo-controlled study of ritodrine therapy.[49] Ritodrine treatment significantly delayed delivery for 24 hours or less; however, it did not significantly modify perinatal outcomes. King and associates conducted a meta-

analysis that involved 16 clinical trials with a total of 890 women, demonstrating that women treated with ritodrine had significantly fewer deliveries within 24 and 48 hours of the start of therapy.[219] However, a statistically significant decrease in the incidence of respiratory distress syndrome, birth weight less than 2500 gm, and perinatal death were not demonstrated. These studies were completed before the use of antenatal steroid therapy became widespread.

Ritodrine can be administered IV or PO. Treatment usually begins with IV infusion. The patient should be closely monitored for fluid balance, cardiac status, and electrolytes (including potassium and glucose), and fetal monitoring should be used. The initial infusion rate of 100 μg per minute described by Barden and coworkers[24] may be too high. A more recent study by Caritis and colleagues suggests an initial infusion of 50 μg per minute with a maximal rate of 350 μg per minute.[53] With cessation of uterine activity, the rate should be reduced at hourly intervals. Oral ritodrine has a rigorous dosing schedule of 10 mg every 2 hours or 20 mg every 4 hours. The half-life is 1 to 2 hours. Plasma levels are only 27% of those obtained during IV infusion, which suggests that a higher oral dose is needed to maintain adequate plasma levels.[391] Relative contraindications include diabetes mellitus, underlying cardiac disease, use of digitalis, hyperthyroidism, severe anemia, and hypertension.

Many of the maternal side effects are due to stimulation of β-receptors throughout the body. These side effects include tachycardia, hypotension, tremulousness, headache, fever, apprehension, chest tightness or pain, and shortness of breath.[30] Serious maternal cardiopulmonary side effects have also been reported, including pulmonary edema, myocardial ischemia, arrhythmia, and maternal death.[238] Pulmonary edema may occur in about 4% of patients receiving parenteral ritodrine. Predisposing factors associated with this complication include a multiple gestation, positive fluid balance, blood transfusion, anemia, infection, polyhydramnios, and underlying cardiac disease. Pulmonary edema probably results from overhydration and an activation of the renin-angiotensin system, resulting in an increase in aldosterone, which causes salt and water retention. If untreated, the pulmonary edema can progress to adult respiratory distress syndrome. The associated use of corticosteroids has been implicated in the development of pulmonary edema. The two most commonly used antepartum steroids, betamethasone and dexamethasone, have minimal mineralocorticoid activity; hence, it is unlikely that these drugs contribute to pulmonary edema.[181] Peripartum heart failure has been reported with long-term use of β-sympathomimetics.[239] Maternal mortality has been reported with IV ritodrine therapy and is associated with pulmonary edema or arrhythmia.[24, 265] A baseline electrocardiogram should be obtained before the start of therapy, and therapy should be discontinued with a heart rate greater than 130 beats per minute or systolic blood pressure less than 90 mm Hg.

Metabolic effects of ritodrine include hypokalemia, resulting from an increase in insulin and glucose concentrations, that drives potassium intracellularly and resolves within 24 hours of discontinuing therapy. Total body potassium remains unchanged. Elevated serum glucose levels are due to an increase in cyclic adenosine monophosphate, with peak levels achieved 3 hours after initiation of treatment. Serum insulin levels also increase in response to the serum glucose elevation and as a direct effect of β_2 stimulation of the pancreas.[181] β_1 stimulation results in lipolysis and mobilization of free fatty acids, acetoacetate, and β-hydroxybutyrate.[403] In patients with diabetes, diabetic ketoacidosis may occur if blood sugar concentrations are not controlled.[429]

Initial studies evaluating long-term exposure to β-sympathomimetics demonstrate no differences in Apgar scores, head circumference, or neurologic status in terms of developmental delay and behavioral differences.[167, 199] Fetal cardiac complications have been reported. These medications readily cross the placental barrier, achieving concentrations in the fetus similar to those in maternal serum.[160] Elevation in the baseline fetal heart rate is seen, as well as a questionable increase in heart rate variability. A wide range of complications has been described, including rhythm disturbances, such as supraventricular tachycardia and atrial flutter. These complications usually resolve within a few days to 2 weeks after cessation of therapy.[46, 186] Septal hypertrophy of the fetus, antenatally and postnatally, has been described with maternal ritodrine treatment. The degree of hypertrophy correlates with the duration of therapy, and hypertrophy usually resolves within 3 months after birth.[336]

Other, more serious fetal complications have included hydrops fetalis, pulmonary edema, and extrauterine cardiac failure.[46] Fetal stillbirth, neonatal death, and a histologic finding of myocardial ischemia have been reported.[43, 244, 336] Neonatal hypoglycemia is another potential complication with β-sympathomimetics, usually developing when delivery occurs within 2 days of treatment. The hypoglycemia is transient and results in medication-induced hyperinsulinemia.[110] Neonatal periventricular-intraventricular hemorrhage may be increased with β-sympathomimetic therapy. In a retrospective study of 2827 women delivering preterm, there was a twofold increase in hemorrhage in fetuses who received betamimetics.[159] Overall, ritodrine has fallen out of favor as a primary tocolytic agent, largely as a result of these potential complications.

TERBUTALINE. Terbutaline is the most commonly used β_2 selective betamimetic agent. It was initially studied by Ingemarsson who randomly assigned 30 patients with preterm labor to IV terbutaline therapy rather than a placebo, demonstrating an 80% success rate compared with 20% for the placebo.[206] Unfortunately, as with studies of other tocolytic agents, subsequent studies of terbutaline have not reported similarly high success rates.[76, 197] One possible mechanism for the failure of long-term treatment with β-sympathomi-

metics is desensitization or downregulation of responsiveness to these agents.[32] The use of a low-dose SC infusion pump attempts to overcome this problem. Terbutaline is often administered SC in 250-μg doses every 20 to 30 minutes (four to six doses) as the first-line tocolytic agent for preterm labor. It has been effective in arresting premature labor but not preventing preterm birth.[60] Lam and associates compared the use of the terbutaline pump with PO terbutaline therapy.[235] The average duration of therapy before breakthrough of preterm labor was 9 weeks with the pump and 2 weeks with PO terbutaline. Total daily drug dosage was considerably lower (3 versus 30 mg per day).[235] Guinn and associates conducted a prospective, double-blind, randomized clinical trial comparing terbutaline pump maintenance therapy to placebo.[162] These investigators demonstrated no significant differences in the preterm delivery rate or neonatal outcomes between the women treated with terbutaline pump and those treated with placebo.

Terbutaline can be administered via PO, SC, or IV routes. When it is administered IV, the protocol includes careful monitoring of the fetus, fluid balance, cardiac status, and electrolytes. The initial infusion is 5 to 10 μg per minute, with the rate gradually increased every 10 to 15 minutes to a maximum of 80 μg per minute.[431] PO terbutaline undergoes significant intestinal tract first-pass metabolism, resulting in a bioavailability that ranges from 10% to 15%.[337] The mean half-life of terbutaline is 3.7 hours, with increased clearance in pregnant patients.[261] The usual PO doses range from 2.5 to 5 mg every 4 to 6 hours, titrated by patient response and maternal pulse.[52, 431]

Maternal side effects and complications are similar to those stated for ritodrine. Terbutaline seems to affect the maternal heart rate less than ritodrine when administered IV.[52] Both PO and IV forms of terbutaline are more diabetogenic than ritodrine.[269, 431] SC administration of terbutaline by the pump does not appear to increase the risk of gestational diabetes, but it does cause elevations in blood glucose levels in patients with diabetes.[250] Neonatal effects of maternally administered terbutaline are similar to those of ritodrine.

Magnesium Sulfate

Magnesium sulfate is one of the most commonly used tocolytic agents. Use of magnesium sulfate as a tocolytic agent was first described by Steer and Petrie in a randomized study of 71 patients with preterm labor.[405] Patients were allocated to IV infusion of either magnesium or ethanol or to a placebo of IV dextrose in water. The magnesium group received a 4-gm bolus followed by a maintenance infusion of 2 gm per hour. The success rate, defined by the absence of contractions for 24 hours, was 77% for magnesium versus 45% for ethanol and 44% for the placebo.[405] Miller and colleagues conducted a randomized comparison of magnesium and terbutaline, demonstrating that magnesium had efficacy similar to terbutaline but fewer side effects.[300] In contrast to IV magnesium sulfate for tocolysis, PO magnesium therapy is not effective for the treatment of preterm labor.[276, 365, 367]

Magnesium affects uterine activity by decreasing the release of acetylcholine at the neuromuscular junction, resulting in decreased amplitude of motor endplate potential and, hence, decreased sensitivity. Magnesium also causes an increase in cyclic adenosine monophosphate, altering the amount of calcium pumped out of myometrial cells,[275] as well as possibly blocking entry of calcium into cells.[89]

Magnesium sulfate is administered IV and is normally given as an initial bolus of 4 to 6 gm over 30 minutes, followed by a maintenance infusion of 1 to 4 gm per hour. Magnesium is excreted almost exclusively by the kidneys. Approximately 75% of the infused dose of magnesium is excreted during the infusion, and 90% is excreted by 24 hours.[87] Magnesium is reabsorbed at the renal level by a transport-limited mechanism; therefore, the glomerular filtration rate significantly affects excretion. On the basis of in vitro studies, serum magnesium levels of 5 to 8 mg/dL are considered to be therapeutic for inhibiting myometrial activity.[6] Once cessation of uterine activity is achieved, the patient is maintained at the lowest possible rate for 12 to 24 hours and weaned off as tolerated.

Maternal side effects secondary to magnesium sulfate are typically dose related. Common side effects noted with the use of magnesium sulfate include flushing, nausea, headache, drowsiness, and blurred vision. Constant monitoring of deep tendon reflexes and serum magnesium levels is mandatory to avoid toxicity. Deep tendon reflexes diminish when serum magnesium levels reach or exceed 12 mg/dL (10 mEq/L). Significant respiratory depression can occur as serum levels reach 14 to 18 mg/dL (12 to 14 mEq/L), and cardiac arrest may occur with levels greater than 18 mg/dL (15 mEq/L).[89] In general, respiratory depression does not occur before loss of deep tendon reflexes. The toxic effects of high magnesium levels can be rapidly reversed with the infusion of 1 gm of calcium gluconate.

Absolute contraindications to the use of magnesium sulfate include myasthenia gravis or heart block. Relative contraindications include underlying renal disease or recent myocardial infarction or use of calcium channel blockers. Concurrent use of calcium channel blockers and magnesium sulfate can result in profound hypotension and should be avoided.[29, 231] Pulmonary edema has been reported to have an incidence rate of approximately 1%.[107] The risk for pulmonary edema is increased in patients with multiple gestation and those receiving combined tocolytic therapy. Because of the potential risk of fluid overload and the subsequent development of pulmonary edema, periodic assessment of fluid balance is essential.

Magnesium readily crosses the placenta, achieving fetal steady-state levels within hours of treatment. Fetal heart rate variability is unaffected by maternal magnesium treatment.[404] No significant alterations in neurologic states or Apgar scores have been reported

with mean umbilical cord concentrations of 3.6 mg/dL.[157] At a cord concentration between 4 and 11 mg/dL, respiratory depression and motor depression have been seen.[351] Long-term use of magnesium (more than 7 days) has been reported to cause fetal bone loss in the proximal humerus, involving 6 of 11 fetuses in comparison with fetuses in the control group.[196] No other studies have reported this finding to date. Serum calcium levels in the fetus and newborn are unchanged or minimally reduced.[86] In summary, overall neonatal side effects and complications with magnesium are minimal compared with β-sympathomimetic therapy.

One interesting and potentially beneficial effect of magnesium sulfate is the potential for reduced neonatal mortality and neurologic morbidity. Three observational reports have suggested that antenatal magnesium sulfate treatment for preterm labor or preeclampsia is associated with a decreased risk for cerebral palsy in infants of very low birth weight.[328, 179, 390] Grether and coworkers conducted a case-control study that demonstrated that magnesium sulfate tocolysis was associated with a decreased risk of mortality (adjusted odds ratio, 0.09; 95% confidence interval, 0.01 to 0.93).[158] A large, prospective multicenter trial is presently ongoing to further explore the potential neonatal benefits of antenatal magnesium sulfate therapy.

Prostaglandin Synthetase Inhibitors

Prostaglandins appear to play a pivotal role in the pathway leading to preterm labor and delivery; therefore, attempts to interrupt this cascade of events are of utmost importance. Prostaglandins are 20-carbon cyclopentane carboxylic acids derived from membrane phospholipids (primarily arachidonic acid) via the enzymatic action of phospholipase A and cyclooxygenase (prostaglandin synthetase). Because a number of drugs that inhibit the action of prostaglandin synthetase are available (e.g., aspirin, ibuprofen, indomethacin, sulindac), this pathway represents a key target for pharmacologic intervention. Of these drugs, indomethacin has been the most extensively studied.

INDOMETHACIN. Indomethacin was first used as a tocolytic agent by Zuckerman and associates who administered it to 50 patients with preterm labor.[446] Tocolysis was achieved in 40 of the 50 patients for at least 48 hours. The first prospective, randomized, double-blind, placebo-controlled study was performed by Niebyl and colleagues.[330] In this study of 30 women with preterm labor, only 1 of 15 women in the indomethacin group failed therapy after 24 hours in comparison with 9 of 15 women in the placebo group. Morales and coworkers compared indomethacin with ritodrine in a randomized trial and found similar efficacy at 48 hours and 7 days.[308] Maternal side effects requiring discontinuation of treatment were much more common in the ritodrine group (24% versus 0%). No differences in fetal side effects were noted except for higher serum glucose levels in the ritodrine group. Similar efficacy was noted by the same authors in a comparative trial of indomethacin and magnesium sulfate.[309]

Indomethacin is usually administered PO or PR in divided doses. A loading dose of 50 to 100 mg is followed by a total 24-hour dose not greater than 200 mg. Initial duration of therapy is 48 hours. Indomethacin blood concentrations usually peak 1 to 2 hours after PO administration, whereas PR administration is associated with levels that peak slightly sooner.[7] Approximately 90% of the drug is protein bound and is excreted by the kidneys unchanged.[416] Indomethacin readily crosses the placenta, equilibrating with maternal concentrations 5 hours after administration. The half-life is approximately 15 hours in the term neonate and somewhat shorter in the preterm neonate.[37]

Most studies have limited the use of indomethacin to 24 to 48 hours' duration because of concerns regarding the development of oligohydramnios and ductal constriction, which may lead to fetal pulmonary hypertension and persistent fetal circulation.[50, 270, 305] If longer therapy is required, close fetal monitoring is indicated, including weekly amniotic fluid indexes and ductal velocities examining for ductal constriction or closure. If the amniotic fluid volume (measured as the fluid depth in the four quadrants of the uterus) falls below 5 cm or if the pulsatility index of the ductus arteriosus is less than 2 cm per second, discontinuation of therapy should be considered. Several long-term studies have evaluated the efficacy and safety of this drug. One study involving 31 fetuses exposed to indomethacin for an average of 44 days compared outcomes to appropriately matched control fetuses and found no statistically significant differences in outcome.[128]

Maternal contraindications to indomethacin use include peptic ulcer disease; allergies to indomethacin or related compounds; hematologic, hepatic, or renal dysfunction; and drug-induced asthma. Fetal contraindications include pre-existing oligohydramnios, a gestational age older than 32 weeks, and congenital fetal heart disease in which the fetus is dependent on the ductus arteriosus for circulation. Major maternal side effects are minimal and infrequent. Gastrointestinal upset may occur, but it can be relieved by either taking the medication with meals or using an antacid.

Several fetal side effects have been reported with the use of indomethacin (see Chapter 11, Part One). Oligohydramnios has been associated with indomethacin.[50, 221] Fetal urine output has been shown to decrease following administration of indomethacin. Within 24 hours after discontinuation of indomethacin therapy, however, urine output returns to baseline levels, indicating a role for prostaglandins in urine production.[50, 221] Examining the effect on renal artery blood flow, Mari and associates found no change in the pulsatility index in 17 fetuses during the first 24 hours of indomethacin therapy.[273] This finding suggests that renal artery constriction and a decrease in blood flow were not responsible for the reduction in

urine output. Therapy for more than 7 days eventually results in the development of oligohydramnios.[222] The onset of oligohydramnios seems to vary from one patient to another and is somewhat unpredictable; therefore, the amniotic fluid index should be followed while the patient is receiving therapy. Resolution usually occurs within 48 hours of discontinuation of treatment. Persistent anuria, neonatal death, and renal microcystic lesions have been reported with prenatal indomethacin exposure.[426] Most of these infants were exposed to doses greater than 200 mg per day for up to 36 weeks of gestation with inadequate amniotic fluid assessment.[426]

Another important potential complication is the development of ductal constriction or closure with prenatal indomethacin exposure. It is theorized that ductal constriction or closure leads to the diversion of right ventricular blood flow into the pulmonary vasculature. With time, this diversion causes pulmonary arterial hypertrophy. After birth, relative pulmonary hypertension can cause shunting of blood through the foramen ovale and away from the lungs, resulting in persistent fetal circulation (see Chapter 43). This complication has been described with long-term indomethacin therapy but not in fetuses exposed to the drug for less than 48 hours.[36, 128]

Development of ductal constriction identified by Doppler echocardiography in human fetuses was first described by Huhta and colleagues.[198] Moise and co-workers detected ductal constriction in 7 of 14 fetuses exposed in utero, with the change seen up to 72 hours after initiation of treatment.[305] There was no correlation with maternal drug levels, and the constrictions resolved within 24 hours after treatment was stopped. No cases of persistent fetal circulation were reported. The observed effects on ductal constriction have been shown to increase with advancing gestational age.[306] At 32 weeks' gestation, 50% of fetuses will demonstrate constriction. On the basis of these data, indomethacin therapy should be discontinued by 32 weeks at the latest.

Another reported complication is an increased risk of necrotizing enterocolitis in fetuses exposed to indomethacin prenatally and who are delivered at less than 30 weeks. Norton and associates performed a retrospective case-control study of 57 fetuses that were delivered at younger than 30 weeks' gestation following recent exposure to indomethacin and compared them with 57 matched control fetuses.[333] In this case-control study, the incidence rate of necrotizing enterocolitis was 29% in the indomethacin group versus 8% in the control group. Additionally, a statistically higher incidence of grades II to IV intraventricular hemorrhage and patent ductus arteriosus was noted in the indomethacin treatment group.[333] No correlations were made with regard to duration of treatment or the time frame of exposure to indomethacin in relation to delivery. Although these results are of concern, when used with the appropriate caution (less than 48 hours of therapy, fetuses younger than 30 to 32 weeks' gestation), indomethacin appears to be a relatively safe and effective tocolytic agent.

SULINDAC. Sulindac is another prostaglandin synthetase inhibitor that is closely related to indomethacin in structure, and it has been reported to have fewer side effects when used for tocolysis.[360] Preliminary experiences, however, indicate that PO sulindac therapy may not be very useful in the prevention of preterm birth.[54] Kramer and colleagues conducted a randomized, double-blind study to evaluate the comparative effects of sulindac and terbutaline on fetal urine production and amniotic fluid volume.[227] Sulindac administration resulted in a significant decrease in fetal urine flow and amniotic fluid volume. Additionally, two fetuses developed severe ductal constriction. Thus, sulindac can cause many of the fetal side effects associated with indomethacin.

Calcium Channel Blockers

Calcium channel blockers are agents that antagonize or normalize excessive transmembrane calcium influx, thus controlling muscle contractility and pacemaker activity in cardiac, vascular, and uterine tissue.[120] To date, most clinical investigations that evaluate the use of calcium channel blockers for the treatment of preterm labor have used nifedipine. Ulmsten and coworkers first reported the use of nifedipine for the treatment of preterm labor in a study involving 10 patients, with resultant cessation of uterine activity for 3 days in all patients during treatment.[423] In a subsequent randomized, controlled study, Read and colleagues reported that the nifedipine group had a significantly longer time interval from presentation to delivery than either a ritodrine or a placebo control group.[362] Ferguson and associates demonstrated that nifedipine was as effective as ritodrine in prolonging pregnancy but that it had far fewer side effects that required discontinuation of therapy.[117]

Nifedipine can be administered in PO or SL form. It is rapidly absorbed by the gastrointestinal tract with detectable blood levels attained within 5 minutes of SL administration.[355] Nifedipine readily crosses the placenta, and serum concentrations of the fetus and the mother are comparable.[374] An initial loading dose of 20 mg PO is typically given, followed by 10 to 20 mg every 6 to 8 hours. Up to 30 mg can be administered per dose, but this dosage may result in more side effects. The SL form is usually not used for treatment of preterm labor because it acts more rapidly than the PO form and can cause acute hypotension.

Contraindications to the use of nifedipine, or any of the calcium channel blockers, include hypotension, congestive heart failure, aortic stenosis, and pre-existing peripheral edema. Concurrent use of calcium channel blockers and magnesium sulfate can result in profound hypotension and should be avoided. Maternal side effects from calcium channel blockers result from the potent vasodilatory effects. These side effects can include dizziness, lightheadedness, flushing, headache, and peripheral edema. The incidence rate of these side effects is approximately 17%, whereas severe effects resulting in the discontinuation of therapy occur in 2% to 5% of patients.[410]

Studies evaluating the fetal effects of calcium channel blocker therapy have been limited to date. One concern is the potential adverse effect calcium channel blockers may have on uteroplacental blood flow, which has been reported in animal studies.[171] Several reports have examined uteroplacental blood flow in patients receiving nifedipine.[272, 312] These studies have demonstrated no significant adverse effects on fetal or uteroplacental blood flow during treatment.[272, 312] Additional studies are needed to more completely evaluate the potential fetal effects of calcium channel blocker therapy. The role of the calcium channel blockers for the treatment of preterm labor remains to be defined.

Oxytocin Antagonists

Oxytocin antagonists have recently been set forth as a novel category of agents that may be useful for the treatment of preterm labor. Because preterm labor may result from early gap junction formation coupled with a rise in oxytocin receptor concentration, oxytocin may be a pivotal hormone in the evolution of parturition.[21, 125] Oxytocin has been shown to be intimately involved in the physiologic pathways that lead to both term[445] and preterm labor.[44] Because oxytocin may bring about the terminal event in a variety of pathophysiologic pathways that lead to preterm delivery, it involves an important central pathway that may be amenable to therapeutic intervention. Because the primary cellular targets for oxytocin are the myometrium and decidua, oxytocin antagonists have the theoretical benefit of being highly organ specific and, thus, having minimal potential for adverse side effects.

Oxytocin antagonists have been shown to effectively inhibit oxytocin-induced uterine contractions in both in vitro and in vivo animal models. The initial human experience with oxytocin antagonist therapy came from several small, uncontrolled studies from the late 1980s.[3, 12] Akerlund and coworkers reported on a series of 13 patients who received a short-term infusion of an oxytocin antagonist that resulted in inhibition of premature labor in all patients; however, 10 of the patients subsequently required treatment with β-agonists.[3] Similarly, Andersen and colleagues reported their experience with 12 patients between 27 and 33 weeks' gestation who were treated with a competitive oxytocin receptor antagonist for 1.5 to 13 hours. Of the 12 patients treated in this case series, 9 had arrest of contractions and remaining 3 patients had no change in contraction frequency.[12]

The most studied oxytocin antagonist is atosiban. Atosiban is a nonapeptide oxytocin analogue that competitively antagonizes the oxytocin-vasopressin receptor and is capable of inhibiting oxytocin-induced uterine contractions. Standard dosing recommendations are for a single initial IV bolus of 6.75 mg of atosiban, followed by an IV infusion at 300 μg per minute for the first 3 hours, then 100 μg per minute for up to 18 hours. Maintenance therapy can be implemented at a rate of 30 μg per minute via continuous infusion.

Several prospective, randomized, blinded clinical trials have demonstrated that atosiban is effective in diminishing uterine contractions in women with threatened preterm birth without causing significant maternal fetal or neonatal adverse effects. Goodwin and associates demonstrated that a 2-hour infusion of atosiban significantly decreased contraction frequency compared with placebo.[150] Romero and colleagues, in a prospective, randomized, double-blind, placebo-controlled multicenter investigation of 501 women with documented preterm labor, demonstrated that atosiban is significantly more effective than placebo in delaying delivery 24 hours, 48 hours, and 7 days.[385] However, the median duration from start of therapy to delivery or treatment failure was not significantly different between the study groups, nor were perinatal outcomes. Moutquin and associates compared atosiban to ritodrine for the treatment of preterm labor.[304] In this multicenter, double-blind, randomized, controlled trial of 212 women with documented preterm labor, the investigators demonstrated comparable tocolytic efficacy of atosiban and conventional ritodrine therapy; however, atosiban was associated with fewer adverse side effects. Similarly, no differences were noted between the groups with respect to neonatal outcomes. The potential use of atosiban for maintenance therapy in patients with arrested preterm labor has also recently been evaluated. Valenzuela and colleagues reported experience from a multicenter, double-blind, placebo-controlled trial of 513 women with arrested preterm labor.[425] Median time from start of maintenance therapy to first recurrence of labor was significantly longer for women treated with atosiban (32.6 days) than for placebo-treated women (27.6 days).

These data suggest that atosiban may be useful in delaying delivery 24 to 48 hours in the setting of preterm labor; however, this delay appears to have minimal affect on neonatal outcomes. Atosiban represents a new approach to the treatment of preterm labor. Further studies are needed to more clearly elucidate the role of the oxytocin antagonists into the therapeutic armamentarium for preterm labor.

Nitric Oxide Donors

Nitric oxide is a potent endogenous hormone that facilitates smooth muscle relaxation in the vasculature, the gut, and the uterus. Recently, interest has arisen regarding the potential use of nitric oxide donors (e.g., nitroglycerin, glycerol trinitrate) as a potential tocolytic therapy. Lees and coworkers compared transdermal glycerol trinitrate to ritodrine for tocolysis in a randomized investigation of 245 women with documented preterm labor between 24 and 36 weeks of gestation.[243] These investigators found no significant differences between glycerol trinitrate and the ritodrine with respect to tocolytic effect and neonatal outcomes. Use of glycerol trinitrate, however,

was associated with fewer maternal side effects. Clavin and associates provided further insights into the potential use of nitric oxide donors for the treatment of preterm labor.[67] Thirty-four women in preterm labor were randomized to tocolysis with either IV nitroglycerin or magnesium sulfate. No difference in the tocolytic efficacy was noted between the two treatments; however, 3 of the 15 women who received nitroglycerin experienced severe hypotension.[67] Similarly, El-Sayed and colleagues evaluated 31 women with documented preterm labor prior to 35 weeks of gestation in a randomized comparison of IV nitroglycerin and magnesium sulfate.[109] Tocolytic failures (tocolysis at 12 hours or later) were significantly more common in women treated with nitroglycerin than in women treated with magnesium sulfate. Importantly, 25% of the women treated with nitroglycerin experienced significant hypotension that required discontinuation of treatment. Given the potential profound hemodynamic effects of these nitric oxide donors on the central and peripheral circulations, these agents should be used with caution in the pregnant patient. Clinical use of these agents for the treatment of preterm labor remains experimental.

ANTIBIOTICS

As previously discussed, preterm labor, especially before 30 weeks of gestation, has been associated with occult upper genital tract infection. Many of the bacterial species involved in this occult infection are capable of inciting an inflammatory response, which ultimately may culminate in preterm labor and delivery.[28, 287] It is on this basis that antibiotics have been suggested as a potential therapy for the treatment or prevention of spontaneous preterm birth.

Elder and coworkers provided the first insights into the potential use of antibiotics to prevent preterm birth.[105] They demonstrated that treatment of nonbacteriuric, asymptomatic pregnant patients with daily tetracycline therapy, as part of an ongoing randomized treatment study of bacteriuria in pregnancy, resulted in fewer preterm births.[105] Subsequent prospective trials of antibiotics in women colonized with *Chlamydia* species, *Ureaplasma* species, and GBS have shown no significant decrease in preterm birth.[111, 112, 223] Recently, however, the association of bacterial vaginosis with preterm birth has prompted renewed interest in the potential use of antibiotics to prevent preterm birth in asymptomatic women. Several prospective antibiotic trials have demonstrated that antenatal treatment of bacterial vaginosis in asymptomatic women at high risk for spontaneous preterm delivery may reduce the subsequent spontaneous preterm delivery rate.[178, 310] Hauth and associates conducted a prospective, randomized, double-blind, placebo-controlled study of 624 women who were identified as being at risk for preterm delivery (e.g., history of previous preterm birth or prepregnancy weight less than 50 kg).[178] These women were randomized to groups being treated with metronidazole 250 mg three times daily for 7 days, erythromycin 333 mg three times daily for 14 days, or placebo. These investigators observed a significant reduction in the rate of preterm birth (49% versus 31%) in subjects with bacterial vaginosis who received antibiotic treatment; however, antibiotic treatment of women without bacterial vaginosis was associated with a significant *increase* in the rate of preterm birth (13.4% versus 4.8%; *P* = .02).[178] Carey and colleagues evaluated the potential use of metronidazole to prevent preterm birth in a prospective, randomized, placebo-controlled study of 1704 low-risk asymptomatic women with bacterial vaginosis.[51] Results from this investigation revealed that treatment of asymptomatic bacterial vaginosis in women at low risk does not reduce the risk for preterm delivery or adverse perinatal outcomes. Based on these data it appears that screening and treatment of bacterial vaginosis in women at high risk for preterm delivery may be an effective treatment to prevent preterm birth. Nondiscriminative screening and treatment of asymptomatic women at low risk does not appear to offer any clear benefit.

In contrast to these data, data reporting on the use of antibiotics for the treatment of documented preterm labor has shown mixed results.[220] Whereas several prospective, randomized trials using antibiotics (ampicillin alone or with metronidazole) to treat documented preterm labor have demonstrated increased pregnancy prolongation and reduced neonatal morbidities,[323, 332, 408] a recent Cochrane meta-analysis summarizing eight of the randomized, controlled clinical trials comparing antibiotic therapy to placebo for the treatment of documented preterm labor demonstrated no difference between placebo and antibiotic treatment with regard to preterm delivery rate, mean pregnancy prolongation, and the incidence of respiratory distress syndrome or neonatal sepsis.[220] Antibiotics were significantly associated with a decreased risk for maternal infection and neonatal necrotizing enterocolitis. Importantly, however, antibiotic use was associated with an increase in perinatally related mortality (odds ratio, 3.47; 95% confidence interval, 1.05 to 11.38). Clearly, further studies are needed to evaluate novel antibiotic regimens and strategies for the treatment of women with preterm labor.

One important use of antibiotics in the setting of preterm delivery is in relation to PPROM. Numerous investigations have shown that the use of a variety of antibiotics in the setting of PPROM can result in increased latency period from the time of membrane rupture to the time of delivery. Recently, Mercer and coworkers reported on a large, prospective, randomized clinical investigation conducted through the NICHD/MFMU network designed to address more clearly the neonatal benefits of antenatal antibiotic use in women with PPROM.[293] For this investigation, 614 women with PPROM were randomized to treatment with either IV ampicillin (2 gm every 6 hours) or erythromycin (250 mg every 6 hours) for 48 hours followed by PO amoxicillin (250 mg every 8 hours) and erythromycin base (333 mg every 8 hours) for 5 days or a matched placebo treatment regimen. In addition to significantly increasing the latency period,

the use of antibiotics in this investigation resulted in a significant reduction in the incidence of respiratory distress syndrome, necrotizing enterocolitis, and composite neonatal morbidity (defined as any of the following: fetal or infant death, respiratory distress, severe intraventricular hemorrhage, stage II or III necrotizing enterocolitis, or sepsis within 72 hours of birth).[293] These results clearly depict the benefits of antibiotic use in the patient population.

CORTICOSTEROIDS

The use of antenatal corticosteroids for the prevention of neonatal respiratory distress syndrome stems from the original animal work by Liggins and Howie in the late 1960s (see Chapter 11, Part One, and Chapter 42). They observed that gravid sheep that had received glucocorticoids to induce preterm labor gave birth to lambs that had accelerated fetal lung maturity and decreased respiratory problems at birth. To follow up on this interesting observation, these investigators conducted the first trial of antenatal glucocorticoid therapy in humans and found that antenatal glucocorticoid administration (12 mg of betamethasone on two occasions 24 hours apart) resulted in a significant decrease in the incidence of respiratory distress syndrome with an associated decrease in perinatal mortality in newborns born before 34 weeks.[247] Interestingly, the observed effect was noted only if delivery occurred after more than 24 hours had elapsed from the first dose and less than 7 days after treatment.

Since that landmark study was published, over 15 additional prospective, randomized, controlled trials have confirmed the decrease in neonatal respiratory distress syndrome related to antenatal administration of glucocorticoids (either betamethasone or dexamethasone). Crowley conducted a meta-analysis of 15 randomized, controlled trials confirming that antenatal glucocorticoid therapy significantly decreased the incidence and severity of neonatal respiratory distress syndrome.[83, 84] Neonatal mortality also was reduced significantly, as well as the incidence of intraventricular hemorrhage and necrotizing enterocolitis. The optimal window for these benefits appeared to be maximal if delivery occurred more than 24 hours after starting treatment but within 7 days.

In spite of these data, antenatal corticosteroids remained underused throughout the 1980s and early 1990s, and the NIH convened a Consensus Development Conference on Antenatal Steroids in 1994 to review the potential risks and benefits of antenatal corticosteroid therapy.[326] Overall, the panel concluded that sufficient data demonstrate that antenatally administered corticosteroids (betamethasone or dexamethasone) significantly reduce the incidence or severity of respiratory distress syndrome, intraventricular hemorrhage, and potentially necrotizing enterocolitis.[326] The panel recommended that all women with fetuses who are between 24 and 34 weeks' gestation at risk for preterm delivery and who are eligible for tocolytic therapy should be considered candidates for antenatal corticosteroid treatment. Additionally, given that treatment for less than 24 hours was significantly associated with a decreased risk for respiratory distress syndrome, intraventricular hemorrhage, and mortality, the panel concluded that steroids should be administered unless delivery is imminent. For women with PPROM, treatment was recommended at less than 30 to 32 weeks because of the high risk of intraventricular hemorrhage. Unresolved issues include the efficacy and safety of repeated steroid dosing, the appropriate dosing and efficacy in multiple gestation and the potential to enhance fetal lung maturation in fetuses beyond 34 weeks' gestation. Recent studies demonstrating worse outcomes in newborns whose mothers received multiple courses of corticosteroids strongly suggest that the practice of giving repetitive weekly courses until 34 weeks be discontinued unless data from randomized clinical trials demonstrate benefit for this practice.[101, 123, 444]

Long-term follow-up on infants exposed in utero to antenatal corticosteroid therapy at 3 and 6 years has not demonstrated any adverse effect on growth, physical development, motor or cognitive skills, or school progress.[68, 262] Hence, a single course of corticosteroids appears to be an efficacious and safe treatment modality to improve neonatal outcomes in patients with preterm delivery.

The commonly used steroids for the enhancement of fetal maturity are betamethasone (12 mg IM every 24 hours, 2 doses) and dexamethasone (6 mg IV every 6 hours, 4 doses). These two glucocorticoids have been identified as the most efficacious because they readily cross the placental barrier to reach the fetal compartment and have long half-lives and limited mineralocorticoid activity.

THYROTROPIN-RELEASING HORMONE

The potential use of thyrotropin-releasing hormone (TRH) to enhance fetal pulmonary maturation was initially proposed based on animal studies that demonstrated that triiodothyronine (T_3) enhances surfactant synthesis (see Chapter 42). Prenatally administered TRH crosses the placental barrier and reaches the fetus, resulting in increased T_3 and prolactin biosynthesis. Concurrent administration of glucocorticoid and T_3 has been shown to be more effective than glucocorticoid alone to accelerate surfactant and to improve lung compliance in the lamb.[389] Several studies have demonstrated enhanced fetal lung maturation with the combined use of TRH and glucocorticoids compared with glucocorticoid treatment alone.[22, 224] Ballard and associates conducted a prospective, randomized trial of TRH and glucocorticoid versus glucocorticoid alone in gestations less than 32 weeks.[22] When one full course of treatment was given and delivery occurred within 10 days, the two treatment groups had no difference in the incidence of respiratory distress syndrome in newborns weighing less than 1500 gm. However, the incidence of chronic lung disease was 18% in the combined therapy group versus 44% in the glucocorticoid therapy alone group

($P < .01$), and fewer cases of chronic lung disease or death (19% versus 38%; $P < .01$) occurred with combined treatment. No short-term adverse effects were noted.

To further evaluate the potential benefit of TRH, Ballard and associates conducted a subsequent prospective, placebo-controlled study of 996 women randomized to treatment with TRH and glucocorticoid or with placebo and glucocorticoid.[23] Results from this investigation, in contrast with the findings from their original study, demonstrated that antenatal TRH and glucocorticoid offered no additional benefit with respect to neonatal morbidity and mortality as compared with glucocorticoid treatment alone. Similar findings were noted with data from the Australian ACROBAT trial in which 1234 women were randomized to receive either TRH with corticosteroids or corticosteroids alone.[85] This study failed to demonstrate any beneficial effects from the use of TRH. In fact, the incidence of respiratory distress syndrome was actually increased in the patients who received the combined treatment. Additionally, the investigators observed that 7% of the mothers became overtly hypertensive as a result of the TRH therapy. These investigators concluded that using TRH to augment fetal maturation appears to offer little benefit, while causing potential harmful maternal and neonatal effects; hence, the use of TRH is not recommended.

PHENOBARBITAL AND VITAMIN K

Until recently, antenatal maternal treatment with phenobarbital, vitamin K, or both was thought to reduce the incidence of intraventricular hemorrhage. This assumption was based on a series of reports that observed benefit from this therapy; however, these reports failed to control for the use of corticosteroids, which have been shown to significantly decrease the incidence of intraventricular hemorrhage.[292] In an attempt to answer more definitively the question of the potential benefit of phenobarbital and vitamin K for the prevention of intracranial hemorrhage, Thorp and colleagues conducted a prospective, randomized, placebo-controlled study of 372 women at risk for preterm birth.[414] Patients were randomized to receive either placebo or treatment with phenobarbital and vitamin K. These investigators found no difference between the two treatment groups with regard to the incidence of grade III and grade IV intraventricular hemorrhage in newborns less than 34 weeks' gestation. Similarly, Shankaran and coworkers conducted a prospective, placebo-controlled clinical trial of 610 women with threatened preterm delivery.[397] Women were randomized to either treatment with antenatal phenobarbital or a placebo group. The results from this investigation demonstrated that antenatal phenobarbital does not decrease the risk of intracranial hemorrhage (see Chapter 11, Part One). Hence, based on the available literature, it appears that neither phenobarbital nor vitamin K offer significant advantage for the prevention of intraventricular hemorrhage above that observed with the use of antenatal corticosteroids.

SUMMARY

In this chapter, we reviewed in detail the epidemiology and pathophysiology of preterm labor, as well as the therapeutic strategies used for prevention and treatment. In spite of our efforts thus far, preterm labor and delivery remains a significant clinical problem globally, accounting for a substantial amount of all neonatal morbidity and mortality. Although we have gained important insights into the pathophysiology of preterm labor over the past several decades, effective therapeutic interventions to decrease spontaneous preterm delivery have not been discovered. Clearly, the development of effective screening tools to identify patients at greatest risk for spontaneous preterm delivery is important for the development of novel therapeutic strategies. As our insights into the diverse etiologies of spontaneous preterm labor evolve, these strategies may lead to a significant reduction in the incidence of spontaneous preterm delivery, with concomitant improvement in perinatal morbidity and mortality rates. Clearly, ongoing research is needed to further explore the pathophysiology of spontaneous preterm delivery and potential therapeutic approaches to deal with this important clinical problem.

■ REFERENCES

1. Abel MH, et al: Suppression of concentration of endometrial prostaglandin in early intrauterine and ectopic pregnancy in women. J Endocrinol 85:379, 1980.
2. Advance Report of Final Natality Studies. Monthly Vital Statistics Report. Washington, DC, National Center for Health Statistics, 1989.
3. Akerlund M, et al: Inhibition of uterine contractions of premature labour with an oxytocin analogue. Results from a pilot study. Br J Obstet Gynaecol 94:1040, 1987.
4. Alberman E, Stanley F: Guidelines to the Epidemiological Approach. In Stanley F, Alberman E (eds): Clinics in Developmental Medicine, No. 87, The Epidemiology of the Cerebral Palsies. Lavenham, Suffolk, Great Britain, Spastics International Medical Publications/Lavenham Press Ltd, 1984, p 27.
5. Allen MC, et al: The limit of viability—Neonatal outcome of infants born at 22 to 25 weeks' gestation. N Engl J Med 329:1597, 1993.
6. Altura BM, et al: Mg^{+2}-Ca^{+2} interacts in contractility of smooth muscle: Magnesium versus organic calcium-channel blockers on myogenic tone and agonist-induced responsiveness of blood vessels. Can J Physiol Pharmacol 65:729, 1987.
7. Alvan G, et al: Pharmacokinetics of indomethacin. Clin Pharmacol Ther 18:364, 1976.
8. American College of Obstetricians and Gynecologists Committee on Obstetric Practice: Committee Opinion No. 173, June 1996, Washington, DC.
9. Amstey MS, et al: Asymptomatic gonorrhea and pregnancy. J Am Vener Dis Assoc 33:14, 1976.
10. Anderson PJ, et al: Non-protein-bound estradiol and progesterone in human peripheral plasma before labor and delivery. J Endocrinol 104:7, 1985.
11. Anderson HF, et al: Prediction of risk for preterm delivery by ultrasonographic measurement of cervical length. Am J Obstet Gynecol 163:859, 1990.
12. Andersen LF, et al: Oxytocin receptor blockade: A new principle in the treatment of preterm labor? Am J Perinatol 6:196, 1989.
13. Andrews WW, et al: Preterm labor: Emerging role of genital tract infections. Infect Agents Dis 4:196, 1995.
14. Andrews WW, et al: Amniotic fluid interleukin-6: Correlation with upper genital tract microbial colonization and gestational age in women delivered after spontaneous labor versus indicated delivery. Am J Obstet Gynecol 173:606, 1995.
15. Andrews WW, et al: The preterm prediction study: Association of mid-trimester genital chlamydia infection and subsequent spontaneous preterm birth. Am J Obstet Gynecol 176:S55, 1997.
16. Andrews WW, et al: Second-trimester cervical ultrasound: Associations with increased risk for recurrent early spontaneous delivery. Obstet Gynecol 95:222, 2000.
17. Armer TL, et al: Intraamniotic infection in patients with intact membranes and preterm labor. Obstet Gynecol Surv 46:589, 1991.
18. Ascarelli MH, et al: Use of fetal fibronectin in clinical practice. Obstet Gynecol Surv 52:S1, 1997.
19. Athayde N, et al: Matrix metalloproteinases-9 in preterm and term human parturition. J Matern Fetal Med 8:213, 1999.
20. Bakketeig LS, et al: Epidemiology of preterm birth: Results from a longitudinal study of births in Norway. In Elder MG, et al (eds): Preterm Labor. London, Butterworths, 1981.
21. Balducci J, et al: Gap junction formation in human myometrium: A key to preterm labor? Am J Obstet Gynecol 168:1609, 1993.
22. Ballard RA, et al: Respiratory disease in very-low-birth weight infants after prenatal thyrotropin-releasing hormone and glucocorticoid. Lancet 339:510, 1992.
23. Ballard RA, et al: Antenatal thyrotropin-releasing hormone to prevent lung disease in preterm infants. North American Thyrotropin-Releasing Hormone Group. N Engl J Med 338:493, 1998.
24. Barden TP, et al: Ritodrine hydrochloride: A beta-mimetic agent for use in preterm labor. I. Pharmacology, clinical history, administration, side effects, and safety. Obstet Gynecol 56:1, 1980.
25. Bashore RA, et al: Plasma unconjugated estriol values in high risk pregnancy. Am J Obstet Gynecol 128:371, 1997.
26. Beischer N, et al: Urinary oestriol assay for monitoring fetoplacental function. Aust N Z J Obstet Gynaecol 31:1, 1991.
27. Beischer N, et al: The biochemistry and clinical application of urinary oestriol measurement during late pregnancy in the 1990's. Aust N Z J Obstet Gynaecol 35:151, 1995.
28. Bejar R, et al: Premature labor: II. Bacterial sources of phospholipase. Obstet Gynecol 57:479, 1981.
29. Ben-Ami M, et al: The combination of magnesium sulphate and nifedipine: A cause of neuromuscular blockade. Br J Obstet Gynaecol 101:262, 1994.
30. Beneditti TJ: Maternal complications of parenteral beta-sympathomimetic therapy for preterm labor. Am J Obstet Gynecol 145:1, 1983.
31. Benirschke K, et al: Intrauterine bacterial infection of the newborn infant. J Pediatr 54:11, 1959.
32. Berg G, et al: β-Adrenergic receptors in human myometrium during pregnancy: Changes in the number of receptors after β-mimetic treatment. Am J Obstet Gynecol 151:392, 1985.
33. Berkowitz GS, et al: Corticotropin-releasing factor and its binding protein: Maternal serum levels in term and preterm deliveries. Am J Obstet Gynecol 174:1477, 1996.
34. Berman SM, et al: Low birth weight, prematurity and postpartum endometritis: Association with prenatal cervical Mycoplasma hominis and Chlamydia trachomatis infections. JAMA 257:189, 1987.
35. Bernstein PS, et al: Beta-human chorionic gonadotropin in cervicovaginal secretions as a predictor of preterm delivery. Am J Obstet Gynecol 179:870, 1998.
36. Besinger RE, et al: Randomized comparative trial of indomethacin and ritodrine for the long-term treatment of premature labor. Am J Obstet Gynecol 164:981, 1991.
37. Bhat R, et al: Disposition of indomethacin in preterm infants. J Pediatr 95:313, 1979.

38. Bieniarz J, et al: Inhibition of uterine contractility in labor. Am J Obstet Gynecol 111:874, 1971.

39. Block BSB, et al: Preterm delivery is not predicted by serial plasma estradiol and progesterone concentration measurements. Am J Obstet Gynecol 150:716, 1984.

40. Blondel B, et al: Home uterine activity monitoring in France. A randomized controlled trial. Am J Obstet Gynecol 167:424, 1992.

41. Bobitt JR, et al: Amniotic fluid infection as determined by transabdominal amniocentesis in patients with intact membranes in premature labor. Am J Obstet Gynecol 140:947, 1981.

42. Bobitt JR, et al: Perinatal complications in group B streptococcal carriers: A longitudinal study of prenatal patients. Am J Obstet Gynecol 151:711, 1985.

43. Bohm N, et al: Focal necrosis, fatty degeneration and subendocardial nuclear polyploidization in the myocardium of newborns. Eur J Pediatr 109:687, 1986.

44. Bossmar T, et al: Receptors for and myometrial responses to oxytocin and vasopressin in preterm and term human pregnancy: Effects of the oxytocin antagonist atosiban. Am J Obstet Gynecol 171:1634, 1994.

45. Branch W: Operations for cervical incompetence. Clin Obstet Gynecol 29:240, 1986.

46. Brosset P, et al: Cardiac complications of ritodrine in mother and baby. Lancet 1:1461, 1982.

47. Brumfield CG, et al: Amniotic fluid α-fetoprotein levels and pregnancy outcome. Am J Obstet Gynecol 157:822, 1987.

48. Burrus DR, et al: Fetal fibronectin, interleukin-6, and C-reactive protein are useful in establishing prognostic subcategories of idiopathic preterm labor. Am J Obstet Gynecol 173:1258, 1995.

49. Canadian Preterm Labor Investigators Group: The treatment of preterm labor with beta-adrenergic agonist ritodrine. N Engl J Med 327:308, 1992.

50. Cantor B, et al: Oligohydramnios and transient neonatal anuria: A possible association with the maternal use of prostaglandin synthetase inhibitors. J Reprod Med 24:220, 1980.

51. Carey JC, et al: Metronidazole to prevent preterm delivery in pregnant women with asymptomatic bacterial vaginosis. National Institute of Child Health and Human Development Network of Maternal-Fetal Medicine Units. N Engl J Med 342:534, 2000.

52. Caritis SN, et al: A double-blind study comparing ritodrine and terbutaline in the treatment of preterm labor. Am J Obstet Gynecol 150:7, 1984.

53. Caritis SN, et al: Pharmacokinetics of ritodrine administered intravenously: Recommendations for changes in the current regimen. Am J Obstet Gynecol 162:429, 1990.

54. Carlan SJ, et al: Outpatient oral sulindac to prevent recurrence of preterm birth. Obstet Gynecol 85:769, 1995.

55. Carr-Hill RA, Hall MH: The repetition of spontaneous preterm labour. Br J Obstet Gynecol 92:921, 1985.

56. Casey ML, et al: Endocrinology of preterm birth. Clin Obstet Gynecol 27:562, 1984.

57. Casey ML, et al: Biomolecular processes in the initiation of parturition: Decidual activation. Clin Obstet Gynecol 31:538, 1988.

58. Casey ML, et al: The formation of cytokines in human decidua: The role of decidua in the initiation of both term and preterm labor [abstract]. Proceedings of the Society of Gynecologic Investigations, Baltimore, 1988.

59. Casey ML, et al: The role of a fetal-maternal paracrine system in the maintenance of a pregnancy and the initiation of parturition: Fetal and neonatal development. Ithaca, NY, Perinatology Press, 1989.

60. Casper RF, et al: Myometrial desensitization to continuous but not to intermittent β-adrenergic agonist infusion in the sheep. Am J Obstet Gynecol 154:301, 1986.

61. Caspi E, et al: The outcome of pregnancy after gonadotropin therapy. Br J Obstet Gynaecol 83:967, 1976.

62. Cassell G, et al: Chorioamnion colonization: Correlation with gestational age in women delivered following spontaneous labor versus indicated delivery. Am J Obstet Gynecol 168:425, 1993.

63. Cassell G, et al: Isolation of microorgansisms from the chorioamnion is twice that from amniotic fluid at cesarean delivery in women with intact membranes. Am J Obstet Gynecol 168:424, 1993.

64. Centers for Disease Control and Prevention: Prevention of perinatal group B streptococcal disease: A public health perspective. MMWR Morb Mortal Wkly Rep 45 (RR-7):1, 1996.

65. Challis JR, et al: Current topic: The placental corticotrophin-releasing hormone-adrenocorticotrophin axis. Placenta 16:481, 1995.

66. Chung C, et al: Induced abortion and spontaneous fetal loss in subsequent pregnancies. Am J Public Health 72:548, 1982.

67. Clavin DK, et al: Comparison of intravenous magnesium sulfate and nitroglycerin for preterm labor. Am J Obstet Gynecol 174:307, 1996.

68. Collaborative Group on Antenatal Steroid Therapy: Effects of antenatal dexamethasone administration in the infant: Long-term follow up. J Pediatr 104:259, 1984.

69. Collaborative Home Uterine Monitoring Study (CHUMS) Group: A multicenter randomized trial of home uterine activity monitoring. Am J Obstet Gynecol 172:253, 1995.

70. Committee to Study the Prevention of Low Birthweight, Division of Health Promotion and Disease Prevention, Institute of Medicine: Preventing Low Birthweight. Washington, DC, National Academy Press, 1985.

71. Copper RL, et al: Warning symptoms, uterine contractions, and cervical examination findings in women at risk of preterm delivery. Am J Obstet Gynecol 162:748, 1990.

72. Copper RL, et al: A multicenter study of preterm birth weight and gestational age specific neonatal mortality. Am J Obstet Gynecol 168:78, 1993.

73. Copper RL, et al: Cervical examination and tocodynamometry at 28 weeks' gestation: Prediction of spontaneous preterm birth. Am J Obstet Gynecol 172:666, 1995.

74. Copper RL, et al: The prematurity prediction study: Maternal stress is associated with spontaneous preterm birth at less than thirty-five weeks' gestation. National Institute of Child Health and Human Development Maternal-Fetal Medicine Units Network. Am J Obstet Gynecol 175:1286, 1996.

75. Cotch MF, et al: Trichomonas vaginalis associated with low birth weight and preterm delivery. The Vaginal Infections and Prematurity Study Group. Sex Transm Dis 24:353, 1997.

76. Cotton DB, et al: Comparison of magnesium sulfate, terbutaline, and a placebo for inhibition of preterm labor: A randomized study. J Reprod Med 29:92, 1984.

77. Cousins L: Cervical incompetence. In Creasy RK, et al (eds): Maternal-Fetal Medicine: Principles and Practice. New York, WB Saunders, 1984.

78. Cousins LM, et al: Serum progesterone and estradiol-17 levels in premature and term labor. Am J Obstet Gynecol 127:612, 1977.

79. Cox SM, et al: Decidual activation is synchronous with spontaneous parturition and with bacterial endotoxin (lipopolysaccharide [LPS]-induced preterm labor) [abstract]. Proceedings of the Society of Gynecologic Investigations, Baltimore, 1988.

80. Cox SM, et al: Accumulation of interleukin-1beta and interleukin-6 in amniotic fluid: A sequela of labour at term and preterm. Hum Reprod Update 3:517, 1997.

81. Creasy RK, et al: System for predicting spontaneous preterm birth. Obstet Gynecol 55:692, 1980.

82. Creasy RK. Preterm birth prevention: Where are we? Am J Obstet Gynecol 168:1223, 1993.

83. Crowley P: The effects of corticosteroid administration before preterm delivery: An overview of the evidence from controlled trials. Br J Obstet Gynaecol 97:4, 1990.

84. Crowley P: Prophylactic corticosteroids for preterm birth. Cochrane Database Syst Rev 2:CD000065, 2000.

85. Crowther CA, et al: Australian collaborative trial of antenatal thyrotropin-releasing hormone (ACROBAT) for prevention of neonatal respiratory disease. Lancet 345:877, 1995.

86. Cruikshank DP, et al: Effects of magnesium sulphate treatment on perinatal calcium metabolism. Am J Obstet Gynecol 134:243, 1979.

87. Cruikshank DP, et al: Urinary magnesium, calcium, and phosphate excretion during magnesium sulphate infusion. Obstet Gynecol 58:430, 1981.

88. Daikoku NH, et al: Premature rupture of membranes and spontaneous preterm labor: Maternal endometritis risks. Obstet Gynecol 59:13, 1982.

89. D'Alton M: Preterm labor. In Oxorn H (ed): Human Labor and Birth, 5th ed. Norwalk, Conn, Appleton-Century-Crofts, 1986.

90. Dammann O, et al: Maternal intrauterine infection, cytokines, and brain damage in the preterm newborn. Ped Res 42:1, 1996.

91. Darne J, et al: Saliva oestriol, oestradiol, oestrone, and progesterone levels in pregnancy: Spontaneous labour at term is preceded by a rise in the saliva oestriol:progesterone ratio. Br J Obstet Gynaecol 94:227, 1987.

92. Darne J, et al: Increased saliva oestriol to progesterone ratio before idiopathic preterm delivery: A possible predictor for preterm labour? Br Med J 294:270, 1987.

93. Davis RO, et al: Elevated levels of midtrimester maternal serum α-fetoprotein are associated with preterm delivery but not with fetal growth retardation. Am J Obstet Gynecol 167:596, 1992.

94. Dooley SL, et al: Urinary estriols in diabetic pregnancy: A reappraisal. Obstet Gynecol 64:469, 1984.

95. Dor J, et al: Elective cervical suture of twin pregnancies diagnosed ultrasonically in the first trimester following induced ovulation. Gynecol Obstet Invest 13:55, 1982.

96. Dray F, et al: Primary prostaglandins in amniotic fluid in pregnancy and spontaneous labor. Am J Obstet Gynecol 126:13, 1976.

97. Dudley DJ, et al: Biosynthesis of interleukin-6 by cultured human chorion laeve cell: Regulation by cytokines. J Clin Endocrinol Metab 75:1081, 1992.

98. Dudley DJ, et al: Decidual cell biosynthesis of interleukin-6: Regulation by inflammatory cytokines. J Clin Endocrinol Metab 74:884, 1992.

99. Dudley DJ: Immunoendocrinology of preterm labor: The link between corticotropin-releasing hormone and inflammation. Am J Obstet Gynecol 180:S251, 1999.

100. Duenhoelter JH, et al: An analysis of the utility of plasma immunoreactive estrogen measurements in determining delivery time of gravidas with a fetus considered at high risk. Am J Obstet Gynecol 125:889, 1976.

101. Dunlop SA, et al: Repeated prenatal corticosteroids delay myelination in the ovine central nervous system. J Matern Fetal Med 6:309, 1997.

102. Dyson DC, et al: Prevention of preterm birth in high-risk patients: The role of education and provider contact versus home uterine monitoring. Am J Obstet Gynecol 164:756, 1991.

103. Dyson DC, et al: Monitoring women at risk for preterm labor. N Engl J Med 338:15, 1998.

104. Ekwo EE, et al: Unfavorable outcome in penultimate pregnancy and premature rupture of membranes in successive pregnancy. Obstet Gynecol 80:166, 1992.

105. Elder HA, et al: The natural history of asymptomatic bacteriuria during pregnancy: The effect of tetracycline on the clinical course and outcome of pregnancy. Am J Obstet Gynecol 111:441, 1971.

106. Ellenberg J, et al: Birth weight and gestational age in children with cerebral palsy or seizure disorders. Am J Dis Child 133:1044, 1979.

107. Elliot JP, et al: Magnesium sulfate as a tocolytic agent. Am J Obstet Gynecol 147:277, 1983.

108. Elliott B, et al: Maternal gonococcal infection as a preventable factor for low birth weight. J Infect Dis 161:531, 1990.

109. El-Sayed YY, et al: Randomized comparison of intravenous nitroglycerin and magnesium sulfate for treatment of preterm labor. Obstet Gynecol 93:79, 1999.

110. Epstein MF, et al: Neonatal hypoglycemia after beta-sympathomimetic tocolytic therapy. J Pediatr 94:449, 1979.

111. Eschenbach DA, et al: Bacterial vaginosis during pregnancy. An association with prematurity and postpartum complications. Scand J Urol Nephrol Suppl 86:213, 1984.

112. Eschenbach DA, et al: A randomized placebo-controlled trial of erythromycin for the treatment of *Ureaplasma urealyticum* to prevent premature delivery. Am J Obstet Gynecol 164:734, 1991.

113. Evaldson GR, et al: Premature rupture of the membranes and ascending infection. Br J Obstet Gynaecol 89:793, 1982.

114. Fadalti M, et al: Placental corticotropin-releasing factor. An update. Ann N Y Acad Sci 900:89, 2000.

115. Fedrick J, et al: Factors associated with spontaneous preterm birth. Br J Obstet Gynaecol 83:342, 1976.

116. Feinberg FR, Kliman JH: Fetal fibronectin and preterm labor. N Engl J Med 172:134, 1992.

117. Ferguson JE II, et al: A comparison of tocolysis with nifedipine or ritodrine: Analysis of efficacy and maternal, fetal, and neonatal outcome. Am J Obstet Gynecol 163:105, 1990.

118. Fiscella K: Race, perinatal outcome, and amniotic infection. Obstet Gynecol Surv 51:60, 1996.

119. Fiscella K: Racial disparities in preterm births: The role of urogenital infections. Public Health Rep 111:104, 1996.

120. Fleckenstein A: History of calcium antagonists. Circ Res 52(Suppl 1):3, 1983.

121. Fortunato SJ, et al: MMP/TIMP imbalance in amniotic fluid during PPROM: An indirect support for endogenous pathway to membrane rupture. J Perinat Med 27:362, 1999.

122. Foulon W, et al: Markers of infection and their relationship to preterm delivery. Am J Perinatol 12:208, 1995.

123. French NP, et al: JP Repeated antenatal corticosteroids: Size at birth and subsequent development. Am J Obstet Gynecol 180:114, 1999.

124. Fuchs F, et al: Treatment of threatened premature labor with large doses of progesterone. Am J Obstet Gynecol 79:173, 1960.

125. Fuchs AR, et al: Oxytocin receptors and human parturition: A dual role for oxytocin in the initiation of labor. Science 215:1396, 1982.

126. Fuchs AR, et al: Endocrinology of human parturition: A review. Br J Obstet Gynaecol 91:948, 1984.

127. Garfield RE, et al: Appearance of gap junctions in the myometrium of women during labor. Am J Obstet Gynecol 140:254, 1981.

128. Gerson A, et al: Safety and efficacy of long-term tocolysis with indomethacin. Am J Perinatol 7:71, 1990.

129. Gibbs RS, et al: A review of premature birth and subclinical infection. Am J Obstet Gynecol 166:1515, 1992.

130. Gilstrap LC III, et al: Survival and short-term morbidity of the premature neonate. Obstet Gynecol 65:37, 1985.

131. Goepfert AR, et al: Prediction of prematurity. Curr Opin Obstet Gynecol 8:417, 1996.

132. Goepfert AR, et al: The preterm prediction study: Association between cervical interleukin-6, fetal fibronectin, and spontaneous preterm birth. Am J Obstet Gynecol 176:S6, 1997.

133. Goldenberg RL, et al: Bed rest in pregnancy. Obstet Gynecol 84:131, 1994.

134. Goldenberg RL, et al: The preterm prediction study: Fetal fibronectin, bacterial vaginosis, and peripartum infection. Obstet Gynecol 87:656, 1996.

135. Goldenberg RL, et al: Plasma ferritin and pregnancy outcome. Am J Obstet Gynecol 175:1356, 1996.

136. Goldenberg RL, et al: The preterm prediction study: Fetal fibronectin testing and spontaneous preterm birth. Obstet Gynecol 87:643, 1996.

137. Goldenberg RL, et al: Sexually transmitted diseases and adverse outcomes of pregnancy. Clin Perinatol 24:23, 1997.

138. Goldenberg RL, et al: The preterm prediction study: Patterns of cervicovaginal fetal fibronectin as predictors of spontaneous preterm delivery. Am J Obstet Gynecol 177:8, 1997.

139. Goldenberg RL, et al: Plasma alkaline phosphatase and pregnancy outcome. J Matern Fet Med 6:140, 1997.

140. Goldenberg RL, et al: Plasma ferritin, PROM and pregnancy outcome. Am J Obstet Gynecol 179:1599, 1998.

141. Goldenberg RL, et al: Markers of preterm birth. Prenat Neonat Med 3:43, 1998.

142. Goldenberg RL, et al: The prematurity prediction study: The value of new vs standard risk factors in predicting early and all spontaneous preterm births. NICHD MFMU Network. Am J Public Health 88:233, 1998.

143. Goldenberg RL, et al: Prevention of premature birth. N Engl J Med 339:313, 1998.

144. Goldenberg RL, et al: The preterm prediction study: Cervical lactoferrin, other markers of lower genital tract infection, and preterm birth. Am J Obstet Gynecol 182:631, 2000.

145. Goldenberg RL, et al: The preterm prediction study: Granulo-

cyte colony stimulating factor and spontaneous preterm birth. Am J Obstet Gynecol 182:625, 2000.

146. Goldenberg RL, et al: Intrauterine Infection and preterm delivery. N Engl J Med 342:1500, 2000.

147. Goldenberg RL, et al: Toward a multiple marker test for spontaneous preterm birth (SPB). Am J Obstet Gynecol 182:S12, 2000.

148. Gomez R, et al: Ultrasonographic examination of the uterine cervix is better than cervical digital examination as a predictor of the likelihood of premature delivery in patients with preterm labor and intact membranes. Am J Obstet Gynecol 171:956, 1994.

149. Goodlin RC, et al: The significance and diagnosis of maternal hypovolemia. Semin Perinatol 5:163, 1981.

150. Goodwin TM, et al: The effect of the oxytocin antagonist atosiban on preterm uterine activity in the human. Am J Obstet Gynecol 170:474, 1994.

151. Grant AM: Cervical cerclage: Evaluation studies. Proceedings of a Workshop on Prevention of Preterm Birth, Paris, INSERM, 1986.

152. Grant AM, et al: Final report of the Medical Research Council/Royal College of Obstetricians and Gynaecologists multicentre randomized trial of cervical cerclage. Br J Obstet Gynaecol 100:516, 1993.

153. MRC/RCOG Working Party on Cervical Cerclage: Final report of the Medical Research Council/Royal College of Obstetricians and Gynaecologists multicenter randomized trial of cervical cerclage. Br J Obstet Gynaecol 100:516, 1993.

154. Gravett MG, et al: Independent associations of bacterial vaginosis and *Chlamydia trachomatis* infections with adverse pregnancy outcome. JAMA 256:1899, 1986.

155. Gravett MG, et al: Preterm labor associated with subclinical amniotic fluid infections and with bacterial vaginosis. Obstet Gynecol 67:229, 1986.

156. Gray DJ, et al: Adverse outcome in pregnancy following amniotic fluid isolation of Ureaplasma urealyticum. Prenat Diagn 12:111, 1992.

157. Green KW, et al: The effects of maternally administered magnesium sulfate on the neonate. Am J Obstet Gynecol 146:29, 1983.

158. Grether JK, et al: Magnesium sulfate tocolysis and risk of neonatal death. Am J Obstet Gynecol 178:1, 1998.

159. Groome LJ, et al: Neonatal periventricular-intraventricular hemorrhage after maternal β-sympathomimetic tocolysis. Am J Obstet Gynecol 167:873, 1992.

160. Gross TJ, et al: Maternal and fetal plasma concentration of ritodrine. Obstet Gynecol 65:793, 1985.

161. Guinn DA, et al: Management options in women with preterm uterine contractions: A randomized clinical trial. Am J Obstet Gynecol 177:814, 1997.

162. Guinn DA, et al: Terbutaline pump maintenance therapy for prevention of preterm delivery: A double-blind trial. Am J Obstet Gynecol 179:874, 1998.

163. Guzick DS, et al: The association of chorioamnionitis with preterm delivery. Obstet Gynecol 65:11, 1985.

164. Hack M, et al: Outcomes of extremely immature infants—A perinatal dilemma. N Engl J Med 329:1649, 1993.

165. Hack M, et al: School-age outcomes in children with birth weights under 750 g. N Engl J Med 331:753, 1994.

166. Hack M, et al: Outcomes of children of extremely low birthweight and gestational age in the 1990's. Early Hum Dev 53:193, 1999.

167. Hadders-Algra M, et al: Long-term follow-up of children prenatally exposed to ritodrine. Br J Obstet Gynaecol 93:156, 1986.

168. Hagerman DD: Clinical use of plasma total estriol measurements in late pregnancy. J Repro Med 23:179, 1979.

169. Hammed C, et al: Silent chorioamnionitis as a cause of preterm labor refractory to tocolytic therapy. Am J Obstet Gynecol 149:726, 1984.

170. Hanssens MC, et al: Sex steroid hormone concentrations in preterm labour and the outcome of treatment with ritodrine. Br J Obstet Gynaecol 85:411, 1978.

171. Harake B, et al: Nifedipine: Effects on fetal and maternal hemodynamics in pregnant sheep. Am J Obstet Gynecol 157:1003, 1987.

172. Harger JH: Cervical cerclage: Patient selection, morbidity and success rates. Clin Perinatol 10:321, 1983.

173. Harger JH, et al: Etiology of recurrent pregnancy losses and outcome of subsequent pregnancies. Obstet Gynecol 62:574, 1983.

174. Harger JH, et al: Risk factors for preterm premature rupture of fetal membranes: A multicenter case-control study. Am J Obstet Gynecol 163:130, 1990.

175. Harrison HR, et al: Cervical *Chlamydia trachomatis* and mycoplasmal infections in pregnancy: Epidemiology and outcomes. JAMA 247:1585, 1983.

176. Hastings MJG, et al: Group B streptococcal colonization and the outcome of pregnancy. J Infect 12:23, 1986.

177. Hauth JC, et al: Infection-related risk factors predictive of spontaneous preterm labor and birth. Prenat Neonat Med 3:86, 1998.

178. Hauth JC, et al: Reduced incidence of preterm delivery with metronidazole and erythromycin in women with bacterial vaginosis. N Engl J Med 333:1732, 1995.

179. Hauth JC, et al: Reduction of cerebral palsy with maternal MgSO$_4$ treatment in newborns weighing 500–1000 g. Am J Obstet Gynecol 172:419, 1995.

180. Hay PE, et al: Abnormal bacterial colonization of the genital tract and subsequent preterm delivery and late miscarriage. Brit Med J 308:295, 1994.

181. Haynes RC, et al: Adrenocorticotropic hormone: Adrenocorticosteroids and their synthetic analogs—inhibitors of adrenocortical steroid biosynthesis. In Goodman LS, et al (eds): The Pharmacologic Basis of Therapeutics, 5th ed. New York, Macmillan, 1975.

182. Heffner LJ, et al: Clinical and environmental predictors of preterm labor. Obstet Gynecol 81:750, 1993.

183. Heinonen PK, et al: Reproductive performance of women with uterine anomalies. Acta Obstet Gynecol Scand 61:157, 1982.

184. Helfgott AW, et al: Is hydration and sedation beneficial in the treatment of threatened preterm labor? A preliminary report. J Matern Fetal Med 3:37, 1994.

185. Hercz P, et al: Change of serum HPL level in maternal vein, umbilical cord vein and artery in mature and premature labour. Eur J Obstet Gynecol Repro Bio 24:189, 1987.

186. Hermansen MC, et al: Neonatal supraventricular tachycardia following prolonged maternal ritodrine administration. Am J Obstet Gynecol 149:798, 1984.

187. Herron M, et al: Evaluation of a preterm birth prevention program: Preliminary report. Obstet Gynecol 59:452, 1982.

188. Hewitt BG, et al: A review of the obstetric and medical complications leading to the delivery of infants of very low birth weight. Med J Aust 149:234, 1988.

189. Hill GB: The microbiology of bacterial vaginosis. Am J Obstet Gynecol 169:450, 1993.

190. Hill GB: Preterm birth: Associations with genital and possibly oral microflora. Ann Periodontol 3:222, 1998.

191. Hillier SL, et al: A case-control study of chorioamnionic infection and histologic chorioamnionitis in prematurity. N Engl J Med 319:972, 1988.

192. Hillier SL, et al: Microbiologic causes and neonatal outcomes associated with chorioamnion infection. Am J Obstet Gynecol 165:955, 1991.

193. Hillier SL, et al: The relationship of amniotic fluid cytokines and preterm delivery, amniotic fluid infection, histologic chorioamnionitis, and chorioamnion infection. Obstet Gynecol 81:941, 1993.

194. Hillier SL, et al: Association between bacterial vaginosis and preterm delivery of a low-birth-weight infant. The Vaginal Infections and Prematurity Study Group. N Engl J Med 333:1737, 1995.

195. Holbrook RH Jr, et al: Evaluation of a risk-scoring system for prediction of preterm labor. Am J Perinatol 6:62, 1989.

196. Holcomb WL, et al: Magnesium tocolysis and neonatal bone abnormalities. Obstet Gynecol 78:611, 1991.

197. Howard TE, et al: A double-blind randomized study of terbutaline in premature labor. Mil Med 12:4, 1982.

198. Huhta JC, et al: Detection and quantitation of constriction of the fetal ductus arteriosus by Doppler echocardiography. Circulation 2:406, 1987.

199. Huisjes HJ, et al: Neonatal outcome after treatment with rito-drine: A controlled study. Am J Obstet Gynecol 147:250, 1983.
200. Iams JD, et al: A prospective random trial of home uterine activity monitoring in pregnancies at increased risk of preterm labor. Am J Obstet Gynecol 157:638, 1987.
201. Iams JD, et al: Cervical sonography in preterm labor. Obstet Gynecol 84:40, 1994.
202. Iams JD, et al: Fetal fibronectin improves the accuracy of diagnosis of preterm labor. Am J Obstet Gynecol 173:141, 1995.
203. Iams J, et al: The length of the cervix and the risk of spontaneous premature delivery. N Engl J Med, 334:567, 1996.
204. Iams JD, et al: Prediction of preterm birth with ambulatory measurement of uterine contraction frequency. Am J Obstet Gynecol 178:S2, 1998.
205. Iams JD, et al: Uterine contraction frequency and preterm birth. Am J Obstet Gynecol 178:S188, 1998.
206. Ingemarsson I: Effect of terbutaline on premature labor. Am J Obstet Gynecol 125:520, 1976.
207. Inglis SR, et al: Detection of tumor necrosis-α, interleukin-6, and fetal fibronectin in the lower genital tract during pregnancy: Relation to outcome. Am J Obstet Gynecol 171:5, 1994.
208. Jones JM, et al: The outcome of pregnancy after cone biopsy of the cervix: A case-control study. Br J Obstet Gynaecol 86:913, 1979.
209. Kanayama N, et al: Collagen types in normal and prematurely ruptured amniotic membranes. Am J Obstet Gynecol 153:899, 1985.
210. Kanayama N, et al: The relationship between granulocyte elastase like activity of cervical mucus and cervical maturation. Acta Obstet Gynecol Scand 70:29, 1991.
211. Kass EH: Bacteriuria and pyelonephritis of pregnancy. Arch Intern Med 105:194, 1960.
212. Katz M, et al: Initial evaluation of an ambulatory system for home monitoring and transmission of uterine activity data. Obstet Gynecol 66:273, 1985.
213. Katz M, et al: Assessment of uterine activity in ambulatory patients at high risk of preterm labor and delivery. Am J Obstet Gynecol 154:44, 1986.
214. Katz M, et al: Early signs and symptoms of preterm labor. Am J Obstet Gynecol 262:230, 1990.
215. Kaufman RH, et al: Genital tract anomalies associated with in utero exposure to diethylstilbestrol. Isr J Med Sci 14:347, 1978.
216. Kaufman RH, et al: Upper genital tract abnormalities and pregnancy outcome in diethylstilbestrol-exposed progeny. N Engl J Med 313:1322, 1985.
217. Keirse MJ: Progestogen administration in pregnancy may prevent preterm delivery. Br J Obstet Gynaecol 97:149, 1990.
218. Kelly RW, et al: Choriodecidual production of interleukin-8 and mechanism of parturition. Lancet 339:776, 1992.
219. King JF, et al: Beta-mimetics in preterm labour: An overview of randomized, controlled trials. Br J Obstet Gynaecol 95:211, 1988.
220. King J, et al: Antibiotics for preterm labour with intact membranes. Cochrane Database Syst Rev 2:CD000246, 2000.
221. Kirshon B, et al: Influence of short-term indomethacin therapy on fetal urine output. Obstet Gynecol 72:51, 1988.
222. Kirshon B, et al: Long-term indomethacin therapy decreases fetal urine output and results in oligohydramnios. Am J Perinatol 8:86, 1991.
223. Klebanoff MA, et al: Outcome of the Vaginal Infections and Prematurity Study: Results of a clinical trial of erythromycin among pregnant women colonized with group B streptococci. Am J Obstet Gynecol 172:1540, 1995.
224. Knight DB, et al: A randomized controlled trial of antepartum thyrotropin-releasing hormone and betamethasone in the prevention of respiratory disease in preterm infants. Am J Obstet Gynecol 171:11, 1994.
225. Korn AP, et al: Plasma cell endometritis in women with symptomatic bacterial vaginosis. Obstet Gynecol 85:387, 1995.
226. Kossmann JC, et al: Characterization of specific steroid binding in human amnion at term. Biol Reprod 27:320, 1982.
227. Kramer W, et al: Randomized, double-blind study comparing sulindac to terbutaline: Fetal renal and amniotic fluid effects. Am J Obstet Gynecol 174:244, 1996.
228. Krohn MA, et al: Vaginal bacteroides species are associated with an increased rate of preterm delivery among women in preterm labor. J Infect Dis 164:88, 1991.
229. Krohn MA, et al: The genital flora of women with intraamniotic infection. J Inf Dis 171:1475, 1995.
230. Kurki T, et al: Bacterial vaginosis in early pregnancy and pregnancy outcome. Obstet Gynecol 80:173, 1992.
231. Kurtzman JL, et al: Do nifedipine and verapamil potentiate the cardiac toxicity of magnesium sulfate? Am J Perinatol 10:450, 1993.
232. Kurtzman JL, et al: Transvaginal versus transperineal ultrasound: A blinded comparison in the assessment of cervical length at mid-gestation. Am J Obstet Gynecol 178:S15, 1998.
233. Kushnir O, et al: Transvaginal sonographic measurement of cervical length: Evaluation of twin pregnancies. J Repro Med 40:380, 1995.
234. La Gamma E, et al: Failure of delayed oral feedings to prevent necrotizing enterocolitis. Am J Dis Child 139:385, 1985.
235. Lam F, et al: Use of the subcutaneous terbutaline pump for long-term tocolysis. Obstet Gynecol 72:810, 1988.
236. Lamont RF, et al: Spontaneous early preterm labour associated with abnormal genital bacterial colonization. Br J Obstet Gynaecol 93:804, 1986.
237. Lamont RF, et al: The role of mycoplasmas, ureaplasmas and chlamydiae in the genital tract of women presenting in spontaneous early preterm labour. J Med Microbiol 24:253, 1987.
238. Lamont R: The contemporary use of beta-agonists. Br J Obstet Gynaecol 100:890, 1993.
239. Lampert MB, et al: Peripartum heart failure associated with prolonged tocolytic therapy. Am J Obstet Gynecol 168:493, 1993.
240. Lands AM, et al: Differentiation of receptor systems by sympathomimetic amines. Nature 214:597, 1967.
241. Lazar P, et al: Multicentered controlled trial of cervical cerclage in women at moderate risk of preterm delivery. Br J Obstet Gynaecol 91:724, 1984.
242. Leake RD, et al: Pharmacokinetics of oxytocin in the human subject. Obstet Gynecol 56:701, 1980.
243. Lees CC, et al: Glyceryl trinitrate and ritodrine in tocolysis: An international multicenter randomized study. GTN Preterm Labour Investigation Group. Obstet Gynecol 94:403, 1999.
244. Lenke R, et al: Sudden unforeseen fetal death in a woman being treated for premature labor. J Reprod Med 29:872, 1984.
245. Leung TN, et al: Elevated mid-trimester maternal corticotrophin-releasing hormone levels in pregnancies that delivered before 34 weeks. Br J Obstet Gynaecol 106:1041, 1999.
246. Leviton A, et al: White matter damage in preterm newborns—an epidemiologic perspective. Early Hum Dev 24:1, 1990.
247. Liggins GC, et al: A controlled trial of antepartum glucocorticoid treatment for the prevention of RDS in premature infants, Pediatrics 50: 515, 1972.
248. Liggins GC: Ripening of the cervix. Semin Perinatol 2:261, 1978.
249. Lin TJ, et al: Metabolic clearance of progesterone in the menstrual cycle. J Clin Endocrinol Metab 35:879, 1972.
250. Lindenbaum C, et al: Maternal glucose intolerance and the subcutaneous terbutaline pump. Am J Obstet Gynecol 166:925, 1992.
251. Linn S, et al: The relationship between induced abortion and outcome of subsequent pregnancies. Am J Obstet Gynecol 146:136, 1983.
252. Lipshitz J, et al: Uterine and cardiovascular effects of beta-2 selective sympathomimetic drugs administered as an intravenous infusion. S Afr Med J 50:1973, 1976.
253. Lockwood CJ, et al: Fetal fibronectin in cervical and vaginal secretions defines a patient population at high risk for preterm delivery. N Engl J Med 325:669, 1991.
254. Lockwood CJ, et al: Fetal fibronectin predicts preterm deliveries in asymptomatic patients [abstract]. Am J Obstet Gynecol 168:311, 1993.
255. Lockwood CJ, et al: New approaches to the prediction of preterm delivery. J Perinat Med 22:441, 1994.
256. Lockwood CJ, et al: Increased interleukin-6 concentrations in cervical secretions are associated with preterm delivery. Am J Obstet Gynecol 171:1097, 1994.

257. Lu G, et al: Current concepts on the pathogenesis and markers of preterm births. Clin Perinatol 27:263, 2000.

258. Ludmir J, et al: A prospective study of cerclage in the DES-exposed pregnant patient [abstract]. Paper presented at the Society of Perinatal Obstetricians Meeting, 1987, Orlando, Fla.

259. Ludmir J, et al: Poor perinatal outcome associated with retained cerclage in patients with premature rupture of membranes. Obstet Gynecol 84:823, 1994.

260. Lundin-Schiller S, et al: Prostaglandin production by human chorion laeve cells in response to inflammatory mediators. Placenta 12:353, 1991.

261. Lyrenas S, et al: Pharmacokinetics of terbutaline during pregnancy. Eur J Clin Pharmacol 29:619, 1986.

262. MacArthur BA, et al: School progress and cognitive development of 6-year-old children whose mothers were treated with betamethasone. Pediatrics 70:99, 1982.

263. MacGregor SN, et al: Cocaine use during pregnancy: Adverse perinatal outcome. Am J Obstet Gynecol 157:686, 1987.

264. MacKenzie LW, et al: Effects of estradiol-17beta and prostaglandins on rat myometrial gap junctions. Prostaglandins 26:925, 1983.

265. Maclennan FM, et al: Fatal pulmonary oedema associated with the use of ritodrine in pregnancy: Case report. Br J Obstet Gynaecol 92:703, 1985.

266. Main DM, et al: Prospective evaluation of a risk scoring system for predicting preterm delivery in black inner city women. Obstet Gynecol 69:61, 1987.

267. Main DM: The epidemiology of preterm birth. Clin Obstet Gynecol 31: 521, 1988.

268. Main DM, et al: Intermittent weekly contraction monitoring to predict preterm labor in low-risk women: A blinded study. Obstet Gynecol 72:757, 1988.

269. Main EK, et al: Chronic oral terbutaline tocolytic therapy is associated with maternal glucose intolerance. Am J Obstet Gynecol 157:664, 1987.

270. Manchester D, et al: Possible association between maternal indomethacin therapy and primary pulmonary hypertension of the newborn. Am J Obstet Gynecol 126:467, 1976.

271. Marbury MC, et al: Work and pregnancy. J Occup Med 26:415, 1984.

272. Mari G, et al: Doppler assessment of the fetal and uteroplacental circulation during nifedipine therapy for preterm labor. Am J Obstet Gynecol 161:1514, 1989.

273. Mari G, et al: Doppler assessment of the renal blood flow velocity waveform during indomethacin therapy for preterm labor and polyhydramnios. Obstet Gynecol 75:199, 1990.

274. Martin DH, et al: Prematurity and perinatal mortality in pregnancies complicated by maternal Chlamydia trachomatis infections. JAMA 247:1585, 1982.

275. Martin RW, et al: Oral magnesium for tocolysis. In Petrie RH (ed): Perinatal Pharmacology. Oradell, NJ, Medical Economics, 1989.

276. Martin RW, et al: Oral magnesium and the prevention of preterm labor in a high-risk group of patients. Am J Obstet Gynecol 166:144, 1992.

277. Martius J, et al: Relationships of vaginal lactobacillus species, cervical Chlamydia trachomatis, and bacterial vaginosis to preterm birth. Obstet Gynecol 71:89, 1988.

278. Maudsley RF, et al: Placental inflammation and infection: A prospective bacteriologic and histologic study. Am J Obstet Gynecol 95:648, 1966.

279. Maymon R, et al: Placental isoferritin measured by a specific monoclonal antibody as a predictive marker for preterm contraction outcome. Obstet Gynecol 74:597, 1989.

280. McClean M, et al: Prediction and early diagnosis of preterm labor: A critical review. Obstet Gynecol Surv 48:2091, 1993.

281. McCormick MC: The contribution of low birth weight to infant mortality and childhood morbidity. N Engl J Med 312:82, 1985.

282. McDonald HM, et al: Vaginal infection and preterm labour. Br J Obstet Gynecol 98:427, 1991.

283. McDonald HM, et al: Prenatal microbiological risk factors associated with preterm birth. Br J Obstet Gynecol 99:190, 1992.

284. McDonald HM, et al: Impact of metronidazole therapy on preterm birth in women with bacterial vaginosis flora (Gardnerella vaginalis): A randomised, placebo controlled trial. Br J Obstet Gynaecol 104:1391, 1997.

285. McDowall M, et al: Employment during pregnancy and infant mortality. Population Trends 26:12, 1981.

286. McGarrigle HHG, et al: Increasing saliva (free) oestriol to progesterone ratio in late pregnancy: A role for oestriol in initiating spontaneous labour in man? Br Med J 289:457, 1984.

287. McGregor JA, et al: Association of cervico-vaginal infections with increased vaginal fluid phospholipase A2 activity. Am J Obstet Gynecol 167:1588, 1988.

288. McGregor JA, et al: Salivary estriol as risk assessment for preterm labor: A prospective trial. Am J Obstet Gynecol 173:1337, 1995.

289. Meis PJ, et al: Causes of low birthweight births in public and private patients. Am J Obstet Gynecol 156:1165, 1987.

290. Meis PJ, et al: Regional program for prevention of premature birth in northwest North Carolina. Am J Obstet Gynecol 157:550, 1987.

291. Meis P, et al: Vaginal infections and spontaneous preterm birth. Am J Obstet Gynecol 172:548, 1995.

292. Ment L, et al: Antenatal steroids, delivery, mode and intraventricular hemorrhage in preterm infants. Am J Obstet Gynecol 172:795, 1995.

293. Mercer BM, et al: Antibiotic therapy for reduction of infant morbidity after preterm premature rupture of the membranes. A randomized controlled trial. National Institute of Child Health and Human Development Maternal-Fetal Medicine Units Network. JAMA 278:989, 1997.

294. Mercer BM, et al: The preterm prediction study: Effect of gestational age and cause of preterm birth on subsequent obstetric outcome. National Institute of Child Health and Human Development Maternal-Fetal Medicine Units Network. Am J Obstet Gynecol 181:1216, 1999.

295. Merkatz JR, et al: Ritodrine hydrochloride: A beta-mimetic agent for use in preterm labor. II. Evidence of efficacy. Obstet Gynecol 56:7, 1980.

296. Meyer RE, et al: Maternal serum placental alkaline phosphatase level and risk for preterm delivery. Am J Obstet Gynecol 173:181, 1995.

297. Milewich L, et al: Initiation of human parturition. VII. Partial characterization of progesterone-metabolizing enzymes of human amnion and chorion laeve. J Steroid Biochem 11:1577, 1979.

298. Miller HC, et al: Maternal factors in the incidence of low birthweight infants among black and white mothers. Pediatr Res 12:1016, 1978.

299. Miller JM, et al: Bacterial colonization of amniotic fluid from intact fetal membranes. Am J Obstet Gynecol 136:796, 1980.

300. Miller JM, et al: A comparison of magnesium sulfate and terbutaline for the arrest of premature labor. J Reprod Med 27:348, 1982.

301. Mitchell MD, et al: Specific production of prostaglandin E by human amnion in vitro. Prostaglandins 15:377, 1978.

302. Mitchell MD, et al: Prostaglandin biosynthesis by human decidual cells: Effects of inflammatory mediators. Prostaglandins Leukot Essent Fatty Acids 41:35, 1990.

303. Mitchell MD, et al: Interleukin-6 stimulates prostaglandin production by human amnion and decidual cells. Eur J Pharmacol 192:189, 1991.

304. Moutquin JM, et al: Double-blind, randomized, controlled trial of atosiban and ritodrine in the treatment of preterm labor: A multicenter effectiveness and safety study. Am J Obstet Gynecol 182:1191, 2000.

305. Moise KJ, et al: Indomethacin in the treatment of premature labor: Effects on the fetal ductus arteriosus. N Engl J Med 319:327, 1988.

306. Moise KJ: Effect of advancing gestational age on the frequency of fetal ductal constriction in association with maternal indomethacin use. Am J Obstet Gynecol 168:1350, 1993.

307. Moller M, et al: Rupture of fetal membranes and premature delivery associated with group B streptococci in urine of pregnant women. Lancet 2:69, 1984.

308. Morales WJ, et al: Efficacy and safety of indomethacin versus ritodrine in the management of preterm labor: A randomized study. Obstet Gynecol 74:567, 1989.

309. Morales WJ, et al: Efficacy and safety of indomethacin compared with magnesium sulfate in the management of preterm labor: A randomized study. Am J Obstet Gynecol 169:97, 1993.

310. Morales WJ, et al: Effect of metronidazole in patients with preterm birth in preceding pregnancy and bacterial vaginosis: A placebo-controlled, double-blind study. Am J Obstet Gynecol 171:345, 1994.

311. Moran DJ, et al: Lack of normal increase in saliva estriol/progesterone ratio in women with labor induced at 42 weeks' gestation. Am J Obstet Gynecol 167:1563, 1992.

312. Moretti MI, et al: The effect of nifedipine therapy on fetal and placental Doppler waveforms in preeclampsia remote from term [abstract]. Proceedings of the Society of Gynecologic Investigations, St. Louis, 1990.

313. Moroz C, et al: Difference in the placental ferritin levels measured by a specific monoclonal antibody enzymoassay in preterm and term delivery. Clin Exp Immunol 69:702, 1987.

314. Morrison JC, et al: Prevention of preterm birth by ambulatory assessment of uterine activity: A randomized study. Am J Obstet Gynecol 156:536, 1987.

315. Morrison JC, et al: Oncofetal fibronectin in patients with false labor as a predictor of preterm delivery. Am J Obstet Gynecol 168:538, 1993.

316. Mortensen OA, et al: Prediction of preterm birth. Acta Obstet Gynecol Scand 66:507, 1987.

317. Mou SM, et al: Multicenter randomized clinical trial of home uterine monitoring for detection of preterm labor. Am J Obstet Gynecol 165:858, 1991.

318. Mueller-Heubach E, et al: Evaluation of risk scoring in a preterm birth prevention study of indigent patients. Obstet Gynecol 160:829, 1989.

319. Mueller-Heubach E, et al: Histologic chorioamnionitis and preterm delivery in different patient populations. Obstet Gynecol 75:622, 1990.

320. Muran D, et al: Myomas of the uterus in pregnancy: Ultrasonographic follow-up. Am J Obstet Gynecol 138:16, 1980.

321. Murphy JF, et al: Employment in pregnancy: Prevalence, maternal characteristics, perinatal outcomes. Lancet 1:1163, 1984.

322. Murtha AP, et al: Maternal serum interleukin-6 concentration as a marker for impending preterm delivery. Obstet Gynecol 91:161, 1998.

323. Nadisauskiene R, et al: Ampicillin in the treatment of preterm labor: A randomised, placebo-controlled study. Gynecol Obstet Invest 41:89, 1996.

324. Nageotte MP, et al: Quantitation of uterine activity preceding preterm, term, and postterm labor. Am J Obstet Gynecol 158:1254, 1988.

325. Nageotte MP, et al: Oncofetal fibronectin in patients at increased risk for preterm delivery [abstract]. Am J Obstet Gynecol 166:274, 1992.

326. National Institutes of Health (NIH) Consensus Development Conference: Effect of corticosteroids for fetal maturation on perinatal outcomes. Am J Obstet Gynecol 173:246, 1995.

327. Nelson KB, et al: Antecedents of cerebral palsy. Multivariate analysis of risk. N Engl J Med 315:81, 1986.

328. Nelson KB, et al: Can magnesium sulfate reduce the risk of cerebral palsy in very-low birthweight infants? Pediatrics 95:263, 1995.

329. Newman RB, et al: Maternal perception of prelabor uterine activity. Obstet Gynecol 68:765, 1986.

330. Niebyl JR, et al: The inhibition of premature labor with indomethacin. Am J Obstet Gynecol 136:1014, 1980.

331. Nishihira J, et al: Mass spectrometric evidence for the presence of platelet-activating factor in human amniotic fluid during labor. Lipids 19:907, 1984.

332. Norman K, et al: Ampicillin and metronidazole treatment in preterm labour: A multicentre, randomised controlled trial. Br J Obstet Gynaecol 101:404, 1994.

333. Norton ME, et al: Neonatal complications after the administration of indomethacin for preterm labor. N Engl J Med 329:1602, 1993.

334. Norwitz ER, et al: The control of labor. N Engl J Med 341:660, 1999.

335. Novy MJ, et al: Plasma concentrations of prostaglandin $F_{2\ \text{alpha}}$ and prostaglandin E_2 metabolites after transabdominal and transvaginal cervical cerclage. Am J Obstet Gynecol 156:1543, 1987.

336. Nuchpuckdee P, et al: Ventricular septal thickness and cardiac function in neonates after in utero ritodrine exposure. J Pediatr 109:687, 1986.

337. Nyberg L: Pharmacokinetic parameters of terbutaline in healthy men: An overview. Eur J Respir Dis 65(Suppl 134):149, 1984.

338. Okazaki T, et al: Initiation of human parturition. XII. Biosynthesis and metabolism of prostaglandins in human fetal membranes and uterine decidua. Am J Obstet Gynecol 139:373, 1981.

339. Okitsu O, et al: Early prediction of preterm delivery by transvaginal ultrasonography. Ultrasound Obstet Gynecol 2:402, 1992.

340. Ovlisen G, et al: Treatment of threatened premature labor with 6α-methyl-17α-acetoxyprogesterone. Am J Obstet Gynecol 79:172, 1960.

341. Owen J, et al: Evaluation of a risk scoring system as a predictor of preterm birth in an indigent population. Am J Obstet Gynecol 163:873, 1990.

342. Owen J, et al: Endovaginal sonography at 16–18 weeks pf gestation predicts subsequent spontaneous preterm delivery in high-risk women. J Soc Gynecol Invest 7:189A, 2000.

343. Padayachi T, et al: Changes in amniotic fluid prostaglandins with oxytocin-induced labor. Obstet Gynecol 68:610, 1986.

344. Pankuch GA, et al: Placental microbiology and histology and the pathogenesis of chorioamnionitis. Obstet Gynecol 64:802, 1984.

345. Papiernik E, et al: Prevention of preterm births: A perinatal study in Haguenau, France. Pediatrics 76:154, 1985.

346. Papiernik E, et al: Precocious cervical ripening and preterm labor. Obstet Gynecol 67:238, 1986.

347. Parisi VM: Cervical incompetence and preterm labor. Clin Obstet Gynecol 31:585, 1988.

348. Parulekar SG, et al: Dynamic incompetent cervix uteri. J Ultrasound Med 7:481, 1988.

349. Peaceman AM, et al: Fetal fibronectin as a predictor of preterm birth in patients with symptoms: A multicenter trial. Am J Obstet Gynecol 177:13, 1997.

350. Petraglia F, et al: Peptide signaling in human placenta and membranes: Autocrine, paracrine and endocrine mechanisms. Endocrinol Rev 17:156, 1996.

351. Petrie RH, et al: Tocolysis using magnesium sulfate. Semin Perinatol 5:266, 1981.

352. Pircon RA, et al: Controlled trial of hydration and bed rest versus bed rest alone in the evaluation of preterm uterine contractions. Am J Obstet Gynecol 161:775, 1989.

353. Polk BF, et al: Association of Chlamydia trachomatis and Mycoplasma hominis with intrauterine growth retardation and preterm delivery. Am J Epidemiol 129:1247, 1989.

354. Quatero HWP, et al: Placental corticotropin releasing factor may modulate human parturition. Placenta 10:439, 1989.

355. Raemsch KD, et al: Pharmacokinetics and metabolism of nifedipine. Hypertension 5(Suppl II):18, 1983.

356. Rajabi M, et al: High levels of serum collagenase in premature labor: A potential biochemical marker. Obstet Gynecol 69:179, 1987.

357. Ramin KD, et al: Ultrasound assessment of cervical length in triplet pregnancies. Am J Obstet Gynecol 180:1442, 1999.

358. Ramsey PS, et al: Elevated cervical ferritin levels at 24 weeks gestation are associated with spontaneous preterm birth in asymptomatic pregnant women. J Soc Gynecol Invest 7:190A, 2000.

359. Ramsey PS, et al: Maternal infections and their consequences. In McIntyre J, Newell ML (eds): Congenital and Perinatal Infections. Cambridge, Cambridge University Press, 2000, p 32.

360. Rasanen J, et al: Fetal cardiac function and ductus arteriosus during indomethacin and sulindac therapy for threatened preterm labor: A randomized study. Am J Obstet Gynecol 172:70, 1995.

361. Rauramo I, et al: Antepartum fetal heart rate variability and intervillous placental blood flow in association with smoking. Am J Obstet Gynecol 146:967, 1983.

362. Read MD, et al: The use of a calcium antagonist (nifedipine) to suppress preterm labour. Br J Obstet Gynaecol 93:933, 1986.
363. Regan JA, et al: Premature rupture of membranes, preterm delivery, and group B streptococcal colonization of mothers. Am J Obstet Gynecol 141:184, 1981.
364. Reis FM, et al: Putative role of placental corticotropin-releasing factor in the mechanisms of human parturition. J Soc Gynecol Invest 6:109, 1999.
365. Ricci JM, et al: Oral tocolysis with magnesium chloride: A randomized controlled prospective clinical trial. Am J Obstet Gynecol 165:603, 1991.
366. Richey SD, et al: The correlation between transperineal sonography and digital examination in the evaluation of the third-trimester cervix. Obstet Gynecol 85:745, 1995.
367. Ridgeway LE, et al: A prospective randomized comparison of oral terbutaline and magnesium oxide for the maintenance of tocolysis. Am J Obstet Gynecol 163:879, 1990.
368. Riduan JM, et al: Bacterial vaginosis and prematurity in Indonesia: Association in early and late pregnancy. Am J Obstet Gynecol 169:175, 1993.
369. Riemer RK, et al: Rabbit uterine oxytocin receptors and in vitro contractile response: Abrupt changes at term and the role of eicosanoids. Endocrinology 119:699, 1986.
370. Rizzo G, et al: Interleukin-6 concentrations in cervical secretions identify microbial invasion of the amniotic cavity in patients with preterm labor and intact membranes. Am J Obstet Gynecol 175:812, 1996.
371. Roberts JS, et al: Oxytocin-stimulated release of prostaglandin F2alpha from ovine endometrium in vitro: Correlation with estrous cycle and oxytocin-receptor binding. Endocrinology 99:1107, 1976.
372. Robertson PA, et al: Neonatal morbidity according to gestational age and birth weight from five tertiary centers in the United States, 1983–1986. Am J Obstet Gynecol 166:1629, 1992.
373. Robinson J, et al: Salivary oestriol in normal pregnancy. Lancet 1:1111, 1981.
374. Rogers RC, et al: Oral nifedipine pharmacokinetics in pregnancy-induced hypertension [abstract]. Proceedings of the Society of Perinatal Obstetricians, Houston, 1990.
375. Romero R, et al: Infection and labor: The detection of endotoxin in amniotic fluid. Am J Obstet Gynecol 157:815, 1987.
376. Romero R, et al: Prostaglandin concentrations in amniotic fluid of women with intraamniotic and preterm labor. Am J Obstet Gynecol 157:1461, 1987.
377. Romero R, et al: Infection and preterm labor. Clin Obstet Gynecol 31:553, 1988.
378. Romero R, et al: The microbiologic significance of pathologic placental chorioamnionitis. Proceedings of the Society of Perinatal Obstetricians, Las Vegas, 1988.
379. Romero R, et al: Endotoxin stimulates prostaglandin E2 production by human amnion. Obstet Gynecol 71:227, 1988.
380. Romero R, et al: Labor and infection. II. Bacterial endotoxin in amniotic fluid and its relationship to the onset of preterm labor. Am J Obstet Gynecol 158:1044, 1988.
381. Romero R, et al: Amniotic fluid concentrations of prostaglandin F2alpha, 13,14-dihydro-15-keto-11,16 cycloprostaglandin E2 (PGEM-II) in preterm labor. Prostaglandins 37:149, 1989.
382. Romero R, et al: Meta-analysis of the relationship between asymptomatic bacteriuria and preterm delivery/birth weight. Obstet Gynecol 73:576, 1989.
383. Romero R, et al: The prevalence, microbiology, and clinical significance of intraamniotic infection in twin gestations with preterm labor. Am J Obstet Gynecol 163:757, 1990.
384. Romero R, et al: Two thirds of spontaneous abortions/fetal deaths after midtrimester genetic amniocentesis are the result of a pre-existing subclinical inflammatory process of the amniotic cavity. Am J Obstet Gynecol 172:261, 1995.
385. Romero R, et al: An oxytocin receptor antagonist (atosiban) in the treatment of preterm labor: A randomized, double-blind, placebo-controlled trial with tocolytic rescue. Am J Obstet Gynecol 182:1173, 2000.
386. Rosen MG, et al: The incidence of cerebral palsy. Am J Obstet Gynecol 167:417, 1992.
387. Ross SM, et al: *Trichomonas* infection in pregnancy—Does it affect perinatal outcome? S Afr Med J 63:566, 1983.
388. Rush RW, et al: A randomized controlled trial of cervical cerclage in women at moderate risk of preterm delivery. Br J Obstet Gynaecol 91:731, 1984.
389. Schellenberg JC, et al: Synergistic hormonal effects on lung maturation in sheep. Am J Physiol 65:94, 1988.
390. Schendel DE, et al: Prenatal magnesium sulfate exposure and the risk of cerebral palsy on mental retardation among very-low-birthweight children age 3 to 5 years. JAMA 276:1805, 1996.
391. Schiff E, et al: Currently recommended oral regimens for ritodrine tocolysis result in extremely low plasma levels. Am J Obstet Gynecol 169:1059, 1993.
392. Schneider JM, et al: Screening for fetal and neonatal risk in the postdate pregnancy. Am J Obstet Gynecol 131:473, 1978.
393. Schneider KTM, et al: Premature contractions: Are they caused by maternal standing? Acta Genet Med Gemellol (Roma) 34:175, 1985.
394. Scholl TO: High third-trimester ferritin concentration: Associations with very preterm delivery, infection, and maternal nutritional status. Obstet Gynecol 92:161, 1998.
395. Schuly KF, et al: Measures to prevent cervical injury during suction and curettage abortion. Lancet 1:1182, 1983.
396. Schwarz BE, et al: Initiation of human parturition. V. Progesterone binding substance in fetal membranes. Obstet Gynecol 48:685, 1976.
397. Shankaran S, et al: The effect of antenatal phenobarbital therapy on neonatal intracranial hemorrhage in preterm infants. N Engl J Med 337:466, 1997.
398. Shiono PH, et al: Smoking and drinking during pregnancy. JAMA 255:82, 1986.
399. Simpson JL, et al: Associations between adverse perinatal outcome and serially obtained second- and third-trimester maternal serum α-fetoprotein measurements. Am J Obstet Gynecol 173:1742, 1995.
400. Skinner KA, et al: Changes in the synthesis and metabolism of prostaglandin by human fetal membranes and decidua at labor. Am J Obstet Gynecol 171:141, 1984.
401. Smith CV, et al: Transvaginal sonography of cervical width and length during pregnancy. J Ultrasound Med 11:465, 1992.
402. Sonek JD, et al: Measurement of cervical length in pregnancy: Comparison between vaginal ultrasonography and digital examination. Obstet Gynecol 76:172, 1990.
403. Spellacy WN, et al: The acute effects of ritodrine infusion on maternal metabolism: Measurements of levels of glucose, insulin, glucagon, triglycerides, cholesterol, placental lactogen, and chorionic gonadotropin. Am J Obstet Gynecol 131:637, 1978.
404. Stallworth JC, et al: The effect of magnesium sulfate on fetal heart rate variability and uterine activity. Am J Obstet Gynecol 140:702, 1981.
405. Steer CM, et al: A comparison of magnesium sulfate and alcohol for the prevention of premature labor. Am J Obstet Gynecol 129:1, 1977.
406. Stevenson DK, et al: Very low birth weight outcomes of the National Institute of Child Health and Human Development Neonatal Research Network, January 1993 through December 1994. Am J Obstet Gynecol 179:1632, 1998.
407. Stillman RJ: In utero exposure to diethylstilbestrol: Adverse effects on the reproductive performance in male and female offspring. Am J Obstet Gynecol 142:905, 1982.
408. Svare J, et al: Ampicillin-metronidazole treatment in idiopathic preterm labour: A randomised controlled multicentre trial. Br J Obstet Gynaecol 104:892, 1997.
409. Sweet RL, et al: Chlamydia trachomatis infection and pregnancy outcome. Am J Obstet Gynecol 156:824, 1987.
410. Talbert RL, et al: Update on calcium-channel blocking agents. Clin Pharm 2:403, 1983.
411. Tamby Raja RL, et al: Endocrinology of normal pregnancy and premature labour. New Zeal Med J 86:89, 1977.
412. Tamura T, et al: Serum ferritin: A predictor of early spontaneous preterm delivery. Obstet Gynecol 87:360, 1996.
413. Thomsen AC, et al: Antibiotic elimination of group B streptococci in urine in prevention of preterm labour. Lancet 1:591, 1987.
414. Thorp JA, et al: Combined antenatal vitamin K for preventing

intracranial hemorrhage in newborns less than 34 weeks' gestation. Am J Obstet Gynecol 86:1, 1995.

415. Torfs CP, et al: Prenatal and perinatal factors in the etiology of cerebral palsy. J Pediatr 116:615, 1990.

416. Trager A, et al: The pharmacokinetics of indomethacin in pregnant and parturient women and in their newborn infants. Zentralbl Gynakol 95:635, 1973.

417. Trautman MS, et al: Amnion cell biosynthesis of interleukin-8: Regulation of cytokines. J Cell Physiol 153:38, 1992.

418. Tropper PJ, et al: Corticotropin releasing hormone concentrations in umbilical cord blood of preterm fetuses. J Dev Physiol 18:81, 1992.

419. Tu FF, et al: Prenatal plasma matrix metalloproteinases-9 levels to predict spontaneous preterm birth. Obstet Gynecol 92:446, 1998.

420. Tucker JM, et al: Etiologies of preterm birth in an indigent population: Is prevention a logical expectation? Obstet Gynecol 177:343, 1991.

421. Tucker JM, et al: Etiologies of preterm birth in an indigent population: Is prevention a logical expectation? Obstet Gynecol 77:343, 1991.

422. Turnbull AC, et al: Significant fall in progesterone and rise in estradiol levels in human peripheral plasma before onset of labour. Lancet 11:110, 1974.

423. Ulmsten U, et al: Treatment of premature labor with the calcium antagonist nifedipine. Arch Gynecol 229:1, 1980.

424. Vadillo-Ortega F, et al: Increased matrix metalloproteinase activity and reduced tissue inhibitor of metalloproteinases-1 levels in amniotic fluids from pregnancies complicated by premature rupture of membranes. Am J Obstet Gynecol 174:1371, 1996.

425. Valenzuela GJ, et al: Maintenance treatment of preterm labor with the oxytocin antagonist atosiban. The Atosiban PTL-098 Study Group. Am J Obstet Gynecol 182:1184, 2000.

426. van der Heijden BJ, et al: Persistent anuria, neonatal death, and renal microcystic lesions after prenatal exposure to indomethacin. Am J Obstet Gynecol 171:617, 1994.

427. Vermont-Oxford Trials Network: Very low birth weight outcomes for 1990. Investigators of the Vermont-Oxford Trials Network. Pediatrics 91:540, 1993.

428. Vohr BR, et al: Neurodevelopmental and functional outcomes of extremely low birth weight infants in the national institute of child health and human development neonatal research network, 1993–1994. Pediatrics 105:1216, 2000.

429. Wager J, et al: Metabolic and circulatory effects of intravenous and oral salbutamol in late pregnancy in diabetic and non-

diabetic women. Acta Obstet Gynecol Scand (Suppl) 108:41, 1982.

430. Wahbeh CJ, et al: Intra-amniotic bacterial colonization in premature labor. Am J Obstet Gynecol 148:739, 1984.

431. Wallace RL, et al: Inhibition of premature labor by terbutaline. Obstet Gynecol 51:387, 1978.

432. Warren WB, et al: Elevated maternal plasma corticotropin releasing hormone levels in pregnancies complicated by preterm labor. Am J Obstet Gynecol 166:1198, 1992.

433. Watts DH, et al: The association of occult amniotic fluid infection with gestational age and neonatal outcome among women in preterm labor. Obstet Gynecol 79:351, 1992.

434. Weibel DR, et al: Evaluation of amniotic fluid in preterm labor with intact membranes. J Reprod Med 30:777, 1985.

435. Wen SW, et al: Intrauterine growth retardation and preterm delivery: Prenatal risk factors in an indigent population. Am J Obstet Gynecol 162:213, 1990.

436. Wenstrom KD, et al: Elevated second-trimester human chorionic gonadotropin levels in association with poor pregnancy outcome. Am J Obstet Gynecol 171:1038, 1994.

437. Wenstrom KD, et al: Elevated amniotic fluid interleukin-6 levels at genetic amniocentesis predict subsequent pregnancy loss. Am J Obstet Gynecol 175:830, 1996.

438. Wenstrom KD, et al: Elevated second-trimester amniotic fluid interleukin-6 levels predict preterm delivery. Am J Obstet Gynecol 178:546, 1998.

439. White CP, et al: Premature delivery and group B streptococcal bacteriuria. Lancet 2:586, 1984.

440. Wolfe CDA, et al: The rate of rise in corticotropin releasing factor and endogenous digoxin-like immunoreactivity in normal and abnormal pregnancies. Br J Obstet Gynaecol 97:832, 1990.

441. Woods FR Jr, et al: Effect of cocaine on uterine blood flow and fetal oxygenation. JAMA 157:957, 1987.

442. Yoon BH, et al: High expression of interleukin-6, interleukin-1β, and tumor necrosis factor-α in periventricular leukomalacia. Am J Obstet Gynecol 174:399, 1996.

443. Yawn BP, et al: Preterm birth prevention in a rural practice. JAMA 262:230, 1990.

444. Yunis KA, et al: Transient hypertrophic cardiomyopathy in the newborn following multiple doses of antenatal corticosteroids. Am J Perinatol 16:17, 1999.

445. Zeeman GG, et al: Oxytocin and its receptor in pregnancy and parturition: Current concepts and clinical implications. Obstet Gynecol 89:873, 1997.

446. Zuckerman H, et al: Inhibition of human premature labor by indomethacin. Obstet Gynecol 44:787, 1974.

17 Fetal Effects of Autoimmune Disease

Neil K. Kochenour

The immune system is a complex integrated system with the primary function of protecting the body from infection. The intact immune system discriminates between foreign substances, which it attempts to destroy, and an individual's tissues, which it tolerates. When this system functions abnormally, individuals react against their own tissues. This process has been termed *autoimmunity*, and pregnancy provides a unique situation for this process. It involves not only the mother but also the fetus, which may be affected indirectly by the mother's autoimmune disease. The fetus may also be affected directly: the IgG antibody crosses the placenta and, if directed against a fetal antigen, may cause damage directly to the fetus (e.g., in autoimmune thrombocytopenia purpura). The fetus may be affected indirectly if an autoantibody affects the uterus or placenta, such as with two antiphospholipid antibodies, lupus anticoagulant antibody and anticardiolipin antibody.

AUTOIMMUNE THROMBOCYTOPENIC PURPURA

Autoimmune thrombocytopenic purpura (ATP) is an autoimmune disorder that is frequently encountered during pregnancy (see Chapter 44). The diagnosis of ATP is made according to established criteria: normal hematocrit and hemoglobin values and normal white blood cell count (unless there has been a recent hemorrhage); normal bone marrow with adequate or increased amount of megakaryocytes; a blood smear showing an increased percentage of large platelets; normal clotting studies; and no other obvious cause for thrombocytopenia. The presence of platelet-associated antibodies supports the diagnosis of ATP. Unfortunately, the criteria used to establish the diagnosis of ATP in pregnancy vary from study to study, with few studies using the presence of a normal or megakaryocytic bone marrow as diagnostic in all patients. The concept of essential thrombocytopenia in pregnancy further compounds the problem of diagnosis. It is possible and likely that many patients considered to have ATP in past studies actually had essential thrombocytopenia of pregnancy. Burrows and colleagues reported thrombocytopenia (platelet count less than 150,000/mL^3) in 500 (7.6%) of 6715 consecutive deliveries.[8] Of these, more than 75% had essential thrombocytopenia.

Corticosteroids provide the primary therapy for ATP, and in the absence of contraindications, they are used initially. For patients who do not respond to corticosteroids, splenectomy is frequently indicated.

Most of the literature supports the thesis that the overall course and severity of ATP are not affected significantly by pregnancy. Because the human placenta actively transports IgG antibodies of all types, the most serious clinical problem in the management of pregnant patients with ATP involves the placental transfer of the maternal antiplatelet antibody, which can result in fetal thrombocytopenia. Even a woman with a previous splenectomy for treatment of her disease can have high levels of the antibody that causes a shortened platelet life span, resulting in thrombocytopenia in both the mother and fetus.

Although the most feared perinatal complication of ATP is intracranial hemorrhage (a condition considered to be more likely in a thrombocytopenic fetus undergoing vaginal delivery), the evidence for it is scanty. Nevertheless, considerable effort has been directed toward identification of the fetus with thrombocytopenia so that a planned cesarean section can be performed. Unfortunately, reliable predictors of fetal platelet count have not been found. However, pregnant women with no antecedent splenectomy or severe thrombocytopenia during pregnancy have a very low risk of severe fetal thrombocytopenia.[38] Recent evidence also suggests that women with ATP who have HLA-DRB3 phenotype seem to be protected against giving birth to a severely thrombocytopenic newborn. Although those having HLA-DRB2 and HLA-DRB5 phenotypes may have a higher risk of delivering fetuses with thrombocytopenia,[16] the precise identification of the fetus with thrombocytopenia requires knowledge of the fetal platelet count.

Clinicians have developed three strategies for deciding the mode of delivery for patients with ATP.[1, 23, 24, 33] None is clearly superior, and all have favorable and unfavorable aspects. Several authors have advocated the use of fetal scalp sampling in labor to determine the fetal platelet count.[31] If the platelet count is greater than 50,000/mL^3, vaginal delivery is attempted; if it is less than 50,000/mL³, a cesarean section is performed. This assay has the advantages of carrying a low risk to the mother and fetus and of being widely available and inexpensive. The major drawback is an incidence of falsely low platelet counts, resulting in unnecessary cesarean birth.

Some groups perform cordocentesis before the onset of labor to determine the fetal platelet count. This procedure is usually performed after fetal maturity is ensured. If the fetal platelet count is greater than 50,000/mL³, vaginal delivery is deemed safe and induction is initiated. This method avoids some of the pitfalls of fetal scalp sampling. The fetal platelet count is accurate, and falsely low determinations have not been reported. However, cordocentesis is not always easily accomplished, and the skills required to obtain the sample are more sophisticated than those needed to obtain a fetal scalp sample. The most serious potential complications of cordocentesis are hemorrhage from the cord or puncture site and cord spasm with fetal bradycardia. Although procedure-related complications are rare, they appear to occur in 1% to 2% of patients. The risk of complications with cordocentesis in fetuses proved to have thrombocytopenia is unknown because only a small number of successful cordocenteses with platelet counts less than 50,000/mL³ as a result of ATP have been reported.

A third approach to delivery in cases of maternal ATP is expectant management, with cesarean section performed for only the usual obstetric reasons. This approach is based on the absence of the clear superiority of the other two approaches and the apparently low risk of adverse fetal outcome.

Platelet transfusion in patients with ATP is generally used therapeutically as a temporary measure in life-threatening situations or prophylactically as part of preoperative preparation. The survival of transfused platelets in patients with ATP is short. Repeated fetal platelet transfusion for patients with ATP is not practical, although it may be an alternative therapy for fetal alloimmune thrombocytopenia when platelet-specific antigens are identified and platelets free of that antigen can be infused.[14] The introduction of high-dose IV IgG therapy in the management of ATP has raised hopes that the effect of the immunoglobulin will extend transplacentally to the fetus.[15, 26, 28, 37] To date, however, the fetal platelet response has not been as predictable as the maternal response. The fetal risk in pregnancies complicated by ATP still has not been defined clearly.

ANTIPHOSPHOLIPID ANTIBODIES

Two antiphospholipid antibodies, lupus anticoagulant (LAC) antibody and anticardiolipin antibody (ACA), are associated with first-trimester spontaneous abortions, intrauterine growth retardation, and fetal death.[4-6] These two closely related antibodies have been found in patients with systemic lupus erythematosus (SLE), with other autoimmune disorders, and with no apparent disease. The antibodies are usually of the IgG type, but they may be of the IgM type. Branch and associates have suggested that testing for antiphospholipid antibodies other than LAC antibody and ACA is not clinically useful in the evaluation of recurrent pregnancy loss.[7]

The presence of LAC antibody is suggested by prolongation of the activated partial thromboplastin time or other phospholipid-dependent coagulation tests. It is measured indirectly by the prolongation of clotting time and the failure to correct to a near-normal value after the addition of an equal volume of normal plasma. However, ACAs are identified by immunoassays such as the enzyme-linked immunosorbent assay or a radioimmunoassay.[18] The relationship between these two antibodies is unclear.[19, 20] Although some have suggested that they are identical antibodies, others have not found such a close correlation. Several reports identify patients with one or the other antibody but not with both.

Numerous studies have identified a high frequency of pregnancy loss in women with LAC antibody.[5] Although less well studied, the fetal death rate among women with ACA is also high. In a study of 21 pregnant patients with SLE, Lockshin and coworkers found that the presence of ACA was the most sensitive predictor of fetal distress or death,[27] but not all patients with ACA have an adverse pregnancy outcome. Apparently, low levels of this antibody do not increase perinatal risk. Cowchock and colleagues identified 19 women who had persistently positive tests for antiphospholipid antibodies but were considered to be low risk because they had none of the associated signs or symptoms of antiphospholipid antibody syndrome.[12] In a randomized trial comparing low-dose aspirin with usual care, the investigators concluded that the treatment of pregnant women with antiphospholipid antibodies who are otherwise at low risk cannot be justified on the basis of the available evidence.

A number of immunopathologic mechanisms have been postulated for the action of the antiphospholipid antibodies. At present, the most attractive hypothesis involves antibody-mediated inhibition of prostacyclin (prostaglandin I₂ [PGI₂]) production. PGI₂ produced and released by the vascular endothelium is a potent vasodilator and inhibitor of platelet aggregation that is believed to be important for the maintenance of normal vascular patency. Thromboxane A₂, a prostaglandin produced by platelets, is a vasoconstrictor that promotes platelet aggregation. It has been postulated that LAC antibody inhibits PGI₂ production by binding to the endothelial cell membranes and by interfering with the release of the phospholipid precursors of prostaglandin production.[29] In addition to the inhibition of PGI₂ production by the vascular epithelium, LAC antibody also interacts with the phospholipid fraction of platelets.

Several therapeutic regimens have been suggested for treating patients with antiphospholipid antibodies. The first successful therapy was a combination of prednisone and low doses of aspirin. More recently, successful therapy has been reported with a combination of heparin and low doses of aspirin.[5] Therapy with corticosteroids and heparin, however, is associated with significant complications. The incidence of preterm delivery appears to be increased with corticosteroid therapy. Gestational diabetes and pregnancy-induced hypertension appear to be more frequent in patients treated with corticosteroids than in those treated with heparin. However, heparin therapy is not without risk. The most common significant risk is heparin-induced osteoporosis. Heparin is also associated with an uncommon idiosyncratic thrombocytopenia. The concomitant use of corticosteroids and heparin is to be avoided if at all possible.

The available evidence indicates that the combination of heparin with low-dose aspirin is the most effective therapy for patients with antiphospholipid antibodies.[13, 25] Several cases of severe osteoporosis with fractures occurring in women with antiphospholipid antibody syndrome who were treated with this regimen have been reported. However, the combination of these two medications has not been shown to be better than either alone in achieving a live infant. Although pregnancy outcome has been improved in treated patients, no uniformly successful therapy exists for patients with antiphospholipid antibodies. On the basis of case reports, IV infusion of γ-globulin (IVIG) appears to be effective additional treatment in cases in which standard therapy has failed. The place for the addition of IVIG as a standard therapy has not been defined, but corticosteroid-resistant thrombocytopenia complicating antiphospholipid antibody syndrome may be one indication for primary treatment with IVIG and low-dose aspirin.[13, 17]

ANTIBODIES AGAINST RIBONUCLEOPROTEIN ANTIGENS

Neonatal lupus syndrome is a rare condition characterized by *congenital heart block,* transient cutaneous lupus, or both.[10, 22, 30] Congenital heart block is the only aspect of neonatal lupus syndrome that is life-threatening. It may result in fetal death, but more commonly it results in neonatal cardiac morbidity or death. A typical antenatal presentation includes a fixed fetal heart rate of 50 to 60 beats per minute, often with nonimmune hydrops. (See Chapter 43.)

A specific association between neonatal lupus syndrome and maternal antinuclear antibodies directed against the soluble tissue ribonucleoprotein antigens SSA/Ro and SSB/La has been found.[32, 34, 36] The SSA antigen is a soluble nuclear antigen, and the Ro antigen is a soluble cytoplasmic antigen. Although the antigens Ro and La were described independently, subsequent studies have shown that they are immunologically identical. Anti-SSA/Ro and anti-SSB/La are IgG autoantibodies to the soluble tissue ribonucleoprotein antigens. Anti-SSA/Ro is present in more than 40% of patients with Sjögren syndrome, in 20% to 25% of those with SLE, and in approximately 5% of those with rheumatoid arthritis. It is rare in patients without connective tissue disease.

It is not clear whether anti-SSA/Ro is responsible for congenital heart block, is involved in another aspect of the pathophysiologic process, or serves as a marker for complete congenital heart block. Not all children born to women with anti-SSA/Ro have congenital heart block. Tissue antigen variation in a child may be relevant because only one member of dizygous twins born to a mother with anti-SSA/Ro in her serum was affected. Perhaps pathophysiologic changes are of varying degrees and produce heart block only when severe. Infants with complete heart block have the cardiac histopathologic features of fibrosis that cause an interruption of the conduction system, fibrotic replacement of the sinoatrial and atrioventricular nodes, and calcification suggestive of earlier inflammation.

The current postdelivery mortality rate in infants with congenital heart block is approximately 25%. At present, no successful in utero therapy exists.[2] If the fetal cardiac conduction system is destroyed, administering medication to the mother in an effort to increase the fetal heart rate will not be successful. In a fetus with severe hydrops, the only hope for improvement of cardiac output is to increase the contractility of the heart with medication or to provide electrical pacing of the heart to increase the heart rate. Although in utero pacemaker placement has been attempted, no successful cases have been reported to date.

MYASTHENIA GRAVIS

Myasthenia gravis, a chronic autoimmune disease, involves the neuromuscular junction, and it is most commonly seen in women in their reproductive years (see Chapter 38, Part Seven). The disease is characterized by progressive fatigue and weakness, typically of the extraocular facial, pharyngeal, and respiratory muscles. Antibodies (generally IgG but possibly IgM) to human acetylcholine receptors are detectable in up to 90% of patients with myasthenia gravis. The serum concentration of acetylcholine antibodies correlates poorly with the severity of the muscular weakness. Rather, the severity of the disease depends on the ability of this antibody to induce accelerated degradation or blockade of the acetylcholine receptor in the skeletal muscles.

The clinical course during pregnancy varies, but a tendency exists for exacerbation, especially during the puerperium. Although most antibodies produced in patients with myasthenia gravis are IgG and cross the placenta, the apparent fetal effects of the antibody are small. Mothers with this disease usually report normal fetal movement; however, arthrogryposis has been reported in several of their infants.[21] Polyhydramnios, which may be expected on the basis of decreased fetal swallowing, has not been a reported feature of this disease. Neonatal myasthenic signs (e.g., flat facies, weak suckling, feeble crying, respiratory distress),[3] all of which respond to anticholinesterase medication, develop in 10% to 20% of infants born to women with myasthenia gravis. The disorder usually begins 12 to 48 hours after birth and may last 10 to 15 weeks (mean, 3 weeks). The delay in onset of symptoms in the newborn has been attributed to the falling levels of protective α-fetoprotein and the presence of a residual anticholinesterase drug from the mother. Although most infants respond to anticholinesterase medication, a small group of patients are severely affected and no therapies have been consistently effective. Tagher and associates described the use of IV-administered immunoglobulin in addition to conventional modalities in a neonate with severe neonatal myasthenia gravis.[35] Despite aggressive management, the child had a prolonged period of weakness and required intensive care.

HERPES GESTATIONIS

Herpes gestationis is a rare autoimmune disease that appears during pregnancy or in the immediate postpartum period. It usually presents with intensely pruritic urticarial plaques.[9] The incidence has been estimated at approximately 1 in 50,000 pregnancies. Cutaneous involvement of the newborn with herpes gestationis is uncommon, reportedly occurring in 2% to 10% of neonates. Usually, these infants have had a very limited cutaneous involvement. Chen and coworkers reported the case of a mother and neonate with confirmed herpes gestationis, both of whom had extensive cutaneous involvement.[11] Systemic steroids are the mainstay of therapy for mothers to relieve pruritus and to suppress the eruption.

MATERNAL THYROTOXICOSIS

(See Chapter 11, Part One.)

SUMMARY

Autoimmunity clearly is recognized as important in many diseases, and when it is present during pregnancy, the fetus frequently is involved. Sometimes the autoimmune response is very specific, with one antibody directed against a precise organ (as with myasthenia gravis). In other instances, such as SLE, the autoimmune response is very broad and may involve several organs. However, even in SLE, specific autoantibodies (the antiphospholipid antibodies LAC and ACA, anti-SSA/Ro antibody and their targets) have been characterized. Therapy most commonly is directed at decreasing the production of the antibody and occasionally at decreasing its end-organ effect. Because the maternal disease activity frequently is not well correlated with the fetal effects, methods of assessing fetal status are important. Unfortunately, current methods of assessing fetal effects of autoimmune disease are frequently less accurate than what is desirable.

■ REFERENCES

1. Ayromlooi J: A new approach to the management of immunologic thrombocytopenic purpura in pregnancy. Am J Obstet Gynecol 130:235, 1978.
2. Barclay C, et al: Successful pregnancy following steroid therapy and plasma exchange in a woman with anti-Ro (SSA) antibodies: Case report. Br J Obstet Gynaecol 94:369, 1987.
3. Barlow CF: Neonatal myasthenia gravis. Am J Dis Child 135:209, 1981.
4. Branch DW: Immunologic disease and fetal death. Clin Obstet Gynecol 30:295, 1987.
5. Branch DW: Antiphospholipid syndrome: Laboratory concerns, fetal loss, and pregnancy management. Semin Perinatol 15:230, 1991.
6. Branch DW, et al: Obstetric complications associated with the lupus anticoagulant. N Engl J Med 313:1322, 1985.
7. Branch DW, et al: Antiphospholipid antibodies other than lupus anticoagulant and anticardiolipin antibodies in women with recurrent pregnancy loss, fertile controls, and antiphospholipid syndrome. Obstet Gynecol 89(4):549, 1997.
8. Burrows RF, et al: Thrombocytopenia at delivery: A prospective survey of 6715 deliveries. Am J Obstet Gynecol 162:731, 1990.
9. Carruthers JA: Herpes gestationis: Clinical features of immunologically proved cases. Am J Obstet Gynecol 131:865, 1978.
10. Chameides L, et al: Association of maternal systemic lupus erythematosus with congenital heart block. N Engl J Med 297:1204, 1977.
11. Chen SH, et al: Herpes gestationis in a mother and child. J Am Acad Dermatol 40:847, 1999.
12. Cowchock S, et al: Do low-risk pregnant women with antiphospholipid antibodies need to be treated? Am J Rep Immunol 39:125, 1998.
13. Cowchock S: Prevention of fetal death in the antiphospholipid antibody syndrome. Lupus 5:467, 1996.
14. Daffos F, et al: Prenatal treatment of alloimmune thrombocytopenic purpura. Lancet 2:632, 1984.
15. Davies SV, et al: Transplacental effect of high-dose immunoglobulin in idiopathic thrombocytopenia (ITP). Lancet 1:1098, 1986.
16. Gandemer V, et al: Pregnancy-associated autoimmune neonatal thrombocytopenia: Role of maternal HLA genotype. Br J Haematol 104:878, 1999.
17. Gordon C, et al: Use of intravenous immunoglobulin therapy in pregnancy in systemic lupus erythematosus and antiphospholipid antibody syndrome. Lupus 7:429, 1998.
18. Harris EN, et al: Anticardiolipin antibodies: Detection by radioimmunoassay and association with thrombosis in systemic lupus erythematosus. Lancet 2:1211, 1983.
19. Harris EN, et al: Anticardiolipin antibodies and lupus anticoagulant. Lancet 2:1099, 1984.
20. Harris EN, et al: Crossreactivity of antiphospholipid antibodies. J Clin Lab Immunol 16:1, 1985.
21. Holmes LB, et al: Contractures in a newborn infant in a mother with myasthenia gravis. J Pediatr 96:1067, 1980.
22. Kasinath BS, et al: Delayed maternal lupus after delivery of offspring with congenital heart block. Arch Intern Med 142:2317, 1982.
23. Kelton JG: Management of the pregnant patient with idiopathic thrombocytopenic purpura. Ann Intern Med 99:796, 1983.
24. Kelton JG, et al: The prenatal prediction of thrombocytopenia in infants of mothers with clinically diagnosed immune thrombocytopenia. Am J Obstet Gynecol 144:449, 1982.
25. Kutteh WH: Antiphospholipid antibody-associated recurrent pregnancy loss: Treatment with heparin and low-dose aspirin to low-dose aspirin alone. Am J Obstet Gynecol 174(5):1584, 1996.
26. Lavery JP, et al: Immunologic thrombocytopenia in pregnancy: Use of antenatal immunoglobulin therapy—case report and review. Obstet Gynecol 66:41S, 1985.
27. Lockshin MD, et al: Antibody to cardiolipin as a predictor of fetal distress or death in pregnant patients with systemic lupus erythematosus. N Engl J Med 313:152, 1985.

28. Mizunuma H, et al: A new approach to idiopathic thrombocytopenic purpura during pregnancy by high-dose immunoglobulin G infusion. Am J Obstet Gynecol 148:218, 1984.

29. Pierro E, et al: Antiphospholipid antibodies inhibit prostaglandin release by decidual cells of early pregnancy: Possible involvement of extracellular secretory phospholipase A_2. Fertil Steril 71(2):342, 1999.

30. Scheib JS, et al: Congenital heart block in successive pregnancies: A case report and evaluation of risk with therapeutic consideration. Obstet Gynecol 73:481, 1989.

31. Scott JR, et al: Fetal platelet counts in the obstetric management of immunologic thrombocytopenic purpura. Am J Obstet Gynecol 136:495, 1980.

32. Scott JS, et al: Connective-tissue disease, antibodies to ribonucleoprotein, and congenital heart block. N Engl J Med 309:209, 1983.

33. Silver RM, et al: Autoimmune disease in pregnancy. Bailliere's Clin Obstet Gynaecol 6:565, 1992.

34. Steier JA, et al: Fetal heart block, anti-SSA and anti-SSB antibodies. Acta Obstet Gynecol Scand 66:737, 1987.

35. Tagher RJ, et al: Failure of intravenously administered immunoglobulin in the treatment of neonatal myasthenia gravis. J Pediatr 134:233, 1999.

36. Taylor PV, et al: Maternal antibodies against fetal cardiac antigens in congenital complete heart block. N Engl J Med 315:667, 1986.

37. Tchernia G, et al: Management of immune thrombocytopenia in pregnancy: Response to infusions of immunoglobulins. Am J Obstet Gynecol 148:225, 1984.

38. Valat AS, et al: Relationships between severe neonatal thrombocytopenia and maternal characteristics in pregnancies associated with autoimmune thrombocytopenia. Br J Haematol 103:397, 1998.

18 Obstetric Management of Multiple Gestation

Neil K. Kochenour

Twins normally occur in approximately 1 in 89 pregnancies, and triplets occur in approximately 1 in 7921 pregnancies. The frequency of multiple births of a higher number can be estimated by applying the Hellin hypothesis, in which the frequency (F) of births of infants can be expressed by

$$F = 89^{(N - 1)}$$

For example, for quadruplets, N equals 4 and F equals 89^3, so that quadruplets occur in approximately 1 in 704,969 pregnancies.

The frequency of monozygous (MZ) twinning apparently is constant throughout the world (3.5 per 1000), whereas the frequency of dizygous (DZ) twinning increases with advancing maternal age, increases by parity, and varies with race. In the United States, the widespread use of ovulation-inducing medication and in vitro fertilization have increased further the incidence of multiple gestation. The use of clomiphene has increased the rate of twinning in the range of 6% to 8% of such pregnancies, and gonadotropin therapy has increased the frequency of multiple gestation even more.[10, 51]

For centuries, multiple births have been regarded with mysticism, awe, and apprehension,[5] and the concern is well placed. Multiple births account for disproportionately high rates of perinatal morbidity and mortality caused primarily by the increased likelihood of low birth weight, which is the result of prematurity, intrauterine growth retardation, or both.[6, 46] Congenital malformations, abnormal presentation, and prolapsed umbilical cord also contribute to the excessive risk. In addition, the maternal risk is increased by polyhydramnios, preeclampsia, placenta previa, postpartum hemorrhage, and anemia, which are all more common in multiple gestation than in singleton pregnancies.

The perinatal death rate for twin gestations is approximately four times that for singleton pregnancies, and it increases correspondingly for gestations of a higher number. The perinatal death rate for MZ twins is approximately 2.5 times that of DZ twins,[7] with that of MZ twins estimated to be as high as 50% (see Chapter 23).[9]

McKeown and colleagues found that the mean birth weight of singleton offspring with a mean gestational age of 280 days is approximately 3400 gm; the mean birth weight of twins with a mean gestational age of 262 days is approximately 2400 gm.[36] Triplets have a mean birth weight of 1800 gm and an average gestation of 247 days. Caspi and associates precisely ascertained the time of ovulation for 111 pregnancies in women whose ovulation had been induced.[10] The average length of gestation in twins was 35 completed weeks; the average length of gestation in triplets was 33 completed weeks.

The possible long-term disadvantages that result from multiple gestation remain somewhat controversial. In Norway, Nilsen and coworkers evaluated the physical and intellectual development of male twins at 18 years of age.[38] Compared with singletons, twice as many male twins were found to be physically unfit for military service. The authors attributed this finding to preterm delivery rather than to twinning per se. Notably, general intelligence apparently was not affected. Babson and colleagues studied MZ twins who were dissimilar in size at birth and found that an undersized twin remained inferior to the other twin in both growth and intelligence into adult life.[3]

Several significant maternal complications occur more frequently with multiple gestation because greater maternal physiologic adaptation to pregnancy is required.[47, 52] Pregnant women with heart disease must adjust to a maternal blood volume increase of 50% to 60% late in pregnancy, compared with a 40% to 50% maternal blood volume increase with a singleton pregnancy.

In a study of 959 consecutive twin gestations, Kovacs and colleagues found that twins had an 83% incidence of antenatal complications, compared with a 32% incidence in singleton gestations.[31] This increased complication rate reflects the higher frequency of three complications: preterm labor, pregnancy-induced hypertension, and fetal death. Recent data indicate that although gestational hypertension, preeclampsia, and eclampsia all occur more commonly in twin pregnancy, they do not lead to significant growth retardation or discordant fetal growth.[8]

EVALUATION AND DIAGNOSIS

Historically, many twin gestations were not recognized until the time of labor (up to 40% to 50% in some studies), which undoubtedly contributed to the increased morbidity and mortality rates. With the availability of diagnostic ultrasound, diagnosis is now made earlier and more frequently.

The use of ovulation-inducing drugs or the implantation of multiple ova with in vitro fertilization always raises the question of multiple gestation. However, other factors should alert a physician to this possibility: a significant discrepancy between menstrual age and size of the uterus (more than 75% of women who subsequently deliver twins have a uterine measurement 4 cm or greater than is indicated for the weeks of gestation); auscultation of two or more heartbeats that differ by more than 10 beats per minute; severe nausea and vomiting and a uterus larger than expected early in pregnancy; an elevated maternal serum α-fetoprotein level early in the second trimester; and anemia late in pregnancy that is unresponsive to the customary iron and multiple vitamin therapy. The early diagnosis of multiple gestation is one of the advantages of maternal serum α-fetoprotein screening.

Whenever multiple gestation is suspected, ultrasound examination should be used to establish the diagnosis. A carefully performed ultrasound examination should detect all sets of twins and identify the presence of one or two amniotic sacs. However, as the number of fetuses increases, the diagnostic accuracy in determining the number of fetuses and the morphometric measurements decreases. When ultrasound examination identifies a twin gestation, careful attention should be paid to placental localization, fetal sex, and membrane thickness. In many instances, the chorionicity of the twins can be established. Chorionicity may be important in later management, may help explain differences in fetal growth patterns, and may aid in diagnosing the twin-twin transfusion syndrome, which is present only in monochorionic twins.

ANTEPARTUM MANAGEMENT

The ultimate goals of reducing perinatal morbidity and mortality rates associated with multiple gestations can be realized by (1) providing an optimum intrauterine environment to ensure fetal growth potential, (2) decreasing the number of very premature infants, (3) identifying the fetuses that are not thriving in the intrauterine environment so as to deliver them before impairment, (4) avoiding fetal trauma during labor and delivery, and (5) providing experienced neonatal care at delivery. As soon as multiple gestation is recognized, the patient should be informed of her high-risk status and about the optimum care required to increase the chances of a good perinatal outcome. Dietary supplementation and counseling should be provided to ensure that dietary needs are met. Although an adequate diet usually supplies the required folate, most authorities recommend folic acid supplementation for women with multiple gestation, as well as iron supplementation.

Numerous methods have been attempted to decrease the incidence of prematurity.[54] Several retrospective studies suggest that bed rest may be of value in the management of twin pregnancies; some suggest that delivery is delayed as a consequence of bed rest.[30, 37, 43] Although other studies do not confirm this finding, some authors suggest that birth weight is increased by bed rest, even if the duration of the pregnancy is not prolonged.[28]

Several prospective, randomized trials have failed to confirm the benefit of hospitalization early in the third trimester of twin gestation.[48] Hospitalization trials have been criticized because (1) patients were hospitalized at 32 weeks' gestation even though retrospective studies suggest that bed rest should begin during the second trimester of pregnancy in order to be of value, and (2) the stress of hospitalization itself may counteract any beneficial effects of bed rest. Whether bed rest is effective and, if it is, how strictly and at what stage of gestation it should be instituted are still not clear. For pregnancies with more than two fetuses, conventional wisdom suggests that bed rest be used liberally; most physicians recommend hospitalization early in the third trimester.

The role of periodic cervical examination in the management of multiple gestation is not well defined. Studies on the management of multiple gestation at high risk of premature labor have suggested that frequent cervical examinations do not predispose the patient to premature rupture of the membranes or infection. However, these examinations do identify patients with premature effacement or dilatation of the cervix, resulting in a more aggressive approach to limiting activity and planning for early hospitalization or tocolysis.[26] Although the prophylactic use of β-sympathomimetic drugs to decrease the incidence of preterm labor has been recommended in multiple gestation, prospective, randomized trials using relatively small doses of these medications have failed to establish any benefit.[35, 40, 49] Serial injections of 17α-hydroxyprogesterone caproate and the prophylactic placement of a cervical cerclage have been advocated to prevent prematurity. Again, there is no evidence that either of these therapies is effective (see Chapter 16).[23]

Surfactant production as measured by the lecithin-sphingomyelin ratio and phosphatidylglycerol in the amniotic fluid is usually similar in the twins when their growth is similar.[50] In multiple gestation with the presence of discordant growth, however, pulmonary maturation may differ markedly among fetuses. Ultrasound, with its capability of measuring multiple morphologic parameters, has resulted in the ability to monitor fetal growth throughout gestation. Although fetal growth during the first two trimesters is similar for singleton and multiple gestations, the growth of multiple fetuses during the third trimester, as determined either by ultrasound parameters or by birth weight, is less than the growth of comparable singleton fetuses.[27, 33] In general, the greater the number of fetuses, the greater the probability of growth retardation. In addition to the generally decreased fetal growth observed in multiple gestation, occasionally one or more multiple fetuses shows more severe growth retardation.[25]

Several studies have demonstrated that twins of dissimilar size are at increased risk in the prenatal, intrapartum, and neonatal periods. The prenatal diagnosis of discordance is sometimes difficult.[22] A number of investigators have studied the value of real-time ultrasonography, umbilical artery velocimetry, or both methods to identify discordant twins.[18, 21, 24, 39] It appears that estimation of fetal weight by ultrasound is the best test to identify discordant growth prenatally. The ability of umbilical artery Doppler velocimetry to identify discordant growth has yet to be demonstrated.

Once the diagnosis of multiple gestation has been made, serial ultrasound examinations should be performed to assess fetal growth.[14, 16] Additionally, fetal well-being should be assessed regularly. Urinary and serum estriol and human placental lactogen measurements, which were not effective in evaluating multiple gestation, have been replaced by biophysical methods such as the nonstress test and the biophysical profile. The use of ultrasound and nonstress tests has greatly improved the ability to identify a fetus in jeopardy. Recent evidence suggests that twin fetuses do not thrive in utero beyond 40 weeks; however, the data available do not permit an accurate assessment of the risk inherent in twin gestations continuing beyond 40 weeks.

The antepartum death of one twin, an uncommon occurrence, is associated more commonly with MZ twinning. Maternal disseminated intravascular coagulation has been described after the prolonged death of one twin in utero.[5, 19, 45, 55] A syndrome in which multicystic encephalomalacia develops in the surviving fetus is the subject of a number of reports.[2, 34] The live-born co-twin of a fetus that died in utero is at increased risk of cerebral impairment, with an overall risk of 20%. The gestational-age–specific prevalence of cerebral palsy after fetal death of the co-twin is much higher than that reported for the general twin population.[41]

One postulated mechanism for this complication is that thromboplastic proteins from the dead twin are transferred into the survivor's circulation, resulting in intravascular coagulation. More recently it has been proposed that massive blood transfer from the survivor into the more relaxed circulation of the dead monochorionic twin may occur through vascular anastomosis. The frequency of either of these severe complications is unknown. Their occurrence underscores the importance of continued careful evaluation when one fetus of a multiple gestation dies in utero.

INTRAPARTUM MANAGEMENT

Intrapartum management of multiple gestation begins as soon as the diagnosis is made. Plans should include delivery at an institution with the facilities and personnel that can provide adequately for the number of infants anticipated. The mother should be informed of the signs and symptoms of preterm labor and encouraged to report their occurrences immediately. Medical personnel responsible for the mother's care should be apprised of her high-risk status. If the patient begins premature labor, the decision must be made whether to inhibit labor. Such a decision should be based on the gestational age of the fetuses, any associated pregnancy complications, the degree of cervical dilatation, the state of the membranes, the well-being of the fetuses as assessed by fetal monitoring, and the potential complications of the tocolytic agent. Because of the maternal cardiovascular adaptations in multiple gestation, the maternal complications with β-sympathomimetic medications are increased.

When delivery is anticipated, the presentations of the fetuses must be determined. The use of real-time ultrasound is preferred for making this determination. If there is any confusion about the presentation, a single x-ray film may be helpful. With twins, all possible combinations of fetal positions occur. The principal controversy in intrapartum management of twin gestation relates to the planned route of delivery, particularly because this consideration is influenced by fetal malpresentation and prematurity. Vertex-vertex pairing occurs in approximately 40% of twins presenting intrapartum, leaving 60% of the cases with one or both twins in a malpresentation. Vertex A/breech B pairing is second in frequency (approximately 25%).

Before 1970, the standard obstetric practice was to manage a twin labor according to the presentation of the first twin, with the delivery of the second twin managed by maneuvers appropriate to the presentation encountered (often by breech extraction). Cesarean section rates with this approach were lower than those for singleton pregnancy at the time. During this era, studies reported an increased neonatal morbidity and mortality risk for twin B, generally with some evidence of an additional risk because of the malpresentation of this twin. Based on this evidence, routine cesarean section was recommended for twins presenting in other than the vertex-vertex position. By the end of the 1970s, this recommendation became widespread practice in the United States.

Notably, case reports before 1976 had in common a low rate of antepartum twin diagnosis (typically fewer than 50% were diagnosed before the onset of labor, and 33% or more were diagnosed only after the delivery of the first twin). Most twin studies since that time have not shown a different mortality risk between twins A and B, which is most likely explained by the much improved rates of antepartum diagnosis and intrapartum monitoring.[15] (That which is not diagnosed cannot be managed specifically or safely.) Evidence shows that the increased risk frequently attributed to twin B occurs principally in the fetus identified late in gestation. Because we can provide intrapartum monitoring of both twins and make optimum preparations for twin delivery, it is reasonable to re-evaluate outcome statistics, because they might influence the choice and planned route of delivery.

With twins older than 33 weeks' gestation who have an estimated fetal weight greater than 1800 gm, a vaginal delivery for vertex-vertex twins is indicated unless some other obstetric circumstance argues against it. In twins older than 33 weeks' gestation or whose fetal weight is greater than 1800 gm, a cesarean section is the most common mode of delivery for a vertex-nonvertex presentation. However, several studies support the safety of vaginal delivery of twin B.[11, 12, 32, 44] In a study by Acker and coworkers that included only uncomplicated pregnancies and labors, 76 second twins weighing more than 1499 gm who were delivered by breech extraction were compared with 74 nonvertex second twins of similar weight who were delivered by cesarean section.[1] No significant differences in low 5-minute Apgar scores or observed morbidity were found in the two groups.

Chervenak and colleagues analyzed neonatal mortality and morbidity rates for 362 twin pairs in 1985.[13] Only 4.7% of these twin gestations were undiagnosed before delivery. Of the vertex-nonvertex pairs, 71% were delivered vaginally. Excluding congenital anomalies incompatible with life, the investigators found no differences in fetal deaths, 5-minute Apgar scores, respiratory distress syndrome, and intraventricular hemorrhage in twin B of vertex-vertex presentations and twin B of vertex-nonvertex presentations who weighed more than 1500 gm.

When the twin gestation period is less than 33 weeks or the estimated fetal weight is less than 1800 gm, most clinicians favor planned vaginal delivery with a vertex-vertex presentation. Although recent evidence favors consideration of breech vaginal delivery for the mature second twin, extrapolated risk data for the premature singleton breech are convincing that cesarean section is the safest choice for the small second twin in presentations other than vertex. If the gestation period is less than 33 weeks or the estimated fetal weight is less than 1800 gm and twin A is in the breech presentation, the delivery should be performed by cesarean section (Fig. 18–1).[4]

If vaginal delivery is attempted, both fetuses should be monitored continuously during labor and preparation should be made for immediate cesarean delivery should it become necessary. The second fetus should be monitored continuously after delivery of the first twin even if the vaginal route of delivery is selected. Appropriate medical personnel must be present to provide immediate care to the infants. Moreover, careful examination of the placenta is important, especially if evidence of twin-twin transfusion is sought. For three or more fetuses, the preferred route of delivery is by cesarean section.

A high perinatal mortality rate is associated with twin-twin transfusion syndrome diagnosed late in the second trimester of pregnancy (see Chapters 23 and 44).[20] Commonly, severe polyhydramnios is present in one twin, with resultant nonimmune hydrops and

FIGURE 18–1. Protocol for delivery management.

growth retardation with severe oligohydramnios in the donor twin. Although no uniformly successful therapy for this condition is currently available, repeated amniocentesis is advocated by some.[42] Recent Australian data indicate that increased gestational age at delivery, the presence of umbilical artery diastolic flow, and a prolonged interval from final amnioreduction were positively associated with the delivery of live fetuses without complications.[17] The use of laser therapy to obliterate the anastomotic sites has been reported. This procedure is possible when the placenta implants posteriorly.[53] Fetoscopic laser coagulation of the placental anastomoses in severe midtrimester twin-twin transfusion is a potentially corrective and effective, minimally invasive procedure (see Chapter 11, Part Two.) Doppler investigation of the umbilical and fetal circulations provides important information on fetal condition, prognosis, and therapeutic effects of the intervention.[56]

SUMMARY

The patient with a multiple gestation is at risk of increased perinatal morbidity and of a number of maternal complications. Pregnancy management should be directed toward achieving an optimum intrauterine environment, decreasing the incidence of prematurity, evaluating fetal growth and well-being, avoiding traumatic delivery, and providing skilled neonatal care.

■ REFERENCES

1. Acker D, et al: Delivery of the second twin. Obstet Gynecol 59:710, 1982.
2. Anderson RL, et al: Central nervous system damage and other anomalies in surviving fetus following second-trimester ante-

natal death of co-twin: Report of four cases and literature review. Prenat Diagn 10:513, 1990.

3. Babson SG, et al: Growth and development of twins dissimilar in size at birth. N Engl J Med 289:937, 1973.

4. Barrett JM, et al: The effect of type of delivery upon neonatal outcome in premature twins. Am J Obstet Gynecol 143:360, 1982.

5. Benirschke K: Intrauterine death of a twin: Mechanisms, implications for surviving twin, and placental pathology. Semin Diagn Pathol 10:222, 1993.

6. Benirschke K, et al: Multiple pregnancy. N Engl J Med 288:1276, 1973.

7. Bronsteen R, et al: Classification of twins and neonatal morbidity. Obstet Gynecol 74:98, 1989.

8. Campbell DM, MacGillivray I: Preeclampsia in twin pregnancies: Incidence and outcome. Hypertens Pregnancy 18:197, 1999.

9. Carr SR, et al: Survival rates of monoamniotic twins do not decrease after 30 weeks' gestation. Am J Obstet Gynecol 163:719, 1990.

10. Caspi E, et al: The outcome of pregnancy after gonadotropin therapy. Br J Obstet Gynaecol 83:967, 1976.

11. Cetrulo CL: The controversy of mode of delivery of twins: The intrapartum management of twin gestation. Semin Perinatol 10:39, 1986.

12. Chervenak FA, et al: Is routine cesarean section necessary for vertex-breech and vertex-transverse twin gestations? Am J Obstet Gynecol 148:1, 1984.

13. Chervenak FA, et al: Intrapartum management of twin gestation. Obstet Gynecol 65:119, 1985.

14. Crane JP, et al: Ultrasonic growth patterns in normal and discordant twins. Obstet Gynecol 55:678, 1980.

15. Crawford JS: A prospective study of 200 consecutive twin deliveries. Anaesthesia 42:33, 1987.

16. D'Alton ME, et al: Antepartum management of twin gestation: Ultrasound. Clin Obstet Gynecol 33:42, 1990.

17. Dickinson JE, Evans SF: Obstetric and perinatal outcomes from the Australian and New Zealand twin-twin transfusion syndrome registry. Am J Obstet Gynecol 182:706, 2000.

18. Divon MY, et al: Discordant twins: A prospective study of the diagnostic value of real-time ultrasonography combined with umbilical artery velocimetry. Am J Obstet Gynecol 161:757, 1989.

19. Enbom JA: Twin pregnancy with intrauterine death of one twin. Am J Obstet Gynecol 152:424, 1985.

20. Erskine RLA, et al: Antenatal diagnosis of placental anastomosis in a twin pregnancy using Doppler ultrasound. Br J Obstet Gynaecol 93:955, 1986.

21. Giles WB, et al: Fetal umbilical artery flow velocity-time waveforms in twin pregnancies. Br J Obstet Gynaecol 92:490, 1985.

22. Haney AF, et al: Significance of biparietal diameter differences between twins. Obstet Gynecol 51:609, 1978.

23. Hartikainen-Sorri AL, et al: Inefficacy of 17-hydroxyprogesterone caproate in the prevention of prematurity in twin pregnancy. Obstet Gynecol 56:692, 1980.

24. Hastie SJ, et al: Prediction of the small for gestational age twin fetus by Doppler umbilical artery waveform analysis. Obstet Gynecol 74:730, 1989.

25. Houlton MCC: Divergent biparietal diameter growth rates in twin pregnancies. Obstet Gynecol 49:542, 1977.

26. Houlton MCC, et al: Factors associated with preterm labour and changes in the cervix before labour in twin pregnancy. Br J Obstet Gynaecol 89:190, 1982.

27. Iffy L, et al: The rate of early intrauterine growth in twin gestation. Am J Obstet Gynecol 146:970, 1983.

28. Jeffrey RL, et al: Role of bed rest in twin gestation. Obstet Gynecol 43:822, 1974.

29. Kogan MD, et al: Trends in twin birth outcomes and prenatal care utilization in the United States. JAMA 284:335, 2000.

30. Komaromy B, et al: The value of bed rest in twin pregnancies. Int J Gynaecol Obstet 15:262, 1977.

31. Kovacs BW, et al: Twin gestations. I. Antenatal care and complications. Obstet Gynecol 74:313, 1989.

32. Laros RK Jr, et al: Management of twin pregnancy: The vaginal route is still safe. Am J Obstet Gynecol 158:1330, 1988.

33. Leveno KJ, et al: Sonar cephalometry in twins: A table of biparietal diameters for normal twin fetuses and a comparison with singletons. Am J Obstet Gynecol 135:727, 1979.

34. Liu S, et al: Intrauterine death in multiple gestation. Acta Genet Med 41:5, 1992.

35. Marivate M, et al: Effect of prophylactic outpatient administration of fenoterol on the time of onset of spontaneous labor and fetal growth rate in twin pregnancy. Am J Obstet Gynecol 128:707, 1977.

36. McKeown T, et al: Observations on fetal growth in multiple pregnancy in man. J Endocrinol 5:387, 1952.

37. Misenhimer HR, et al: Effects of decreased prenatal activity in patients with twin pregnancy. Obstet Gynecol 51:692, 1978.

38. Nilsen ST, et al: Male twins at birth and 18 years later. Br J Obstet Gynaecol 91:122, 1984.

39. Nimrod C, et al: Doppler ultrasound prediction of fetal outcome in twin pregnancies. Am J Obstet Gynecol 156:402, 1987.

40. O'Connor MC, et al: Double-blind trial of ritodrine and placebo in twin pregnancy. Br J Obstet Gynaecol 86:706, 1979.

41. Pharoah PO, Adi Y: Consequences of in-utero death in a twin pregnancy. Lancet 335:1597,2000.

42. Pinette MG, et al: Treatment of twin/twin transfusion syndrome. Obstet Gynecol 82:841, 1993.

43. Powers WF, et al: Bed rest in twin pregnancy: Identification of a critical period and its cost implications. Am J Obstet Gynecol 134:23, 1979.

44. Rabinovici J, et al: Randomized management of the second nonvertex twin: Vaginal delivery or cesarean section. Am J Obstet Gynecol 156:52, 1987.

45. Romero R, et al: Prolongation of a preterm pregnancy complicated by death of a single twin in utero and disseminated intravascular coagulation. N Engl J Med 310:772, 1984.

46. Ron-El R, et al: Triplet and quadruplet pregnancies and management. Obstet Gynecol 57:458, 1981.

47. Rovinsky JJ, et al: Cardiovascular hemodynamics in pregnancy. III. Cardiac rate, stroke volume, total peripheral resistance, and central blood volume in multiple pregnancy: Synthesis of results. Am J Obstet Gynecol 95:787, 1966.

48. Saunders MC, et al: The effects of hospital admission for bed rest on the duration of twin pregnancy: A randomised trial. Lancet 2:793, 1985.

49. Skjaerris J, et al: Prevention of prematurity in twin pregnancy by orally administered terbutaline. Acta Obstet Gynecol Scand 108(Suppl):39, 1982.

50. Spellacy WN, et al: Amniotic fluid L/S ratio in twin gestation. Obstet Gynecol 50:66, 1978.

51. Tough SC, et al: Effect of in utero fertilization on low birth weight, preterm delivery, and multiple birth. J Pediatr 136:618, 2000.

52. Veille JC, et al: Maternal cardiovascular adaptations to twin pregnancy. Am J Obstet Gynecol 153:261, 1985.

53. Ville Y, et al: Preliminary experience with endoscopic laser surgery for severe twin-twin transfusion syndrome. N Engl J Med 332:224, 1995.

54. Weekes ARL, et al: The relative efficacy of bed rest, cervical suture, and no treatment in the management of twin pregnancy. Br J Obstet Gynaecol 84:161, 1977.

55. Yoshioka H, et al: Multicystic encephalomalacia in a liveborn twin with a stillborn macerated co-twin. J Pediatr 95:798, 1979.

56. Zikulnig L, et al: Prognostic factors in severe twin-twin transfusion syndrome treated by endoscopic laser surgery. Ultrasound Obstet Gynecol 14:380, 1999.

Post-term Pregnancy

Neil K. Kochenour

The post-term pregnancy, a pregnancy that persists longer than 280 days after ovulation, dramatically illustrates the importance of a precise determination of gestational age. For women with 28-day cycles who normally ovulate on approximately day 14, a post-term pregnancy begins at 42 weeks after the onset of the last menstrual period. Although this definition includes approximately 10% of all pregnancies, some pregnancies are actually not post-term but instead are the result of ovulation after the 14th day or an error in the estimation of gestational age. A pregnancy that persists longer than 42 weeks' gestation is termed *postdate* or *post-term*, and the infant who is born at this time is labeled *postmature* or *dysmature*. The term "dysmature," however, emphasizes that the fetus need not be postmature to have the characteristic features of postmaturity, which most obstetricians identify as a result of placental insufficiency.

Although knowledge about the mechanism of parturition has increased rapidly, why some pregnancies are abnormally prolonged is not clear. Several uncommon conditions, such as anencephaly and placental sulfatase deficiency, are associated with prolonged gestations. In anencephalic fetuses, those without a pituitary gland frequently have prolonged gestation.[29] Until the mechanism governing the onset of normal parturition in humans is clearly understood, the causes of prolonged gestation probably will remain elusive. Evidence that the fetus itself plays an important role in the onset of labor is accumulating; the post-term pregnancy may be of fetal origin.

The fetus of a post-term pregnancy continues to grow in utero and is unusually large at birth, but if the uterine environment is unfavorable for fetal growth, the infant appears at birth to have lost considerable weight (especially from the loss of subcutaneous fat and muscle mass). Although the large infant is at greater risk of birth trauma,[35] the small dysmature infant is at the greatest risk of fetal distress during labor and of neonatal morbidity. These pregnancies frequently are accompanied by oligohydramnios and thick meconium, which carry an increased risk of meconium aspiration.

Although the dysmature infant born post-term was recognized early in this century, it was not until 1945

that the clinical findings characteristic of these infants (wasting and staining of the skin, nails, and umbilical cord) were organized into a syndrome by Clifford.[5] In 1963, Browne emphasized the significance of this condition when he reported that the perinatal mortality rate doubled by 43 weeks' gestation and tripled by 44 weeks' gestation compared with the perinatal mortality rate at 39 to 41 weeks' gestation (Fig. 19–1).[1]

Other pregnancy variables affect the risk of prolonged pregnancy.[36] Maternal hypertension during pregnancy in a woman of advanced age appears to result in an earlier and more rapid increase in the

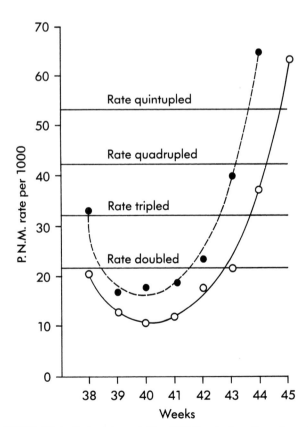

FIGURE 19–1. Perinatal mortality (PNM) rate for all prolonged pregnancies *(solid line)* and for prolonged pregnancies in patients with preeclampsia *(hatched line)*. (From Browne JCM: Postmaturity. Am J Obstet Gynecol 85:573, 1963.)

perinatal mortality rate after 42 weeks' gestation. Clifford suggested that fetal postmaturity is limited to the primigravid woman.[6] However, although the perinatal mortality rate in the multigravid woman after 42 weeks' gestation is lower than in the primigravid woman, there is still an increased risk.

MANAGEMENT

Management of the post-term pregnancy has been the subject of considerable investigation and debate.* Unfortunately, most reports have described the results of specific management protocols,[10, 15] using a given antepartum fetal surveillance test to identify the fetus at risk. Although no consensus has emerged for the ideal management of postmaturity, numerous protocols have been devised. All protocols address the following issues, which make the management of this condition difficult:

- An important principle of prenatal care is the accurate determination of gestational age; however, it is not always possible, and a pregnancy may not be as advanced as is thought.
- Even after 280 days of gestation, most fetuses are not in jeopardy.
- Current methods for fetal surveillance are not totally reliable for identifying the fetus at risk of fetal death or serious morbidity.
- No safe, consistently effective method of cervical ripening is currently available.
- Induction of labor is not always successful, and induced labors usually last longer than spontaneous labors.
- Cesarean delivery increases maternal risk.

Traditionally, with a well-established gestational age, the concern about a post-term pregnancy begins at approximately 42 weeks' gestation. However, Guidetti and colleagues suggested that the adverse perinatal outcome associated with pregnancies of more than 42 weeks' gestation may also be present in pregnancies of 41 to 42 weeks' gestation, and they recommended that post-term fetal testing begin at 41 weeks' gestation.[16] If the cervix is favorable for induction at 42 weeks, many obstetricians recommend induction of labor. Labor in a patient with a favorable cervix is successful 95% of the time. Labor can be induced by administering IV oxytocin or by rupturing the membranes and administering oxytocin only if labor does not begin spontaneously.

What should be done for the patient with well-established dates but an unfavorable cervix is more controversial. The introduction of prostaglandin E_2 intracervical gel has made induction of labor with an unfavorable cervix a reasonable option for the management of the post-term pregnancy. Several prospective, randomized trials have compared induction of labor after cervical ripening with prostaglandin E_2 gel and intensive fetal surveillance until the onset of

spontaneous labor in the management of the post-term pregnancy. Two large, multicenter trials were undertaken. The National Institute of Child Health and Human Development Network of Maternal-Fetal Medicine Units reported a study of 440 women with uncomplicated pregnancy at 41 weeks' gestation who were randomly assigned either to immediate induction of labor ($n = 265$) or to expectant management ($n = 175$).[28] Patients in the expectant management group underwent nonstress testing and amniotic fluid volume assessment twice a week. Patients in the induction group underwent induction within 24 hours of randomization. For an evaluation of the efficacy of intracervical prostaglandin E_2 gel, patients in the induction group were randomly assigned in a 2:1 scheme to receive either 0.5 mg of prostaglandin E_2 gel or placebo gel intracervically 12 hours before induction of labor with oxytocin. There were no differences in mean birth weight or the frequency of macrosomia between the two groups. Regardless of parity, prostaglandin E_2 intracervical gel was not more effective than placebo in ripening the cervix. The cesarean delivery rate was not significantly different in the expectant (18%), prostaglandin E_2 gel (23%), or placebo gel (18%) groups. The authors concluded that both management schemes are acceptable when considering perinatal morbidity or death. Recent data suggest that application of prostaglandin E_2 gel in women with post-term pregnancies and unfavorable cervices may reduce the induction rate.[23]

The Canadian Multicenter Post-term Pregnancy Trial Group studied 3407 women with uncomplicated pregnancies at 41 or more weeks' duration. The women were randomly assigned to undergo induction of labor or to have serial antenatal monitoring and undergo spontaneous labor unless there was evidence of fetal or maternal compromise, in which case labor would be induced and cesarean section performed. In the induction group, labor was induced by the intracervical application of prostaglandin E_2. Serial antenatal monitoring consisted of fetal kick counts, nonstress tests, and assessment of amniotic fluid. Among the 1701 women in the induction group, 21.2% underwent cesarean section, compared with 24.5% of the 1706 women in the monitored group ($P = .03$). This difference existed because fewer cesarean sections were performed as a result of fetal distress among the women in the induction group (5.7% versus 8.3%; $P = .003$). The frequency of neonatal morbidity was similar in the two groups. When two infants with lethal congenital anomalies were excluded, there was no significant difference in the number of perinatal deaths between the groups. These authors concluded that the rate of cesarean section is lower with induction of labor than with serial antenatal monitoring. The perinatal mortality and neonatal morbidity rates are similar with the two management approaches. Therefore, it appears that both strategies are acceptable methods for managing the post-term pregnancy. There may be a small decrease in the number of cesarean sections with an aggressive ap-

---

*References 2, 3, 7–9, 14, 17, 19, 30, 31, 33.

proach to induction of labor rather than with expectant management.

When patients have uncertain dates and the pregnancy is suspected of being post-term, management tends to be more conservative than when dates are well established. In the absence of any identifying complication of pregnancy and with an adequate amount of amniotic fluid volume and demonstrated fetal well-being, the risk posed by intervention is probably greater than the risk posed by possible post-term gestation.

FETAL SURVEILLANCE

(See also Chapter 9.)

Antepartum fetal surveillance has proved to be essential in the post-term pregnancy. However, no single test is optimum for all high-risk situations, and no single test has proved to be completely reliable in identifying a compromised fetus in the post-term pregnancy.[21]

Biochemical Methods

Historically, the most common biochemical test for fetal well-being is the measurement of maternal serum or urinary estriol.[37] Although these tests have been replaced almost universally by biophysical measurements, estriol measurements in the post-term pregnancy are reliable for identifying a fetus at risk.[20] The incidence of dysmaturity in patients born after 42 weeks' gestation is approximately 50% when the mother has low estriol levels. Conversely, the chance of delivering a dysmature infant when estriol levels are in the normal range is small.

Biophysical Methods

Fetal movement is one of the oldest variables used in evaluating the condition of a fetus. Maternal assessment of fetal movement is simple, universally available, convenient, inexpensive, and reasonably accurate as a predictor of fetal well-being. Fetal movement as perceived by the mother is frequently used with other measures of fetal well-being in patients at high risk. The confirmation of numerous studies that acceleration of the fetal heart rate in association with fetal movement is a good predictor of fetal well-being forms the basis of the nonstress test (NST). In most high-risk situations, this test is performed at weekly intervals. However, the evidence indicates that a 1-week interval between NSTs is too long to permit detection of all fetuses at risk in post-term pregnancies.[12] Miyazaki and associates reported an 8% incidence of nonreactive NSTs in a group of 125 women with post-term pregancies.[27] Of significance, the presence of spontaneous decelerations, even with the reactive NST, is ominous in patients with post-term pregnancy.

In 1985, Phelan and coworkers stressed the importance of assessing the amniotic fluid volume in conjunction with giving an NST in the evaluation of patients with post-term pregnancies.[32] They found that real-time ultrasound estimates of adequate amniotic fluid volumes were a reliable predictor of fetal well-being in post-term pregnancies. The lower the estimated amniotic fluid volume, the greater the incidence of antepartum fetal heart rate tests indicating decelerations or bradycardias.

An analysis of the patterns of fetal heart rate decelerations during labor led to the identification of late decelerations as a presumptive sign of in utero placental insufficiency. Subsequent research demonstrated that late decelerations result from impaired oxygen transfer across the placenta. With each uterine contraction, blood flow decreases, or stops, resulting in a diminished respiratory gas exchange between the mother and the fetus. This observation led to the development of the contraction stress test (CST). A CST is performed by inducing contractions by the administration of IV oxytocin or by nipple stimulation. The fetal heart rate is monitored externally. Theoretically, late decelerations during the CST (a positive CST result) depict a fetus at risk. Conversely, the absence of repetitive late decelerations (a negative CST result) is indicative of fetal well-being. Experience has demonstrated that fetal death resulting from placental insufficiency within 1 week of a negative CST result is extremely rare. However, approximately 25% of fetuses with a positive CST result whose mothers are allowed to labor show no evidence of late decelerations during the intrapartum period.

Freeman and colleagues recommended the CST as the primary method of fetal surveillance in pregnancies continuing beyond 280 days.[13] In a series of 679 post-term pregnancies, no perinatal deaths occurred, and perinatal morbidity was no greater than in the control population; 75% of the women with post-term pregnancies went into spontaneous labor.

Evaluation with several biophysical parameters may predict fetal death better. The biophysical profile consists of five variables: the NST, fetal breathing movements, fetal tone, fetal movements, and quantitative evaluation of the amniotic fluid[25] (see Chapter 9). An advantage of the biophysical profile in the management of post-term pregnancies is that it evaluates the amount of the amniotic fluid. After studying 727 women with post-term pregnancies, Leveno concluded that the cause of fetal distress in post-term pregnancies is typically oligohydramnios, which results in cord compression, rather than placental insufficiency.[22] Many obstetricians have found that the presence of oligohydramnios is a good predictor of fetal compromise and an indication for delivery in the women with a post-term pregnancy.

Johnson and associates used twice-weekly biophysical profiles as a method of fetal surveillance in post-term pregnancies.[18] In an analysis of 307 consecutive post-term pregnancies they demonstrated that if patients had normal profiles, waiting for spontaneous labor resulted in healthy neonates and a much lower cesarean delivery rate (15% for cesarean delivery versus 42% for prophylactic induction).

Routine ultrasound screening for macrosomia has

been recommended as part of the management of post-term pregnancies. In 317 consecutive patients with prolonged pregnancies under fetal surveillance at more than 41 weeks' gestation, Chervenak and coworkers found a 25% incidence of macrosomia at 41 weeks' gestation.[4] A significant increase was found in the incidence of cesarean section for macrosomic fetuses compared with nonmacrosomic fetuses.

INTRAPARTUM MANAGEMENT

The fetus of a post-term pregnancy is more susceptible to stress during labor than the fetus of a normal pregnancy. Women with post-term pregnancy should be cautioned to come to the hospital as soon as labor begins. Continuous electronic fetal monitoring should be used throughout labor.[26] If real-time ultrasound is available, the amount of amniotic fluid should be evaluated. Whether to rupture membranes is controversial. Although reducing the amount of amniotic fluid by amniotomy certainly can increase the possibility of cord compression, amniotomy usually identifies the presence of thick meconium, which is important for several reasons:

- Thick meconium is evidence of fairly recent fetal stress.
- If aspirated by the fetus, thick meconium can lead to a syndrome associated with a high perinatal mortality rate (see Chapter 42, Part Five).
- In the presence of thick meconium, abnormal heart rate tracings are even more ominous.

Moreover, the rupture of the membranes allows placement of an internal fetal electrode to provide more accurate information than the external system allows.

Biochemical monitoring with fetal scalp blood sampling can be helpful in the intrapartum evaluation of the fetus. Post-term fetuses are particularly vulnerable at the time of delivery. The aspiration of meconium can be minimized by suctioning the fetus as soon as the head is delivered and before delivery of the thorax. In the presence of hypoxemia and dysmaturity, the post-term infant may be at considerable risk of experiencing the adverse effects of asphyxia. Finally, hypoglycemia may be a manifestation of depleted nutrient stores caused by postmaturity.

LONG-TERM FOLLOW-UP

Studies of the subsequent development of fetuses from prolonged pregnancies are difficult to evaluate. Most authors have not separated dysmature neonates from those showing no effects of prolonged pregnancy. In Lovell's 1-year study,[24] a group of 106 postmature infants was compared with a group of non-postmature, matched control subjects. The post-term pregnancies resulted in a higher incidence of fetal distress during labor and of abnormal neurologic signs during the first few days of life. During the first year of life, an increased number of severe illnesses and sleep deficits were present, and at 1 year an increased proportion of the infants from the post-term pregnancies demonstrated low social quotients. Unfortunately, the author did not compare neonates showing evidence of dysmaturity with neonates in the post-term group showing no evidence of dysmaturity.

Field and colleagues reported the outcome for a group of 40 dysmature offspring born post-term.[11] The Bayley Scales of Infant Development motor scores of the postmature infants were equivalent to those of control infants by 8 months of age, but the mental scores were slightly lower. In a prospective study by Shime and associates,[34] 129 children born after prolonged pregnancies were compared with 184 control children born at term. No differences were found between the two groups with respect to IQ scores, physical milestones, or intercurrent illnesses at 1 or 2 years of age. These investigators differentiated between prolonged pregnancies resulting in so-called normal infants and those resulting in infants with dysmaturity. The only significant differences were notably greater locomotor and IQ subscores at year 2 for the combined group of term infants than for the combined group of infants born after a prolonged pregnancy.

SUMMARY

The post-term pregnancy is associated with increased perinatal morbidity and mortality rates. Management begins with the accurate determination of gestational age. At 42 weeks' gestation (some suggest earlier), induction of labor should be considered in a woman with a favorable cervix. If the cervix is unfavorable for induction, intensive fetal surveillance should begin. Of significance is a marked decrease in the amount of amniotic fluid, which is an especially ominous sign in these pregnancies. The postmature fetus is susceptible to hypoxic damage before and during labor and to meconium aspiration during labor and at the time of delivery. Although the optimum management of this condition has not been determined, a number of clinical protocols have been shown to reduce considerably the perinatal morbidity and mortality rates of the post-term pregnancy.

■ REFERENCES

1. Browne JCM: Postmaturity. Am J Obstet Gynecol 85:573, 1963.
2. Buttino LT, et al: Intracervical prostaglandin in postdate pregnancy: A randomized trial. J Reprod Med 35:155, 1990.
3. Cario GM: Conservative management of prolonged pregnancy using fetal heart rate monitoring only: A prospective study. Br J Obstet Gynaecol 91:23, 1984.
4. Chervenak JL, et al: Macrosomia in the postdate pregnancy: Is routine ultrasonographic screening indicated? Am J Obstet Gynecol 161:753, 1989.
5. Clifford SH: Clinical significance of yellow staining of the vernix caseosa, skin, nails, and umbilical cord. Am J Dis Child 69:327, 1945.
6. Clifford SH: Post maturity—with placental dysfunction. J Pediatr 44:1, 1954.

7. Devoe LD, et al: Postdates pregnancy—assessment of fetal risk and obstetric management. J Reprod Med 28:576, 1983.
8. Dyson DC, et al: Management of prolonged pregnancy: Induction of labor versus antepartum fetal testing. Am J Obstet Gynecol 156:928, 1987.
9. Eden RD, et al: Comparison of antepartum testing schemes for the management of the postdate pregnancy. Am J Obstet Gynecol 144:683, 1982.
10. Elliott JP, et al: The use of breast stimulation to prevent postdate pregnancy. Am J Obstet Gynecol 149:628, 1984.
11. Field TM, et al: Developmental effects of prolonged pregnancy and the postmaturity syndrome. J Pediatr 90:836, 1977.
12. Fleischer A, et al: Antepartum nonstress test and the postmature pregnancy. Obstet Gynecol 66:80, 1985.
13. Freeman RK, et al: Postdate pregnancy: Utilization of contraction stress testing for primary fetal surveillance. Am J Obstet Gynecol 140:128, 1981.
14. Granados JL: Survey of the management of postterm pregnancy. Obstet Gynecol 63:651, 1984.
15. Guidetti DA, et al: Fetal umbilical artery flow velocimetry in postdate pregnancies. Am J Obstet Gynecol 157:1521, 1987.
16. Guidetti DA, et al: Postdate fetal surveillance: Is 41 weeks too early? Am J Obstet Gynecol 161:91, 1989.
17. Hannah ME, et al: Induction of labor as compared with serial antenatal monitoring in postterm pregnancy. N Engl J Med 326:1587, 1992.
18. Johnson JM, et al: Biophysical profile scoring in the management of the postterm pregnancy: An analysis of 307 patients. Am J Obstet Gynecol 154:269, 1986.
19. Knox GE, et al: Management of prolonged pregnancy: Results of a prospective randomized trial. Am J Obstet Gynecol 134:376, 1979.
20. Kochenour NK: Estrogen assay during pregnancy. Clin Obstet Gynecol 25:659, 1982.
21. Kohouzami VA, et al: Comparison of urinary estrogens, contraction stress tests and nonstress tests in the management of postterm pregnancy. J Reprod Med 28:189, 1983.
22. Leveno KJ: Prolonged pregnancy. 1. Observations concerning the causes of fetal distress. Am J Obstet Gynecol 150:465, 1984.
23. Lien JM, et al: Antepartum cervical ripening: Applying prostaglandin E2 gel in conjunction with scheduled nonstress tests in postdate pregnancies. Am J Obstet Gynecol 179:453, 1998.
24. Lovell KE: The effect of postmaturity on the developing child. Med J Aust 1:13, 1973.
25. Manning FA, et al: Fetal biophysical profile scoring: A prospective study in 1,184 high-risk patients. Am J Obstet Gynecol 140:289, 1981.
26. Miller FC, et al: Intrapartum assessment of the postdate fetus. Am J Obstet Gynecol 141:516, 1981.
27. Miyazaki FS, et al: False reactive nonstress tests in postterm pregnancies. Am J Obstet Gynecol 140:269, 1981.
28. National Institute of Child Health and Human Development Network of Maternal-Fetal Medicine Units: A clinical trial of induction of labor versus expectant management in postterm pregnancy. Am J Obstet Gynecol 170:716, 1994.
29. Nwosu UC, et al: Possible adrenocortical insufficiency in postmature neonates. Am J Obstet Gynecol 122:969, 1975.
30. Owen J, et al: A randomized, double-blind trial of prostaglandin E_2 gel for cervical ripening and meta-analysis. Am J Obstet Gynecol 165:991, 1991.
31. Phelan JP, et al: Continuing role of the nonstress test in the management of postdate pregnancy. Obstet Gynecol 64:624, 1984.
32. Phelan JP, et al: The role of ultrasound assessment of amniotic fluid volume in the management of the postdate pregnancy. Am J Obstet Gynecol 151:304, 1985.
33. Rayburn WF, et al: Antepartum prediction of the postmature infant. Obstet Gynecol 60:148, 1982.
34. Shime J, et al: The influence of prolonged pregnancy on infant development at one and two years of age: A prospective controlled study. Am J Obstet Gynecol 154:341, 1986.
35. Spellacy WN, et al: Macrosomia—maternal characteristics and infant complications. Obstet Gynecol 66:158, 1985.
36. Stubblefield PG, et al: Perinatal mortality in term and postterm births. Obstet Gynecol 56:676, 1980.
37. Yeh S, et al: Plasma unconjugated estriol as an indicator of fetal dysmaturity in postterm pregnancy. Obstet Gynecol 62:22, 1983.

20

Erythroblastosis Fetalis

Andrée M. Gruslin

Thomas R. Moore

HISTORICAL BACKGROUND

Although Hippocrates initially described features of erythroblastosis fetalis in 400 BC, the first clinical report of this disorder is attributed to a French midwife who delivered twins in 1609. The first twin was hydropic and stillborn; the second was severely jaundiced and later died of kernicterus.

Diamond and colleagues noted the presence of extramedullary erythropoiesis along with erythroblastosis and red blood cell hemolysis in 1932.[15] The pathophysiology underlying these findings remained unclear until 1940, when Landsteiner and associates discovered the Rh antigen.[34] By injecting blood from the *Macaca mulatta* (rhesus monkey) into guinea pigs and rabbits, they obtained red blood cell antiserum that, when injected into other rhesus monkeys, provoked red cell agglutination. Agglutination was the direct result of the presence of an antigen they called *rhesus* (Rh). Subsequently, in 1941, Levine and coworkers observed that the exposure of a woman who is RhD (rhesus blood group; D antigen) negative to cells that are RhD positive led to the formation of antibodies responsible for red cell hemolysis.[35]

In 1948, Wiener postulated that transplacental passage of RhD-positive fetal blood into the maternal circulation could trigger the production of antibodies against fetal cells.[66] This process was later confirmed by Chow in the mid-1950s.[10]

Improved understanding of the pathophysiology of erythroblastosis fetalis allowed Finn and colleagues,[18] in 1961, to propose the administration of anti-D antibodies to nonimmunized mothers, immediately postpartum, to prevent maternal antibody production by eliminating any fetal cells entering the maternal circulation. Clarke and associates studied a group of male volunteers who were RhD negative,[11] sensitized through previous injection of Rh-positive red cells. Half of this group had also received anti-D IgM. IgM was used (as opposed to IgG) because anti-A and anti-B were known to be IgMs. The ineffectiveness of IgM became very obvious through the production of antibodies in a high percentage of both control and treatment subjects. Another study was initiated using IgG, the efficacy of which had been previously demonstrated in vitro by Stern and associates.[61] Successful protection from isoimmunization was accomplished in 18 of 21 study subjects.[11]

Subsequently, Freda and coworkers,[22] using whole serum, studied the efficacy of specific anti-D IgG in RhD-negative male volunteers from the Sing Sing correctional facility, Ossining, New York. Ten inmates received monthly injections with RhD-positive cells for 5 months. Five subjects in the treatment group also received a dose of anti-D IgG before each RhD-positive red blood cell injection. Sensitization was prevented in all volunteers who had been cotreated with anti-D IgG, whereas four of five control subjects produced anti-D antibodies. This result provided clear evidence of effective prophylaxis against sensitization by administration of anti-D IgG before exposure to RhD-positive red cells.

Unfortunately, because of the unpredictability of maternal exposure to RhD-positive cells during pregnancy, this cotreatment form of prophylaxis would be difficult to apply clinically. Therefore, a second series of injections was conducted in a different group of 20 male inmate volunteers, to whom prophylaxis was administered about 72 hours after exposure to RhD-positive cells. However, because it was feared that a strictly timed protocol might promote a prison break, Freda and coworkers used a variable period for postexposure injection of anti-D IgG, up to a maximum of 72 hours.[22] It is of interest that this injection schedule, based on prison logistics, remains the basis for the recommended schedule of anti-D administration even today. Fortunately, postexposure prophylaxis was equally successful in preventing sensitization. This work inspired subsequent British and American trials among pregnant women, which further established the safety and efficacy of anti-D IgG administration.[6, 21, 62]

GENETICS OF THE Rh SYSTEM

The Rh blood group system includes antigens encoded by two genes localized on chromosome

1p36.13–p34.3. The *RhD* gene codes for the red blood cells' D antigen, and it is linked to a highly homologous region, RhCcEe. Although this system comprises over 40 discrete antigens, only 5 of them are clinically relevant: D, C, c, E, and e. Of these, only the D antigen has no antithetical counterpart. Although most blood group alleles arise through point mutations (e.g., RhE/e), this does not appear to be the case for individuals who are D negative. Indeed, in this situation, absence of the entire RhD polypeptide has been demonstrated, suggesting that gene deletion is responsible for the D-negative phenotype. The complete absence of the peptide is thought to be partly responsible for the high immunogenicity of the D antigen.

The unraveling of the molecular basis of the Rh system has recently led to the development of techniques that allow Rh typing for not only paternal but also fetal genotyping. Polymerase chain reaction (PCR) determination of paternal RhD status can facilitate counseling and dictate the need for intervention, because paternal heterozygosity is associated with a 50% risk of fetal RhD negativity, whereas homozygosity always produces an RhD-positive conceptus, and the fetus will therefore be unaffected.

A PCR-based technique has also been developed and used for fetal typing using amniocytes or villi, allowing diagnosis in the first trimester.[1, 2, 38, 63] More recently, successful preimplantation typing using single blastomere analysis was reported.[3] This method, based on simultaneous amplification of an RhD-specific sequence and an internal control in single cells, allowed the selective transfer of only RhD-negative embryos.

The application of these molecular methods is probably one of the more important recent advances in the field of Rh disease, and in the future, it will likely contribute to major reductions in unnecessary intervention and further prevention of the disease through embryo selection.

PATHOPHYSIOLOGY OF RhD ISOIMMUNIZATION

SENSITIZATION

Erythroblastosis fetalis is characterized by fetal red blood cell hemolysis that results from the presence of anti-D maternal antibodies in the fetal circulation. The isoimmunization process occurs initially because of exposure of the mother who is RhD negative to red cells that are RhD positive. This exposure may occur (1) after transfusion of unmatched blood, (2) in association with parturition or abortion, or (3) during pregnancy through asymptomatic transplacental passage of RhD-positive fetal cells. Fetomaternal transfusion has been documented in 7%, 16%, and 29% of patients in their first, second, and third trimesters, respectively.[12] In the peripartum period, the incidence of fetomaternal hemorrhage can be as high as 50%.[13] It is essential to emphasize the potential for maternal sensitization as early as the first trimester in association with miscarriage or ectopic pregnancy. As few as 0.2 mL of fetal cells are sufficient to cause maternal anti-D sensitization.[13]

The clinician should be aware of other potential sensitizing events (Table 20–1), including elective pregnancy terminations (5% risk of fetomaternal hemorrhage), amniocentesis, chorionic villus sampling, cordocentesis, external cephalic version, and even IV drug abuse, in which women who are Rh negative share needles with partners who are Rh positive. In fact, it is in a group of IV drug abusers that Bowman and colleagues have observed the severest cases of fetal Rh disease, possibly as a consequence of repetitive maternal exposure to the RhD antigen.[8]

Surprisingly, maternal exposure to RhD-positive cells does not always result in sensitization. In some cases, this circumstance may be explained by the protection conferred by ABO blood group incompatibility. Under those conditions, hemolysis activated by the ABO system destroys all fetal cells present in the maternal circulation. As a result, the RhD antigen is never "seen" by the Rh system; therefore, no immune reaction is elicited. With ABO incompatibility, the risk of Rh isoimmunization is reduced from 16% to between 1% and 2%.[41]

In most instances, however, exposure triggers the production of IgM, which constitutes a slow and weak response. Because of high molecular weight, IgM does not cross the placenta and thus has no effect on the fetus. However, the second exposure to RhD leads to the production of IgG, which, because of its lower molecular weight, readily crosses the placenta and enters the fetal circulation. Placental antibody transfer occurs in two steps.[50] Initially, IgGs undergo pinocytosis into endosomes and bind to Fc receptors with a high degree of affinity. Subsequently, the IgG-Fc complex is transported in vesicles to the basolateral surface of the placenta, where the IgG is released. This process, although present early in gestation, is known to increase significantly after 22 weeks as manifested by an exponential rise in fetal IgG levels until term. This rise in fetal concentration of IgG reflects a maturation in immunoglobulin transfer. Once in the fetal circulation, IgG antibodies bind to the RhD antigens on the fetal red cell membranes, and such antibody-coated fetal red cells adhere to macrophages, forming rosettes and leading ultimately to hemolysis and macrophage phagocytosis.

The underlying pathophysiology of RhD sensitization as described, however, is under the influence of various other factors. Discrepancies between maternal titer and severity of fetal disease have been reported, and mothers with marked sensitization have delivered infants with mild disease. These results may be explained by the presence of inhibitory antibodies in maternal sera. More specifically, HLA-DR antibodies have been shown in vitro to inhibit monocyte lytic activity against red cells, thereby preventing significant hemolysis.[58] Studies have reported that these antibodies were detected in a majority of women presenting with the clinical picture described here.[16] These antibodies presumably would cross the pla-

TABLE 20–1 INDICATIONS FOR Rh PROPHYLAXIS

INDICATION	JUSTIFICATION	DOSAGE (μg)	
		1st Trimester	**2nd/3rd Trimester**
Spontaneous abortion/IUFD	2%–3% Sensitization	50	300
Therapeutic abortion	4%–5% Sensitization	50	300
Ectopic pregnancy	2%–5% Sensitization	50	300
Chorionic villus sampling	50% FMH	50	300
Amniocentesis	10% FMH	300	300
Percutaneous umbilical blood sampling	40% FMH	300	300
Abruptio placentae/placenta previa	Variable	300	300
Antepartum vaginal bleeding	Variable	300	300
External cephalic version	Variable	N/A	300
Trauma	Variable	300	300
Pregnancy (28 weeks/postpartum)	7%–8% Sensitization* 15% Sensitization†	N/A	300
Delivery	50% FMH	N/A	300

FMH, fetomaternal hemorrhage; IUFD, intrauterine fetal demise.
*First pregnancy.
†Second pregnancy.

centa and inhibit destruction of fetal red cells by macrophages through the formation of a complex on the membranes of these macrophages, resulting in receptor blockage.

Characteristics of the antibody, such as subclass, concentration, and specificity, also modulate the maternal-fetal response. For instance, IgG3 appears to have a more important role than IgG1; in vitro experiments have demonstrated greater adherence as well as phagocytic and lytic activities for IgG3 than IgG1.[33] In addition, the severity of hemolysis is related to antibody concentration, and this appears to depend on maternal HLA phenotype. For example, HLA-DQB1 allele 0201 may play a particular role, given its markedly higher frequency in women with higher anti-D titers than in those with lower anti-D titers (77% versus 20%).[28] As mentioned earlier, antibody specificity against cells of erythroid lineage is also an important determinant of disease severity, as is antigen density. Indeed, for marked hemolysis to occur, the antigen must be distributed in significant amounts on fetal red cells; therefore, the maturation of expression of these antigens is important. For example, D antigen is known to be present by 4 to 6 weeks' gestation, thereby allowing hemolysis to be initiated at an early stage. By contrast, other antigens, such as A and B, are sparingly distributed on these same red cells, partly explaining the milder degrees of disease severity seen in these situations.

HYDROPS FETALIS

The progressive immunologic destruction of red blood cells must be matched by fetal erythropoiesis if anemia is to be avoided. More reticulocytes and immature red cell forms appear in the circulation of affected fetuses. With an increasing IgG titer and increasing severity of hemolysis, extramedullary tis-

sues (liver, spleen) are recruited for erythropoiesis. Erythroblastosis results in severe cases. The outcome for the fetus depends on the relative severity of antibody-mediated hemolysis versus erythropoietic capability. In the extreme, severe anemia leads to fetal hydrops and death (see also Chapter 21). This sequence of events was demonstrated by Nicolaides and associates in a group of 127 isoimmunized pregnancies at 17 to 36 weeks' gestation.[43] Moderate fetal anemia was associated with reticulocytosis, whereas markedly decreased hemoglobin concentrations (7 gm/dL) were associated with erythroblastosis.

Despite efforts at increased erythropoiesis, overwhelming hemolysis may result in profound anemia. Fortunately, through marked increases in cardiac output, the fetus typically maintains pH and partial pressure of oxygen and carbon dioxide within normal limits until a hemoglobin deficit of 7 gm/dL is reached. At this point, the high concentrations of lactic acid exceed the placental clearance capacity and lactic acidosis develops. A hematocrit of 15% appears to be a critical level below which compensatory mechanisms are usually insufficient, leading to the onset of hydrops.[42] Signs of hydrops include pericardial and pleural effusions, ascites, skin edema, hepatosplenomegaly, polyhydramnios, and placental thickening (Fig. 20–1). Although it has been reported that hydrops could develop with a hemoglobin deficit of 7 gm/dL, that finding should be evaluated in the context of gestational age. This approach is supported by a recent report including 111 fetuses at risk for anemia.[39] A clear increase in median values of hemoglobin was noted with advancing gestational age, from 10.6 gm/dL at 18 weeks to 13.8 gm/dL at 40 weeks. Given these significant variations, deficits in hemoglobins need to be interpreted carefully because they have different meanings at different gestational ages. Indeed, it has been suggested that the use of a hemo-

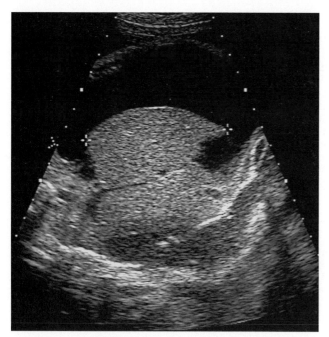

FIGURE 20–1. Transverse section of the fetal abdomen demonstrating marked liver enlargement (indicated by caliper) as well as the presence of marked ascites.

globin value of less than 0.5 times the median for gestational age would appear to be more appropriate for identifying fetuses at significant risk of hydrops.

The exact pathophysiologic mechanism for hydrops is still unclear. Three mechanisms have been proposed: high-output cardiac failure, liver dysfunction, and fetal hypoxemia. Many believe that a combination of these factors is involved. It is likely that, with worsening anemia, hemodynamic demands exceed cardiac reserves, resulting in heart failure, fetal hypoxemia, and high systemic venous pressure. These conditions cause endothelial damage, followed by extravascular protein leakage, which results in accumulation of fluid in various body cavities.

This hypothesis is strongly supported by the work of Nicolaides and associates, who studied 17 isoimmunized fetuses between 18 and 25 weeks of gestation.[42] They demonstrated hypoalbuminemia in six of seven hydropic fetuses and in only two nonhydropic fetuses. More importantly, the ascitic fluid albumin and total protein concentrations were more than 50% of their corresponding plasma levels, suggesting extravascular loss through endothelial damage.

Hypoproteinemia may also result from decreased hepatic synthesis caused by liver infiltration by erythroblasts. Crowding of hepatic structures leads to portal hypertension and hepatic ischemia. Current data also support this explanation. Nicolini and coworkers measured liver enzymes in 25 fetuses with severe Rh disease and compared the results with those of 17 fetuses in a control group.[47] Levels of aspartate and alanine aminotransferases were more elevated in hydropic fetuses than in Rh-sensitized nonhydropic fetuses, although an overlap was observed between hydropic and nonhydropic cases. The authors also observed a positive correlation between nucleated red blood cell counts (a reflection of extramedullary erythropoiesis) and levels of aspartate aminotransferase, which suggests that liver infiltration by erythropoietic cells can cause hepatic dysfunction.

FIRST-TRIMESTER AND PREIMPLANTATION DIAGNOSIS

When alloimmunization is a risk factor and the father is an RhD heterozygote, fetal disease, depending on fetal genotype, is a possibility. Recent advances in our understanding of the molecular genetics of the Rh system have led to the design of new techniques that are applicable to the very early specifying of genotype. These techniques have made it possible to determine the fetal RhD status during the first trimester with great accuracy and, more recently, have also allowed preimplantation diagnosis, thereby completely preventing the disease through selective transfer of RhD-negative embryos.

Indeed, Fisk and colleagues reported the use of PCR in fetal RhD typing.[19] They obtained amniotic fluid from five women and chorionic villi from one. All women were RhD negative with partners who were heterozygous for the RhD antigen. When PCR was used to amplify DNA samples, four fetuses were shown to be Rh positive. In the two remaining fetuses, Rh negativity was correctly diagnosed. The diagnoses were confirmed serologically after delivery. A more recent review of 500 cases reported sensitivity of 98.7% and specificity of 100% when using PCR typing of amniotic cells.[63] These genetic techniques provide patients with options such as termination and aggressive early assessment and therapy. They also avoid the need for further procedures in fetuses who are Rh negative. The benefits of the information obtained along with the accuracy of the methods used have greatly contributed to the implementation of prenatal genotyping in obstetric practice. The clinician must, however, remember the risk of fetomaternal hemorrhage with chorionic villus sampling and weigh this risk against the benefits of fetal Rh typing. More data on how to avoid the risk are emerging, pointing to the potential role of isolation of fetal cells from maternal circulation with their subsequent typing. Using fluorescence in situ hybridization (FISH) and PCR in combination, Sekizawa and coworkers successfully retrieved 101 fetal nucleated erythrocytes from four subjects and correctly predicted fetal gender and Rh status.[56] At present, this approach remains investigational, but it appears promising and may ultimately allow noninvasive early diagnosis by maximizing genetic information available from even a single cell.

The possibility of preimplantation diagnosis of Rh genotype has also been investigated. Avner and coworkers have reported using single blastomere analysis and applying PCR to determine RhD status of two of three embryos studied, leading to their selection for in utero transfer.[3] Although pregnancies were not achieved, the technology described may well represent an increasingly important future preventive approach, especially in cases of severely sensitized women who have a very high risk of marked fetal anemia and hydrops in any of their future pregnancies.

MANAGEMENT

Rh IMMUNOGLOBULIN PROPHYLAXIS

Although the formation of RhD antibodies in the mother can be prevented by the administration of Rh immune globulin, the exact mechanism by which these antibodies are formed is not well understood. Several theories have been proposed. Most likely, anti-D IgG in the maternal circulation binds to the fetal red cells carrying the RhD antigen. Subsequently, immunoglobulin-bound red cells are lysed through complement fixation; phagocytosis by macrophages also contributes to the elimination of RhD antigenic sites. There may be an additional effect, accomplished by trapping the IgG-coated red blood cells in the spleen and lymph nodes, in which a central suppressive effect may be achieved. As a result, further production of antibodies is suppressed, and all existing antibodies are actively destroyed.

The use of Rh IgG prophylaxis is indicated in the management of all nonimmunized pregnant women who are Rh negative. Current recommendations include routine administration at 28 weeks to all pregnant women who are RhD negative and within 72 hours postpartum for those with an infant who is RhD positive.[27] Use of the 28-week dose has been demonstrated by Bowman and coworkers[6] to reduce third-trimester sensitization from 1.8% to less than 0.11%. The standard dose, 300 µg, is based on the amount of IgG that will provide protection for up to 30 mL of fetal blood (15 mL of packed fetal cells). This dose provides satisfactory prophylaxis for 99% of all term deliveries. In a few cases, a greater amount of fetal blood will enter the maternal circulation. In women at high risk, a Kleihauer-Betke smear test can be performed to quantitate the fetal blood present. For every 30 mL of fetal blood detected, an additional 300 µg dose can be administered. High-risk conditions include abruptio placentae, placenta previa, and manual placental removal.

Because the half-life of Rh IgG is 21 to 30 days, the 28-week injection should be protective until term. One should then give Rh IgG to an infant who is Rh positive within 72 hours of delivery, because a protective effect has been documented if the treatment is given within that period. Because this ideal interval has been determined empirically, Rh IgG still can be administered up to 13 days after exposure for partial protection. Situations mandating Rh prophylaxis are summarized in Table 20–1.

The present practice of obtaining Rh IgG from pooled donors' sera raises the issue of transmission of human immunodeficiency virus and hepatitis B and C viruses. Fortunately, it appears that the tech-

nique used (cold alcohol fractionation) destroys these types of viruses. Additionally, all donors are now tested for these viruses; so far, no cases of transmission of human immunodeficiency virus or hepatitis B virus have been reported to have resulted from the administration of Rh IgG. However, isolated cases of hepatitis C transmission have been reported in Europe, before universal screening of donors.[51]

To eliminate this potential risk and to ensure a continuous supply of Rh IgG, researchers are directing their efforts toward the development of monoclonal anti-D antibodies.[32] However, preliminary data indicate that monoclonal anti-D may be less effective than IgG obtained from multiple donors. Recent investigations have suggested that the use of a combination of at least IgG1 and IgG3 may be necessary. Thus far, phase I trials have shown promising results. In a small group of volunteers, administration of two monoclonal antibodies, BRAD 3(IgG3) and BRAD 5 (IgG1), produced from lymphoblastoid cell lines, protected them from mounting a primary anti-D response to D-positive red blood cells.[32] The data indicate a clear need for further research in this area.

Finally, a special circumstance should be mentioned: the case of the mother who is D[u] positive (positive for weak RhD). The basis for such a weak D antigen expression is the presence, on the opposite chromosome, of C and E antigens. In most instances, these patients are actually genetically RhD positive and therefore have no risk of isoimmunization. More rarely, a patient is reported to be D mosaic. These individuals are missing a portion of epitope of the D antigen, and although they can form anti-D antibodies, hemolytic disease in the fetus does occasionally occur.

SCREENING

Antenatal management of the pregnant woman who is Rh-negative, as summarized in Figure 20–2, begins with screening. The efficient identification of pregnancies in which there is a risk of Rh isoimmunization requires that all patients undergo an indirect Coombs test in the first trimester. This allows detection of RhD antibodies as well as other atypical antigens that may also cause hydrops. It is important that all women of reproductive age know their own RhD status and

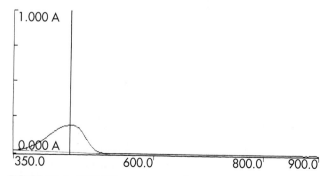

FIGURE 20–2. ΔOD-450 measurement by spectrophotometry at 32 weeks of Rh-sensitized pregnancy.

understand the procedures to be followed should they become pregnant.

Patients demonstrating sensitization to RhD should have their anti-D titer evaluated by a reliable laboratory because the risk of severe disease correlates roughly with the amount of IgG passing transplacentally to the fetus. Although each laboratory should set guidelines based on local experience, anti-D titers of 1:8 rarely, if ever, result in significant fetal jeopardy. In these cases, monthly maternal titer assessment is adequate follow-up. However, if the titer exceeds 1:8 or 1:16, invasive evaluation may be required.

The timing of the first amniocentesis or cordocentesis should be determined with consideration of titer as well as obstetric history. Low titers (1:8 to 1:16) in the first sensitized pregnancy may be evaluated by amniocentesis beginning at 26 to 28 weeks. However, a woman with a prior pregnancy with fetal hydrops or fetal death before 18 to 20 weeks may require cordocentesis as early as 22 weeks. In general, if titers are equal to or greater than 1:128, the first procedure should be performed at 20 to 24 weeks' gestation.

Traditionally, antenatal management of fetuses at risk of erythroblastosis fetalis has relied on the careful follow-up of anti-D titers. However, discrepancies between the titer and severity of the fetal disease continue to occur often on the basis of the lack of correlation between antibody titration, concentration, and biologic activity in vivo. Therefore, several new assays have been designed to further improve the appropriate identification of fetuses at risk. These can be divided into quantitative and cellular (functional) assays.

Quantitative Assays

Quantitative tests, using technologies such as ELISA, flow cytometry, or radioimmunoassay, attempt to measure binding of anti-D IgG to red blood cells in maternal serum. So far, several authors have demonstrated that quantification of antibodies, using AutoAnalyzer (U.K.), appears to better discriminate affected fetuses from unaffected fetuses, although difficulties at establishing a threshold beyond which severe hemolytic disease will occur still remain. Flow cytometry, although helpful in distinguishing subclasses of antibody present, is generally not believed to be useful as a screening test.

Functional Assays

Cellular assays aim to measure the biologic activity of antibodies by determining their ability to promote interactions between D-positive red cells and effector cells. This is achieved by sensitizing erythrocytes with maternal antibodies and subsequently incubating them with effector cells (e.g., monocytes). Interaction of these two cells in the form of binding, lysis, and phagocytosis is measured by different assays. For example, the chemiluminescence test measures the metabolic response of monocyte activation in the form of a light emission as produced subsequent to respira-

tory bursts associated with their interaction with erythrocytes. The monocyte monolayer assay measures the adherence and phagocytosis of red cells by monocytes. Finally, the antibody-dependent cellular cytotoxicity (ADCC) assay measures lysis of radiolabeled, coated erythrocytes.

The value of these assays has been evaluated retrospectively and prospectively. The chemiluminescence test has recently been applied to a population of 132 sensitized pregnant women.[26] Results showed that this assay was superior to antibody quantification (AutoAnalyzer) in predicting need for invasive testing and that a cutoff value of over 30% identified all cases of hemolysis. Although it would appear from the data that chemiluminescence may be helpful to improve appropriate identification of affected infants, chemiluminescence has had a limited role in predicting unaffected infants.

Studies using monocyte monolayer assays have resulted in controversial data. Although some have reported appropriate identification of affected cases in 95% using a cutoff of 20%, others have not been able to reproduce these findings.[25]

ADCC assays have been more extensively studied, and even applied clinically in the Netherlands, because of their ability to correctly predict unaffected infants when results remain under a given threshold.[17]

Although none of these assays are in routine clinical use in North America, more data are emerging to suggest that they may contribute significantly to better identification of the fetus at risk for hemolysis, therefore, directing invasive diagnosis and treatment more appropriately. Several authors have indeed suggested that these assays be incorporated into a structured approach in the evaluation of Rh isoimmunization.[25] For instance, once sensitization using titers has been identified, chemiluminescence and ADCC assays can be used to assess the risk of fetal disease further and to predict severity more accurately, which, in turn, may help to avoid or delay invasive procedures or to target for early diagnosis and treat the fetus who is at greater risk. Because both approaches theoretically may improve fetal-maternal outcome, it is worthwhile to pursue a more accurate and structured approach toward the proper identification of unaffected and affected fetuses.

SPECTROPHOTOMETRY

Optical Density of Amniotic Fluid

A scheme for assessing the severity of fetal hemolysis was first developed by Liley in 1961.[37] Using spectrophotometry, the examiner measures the change in optical density (ΔOD) at 450 nm, which reflects the concentration of bilirubin in amniotic fluid. From this change, an estimate of the fetal hemolytic process can be made. Quantification of this increase in OD at 450 nm is obtained by connecting OD values at 375 and 525 nm, then measuring the distance between this line and the rise in OD at 450 nm (see Figs. 20–2 and 20–3).

Liley collected these data initially from 101 Rh-isoimmunized pregnant women between 27 and 41 weeks of gestation.[37] By plotting the ΔOD at 450 (ΔOD-450) nm versus gestational age on semilogarithmic paper, he defined three zones that correlated with disease severity. Zone 1 predicts an unaffected fetus or a minimally affected infant with a 10% risk of need for postnatal exchange transfusion. Zone 2 correlates with moderate disease. Zone 3 indicates a high degree of hemolysis and is correlated with fetal or neonatal death unless delivery or transfusion is accomplished. Predictive power is improved further by dividing zone 2 into two: a lower zone (20% risk of exchange transfusion) and an upper zone (80% risk of exchange transfusion), for a total of four zones.

Readings falling into zone 1 or lower zone 2 should be repeated within 2 to 4 weeks. Upper zone 2 values deserve follow-up in 1 week. For values within upper zone 2 or reaching zone 3, fetal blood sampling and fetal transfusion or delivery, depending on gestational age, are recommended.

Unfortunately, since Liley's pioneering work, several problems with using this amniotic fluid density measurement to assess the degree of fetal anemia have arisen. For example, meconium or blood contamination of amniotic fluid may obscure the 450 nm reading, making determination of the peak value impossible. More importantly, the predictability of ΔOD-450 nm values obtained in the second trimester have been questioned. The original data obtained by Liley were from pregnancies between 27 and 41 weeks because in utero management or delivery of fetuses less than 27 weeks' gestation was not feasible in 1961. Today, however, availability of treatment options for fetuses as young as 20 to 22 weeks' gestation has required an extrapolation of the Liley zones to as early as 18 weeks' gestation. Nevertheless, simple retrograde extension of zone boundaries may not be appropriate. To assess the validity of this extrapolation, Nicolaides and associates compared hematrocrits of umbilical cord blood obtained from 50 RhD-isoimmunized fetuses at 18 to 25 weeks' gestation and determined the peak ΔOD-450 nm of amniotic fluid obtained simultaneously.[44] A control group consisted of 475 amniotic fluid samples and 153 blood samples obtained from unaffected pregnancies between 16 and 36 weeks. Their results revealed a significant inaccuracy of ΔOD-450 nm values in the prediction of severity of isoimmunization between 18 and 25 weeks. In fact, no identifiable cutoff level for ΔOD-450 nm could discriminate between mildly and severely affected fetuses. Fortunately, the results did confirm the accuracy of amniocentesis for predicting severe disease after 27 weeks. Subsequent to this, Queenan and co-workers pooled their data on amniotic fluid bilirubin concentrations as obtained during genetic amniocenteses and created a new graph.[52] Their observations confirmed the predictability of this testing in the late second and third trimesters and further suggested that extrapolation to 20 weeks of gestation, using flattened curves, was more appropriate in identifying affected fetuses early on. However, in a more recent comparative study of the Queenan and Liley curves, Spinnato and colleagues questioned the performance of the Queenan curve and suggested that it frequently overestimated the risk.[60] Although some methodological questions were raised about Spinnato and colleagues' study—for example, the inclusion of patients sensitized to antigens other than D—it pointed to some potential difficulties in interpretation of results obtained early in the second trimester.

Modified Liley Curve

To avoid the inaccuracies mentioned above, use of a modified curve (Fig. 20–3) that provides prognostic information is recommended. The four typical zones are depicted (zone 1, lower zone 2, higher zone 2, and zone 3), but from 19 to 28 weeks, an upper limit of normal ΔOD-450 values for these gestations is defined, consistent with the observation of Nicolaides and associates.[44] The curve also delineates an upper zone in which intrauterine transfusion is necessary. The improved predictability in this modified chart relies on the flattening of the curve between 19 and 28 weeks, setting the upper limit of normal at a much lower value than would be expected if the original curve were simply extrapolated.

The findings described earlier suggest that, in certain instances, fetal blood sampling rather than amniocentesis may be needed to evaluate fetal hematocrit before 27 weeks. However, the convenience of direct umbilical blood sampling must be weighed against the risks of fetomaternal hemorrhage (50% incidence)[4] and of provoking increased maternal antibody production. The risk of fetal death (1%) associated with cordocentesis is,[55] of course, much greater than that associated with amniocentesis (1 in 300).

ULTRASOUND

Rh Isoimmunization

High-resolution ultrasound is an essential adjunct in the assessment of isoimmunized pregnancies, allowing documentation of extent, progression of disease, and early detection of hydrops. Additionally, ultrasound guidance is indispensable in interventions such as fetal blood sampling and transfusion. Finally, ultrasound assessment of fetal behavior (the biophysical profile) provides important evidence of fetal well-being (see Chapter 9).

Ultrasound evaluation in cases of Rh isoimmunization requires a thorough examination of fetal anatomy, placental morphologic features, and amniotic fluid volume. The fetus should be examined for the presence of hydrops (skin edema, ascites, pericardial and pleural effusion, and hepatosplenomegaly). Early signs of ascites include visualization of both sides of the bowel wall and lucent outlining of organs such as the bladder and stomach.[54] Approximately 30 mL of free peritoneal fluid is associated with this finding. With further fluid accumulation, a clear rim appears adjacent to the fetal bladder; this correlates with the

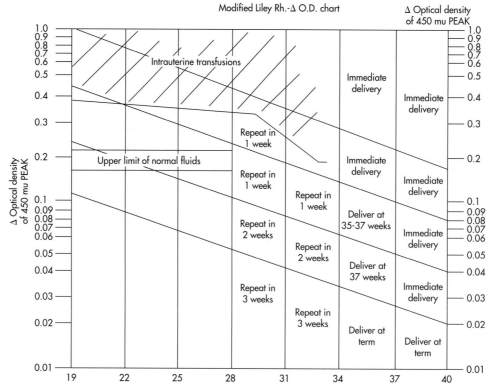

FIGURE 20–3. Modified Liley curve with improved predictability from ΔOD-450 readings in early gestation. Gestational age in weeks is shown on the horizontal axis.

presence of 50 mL of fluid. Marked ascites (100 mL) is frequently accompanied by findings of fetal skin edema and is particularly evident in the scalp, the extremities, and the abdominal wall.

Hepatosplenomegaly, reflecting increased extra-medullary erythropoiesis, may be detected through increasing abdominal circumference measurements (see Fig. 20–1). Vintzileos and colleagues proposed that liver enlargement may represent one of the earliest findings of significant fetal anemia.[65] Similarly, worsening of fetal hemolysis is associated with gradual thickening of the placenta, and a cross section greater than 4 cm thick is associated with significant anemia (Fig. 20–4). Cardiomegaly also may be visible given the demands on the myocardium necessary to maintain perfusion (Fig. 20–5). Finally, a quantitative examination of amniotic fluid volume may provide important clues of early fetal anemia. Initially, subjectively increased fluid volume is seen and may be followed by polyhydramnios. Further deterioration is later manifested by oligohydramnios, an ominous finding dictating intervention, especially when it is associated with signs of hydrops.

Prediction of Anemia

Fetal blood sampling provides the most accurate determination of fetal hematocrit. Such invasive procedures, however, carry a significant fetal loss rate; therefore, investigators have attempted to use ultrasound to predict the degree of anemia. The course

of deteriorating erythroblastosis fetalis is marked by polyhydramnios, followed by placentomegaly, hepatomegaly, ascites, and, finally, generalized fetal hydrops.

Hoping to identify one of these signs or a specific sequence of events as a predictor for the severity of anemia, Chitkara and coworkers evaluated 15 isoimmunized pregnancies with fetal blood sampling and various ultrasound parameters.[9] Their findings revealed that only frank hydrops was predictive of se-

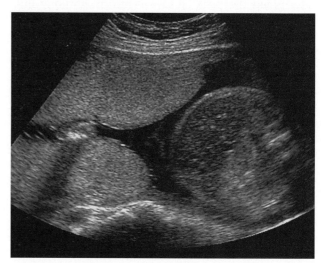

FIGURE 20–4. Significant placentomegaly (left) at 26 weeks, which was shortly followed by the development of hydrops.

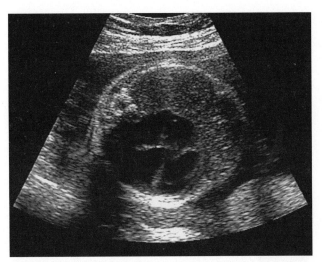

FIGURE 20–5. Transverse view of fetal thorax demonstrating profound cardiomegaly as the fetus attempted to compensate for the severe anemia.

vere fetal anemia (hematocrit, less than 15%). Nicolaides and associates[46] reported similar results from a series of 50 isoimmunized pregnancies, demonstrating poor predictive power of placental thickness and amniotic fluid volume. Reece and associates then compared ultrasound and analysis of ΔOD-450 nm amniotic fluid in the prediction of neonatal complications of isoimmunization (i.e., need for exchange transfusion, organomegaly, ascites, and neonatal death).[53] Their results demonstrated consistently poor predictive power when ultrasound, ΔOD-450 values, or a combination of both modalities was used. Small studies have also correlated splenic size to severe anemia with varying success and have explained their observations of splenomegaly by the need for extramedullary hematopoiesis in cases of severe anemia.

Doppler flow analysis offers a noninvasive tool that may be useful in identifying the anemic fetus as fetal cardiac output rises progressively and hematocrit falls. Unfortunately, formulas derived to predict fetal hematocrit have to date been too inaccurate for clinical use. With evolving experience and use of sophisticated technologies, Iskaros and coworkers demonstrated recently in a prospective study that serial measurements of maximum velocity of umbilical vein flow correlated to some degree with fetal hematocrit and predicted the need for postnatal exchange transfusion in 6 of 7 cases.[30] Importantly, their data also suggested that elevation in maximum velocity of umbilical vein flow preceded hepatosplenomegaly. A new splenic artery Doppler velocimetry index also was established and studied in a small population of sensitized pregnant women.[5] Results showed that a normal Doppler angle in the main splenic artery is predictive of a decreased risk of severe anemia, whereas a smaller angle might be more reflective of a rapid deceleration phase owing to the hyperdynamic fetal state caused by the anemia. Application of this Doppler index in this very small study resulted in a sensitivity of 100% and a false positive rate of 8.8%

in the diagnosis of severe anemia in nonhydropic fetuses. The Collaborative Group for Doppler Assessment of the Blood Velocity in Anemic Fetuses recently reported their experience with the use of peak velocity measurements of the middle cerebral artery (MCA) in the prediction of moderate to severe anemia.[39] This particular vessel was selected because it has been well established that cerebral arteries respond rapidly to hypoxemia by increasing blood flow velocity in order to optimize brain perfusion. In addition, it also has been shown that as fetal hematocrit rises, peak systolic velocity in the MCA decreases. A group of 111 fetuses at risk of anemia from maternal red cell isoimmunization were studied using these physiologic observations. Peak velocity measurements of the MCA were compared to the severity of anemia, and using a cutoff value of 1.5 times the median (because these values change with advancing gestational age), all fetuses with moderate and severe anemia were correctly identified (Fig. 20–6).

Given a sensitivity of 100% in the prediction of moderate and severe anemia and a false positive value of 12%, the authors concluded that measurement of peak velocity in fetal MCAs was an accurate and noninvasive tool for the identification of the fetus at risk, thereby improving the identification of those requiring invasive procedures such as transfusions. Widespread use of this technique may contribute to further decreasing the number of fetuses exposed to invasive diagnostic approaches, such as cordocentesis, reducing fetal losses directly related to the procedure itself. These encouraging results should prompt further prospective investigation when these noninvasive modalities are used.

SUPPRESSIVE THERAPY

Intravenous Immunoglobulin

Although most fetuses with severe RhD hemolytic disease are treated successfully with intrauterine transfusions, some cannot be, owing to a very young gestational age or technical difficulties, which make access to the umbilical vessels impossible. In those instances, an adjunct may be helpful in delaying the transfusion until it is technically possible. Maternal administration of IV immunoglobulin (IVIG) has been proposed as an adjunct because it might lead to feedback inhibition of maternal antibody synthesis, blockade of reticuloendothelial Fc receptors, or blockade of placental antibody transport.[20] So far, although the mechanism of action of IVIG remains unclear, early studies are showing promising results. Indeed, maternal IVIG administration has been shown retrospectively and prospectively in small studies to be associated with improved outcomes in index pregnancies compared with previous ones and with significant delays in need for intrauterine transfusions.[20]

Unfortunately, the cost of IVIG remains an important limiting factor and restrains its use significantly. At this time, given limited available data and financial constraints, maternal IVIG administration

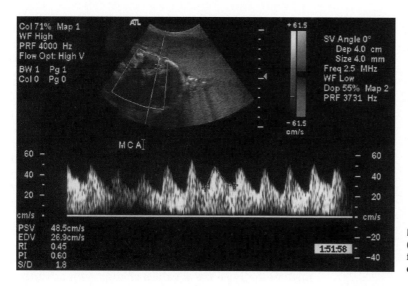

FIGURE 20–6. Measurement of peak systolic velocity (PSV) in the middle cerebral artery of an anemic fetus. As seen, PSV was 48.5 cm per second, which exceeds 1.55 times the median expected at 26 weeks.

should remain an adjunct to intravascular transfusions or be used only in cases in which transfusions are technically impossible. However, the encouraging results provided by the early studies suggest that this therapy warrants further prospective evaluation.

FETAL TRANSFUSION

Intravascular Transfusion

One of the most significant advances in the management of erythroblastosis fetalis has been the development of fetal transfusion techniques. In 1963, Liley inadvertently punctured the fetal peritoneal cavity during an attempted amniocentesis. On that day, as stated so eloquently by his daughter, "he punctured not only the uterus and the fetal abdomen but also the conceptual barrier that the fetus was beyond the reach of treatment."[36] Indeed, he exploited this accident by successfully performing the first intraperitoneal transfusion of red cells. These cells are subsequently absorbed via the subdiaphragmatic lymphatics to reach the venous circulation. However, this process can be significantly impeded by the presence of hydrops. In 1984, Rodeck and colleagues introduced intravascular transfusion (IVT) facilitated by fetoscopy.[54] The high rate of fetal loss with fetoscopy (10% to 12%) led to the use of ultrasound to guide access to the fetal umbilical circulation. The risk of fetal death in nonhydropic fetuses with ultrasound-guided transfusion is now approximately 2%.[31, 55]

Intravascular transfusion involves maternal premedication with relaxants, prophylactic antibiotics, and, at times, tocolytic agents or steroids. After premedication, ultrasound is used to locate the best access site, which is usually at the umbilical insertion into the placenta. If this site cannot be used, other areas can be sampled, including the cord insertion in the fetal abdomen, a free loop of cord, or the hepatic portion of the umbilical vein. Intracardiac sampling also has been reported. Occasionally, the combination of intraperitoneal and intravascular approaches has been used in an attempt to delay the next transfusion

by creating a reservoir of red cells in the peritoneal cavity.

Once the area to be sampled has been identified, the maternal abdomen is cleaned aseptically, and a 20- or 22-gauge needle is introduced through the maternal abdomen into the target vessel. Once the needle is in place, a depolarizing agent may be injected to induce fetal paralysis. A sample of fetal blood is obtained and immediately analyzed for hemoglobin, hematocrit, and blood type. The fetal source of blood can be verified by mean corpuscular volume because the fetal value is 100 to 120 μm^3 and the adult value is approximately 90 μm^3.

A hematocrit less than 30% indicates the need for transfusion because this finding represents significant anemia (a value of 30% is equivalent to less than the 2.5th percentile in fetuses older than 20 weeks' gestation). Group O Rh-negative blood is used for transfusion. Many centers use irradiated blood to prevent graft-versus-host disease; however, Bowman and coworkers reported 275 survivors who had transfusions with nonirradiated blood without disease.[7] The goal is to reach a fetal hematocrit of 40% (and up to 60% depending on the institution), with the amount of blood necessary varying according to initial hematocrit and fetal weight. To minimize potential increases in fetal blood viscosity, a transfusion hematocrit of 90% is used, and post-transfusion fetal hematocrit should not exceed 55%. Although different centers use different target hematocrits, values of approximately 40% are acceptable by most, because they are more physiologic (at term, a normal fetal hematocrit is around 45%). Though formulas and nomograms have been designed to calculate the volume needed to obtain a reasonable hematocrit,[45] many prefer to determine the hematocrit intermittently during the transfusion and to adjust the amount to be transfused.

During the IVT, an ultrasonographer observes the fetal heart rate. Also, one can easily visualize the turbulence of blood flow within the umbilical vessel as evidence of flow continuity. During this time, an increase in umbilical venous pressure by 1.7 to 4.6 mm Hg has been documented to occur along with a 25% decrease in cardiac output.[55] This result may be explained by an increased afterload owing to the increased viscosity that causes the fetus to decrease its stroke volume and cardiac output. These parameters return gradually to their baseline; for cardiac output, this is accomplished within 24 hours. At completion of the procedure, a sample of fetal blood is obtained to determine a final hematocrit. The needle is withdrawn, and the fetal heart rate monitored until it is reassuring. Complications related to IVT are fairly uncommon in experienced hands. The procedure-related fetal loss rate is reported to be from 1% to 2%. Other risks are detailed in Table 20–2; however, the incidence of fetomaternal hemorrhage (50%) associated with IVT deserves special mention.

Intraperitoneal Transfusion

As mentioned earlier, intraperitoneal transfusion (IPT) was first performed in 1963 and significantly contributed to improved survival of fetuses affected by Rh disease (i.e., anemic). IPT is technically less difficult than IVT, but it is less effective, especially in the hydropic fetus. Technically, ultrasound is used to direct a 20-gauge needle into the fetal peritoneal cavity; a location just above the bladder is ideal. Proper placement of the needle is ascertained by injecting saline solution before the blood is transfused. The blood volume necessary to obtain the targeted hemoglobin value must be carefully calculated to avoid excessive intraperitoneal pressure associated with overtransfusion, which can impede umbilical vein blood flow and ultimately lead to fetal death.[48] Bowman and coworkers reported a simple equation for ITP volume[7]: Transfused volume mL = (weeks' gestation − 20) × 10 mL. In addition to the lack of direct observation of fetal hematocrit, there are other inherent difficulties with IPT. Hydropic fetuses, for example, may not benefit from IPT because of compromised ability to absorb red blood cells through the lymphatic vessels. Bowman and coworkers also reported a 20% spontaneous labor rate after IPT.[4] Finally, the daily absorption of red cells in the nonhydropic fetus is limited to 10% to 12%, leading to slow recovery from severe anemia.

The IPT procedure remains useful in cases in which the caliber of the umbilical vessels does not allow placement of the needle for transfusion or when IVT is technically impossible because of the location of the cord insertion and the fetal position. Some also advocate its use because of the slower post-transfusion decline in hematocrit compared with that of IVT, requiring fewer procedures. On the basis of available data, IVT remains the procedure of choice, especially in the hydropic fetus. However, IPT should be considered in the special circumstances noted.

The timing of subsequent transfusions depends largely on the hematocrit reached at the completion of the procedure. Grannum and associates[24] observed a daily hematocrit drop of approximately 1% and, therefore, recommend an additional procedure within 1½ to 2½ weeks of the initial one. Bowman and coworkers reported that the average donor hemoglobin attrition rate was 0.4 gm/dL per day, and they give repeated transfusions every 2 to 3 weeks. IPT allows larger transfused volumes and generally needs to be repeated less frequently in an affected pregnancy. In fact, Bowman and coworkers noted that to treat a fetus from age 21 to 34 weeks, fewer than four IPTs are typically required, compared with seven or eight IVTs.

The previously mentioned combination of intraperitoneal and intravascular approaches has been helpful in increasing intervals between transfusions. Indeed, the mean daily decrease in fetal hematocrit was reported to compare favorably with the 1.14%

TABLE 20–2 COMPARISON OF TRANSFUSION TECHNIQUES

	ADVANTAGES	DISADVANTAGES/RISKS
INTRAVASCULAR TRANSFUSION	Allows determination of hematocrit Rapid correction of anemia Only procedure benefiting severely hydropic fetuses Superior survival rates compared with IPT in many studies Rapid reversal of hydrops	Cardiac overload Hemorrhage from venipuncture FMH (40%) Cord hematoma Rapid decline in hematocrit More difficult technique if inexperienced examiner Fetal bradycardia (8%) Fetal loss (2%) Infection Possible increased incidence of porencephalic cyst
INTRAPERITONEAL TRANSFUSION	Technically easy procedure Very effective in absence of hydrops Long-lasting adequate hematocrit requiring fewer interventions	Low success rate in hydrops Possibilities of impairment of venous return if excessive blood is transfused Slow RBC absorption Possible hepatic tear and intra-abdominal organ damage No allowance for determination of hematocrit

FMH, fetomaternal hemorrhage; IPT, intraperitoneal transfusion; RBC, red blood cell.

reported with IVT.[40] In general, in most centers, transfusions are performed every 2 weeks for the first two transfusions, then every 3 to 4 weeks.

The severely anemic fetus presenting in the second trimester sometimes is an exception to this and often benefits from an initial transfusion to a hematocrit of 25%, followed by a second one 48 hours later with a goal of 35%. This approach aims to reduce the volume load to the fetus, thereby reducing risks of demise; it has been demonstrated by Selbing and colleagues that a transfusion volume exceeding 20 mL/kg was associated with lower survival.[57]

During the intervals between interventions, serial fetal biophysical assessments are recommended, with monitoring for any evidence of deterioration, such as the development of polyhydramnios or hydrops.

TIMING OF DELIVERY

Disease severity and gestational age remain the most significant determinants of the timing of delivery. Generally, no fetal or maternal benefit is gained by continuing the pregnancy beyond 36 to 38 weeks; in fact, continuation may be detrimental to the fetus. In general, the last transfusion is performed at around 35 weeks, when there is a reasonable chance of pulmonary maturity and an amniocentesis to determine lung maturity can be performed. Both lecithin-sphingomyelin ratio and phosphatidylglycerol levels should be assessed, but results may be altered by the presence of bilirubin in the amniotic fluid. If a mature profile is obtained, delivery is preferable. Otherwise, delivery can be planned in 2 to 3 weeks.

The site of delivery also deserves mention. A fetus in the low-risk group (Liley zone 1) may be delivered in a hospital with availability of exchange transfusion, which is needed in 10% of cases. Moderately or severely affected fetuses need expert neonatal care because their presentation may be complicated by hydrops and prematurity; therefore, a tertiary care center is the location of choice for the birth of these infants.

OUTCOME

SHORT-TERM

Because of more sophisticated ultrasound technology and improved operator skills and techniques in neonatal care, perinatal survival after in utero transfusions has improved significantly. This improvement was well demonstrated in a summary of studies using direct fetal IVTs. A total of 411 fetuses were included, and the overall survival rate was 84%.[55] The data further revealed, as suspected, that fetuses with severe anemia but no hydropic features were five times more likely to survive than those with hydrops. Indeed, the nonhydropic survival rate was 94%, but it decreased to 74% for hydropic fetuses.

Two more recent series have confirmed these data. Janssens and coworkers have described 92 fetuses who underwent in utero transfusions and reported an overall survival rate of 83.7%.[31] Similarly, in a series of 43 fetuses, an overall survival rate of 81% was achieved.[23] Once again, the influence of hydrops on outcome was demonstrated through an important difference in perinatal mortality (4 out of 11 for hydropic fetuses versus 4 out of 32 for nonhydropic fetuses).

Once delivered, the neonate should be examined thoroughly to establish the need for further therapy. Because fetal transfusion appears to suppress hematopoiesis, many neonates require transfusions. Indeed, in Janssens and coworkers' study,[31] such suppression was confirmed by demonstrating a positive correlation between the number of intrauterine transfusions and the number of postnatal transfusions. However, a negative correlation existed between the number of intrauterine transfusions and the number of exchange transfusions, as well as the need for phototherapy, which suggests that, although appropriate in utero treatment appears to optimize immediate neonatal hematologic conditions and to improve survival, it suppresses erythropoiesis. This belief is further supported by low reticulocyte counts, low levels of erythropoietin and erythroid hyperplasia of bone marrow. Therefore, it is important to continue surveillance of these infants for a period of 8 to 10 weeks with follow-up of hematocrit and reticulocyte count. Administration of recombinant erythropoietin appears to be promising in this population, but criteria have yet to be established.[14, 49] At this time, symptomatic infants displaying poor weight gain or lethargy or asymptomatic infants with hemoglobin of 6 gm/dL or less often are transfused.

LONG-TERM

More data are now emerging on long-term outcome of fetuses transfused in utero. Although information is still limited and should be interpreted with caution, it appears to be reassuring. Indeed, even in those having severe disease, most infants seem to achieve normal neurodevelopment. This belief was well demonstrated in a series of 40 children, followed until 62 months of age.[29] The 22 infants who were assessed between 9 and 18 months showed a normal global developmental quotient; the 11 followed until 62 months displayed normal cognitive abilities. Only one case of severe bilateral deafness and one case of right spastic hemiplegia were diagnosed. Both infants were delivered by emergency cesarean section, the first because of severe hydrops at 32 weeks and the second because of fetal distress and premature rupture of membranes at 34 weeks. Interestingly, there was no correlation between the global development quotient and the severity of disease, including presence of hydrops and number of transfusions. This information, combined with a 4.5% incidence of major neurologic handicaps, supports the continued use of IVTs.

A larger series of 92 fetuses was recently reported with outcomes on 69 infants from 6 months to 6 years of age.[31] In this group, most children were found to have no significant general health problems, but 56% had frequent respiratory tract infections. As a result, there was a certain degree of hearing loss in 5 children, and 3 children had otherwise unexplained hearing disability. A 17% incidence of motor or speech delay was noted in those in early childhood, but for most children, these conditions were resolved with physical or speech therapy. Of the 69 children tested, 64 had no neurologic abnormalities and 92.8% had normal developmental outcome.

Once again, outcome was not correlated with presence of hydrops, but the risk of neurologic abnormalities was significantly greater in fetuses exposed to perinatal asphyxia and in those with lower cord blood hemoglobin levels.

Even longer term follow-up data are now available. In a recent study by Grab and associates, 30 children were followed for up to 6 years of age.[23] All children were able to attend regular primary school and only two survivors displayed mild sensorineurologic disabilities. One suffered slight speech delay; the other was delivered at 29 weeks by an emergency cesarean because of persistent bradycardia following a transfusion and initially showed mild psychomotor disabilities, though further neurologic evaluations were normal at the age of 6. Interestingly, both children were nonhydropic in utero, and no cases of either moderate or severe neurologic disabilities were observed even in the presence of very severe disease and hydrops.

Although these results are encouraging, difficulties in appropriate follow-up of all children remain a problem, which is partly why the data should be interpreted carefully. Very few studies have been able to describe outcomes for all children, raising the possibility that those lost to follow-up might have had worse outcomes. However, despite this shortcoming, the available data suggest that for most infants, a normal neurodevelopmental outcome can be expected, thereby justifying aggressive treatment of fetuses with severe hemolytic disease including hydrops.

ATYPICAL ANTIGENS

Many other antigen systems are present on the surface of fetal red blood cells. After transfusion of unmatched blood, 1% to 2% of patients acquire antibodies against these so-called *atypical antigens* and face the possibility of isoimmunization in a subsequent pregnancy. Fortunately, antibodies produced against most of these antigens are of the IgM type and are of no consequence to the fetus because they do not cross the placenta. This is the case for anti-Le and anti-P. Other antibodies can cause mild disease for which no treatment is indicated (e.g., Fy, Jk, Lw).

However, Kell, Duffy, Diego, Kidd, MNSs, P, C, c, and E have all been associated with moderate to severe hemolytic disease. Of these, Kell antigen is probably second to RhD in its importance and strength. The Kell blood group system consists of 23

antigens encoded by a single gene on chromosome 7. The strongest immunogens of this system are K1 and K2. However, because 91% of the population is Kell negative and only 5% of those people will develop anti-Kell antibody after an incompatible transfusion, this type of isoimmunization remains relatively uncommon.[29]

Modern approaches to the management of the Kell-sensitized pregnant woman require an understanding of the pathophysiologic principles behind this entity, because this process appears to be different from RhD sensitization. For example, fetuses affected by Kell sensitization compared with RhD have a lower number of circulating reticulocytes and an inappropriately low number of normoblasts for the degree of anemia.[4] In addition, the bilirubin concentration in the amniotic fluid is lower than expected for the degree of anemia, and the antibody titer does not correlate with disease severity. These observations suggest that Kell sensitization leads to suppression of erythropoiesis. In support of this suggestion, Vaughan and colleagues have demonstrated the inhibition of Kell-positive erythroid progenitor cells by anti-Kell antibodies.[64] This inhibition was found to be dose dependent, specific for cells of erythroid lineage. A greater effect was noted on more immature erythroid cells, suggesting a differential importance for Kell antigen at specific stages of erythroid development.

This information has very important implications for the management of Kell-sensitized pregnant women. The initial approach should include paternal Kell genotyping followed by fetal genotyping (chorionic villus sampling or amniocentesis by PCR)[59] if the father is heterozygous. Titers are not generally reliable and hemolysis is not as important as in RhD; therefore, serial amniocentesis for ΔOD-450 measurements may not be very helpful and may even be misleading. Indeed, even low titers and low ΔOD-450 levels have been found in the presence of severe anemia. Suggested approaches consist of early ultrasound surveillance for the development of hydrops with cordocentesis at 20 to 22 weeks to evaluate the degree of anemia. The need for transfusion using this approach can then be re-evaluated every few weeks and transfusion schedules can be established as needed.

■ REFERENCES

1. Avent ND: Antenatal genotyping of the blood groups of the fetus. Vox Sang 74 (Suppl 12):365, 1998.
2. Avent ND, Martin PGP: Kell typing by allele-specific PCR (ASP). Br J Haematol 93:728, 1996.
3. Avner R, et al: Management of rhesus isoimmunization by preimplantation genetic diagnosis. Mol Hum Repro 2(1):60, 1996.
4. Babinszki A, et al: Prognostic factors and management in pregnancies complicated with severe Kell alloimmunization experiences of the last 13 years. Am J Perinatol 15(12):685, 1998.
5. Bahado-Singh R, et al: A new splenic artery Doppler velocimetric index for prediction of severe anemia associated with Rh alloimmunization. Am J Obstet Gynecol 181 1:49, 1999.
6. Bowman JM, et al: Rh isoimmunization during pregnancy: Antenatal prophylaxis. Can Med Assoc J 118:623, 1978.

7. Bowman JM: Hemolytic disease (erythroblastosis fetalis). In Resnick R, et al (eds): Maternal Fetal Medicine Principles and Practice, 3rd ed. Philadelphia, WB Saunders, 1994, p 711.

8. Bowman J et al: Intravenous drug abuse causes Rh immunization. Vox Sang 61:96, 1991.

9. Chitkara U, et al: The role of sonography in assessing severity of fetal anemia in Rh and Kell isoimmunized pregnancies. Obstet Gynecol 71:393, 1988.

10. Chow B: Anemia from bleeding of the fetus into the maternal circulation. Lancet 1:1213, 1954.

11. Clarke CA, et al: Further experimental studies on the prevention of Rh haemolytic disease. BMJ 1:979, 1963.

12. Cohen F, et al: Mechanisms of isoimmunization. I. The transplacental passage of fetal erythrocytes in homospecific pregnancies. Blood 23:621, 1964.

13. Copel JA, et al: Alloimmune disorders and pregnancy. Semin Perinatol 15:251, 1991.

14. Dallacasa P, et al: Erythropoietin course in newborns with Rh hemolytic disease transfused and not transfused in utero. Pediatr Res 40:357, 1996.

15. Diamond LK, et al: Erythroblastosis fetalis and its association with universal edema of the fetus, icterus gravis neonatorum and anemia of the newborn. J Pediatr 1:269,1932.

16. Dooren MC, et al: Protection against immune haemolytic disease of newborn infants by maternal monocyte B reactive IgG alloantibodies. Lancet 339:1067, 1992.

17. Engelfriet CP, et al: International forum. Laboratory procedures for the prediction of the severity of haemolytic disease of the newborn. Vox Sang 69:61, 1995.

18. Finn R, et al: Experimental studies on the prevention of Rh hemolytic disease. BMJ 1:1486, 1961.

19. Fisk NM, et al: Clinical utility of fetal RhD typing in alloimmunized pregnancies by means of polymerase chain reaction on amniocytes or chorionic villi. Am J Obstet Gynecol 171:50, 1994.

20. Flint T, et al: Intravenous immune globulin in the management of severe RhD hemolytic disease. Ostet Gynecol Surv 52:193, 1997.

21. Freda VJ, et al: Prevention of Rh hemolytic disease with Rh immune globulin. Am J Obstet Gynecol 128:45, 1977.

22. Freda VJ, et al: Successful prevention of experimental Rh sensitization in man with an anti-Rh gamma 2 globulin antibody preparation: A preliminary report. Transfusion 4:26, 1964.

23. Grab D, et al: Treatment of fetal erythroblastosis by intravascular transfusions: Outcome at 6 years. Obstet Gynecol 93:165, 1999.

24. Grannum PAT, et al: Prevention of Rh isoimmunization and treatment of the compromised fetus. Semin Perinatol 12:234, 1988.

25. Hadley AG: A Comparison of in vitro tests for predicting the severity of haemolytic disease of the fetus and newborn. Vox Sang. 74 (Suppl 2):375, 1998.

26. Hadley AG, et al: The ability of the chemiluminescence test to predict clinical outcome and the necessity for amniocentesis in pregnancies at risk of haemolytic disease of the newborn. Br J Obstet Gynaecol 105:231, 1998

27. Hartwell EA: Use of Rh immune globulin. ASCP Practice Parameter. Am J Clin Pathol 110:281, 1998.

28. Hilden JO, et al: HLA phenotypes and severe Rh(D) immunization. Tissue Antigens 46:313,1995.

29. Hudon L, et al: Long-term neurodevelopmental outcome after intrauterine transfusion for the treatment of fetal hemolytic disease. Am J Obstet Gynecol 179:858, 1998.

30. Iskaros J, et al: Prospective non-invasive monitoring of pregnancies complicated by red cell alloimmunization. Ultrasound Obstet Gynecol 11:432, 1998.

31. Janssens HM, et al: Outcome for children treated with fetal intravascular transfusions because of severe blood group antagonism. J Pediatr 131:373, 1997.

32. Kumpel BM: Monoclonal anti-D for prophylaxis of RhD haemolytic disease of the newborn. Tranfus Clin Biol 4:351, 1997.

33. Kumpel BM, Hadley AG: Functional interactions of red cells sensitized by IgG1 and IgG3 human monoclonal anti-D with enzyme B modified monocytes and FcR-bearing cell lines. Mol Immunol 27:247, 1990.

34. Landsteiner K, et al: An agglutinable factor in human blood recognized by immune sera for rhesus blood. Proc Soc Exp Biol Med 43:223, 1940.

35. Levine P, et al: Isoimmunization in pregnancy: Its possible bearing on the etiology of erythroblastosis fetalis. JAMA 116:825, 1941.

36. Liley HJ: Rescue in inner space: Management of Rh hemolytic disease. Editorial. J Pediatr 131:340, 1997.

37. Liley AW: Liquor amnii analysis in management of pregnancy complicated by rhesus sensitization. Am J Obstet Gynecol 82:1359, 1961.

38. Lipitz S, et al: Obstetrics outcomes after RhD and Kell testing. Human Reproduction 13:1472, 1998.

39. Mari G: Noninvasive diagnosis by Doppler ultrasonography of fetal anemia due to maternal red-cell alloimmunization. N Engl J Med 342:9, 2000.

40. Moise KJ, et al: Comparison of four types of intrauterine transfusion. Effect on fetal hematocrit. Fetal Ther 4:126, 1989.

41. Nevanlinna HR, et al: The influence of mother-child ABO incompatibility on Rh immunization. Vox Sang 1:26, 1965.

42. Nicolaides KH, et al: The relationship of fetal plasma protein concentration and hemoglobin level to the development of hydrops in rhesus isoimmunization. Am J Obstet Gynecol 152:341, 1985.

43. Nicolaides KH, et al: Erythroblastosis and reticulocytosis in anemic fetuses. Am J Obstet Gynecol 159:1063, 1988.

44. Nicolaides KH, et al: Have Liley charts outlived their usefulness? Am J Obstet Gynecol 155:90, 1986.

45. Nicolaides KH, et al: Measurement of human fetoplacental blood volume in erythroblastosis fetalis. Am J Obstet 157:50, 1987.

46. Nicolaides KH, et al: Failure of ultrasonographic paramaters to predict the severity of fetal anemia in Rhesus isoimmunization. Am J Obstet Gynecol 158:920, 1988.

47. Nicolini U, et al: Fetal liver dysfunction in Rh alloimmunization. Br J Obstet Gynecol 98:287, 1991.

48. Nicolini U, et al: Pathophysiology of pressure changes during intrauterine transfusion. Am J Obstet Gynecol 160:1139, 1989.

49. Ovali F, et al: Management of late anemia in rhesus hemolytic disease: Use of recombinant human erythropoietin (a pilot study). Pediatr Res 39:831, 1995.

50. Palfi M, et al: Placental transport of maternal immunoglobulin G in pregnancies at risk of Rh(D) hemolytic disease of the newborn. Am J Reprod Immunol 19:323, 1998.

51. Power JP, et al: Hepatitis C viraemia in recipients of Irish intravenous anti-D immunoglobulin. Lancet 344:1166, 1994.

52. Queenan JT, et al: Deviation in amniotic fluid optical density at a wavelength of 450nm in Rh-immunized pregnancies from 14 to 40 weeks' gestation. A proposal of clinical management. Am J Obstet Gynecol 168:1370, 1993.

53. Reece EA, et al: Ultrasonography versus amniotic fluid spectral analysis: Are they sensitive enough to predict neonatal complications associated with isoimmunization? Obstet Gynecol 74: 357, 1989.

54. Rodeck CH, et al: The management of severe rhesus isoimmunization by fetoscopic intravascular transfusion. Am J Obstet 150:769, 1984.

55. Schumacher B, Moise KJ. Fetal transfusion for red blood cell alloimmunization in pregnancy. Obstet Gynecol 88:137, 1996.

56. Sekizawa A, et al: Fetal cell recycling: Diagnosis of gender and RhD genotype in the same fetal cell retrieved from maternal blood. Am J Obstet Gynecol 181:1237, 1999.

57. Selbing A, et al: Intrauterine intravascular transfusions in fetal erythroblastosis: The influence of net transfusion volume on fetal survival. Acta Obstet Gynecol Scand 72:20, 1993.

58. Shepard SL, et al: Inhibition of the monocyte chemiluminescent response to anti-D sensitized red cells by FcX receptor I-blocking antibodies which ameliorate the severity of haemolytic disease of the newborn. Vox Sang 70:157, 1996.

59. Soohee L, et al: Prenatal diagnosis of Kell blood group genotypes: KEL1 and KEL2. Am J Obstet Gynecol 175:455, 1996.

60. Spinnato JA, et al: Hemolytic disease of the fetus: A comparison of the Queenan and extended Liley methods. Obstet Gynecol 92:441, 1998.

61. Stern K, et al: Experimental isoimmunization to hemoantigens in man. J Immunol 87:189, 1961.

62. Tovy LAD, et al: The Yorkshire antenatal anti-D immunoglobulin trial in primiparidae. Lancet 2:244, 1983.

63. Van den Veyver LB, Moise KJ: Fetal RhD typing by polymerase

chain reaction in pregnancies complicated by Rhesus alloimmunization. Obstet Gynecol 88:1061, 1996.

64. Vaughan JL, et al: Inhibition of erythroid progenitor cells by anti-Kell antibodies in fetal alloimune anemia. N Engl J Med 338:798, 1998.

65. Vintzileos AM, et al: Fetal liver ultrasound measurements in isoimmunized pregnancies. Obstet Gynecol 68:162, 1986.

66. Wiener AS: Diagnosis of treatment of anemia of the newborn caused by occult transplacental hemorrhage. Am J Obstet Gynecol 56:717, 1948.

21 | Amniotic Fluid and Nonimmune Hydrops Fetalis

Richard B. Wolf

Thomas R. Moore

Amniotic fluid surrounds and protects the developing embryo throughout gestation and provides an indirect measure of fetal well-being. Although the precise mechanisms involved in the regulation of amniotic fluid volume are not completely understood, it is clear that abnormalities of amniotic fluid volume are associated with abnormal fetal and maternal vascular volumes. By understanding the dynamics of amniotic fluid pathways and the normal exchange of water and solutes between the fetus and the amniotic fluid, one can appreciate the physiologic basis of the clinical conditions oligohydramnios and polyhydramnios. Nonimmune hydrops fetalis, an associated condition of fetal fluid overload, also is discussed in this chapter. Immune hydrops fetalis, which produces erythroblastosis fetalis, is discussed in Chapter 20.

AMNIOTIC FLUID DYNAMICS

The pathways of amniotic fluid have long been misunderstood. It was formerly believed that the majority of amniotic fluid was passed into the amniotic cavity as a transudate from the maternal vessels. Fetal urination was believed to be an unlikely source of amniotic fluid production because it was "unreasonable to suppose that nature would have an individual floating in and drinking its own excreta."[42] Modern concepts in amniotic fluid dynamics involve numerous pathways for movement of amniotic fluid and solutes, including fetal swallowing, urination, respiratory secretions, and transport within and across the fetal membranes.

COMPOSITION

Although amniotic fluid contains 98% to 99% water,[13] its composition changes with gestation. In early pregnancy, amniotic fluid is isotonic, with maternal serum representing its probable origin as a transudate from maternal or fetal tissues.[17] As the fetal skin becomes keratinized and as renal function matures, amniotic fluid osmolality declines from 290 mOsm/kg in the first trimester to approximately 255 mOsm/kg near

term.[54] Amniotic fluid creatinine, urea, and uric acid concentrations increase in the latter two thirds of gestation. Proteins, in the form of albumin, provide a minor source of nutrition for the developing fetus. Near term the amniotic fluid contains desquamated fetal cells, hair, vernix caseosa, and, possibly, meconium.

VOLUME

During pregnancy, approximately 6 L of water accumulate in the gravid women. The majority of this fluid is associated with growth of the conceptus: 2800 mL in the fetus, 400 mL in the placenta, and 700 to 800 mL of amniotic fluid.[158, 160] The remainder of the fluid is associated with the uterus (800 mL), breasts (500 mL), and maternal blood volume expansion (850 mL).[160] Despite complex osmotic, electrostatic, and hydrostatic forces, amniotic fluid volume is highly regulated, gradually rising in the first trimester, stabilizing in the second trimester, and declining late in the third trimester.

In a meta-analysis of 12 studies of direct measurement or dye dilution technique comprising 705 normal pregnancies, Brace and Wolf showed that amniotic fluid volume increased steadily in early gestation and remained relatively stable between 22 and 39 weeks, averaging 750 to 800 mL (Fig. 21–1).[15] Amniotic fluid declined thereafter by 8% per week, and the mean volume was approximately 500 mL by 42 weeks. From this curve, it can be understood that variation is modest in the low end of the curve (5th percentile, 300 mL) but relatively marked in the upper end (95th percentile, 1750 mL).

PRODUCTION AND REGULATION

Amniotic fluid turnover has not been investigated fully in early gestation, but studies of amniotic fluid turnover in the second half of pregnancy show that the bulk of amniotic fluid is produced by fetal urination and removed by fetal swallowing.[55, 159] A significant amount of fluid also is produced from secretions of the respiratory tract, with lesser amounts coming

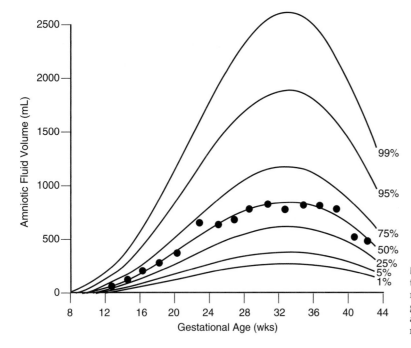

FIGURE 21–1. Amniotic fluid as a function of gestational age. Dots are means for 2-week intervals. Lines represent percentiles calculated from polynomial regression. (Modified from Brace RA, Wolf EJ: Normal amniotic fluid volume changes throughout pregnancy. Am J Obstet Gynecol 161:382, 1989.)

from nasopharyngeal secretions. As shown in Figure 21–2, excess fluid is reabsorbed via intramembranous and transmembranous routes.[53]

Rabinowitz and colleagues estimated that amniotic fluid production by fetal urination increases from 120 mL per day (5 mL per hour) at 20 weeks to 1200 mL per day (50 mL per hour) at term.[147] The investigators used serial ultrasound measurements of the fetal bladder, taken every 2 to 5 minutes, to calculate the rate of urine production.[147] Previous studies had shown urine production to be approximately one half of the amount calculated by Rabinowitz and colleagues,[92, 190] but the earlier studies involved less frequent observations and may have underestimated the rate of production. The true rate is probably some-

where between those values, with near-term urine flow at approximately 700 to 900 mL per day.[71] Urine production is decreased in women whose pregnancies are complicated by intrauterine growth restriction (IUGR).[92, 190] However, low urine output is not associated with lower Apgar scores, pH less than 7.25, or late decelerations in labor.[190] Further, there appears to be no correlation between fetal weight and urine production in women with normal pregnancies.[92, 190]

Fetal lungs are known to secrete approximately 300 to 400 mL of fluid per day, influenced by chloride ion exchange across the pulmonary epithelium.[68, 105] However, the fetus swallows approximately one half of this fluid before it enters the amniotic cavity.[16] Amniotic fluid is prevented from re-entering the lungs by the closed larynx, producing a net efflux of fluid.[69] Thus, the net amount entering the amniotic fluid from the lungs is approximately 150 to 200 mL per day. Fetal breathing movements are known to diminish late in gestation,[24] which may account partially for decreased amniotic fluid volume near term.

Fetal swallowing begins as early as 8 to 11 weeks and increases with gestational age,[18] facilitating removal of amniotic fluid. In animal studies, swallowing accounts for removal of approximately 1000 mL per day near term, and the amount removed increases from 100 mL/kg per day to 500 mL/kg per day over the last third of gestation.[174] In early human studies of normal, near-term fetuses, ingested amniotic fluid ranged from 210 to 840 mL per day (average, 565 mL), amounting to almost 5% to 10% of the fetal body weight.[142, 143]

Excess fluid not removed by fetal swallowing is reabsorbed into the fetal circulation via the intramembranous pathway, which is capable of absorbing large quantities of fluid.[54] In animal studies in which the fetal esophagus was ligated, amniotic fluid was found

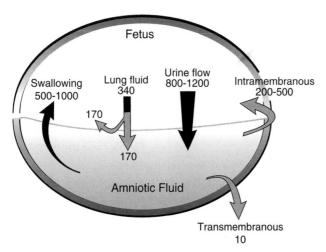

FIGURE 21–2. Pathways for daily fluid production and removal between the fetus and amniotic fluid compartments (measured in mL). (From Gilbert WM, et al: Amniotic fluid dynamics. Fetal Med Rev 3:89, 1991. Reprinted with permission of Cambridge University Press.)

to be near normal 2 to 3 weeks later.[107, 189] In sheep, Gilbert and Brace demonstrated rapid absorption of intra-amniotic water into the fetal circulation via fetal vessels on the surface of the placenta.[53] Other sites of potential fluid exchange include the nasopharyngeal mucosae, though it is unlikely this adds significantly to the overall fluid volume dynamics.[17]

CLINICAL DETERMINATION OF AMNIOTIC FLUID VOLUME

Assessment of the amniotic fluid volume is important because variation above or below normal is associated with an increased incidence of perinatal morbidity and mortality.[27, 28, 165] The methods for ultrasound assessment of amniotic fluid volume have been recently reviewed.[117] The ideal method for assessing amniotic fluid volume should be reproducible and clinically efficient, as well as have a high predictive value. The methods available include subjective estimation, maximum vertical pocket measurement, and amniotic fluid index measurement.

SUBJECTIVE ESTIMATION

Subjective estimation of amniotic fluid as being normal, reduced, or absent has been correlated with fetal outcome.[35] This method is based on the presence or absence of echolucent pockets between the fetal limbs and the fetal trunk or uterine wall. Pregnant women with reduced or absent amniotic fluid have an increased incidence of meconium-stained fluid, fetal acidosis, and birth asphyxia of the fetus or infant. Subjective scoring systems have been proposed,[59, 113] but the predictive ability of subjective methods varies widely and depends on the experience of the sonographer.[65]

MAXIMUM VERTICAL POCKET MEASUREMENT

Initial quantitative assessments of amniotic fluid volume included amniotic fluid pocket width.[99] *Decreased amniotic fluid volume*, when the widest pocket visualized is less than 1 cm, was associated with IUGR, and perinatal morbidity was increased 10-fold. However, this method was later criticized as being relatively insensitive in predicting poor perinatal outcome.[76] Chamberlain and associates later showed that using the *maximum vertical pocket* (MVP) was more predictive of poor outcome. They defined oligohydramnios as MVP of less than 2 cm and polyhydramnios as MVP of 8 cm or greater (Table 21–1).[27, 28]

AMNIOTIC FLUID INDEX MEASUREMENT

The *amniotic fluid index* (AFI) is currently the most widely used clinical method for determining amniotic fluid volume. The AFI is calculated as the mathematical sum of the deepest vertical pockets from each of four quadrants of the uterus, using the maternal umbilicus as the central reference point.[131] The AFI correlates closely with actual amniotic fluid volume

TABLE 21–1   DIAGNOSTIC CATEGORIES BY MAXIMUM VERTICAL POCKET (MVP) MEASUREMENT

AMNIOTIC FLUID VOLUME	MVP VALUE	PATIENTS
Polyhydramnios	≥ 8.0 cm	3%
Normal	>2–<8 cm	94%
Moderate oligohydramnios	≥1–≤2 cm	2%
Severe oligohydramnios	<1 cm	1%

Modified from Chamberlain PF, et al: Ultrasound evaluation of amniotic fluid volume I: The relationship of marginal and decreased amniotic fluid volumes to perinatal outcome. Am J Obstet Gynecol 150:245, 1984.

as determined by dye dilution technique, though it tends to overestimate actual amniotic fluid volume at the upper end of its extreme (Fig. 21–3).[34] Still, the AFI is superior to single MVP techniques in identifying patients with abnormal volumes of amniotic fluid.[115] Further, the AFI is a relatively simple technique with good intra- and interobserver correlation.[20, 151] Using this technique, severe oligohydramnios is defined as an AFI of 5 cm or less and polyhydramnios as an AFI of 25 cm or more.[22, 115, 131, 132]

In a large study of 791 normal pregnancies, Moore and Cayle established the mean and outer boundaries (5th and 95th percentiles, respectively) from 16 to 42 weeks' gestation.[114] As shown in Figure 21–4, the shape of the AFI curve is similar to that from Brace and Wolf,[15] as determined from direct amniotic fluid measurements (see Fig. 21–1). Throughout most of the pregnancy, the mean is approximately 15 cm, gradually declining after 33 weeks. The average AFI near term is 12 cm, with the 95th percentile (polyhydramnios) being approximately 20 cm and the 5th percentile (oligohydramnios) being approximately 7 cm. Note that the absolute maximum normal AFI is less than 25 cm. Typical limits for amniotic fluid assessment by AFI are shown in Table 21–2.[116] A normal AFI is illustrated in Figure 21–5.

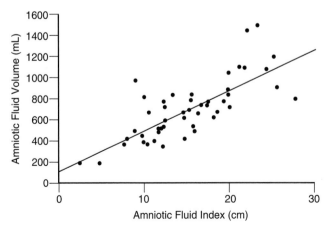

FIGURE 21–3. Correlation of amniotic fluid index to actual amniotic fluid volume determined by dye dilution technique. (Modified from Croom CS, et al: Do semiquantitative amniotic fluid indexes reflect actual volume? Am J Obstet Gynecol 167:995, 1992.)

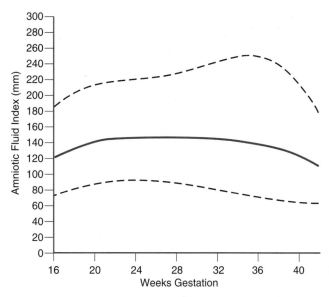

FIGURE 21–4. Amniotic fluid index. Four-quadrant sum of deepest vertical pockets (measured in mm). Solid line indicates the median values. Upper and lower dashed lines are the 95th and 5th percentiles, respectively. (Adapted from Moore TR, Cayle JE: The amniotic fluid index in normal human pregnancy. Am J Obstet Gynecol 162:1168, 1990.)

ABNORMALITIES OF AMNIOTIC FLUID VOLUME

CLINICAL ASSOCIATIONS WITH POOR PERINATAL OUTCOME

Increased Perinatal Morbidity and Mortality

Pregnancies complicated by extremes of amniotic fluid volume are associated with increased morbidity and mortality.[165] In a study involving 7582 high-risk obstetric referral patients, Chamberlain and associates[27, 28] measured the amniotic fluid using the MVP technique. The corrected *perinatal mortality* (PNM) rate for patients with normal amniotic fluid volume was 1.97 in 1000. In patients with polyhydramnios, the PNM rate was 4.12 in 1000; in patients with oligohydramnios, the PNM rate increased over 50-fold to 109.4 in 1000. In Mercer and Brown's series of patients with oligohydramnios, more than 80% of cases resulted in poor perinatal outcome.[104] In those with anhydramnios (absent amniotic fluid), the PNM rate was 88%, compared with 11% for those with moderate oligohydramnios.[113] The sonographic appearance of anhydramnios is illustrated in Figure 21–6. Jacoby and Charles noted a 34% PNM rate in their series of 156 patients diagnosed with polyhydramnios at the time of delivery.[83] Of these deaths, 48% were due to congenital anomalies (mostly anencephaly). In a series by Hill and coworkers, after correcting for lethal congenital anomalies, the PNM rate for polyhydramnios diagnosed before delivery was 58.8 in 1000.[75]

Polyhydramnios increases maternal and neonatal morbidity and is associated with diabetes, congenital anomalies, and multiple gestation.[75, 133] Deliveries are

TABLE 21–2 DIAGNOSTIC CATEGORIES BY AMNIOTIC FLUID INDEX (AFI) MEASUREMENT

AMNIOTIC FLUID VOLUME	AFI VALUE	PATIENTS
Polyhydramnios	≥25 cm	2%
Normal	>8–<25 cm	76%
Moderate oligohydramnios	≥5–≤8 cm	20%
Severe oligohydramnios	<5 cm	2%

Modified from Moore TR: Oligohydramnios. Contemp Obstet Gynecol 41(9):15, 1996.

complicated by malpresentation in 20% of cases,[83] and the chances of chromosomal abnormalities are increased 5- to 30-fold compared with patients with normal fluid volume.[6, 19] Preterm delivery also is prevalent in those with polyhydramnios, with 18.9% of fetuses delivered before 37 weeks' gestation in one series.[100] Even after correcting for specific causes, such as diabetes and congenital anomalies, idiopathic polyhydramnios is associated with higher rates of malpresentation, macrosomatia, and cesarean delivery.[125]

Perinatal morbidity associated with oligohydramnios is increased with higher rates of meconium-stained amniotic fluid, fetal distress, and low Apgar scores.[152] IUGR (birth weight less than 10th percentile for gestational age at delivery) also is common in pregnancies with oligohydramnios.[36, 74, 99] Operative intervention for fetal distress in labor is three times more likely in women with oligohydramnios than in those with normal amniotic fluid.[36, 62] Even in the absence of IUGR or fetal anomaly, the patient with idiopathic oligohydramnios is three times more likely to deliver preterm[50] and 30 times more likely to be induced for fetal indications than those with normal amniotic fluid volume.[148]

Increased Congenital Anomalies

Congenital anomalies are present in approximately 20% of patients with polyhydramnios.[75, 83, 145] The most common congenital anomalies associated with polyhydramnios are those that inhibit fetal swallowing: gastrointestinal obstruction (e.g., esophageal or duodenal atresia) and intracranial anomalies (e.g., anencephaly).[40] The risk of fetal anomaly correlates with the degree of polyhydramnios, with marked polyhydramnios (MVP greater than 16 cm) increasing the risk of anomaly to nearly 90%.[40]

Oligohydramnios is generally associated with genitourinary tract anomalies that inhibit urination (e.g., renal agenesis, polycystic kidneys, urinary obstruction).[120, 166] In a series by Bastide and colleagues, the incidence of major congenital anomalies in fetuses of women with severe oligohydramnios was approximately 13%.[8] Prolonged oligohydramnios, particularly during the critical period of fetal pulmonary development, can cause pulmonary hypoplasia.[128, 179] Positional deformities (e.g., skeletal and facial abnormalities) also are common in chronic oligohydram-

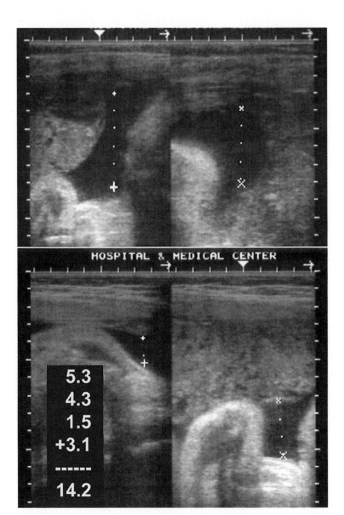

FIGURE 21–5. Normal four-quadrant amniotic fluid index, totaling 142 mm.

nios.[122, 140] The sonographic appearance of posterior urethral valves with megacystis is shown in Figure 21–7.

Uteroplacental Insufficiency

Oligohydramnios may be indicative of poor placental function. Because placental function and maternal hydration determine fetal urinary output,[117] oligohydramnios is frequently associated with IUGR, intrapartum asphyxia, and fetal death. In a Doppler imaging study by Cruz and coworkers,[37] patients with oligohydramnios and intact membranes were found to have higher flow resistance in the uterine and umbilical arteries than that in patients with normal amniotic fluid volumes. Nicolaides and associates noted that urine production in growth-restricted fetuses was decreased and that it correlated with the degree of fetal hypoxemia.[121] This result is perhaps an endocrine response to intrauterine stress with increased vasopressin secretion,[134] shunting blood flow preferentially to the fetal heart and central nervous system and away from the kidneys.[126]

In post-term pregnancies, amniotic fluid volume is more predictive of fetal distress than is fetal heart rate

tracing,[175] with women with adequate amniotic fluid volume having significantly better perinatal outcome than those without adequate amniotic fluid.[43, 129] Oligohydramnios in post-term pregnancies is associated with a fourfold increase in cesarean deliveries, mostly for fetal distress.[36]

OLIGOHYDRAMNIOS

The diagnostic study and clinical management of oligohydramnios should be directed toward diagnosing lethal fetal anomalies, identifying uteroplacental insufficiency, evaluating for premature rupture of membranes (PROM), and correcting or alleviating remediable underlying conditions. Moderate oligohydramnios is defined as an AFI of less than 8 cm or the absence of an amniotic fluid pocket at least 2 cm in depth; severe oligohydramnios is defined as an AFI of less than 5 cm[130] or an MVP less than 1 cm.[27] The diagnosis of oligohydramnios should be confirmed by repeating the measurement several times, averaging the result, and comparing it to normal values appropriate for that gestational age.[20]

Etiology

Conditions associated with oligohydramnios are shown in Box 21–1. In a series by Shenker and colleagues, the most common cause of oligohydramnios was PROM (50%), followed by IUGR (18%) and congenital anomalies (14%).[163] Genitourinary malformations include renal agenesis, cystic dysplasia of the kidneys, and obstructive uropathies, including ureteropelvic junction syndrome and posterior urethral valve syndrome.

Oligohydramnios can be the result of maternal ingestion of certain medications. The most significant

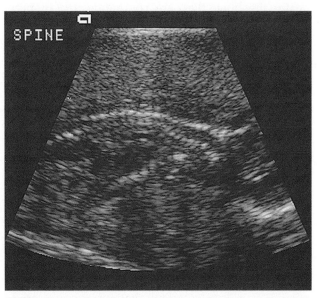

FIGURE 21–6. Anhydramnios. Note complete absence of amniotic fluid.

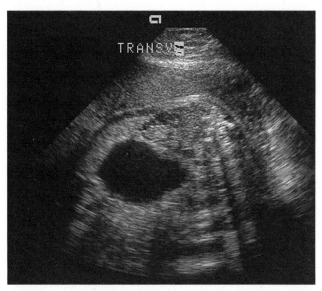

FIGURE 21–7. Posterior urethral valve syndrome. Male fetus with "keyhole" bladder on ultrasound. Note absence of amniotic fluid.

medications are the prostaglandin synthetase inhibitors that are used to inhibit labor, reduce polyhydramnios, and relieve pain.[73, 88] These medications reduce the fetal glomerular filtration rate, resulting in decreased fetal urine output and in oligohydramnios in up 70% of patients.[72] They may also decrease uteroplacental perfusion and cause the ductus arteriosus to close prematurely.[88] Although these effects are reversible,[58] patients maintained on indomethacin for over 72 hours should be evaluated with semiweekly amniotic fluid assessments and fetal echocardiography. Angiotensin-converting enzyme (ACE) inhibitors also have been implicated as causing oligohydramnios, presumably secondary to severe fetal hypotension.[39, 67] In addition, ACE inhibitors are associated with producing prolonged neonatal anuria, renal anomalies, ossification defects in the fetal skull, and death; therefore, they are contraindicated in pregnancy.[135]

Diagnostic Evaluation

RULE OUT RUPTURED MEMBRANES. A sterile speculum examination should be performed on any patient suspected of having PROM. However, these exams are often negative or equivocal, frequently making it difficult to diagnose chronic fluid leakage as the cause of low amniotic fluid. Still, if a normal-sized fetal bladder is observed on ultrasound with concomitant severe oligohydramnios, the likelihood of PROM is high.

ASSESS FETAL ANATOMY. Renal and ureteral anomalies are the most common causes of severe oligohydramnios in the absence of ruptured membranes.[120, 166] However, cardiac, skeletal, and central nervous system anomalies may coexist with primary renal anomalies.[102] Therefore, a careful anatomic survey should be performed to rule out congenital anomalies, pay-

ing close attention to the renal parenchyma, dimensions of the renal pelvis, and morphologic features of the fetal urinary bladder. In addition, renal anomalies may be associated with aneuploidy,[124, 168] so evaluation for other signs of aneuploidy (i.e., trisomies 21 and 18) should be included, and genetic amniocentesis should be considered. With bilateral renal agenesis, there is virtual anhydramnios from 16 weeks onward. Identification of the absence of renal arteries on power Doppler imaging (Fig. 21–8) may be necessary to document renal agenesis because the fetal adrenals can become hypertrophied and resemble renal structures.[161, 162] Conversely, polycystic renal disease and obstructive uropathy (e.g., ureteropelvic junction obstruction) may not become evident until the late second trimester. Unilateral disease rarely causes significant decreases in amniotic fluid.

ASSESS FETAL GROWTH. Oligohydramnios is known

■ **BOX 21–1**

PRINCIPAL DIAGNOSES ASSOCIATED WITH OLIGOHYDRAMNIOS

Fetal
Chromosomal abnormalities
Congenital anomalies
    Genitourinary (renal agenesis, polycystic or
        multicystic dysplastic kidneys, ureteral or
        urethral obstruction)
Intrauterine growth restriction
Intrauterine fetal demise
Postmaturity
Rupture of membranes (occult or overt)
    Preterm
    Prolonged

Maternal
Uteroplacental insufficiency
    Autoimmune condition
        Antiphospholipid antibodies, collagen vascular
            disease
    Maternal hypertension
    Diabetic vasculopathy
    Maternal hypovolemia
    Preeclampsia/pregnancy-induced hypertension
Medications
    Prostaglandin synthetase inhibitors
    Angiotensin-converting enzyme inhibitors

Placental
Chronic abruption
Placental crowding in multiple gestation
Twin-twin transfusion

Idiopathic

Modified from Peipert JF, Donnenfeld AE: Oligohydramnios: A review. Obstet Gynecol Surv 46:325, 1991.

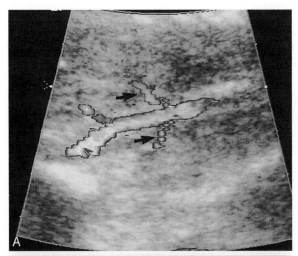

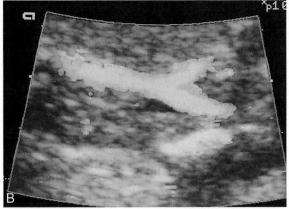

FIGURE 21–8. Bilateral renal agenesis. *A*, Doppler image of normal renal arteries (*arrows*) at 19 weeks' gestation. *B*, Power Doppler image of fetal abdominal aorta and its bifurcation at 20 weeks' gestation, demonstrating bilateral absence of renal arteries. (From Sepulveda W, et al: Accuracy of prenatal diagnosis of renal agenesis with color flow imaging in severe second-trimester oligohydramnios. Am J Obstet Gynecol 173:1788, 1995.)

ASSESS FETAL PULMONARY STATUS. Pulmonary hypoplasia, whether from renal or nonrenal etiology, is a known complication of prolonged oligohydramnios, with a PNM rate exceeding 70%.[7, 150, 164, 173] The risk of developing pulmonary hypoplasia is greatest if oligohydramnios is prolonged and occurs during the canalicular phase of alveolar proliferation, from 16 to 24 weeks of gestation.[108, 128] Hadi and associates showed that the absence of a fluid pocket of at least 2 cm between 20 and 25 weeks of gestation is predictive of impaired survival (30% survival if the pocket is less than 2 cm; 98% if the pocket is 2 cm or greater).[64] The estimated probability of developing pulmonary hypoplasia with oligohydramnios in the second trimester is illustrated in Figure 21–9. Although the precise pathophysiology of pulmonary hypoplasia is unclear, inhibition of fetal breathing,[14] lack of a trophic function of amniotic fluid within the airways,[2] and simple mechanic compression of the chest have been proposed as causes.[173]

Several techniques for evaluation of the fetal chest to predict pulmonary hypoplasia have been proposed.[31, 85, 123] Vintzileos and coworkers reviewed six ultrasonographic parameters for predicting pulmonary hypoplasia and found the highest sensitivity (85%) and specificity (85%) were achieved by calculating the lung area ratio[181]:

$$\frac{\text{Chest area} - \text{Cardiac area}}{\text{Chest Area}} \times 100$$

The normal lung area ratio should be greater than 66% (Fig. 21–10).

Diagnostic Adjuncts

A precise diagnosis is necessary to guide appropriate counseling and treatment of women whose pregnan-

to be associated with IUGR.[74, 99] Therefore, if PROM and congenital anomalies are excluded, IUGR resulting from uteroplacental insufficiency should be considered. Chronic poor placental function may be due to maternal autoimmune disease, hypertension, or vasculopathy.[127] In general, asymmetric IUGR, with the fetal abdomen lagging behind the fetal head in growth, is more predictive of uteroplacental insufficiency, whereas symmetric IUGR is more likely to be due to aneuploidy or congenital anomaly.[102] Doppler studies of uterine and umbilical blood flow may reveal patterns of high resistance in patients with oligohydramnios and IUGR, confirming the diagnosis of placental insufficiency.[94, 157] Because the risk of fetal asphyxia and death are high in oligohydramnios with IUGR,[99] intensive fetal monitoring and hospitalization should be considered in cases diagnosed between 26 and 32 weeks' gestation. Amniocentesis to assess lung maturity should be performed after 32 weeks, and delivery should be undertaken if the lungs are mature.

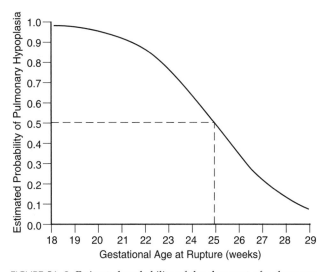

FIGURE 21–9. Estimated probability of development of pulmonary hypoplasia by gestational age in severe oligohydramnios (less than 2 cm maximum vertical pocket). Solid line indicates probability curve. Dashed lines illustrate 50% probability at approximately 25 weeks' gestation. (From Vergani P, et al: Risk factors for pulmonary hypoplasia in second-trimester premature rupture of membranes. Am J Obstet Gynecol 170:1359, 1994.)

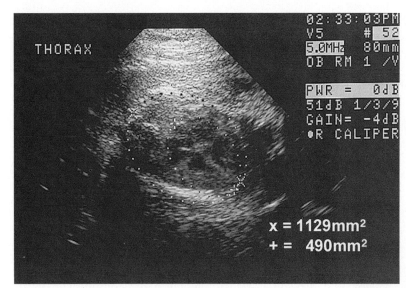

FIGURE 21–10. Decreased lung area–to–chest area ratio, suggestive of pulmonary hypoplasia. The lung area is calculated as $[(1129 - 490) \div 1129] \times 100 = 56.6\%$, and it is clearly reduced.

cies are complicated by oligohydramnios, but decreased amniotic fluid makes ultrasonographic analysis difficult. Amnioinfusion, indigo carmine dye, and furosemide are adjuncts that have been recommended to improve diagnostic capability in oligohydramnios.

AMNIOINFUSION. Infusion of normal saline solution into the amniotic cavity has been used midtrimester to improve ultrasound evaluation in suspected renal agenesis. In a series by Fisk and colleagues, suspected fetal anomalies were confirmed in 90% of patients.[47] However, only 13% of the etiologic diagnoses were changed as a result of information obtained at amnioinfusion. Quetel and associates aspirated a small amount of the fluid instilled for chromosome analysis and were successful in obtaining a karyotype in 70% of patients.[146]

INDIGO CARMINE DYE. Instillation of indigo carmine dye at the time of amnioinfusion can help diagnose PROM if the dye subsequently stains a tampon placed in the vagina.[51] However, most cases of PROM can be diagnosed clinically without this invasive procedure. Methylene blue dye has been reported to cause methemoglobinemia and hemolysis; therefore, it should not be used.[103]

FUROSEMIDE CHALLENGE. Although initially promising as a method for stimulating fetal bladder filling and demonstrating renal function,[191] maternal furosemide has subsequently been found to be inconsistent in its effect.[70] In animal studies, Chamberlain and associates showed that maternally administered furosemide failed to cross the placenta.[29] However, Gilbert and coworkers showed that furosemide injected into the amniotic sac could enter the fetal circulation via the intramembranous route.[56]

Treatment

Management of oligohydramnios depends on the severity of the condition, the underlying cause of the condition, and the gestational age of the patient. In general, mild oligohydramnios can be managed conservatively with frequent biophysical testing and appropriately timed delivery. Severe oligohydramnios may benefit from amnioinfusion, though cases of renal agenesis and other lethal congenital or chromosomal defects require little more than expectant management or termination of the pregnancy. The patient with PROM should deliver if there is evidence of infection; otherwise, the patient can be treated conservatively until the fetus reaches an age of likely lung maturity (older than 34 weeks) or has abnormal biophysical test results. Women with term and post-term pregnancies who have an AFI less than 5 cm or an MVP less than 2 cm have a fetus at high risk of morbidity.[27, 152] Therefore, antepartum testing in these patients should always include twice-weekly AFI evaluation.[188] If the fluid is decreased, delivery should be considered.

MATERNAL HYDRATION. Low amniotic fluid volume has been associated with decreased maternal intravascular volume.[60] However, when Powers and Brace infused isotonic lactated Ringer's irrigation in patients with low AFI, it did not improve the amniotic fluid volume.[141] When diluted (hypotonic) lactated Ringer's irrigation was infused, the maternal serum osmolality was lowered. This result produced an increase in fetal urine production and improved amniotic fluid volume. Oral hydration with plain water also has been shown to improve the AFI of patients with low amniotic fluid by approximately 30%[86]; in patients with normal amniotic fluid, the AFI improved by 16%.[87] Flack and colleagues subsequently demonstrated that hypotonic hydration improved uteroplacental perfusion, which improved amniotic fluid volume.[48] A recent comparison of techniques for maternal hydration showed that PO and IV hypotonic solutions were equally effective at increasing the AFI, with changes in amniotic fluid correlating inversely with changes in maternal osmolality.[44] These results suggest that increasing maternal fluid volume and decreasing maternal osmolality may be effective in improving oligohydramnios.

AMNIOINFUSION. Intrapartum infusion of saline solution into the amniotic cavity has become an accepted practice for patients with a low AFI and repetitive variable fetal heart rate decelerations.[187] Miyazaki and Nevarez demonstrated a dramatic 12-fold reduction in fetal heart rate decelerations in their study using transcervical amnioinfusion, but the procedure did not significantly change the cesarean section rate (18.4% versus 25.5%, P = .55).[106] However, in this study, the AFI was not evaluated as part of the patient's selection. Subsequently, Strong and associates used amnioinfusion in patients with oligohydramnios and achieved a significant reduction in operative delivery for fetal distress by maintaining the AFI at greater than 8 cm.[170] Meconium passage, severe variable decelerations, and end-stage bradycardia also were reduced. Prophylactic amnioinfusion is especially effective in preterm patients with PROM.[118] Transabdominal amnioinfusion also has been used effectively as prophylaxis against fetal distress prior to induction of labor in oligohydramnios at term.[180] However, complications from amnioinfusion, including uterine overdistention,[172] hypertonus,[138] and amniotic fluid embolism[96] warrant using this modality with cautious, close monitoring.

In severe second-trimester oligohydramnios, serial transabdominal amnioinfusion also has been advocated as a therapeutic procedure to prevent pulmonary hypoplasia and to improve outcomes.[47] However, in Fisk and colleagues' limited series of nine patients, only 33% of the neonates survived.[47] Further study is necessary to determine whether repeated amnioinfusion in second-trimester oligohydramnios can improve neonatal outcome.

POLYHYDRAMNIOS

Polyhydramnios (or hydramnios) is a condition of amniotic fluid in excess of 2000 mL at term.[15] In general, patients with polyhydramnios have a better prognosis than those with oligohydramnios,[27, 28] with the clinical management directed toward diagnosing fetal anomalies, correcting underlying maternal conditions (e.g., diabetes), and reducing the amniotic fluid volume in selected circumstances. Clinically, polyhydramnios is defined as an AFI of greater than the 95th percentile for gestational age,[114] over 25 cm at any age,[22] or the presence of any single amniotic fluid pocket 8 cm or more in depth.[28] Polyhydramnios can be diagnosed as early as 16 weeks' gestation, but it is rare before 25 weeks' gestation.[166] Because amniotic fluid normally decreases in the late third trimester,[114] polyhydramnios can be present with an AFI less than 20 cm. An example of polyhydramnios is shown in Figure 21–11. Maternal symptoms of polyhydramnios include dyspnea, edema, increased weight, and distention of the uterus. Perinatal complications include preterm labor, PROM, placental abruption, malpre-

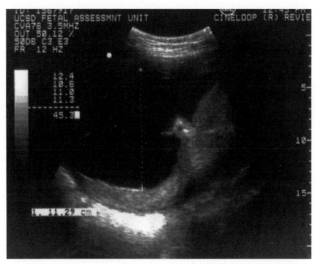

FIGURE 21–11. Polyhydramnios. The amniotic fluid index is 453 mm, and the single largest vertical pocket is greater than 80 mm.

sentation, increased risk of operative delivery, and postpartum hemorrhage.[100, 125]

Etiology

Conditions associated with polyhydramnios are shown in Box 21–2. In several series, polyhydramnios was most often idiopathic, with a frequency ranging from approximately 35% to 65% of cases.[10, 75, 83, 145] Congenital anomalies that interfere with swallowing or intestinal absorption were the next most common associated conditions. The prevalence of congenital anomalies correlates with the severity of polyhydramnios, with a 2.6 times greater incidence of anomalies in severe polyhydramnios (75%) than in mild polyhydramnios (29%).[5] Development of the Rh immune globulin to prevent immune hydrops due to Rh isoimmunization (see Chapter 20) and improved control of diabetes in pregnancy (see Chapter 15) have decreased the incidence of polyhydramnios due to these conditions. Aneuploidy is increased in significant polyhydramnios, and amniocentesis for karyotype should be considered.[19]

Diagnostic Evaluation

ASSESS FETAL ANATOMY. A detailed anatomic ultrasonographic survey should be performed to assess for possible congenital anomalies, paying particular attention to the gastrointestinal system for abnormalities that inhibit swallowing. With proximal obstruction (e.g., esophageal atresia or esophageal compression from diaphragmatic hernia or lung mass), the usual stomach "bubble" is absent. Distal obstruction is viewed as multiple cystic structures in the fetal abdomen (e.g., duodenal atresia may have a characteristic "double bubble" [Fig. 21–12]). Decreased fetal deglutition resulting in polyhydramnios is also associated with anencephaly, trisomy 18, trisomy 21, muscular dystrophies, and skeletal dysplasias. Ultrasound

---

■ **BOX 21–2**

PRINCIPAL DIAGNOSES ASSOCIATED WITH POLYHYDRAMNIOS

Fetal

Chromosomal abnormalities
Congenital anomalies
  Gastrointestinal (duodenal or esophageal atresia, tracheoesophageal fistula, omphalocele, diaphragmatic hernia)
  Craniofacial (anencephaly, holoprosencephaly, hydrocephaly, micrognathia, cleft palate)
  Pulmonary (cystic adenomatoid malformation, chylothorax)
  Cardiac (malformations, arrhythmias)
  Skeletal deformities
Fetal hydrops (immune or nonimmune)
Anemia (fetomaternal hemorrhage)
Constitutional macrosomatia

Maternal

Diabetes mellitus
  Gestational
  Adult onset (type II)

Placental

Chorioangioma
Twin-twin transfusion

Idiopathic

Adapted from Phelan JP, Martin GI: Polyhydramnios: Fetal and neonatal implications. Clin Perinatal 16:987, 1989; Hill LM, et al: Polyhydramnios: Ultrasonically detected prevalence and neonatal outcome. Obstet Gynecol 69:21, 1987; and Ben-Chetrit A, et al: Hydramnios in the third trimester of pregnancy: A change in the distribution of accompanying anomalies as a result of early ultrasonographic prenatal diagnosis. Am J Obstet Gynecol 162:1344, 1990.

---

markers of aneuploidy should be viewed carefully and amniocentesis should be considered.

In patients with multiple gestation and polyhydramnios, twin-twin transfusion should be suspected. Vascular anastomoses can exist in monochorionic placentas, causing a donor-to-recipient flow of blood with subsequent vascular fluid overload and marked polyhydramnios in the recipient twin's sac. The donor twin is typically smaller and fluid restricted, typically appearing "stuck," and can be missed during cursory ultrasound examination.[30] Discordance in amniotic fluid volume often precedes growth disturbances in twins; therefore, serial ultrasound examinations are prudent in monozygotic twins (see Chapter 18).

RULE OUT MATERNAL DIABETES. If the fetal abdominal circumference is markedly greater than the head circumference on ultrasound in a patient with otherwise unexplained polyhydramnios, maternal diabetes

should be suspected and evaluated with a glucose tolerance test (see Chapter 15). Polyhydramnios in diabetes is associated with increased perinatal morbidity and mortality beyond that of diabetes itself, and it is associated with poor glycemic control.[32] Polyhydramnios in these cases is due to the maternal hyperglycemia producing a diuretic effect in the fetus, with subsequent increased urine production.[92] Macrosomia is also linked with polyhydramnios.[11]

Treatment

If polyhydramnios is due to diabetes or erythroblastosis fetalis, the patient should be treated as outlined in Chapters 15 and 20. If nonlethal congenital anomalies are uncovered, appropriate pediatric specialists should be consulted for postnatal treatment. In patients with mild polyhydramnios (AFI of 24 to 40 cm), if there are no chromosomal or anatomic abnormalities and the patient is not diabetic or isoimmunized, the perinatal outcome should be no different than that in patients with normal amniotic fluid volume.[167] In these patients, however, uterine overdistention may stimulate preterm uterine contractions, and labor may ensue. These patients should be counseled on the signs and symptoms of preterm labor and be examined on a weekly or twice-weekly basis for early cervical changes. In women with severe polyhydramnios (AFI over 40 cm), amnioreduction or administration of prostaglandin inhibitors should be considered.

AMNIOREDUCTION. Removal of large volumes of excessive amniotic fluid may prolong pregnancy in patients with severe polyhydramnios. As first demonstrated by Caldeyro-Barcia and coworkers, using transabdominal pressure transducers, amnioreduction

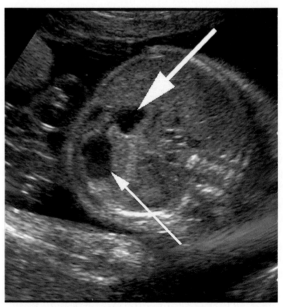

FIGURE 21–12. Duodenal atresia. Note the characteristic double bubble sign within the fetal abdomen, illustrating the fluid-filled stomach (*small arrow*) and duodenum (*large arrow*) on this transverse view of the fetal abdomen.

can reduce the baseline tonus and contractility of the uterus in cases of polyhydramnios[21]; however, amniotic fluid invariably returns, making serial amnioreductions necessary for maternal dyspnea and preterm labor.[136, 145] Most reports in the literature using serial amnioreduction are limited to treatment of polyhydramnios in twin-twin transfusion syndrome. In a series of 200 amnioreductions performed in 94 patients by Elliott and associates,[46] the goal was to restore a normal AFI (less than 25 cm). The median volume removed was 1500 mL (range, 350 to 10,000 mL), with a very low complication rate (1.5%), and delivery was delayed to a median gestational age of 37 weeks. Complications of amnioreduction include labor, abruption, PROM, hypoproteinemia, and infection.

PROSTAGLANDIN SYNTHETASE INHIBITORS. Indomethacin is a potent inhibitor of prostaglandin synthesis that reduces amniotic fluid by decreasing fetal urine production,[88] enhancing fluid reabsorption by the fetal lungs,[169] and increasing transmembranous absorption of excessive amniotic fluid.[98] Reports generally cite a starting dose of 25 mg PO every 6 hours, but doses can range up to 100 mg every 4 to 8 hours, depending on the severity of polyhydramnios and clinical response.[112] The indomethacin treatment should be monitored with twice-weekly ultrasound examination, and treatment should be discontinued once the fluid is reduced by one half to one third of its original volume or when the AFI is less than 20 cm. Indomethacin is effective in reducing the amniotic fluid volume in over 90% of cases of polyhydramnios[89, 112]; however, complications during indomethacin treatment include premature closure of the ductus arteriosus,[110] renal complications,[52] and necrotizing enterocolitis.[177] Chronic ductal closure in utero can produce right-sided hypertension, fetal hydrops, and persistent pulmonary hypertension in the neonate.[38, 109] The risk of ductal constriction is 5% at 27 weeks and increases to almost 50% by 32 weeks[176]; therefore, indomethacin treatment should be discontinued before oligohydramnios results and before 32 weeks to avoid iatrogenic side effects.

NONIMMUNE HYDROPS FETALIS

Hydrops fetalis is a condition of excessive fluid accumulation in the fetus with resultant high morbidity and mortality. In 1943, Potter distinguished *nonimmune hydrops fetalis* (NIHF) from immune hydrops in a group of hydropic neonates whose mothers were Rh positive.[139] Since then, with the development of the Rh immune globulin in the 1960s for the prevention of Rh disease (see Chapter 20), approximately 90% of cases of hydrops fetalis are diagnosed as being due to nonimmune disease.[156, 184] Improvements in ultrasound technology have allowed earlier antenatal diagnosis of conditions that would have otherwise presented as unexplained stillbirth, and those improvements have expanded our understanding of the underlying conditions that cause NIHF. Still, the

prognosis in NIHF is poor with PNM rates that range from 50% to over 90% in several series.[66, 80, 101, 182, 185] Maternal complications include preeclampsia (10% to 20%), malpresentation (24%), and increased rate of cesarean delivery for fetal distress (29%).[61]

Diagnosis

The antenatal diagnosis of NIHF is made by the ultrasonographic finding of fluid accumulation in the fetus or placenta in the absence of a circulating maternal antibody. Specifically, it is defined by identifying excess serous fluid in at least one space (ascites, pleural effusion, or pericardial effusion) accompanied by skin edema (greater than 5 mm thick), or by fluid in two potential spaces without the accompanying edema.[97, 149] Ascites can be detected when a minimum of 50 mL is present in the fetal abdomen.[77] Polyhydramnios and placental thickening (greater than 6 cm thick) also are associated with NIHF.[49] When oligohydramnios develops in NIHF, it is an especially ominous finding.[49, 183] The frequencies of ultrasonographic findings in NIHF are listed in Table 21–3. Typical sonographic findings in NIHF are shown in Figure 21–13.

Pathophysiology

The basic mechanism for the formation of fetal hydrops is an imbalance of interstitial fluid production and lymphatic return. Fluid accumulation in the fetus can be due to (1) congestive heart failure, (2) obstructed lymphatic flow, or (3) decreased plasma osmotic pressure. The fetus is particularly susceptible to interstitial fluid accumulation because of its greater capillary permeability, compliant interstitial compartments, and vulnerability to venous pressures on lymphatic return.[4] Compensatory mechanisms for maintaining homeostasis during hypoxia owing to underlying disease include increased efficiency of oxygen extraction, redistribution of blood flow to the brain and heart, and volume augmentation to enhance cardiac output. Unfortunately, these mechanisms increase venous pressure and ultimately produce interstitial fluid accumulation and characteristic hydropic changes in fetuses. Increased venous pres-

TABLE 21–3 PRINCIPAL ULTRASONOGRAPHIC FINDINGS IN NONIMMUNE HYDROPS FETALIS

FINDING	PATIENTS
Ascites	85%
Scalp edema	59%
Thickened placenta	55%
Body wall edema	52%
Polyhydramnios	48%
Pleural effusion	33%
Pericardial effusion	22%

Adapted from Mahony BS, et al: Severe nonimmune hydrops fetalis: Sonographic evaluation. Radiology 151:757, 1984.

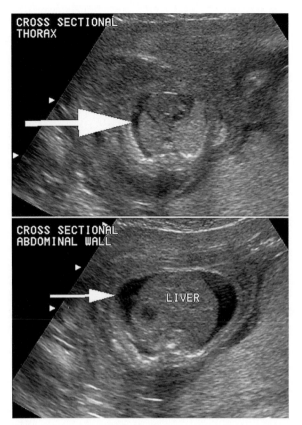

FIGURE 21–13. Classic hydrops fetalis on ultrasound. *A,* Thoracic findings. Note the pericardial effusion, bilateral pleural effusions *(large arrow),* and skin thickening. *B,* Abdominal findings. Note the fetal ascites *(small arrow).*

sure contributes to edema and effusions by increasing the capillary hydrostatic pressure and decreasing the lymphatic return.[111] Further, the hepatic synthesis of albumin may be impaired due to decreased hepatic perfusion and increased extramedullary hematopoiesis. Because albumin acts as the predominant oncotically active plasma protein, hypoalbuminemia increases transcapillary fluid movement at times of circulatory compromise.[4] NIHF typically undergoes a steadily degenerative course, unless the underlying cause is amenable to intrauterine therapy. Although NIHF sometimes resolves spontaneously, cases diagnosed earlier in pregnancy have a worse prognosis than cases diagnosed later in pregnancy.[82, 84]

Etiology

The possible etiologies of NIHF are ever expanding as formerly unknown causes are being reported. The conditions associated with NIHF are presented in Box 21–3. The prognosis depends on the underlying cause, with cardiac tachyarrhythmias that may be controlled by medication carrying the best prognosis. The frequency of diagnoses associated with NIHF is shown in Table 21–4. Cardiovascular malformation or arrhythmia is the most common finding, representing 22% of the total cases. In two series,[137, 171] the etiology

was unable to be determined before or after delivery in 33% of cases.

The ventricles of the fetal heart are generally less compliant than those in later life, so conditions that increase preload or significantly restrict outflow ultimately lead to cardiac stress and right-sided heart failure.[90] Therefore, whether the underlying disease causes low-output failure (e.g., congenital heart block, cardiac anomalies, cardiomyopathy, or intrathoracic masses) or high output failure (e.g., vascular tumors such as chorioangioma or sacrococcygeal teratoma, or vascular anastomoses in twin-twin transfusion), the result is cardiac failure and NIHF.

Anemia owing to infection, intrinsic blood disease, or fetomaternal hemorrhage can cause NIHF. Severe anemia from infection can cause high output failure, and it accounts for approximately 5% to 10% of cases in most series.[77, 171] In the case of human parvovirus B19, anemia is due to bone marrow suppression and aplastic anemia[153]; however, as the fetal immune system matures, the hydrops may spontaneously resolve.[144] Viral infections also can cause myocarditis and hepatitis that further worsen cardiac output and liver function. Intrinsic blood disorders such as α-thalassemia can produce severe fetal anemia. In women of Southeast Asian descent, α-thalassemia is the predominant cause of NIHF and is due to a complete absence of synthesis of the α chain of hemoglobin.[63] Anemia from fetomaternal hemorrhage (e.g., abruption, trauma, or amniocentesis) can be diagnosed by Kleihauer-Betke stain of the maternal blood or by elevated serum α-fetoprotein.[45]

Other etiologies for NIHF include chromosomal abnormalities, intrathoracic masses, and metabolic diseases. Chromosomal anomalies frequently produce cystic hygromas, which are common in fetuses diagnosed with NIHF before 20 weeks.[156] The cystic hygroma itself may cause the hydrops by restricting lymphatic flow and increasing interstitial edema. The most common chromosomal anomaly with cystic hygroma is Turner syndrome (45,XO), though trisomies 21, 18, and 13 are also common among chromosomally abnormal fetuses. These fetuses often have heart defects as well, which contribute to the formation of hydrops.[149] Intrathoracic masses (e.g., cystic adenomatoid malformation, pulmonary sequestration, and diaphragmatic hernia) restrict lymphatic flow and contribute to formation of hydrops. Chylothorax can produce massive pleural effusions, which can result in pulmonary hypoplasia, carrying a 50% mortality rate if polyhydramnios accompanies the effusions.[186] Metabolic diseases (e.g., Gaucher, Tay-Sachs, gangliosidosis) may require parental testing for carrier status or direct fetal blood analysis for diagnosis.

Diagnostic Evaluation

The diagnostic workup of the hydropic fetus should focus on finding the underlying cause. In general, the diagnostic workup should begin with obtaining the maternal history of hereditary or metabolic diseases, diabetes, or anemia; history of exposure to infection;

BOX 21–3

PRINCIPAL DIAGNOSES ASSOCIATED WITH NONIMMUNE HYDROPS FETALIS

High Cardiac Output

Tachyarrhythmia
Twin-twin transfusion
Placental chorioangioma
Intracranial meningeal hemangioendothelioma
Truncus arteriosus
Cavernous hemangioma
Thyrotoxicosis

Genetic Abnormality

Trisomy 21
Trisomy 15
XXXXY syndrome
Turner syndrome (45,XO)
Noonan syndrome
Trisomy 18
Skeletal dysplasia
Arthrogryposis multiplex congenita
Multiple pterygium syndrome

Fetal Anemia

β_1-Glucuronidase deficiency
Congenital leukemia
Hemoglobinopathy (e.g., α-thalassemia)
Hemolytic anemia
Hemorrhagic endovasculitis
Intracerebral hemorrhage
Massive fetomaternal hemorrhage
Methemoglobinemia
Parvovirus

Infection

Toxoplasmosis
Rubella
Cytomegalovirus
Herpes simplex virus
Syphilis
Adenovirus

Vascular Obstruction
Intrathoracic

Chylothorax
Cystic adenomatoid malformation
Diaphragmatic hernia
Intrapericardial teratoma
Mediastinal teratoma
Peribronchial tumor
Pleural effusion
Premature closure of the ductus arteriosus
Premature restriction of the foramen ovale
Pulmonary sequestration
Elsewhere

Absent ductus venosus
Renal vein thrombosis
Hemochromatosis
Umbilical cord torsion

Lymphatic Obstruction

Cystic hygroma
Hypomobility
Congenital myotonic dystrophy

Metabolic Disease

Gaucher disease
GM_1 gangliosidosis, type 1
Hurler syndrome
Mucolipidosis, type 1
Niemann-Pick disease
Lysosomal storage disorders

Idiopathic

---

and use of medication. A detailed ultrasonographic fetal evaluation and maternal laboratory analysis should follow. A systematic approach is imperative with invasive fetal testing, using amniocentesis or cordocentesis to follow, based on initial maternal laboratory results. The recommended workup of a fetus with NIHF is outlined in Box 21–4.

ULTRASOUND. Once the diagnosis for NIHF has been made, a detailed ultrasound examination should be undertaken to determine the etiology and to better grade the prognosis. When structural defects are associated with NIHF, the mortality rate is often 100%.[26] Scoring systems, developed to predict whether anemia is involved,[155] may be useful for objectively assessing progress. Thereafter, serial sonographic examinations are indicated to follow the progression of disease or improvement with treatment.

The anatomy of the fetus should be carefully surveyed for structural malformation. Neural tube defects and intracranial masses or defects should be ruled out. The chest should be evaluated for mass lesions (e.g., cystic adenomatoid malformation, pulmonary sequestration, and diaphragmatic hernia) (Fig. 21–14). Because cardiac anomalies are the most common cause of NIHF,[78, 137] fetal echocardiography should be performed. Echogenic areas within the fetal abdomen may indicate cystic fibrosis, viral infection, hepatic fibrosis, or polycystic kidneys. Echolucent areas may indicate bowel obstruction (e.g., duodenal atresia and volvulus). The fetal skeleton should be evaluated for biometry, and because skeletal dysplasias are associated with hydrops, bone mineralization, shape, and fractures should be noted. Fetal movement should be ascertained, with progressive reduction in fetal movement being predictive of poor outcome that

TABLE 21–4 FREQUENCY OF DIAGNOSES ASSOCIATED WITH NONIMMUNE HYDROPS FETALIS*

	n	%
Cardiovascular malformation/arrhythmia	113	22
Aneuploidy	46	9
Twin-twin transfusion	30	6
Anemia	26	5
Infection	24	5
Pulmonary anomalies	30	6
Abdominal organ anomalies	44	9
Skeletal anomalies	19	4
Multiple system anomalies	13	2
Central nervous system anomalies	11	2
Placental chorioangioma	5	1
Other identifiable causes		1
Idiopathic	146	28

*N = 513.

Adapted from Poeschmann RP, et al: Differential diagnosis and causes of nonimmunological hydrops fetalis: A review. Obstet Gynecol Surv 46:223, 1991.

frequently precedes intrauterine death.[78] The placenta and umbilical cord should be assessed for chorioangiomas, which can lead to hydrops from high output cardiac failure.

LABORATORY TESTING. Maternal blood testing should include blood typing and indirect Coombs antibody screening to rule out immune causes of the fetal hydrops. Congenital fetal infection is evaluated using TORCH titers (*t*oxoplasmosis, *o*ther agents [congenital syphilis, parvovirus B19], *r*ubella, *c*ytomegalovirus, *h*erpes simplex). Fetal anemia is otherwise evaluated with a Kleihauer-Betke stain to evaluate for fetomaternal hemorrhage and hemoglobin electrophoresis if indicated by genetic and family history. Maternal triple screen should be drawn because α-fetoprotein and human chorionic gonadotropin often are elevated in nonimmune hydrops.[12, 45, 154] The results may give some indication of the etiology and prognosis of the NIHF.

FETAL ECHOCARDIOGRAPHY. A complete fetal echocardiogram is necessary to rule out structural cardiac defects and to evaluate the cardiac rate and rhythm.[90] Structural cardiac defects associated with NIHF generally carry a very poor prognosis with PNM rates of 80% to 100%.[3, 33] Areas to be evaluated include the four-chamber view (to rule out hypoplastic ventricle), atrioventricular septum (for septal defects), valves, and outflow tracts. Biventricular width should be measured because outer dimensions higher than the 95th percentile are associated with poor outcome.[23] Masses within the heart (e.g., teratoma, rhabdomyoma) may also be present. Cardiac arrhythmias are best evaluated using M-mode ultrasound; both tachyarrhythmias and bradyarrhythmias are implicated in NIHF. If a fetal arrhythmia is uncovered, it often can be treated and can have the best prognosis of all

---

■ BOX 21–4

ANTENATAL EVALUATION OF NONIMMUNE HYDROPS FETALIS

Maternal History
Age, parity, gestation
Hereditary or metabolic diseases, anemia
Recent infections or contacts
Medication use

Maternal Laboratory Evaluation
Complete blood cell count
Blood type, Rh, indirect Coombs antibody screen
Kleihauer-Betke stain
Syphilis, TORCH and parvovirus B19 titers
Culture for group B streptococcus, *Listeria*
Maternal triple screen
Oral glucose tolerance test
Optional, as indicated:
    Metabolic studies
    Hemoglobin electrophoresis
    G6PD, pyruvate kinase
    Autoimmune screen (SLE, anti-Ro and -La)

Ultrasonography
Identify anatomic abnormalities
Evaluate extent of edema and effusions
Rule out twin gestation
Doppler blood flow assessment

Fetal Echocardiography
Evaluate for cardiac malformation, arrhythmia

Amniocentesis
Karyotype
Culture or PCR for TORCH, parvovirus
Amniotic fluid α-fetoprotein
Restriction endonucleases (thalassemias)
Lecithin-sphingomyelin ratio, phosphatidyl glycerol to evaluate lung maturity

Fetal Blood Sampling
Karyotype
Complete blood cell count
Blood type; hemoglobin electrophoresis
Blood chemistries, albumin, gases
Culture or PCR for TORCH, parvovirus
Metabolic testing (Tay-Sachs, Gaucher, GM_1 gangliosidosis)

Fetal Effusion Sampling
Culture or PCR for TORCH, parvovirus
Protein content
Cell count and cytology

G6PD, glucose-6-phosphate dehydrogenase; PCR, polymerase chain reaction; SLE, systemic lupus erythematosus; TORCH, toxoplasmosis, other agents, rubella, cytomegalovirus, herpes simplex.

Modified from Swain, et al: Prenatal diagnosis and management of nonimmune hydrops fetalis. Aust N Z J Obstet Gynaecol 39:285, 1999.

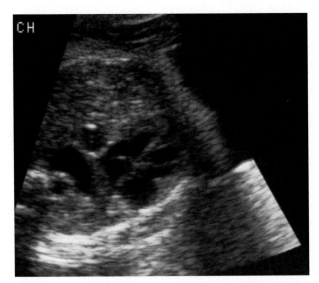

FIGURE 21–14. Diaphragmatic hernia. Transverse image at the level of the fetal heart demonstrating loops of bowel within the left side of the thorax and displacement of the heart to the right.

cases of NIHF.[149] Complete fetal heart block warrants evaluation of maternal connective tissue disease and autoimmune antibodies.

INVASIVE FETAL TESTING. If maternal blood testing and ultrasound evaluation fail to provide a definitive cause for the NIHF, invasive testing may be necessary. Amniocentesis provides amniotic fluid samples for karyotype, viral culture, α-fetoprotein, and metabolic and enzyme analysis. Fluorescent in situ hybridization (FISH) analysis of chromosomes can give preliminary karyotype results within a few days, whereas standard culture technique results may take up to 2 weeks. Similarly, polymerase chain reaction (PCR) studies for viral agents can give rapid results, whereas culture confirmation takes longer. In addition, lung maturity status can be evaluated to help develop plans for delivery.

In cases in which fetal anemia is suspected, cordocentesis for direct fetal blood sampling may be warranted.[79] In addition to giving direct information on chromosomal, metabolic, and hematologic parameters, cordocentesis also provides access for intrauterine treatment. Additionally, identification of specific immunoglobulins and isolation of viral antigens are possible. However, the risk associated with cordocentesis is higher than that of amniocentesis (1% versus 0.3%), and it should be performed by skilled individuals.

POSTNATAL EVALUATION. If the prenatal evaluation has failed to identify the etiology of the NIHF, postnatal evaluation should be undertaken (Box 21–5). Blood samples should be obtained for laboratory analysis similar to antenatal testing: karyotype, complete blood cell count, hemoglobin electrophoresis, and metabolic and chemistry studies. In addition, blood type should be ascertained. Structural defects should be evaluated using skeletal radiographs and ultra-

sound. A dysmorphology or genetic consultation also may be helpful, particularly to determine recurrence risks. In case of intrauterine or neonatal death, autopsy is recommended.

Treatment

In general terms, treatment depends on the underlying cause of NIHF and the gestational age of the fetus. If the fetus is not mature enough to survive outside the womb, conservative management should be undertaken. If the fetus is older than 34 weeks' gestation, has a mature lung profile, or is deteriorating from the effects of NIHF, delivery should be considered (Box 21–6). Otherwise, treatment is restricted to treatment of anemia, cardiac arrhythmia, polyhydramnios, and pleural effusion. Often, in the case of anemia, a single fetal transfusion reverses the signs of hydrops, though serial transfusions may be required. Infection by parvovirus B19 is amenable to intrauterine transfusion,[153] but neonatal stem cell transplantation may be needed for α-thalassemia.[25] Fetomaternal hemorrhage is also treated with intrauterine transfusion.[91] However, if the bleeding is ongoing, delivery may be required. Maternal digitalization may control tachyarrhythmias, but this procedure should be performed in consultation with a pediatric cardiologist. Amnioreduction may be required in the case of excessive polyhydramnios to reduce maternal symptoms and preterm labor. Pleurocentesis may be useful to decrease the incidence of pulmonary hypoplasia, which can complicate large pleural effusions. Occasionally, fetal paracentesis is undertaken to relieve marked ascites in order to allow vaginal delivery and prevent dystocia.[41] However, the hydropic fetus may be less tolerant of hypoxic episodes that can occur in

---

■   **BOX 21–5**

POSTNATAL EVALUATION OF NONIMMUNE HYDROPS FETALIS

Laboratory Evaluation
Complete blood cell count
Blood type, Rh factor
Karyotype
Blood chemistries, metabolic studies
Hemoglobin electrophoresis, if indicated

Radiographic Imaging
Skeletal radiographs
Ultrasonography
  Cardiac
  Thoracic
  Abdominal

Dysmorphology Evaluation

Autopsy

BOX 21–6

MANAGEMENT OF NONIMMUNE HYDROPS
FETALIS

Conservative Management in Hospital

Hospitalize the patient if
  Fetal skin thickening
  Pericardial effusion
  Nonreactive NST
  Biophysical profile ≤6
  Subjective decreased fetal movement
  Gestational age below 32 to 34 weeks
Treat underlying cause, if possible
Administer antenatal corticosteroids
Monitor serial growth and effusion volumes
NST and biophysical profile every 2 or 3 days

Deliver Patient

Gestational age over 34 weeks
Mature fetal lung profile
Biophysical profile persists <6
Maternal compromise (e.g., mirror syndrome)

NST, nonstress test.

---

labor; therefore, cesarean section is often employed for delivery. Still, the parents should be fully informed about the guarded prognosis, regardless of delivery route.

CONSERVATIVE MANAGEMENT. For patients in whom no cause can be ascertained, close observation for fetal decompensation is recommended, especially for gestations less than 32 weeks. The patient should be hospitalized if ultrasonography demonstrates fetal edema or pericardial effusion, or if antenatal testing with nonstress testing (NST) and biophysical profile (BPP) is less than reassuring. During the hospitalization, steroids should be administered to accelerate fetal lung maturity and to reduce the risks of necrotizing enterocolitis and intraventricular hemorrhage. Serial ultrasounds should be performed to follow serial growth and to monitor fluid accumulation, with antepartum testing (NST and BPP) continued every 2 or 3 days. During this time, continued efforts should be undertaken to ascertain the underlying etiology of the NIHF.

DELIVERY INDICATIONS. After 34 weeks' gestation, the best management for the hydropic fetus is delivery; indeed, between 32 and 34 weeks, few therapeutic maneuvers are likely to be of benefit compared with expert neonatal care. A mature fetal lung profile from amniocentesis or degenerating fetal condition warrants an even earlier delivery. However, the premature hydropic infant presents enormous management challenges and has a high PNM rate. Therefore, the optimal timing of delivery should be discussed by the obstetricians, perinatologists, and neonatologists

involved. Additional consultations may be necessary from pediatric surgeons, cardiologists, and cardiothoracic surgeons. In cases of maternal compromise from mirror syndrome (maternal hydrops),[178] a preeclampsia-like disease in mothers of hydropic fetuses, delivery is necessary.

FETAL SURGERY AND EXPERIMENTAL TREATMENT (see Chapter 11, Part Two). Occasionally, a hydropic fetus may be a candidate for in utero surgical intervention, such as repair of diaphragmatic hernia, congenital cystic adenomatoid malformation, or extralobar pulmonary sequestration.[1, 9] Urinary diversion in cases of bladder outlet obstruction also has been used, though long-term prognosis remains poor. Paracentesis and thoracentesis have been attempted, but in Watson and Campbell's series,[185] 27% of the fetuses reaccumulated fluid within 48 hours. Use of a peritoneal shunt in a case of massive ascites of unknown etiology improved the ascites, but the fetus died after developing other signs of NIHF.[57] Treatments with intraperitoneal injections of albumin have been attempted with some promising results. In a series by Maeda and coworkers, 75% of hydropic fetuses without pleural effusion who were treated with intraperitoneal albumin survived.[95] However, more than 90% of fetuses with pleural effusion so treated died. Intravascular injection of albumin also has been attempted, but it has been unsuccessful.[93] Shunts placed to drain pleural effusion also have been attempted, and good survival rates have been noted.[119]

Prognosis

Overall, the prognosis for patients with NIHF is poor, particularly if there are known structural defects or if the cause of NIHF is unknown. In these circumstances, the PNM rate approaches 100%. In cases of tachyarrhythmias, the prognosis is much better, assuming that the mother is treated with antiarrhythmic medications. For all other cases, the PNM rate may exceed 50%. Cases discovered early in pregnancy (before 24 weeks) have a worse prognosis,[101] whereas those discovered late in pregnancy may benefit from delivery and intensive neonatal care. However, most patients deliver preterm, with only 1 in 10 hydropic fetuses delivered after 37 weeks.[185] Indeed, in one large series,[81] 35% were delivered before 28 weeks' gestation, and 60% between 28 and 36 weeks' gestation. Fortunately, the risk of recurrence in a subsequent pregnancy is low, though 10% of patients had recurrent hydrops in one series.[185]

In summary, NIHF is a syndrome of multiple possible etiologies causing fluid overload in the fetus with a common end point of high perinatal morbidity and mortality. Despite meticulous diagnostic study, 33% of cases remain idiopathic, even following delivery. Thoughtfully designed treatment regimens may help some fetuses, but delivery may be the only recourse in cases of degenerating fetal condition. Therefore, antenatal testing should be directed toward identifying potentially viable fetuses, detecting lethal anomalies, and preventing maternal morbidity from unnecessary intervention.

■ REFERENCES

1. Adzick NS, et al: Fetal lung lesions: Management and outcome. Am J Obstet Gynecol 179:884, 1998.
2. Alcorn D, et al: Morphological effects of chronic tracheal ligation and drainage in the fetal lamb lung. J Anat 123:649, 1977.
3. Allan LD, et al: Aetiology of non-immune hydrops: The value of echocardiography. Br J Obstet Gynaecol 93:223, 1986.
4. Apkon M: Pathophysiology of hydrops fetalis. Semin Perinatol 19:437, 1995.
5. Barkin SZ, et al: Severe polyhydramnios: Incidence of anomalies. AJR Am J Roentgen 148:155, 1987.
6. Barnhard Y, et al: Is polyhydramnios in an ultrasonographically normal fetus an indication for genetic evaluation? Am J Obstet Gynecol 173:1523, 1995.
7. Barss VA, et al: Second trimester oligohydramnios, a predictor of poor fetal outcome. Obstet Gynecol 64:608, 1984.
8. Bastide A, et al: Ultrasound evaluation of amniotic fluid: Outcome of pregnancies with severe oligohydramnios. Am J Obstet Gynecol 154:895, 1986.
9. Benacerraf BR, Frigoletto FD Jr: In utero treatment of a fetus with diaphragmatic hernia complicated by hydrops. Am J Obstet Gynecol 155:817, 1986.
10. Ben-Chetrit A, et al: Hydramnios in the third trimester of pregnancy: A change in the distribution of accompanying anomalies as a result of early ultrasonographic prenatal diagnosis. Am J Obstet Gynecol 162:1344, 1990.
11. Benson CB, et al: Amniotic fluid volume in large-for-gestational-age fetuses of nondiabetic mothers. J Ultrasound Med 10:149, 1991.
12. Bernstein IM, Capeless EL: Elevated maternal serum alpha-fetoprotein and hydrops fetalis in association with fetal parvovirus B-19 infection. Obstet Gynecol 74:456, 1989.
13. Blackburn ST, Loper DL: The prenatal period and placental physiology. In Blackburn ST, Loper DL (eds): Maternal, Fetal, and Neonatal Physiology: A Clinical Perspective. Philadelphia, WB Saunders, 1992, p 36.
14. Blott M, Greenough A: Neonatal outcome after prolonged rupture of the membranes starting in the second trimester. Arch Dis Child 63:1146, 1988.
15. Brace RA, Wolf EJ: Normal amniotic fluid volume changes throughout pregnancy. Am J Obstet Gynecol 161:382, 1989.
16. Brace RA: Swallowing of lung liquid and amniotic fluid by the ovine fetus under normoxic and hypoxic conditions. Am J Obstet Gynecol 171:764, 1994.
17. Brace RA: Physiology of amniotic fluid volume regulation. Clin Obstet Gynecol 40:280, 1997.
18. Brace RA: Dynamics and disorders of amniotic fluid. In Creasy RK, Resnik R (eds): Maternal Fetal Medicine, 4th ed. Philadelphia, WB Saunders, 1999, p 632.
19. Brady K, et al: Risk of chromosomal abnormalities in patients with idiopathic polyhydramnios. Obstet Gynecol 79:234, 1992.
20. Brunner JP, et al: Intraobserver and interobserver variability of the amniotic fluid index. Am J Obstet Gynecol 168:1309, 1993.
21. Caldeyro-Barcia R, et al: Uterine contractility in polyhydramnios and the effects of withdrawal of the excess of amniotic fluid. Am J Obstet Gynecol 73:1238, 1957.
22. Carlson DE, et al: Quantifiable hydramnios: Diagnosis and management. Obstet Gynecol 75:989, 1990.
23. Carlson DE, et al: Prognostic indicators of the resolution of nonimmune hydrops fetalis and survival of the fetus. Am J Obstet Gynecol 163:1785, 1990.
24. Carmichael L, et al: Fetal breathing, gross body movements, and maternal and fetal heart rates before spontaneous labor at term. Am J Obstet Gynecol 148:675, 1984.
25. Carr S, et al: Intrauterine therapy for homozygous alpha-thalassemia. Obstet Gynecol 85:876, 1995.
26. Castillo RA, et al: Nonimmune hydrops fetalis: Clinical experience and factors related to a poor outcome. Am J Obstet Gynecol 155:812, 1986.
27. Chamberlain PF, et al: Ultrasound evaluation of amniotic fluid volume I: The relationship of marginal and decreased amniotic fluid volumes to perinatal outcome. Am J Obstet Gynecol 150:245, 1984.
28. Chamberlain PF, et al: Ultrasound evaluation of amniotic fluid volume II: The relationship of increased amniotic fluid volume to perinatal outcome. Am J Obstet Gynecol 150:250, 1984.
29. Chamberlain PF, et al: Ovine fetal urine production following maternal intravenous furosemide administration. Am J Obstet Gynecol 151:815, 1985.
30. Chescheir NC, Seeds JW: Polyhydramnios and oligohydramnios in twin gestations. Obstet Gynecol 71:882, 1988.
31. Chitkara U, et al: Prenatal sonographic assessment of the fetal thorax: Normal values. Am J Obstet Gynecol 156:1069, 1987.
32. Cousins L: Pregnancy complications among diabetic women: Review 1965–1985. Obstet Gynecol Surv 42:140, 1987.
33. Crawford DC, et al: Prenatal detection of congenital heart disease: factors affecting obstetric management and survival. Am J Obstet Gynecol 159:352, 1988.
34. Croom CS, et al: Do semiquantitative amniotic fluid indexes reflect actual volume? Am J Obstet Gynecol 167:995, 1992.
35. Crowley P: Non quantitative estimation of amniotic fluid volume in suspected prolonged pregnancy. J Perinat Med 8:249, 1980.
36. Crowley P, et al: The value of ultrasound measurement of amniotic fluid volume in the management of prolonged pregnancies. Br J Obstet Gynecol 91:444, 1984.
37. Cruz AC, et al: Continuous-wave Doppler ultrasound and decreased amniotic fluid volume in pregnant women with intact or ruptured membranes. Am J Obstet Gynecol 159:708, 1988.
38. Csaba IF, et al: Relationship of maternal treatment with indomethacin to persistence of fetal circulation syndrome. J Pediatr 92:484, 1978.
39. Cunniff C, et al: Oligohydramnios sequence and renal tubular malformation associated with maternal enalapril use. Am J Obstet Gynecol 162:187, 1990.
40. Damato N, et al: Frequency of fetal anomalies in sonographically detected polyhydramnios. J Ultrasound Med 12:11, 1993.
41. De Crespigny LC, et al: Fetal abdominal paracentesis in the management of gross fetal ascites. Aust N Z J Obstet Gynaecol 20:228, 1980.
42. DeLee JB: Physiology of pregnancy: Development of the ovum. In The Principles and Practice of Obstetrics. Philadelphia, WB Saunders, 1913, p 28.
43. Divon MY, et al: Longitudinal measurement of amniotic fluid index in postterm pregnancies and its association with fetal outcome. Am J Obstet Gynecol 172:142, 1995.
44. Doi S, et al: Effect of maternal hydration on oligohydramnios: A comparison of three volume expansion methods. Obstet Gynecol 92:525, 1998.
45. Downing GJ, et al: Nonimmune hydrops fetalis caused by a massive fetomaternal hemorrhage associated with elevated maternal serum alpha-fetoprotein levels. A case report. J Reprod Med 35:444, 1990.
46. Elliott JP, et al: Large-volume therapeutic amniocentesis in the treatment of hydramnios. Obstet Gynecol 84:1025, 1994.
47. Fisk NM, et al: Diagnostic and therapeutic transabdominal amnioinfusion in oligohydramnios. Obstet Gynecol 78:270, 1991.
48. Flack NJ, et al: Acute maternal hydration in third-trimester oligohydramnios: Effect on amniotic fluid volume, uteroplacental perfusion, and fetal blood flow and urine output. Am J Obstet Gynecol 173:1186, 1995.
49. Fleischer AC, et al: Hydrops fetalis: Sonographic evaluation and clinical implications. Radiology 141:163, 1981.
50. Garmel SH, et al: Oligohydramnios and the appropriately grown fetus. Am J Perinatol 14:359, 1997.
51. Gembruch U, Hansmann M: Artificial instillation of amniotic fluid as a technique for the diagnostic evaluation of cases of oligohydramnios. Prenat Diagn 8:33, 1988.
52. Gerson A, et al: Treatment of polyhydramnios with indomethacin. Am J Perinatol 8:97, 1991.
53. Gilbert WM, Brace RA: The missing link in amniotic fluid regulation: Intramembranous absorption. Obstet Gynecol 74:748, 1989.

54. Gilbert WM, et al: Amniotic fluid dynamics. Fetal Med Rev 3:89, 1991.

55. Gilbert WM, Brace RA: Amniotic fluid volume and normal flows to and from the amniotic cavity. Semin Perinatol 17:150, 1993.

56. Gilbert WM, et al: Potential route for fetal therapy: Intramembranous absorption of intraamniotically injected furosemide. Am J Obstet Gynecol 172:1471, 1995.

57. Goldberg JD, et al: Prenatal shunting of fetal ascites in nonimmune hydrops fetalis. Am J Perinatol 3:92, 1986.

58. Goldenberg RL, et al: Indomethacin-induced oligohydramnios. Am J Obstet Gynecol 160:1196, 1989.

59. Goldstein RB, Filly R: Sonographic estimation of amniotic fluid volume: Subjective assessment versus pocket measurements. J Ultrasound Med 7:363, 1988.

60. Goodlin RC, et al: Relationship between amniotic fluid volume and maternal plasma volume expansion. Am J Obstet Gynecol 146:505, 1983.

61. Graves GR, Baskett TF: Nonimmune hydrops fetalis: Antenatal diagnosis and management. Am J Obstet Gynecol 148:563, 1984.

62. Grubb DK, Paul RH: Amniotic fluid index and prolonged antepartum fetal heart rate decelerations. Obstet Gynecol 79:558, 1992.

63. Guy G, et al: Alpha-thalassemia hydrops fetalis: Clinical and ultrasonographic considerations. Am J Obstet Gynecol 153:500, 1985.

64. Hadi HA, et al: Premature rupture of the membranes between 20 and 25 weeks' gestation: Role of amniotic fluid volume in perinatal outcome. Am J Obstet Gynecol 170:1139, 1994.

65. Halperin ME, et al: Reliability of amniotic fluid volume estimation from ultrasonograms: Intraobserver and interobserver variation before and after the establishment of criteria. Am J Obstet Gynecol 153:264, 1985.

66. Hansmann M, et al: New therapeutic aspects in nonimmune hydrops fetalis based on four hundred and two prenatally diagnosed cases. Fetal Ther 4:29, 1989.

67. Hanssens M, et al: Fetal and neonatal effects of treatment with angiotensin-converting enzyme inhibitors in pregnancy. Obstet Gynecol 78:128, 1991.

68. Harding R, et al: Composition and volume of fluid swallowed by fetal sheep. Q J Exp Physiol 69:487, 1984.

69. Harding R, et al: Influence of upper respiratory tract on liquid flow to and from fetal lungs. J Appl Physiol 61:68, 1986.

70. Harman CR: Maternal furosemide may not provoke urine production in the compromised fetus. Am J Obstet Gynecol 150:322, 1984.

71. Hedriana HL, Moore TR: Accuracy limits of ultrasonographic estimation of human fetal urinary flow rate. Am J Obstet Gynecol 171:989, 1994.

72. Hendricks SK, et al: Oligohydramnios associated with prostaglandin synthetase inhibitors in preterm labour. Br J Obstet Gynecol 97:312, 1990.

73. Hickok DE, et al: The association between decreased amniotic fluid volume and treatment with nonsteroidal anti-inflammatory agents for preterm labor. Am J Obstet Gynecol 160:1525, 1989.

74. Hill LM, et al: Oligohydramnios: Ultrasonically detected incidence and subsequent fetal outcome. Am J Obstet Gynecol 147:407, 1983.

75. Hill LM, et al: Polyhydramnios: Ultrasonically detected prevalence and neonatal outcome. Obstet Gynecol 69:21, 1987.

76. Hoddick WK, et al: Ultrasonographic determination of qualitative amniotic fluid volume in intrauterine growth retardation: Reassessment of the 1 cm rule. Am J Obstet Gynecol 149:758, 1984.

77. Holzgreve W, et al: Investigation of nonimmune hydrops fetalis. Am J Obstet Gynecol 150:805, 1984.

78. Holzgreve W, et al: Nonimmune hydrops fetalis: Diagnosis and management. Semin Perinatol 9:52, 1985.

79. Hsieh FJ, et al: Percutaneous ultrasound-guided fetal blood sampling in the management of nonimmune hydrops fetalis. Am J Obstet Gynecol 157:44, 1987.

80. Hutchison AA, et al: Nonimmunologic hydrops fetalis: A review of 61 cases. Obstet Gynecol 59:347, 1982.

81. Im SS, et al: Nonimmunologic hydrops fetalis. Am J Obstet Gynecol 148:566, 1984.

82. Iskaros J, et al: Outcome of nonimmune hydrops fetalis diagnosed during the first half of pregnancy. Obstet Gynecol 90:321, 1997.

83. Jacoby HE, Charles D: Clinical conditions associated with hydramnios. Am J Obstet Gynecol 94:910, 1966.

84. Jauniaux E: Diagnosis and management of early non-immune hydrops fetalis. Prenat Diagn 17:1261, 1997.

85. Johnson A, et al: Ultrasonic ratio of fetal thoracic to abdominal circumference: An association with fetal pulmonary hypoplasia. Am J Obstet Gynecol 157:764, 1987.

86. Kilpatrick SJ, et al: Maternal hydration increases amniotic fluid index. Obstet Gynecol 78:1098, 1991.

87. Kilpatrick SJ, Safford KL: Maternal hydration increases amniotic fluid index in women with normal amniotic fluid. Obstet Gynecol 81:49, 1993.

88. Kirshon B, et al: Influence of short-term indomethacin therapy on fetal urine output. Obstet Gynecol 72:51, 1988.

89. Kirshon B, et al: Indomethacin therapy in the treatment of symptomatic polyhydramnios. Obstet Gynecol 75:202, 1990.

90. Kleinman CS, et al: Fetal echocardiography for evaluation of in utero congestive heart failure: A technique for the study of nonimmune fetal hydrops. N Engl J Med 306:568, 1982.

91. Kohlenberg CF, Ellwood DA: Fetomaternal haemorrhage treated with intravascular transfusion: A late complication of amniocentesis? Br J Obstet Gynaecol 101:912, 1994.

92. Kurjak A, et al: Ultrasonic assessment of fetal kidney function in normal and complicated pregnancies. Am J Obstet Gynecol 141:266, 1981.

93. Lingman G, et al: Albumin transfusion in non-immune fetal hydrops: Doppler ultrasound evaluation of the acute effects on blood circulation in the fetal aorta and the umbilical arteries. Fetal Ther 4:120, 1989.

94. Lombardi SJ, et al: Umbilical artery velocimetry as a predictor of adverse outcome in pregnancies complicated by oligohydramnios. Obstet Gynecol 74:338, 1989.

95. Maeda H, et al: Intrauterine treatment on non-immune hydrops fetalis. Early Hum Dev 29:241, 1992.

96. Maher JE, et al: Amniotic fluid embolism after saline amnioinfusion: Two cases and review of the literature. Obstet Gynecol 83:851, 1994.

97. Mahony BS, et al: Severe nonimmune hydrops fetalis: Sonographic evaluation. Radiology 151:757, 1984.

98. Mamopoulos M, et al: Maternal indomethacin therapy in the treatment of polyhydramnios. Am J Obstet Gynecol 162:1225, 1990.

99. Manning FA, et al: Qualitative amniotic fluid volume determination by ultrasound: Antepartum detection of intrauterine growth retardation. Am J Obstet Gynecol 139:254, 1981.

100. Many A, et al: The association between polyhydramnios and preterm delivery. Obstet Gynecol 86:389, 1995.

101. McCoy MC, et al: Non-immune hydrops after 20 weeks' gestation: Review of 10 years' experience with suggestions for management. Obstet Gynecol 85:578, 1995.

102. McCurdy CM Jr, Seeds JM: Oligohydramnios: Problems and treatment. Semin Perinatol 17:183, 1993.

103. McEnerney JK, McEnerney LN: Unfavorable outcome after intraamniotic injection of methylene blue. Obstet Gynecol 61:35S, 1983.

104. Mercer LJ, Brown LG: Fetal outcome with oligohydramnios in the second trimester. Obstet Gynecol 67:840, 1986.

105. Mescher EJ, et al: Ontogeny of tracheal fluid, pulmonary surfactant and plasma corticosteroids in the fetal lamb. J Appl Physiol 39:1017, 1975.

106. Miyazaki FS, Nevarez F: Saline amnioinfusion for relief of repetitive variable decelerations: A prospective randomized trial. Am J Obstet Gynecol 153:301, 1985.

107. Minei LJ, Suzuki K: Role of fetal deglutition and micturition in the production and turnover of amniotic fluid in the monkey. Obstet Gynecol 48:177, 1976.

108. Moessinger AC, et al: Oligohydramnios-induced lung hypoplasia: The influence of timing and duration in gestation. Pediatr Res 20:951, 1986.

109. Mogilner BM, et al: Hydrops fetalis caused by maternal indomethacin treatment. Acta Obstet Gynecol Scand 61:183, 1982.

110. Moise KJ Jr, et al: Indomethacin in the treatment of premature labor: Effects on the fetal ductus arteriosus. N Engl J Med 319:327, 1988.

111. Moise KJ Jr, et al: Do abnormal Starling forces cause fetal hydrops in red blood cell alloimmunization? Am J Obstet Gynecol 167:907, 1992.

112. Moise KJ Jr: Polyhydramnios. Clin Obstet Gynecol 40:266, 1997.

113. Moore TR, et al: The reliability and predictive value of an amniotic fluid scoring system in severe second-trimester oligohydramnios. Obstet Gynecol 73:739, 1989.

114. Moore TR, Cayle JE: The amniotic fluid index in normal human pregnancy. Am J Obstet Gynecol 162:1168, 1990.

115. Moore TR: Superiority of the four-quadrant sum over the single-deepest-pocket technique in ultrasonographic identification of abnormal amniotic fluid volumes. Am J Obstet Gynecol 163:762, 1990.

116. Moore TR: Oligohydramnios. Contemp Obstet Gynecol 41(9): 15, 1996.

117. Moore TR: Clinical assessment of amniotic fluid. Clin Obstet Gynecol 40:303, 1997.

118. Nageotte MP, et al: Prophylactic intrapartum amnioinfusion in patients with preterm premature rupture of membranes. Am J Obstet Gynecol 153:557, 1985.

119. Negishi H, et al: Outcome of non-immune hydrops fetalis and a fetus with hydrothorax and/or ascites: With some trials of intrauterine treatment. J Perinat Med 25:71, 1997.

120. Newbould MJ, et al: Oligohydramnios sequence: The spectrum of renal malformations. Br J Obstet Gynecol 101:598, 1994.

121. Nicolaides KH, et al: Relation of rate of urine production to oxygen tension in small-for-gestational-age fetuses. Am J Obstet Gynecol 162:387, 1990.

122. Nimrod C, et al: The effect of very prolonged membrane rupture on fetal development. Am J Obstet Gynecol 148:540, 1984.

123. Nimrod C, et al: Ultrasound prediction of pulmonary hypoplasia. Obstet Gynecol 68:495, 1986.

124. Nyberg DA, et al: Age-adjusted ultrasound risk assessment for fetal Down's syndrome during the second trimester: Description of the method and analysis of 142 cases. Ultrasound Obstet Gynecol 12:8, 1998.

125. Panting-Kemp A, et al: Idiopathic polyhydramnios and perinatal outcome. Am J Obstet Gynecol 181:1079, 1999.

126. Peeters LLH, et al: Blood flow to fetal organs as a function of arterial oxygen content. Am J Obstet Gynecol 135:637, 1979.

127. Peipert JF, Donnenfeld AE: Oligohydramnios: A review. Obstet Gynecol Surv 46:325, 1991.

128. Perlman M, Levin M: Fetal pulmonary hypoplasia, anuria, and oligohydramnios: Clinicopathologic observations and review of the literature. Am J Obstet Gynecol 118:1119, 1974.

129. Phelan JP, et al: The role of ultrasound assessment of amniotic fluid volume in the management of the postdate pregnancy. Am J Obstet Gynecol 151:304, 1985.

130. Phelan JP, et al: Amniotic fluid volume assessment with the four-quadrant technique at 36–42 weeks' gestation. J Reprod Med 32:540, 1987.

131. Phelan JP, et al: Amniotic fluid measurements during pregnancy. J Reprod Med 32:601, 1987.

132. Phelan JP, Martin GI: Polyhydramnios: Fetal and neonatal implications. Clin Perinatol 16:987, 1989.

133. Phelan JP, et al: Polyhydramnios and perinatal outcome. J Perinatol 10:347, 1990.

134. Piacquadio KM, et al: Role of vasopressin in mediation of fetal cardiovascular response to acute hypoxia. Am J Obstet Gynecol 163:1294, 1990.

135. Piper JM, et al: Pregnancy outcome following exposure to angiotensin-converting enzyme inhibitors. Obstet Gynecol 80:429, 1992.

136. Pitkin RM: Acute polyhydramnios recurrent in successive pregnancies: Management with multiple amniocenteses. Obstet Gynecol 48:42, 1976.

137. Poeschmann RP, et al: Differential diagnosis and causes of nonimmunological hydrops fetalis: A review. Obstet Gynecol Surv 46:223, 1991.

138. Posner MD, et al: The effect of amnioinfusion on uterine pressure and activity: A preliminary report. Am J Obstet Gynecol 163:813, 1990.

139. Potter EL: Universal edema of the fetus unassociated with erythroblastosis. Am J Obstet Gynecol 46:130, 1943.

140. Potter EL: Facial characteristics of infants with bilateral renal agenesis. Am J Obstet Gynecol 51:885, 1946.

141. Powers DR, Brace RA: Fetal cardiovascular and fluid responses to maternal volume loading with lactated Ringer's or hypotonic solution. Am J Obstet Gynecol 165:1504, 1991.

142. Pritchard JA: Deglutition by normal and anencephalic fetuses. Obstet Gynecol 25:289, 1965.

143. Pritchard JA: Fetal swallowing and amniotic fluid volume. Obstet Gynecol 28:606, 1966.

144. Pryde PG, et al: Spontaneous resolution of nonimmune hydrops fetalis secondary to human parvovirus B19 infection. Obstet Gynecol 79:859, 1992.

145. Queenan JT: Recurrent acute polyhydramnios. Am J Obstet Gynecol 106:625, 1970.

146. Quetel TA, et al: Amnioinfusion: An aid in the ultrasonographic evaluation of severe oligohydramnios in pregnancy. Am J Obstet Gynecol 167:333, 1992.

147. Rabinowitz R, et al: Measurement of fetal urine production in normal pregnancy by real-time ultrasonography. Am J Obstet Gynecol 161:1264, 1989.

148. Roberts D, et al: The fetal outcome in pregnancies with isolated reduced amniotic fluid volume in the third trimester. J Perinat Med 26:390, 1998.

149. Romero R, et al: Nonimmune hydrops fetalis. In Romero R, et al (eds): Prenatal Diagnosis of Congenital Anomalies. Norwalk, Conn, Appleton & Lange, 1988, p 414.

150. Rotschild A, et al: Neonatal outcome after prolonged preterm rupture of the membranes. Am J Obstet Gynecol 162:46, 1990.

151. Rutherford SE, et al: Four-quadrant assessment of amniotic fluid volume: Interobserver and intraobserver variation. J Reprod Med 32:587, 1987.

152. Rutherford SE, et al: The four-quadrant assessment of amniotic fluid volume: An adjunct to antepartum fetal heart rate testing. Obstet Gynecol 70:353, 1987.

153. Sahakian V, et al: Intrauterine transfusion treatment of nonimmune hydrops fetalis secondary to human parvovirus B19 infection. Am J Obstet Gynecol 164:1090, 1991.

154. Saller DN Jr, et al: The detection of non-immune hydrops through second-trimester maternal serum screening. Prenat Diagn 16:431, 1996.

155. Saltzman DH, et al: Sonographic evaluation of hydrops fetalis. Obstet Gynecol 74:106, 1989.

156. Santolaya J, et al: Antenatal classification of hydrops fetalis. Obstet Gynecol 79:256, 1992.

157. Sarno AP Jr, et al: Intrapartum Doppler velocimetry, amniotic fluid volume, and fetal heart rate as predictors of subsequent fetal distress. I. An initial report. Am J Obstet Gynecol 161:1508, 1989.

158. Seeds AE: Water metabolism of the fetus. Am J Obstet Gynecol 92:727, 1965.

159. Seeds AE: Current concepts of amniotic fluid dynamics. Am J Obstet Gynecol 138:575, 1980.

160. Seitchik J: Water and electrolyte metabolism in normal pregnancy. Clin Obstet Gynecol 7:185, 1964.

161. Sepulveda W, et al: Accuracy of prenatal diagnosis of renal agenesis with color flow imaging in severe second-trimester oligohydramnios. Am J Obstet Gynecol 173:1788, 1995.

162. Sepulveda W, et al: Sirenomelia sequence versus renal agenesis: Prenatal differentiation with power Doppler ultrasound. Ultrasound Obstet Gynecol 11:445, 1998.

163. Shenker L, et al: Significance of oligohydramnios complicating pregnancy. Am J Obstet Gynecol 164:1597, 1991.

164. Shipp TD, et al: Outcome of singleton pregnancies with severe oligohydramnios in the second and third trimesters. Ultrasound Obstet Gynecol 7:108, 1996.

165. Shmoys SM, et al: Amniotic fluid index: An appropriate predictor of perinatal outcome. Am J Perinatol 7:266, 1990.

166. Sivit CJ, et al: The sonographic evaluation of fetal anomalies in oligohydramnios between 16 and 30 weeks gestation. AJR Am J Roentgenol 146:1277, 1986.

167. Smith CV, et al: Relation of mild idiopathic polyhydramnios to perinatal outcome. Obstet Gynecol 79:387, 1992.

168. Sohl BD, et al: Utility of minor ultrasonographic markers in the prediction of abnormal fetal karyotype at a prenatal diagnostic center. Am J Obstet Gynecol 181:898, 1999.

169. Stevenson KM, Lumbers ER: Effects of indomethacin on fetal renal function, renal and umbilicoplacental blood flow and lung liquid production. J Dev Physiol 17:257, 1992.

170. Strong TH, et al: Prophylactic intrapartum amnioinfusion: A randomized clinical trial. Am J Obstet Gynecol 162:1370, 1990.

171. Swain S, et al: Prenatal diagnosis and management of nonimmune hydrops fetalis. Aust N Z J Obstet Gynaecol 39:285, 1999.

172. Tabor BL, Maier JA: Polyhydramnios and elevated intrauterine pressure during amnioinfusion. Am J Obstet Gynecol 156:130, 1987.

173. Thomas IT, Smith DW: Oligohydramnios, cause of the nonrenal features of Potter's syndrome, including pulmonary hypoplasia. J Pediatr 84:811, 1974.

174. Tomada S, et al: Amniotic fluid volume and fetal swallowing rate in sheep. Am J Physiol 249:R133, 1985.

175. Tongsong T, Srisomboon J: Amniotic fluid volume as a predictor of fetal distress in postterm pregnancy. Int J Gynaecol Obstet 40:213, 1993.

176. Van den Veyver IB, et al: The effect of gestational age and fetal indomethacin levels on the incidence of constriction of the fetal ductus arteriosus. Obstet Gynecol 82:500, 1993.

177. Vanhaesebrouck P, et al: Oligohydramnios, renal insufficiency, and ileal perforation in preterm infants after intrauterine exposure to indomethacin. J Pediatr 113:738, 1988.

178. Van Selm M, et al: Maternal hydrops syndrome: A review. Obstet Gynecol Surv 46:785, 1991.

179. Vergani P, et al: Risk factors for pulmonary hypoplasia in second-trimester premature rupture of membranes. Am J Obstet Gynecol 170:1359, 1994.

180. Vergani P, et al: Transabdominal amnioinfusion in oligohydramnios at term before induction of labor with intact membranes: A randomized clinical trial. Am J Obstet Gynecol 175:465, 1996.

181. Vintzileos AM, et al: Comparison of six different ultrasonographic methods for predicting lethal fetal pulmonary hypoplasia. Am J Obstet Gynecol 161:606, 1989.

182. Wafelman LS, et al: Nonimmune hydrops fetalis: Fetal and neonatal outcome during 1983–1992. Biol Neonate 75:73, 1999.

183. Wallenburg HC, Wladimiroff JW: The amniotic fluid. II. Polyhydramnios and oligohydramnios. J Perinat Med 5:233, 1977.

184. Warsof SL, et al: Immune and non-immune hydrops. Clin Obstet Gynecol 29:533, 1986.

185. Watson J, Campbell S: Antenatal evaluation and management in nonimmune hydrops fetalis. Obstet Gynecol 67:589, 1986.

186. Weber AM, Philipson EH: Fetal pleural effusion: A review and meta-analysis for prognostic indicators. Obstet Gynecol 79:281, 1992.

187. Wenstrom K, et al: Amnioinfusion survey: Prevalence, protocols, and complications. Obstet Gynecol 86:572, 1995.

188. Wing DA, et al: How frequently should the amniotic fluid index be performed during the course of antepartum testing? Am J Obstet Gynecol 174:33, 1996.

189. Wintour EM, et al: Regulation of amniotic fluid volume and composition in the ovine fetus. Obstet Gynecol 52:689, 1978.

190. Wladimiroff JW, Campbell S: Fetal urine-production rates in normal and complicated pregnancy. Lancet 1:151, 1974.

191. Wladimiroff JW: Effect of furosemide on fetal urine production. Br J Obstet Gynaecol 82:221, 1975.

22 Perinatal Infections

Tracy A. Cowles

Bernard Gonik

Infection of the female urogenital tract is not an uncommon complication of pregnancy. Responsible organisms include a vast array of viruses, bacteria, and parasites. As in most gynecologic infections, those complicating pregnancy tend to be polymicrobial.

Infectious complications during pregnancy lead to an increase in morbidity and mortality for both patients—the fetus and the mother. Premature rupture of the membranes, premature labor, and preterm delivery can be the result of infection. Pyelonephritis, endometritis, and sepsis are common examples of maternal morbidity. Neonatal infection, occurring at a time when the immature immunologic system is less protective, may predispose to meningitis, pneumonia, sepsis, or death.

Early diagnosis and aggressive treatment of infection during pregnancy may substantially lower the associated morbidity and mortality. In this chapter the discussion focuses on common clinical disorders and specific pathogens causing infection during pregnancy.

CLINICAL DISORDERS

URINARY TRACT INFECTION

Urinary tract infections are the most common medical complications of pregnancy. They may be classified as asymptomatic or symptomatic (acute cystitis or pyelonephritis).

Several physiologic changes occur during pregnancy that may promote the development of symptomatic urinary tract infection. The "physiologic hydronephrosis" of pregnancy, which is the dilatation of the ureters and renal pelves, is the result of decreased muscle tone surrounding the ureters and the mechanical obstruction of the enlarging uterus. Decreased muscle tone in the bladder results in increased capacity and incomplete emptying. These findings predispose to vesicoureteric reflux, which facilitates ascending migration of bacteria. In addition, physicochemical properties of the urine may predispose to symptomatic urinary tract infection. Urinary pH is elevated, glycosuria is common, and excess excretion of estrogen may promote bacteria capable of causing symptomatic urinary tract infection. Certain clinical conditions such as anemia and sickle cell trait have also been reported to predispose to urinary tract bacterial colonization.

Asymptomatic bacteriuria, defined as greater than 100,000 organisms in the urine of a patient who lacks symptoms, is present in 4% to 7% of the pregnant population. The prevalence of bacteriuria is related to lower socioeconomic status, sickle cell trait, and increased parity. Women with neurogenic urinary retention secondary to spinal cord injuries, diabetes mellitus, and structural abnormalities of the urinary tract are also at increased risk. Although pregnant women have about the same prevalence as nonpregnant sexually active women of reproductive age, pregnant women are more likely to develop symptoms of acute infection. As in nonpregnant women, *Escherichia coli* is by far the predominating organism (80% to 90%). *Proteus mirabilis, Klebsiella pneumoniae,* and group B β-hemolytic streptococci (GBS) are also commonly identified pathogens.

The goal of antibiotic treatment for pregnant women with asymptomatic bacteriuria is sterile urine for the remainder of the pregnancy. This is usually accomplished with a short course of a sulfonamide, ampicillin, or nitrofurantoin and monthly culture surveillance. Recurrences are common (approximately one third of patients), and suppressive therapy should be instituted once the culture is again cleared with a short course of antibiotic therapy.[72]

Cystitis in Pregnancy

Acute cystitis occurs in 1.3% of pregnancies and seems to be a separate clinical entity from asymptomatic bacteriuria and acute pyelonephritis. Cystitis, unlike the other two, does not tend to be preceded by bacteriuria in the initial screening cultures, does not recur as frequently, and is not the result of fluorescent-positive, antibody-coated bacteria, suggesting upper tract involvement. The most common pathogen is again *E. coli*, and antibiotic treatment with ampicillin, sulfonamides, or nitrofurantoin is appropriate.

Acute Pyelonephritis in Pregnancy

The incidence of acute pyelonephritis during pregnancy is 1% to 2.5%, with an estimated recurrence rate of 10% to 18% during the same pregnancy. Clinical manifestations include fever, costovertebral angle tenderness, nausea, vomiting, and symptoms of lower urinary tract infection, such as frequency, dysuria, and urgency. The pregnant patient may become quite ill with severe dehydration, transient renal dysfunction, respiratory distress, and septicemia.

The microbiology of pyelonephritis is similar to that described for lower tract disease in pregnancy. Initial antibiotic therapy includes the use of an aminoglycoside or an advanced-generation penicillin or cephalosporin. Therapy can be tailored to the results of the urine culture when these data become available. Clinical response is usually rapid, with 85% of cases showing a decrease in temperature elevation within 48 hours. Recurrence of the pyelonephritis may be as high as 60% if suppressive antimicrobial therapy is not maintained throughout the duration of the pregnancy. Renal calculi and anatomic obstruction can be responsible for a failure to respond to otherwise effective antibiotic treatment. Ultrasonography, limited-exposure intravenous pyelography, or magnetic resonance imaging may be employed in the evaluation of a patient who continues with fever or worsening symptoms.

Acute respiratory distress more frequently complicates the treatment of pyelonephritis in pregnant women. Those with the highest fevers, highest maternal heart rates, and those receiving concomitant tocolytic agents may be at the greatest risk.[97] However, clinical parameters do not clearly delineate women who are at risk for this potentially fatal complication.

The effect of pyelonephritis on the outcome of pregnancy is unclear. In the preantibiotic era, untreated pyelonephritis was associated with a 20% to 50% risk of prematurity. However, antibiotic treatment reduces the risk of preterm delivery significantly. One study reporting on 107 cases of acute pyelonephritis in 103 gravidas noted no increase in prematurity or in infants of low birth weight when compared with a control group.[35] The recognized maternal morbidity and potential perinatal morbidity mandate prompt and appropriate treatment of acute pyelonephritis in the pregnant patient.

PRETERM LABOR AND PREMATURE RUPTURE OF THE MEMBRANES

Prematurity complicates 7% to 10% of all births and is responsible for a disproportionately large fraction of perinatal morbidity and mortality. Although the various mechanisms underlying premature rupture of membranes (PROM) and preterm labor (PTL) are imperfectly understood, there is a growing body of evidence to suggest that between 20% and 40% of preterm birth (PTB) may have intrauterine infection/inflammation as a precipitating factor.

Evidence of the association between PTB and infection includes (1) histologic chorioamnionitis being more common in cases of PTB; (2) clinical infection in mothers and neonates seen more frequently after PTB; (3) several genital tract isolates known to be associated with PTB; (4) 10% to 15% of amniotic fluid cultures from women with PTB being positive; (5) prostaglandin and cytokine production following infection and inflammation; (6) data from animal research; and (7) antibiotics lowering PTB in some clinical trials.[40]

Preterm Premature Rupture of Membranes

Preterm PROM is responsible for one third of preterm births, accounting for 130,000 births in the United States annually.[69] Neonatal morbidity and mortality are associated with gestational age at birth and an increase in infectious complications. Antibiotics have been used in women with preterm PROM to attempt to prolong the time from onset to delivery and decrease infectious morbidity.

A number of trials have been reported in which antibiotics were studied in a randomized, prospective fashion. When taken together, several findings become important. The most significant differences have been found in the length of latent phase or the number of women with a latent phase greater than 1 week. Also a decrease in the incidence of intra-amniotic infection (IAI) has been reported. A decrease in perinatal mortality is difficult to prove, although these studies suggest a trend toward less stillbirth and infant death due to sepsis. Culture-proven neonatal sepsis, respiratory distress syndrome, intraventricular hemorrhage, and pneumonia are seen less frequently when antibiotics are used in preterm PROM.[60, 61] These benefits are more pronounced at the earlier gestational ages (less than 32 weeks' gestation). Between 32 and 36 weeks, it is less obvious that expectant management and antibiotics are as beneficial.

The optimal antibiotic regimen for the patient with preterm PROM has not yet been defined. Initial treatment with broad-spectrum antibiotics such as ampicillin plus erythromycin or an extended-spectrum penicillin or cephalosporin seems warranted. After 48 hours, oral therapy should be continued to finish a week-long course. GBS carriers should be treated with penicillin.

Antibiotics in Preterm Birth Prevention

The use of antibiotics in pregnancies complicated by PTL with intact membranes has likewise been studied. In this clinical scenario, antibiotics do not seem to prolong pregnancy or improve neonatal morbidity.[31] In other situations, antibiotics have been helpful in preventing PTB. *Neisseria gonorrhoeae* and *Chlamydia trachomatis* should routinely be screened for in pregnant women. Treatment will decrease PROM and PTB and improve neonatal birth weight and prevent transmission of these genital tract infections. Screening for and treating bacterial vaginosis in women at high risk for preterm labor also improves pregnancy outcome. It is standard to screen for and treat asymptomatic bacteriuria, which is associated with maternal pyelonephritis and PTB. Although, the treatment of maternal GBS colonization is not recommended, antibiotic treatment for group B streptococcal bacteriuria has been shown to decrease the PTB rate. It is also reasonable to treat symptomatic *Trichomonas vaginalis* infection, although the association with PTB is less consistent.

INTRA-AMNIOTIC INFECTION

Clinically evident intrauterine infection complicates 1% to 10% of pregnancies, leading to an increase in maternal morbidity and perinatal morbidity and mortality. A variety of terms have been used for this clinical entity. In this chapter, the term *intra-amniotic infection* is used to distinguish the overt clinical infection from bacterial colonization of the amniotic fluid or histologic inflammation of the umbilical cord or placenta.

Diagnosis

The clinical diagnosis of IAI is made on the basis of maternal fever, foul odor of the amniotic fluid, and leukocytosis (Box 22–1). Ruptured membranes are invariably present and, along with fever and leukocytosis, are the most common findings. Uterine tenderness and foul-smelling amniotic fluid are more specific but present in a minority of cases.

Laboratory criteria, likewise, tend to be nonspecific. Peripheral blood leukocytosis commonly occurs in normal labor. Maternal bacteremia occurs in only 10% of patients. Positive Gram stains and colony counts of greater than 10^2/mL of amniotic fluid are associated with clinical infection. However, in unselected patients with ruptured membranes, bacteria is often demonstrated in the amniotic fluid despite a lack of clinical evidence of infection.

Clinical risk factors associated with IAI include duration of membrane rupture, transcervical instrumentation, and digital examinations. Patients with premature PROM are more likely to experience IAI.

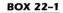

BOX 22–1

CLINICAL DIAGNOSIS OF INTRA-AMNIOTIC INFECTION

Maternal fever
Foul-smelling amniotic fluid
Leukocytosis
Uterine tenderness
Maternal and/or fetal tachycardia

In patients with intact membranes, IAI has been seen occasionally in patients who have undergone amniocentesis or percutaneous umbilical blood sampling and more frequently in patients who have had a cervical cerclage placed.

Blood culture–positive neonatal sepsis is relatively uncommon (8% to 12%), even in the presence of overt maternal IAI.[100] Most cases of early-onset neonatal sepsis begin before delivery. The neonatal response to infection is nonspecific, and diagnosis of sepsis immediately after delivery is difficult. The earliest signs are subtle and include changes in color, tone, activity, and feeding and poor temperature control. Late signs may include dyspnea, apnea, arrhythmias, hepatosplenomegaly, seizures, bulging fontanelles, and irritability. Signs of meningitis or pneumonia or both may follow. Recently, evidence suggestive of an association between IAI and neonatal cerebral palsy has developed, although the relationship is far from understood.[78] Overall, perinatal morbidity and mortality, particularly in the preterm infant, are increased in association with maternal IAI.

Pathophysiology

Before the rupture of membranes and labor, the amniotic cavity is almost always sterile. The cervical mucus, placental membranes, and amniotic fluid provide physical and chemical barriers to bacterial infection. However, there are several ways that bacteria can gain access to the uterine cavity, causing infection. Instrumentation such as during amniocentesis, percutaneous umbilical sampling, and intrauterine transfusion can introduce bacteria into the previously sterile environment. Viral infection most commonly infects the fetus and amniotic fluid by means of hematogenous spread through the placenta and umbilical cord. *Listeria monocytogenes* may cause fulminant IAI by this route. The most likely route of infection associated with IAI, however, is the ascending route.

Recent studies have demonstrated that IAI is a polymicrobial infection, involving aerobic and anaerobic bacteria. When comparing patients in labor with clinical evidence of IAI with matched controls, Gibbs and colleagues found that infected patients had greater numbers of more virulent organisms cultured from their amniotic fluid.[41] Organisms included *Bacteroides* species, 25%; GBS, 12%; other streptococci, 13%; *E. coli*, 10%; and other gram-negative rods. The organisms of bacterial vaginosis, namely, *Gardnerella vaginalis*, *Mycoplasma hominis*, and anaerobes, have also been found in amniotic fluid of women with IAI, suggesting that women with bacterial vaginosis may be more likely to develop IAI. Chlamydia does not seem to contribute to the incidence of IAI.

Maternal Treatment

Antibiotic therapy should be instituted on establishing the diagnosis of IAI. Immediate intrapartum treatment benefits both the mother and the neonate. Broad-spectrum intravenously administered antibiotics (frequently ampicillin and an aminoglycoside) are begun. Cesarean section, although more frequently performed in the presence of IAI, is undertaken only for obstetric indications. Clindamycin or other agents with anaerobic coverage are added to the therapeutic regimen if cesarean section is undertaken, to reduce the risk of antibiotic failure during the postoperative period. Antibiotics should be continued until the patient has been afebrile for 24 to 48 hours. Complications of maternal infection are more frequent after a cesarean section than after vaginal delivery and may include endometritis (up to 30%), wound infection (3% to 5%), sepsis (2% to 4%), pelvic abscess, and septic pelvic thrombophlebitis.[100]

BACTERIAL VAGINOSIS

Bacterial vaginosis is a common disorder, the understanding of which continues to evolve. In 1955, Gardner and Dukes[39] described the classic clinical findings of this vaginitis: (1) a gray-white homogeneous discharge; (2) elevated pH of vaginal discharge to more than 4.5; (3) a fishy amine odor on mixing the discharge with 10% potassium hydroxide; and (4) clue cells on wet preparation. Vaginal culture reveals a variety of organisms, including *Gardnerella vaginalis*, *Mobiluncus* species, a wide range of anaerobic organisms, and *Mycoplasma hominis*. *Lactobacillus*, normally the dominant organism in the vagina and responsible for the low vaginal pH, is absent or present only in low numbers. The prevalence of bacterial vaginosis is 10% to 30% in pregnant women, the majority of whom are asymptomatic. The most common complaint among symptomatic women is malodorous vaginal discharge.

A number of studies have linked bacterial vaginosis with adverse pregnancy outcomes. An increase in PTB associated with PTL or preterm PROM or both has been described along with increases in chorioamnionitis and postpartum endomyometritis.[53, 59] The lower genital tract infection seems to be related to PTB through mechanisms that involve upper tract infection or at least inflammation.[51] Further evidence that supports the association of bacterial vaginosis with PTB comes from trials that indicate that treatment of bacterial vaginosis diagnosed in women at high risk for PTB actually lowered the incidence of PTL and PROM.[46, 57, 66] Among women at low risk for PTB, antibiotic treatment does not seem to lower the PTB rate.[57]

Metronidazole is extremely effective in the treatment of nonpregnant women. However, because of reported carcinogenicity in rodents and mutagenicity in bacteria, clinicians have been reluctant to use this drug during the first trimester of pregnancy. A meta-analysis that reviewed the records of over 200,000 women did not find an association between metronidazole use in the first trimester of pregnancy and birth defects.[14] Ampicillin is curative 40% to 50% of the time, whereas sulfonamides and erythromycin are not significantly more successful than placebo. Intravaginal clindamycin cream and metronidazole gel

have been shown to be efficacious in limited clinical trials. Because of the potential to reduce PTB in populations at high risk, serious consideration should be given to the use of metronidazole in women with bacterial vaginosis.

VIRAL PATHOGENS

HUMAN IMMUNODEFICIENCY VIRUS

(See Chapter 37, Part Four.)

Our understanding of the pathogenesis and treatment of human immunodeficiency virus (HIV) has expanded greatly over recent years:

> A disease that was unknown two decades age, that was untreatable only a decade ago, and whose rate of mother-to-child transmission was immutable just 5 years ago, is now readily diagnosed, treated with increasing effectiveness, and blocked from transmission in the large majority of cases.[64]

It is imperative that clinicians keep abreast of the latest data and literature to provide the best care for the pregnant woman and her offspring.

Epidemiology

Although originally considered an infection confined to male homosexuals, the epidemic of human immunodeficiency virus type 1 (HIV-1) continues to affect an expanding population. The Centers for Disease Control and Prevention (CDC) reported 71,818 cases of acquired immunodeficiency syndrome (AIDS) in women in the United States by the end of 1995. This number accounts for 19% of all U.S. cases. It is assumed that 107,000 to 150,000 U.S. women are currently asymptomatic HIV carriers. The greatest rate of increase in incidence has been in young, heterosexually infected females; in 1995, HIV infection was the third leading cause of death among women aged 25 to 44 years and the leading cause of death among African-American women in this age group.[64]

Screening

The ethics and issues involved in prenatal screening have been hotly debated. Counseling regarding voluntary and confidential screening should be offered as part of routine prenatal care. Because risk-based screening has been an insensitive predictor of infection, the universal offer of antibody testing to all pregnant women is recommended. If the initial enzyme-linked immunosorbent assay is positive, a confirmatory test, most often the Western blot assay for antibodies to specific HIV proteins, is performed. Pretest and post-test counseling should be offered to all those screened; extensive social and medical support services need to be identified for those testing positive.

Clinical Considerations

HIV infection leads to progressive incompetence of the immune system, making the individual susceptible to opportunistic infections and unusual neoplasms. An HIV-infected individual with an opportunistic infection, neoplasia, dementia encephalopathy, or wasting syndrome receives the diagnosis of AIDS. This diagnosis has been expanded to include those with CD4 counts less than 200 CD4 lymphocytes/mm³, cervical cancer, pulmonary tuberculosis, and recurrent pneumonia.

Many clinical studies have attempted to determine both the effects of pregnancy on the course of maternal HIV-related disease and the effects of HIV infection on pregnancy outcome. Although some degree of immunosuppression may occur during pregnancy, this does not seem to alter the disease in pregnant women. The effect of pregnancy on immunologic parameters in HIV-positive women is marginal, and pregnancy does not appear to markedly influence the progression of the HIV infection.

The effect of HIV infection on pregnancy outcome has been difficult to quantify. It appears that this infection is associated with an increase in adverse pregnancy outcome, but the relationship is clouded by uncontrolled and confounded data. There appears to be a fourfold risk of spontaneous abortion but no increase in fetal anomalies. HIV-infected gravidas have an increased odds ratio of about 2 for growth restriction, low birth weight, and PTB. This tendency toward adverse outcomes is less obvious in developed countries. An increase in stillbirth is not seen in developed countries.[10]

Diagnosis and Treatment

An enzyme-linked immunosorbent assay is used for the initial screening. This test relies on a colorimetric change mediated by an antigen-antibody reaction. If it is repeatedly positive, a Western blot test is performed. The Western blot identifies antibodies against specific portions of the virus; it is positive if antibodies to p24, p31, and either gp41 or gp160 are present.

Because of the high viral turnover rate, it has become clear that early institution of multiple, potent antiretroviral agents provides the best long-term control of viral replication. Multiple drug therapy frequently starts with a protease inhibitor and two nucleoside reverse transcriptase inhibitors. In most respects, the pregnant woman should be treated just as her nonpregnant counterpart. If multiple drug therapy is initiated, zidovudine should be included in the regimen because it is the only agent that has been shown to block vertical transmission.[25] When pregnancy and HIV infection are diagnosed simultaneously, the patient may want to finish the first trimester before undertaking potent combination therapy.[15] Appropriate use of combination therapy should drive the viral load to below the limits of detection.[65]

Transmission

Transplacental infection has been well documented. HIV has been directly isolated from the placenta, the amniotic fluid, and early products of conception. HIV is also found in breast milk, and breast feeding is a documented route of late perinatal infection. Because safe infant formula is available in the United States, the Public Health Service has recommended that infected mothers avoid breast milk feeding.[22]

Intrapartum infection of the neonate accounts for 70% to 80% of the vertical transmission. When no efforts are made to block transmission, 25% to 30% of newborns acquire the infection; higher rates have been reported in developing countries and in symptomatic patients. The original evidence that vertical transmission could be reduced came as a result of the AIDS Clinical Trial Group (ACTG) protocol 076. This trial enrolled pregnant women who had no clinical indication for or use of antiretroviral therapy during the current pregnancy and who had CD4-positive counts of more than 200/mm³. The efficacy of zidovudine versus placebo was studied. Preliminary analysis of 364 births showed a 67% reduction in HIV transmission from 25.5% to 8.3%.[25] Because of this information, the trial was stopped and the Public Health Service recommended offering zidovudine to pregnant women at more than 14 weeks of gestation to lower the risk of fetal infection. ACTG 185 demonstrated that similar results could also be obtained in women who had previous exposure to zidovudine or a CD4 count less than 200/mm³.

In addition to the use of medical therapy to reduce vertical transmission, changes in obstetric management have been evaluated. Simple steps, such as reducing the number of episiotomies, the use of instrumentation, and duration of membrane rupture, would seem to reduce the fetal exposure to the virus found in vaginal blood and secretions.

Several studies have suggested that the use of cesarean section before the onset of labor or membrane rupture would independently reduce the rate of transmission.[34, 50] This effect appears to hold up even when antiretroviral therapy was used. A meta-analysis of 15 prospective cohort studies conducted between 1982 and 1996 demonstrated a 10.4% transmission rate with elective cesarean section versus a 19.0% rate with other routes of delivery when antiretroviral agents were not used. With the use of antiretroviral therapy, the rate of transmission was only 2.0% with elective section versus 7.3% for other modes of delivery.[50] However, these studies do not include information on viral load, which influences the transmission rate. It may be that as combination therapy is used, driving viral loads to undetectable levels, that the use of elective cesarean section will add little to the reduction of neonatal infection. And cesarean section is not without its own inherent risk, which may be increased in HIV-infected women. Unfortunately, trials examining the use of cesarean section in women taking potent combination therapy are not feasible because of the large numbers of patients that would be required to demonstrate a difference in transmission rates. For now, the risks of surgical morbidity versus the benefits of cesarean delivery to reduce the risk of neonatal infection will have to be weighed in each individual clinical situation.

Antepartum Management

(See Chapter 11, Part One.)

Antepartum evaluation of the HIV-positive patient should include both clinical and laboratory surveillance for immune dysfunction, disease progression, and opportunistic infection. Evidence of sexually transmitted diseases, such as syphilis, gonorrhea, chlamydia, and herpes simplex virus, should be sought. Baseline serologic markers for toxoplasmosis and cytomegalovirus may be useful in documenting previous exposure and risk for fetal infection. Immune function studies should include a complete blood cell count with differential, CD4 count, and viral load studies each trimester. A tuberculosis skin test should be included with the prenatal laboratory studies, and appropriate controls must be used to detect possible anergy. The patient should have documented prior immunization to hepatitis B, pneumococcus, and influenza or receive appropriate vaccination during pregnancy.

At present, fetal surveillance is limited to traditional studies, including ultrasonography to evaluate fetal growth and other biophysical parameters. Although fetal blood sampling might possibly identify infected fetuses, the use of this modality may increase the risk of infection and is avoided.

Further antenatal management must be individualized to the patient. Opportunistic infections should be aggressively treated. *Pneumocystis carinii* pneumonia is a common AIDS-defining disease with a significant mortality rate. Cervical dysplasia and tuberculosis may also more frequently complicate the pregnancies of HIV-1 infected women.

VARICELLA-ZOSTER

(See Chapter 37, Part Four.)

Varicella-zoster virus (VZV) is a member of the herpesvirus group. Exposure in childhood results in chickenpox, and 85% to 95% of young adults in temperate climates have developed immunity to the virus. Ten to 20 percent of adults experience a reactivation of the virus, developing the painful skin lesions of herpes zoster along one or two adjacent dermatomes, commonly called shingles.[95]

VZV is a highly contagious virus with an incubation period of 13 to 17 days. Children usually experience a 4- to 7-day period in which pruritic, erythematous vesicles cover the head, neck, and trunk. Adults comprise only 2% of chickenpox cases but frequently have a more severe illness. They account for 25% of the mortality, which is primarily due to varicella pneumonia. Pregnant women may be at particularly high risk of death when they develop this complication.[26]

Prevention

A live attenuated varicella vaccine has been developed that can be administered preconceptionally to women who are susceptible to varicella infection. Some recommend routine serologic screening at the first prenatal visit of those without a history of childhood infection.[27] When the vaccine is routinely administered in the postpartum period to those who are seronegative, this screening appears to be a cost-effective way to reduce the morbidity and mortality associated with perinatal infection.[42, 93]

VZV Infections in Pregnancy

Because most pregnant women acquire immunity to VZV in childhood, varicella infection is uncommon in pregnancy. The incidence of varicella in pregnancy has been estimated at 5 per 10,000, and the incidence of zoster, primarily a disease of older people, is assumed to be even less. Even when pregnant women give a negative or uncertain history of childhood varicella infection, serologic testing reveals that approximately 80% of them are immune to VZV.

Varicella-zoster immune globulin (VZIG) has been used in pregnant women who do not have antibody to VZV to prevent or modify the course of the disease. Administration as soon as possible, certainly within 96 hours, after exposure is necessary. Administration is facilitated by already knowing the patient's susceptibility (from prenatal screening) or being able to determine the presence of IgG antibodies within 24 to 48 hours.[85] The ability of VZIG to block vertical transmission is unknown.

Although acyclovir has little effect in the course of uncomplicated varicella in adults, the early use of the antiviral agent in the treatment of varicella pneumonia has been shown to reduce mortality in pregnant patients. An increase in birth defects has not been attributed to the systemic use of acyclovir during pregnancy.

Fetal VZV Infections

A congenital VZV syndrome has been described in infants born to mothers who were infected with the virus in the first half of pregnancy. The physical stigma of the syndrome include scarred, segmental, or dermatomal skin lesions; limb deformities, almost always ipsilateral and distal to the skin lesions; and central nervous system abnormalities, including cortical atrophy, intracranial calcification, chorioretinitis, and optic atrophy.[70] The frequency of defects consistent with congenital VZV syndrome after infection in the first 20 weeks of pregnancy has been reported to range between 0% and 3%, with the highest incidence occurring when maternal infection occurred at between 13 and 20 weeks' gestation.[71] None of these studies reported evidence of this syndrome when maternal infection developed in the second half of pregnancy.

Congenital VZV syndrome can be diagnosed in

utero when structural findings are demonstrated on ultrasonographic evaluation. When polymerase chain reaction (PCR) analysis of placental or fetal specimens is undertaken, it appears that transplacental infection occurs much more commonly (36%) than the full-blown fetal syndrome.[54]

Neonatal VZV Infections

A neonate may acquire a varicella infection in utero without developing the congenital syndrome or be infected postnatally (Table 22–1). Infants exposed to in utero varicella infection during the second half of pregnancy up to 21 days before delivery run a very minimal risk of the congenital VZV syndrome; however, they may develop zoster in infancy. Infants who were exposed to varicella from 20 days before delivery to 6 days before delivery may display serologic evidence or minimal symptoms of chickenpox at birth. Because the time before delivery has allowed the formation and transplacental passage of maternal antibody, these infants are at little risk for severe disease. Infants delivered to mothers who develop varicella less than 5 days before delivery or up to 2 days after delivery are at much higher risk of serious sequelae because they lack the passively acquired maternal antibody. Infants in this circumstance have a 17% chance of manifesting congenital varicella infection with an untreated case-fatality rate of 31%.[54] Immediate administration of VZIG to the infants is therefore recommended after delivery. Antiviral therapy with acyclovir may be helpful in ameliorating disease in these infants.

Birth defects have been occasionally reported in pregnancies complicated by maternal zoster. However, it is doubtful that a significant viremia occurs with zoster in the presence of specific VZV antibodies and therefore unlikely that maternal zoster is responsible for an increase in fetal anomalies.[32]

RUBELLA

(See Chapter 37, Part Four.)

Rubella is a mild viral infection, is confined to the human host, and occurs worldwide. Infection during pregnancy is responsible for miscarriages, stillbirths, and congenital malformations. Late sequelae of congenital infection are frequent. The introduction of the rubella vaccine has greatly reduced but not eliminated the neonatal morbidity associated with infection during pregnancy.[84]

Epidemiology and Clinical Manifestations

Before the introduction of the rubella vaccination in 1969, rubella was most common in 5- to 9-year olds with 85% of 15- to 19-year olds demonstrating immunity. Epidemics occurred at 6- to 9-year intervals, with major pandemics every 10 to 30 years. Maternal rubella infection early in pregnancy frequently results in fetal malformations consistent with the congenital rubella syndrome. The incidence of congenital rubella syndrome in 1970 was 1.8/100,000 live births. The epidemiology of this infection has changed dramatically with the licensure of the live attenuated rubella vaccine. An all-time low of 225 cases of rubella was reported to the CDC in 1988, a 99% decrease since 1969, the year the vaccine was introduced. Cases of congenital rubella syndrome are occasionally reported in the United States after outbreaks of rubella infection. However, it is the goal of the CDC to eradicate the virus in the United States by the diligent use of the rubella vaccine.[77]

The rubella infection is subclinical in 30% of patients. Symptomatic disease is typically mild and occurs 14 to 21 days after infection. A mild prodrome of fever, malaise, and low-grade fever may precede the rash. The rash is macular, begins on the face and neck, proceeds downward, and disappears over 3 to 4 days. Postauricular, suboccipital, and posterior cervical lymphadenopathy are typically present. Diagnosis on clinical grounds is difficult; serologic confirmation of a fourfold increase in antibody titer is required. IgM is present for 4 weeks after the rash. Low or equivocal levels of IgM should be viewed with caution because cross reactivity with human parvovirus IgM has been described.

Maternal-Fetal Transmission

Fetal infection can occur after maternal rubella viremia at any stage of pregnancy. Miller and associates prospectively evaluated 1016 women with confirmed rubella during pregnancy, 407 of whom elected to carry the fetus to term.[62] The risk of congenital infection varied from 81% in the first 12 weeks to 30% with exposure at 23 to 30 weeks and 100% if exposed during the last month of pregnancy. The malformations associated with congenital rubella syndrome are gestational age dependent. Multiple defects occur after very early exposure; almost every fetus exposed during the first month of pregnancy develops abnormally. Cardiac defects almost always follow exposure before 10 weeks of gestation. Deafness will occur after exposure up to 16 weeks of gestation. Congenital defects after exposure after 20 weeks are rare.[99] Reinfection can occasionally occur when a person with

TABLE 22–1 MATERNAL-FETAL TRANSMISSION OF VARICELLA ZOSTER

MATERNAL INFECTION	FETAL INFECTION
First trimester	Congenital VZV syndrome rare
Second and third trimester up to 21 days before delivery	May develop zoster during infancy
20 days until 6 days before delivery	Serologic evidence or minimal symptoms of chickenpox
5 days before delivery to 2 days after delivery	17% chance of acute infection; 31% untreated case mortality rate

documented rubella immunity is re-exposed to the virus.[81] Congenital rubella syndrome has been rarely reported when reinfection occurs before 12 weeks' gestation.[77]

Fetal Infection

The full-blown congenital rubella syndrome includes in descending frequency: hearing loss, mental retardation, cardiac malformation, and ocular defects. Hearing loss is sensorineural and can occur along with other defects or alone in 40% of cases.[90] Mental retardation is common and frequently severe. Cardiac lesions are present in half of infants exposed during the first 2 months of pregnancy. Patent ductus arteriosus is most common (approximately 70%), with pulmonary artery stenosis, aortic valvular stenosis, and tetralogy of Fallot also seen. Ocular abnormalities commonly include congenital cataract, retinopathy, and microphthalmia.

Delayed manifestations of congenital rubella syndrome are also common, occurring in more than 20% of congenitally infected patients. Insulin-dependent diabetes mellitus develops by age 35 in 20% to 40% of individuals with congenital rubella infection. Thyroid disease develops in 5% of these patients. Deafness and eye abnormalities not evident at birth can develop. Progressive rubella panencephalopathy has been described in 12 males who developed progressive encephalopathy leading to death.[90]

Prevention

Despite recommendations for universal immunization, it is estimated that up to 20% of women of reproductive age in the United States are seronegative for rubella. The prevention of congenital rubella syndrome relies heavily on vaccinating susceptible females. The vaccine is a live attenuated vaccine and should not be administered within 3 months before conception or during pregnancy because of theoretical fetal risks. No cases of congenital rubella syndrome have been reported when the vaccine has been administered during this period, although there is a small theoretical risk of congenital infection (0% to 2%).[19]

Because of the high percent of pregnancies affected when exposed to rubella infection, counseling regarding the termination of pregnancy should be offered. Prenatal diagnosis can be made after 20 weeks' gestation when IgM is detected in fetal blood. The presence of virus can also be uncovered by using reverse transcription and nested PCR in either chorionic villus, amniotic fluid, or fetal blood samples.[73, 96]

HERPES SIMPLEX VIRUS

Herpes simplex virus (HSV) infections are common and can be grouped into two serologic subtypes: HSV-1 and HSV-2. The most common clinical manifestation of HSV-1 is pharyngitis and gingivostomatitis, although it may be responsible for genital infection as well. The most common infection caused by HSV-2 is genital herpes. Primary genital herpes infection is usually associated with local lesions and systemic symptoms.

Epidemiology and Clinical Manifestations

It is estimated that over 600,000 new cases occur annually to contribute to a pool of over 20 million cases.[79] The prevalence of HSV infection is dependent on age, sexual activity, and socioeconomic class. Seroepidemiologic studies in obstetric populations show antibody to HSV-2 to be present in 19% to 55% of the patients, depending on the population source.[36]

Until recently, the clinical manifestations of genital HSV infection were used to classify the infection. Primary infection was usually associated with multiple, painful genital vesicles, which proceed to an ulcerative stage frequently accompanied by inguinal adenopathy. Systemic symptoms include fever, malaise, myalgias, headache, and nausea. A first-episode nonprimary infection occurred when the first clinical episode of HSV presented in a patient with existing antibodies to HSV-1 or HSV-2. The clinical course was considered similar to that of recurrent disease. Recurrent disease occurs more frequently after HSV-2 infections; mild local lesions occur and last about half as long as initial lesions, and systemic manifestations are absent.

However, considerable overlap in the clinical manifestation of HSV makes it impossible to distinguish between primary and recurrent disease.[47] Furthermore, 20% to 30% of pregnant women who are seropositive for HSV have never been symptomatic.[13]

Confirmation of the diagnosis in the past depended heavily on viral cultures as antigen detection techniques had lower sensitivities and was not type specific. Recently, PCR techniques and type-specific serologic testing have made the diagnosis more accurate and provide a way to distinguish between the primary and recurrent infection.[8, 12, 79]

Asymptomatic shedding of the virus is not uncommon. It may occur in 3% to 16% of pregnant women and may be as high as 33% in women acquiring the infection during pregnancy.[13] Disseminated herpes infection has been reported in a limited number of pregnant patients; mortality for both mother and fetus approaches 40%. The safety of acyclovir during pregnancy has been fairly well established, and its use is beneficial in severe or disseminated disease.[52, 88] Valacyclovir, which is metabolized to acyclovir, and famciclovir are also used to treat genital HSV. The experience with these drugs in pregnancy is more limited; both are members of the Food and Drug Administration's class B.

Antepartum Screening and Maternal-Fetal Transmission

Transplacental infection is rarely reported. Primary HSV infections during the first trimester seem to increase the frequency of spontaneous abortions, stillbirths, and prematurity. Infants born with suspected in utero infection typically have vesicular skin lesions at the time of birth. Congenital malformations most frequently include microcephaly, intracranial calcifications, and evidence of diffuse brain damage. Primary infection in the later trimesters does not seem to increase the risk of transplacental infection, although these mothers have a longer course of viral shedding and more numerous recurrences and are therefore more likely to expose the neonate during delivery.

The major risk of infection for the neonate is intrapartum exposure to an infected birth canal. Vaginal delivery in the presence of a primary infection results in neonatal infection approximately 50% of the time. Asymptomatic maternal infection has a 33% risk of neonatal infection. Transmission risk drops to 3% to 4% when recurrent lesions are present at vaginal delivery, and the risk of transmission drops to 0.004% in the presence of asymptomatic shedding.[88] Current recommendations include cesarean section before or shortly after rupture of membranes when an active HSV lesion or prodromal symptomatology is present to minimize the neonate's viral exposure.[80]

This strategy does not prevent all cases of neonatal herpes because the majority of infected infants are born to mothers who have never had symptoms.

The prophylactic use of acyclovir in the last weeks of pregnancy to reduce the chance of recurrence necessitating cesarean section has been examined. Although this usage does decrease recurrent infection in those with a primary infection or frequent severe recurrences, it is less obvious that it decreases asymptomatic shedding or recurrent lesions in those with infrequent outbreaks. Oral acyclovir prophylaxis also appears to be more cost effective than simply performing cesarean sections in all women with active lesions without increasing neonatal morbidity.[76, 88]

CYTOMEGALOVIRUS

Cytomegalovirus (CMV) is a ubiquitous virus that infects most people in their lifetime. In adults, primary infection is usually asymptomatic, although approximately 10% will experience a mononucleosis-type syndrome. Reactivation of latent infection can occur with viral shedding in cervical secretions, tears, saliva, urine, and breast milk. The virus can be transmitted to the fetus after primary or recurrent infection. Approximately 10% of the infected infants will be affected at birth, and many will develop sequelae over the first 5 years of life.

Epidemiology and Clinical Manifestations

Acquisition rates of CMV vary inversely with socioeconomic status. Seroepidemiologic studies in the United States indicate that 50% to 60% of pregnant, middle-class women have antibodies to CMV, compared with 70% to 85% of those from lower socioeconomic groups. Two to 2.5 percent of susceptible women will acquire CMV infection during pregnancy.[94] Primary infection is asymptomatic in most healthy individuals; some experience a mononucleosis-like illness with fever, fatigue, and lymphadenopathy.

Seroconversion from IgG-negative to IgG-positive status is the best demonstration of primary infection. IgM only develops in 75% of those with primary infection and may persist up to 18 months. It may also be present in 10% of those with recurrent infection. A fourfold rise in IgG titers also most likely represents primary infection. A smaller rise in IgG titers can be seen in recurrent infection.[11]

Maternal-Fetal Transmission

Vertical transmission can occur after either primary or recurrent CMV infection. One to two percent of all infants born in the United States have documented congenital infection. Congenital CMV infection occurs in 30% to 40% of infants born to mothers experiencing primary CMV infection during pregnancy[94] (Fig. 22–1). The rate of transmission after recurrent infection is probably similar to primary disease, although the percent of infants symptomatic at birth (less than 1%)

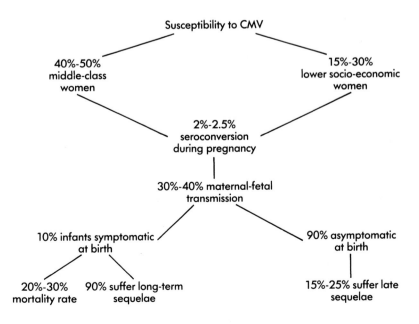

FIGURE 22–1. Maternal-fetal cytomegalovirus transmission.

or developing serious sequelae (5% to 10%) is much lower.[74] Timing of maternal infection may also be critical in that it has been suggested that risk of delivering a symptomatic infant or one who will develop sequelae is higher if maternal infection occurs during the first half of pregnancy.

Fetal and Neonatal Infection

The diagnosis in utero of fetal CMV infection may be suggested on the basis of an abnormal ultrasound evaluation. CMV is a relatively common cause of nonimmune hydrops; intrauterine growth retardation, microcephaly, hepatosplenomegaly, periventricular calcifications, oligohydramnios, and echogenic bowel may also be present. In utero diagnosis may be accomplished by the identification of viral DNA using PCR techniques.

Of infants born with CMV infection, 10% are symptomatic at birth. Infant mortality in this group is 20% to 30%, and most suffer some long-term serious sequelae. Hepatosplenomegaly is the most common clinical finding. Microcephaly is also common and is frequently associated with periventricular calcifications. Optic abnormalities, intellectual impairment, and dental defects are reported. Sensorineural hearing loss develops in 30% of infants symptomatic at birth.

Most infants (more than 90%) identified at birth as being infected are asymptomatic. It has been recently recognized that 15% to 25% of these infants may suffer late sequelae, including neurologic abnormalities, sensorineural hearing loss, and mental retardation.[94] These sequelae are much more likely to follow primary maternal infection.

Prevention of congenital CMV hinges on prevention of maternal infection using such measures of careful hand washing and latex condoms and avoiding contact with children's secretions. CMV vaccines are currently undergoing clinical trials. The use of antiviral agents such as gancyclovir is limited to treating severe infections in newborns or immunocompromised mothers.[68]

HEPATITIS

Hepatitis is a common and highly contagious viral illness. Six distinct types of viral hepatitis exist, each with different implications for the pregnant woman and her fetus.

Hepatitis A

Hepatitis A virus (HAV) is an RNA virus that is responsible for approximately 45% of cases of acute hepatitis. Infection produces a mild, self-limiting illness that does not result in a chronic carrier state. Transmission is by an oral-fecal route subsequent to contaminated food or water; parenteral transmission is rare. Diagnosis is made by identification of IgM-specific antibody, which appears 30 days after exposure and persists for 6 months. Sexual and household contacts should receive intramuscular immunoglobu-

lin and a hepatitis A vaccine. The vaccine is safe for use in pregnant women.

Infection with HAV does not seem to increase the risk of adverse pregnancy outcome. Infants delivered of acutely infected women should receive immunoglobulin to decrease the risk for transmission after delivery.

Hepatitis C

Post-transfusion hepatitis in the absence of markers for HAV and HBV was originally termed non-A, non-B hepatitis (NANBH). Now the structure of the hepatitis C virus (HCV) has been delineated and it is understood that HCV is primarily responsible for parenterally transmitted NANBH. Principal risk factors for HCV transmission are blood and blood product transfusion and the use of illicit intravenous drugs.

HCV is the most common chronic bloodborne infection in the United States. The number of new infections per year has declined from 230,000 in the 1980s to 36,000 in 1996, owing to careful screening of transfused blood products. However, it is estimated that 3.9 million (1.8%) Americans are infected with HCV. Deaths from HCV-related liver disease currently number 8,000 to 10,000 per year; the number is very likely to climb in the next 10 to 20 years as more people reach the age when complications from chronic liver disease occur.[23]

Acute HCV infection occurs after an incubation period of 30 to 60 days; infection is asymptomatic in 75% of patients. Jaundice and nonspecific symptoms may occur 6 to 7 weeks after exposure. Average time for seroconversion is 8 to 9 weeks; 80% seroconvert by 15 weeks and 97% seroconvert by 6 months. Although fulminant infection is rare, chronic liver disease develops in 75% to 85% of patients after HCV infection. The chronic course is slow and insidious, with most patients showing no signs or symptoms of the disease for 10 to 20 years. However, these patients may develop progressive liver disease or cirrhosis, may need a liver transplant, and may die of their disease. An effective vaccine is unlikely to be developed in the near future. Interferon alfa has been shown to decrease detectable levels of viral RNA and normalize alanine aminotransferase levels; however, more than 50% of patients experience relapse when therapy is stopped.

The risk of perinatal transmission of HCV varies and may depend on the HCV viral load. In HIV-negative women, the risk of fetal infection is 5.2% (range: 0% to 33%), whereas in HIV-positive women the risk of transmission is 23.4% (range: 9% to 70%).[33] Maternal HCV antibodies cross the placenta; therefore, newborn screening should be done by testing for HCV RNA at 6 to 12 months of age. The long-term outcome of infected neonates is not yet well understood. Most infants remain viremic and progress to chronic hepatitis. Immunoprophylaxis in the newborn has not been demonstrated to be efficacious. Cesarean section does not provide protection against maternal-fetal transmission and should be performed for routine obstetric indications only. Breast feeding appears to be safe.

Hepatitis E

Although HCV is the primary cause of NANBH in industrialized countries, a second distinct virus, hepatitis E (HEV), is responsible for outbreaks of enterally acquired NANBH in developing countries. Reports of infection with HEV in U.S. citizens traveling abroad and exposed to contaminated food and water have been documented.[18]

Although many cases remain subclinical, the case-fatality rate is higher (1% to 2%) than that seen with HAV (1 to 2/1000). Chronic hepatitis does not seem to be a complication of HEV infection. Acute HEV infection during pregnancy has been associated with an increase in both maternal mortality and adverse pregnancy outcome, including preterm delivery and stillbirth.

Hepatitis G

Hepatitis G (HGV) is an RNA virus related to hepatitis C. It is more prevalent but less virulent than HCV. Diagnosis relies on identification of viral nucleic acids by PCR techniques. HGV commonly occurs in association with HBV, HCV, and HIV infections. A chronic carrier state exists, and perinatal transmission has been documented. Prognosis for infected infants remains to be determined.[30]

Hepatitis B

Of all the viruses that cause acute hepatitis, the one that is responsible for most of the concerns in regard to pregnancy is hepatitis B virus (HBV).

EPIDEMIOLOGY AND CLINICAL MANIFESTATIONS. In the United States, there are over 300,000 new cases of HBV a year, with 12,000 to 20,000 patients becoming chronic carriers. The prevalence of the carrier state varies from a high of 5% to 15% among Alaskan Inuits and Asians to less than 0.5% of the general American population. Approximately 1 million Americans are chronic HBV carriers. Most cases of HBV occur in homosexual or bisexual males, intravenous drug abusers, and the heterosexual partners of infected men. The risk of post-transfusion HBV infection dropped dramatically with the screening of blood donors.

The incubation period for acute HBV varies from 45 to 150 days. At least 50% of healthy adults and children are asymptomatic; an even higher percent of infants infected during the first year of life exhibit no symptoms. Symptoms of acute hepatitis in the adult include anorexia, malaise, weakness, and abdominal pain; clinical signs include jaundice, icterus, hepatic tenderness, and weight loss. The acute course usually runs 3 to 4 weeks, but symptoms may persist up to 6 months. Fulminant hepatitis is a rare occurrence, characterized by acute liver failure, hepatic encephalopathy, coma, and death in 70% to 80% of the patients.

The diagnosis of HBV is based on serologic markers (Fig. 22–2). Surface antigen (HBsAg) is the first marker to appear in acute infection and is present before the onset of clinical symptoms. At about the same time, e antigen (HBeAg) appears. This antigen disappears before clinical symptoms resolve and is usually followed by the antibody (anti-HBe). Antibody to the surface antigen (anti-HBs) appears during the convalescent period, and high titers are an indication of immunity. The core antigen (HBcAg) is not present in serum in insufficient quantities to be clinically useful. The antibody to HBcAg is typically present in the window between detectable HBsAg and anti-HBs.

Approximately 10% of patients with acute HBV infection become chronic carriers. These patients fail to develop anti-HBs, and the HBsAg persists. In chronic active infection, HBeAg may persist for years, followed by the gradual seroconversion to anti-HBe. Asymptomatic carriers are characterized by the presence of HBsAg and anti-HBc with normal results of liver function tests.

MATERNAL-FETAL TRANSMISSION. Acute HBV infection complicates 1 to 2/1000 pregnancies; chronic infection is present in 5 to 15/1000 pregnancies. The transmission rate of the HBV virus from mother to infant varies with the clinical setting (Table 22–2). Women infected with HBV in the first or second trimester rarely pass the infection to the neonate. A transplacental leak of HBV with a maternal-fetal hemorrhage may account for the unusual cases of in utero infection. Most evidence suggests that the neonate is infected at the time of delivery as a consequence of exposure to contaminated blood and genital tract secretions. Infants who are seronegative at birth convert after an incubation period of 2 to 4 months. Women who are infected in the third trimester have

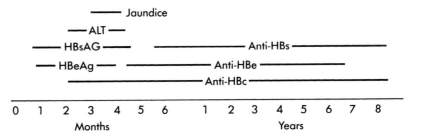

FIGURE 22–2. Clinical and serum markers of hepatitis.

TABLE 22–2   MATERNAL-FETAL
TRANSMISSION OF
HEPATITIS B VIRUS

MATERNAL INFECTION	FETAL INFECTION
Acute first/second trimester	Rare
Acute third trimester	40%–60%
Chronic carrier	
HBsAg⁺/HBeAg⁻	10%–20%
HBsAg⁺/HBeAg⁺	80%–90%

an increased chance (up to 75%) of passing the virus to their infants. The most predictive marker for vertical transmission is the HBeAg; when HBeAg is present, the transmission rate reaches 80% to 90%. In chronic carriers, the additional presence of anti-HBe drops the transmission rate to 10% to 20%.[6]

Most hepatitis infections in infants are asymptomatic, although occasionally fulminant cases are reported. Most infants who are infected at birth will become chronic carriers of HBsAg. Many of these will go on to have adverse sequelae, including cirrhosis, chronic active hepatitis, and primary hepatocellular carcinoma.

PRENATAL SCREENING AND IMMUNIZATION RECOMMENDATIONS. The recognition that immunization at birth would be 85% to 95% effective in prevention of the development of the HBV chronic carrier state in the neonate has prompted prenatal HBV screening of obstetric patients. The CDC and the American College of Obstetrics and Gynecology advocate routine screening of all patients at their first antepartum visit and perhaps repeat screening during the third trimester for those in especially high-risk situations.[21]

The prevention of neonatal hepatitis depends on the prompt administration of immune globulin and hepatitis B vaccination. Hepatitis B immune globulin (HBIG) given at birth reduces infection rates from 94% to 75% and the chronic carrier rate from 91% to 22%. The addition of hepatitis vaccine drops the chronic carrier rate to 0% from 14%.[101] Most authorities recommend HBIG be given within 12 hours of delivery and vaccination begin within the first week of life. In addition to those infants at risk because of the maternal infectious status, the CDC now recommends immunization of all infants, including those born to mothers who are HBsAg negative.

Vaccination of health workers for HBV may prevent many of the 12,000 cases of HBV infection acquired in the workplace as a result of needlestick or splash accidents. Those who have been exposed should also receive HBIG. Pregnancy is not a contraindication to vaccination or administration of HBIG in those at risk of infection.

Hepatitis D

Hepatitis D (HDV) is dependent on coinfection with HBV for replication. Therefore, the epidemiology of HDV is identical to that of HBV. Acute infection can occur in two forms: coinfection and superinfection. Coinfection occurs when the patient simultaneously acquires HBV and HDV; the disease tends to be mild, self-limiting without chronic implications. Superinfection occurs when a chronic carrier of HBV becomes infected with HDV. This occurs in 20% to 25% of chronic carriers and frequently leads to chronic hepatitis, cirrhosis, and portal hypertension with an eventual mortality rate of 25%.

Pregnant patients with hepatitis D (identified by IgM-specific antibody or antigen detection) should receive supportive care with close monitoring of liver function. Transmission to the neonate is rare because neonatal immunoprophylaxis is almost uniformly protective against hepatitis D.

PARVOVIRUS

Parvoviruses are the smallest DNA-containing viruses that infect mammalian cells; the human B19 parvovirus is the only parvovirus found in humans. Infection results in the childhood erythema infectiosum (EI) or fifth disease. Infection is usually mild or asymptomatic in the susceptible gravida; however, it may cause nonimmune hydrops and fetal death.

Epidemiology

EI is primarily a disease of schoolchildren; therefore, the prevalence is age related. In children younger than the age of 5 years, prevalence is less than 5%, rising to 40% by the age of 20. Fifty to 60 percent of women of reproductive age are immune.

The primary mode of transmission is through direct contact with respiratory secretions of viremic patients. The incubation period is 4 to 14 days. There is a seasonal variation to parvovirus infection, with outbreaks more common in the late winter and early spring. Long-term cycles of 4 to 7 years also appear to occur within communities. Although teachers and daycare workers would seem to have the highest occupational risk of acquiring the virus, by far the greatest risk of infection in susceptible individuals is exposure to one's own infected children.[98] Removing pregnant women from the workplace during seasonal case clusters does not seem to be justified.[45]

Clinical Features

One fourth to one third of infected individuals are asymptomatic. Children typically display a reticular, malar rash; this characteristic rash is responsible for the "slapped cheeks" description. The rash may be accompanied by headache, sore throat, and low-grade fever. Joint involvement can occur in children (8%), but acute arthritis is much more common in adults (80%). Frequently, the arthralgias, involving the wrist, hands, ankles, and knees, are the only symptoms that the adult perceives.

Because the parvovirus replicates in and destroys the erythroid precursor cells, a limited erythroid aplasia occurs. This is clinically inapparent (resulting in a 1-gm drop in hemoglobin) in an otherwise healthy adult because its duration of 7 to 10 days is short compared with the red blood cell half-life of 120 days. However, this can become a serious problem for those with chronic anemia, such as sickle cell anemia, or for those immunocompromised individuals who have difficulty clearing the virus.

Viral culture is quite difficult, and diagnosis relies on serologic testing. IgM antibodies develop very rapidly, typically persisting for 2 to 3 months, although occasionally as long as 6 months. IgG antibodies develop several days after the IgM antibodies and remain positive for a lifetime, conferring lifelong immunity. Serologic testing should be considered in patients with known exposure, with symptoms (including acute arthritis), and with nonimmune hydrops. Isolated IgM positivity may mean very recent infection, but follow-up testing should demonstrate IgG seroconversion because false positive IgM findings have been reported.

Fetal Infection

Vertical transmission rates appear to be about 33%. There is very little evidence to suggest that the virus is teratogenic. When infection occurs before 20 weeks' gestation, the fetal loss rate appears to be about 10%. Infection after 20 weeks results in hydrops or fetal death approximately 1% of the time.[56] Hydrops is usually the result of fetal aplastic anemia but may sometimes be caused by acute viral myocarditis. Intrauterine transfusion may be beneficial to some fetuses suffering from severe anemia. Approximately 85% of fetuses who receive a transfusion to correct their anemia will survive.[82] However, about one third of the cases of fetal hydrops will spontaneously resolve with a healthy live-born infant. Long-term studies suggest that development in surviving neonates is normal and excess development delay is not seen.[63, 83]

BACTERIAL AND OTHER PATHOGENS

GONORRHEA

Neisseria gonorrhoeae, a gram-negative diplococcus, is the cause of the most frequently reported communicable disease in the United States. It is found most commonly in the urogenital tract but can infect the pharynx and the conjunctiva; when disseminated it causes sepsis and arthritis. Perinatal complications may include PROM, prematurity, chorioamnionitis, intrauterine growth retardation, neonatal sepsis, and postpartum endometritis.

Epidemiology and Clinical Manifestations

It is estimated that 600,000 new gonorrhea infections occur in the United States every year.

Over 80% of the reported cases occur in individuals in the 15- to 29-year-old age group with an ever-increasing percentage of the cases occurring in adolescents in the 15- to 19-year-old group. In nonpregnant women, uncomplicated anogenital gonorrhea most frequently infects the endocervix but can involve the Skene glands, urethra, Bartholin glands, or anus.

Gonococcal infections in pregnant women tend to be asymptomatic. Most common symptoms when noted are vaginal discharge and dysuria. Cervical cultures are recommended at the first prenatal visit, and repeat cultures in the patient at high risk in the third trimester may be appropriate. The CDC recommendation for treatment reflects the increasing identification of penicillinase-producing *N. gonorrhoeae* species. A single dose of ceftriaxone, 125 mg IM, or cefixime, 400 mg PO, and then azithromycin 1 gm PO or doxycycline 100 mg PO twice a day for 7 days has been recommended. This antibiotic regimen also frequently treats (40% to 60%) concomitant chlamydial infections.[16]

Association with Adverse Pregnancy Outcome

Untreated maternal endocervical gonococcal infection has been associated with such perinatal complications as prematurity, PROM, intrauterine growth retardation, neonatal infection, and postpartum endometritis. These associations are controversial; gonorrhea infection may simply serve as a marker for other confounding variables known to be associated with poor pregnancy outcome.

Neonatal Gonococcal Ophthalmia

(See also Chapters 37 and 51, Part Two.)

The conjunctivitis caused by gonorrhea has been recognized since the late 1800s. The prophylactic use of silver nitrate eyedrops, erythromycin, or tetracycline ointment after delivery lowered the incidence of gonococcal ophthalmia neonatorum from 10% to less than 0.5%. Gonococcal conjunctivitis is usually manifested within 4 days after birth by frank purulent discharge from both eyes. If untreated, the disease can rapidly progress to corneal ulceration, resulting in scarring and blindness. Treatment should include hospitalization, frequent ophthalmic irrigation, and intravenous therapy with ceftriaxone or cefotaxime.[16] The infant should be closely evaluated for evidence of disseminated gonococcal infection. Infants born to mothers with untreated gonorrhea should be empirically treated with a single injection of ceftriaxone.[16]

GROUP B STREPTOCOCCAL INFECTION

The hemolytic streptococci cause a variety of infectious disease and remain a significant cause of perinatal morbidity and mortality. β-Hemolytic streptococci have been divided into subgroups by serotype: A, B, and D, with groups C and G usually reported simply as "beta-hemolytic streptococci, not groups A, B or D." Before the introduction of antibiotics, group A *Streptococcus* was responsible for puerperal sepsis and 75% of maternal mortality due to infection. Today,

GBS causes the majority of the morbidity and mortality: sepsis, pneumonia, and meningitis in the newborn and urinary tract infection, amnionitis with PROM or PTB, and postpartum endometritis in the gravida.[87a]

Epidemiology and Transmission

Asymptomatic vaginal colonization with GBS occurs in 8% to 28% of pregnant women. The reported prevalence of vaginal colonization varies with age (increasing with advancing age), race (highest in African Americans), geographic locale, and gravidity. It also varies with the number of cultures performed, culture media used, and sites cultured (highest from anorectal cultures, lowest from cervical cultures). Colonization can be intermittent or transient, making vaginal culture in the mid trimester an imperfect predictor of culture status at delivery.

Vertical transmission can occur in utero through either ruptured or intact membranes or during passage through an infected birth canal. The risk of transmission has been shown to range from 40% to 70%. Although approximately two thirds of infants born to colonized mothers become asymptomatic colonized carriers themselves, only one symptomatic GBS infection occurs for every 100 colonized infants. Symptomatic infection is divided into early onset with symptoms present at birth or shortly thereafter (incidence: 1.3 to 3/1000 live births) and late onset with symptoms appearing more than 7 days after delivery (incidence: 1 to 1.7/1000 live births).[4]

Because of the discrepancy between infant carrier rates and rates of actual infection, attempts have been made to determine risk factors for neonatal infection. Three factors play a particularly important role in symptomatic GBS in the newborn: prematurity, prolonged rupture of membranes, and intrapartum fever. There is a 10- to 15-fold increase in the risk of early-onset GBS infection in preterm infants. Boyer and colleagues found the attack rate in infants weighing less than 2500 gm to be 7.9/1000 as opposed to 0.6/1000 in term infants.[9] Additionally, the preterm infant develops a more serious disease, with a mortality rate of 28% as compared with the 2% mortality rate found in the term neonate.

Neonatal Infection

(See also Chapter 37, Part Two.)

By definition, early-onset GBS infection appears in the first week of life. However, the majority of infants display symptoms within the first 48 hours and about half are symptomatic at delivery. The three major clinical presentations include septicemia (bacteremia and clinical signs of sepsis), pneumonia (present in 40%), and meningitis (present in 30%). The fulminant form presents with shock, complicated by respiratory distress, and frequently results in death. Neonatal mortality rates ranged from 50% to 70% during the 1970s; however, improvements in neonatal care have placed the current mortality rate in the 5% to 20%

range,[89] with infants of low birth weight or who are preterm having about twice the risk of fatal outcome.

Late-onset GBS begins more insidiously between 1 and 12 weeks of life. Many (30%) of these infants develop meningitis, some with long-term sequelae. The mortality rate, like that for early-onset disease, has decreased over recent years to 2% to 6%.

Maternal Infection

Maternal fever intrapartum is indicative of IAI, which is frequently associated with GBS infection. Histologic evidence of chorioamnionitis and funisitis was present in 81% of the cases in which GBS colonization was associated with preterm PROM. Postpartum endometritis, characterized by high, spiking fever within 12 hours of delivery, tachycardia, chills, and tender uterine fundus, occurs 15% to 25% of the time after PROM and is even higher after cesarean section.[58] Wound infection and sepsis may follow GBS infection. The diagnosis of intrapartum IAI or postpartum infection mandates broad-spectrum antibiotic coverage for suspected polymicrobial infection. Ampicillin is the most frequently used drug to combat GBS; the first- and second-generation cephalosporins, erythromycin, and clindamycin also provide adequate coverage.

Prevention

Infection with GBS remains a problem, and its prevention, a controversy. Major efforts have gone into attempting to block vertical transmission by the administration of prophylactic antibiotics. Little agreement has been reached on the most efficacious strategy. Attempts at washing the vagina with an antiseptic such as chlorhexidine have not changed disease rates. Chemoprophylaxis during pregnancy is also unsuccessful. Administering penicillin intramuscularly to all neonates immediately after delivery may decrease some of the neonatal disease but will inadequately treat and may mask symptoms in those who are the sickest in the first few hours after delivery. Although GBS is easily eradicated from the vagina of pregnant carriers with antibiotics, recolonization from the gastrointestinal tract occurs frequently and the patient may again be GBS positive at the time of delivery. Because of these experiences, most experts believe that intrapartum antibiotic prophylaxis is the best strategy. Deciding which laboring patient should receive prophylaxis remains controversial.

The CDC issued recommendations in 1996 that took into consideration the prevention strategies that had been proposed by the American Academy of Pediatricians and the American College of Obstetricians and Gynecologists in 1992.[1, 2, 20] They suggested that either a culture-based strategy or a risk-based strategy could be cost effective and lower the incidence of GBS infection in the neonate.

The first prevention strategy involves screening all pregnant women at 35 to 37 weeks of gestation with an anogenital culture in selective broth medium. All culture-positive women would receive antibiotic prophylaxis in labor. Women with unknown results or risk factors (e.g., less than 37 weeks, rupture of membranes more than 18 hours, or fever) would also have antibiotic prophylaxis. The risk-based protocol does not involve antepartum cultures but instead involves treating women in labor who have the just-listed risk factors. Regardless of the strategy employed, the CDC recommends prophylaxis for those who have GBS bacteriuria during pregnancy or a previous infant with GBS infection.

Over a 6-year period from 1993 to 1998, there has been a substantial decline in the incidence of GBS disease in newborns, including a major reduction in the excess incidence of these infections in African-American infants. These improvements coincide with the efforts to prevent perinatal disease by the wider use of prophylactic intrapartum antibiotics. As a result, the number of cases of early-onset neonatal disease has fallen from about 1.7 to 0.6 per 1000 live births.

Strategies that involve antibiotic treatment of the newborn have also been studied. Single intramuscular injections of aqueous penicillin administered to the neonate immediately after delivery will prevent gonococcal ophthalmia and drop the incidence of GBS infection. The major drawback to this approach is that the majority of infants developing severe early-onset disease are bacteremic at birth or very shortly thereafter and a single intramuscular dose of penicillin is ineffective and may mask early symptoms. Little consensus exists on the management of asymptomatic infants born to mothers receiving intrapartum antibiotics because of GBS colonization. Management schemes range from expectant observation to a complete workup for sepsis and prophylactic administration of antibiotics.

New avenues of prevention of neonatal GBS infections are being actively explored. The use of a maternal vaccination against a polysaccharide capsule antigen or a universal antigen of the subtypes of GBS may allow placental transfer of antibodies that could reduce or eliminate neonatal infection. Other research is directed at the use of hyperimmune and monoclonal IVIG as adjuvant therapy or prophylaxis for the very preterm neonate.

SYPHILIS

(See Chapter 37, Part Two.)

Descriptions of syphilis and its many manifestations have appeared in the medical literature since the 16th century. The introduction of antibiotics 50 years ago reduced the incidence of congenital syphilis to an all time low of 200 reported cases in 1958. However, a resurgence of primary and secondary syphilis in recent years has caused a concomitant resurgence in neonatal cases.

Epidemiology

From the late 1970s to the mid 1980s the incidence of primary and secondary syphilis rose slowly. Between 1986 and 1990, the epidemiology began to shift dramatically. The incidence of reported primary and secondary cases in women rose 240%, peaking at 20.3 cases per 100,000 population in 1990. Only 3.2 cases per 100,000 were reported in 1997.[87] The incidence of congenital infection has paralleled this rise and fall. The decline may reflect the renewed attention given to syphilis control programs after the epidemic of the 1980s was recognized (Fig. 22–3).

The sudden increase in reported cases in females seems to be related to the practice of trading sex with multiple partners to acquire illicit drugs, especially crack cocaine. Because these partners are frequently anonymous, the traditional syphilis-control strategy of partner notification is ineffective. Many of these women who became pregnant received little or poor prenatal care.[17] The relationship of HIV infection to the acquisition of syphilis is still uncertain.

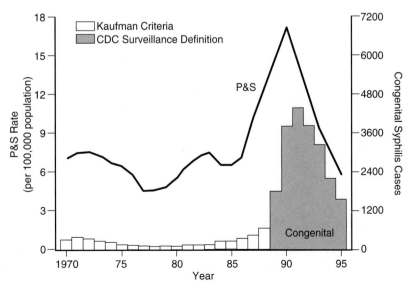

FIGURE 22–3. Congenital syphilis cases in infants younger than 1 year of age and rates of primary and secondary (P&S) syphilis among women in the United States, 1970 to 1995. (From Centers for Disease Control and Prevention, Atlanta, Georgia, Public Health Service, 1996.)

Clinical Manifestations and Diagnosis

After an incubation period of 10 to 90 days from exposure to *Treponema pallidum*, the painless, hard chancre of primary syphilis appears. Although this is readily apparent in males, it is frequently located in the vagina or on the cervix of females and passes unnoticed by the patient. Six weeks to 6 months after the primary inoculation there is involvement of all the major organ systems during the secondary stage. The patient may present with a maculopapular rash of the palms and soles, condyloma latum, and generalized lymphadenopathy. The findings spontaneously clear as the patient enters the latent stage. If untreated, approximately one third of patients will develop tertiary syphilis with involvement of the central nervous and cardiovascular systems and gumma formation.[91]

Clinical diagnosis, especially in pregnant patients, of "the great imitator" may be difficult. Antepartum diagnosis relies on serologic screening using nontreponemal tests such as the Venereal Disease Research Laboratory (VDRL) or the Rapid Plasma Reagin (RPR) tests. False positives occur in 1% to 2% of tests and may be caused by recent febrile illness, subclinical autoimmune disease, or laboratory error. Reactive nontreponemal tests are confirmed by specific antibody tests such as the microhemagglutination assay for antibodies to *T. pallidum* (MHA-TP) or the fluorescent treponemal antibody-absorption (FTA-ABS) test.[49]

Congenital Syphilis

(See also Chapter 37, Part Two.)

Treponemes appear capable of crossing the placenta at any point in pregnancy, and infection can cause preterm delivery, stillbirth, congenital infection, and neonatal death. Congenital syphilis causes fetal or perinatal death in 40% to 50% of the infants affected. Spontaneous abortion and stillbirth may be the result of overwhelming infection of the placenta and resultant nonimmune hydrops. Older literature suggests that transmission occurs in virtually all of infants born to mothers with primary and secondary syphilis, although only half of the infants may be symptomatic. The rate of transmission drops to 40% with early latent (less than 2 years) and 6% to 14% with late latent stages. Even with appropriate antepartum diagnosis and antibiotic treatment of the mother, 11% of infants may demonstrate central nervous system involvement.

Clinical manifestations appearing in the first 2 years of life are referred to as early congenital syphilis, and those appearing later are referred to as late congenital syphilis. Early disease is associated with hemolytic anemia, hepatosplenomegaly, and cutaneous bullous eruptions. Periostitis, osteochondritis, and meningitis are common findings. Late stigmata include periostitis of frontal and parietal bones, Hutchinson teeth, mulberry molars, saddle nose, saber shins, eighth nerve deafness, rhagades, central nervous system abnormalities, and Clutton joints.

Prevention

The prevention of congenital syphilis requires prenatal care, antepartum screening, and appropriate antibiotic therapy. The CDC recommendations state that regardless of gestational age, infected gravidas should be immediately treated with penicillin appropriate for the stage of syphilis as recommended for nonpregnant patients.[16] Patients with a history of penicillin allergy may be treated with penicillin after negative skin testing or penicillin desensitization. Tetracycline is not recommended during pregnancy because of adverse fetal effects. Although erythromycin may be acceptable treatment in adults, it does not cross the placenta readily and may not treat the fetus as well as penicillin. Maternal follow-up includes monthly nontreponemal serologic testing. A rise in titers or lack of a fourfold drop in titers over 3 months indicates a need for re-treatment. All patients should be offered counseling and testing for HIV antibody, owing to the frequent associations of the two infections.

As in nonpregnant patients, treatment of the early stages of syphilis may precipitate the Jarisch-Herxheimer reaction. The typical fever, myalgias, and headaches begin 2 to 4 hours after treatment and last 12 to 48 hours. In addition, uterine contractions, decreased fetal movement, and fetal bradycardia can occur in pregnant patients. Fetal death is more likely to occur during the Jarisch-Herxheimer reaction when the fetus is also affected.[67]

At birth the placenta and cord should be examined by darkfield microscopy for treponemes. Neonatal serum should be examined for IgM. Cerebrospinal fluid evaluation and long bone radiography may be indicated. In the asymptomatic infant at birth, whose mother was appropriately treated and close follow-up is ensured, no antibiotic treatment may be needed. In the asymptomatic infant in which follow-up is doubtful, a single intramuscular dose of benzathine penicillin is recommended. If the infant has active infection or neurosyphilis cannot be excluded, the CDC recommends a 10-day course of intramuscularly or intravenously administered penicillin.[16]

LISTERIOSIS

Listeria monocytogenes is a motile, microaerophilic gram-positive bacillus that infects primarily pregnant women, newborns, the elderly, and immunocompromised individuals. Maternal infection can lead to stillbirth and premature delivery. Neonatal infection is associated with a high morbidity and mortality rate.

Epidemiology

L. monocytogenes is an unusual but important cause of perinatal infection. Cases may be sporadic or occur in epidemics.[28] Many types of mammals and birds harbor the organism, which is viable in manure for long periods of time. Food and dairy products have been implicated as sources of outbreaks.[24]

Maternal Disease and Transmission

Approximately half of women delivering infants infected with *L. monocytogenes* are asymptomatic before and during labor.[55] When symptomatic, they present with a nonspecific flulike syndrome with back pain, fever, malaise, and upper respiratory tract symptoms. Diagnosis is most accurately confirmed with blood or amniotic fluid cultures. Premature labor may accompany these findings.

Transmission is generally believed to be hematogenous with evidence of placental infection. However, some neonates may be infected by ascending infection, even across intact membranes. When listeriosis is diagnosed during pregnancy, treatment with high doses of ampicillin has been suggested.[92]

Fetal and Neonatal Infection

(See also Chapter 37, Part Two.)

Listeriosis septicemia may cause stillbirth or preterm delivery before viability is reached; however, it does not seem to be a cause of recurrent fetal loss. Prematurity, birth weight less than 2500 gm, and evidence of fetal compromise are common. Like neonates with GBS infections, neonates with *L. monocytogenes* infection have either early (less than 4 hours after delivery) or late (1 to 6 weeks after delivery) manifestations. The infants presenting with early-onset disease classically have skin lesions, severe respiratory distress, hepatosplenomegaly, and laboratory evidence of sepsis. These infants are more likely to have mothers who were symptomatic before or during labor. Late-onset disease usually affects term healthy infants with the typical symptoms of bacterial meningitis. Neonatal mortality in early-onset disease ranges from 30% to 60%.[92]

CHLAMYDIAL INFECTION

Chlamydia are obligate intracellular bacteria. The organism depends on the invading cell for its energy supply and destroys the cell with replication. The 15 serotypes of *C. trachomatis* are responsible for three major groups of infection. Serotypes L1, L2, and L3 cause lymphogranuloma venereum; serotypes A, B, Ba, and C cause endemic blinding trachoma, the most common cause of blindness; and the remaining serotypes D through K are sexually transmitted agents that cause inclusion conjunctivitis, newborn pneumonia, urethritis, cervicitis, salpingitis, acute urethral syndrome, and perinatal infections.

Epidemiology and Clinical Manifestations

C. trachomatis is a very common sexually transmitted disease, with more than 4 million infections occurring annually. It is generally believed that 5% to 10% of sexually active women in the United States carry chlamydiae in their cervix. Certain risk groups, such as young, inner-city women, especially African Americans, have a much higher prevalence. In large, prospective studies, the prevalence in pregnant women has ranged from 2% to 25%, depending on the group studied. Forty to sixty percent of women with positive gonorrhea cultures have a concomitant chlamydial infection. The anatomic site in the female genital tract most frequently infected with *C. trachomatis* is the cervix. The ensuing endocervicitis may be asymptomatic or more commonly associated with a hypertrophic cervical erosion and copious mucopurulent discharge containing a high number of polymorphonuclear leukocytes. *C. trachomatis* is a common cause of tubal infertility.

Cell culture has long been the gold standard for diagnosis of chlamydial infection. Recently, rapid nonculture detection kits utilizing conjugated monoclonal antibodies or enzyme immunoassay have been promoted. The performance of only a few of these has been adequately tested in large-scale clinical trials. The treatment of choice in chlamydial infections has been tetracyclines and erythromycin. Erythromycin base or succinate (or ampicillin if gastrointestinal intolerance develops) is used for treatment during pregnancy.

Association with Adverse Pregnancy Outcome

Many studies have attempted to associate endocervical infection with *C. trachomatis* and adverse pregnancy outcome, including prematurity, PROM, intrauterine growth retardation, and postpartum endometritis.

Although some report no association of chlamydial infection with delivery before 37 weeks' gestation, others report odds ratios from 1.6 to 5.4. Berman and Harrison attempt to explain part of this discrepancy by noting a tighter association of prematurity and low birth weight with recent chlamydial infection as demonstrated by the presence of IgM antibodies or IgG seroconversion.[7]

Antepartum treatment of chlamydia during pregnancy appears to improve pregnancy outcome, as suggested by Ryan and associates, who studied 11,544 women, 2433 (21.08%) of whom had a positive *Chlamydia* culture on their first prenatal visit (Table 22–3).[86] Of the women with the positive cultures, 1100 were untreated and 1323 were treated with oral erythromycin or sulfamethoxazole. If untreated, culture-positive patients had a higher incidence of PROM, birth weight less than 2500 gm, and a lower incidence of newborn survival.

Effects on the Newborn

(See also Chapter 37, Part Two.)

Infants delivered vaginally to a woman with a chlamydial infection of the cervix have a 25% to 60% chance of becoming infected themselves. Although uncommon, *C. trachomatis* has been isolated from infants delivered by elective cesarean section despite intact membranes.

Acute neonatal conjunctivitis in the newborn as a result of perinatal exposure to *C. trachomatis* has been

TABLE 22–3 ASSOCIATION OF PREGNANCY OUTCOME AND *CHLAMYDIA TRACHOMATIS*

| | CHLAMYDIA POSITIVE | | CHLAMYDIA NEGATIVE | TOTAL |
	Untreated	Treated		
PROM*	58 (5.2%)	39 (2.9%)	243 (2.7%)	340
Birth weight <2500 gm	218 (19.6%)	145 (11.0%)	1068 (11.7%)	1431
Newborn survival†	1083 (97.6%)	1315 (99.4%)	8973 (98.5%)	11,371
Total numbers	1110	1323	9111	11,544

*Premature rupture of the membranes.
†Defined as survival until hospital discharge.
From Ryan GM: *Chlamydia trachomatis* infection in pregnancy and effect of treatment on outcome. Am J Obstet Gynecol 162:34, 1990.

recognized for some time. This organism is now the leading cause of neonatal conjunctivitis. Of those infants becoming infected with *C. trachomatis* after exposure during delivery, 17.5% to 46.5% will develop this conjunctivitis. When the infants of 230 culture positive mothers received one of the three prophylactic regimens (silver nitrate, tetracycline 1%, or erythromycin 0.5%), no significant difference in the rate of chlamydial conjunctivitis was noted (20%, 11%, and 14%, respectively).[44]

Up to 20% of infants delivered through a cervix infected with chlamydia will develop pneumonia. Infants present between 4 and 11 weeks with signs of congestion and obstruction, little nasal discharge, minimal fever, tachypnea, and a prominent staccato-type cough. Chest radiograph reveals hyperinflated lungs with bilateral interstitial infiltrates. Blood gas analysis frequently shows mild or moderate hypoxia. Approximately 50% of these infants have a history of or concurrent conjunctivitis. Most infants recover quickly on oral erythromycin. Other neonatal clinical manifestations of *C. trachomatis* infection include otitis media, bronchiolitis, and perhaps gastroenteritis.

TOXOPLASMOSIS

(See also Chapter 37, Part Three.)

Toxoplasma gondii is a parasite of felines, although other mammals and some avian species may be infected. The parasite has three distinct life cycle phases: the tachyzoite, tissue cyst, and oocyst. The oocysts are produced in the gastrointestinal tract of the feline and excreted in the feces. Ingestion by humans allows the circulation of the tachyzoites, the ovoid unicellular organisms characteristic of acute infection. Tachyzoites remain viable for hours in extracellular secretions and can be transmitted through blood transfusion or needlestick or across the placenta. Tissue cysts form as early as the eighth day of infection, are commonly located in striated muscle and the brain, and serve as a source of persistent infection for the life of the host. Human infection can also be caused by eating undercooked or raw meat (e.g., beef, lamb, or pork) containing tissue cysts. In immunocompetent adults, acute infection is not dramatic and clinical symptoms, when they do occur, include malaise, fever, rash, splenomegaly, and lymphadenopathy. Permanent immunity develops.[5]

The prevalence of toxoplasmosis ranges from 3%

to 30% in the United States, depending on geography, lifestyle, and pets.[3] Diagnosis of acute maternal infection relies on detection of IgM or rising or high titers of IgG. A variety of tests have been employed to make the diagnosis of fetal infection in utero. Ultrasound evaluation may detect dilation of the ventricles, ascites, hepatomegaly, and intracranial calcifications; however, the majority (80%) of cases will not have ultrasonographic evidence of infection.[75] Fetal blood samples for IgG and IgM and amniotic fluid for culture and mouse inoculation have been traditionally used for fetal diagnosis. However, PCR techniques performed on amniotic fluid samples alone provide equal sensitivity and specificity of the older diagnostic tests with less risk of pregnancy loss.[37] Prevention of maternal disease includes avoidance of undercooked meat, unwashed berries, or vegetables that may have had contact with soil exposed to cat excrement and exposure to litter boxes of potentially infected pets.

Transmission and Neonatal Disease

Intrauterine infection is possible only when the circulating tachyzoites are present to invade the placenta and then infect the fetus. Therefore, vertical transmission is limited to primary infection or reactivation in an immunocompromised host. Latent infection may be reactivated, causing fetal infection in transplant or AIDS patients; it is unlikely to adversely affect pregnancy outcome in healthy gravidas.

The transmission rate increases from 20% to 50% to 65% in the first, second, and third trimesters, respectively.[37, 48] The severity of fetal disease is inversely related to the gestational age at the time of infection. The vast majority of infected infants are asymptomatic at birth, although serious manifestations, such as chorioretinitis, may develop during childhood.[43] Abnormalities in the affected infant can include chorioretinitis, hydrocephaly, microcephaly, mental retardation, hepatosplenomegaly, jaundice, and lymphadenopathy.

The best information on fetal infection with *T. gondii* comes from France, where the prevalence is approximately 10 times that in the United States. There, serologic screening is compulsory. If initially seronegative, the pregnant woman is screened monthly for seroconversion. If untreated, the primarily infected gravida produces a clinically infected infant 13% to 30% of the time. Including the spontaneous abortions that may have been caused by toxoplasmosis infection would raise the transmission rate to 46%. Because of the much lower incidence of toxoplasmosis in this country, routine screening is not recommended.[3]

French women are now treated with spiramycin when acute infection is diagnosed. At 20 to 24 weeks, prenatal diagnosis is attempted by obtaining fetal blood by cordocentesis; amniotic fluid IgG and IgM antibody titers are performed and mice inoculated, looking for signs of infections. If the fetus appears infected, pyrimethamine and either sulfadoxine or sulfadiazine are added to the treatment regimen. Daffos and coworkers reported on 746 documented cases of maternal toxoplasmosis treated in this manner.[29] Congenital infection was demonstrated in 42 infants, 39 of whom were diagnosed antenatally. Twenty-four pregnancies were terminated, and 15 were carried to term. Of the 15 fetuses with congenital toxoplasmosis, all but 2 who had chorioretinitis remained clinically well throughout follow-up. Maternal infection occurred earlier in the pregnancy in fetuses who were aborted, and almost all had ultrasonographic evidence suggestive of toxoplasmosis. Three fetuses of the remaining 702 demonstrated evidence of congenital toxoplasmosis despite negative antepartum studies, 2 with subclinical disease and 1 with meningoencephalitis and chorioretinitis. Thus, prenatal diagnosis is practical and can provide information for those debating pregnancy termination. It appears that the initiation of in utero therapy may reduce the severity of the disease in newborns.[38]

■ REFERENCES

1. American Academy of Pediatrics Committee of Infectious Diseases and Committee on Fetus and Newborn: Guidelines for prevention of group B streptococcal (GBS) infection by chemoprophylaxis. Pediatrics 90:775, 1992.
2. American College of Obstetricians and Gynecologists: Group B streptococcal infections in pregnancy: ACOG's recommendations. ACOG News 37:1, 1993.
3. Bader TJ, et al: Prenatal screening for toxoplasmosis. Obstet Gynecol 90:457, 1997.
4. Baker CJ: Group B streptococcal infections. Clin Perinatol 24:59, 1997.
5. Beazley D, Ergerman R: Toxoplasmosis. Semin Perinatol 22:332, 1998.
6. Beasley RP, et al: The e antigen and vertical transmission of hepatitis B surface antigen. Am J Epidemiol 105:94, 1977.
7. Berman SW, et al: Low birth weight, prematurity and postpartum endometritis: Association with prenatal cervical *Mycoplasma hominis* and *Chlamydia trachomatis* infections. JAMA 257:1189, 1987.
8. Boggess KA, et al: Herpes simplex virus type 2 detection by culture and polymerase chain reaction and relationship to genital symptoms and cervical antibody status during the third trimester of pregnancy. Am J Gynecol Obstet 176:443, 1997.
9. Boyer KM, et al: Antimicrobial prophylaxis of neonatal group B streptococcal sepsis. Clin Perinatol 15:831, 1988.
10. Brocklehurst P, French R: The association between maternal HIV infection and perinatal outcome: A systematic review of the literature and meta-analysis. Br J Obstet Gynaecol 105:836, 1998.
11. Brown H, Abernathy MP: Cytomegalovirus infection. Semin Perinatol 22:260, 1998.
12. Brown ZA: Genital herpes complicating pregnancy. Dermatol Clin 16:805, 1998.
13. Brown ZA, et al: Genital herpes in pregnancy: Risk factors associated with recurrences and asymptomatic viral shedding. Am J Obstet Gynecol 153:24, 1985.
14. Caro-Paton T, et al: Is metronidazole teratogenic? A meta-analysis. Br J Clin Pharmacol 44:179, 1997.
15. Carpenter CCJ, et al: Antiretroviral therapy for HIV infection in 1998: Updated recommendations of the International AIDS Society—USA panel. JAMA 280:78, 1998.
16. Centers for Disease Control: 1998 guidelines for treatment of sexually transmitted diseases. MMWR Morbid Mortal Wkly Rep 47:RR-1, 1998.
17. Centers for Disease Control: Epidemic of congenital syphilis—Baltimore, 1996–1997. MMWR Morbid Mortal Wkly Rep 47:904, 1998.
18. Centers for Disease Control: Hepatitis E among US travelers, 1989–1992. MMWR Morbid Mortal Wkly Rep 42:1, 1993.
19. Centers for Disease Control: Measles, mumps, and rubella-vaccine use and strategies for elimination of measles, rubella, and congenital rubella syndrome and control of mumps: Recommendations of the Advisory Committee on Immunization Practices (ACIP). MMWR Morbid Mortal Wkly Rep 47:RR-8:1, 1988.
20. Centers for Disease Control: Prevention of perinatal group B streptococcal disease: A public health perspective. MMWR Morbid Mortal Wkly Rep 45(RR-7):1, 1996.
21. Centers for Disease Control: Prevention of perinatal transmission of hepatitis B virus: Prenatal screening of all pregnant women for hepatitis B surface antigen. MMWR Morbid Mortal Wkly Rep 37:341, 1988.
22. Centers for Disease Control: Public Health Service Task Force recommendations for the use of antiretroviral drugs in pregnant women infected with HIV-1 for maternal health and for reducing perinatal HIV-1 transmission in the United States. MMWR Morbid Mortal Wkly Rep 47:RR-2, 1998.
23. Centers for Disease Control: Recommendations for prevention and control of hepatitis C virus (HCV) infection and HCV-related chronic disease. MMWR Morbid Mortal Wkly Rep 47:1, 1998.
24. Centers for Disease Control: Update: Multistate outbreak of listeriosis—United States, 1998–1999. MMWR Morbid Mortal Wkly Rep 47:1117, 1999.
25. Centers for Disease Control: Zidovudine for the prevention of HIV transmission from mother to infant. MMWR Morbid Mortal Wkly Rep 43:285, 1994.
26. Chandra PC, et al: Successful pregnancy outcome after complicated varicella pneumonia. Obstet Gynecol 92:680, 1998.
27. Chapman SJ: Varicella in pregnancy. Semin Perinatol 22:339, 1998.
28. Cherubin CE, et al: Epidemiological spectrum and current treatment of listeriosis. Rev Infect Dis 13:1108, 1991.
29. Dafos F, et al: Prenatal management of 746 pregnancies at risk for congenital toxoplasmosis. N Engl J Med 318:271, 1988.
30. Duff P: Hepatitis in pregnancy. Semin Perinatol 22:277, 1998.
31. Egarter C, et al: Adjunctive antibiotic treatment in preterm labor and neonatal morbidity: A meta-analysis. Obstet Gynecol 88:303, 1996.
32. Enders G, et al: Consequences of varicella and herpes zoster in pregnancy: Prospective study of 1739 cases. Lancet 343:1547, 1994.
33. Eriksen NL: Perinatal consequences of hepatitis C. Clin Obstet Gynecol 42:121, 1999.
34. European Mode of Delivery Collaboration: Elective cesarean section versus vaginal delivery in prevention of vertical HIV-1 transmission: A randomized clinical trial. Lancet 353:1035, 1999.
35. Fan YD, et al: Acute pyelonephritis in pregnancy. Am J Perinatol 4:324, 1987.
36. Fleming DT, et al: Herpes simplex virus type 2 in the United States, 1976 to 1994. N Engl J Med 337:1105, 1997.
37. Forestier F, et al: Prenatal diagnosis of congenital toxoplasmosis by PCR: Extended experience. Prenat Diag 18:405, 1998.

38. Foulon W, et al: Treatment of toxoplasmosis during pregnancy: A multicenter study of impact on fetal transmission and children's sequelae at age 1 year. Am J Obstet Gynecol 180:410, 1999.

39. Gardner HL, et al: *Haemophilus vaginalis* vaginitis. Am J Obstet Gynecol 69:962, 1955.

40. Gibbs RS, Eschenbach DA: Use of antibiotics to prevent preterm birth. Am J Obstet Gynecol 177:375, 1997.

41. Gibbs RS, et al: Quantitative bacteriology of amniotic fluid from patients with clinical intra-amniotic infection at term. J Infect Dis 145:1, 1982.

42. Glantz JC, Mushlin AI: Cost-effectiveness of routine antenatal varicella screening. Obstet Gynecol 91:519, 1998.

43. Guerina NG, et al: Neonatal serologic screening and early treatment for congenital *Toxoplasma gondii* infection. N Engl J Med 330:1858, 1994.

44. Hammerschlag MR, et al: Efficacy of neonatal ocular prophylaxis for the prevention of chlamydial and gonococcal conjunctivitis. N Engl J Med 320:769, 1989.

45. Harger JH, et al: Prospective evaluation of 618 pregnant women exposed to parvovirus B19: Risks and symptoms. Obstet Gynecol 91:416, 1998.

46. Hauth JC, et al: Reduced incidence of preterm delivery with metronidazole and erythromycin in women with bacterial vaginosis. N Engl J Med 333:1732, 1995.

47. Hensleigh PA, et al: Genital herpes during pregnancy: Inability to distinguish primary and recurrent lesions clinically. Obstet Gynecol 89:891, 1997.

48. Hohfeld P, et al: Fetal toxoplasmosis: Outcome of pregnancy and infant follow-up after in utero treatment. J Pediatr 115:765, 1989.

49. Hollier LM, Cox SM: Syphilis. Semin Perinatol 22:323, 1998.

50. The International Perinatal HIV Group: The mode of delivery and the risk of vertical transmission of human immunodeficiency virus type 1-A meta-analysis of 15 prospective cohort studies. N Engl J Med 340:977, 1999.

51. Kimberlin DF, Andrews WW: Bacterial vaginosis: Association with adverse pregnancy outcome. Semin Perinatol 22:242, 1998.

52. Kimberlin DF, et al: Pharmacokinetics of oral valacyclovir and acyclovir in late pregnancy. Am J Obstet Gynecol 179:846, 1998.

53. Kurki T, et al: Bacterial vaginosis in early pregnancy and pregnancy outcome. Obstet Gynecol 80:173, 1992.

54. Kustermann A, et al: Prenatal diagnosis of congenital varicella infection. Prenat Diag 16:71, 1996.

55. Lorber B: Listeriosis. Clin Infect Dis 24:1, 1997.

56. Markenson GR, Yancey MK: Parvovirus B19 infections in pregnancy. Semin Perinatol 22:309, 1998.

57. McDonald HM, et al: Impact of metronidazole therapy on preterm birth in women with bacterial vaginosis flora *(Gardnerella vaginalis)*: A randomized, placebo controlled trial. Br J Obstet Gynecol 104:1391, 1997.

58. McKenna DS, Iams JD: Group B streptococcal infections. Semin Perinatol 22:267, 1998.

59. Meis P, et al: The preterm prediction study: Significance of vaginal infections. Am J Obstet Gynecol 173:1231, 1995.

60. Mercer BM: Antibiotic therapy for preterm premature rupture of membranes. Clin Obstet Gynecol 41:461, 1998.

61. Mercer B, et al, for the National Institute of Child Health and Human Development Maternal Fetal Medicine Units Network: Antibiotic therapy for reduction of infant morbidity after preterm premature rupture of the membranes. JAMA 278:989, 1997.

62. Miller E, et al: Consequences of confirmed maternal rubella at successive stages of pregnancy. Lancet 2:781, 1982.

63. Miller E, et al: Immediate and long-term outcome of human parvovirus B19 infection in pregnancy. Br J Obstet Gynaecol 105:174, 1998.

64. Minkoff HL: Human immunodeficiency virus infection in pregnancy. Semin Perinatol 22:293, 1998.

65. Montaner JSG, et al: Antiretroviral treatment in 1998. Lancet 352:1919, 1998.

66. Morales WJ, et al: Effect of metronidazole in patients with preterm birth in preceding pregnancy and bacterial vaginosis: A placebo-controlled, double-blind study. Am J Obstet Gynecol 171:345, 1994.

67. Myles TD, et al: The Jarisch-Herxheimer reaction and fetal monitoring changes in pregnant women treated for syphilis. Obstet Gynecol 92:859, 1998.

68. Nelson CT, Demmler GJ: Cytomegalovirus infection in the pregnant mother, fetus and newborn infant. Clin Perinatol 24:151, 1997.

69. Parry S, Strauss JF: Premature rupture of the fetal membranes. N Engl J Med 338:663, 1998.

70. Paryani SG, et al: Intrauterine infection with varicella-zoster virus after maternal varicella. N Engl J Med 314:1542, 1986.

71. Pastuszak AL, et al: Outcome after maternal varicella infection in the first 20 weeks of pregnancy. N Engl J Med 330:901, 1994.

72. Patterson TF, Andriole VT: Detection, significance and therapy of bacteriuria in pregnancy: Update in the managed health care era. Infect Dis Clin North Am 11:593, 1997.

73. Peltola H, Leinikki P: Rubella gene sequencing as a clinician's tool. Lancet 352:1799, 1998.

74. Piper JM, Wen TS: Perinatal cytomegalovirus and toxoplasmosis: Challenges of antepartum therapy. Clin Obstet Gynecol 42:81, 1999.

75. Puder KS, et al: Ultrasound characteristics of in utero infection. Infect Dis Obstet Gynecol 5:262, 1997.

76. Randolph AG, et al: Acyclovir prophylaxis in late pregnancy to prevent neonatal herpes: A cost effective analysis. Obstet Gynecol 88:603, 1996.

77. Reef SE: Rubella and congenital rubella syndrome. Bull World Health Organ 76:S2:156, 1998.

78. Riggs JW, Blanco JD: Pathophysiology, diagnosis and management of intraamniotic infection. Semin Perinatol 22:251, 1998.

79. Riley LE: Herpes simplex virus. Semin Perinatol 22:284, 1998.

80. Roberts SW, et al: Genital herpes during pregnancy: No lesions, no cesarean. Obstet Gynecol 85:261, 1995.

81. Robinson J, et al: Congenital rubella after anticipated maternal immunity: Two cases and a review of the literature. Pediatr Infect Dis J 13:812, 1994.

82. Rodis JF, et al: Management of parvovirus infection in pregnancy and outcomes of hydrops: A survey of members of the Society of Perinatal Obstetricians. Am J Obstet Gynecol 179:985, 1998.

83. Rodis JF, et al: Long-term outcome of children following maternal human parvovirus B19 infection. Obstet Gynecol 91:125, 1998.

84. Rosa C: Rubella and rubeola. Semin Perinatol 22:318, 1998.

85. Rouse DJ, et al: Management of the presumed susceptible varicella (chickenpox)-exposed gravida: A cost-effectiveness/cost-benefit analysis. Obstet Gynecol 87:932, 1996.

86. Ryan GM, et al: *Chlamydia trachomatis* infection in pregnancy and effect of treatment on outcome. Am J Obstet Gynecol 162:34, 1990.

87. Sanchez PJ, Wendel GD: Syphilis in pregnancy. Clin Perinatol 24:71, 1997.

87a. Schrag SJ, et al: Group B streptococcal disease in the era of intrapartum antibiotic prophylaxis. N Engl J Med 342:15, 2000.

88. Scott LL: Prevention of perinatal herpes: Prophylactic antiviral therapy. Clin Obstet Gynecol 42:134, 1999.

89. Siegel JD: Prophylaxis for neonatal group B *Streptococcus* infections. Semin Perinatol 22:33, 1998.

90. Sever JL, et al: Delayed manifestation of congenital rubella. Rev Infect Dis 7:S164, 1985.

91. Sheffield JS, Wendel GD: Syphilis in pregnancy. Clin Obstet Gynecol 42:97, 1999.

92. Silver HM: Listeriosis during pregnancy. Obstet Gynecol Surv 53:737, 1998.

93. Smith WJ, et al: Prevention of chickenpox in reproductive-age women: Cost-effectiveness of routine prenatal screening with postpartum vaccination of susceptibles. Obstet Gynecol 92:535, 1998.

94. Stango S, et al: Primary cytomegalovirus infection in pregnancy: Incidence, transmission to fetus and clinical outcome. JAMA 256:1904, 1986.

95. Strauss SE, et al: NIH Conference. Varicella-zoster infections: Virology, natural history, treatment and prevention. Ann Intern Med 108:221, 1988.

96. Tanemura M, et al: Diagnosis of fetal rubella infection with reverse transcription and nested polymerase chain reaction: A study of 34 cases diagnosed in fetuses. Am J Obstet Gynecol 174:578, 1996.

97. Towers CV, et al: Pulmonary injury associated with antepartum pyelonephritis: Can patients at risk be identified? Am J Obstet Gynecol 164:974, 1991.

98. Valeur-Jensen AK, et al: Risk factors for parvovirus B19 infection in pregnancy. JAMA 28:1109, 1999.

99. Webster WS: Teratogen update: Congenital rubella. Teratology 58:13, 1988.

100. Yoder PR, et al: A prospective, controlled study of maternal and perinatal outcome after intra-amniotic infection at term. Am J Obstet Gynecol 145:695, 1983.

101. Zanetti AR, et al: Multicenter trial on the efficacy of HBIG and vaccine in preventing perinatal hepatitis B: Final report. J Med Virol 18:327, 1986.

Placental Pathology

Raymond W. Redline

No evaluation of a sick neonate is complete without knowing the status of the organ that has supported the fetus through the preceding gestation—the placenta with its surrounding membranes. The placenta has two opposing functions during gestation. It is both the sole source of all metabolic fuels to the fetus and the sole protection for the fetus against noxious external influences, such as genital microorganisms, the maternal immune system, and the spatial constraints of the uterus. It is therefore important for the neonatologist and the obstetrician to be aware of specific pathogenic sequences of placental lesions that compromise these functions.

This chapter makes no attempt to comprehensively review placental pathology; the reader is referred to two general references.[13, 22] Rather it provides an overview of three topics: (1) optimal use of the pathology service to obtain useful information, (2) an understanding of specific patterns of placental injury in the context of normal form and function, and (3) clinicopathologic correlation (i.e., which lesions are seen in which clinical situations).

OPTIMAL USE OF THE PATHOLOGIST

As just suggested, any infant requiring the care of a neonatologist should have a placental examination. Because not all placentas are submitted to pathology, every obstetric service must have a specific list of situations in which placental examination is indicated. An example of such a list is provided in Box 23–1.[89] Because many sick neonates are transported from other hospitals, there should be a policy to ensure timely placental examination. The best solution is to transport the placenta in a watertight container along with the neonate to the tertiary care center. For various reasons, transport of the tissue specimen itself is sometimes not practical. In these cases, the slides and pathology report from the referring hospital should be requested and reviewed by the pathologist at the hospital where the neonate is to be treated. Whenever possible, placentas should be refrigerated immediately after delivery and delivered without fixative to the pathology laboratory. Specimens maintained in this fashion remain useful as long as 7 days

after delivery. When refrigeration within 1 to 2 hours of delivery is not possible, placentas should be immersed in 2 to 3 volumes of formalin, where they can remain for an indefinite period before examination by the pathologist. An informed evaluation of the placenta requires that the pathologist be aware of the clinical situation. Some mechanism, usually a form, must be established to convey this information. A proper balance should be struck between a totally open-ended form and a tedious checklist. An example of a form that we have found useful in our institution is given in Figure 23–1. Placental diagnosis requires very few special studies. Even bacterial cultures in cases of suspected chorioamnionitis rarely provide useful information beyond that which is available from placental histology and the infant's blood culture. Occasionally, fungal stains of the cord and membranes may be useful for neonatal management. In selected situations a placental karyotype may be of interest. Recent data suggest that some cases of intrauterine fetal demise and idiopathic intrauterine growth retardation (IUGR) may be explained on the basis of chromosomal anomalies confined to placental tissues (confined placental mosaicism).[44, 46, 47, 117]

STRUCTURE, FUNCTION, AND PATHOLOGY

OVERVIEW

At its simplest level the placenta is nothing more than fetal vessels and surrounding connective tissue surrounded by a continuous layer of epithelium, the trophoblast. This fetal vascular bed sits in a pool of maternal blood, the intervillous space, which is continuously filled and drained from below by maternal uterine arteries and veins (Fig. 23–2). The same unit of structure is repeated in the membranes in an attenuated form. Early in pregnancy the fetal vasculature and maternal intervillous space involute in that portion of the gestational sac destined to become the membranes, leaving a tough shell of fetal connective tissue and placental trophoblast in contact with the maternal uterus. Detailed knowledge of each of these anatomic compartments and their reaction patterns in

---

■ **BOX 23–1**

INDICATIONS FOR PLACENTAL
EXAMINATION

Neonatal

- Prematurity
- Intrauterine growth retardation
- Unexpected adverse outcome
- Congenital anomalies
- Suspicion of fetal infection
- Fetal hydrops
- Fetal hematologic abnormalities

Obstetric

- Intrauterine fetal demise
- Maternal disease or maternal death
- Signs of maternal infection
- Gestational hypertension
- Oligohydramnios or polyhydramnios
- Antepartum hemorrhage (acute and/or chronic)
- Postpartum hemorrhage
- Abnormal biophysical or biochemical monitoring
- In utero therapy
- Abnormal placenta noted at delivery

---

abnormal pregnancies provides the basis for understanding placental pathology.

Considering the fetal circulation first, the placenta is perfused by a pair of umbilical arteries and drained by a single umbilical vein. Because there is an arterial anastomosis near the umbilical cord insertion site, the fetus is not handicapped if one of the arteries is absent or occluded. The vein, on the other hand, is the sole supply of oxygenated placental blood for the fetus. It also has the thinnest wall and is the easiest to collapse of the three umbilical vessels. Large arteries and veins branching off the umbilical vessels transmit blood through the connective tissue of the primary and secondary stem villi to the terminal villous units where gas exchange occurs. Decreased flow in these vessels leads to luminal occlusion (fibromuscular sclerosis) and involution of the distal vascular bed (avascular villi).[32] This reaction is global in placentas from stillborn fetuses and focal in live-born infants with placental thrombi (Fig. 23–3A). Each terminal villous unit consists of a central tertiary stem villus and several surrounding terminal villi. Tertiary

stem villi have at least one arteriole that directly regulates flow to the terminal villous capillary bed. Obliteration, stenosis, or spasm of these arterioles can profoundly impact gas exchange.[31, 35, 97] Finally, terminal villi have a capillary bed that can sustain microvascular damage, leading to villous edema[76] or stromal hemorrhage,[33] or undergo reactive hyperplasia (chorangiosis) in response to hypoxia or other local stimuli.[4]

Turning to the maternal circulation, it is important to emphasize that adequate placental perfusion depends on pregnancy-related increases in maternal intravascular volume and decreases in maternal vascular tone.[74] Maternal conditions such as renal disease, essential hypertension, and collagen-vascular disease can cause *chronic uteroplacental underperfusion* by interfering with these systemic accommodations to pregnancy. To ensure adequate perfusion of the intervillous space the human placenta has evolved a mechanism for remodeling and enlarging uteroplacental arteries.[82, 85] Placental trophoblast grows down the lumen of these vessels, invades the vascular wall, and replaces the smooth muscle layer with a noncontractile layer of fibrinoid matrix. Failure to execute this entire sequence may compromise baseline perfusion and leave uteroplacental vessels susceptible to spasm, degeneration, and rupture. These abnormalities are believed to play an important role in the pathogenesis of preeclampsia and abruptio placentae.[19] It is also important that maternal blood contacts a nonadhesive trophoblastic cell membrane to prevent activation of the coagulation system. Another maternal disorder associated with uteroplacental underperfusion is the antiphospholipid antibody syndrome. Recent data indicate that the anionic phospholipid binding protein annexin-V plays an important role in preventing the assembly of active coagulation factor complexes on the trophoblast cell membrane.[86] Antiphospholipid antibodies have been shown to displace annexin-V from the cell surface, thereby accounting for preeclamptic-like pathology in affected pregnancies.

Intervening between the fetal and maternal circulations are the tissues sometimes referred to as the interhemal membrane. These include syncytiotrophoblast, the trophoblast basement membrane, and intravillous connective tissue. One important trophoblastic reaction pattern that can reduce the diffusion distance across the interhemal membrane is syncytial knotting, an adaptive response to hypoxia (see Fig. 23–3C). This elegant mechanism, which has been substantiated by in vitro organ culture studies, consists

---

Sheet filled out M.D. (printed name) _____

Gestational Age (best estimate): _____

Ob Index: G____ Full Term _____ Prem ____ Ab ____ Lvg ____

Maternal History:

Baby (weight, Apgars, malformations, other): _____

Any specific questions about this placenta?

FIGURE 23–1. Placental data sheet used to transmit clinical history to the pathologist. Each item is widely spaced on the actual full-page form to provide sufficient space for free text.

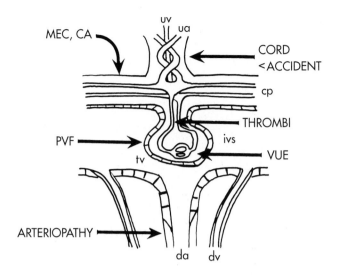

FIGURE 23–2. Schematic diagram of a functional unit in the placenta with sites and patterns of injury indicated by arrows. Deoxygenated fetal blood enters via umbilical arteries (ua) and flows through chorionic plate (cp) and stem villous arteries before entering terminal villi (tv). Flow into capillaries is regulated by stem villous arterioles. Postcapillary venules combine to form stem villous and chorionic plate veins, which drain to a single umbilical vein (uv) that carries oxygenated blood to the fetus. Maternal blood enters the intervillous space (ivs) via decidual arteries (da) lined with trophoblast *(hatched lines)* and drains through unmodified decidual veins (dv). Decidual arteriopathy (ARTERIOPATHY) restricts maternal perfusion of the intervillous space. Perivillous fibrin (PVF) coats villous trophoblast *(hatched lines)*, preventing gas exchange. Villitis of unknown etiology (VUE) expands the villous stroma, increasing the diffusion distance. Cord accidents compress the umbilical vessels, causing a global decrease in fetoplacental circulation. Meconium (MEC) and chorioamnionitis (CA) may decrease villous perfusion by damaging fetal vessels in the chorionic plate. Fetal thrombotic vasculopathy (THROMBI) similarly decreases the distal fetal vascular bed.

of a clustering of syncytiotrophoblast nuclei at one pole of the villus, leading to attenuation of the cytoplasmic barrier to gas exchange around the remaining circumference.[64, 111] Because trophoblast and especially syncytial knots are in direct contact with maternal blood, they can be easily dislodged, as attested to by their common presence in the lungs at autopsy in cases of maternal death. Although a mechanism for villous repair and re-epithelialization exists,[79] it is inevitable that some of these traumatic events will cause villous hemorrhage and fetomaternal transfusion. Cell traffic also occurs in the opposite direction (maternofetal transfusion).[106] When maternal inflammatory cells cross the trophoblastic barrier they may participate in an allograft-type response against fetal antigens in the villi. This process is believed to occur in *villitis of unknown etiology (VUE)*, and the resulting chronic inflammation increases diffusion distance[92] (see Fig. 23–3D). Another process increasing diffusion distance is *massive perivillous fibrin deposition ("maternal floor infarction")*, an idiopathic accumulation of trophoblast-derived extracellular matrix material that surrounds terminal villi compromising both intervillous circulation and gas exchange[66] (see Fig. 23–3B).

The final placental compartment to be discussed is the fluid-filled sac of membranes, which must rupture to allow vaginal delivery. In theory, membranes may prematurely rupture for one of two reasons: increased luminal pressure or weakening of their normal structural integrity. Increased pressure can be caused by premature contractions, cervical dilation, or polyhydramnios. Structural integrity may be compromised by trauma, inflammatory responses associated with ascending bacterial infection, or ischemic necrosis caused by premature placental separation (abruption). The amniotic fluid contained within the sac is predominantly derived from fetal urine, and its volume may in some cases reflect fetal fluid balance.[16] *Chronic uteroplacental underperfusion* can therefore lead to fetal hypovolemia and oligohydramnios in the absence of membrane rupture or fetal urinary tract anomalies. Oligohydramnios, regardless of its underlying cause, may lead to umbilical cord compression in the short

term,[59] limb deformities in the intermediate term,[108] and failure of adequate lung growth in the long term[115] (see Chapter 21). Placental membranes can also incorporate various exogenous substances suspended in the amniotic fluid, some of which, such as meconium and bacterial products, may damage both the membranes and the underlying fetal vessel wall.[6, 7, 43] A third exogenous substance found in membranes is hemosiderin, which can be an indicator of chronic peripheral separation (chronic abruption).[93]

MATERNAL VASCULAR PATHOLOGY

Muscularized maternal arteries supplying the intervillous space are susceptible to stenosis, occlusion, or rupture. Stenosis leads to *chronic uteroplacental underperfusion*, which is characterized by low placental weight, increased syncytial knotting, and focal villous agglutination (microinfarction) particularly in "watershed zones" between spiral arteries.[72, 73] Total occlusion causes villous infarction.[116] Although experimental studies have shown that up to 20% to 25% of villous parenchyma can be infarcted without acute fetal compromise,[32] these studies fail to account for the impaired status of the remaining placenta in most maternal vasculopathic disorders. Rupture of maternal arteries *(acute abruption)* may occasionally be attributed to trauma but is more commonly an ischemia-reperfusion injury with secondary rupture of the injured vascular wall. The common association of abruption with vasoactive drugs such as nicotine and especially cocaine is consistent with this pathogenesis.[2, 21, 75] *Chronic abruption* may also occur and presents pathologically as chronic peripheral separation, which is characterized by diffuse chorioamnionic hemosiderin deposition and placental circumvallation.[14, 40, 78, 96] Most evidence to date suggests that chronic abruption represents venous rather than arterial hemorrhage. Because muscular arteries are incompletely remodeled in preeclampsia, maternal vascular lesions of all types are especially frequent in this disorder. However, identical lesions may be seen with idiopathic IUGR, antiphospholipid antibody syndrome,

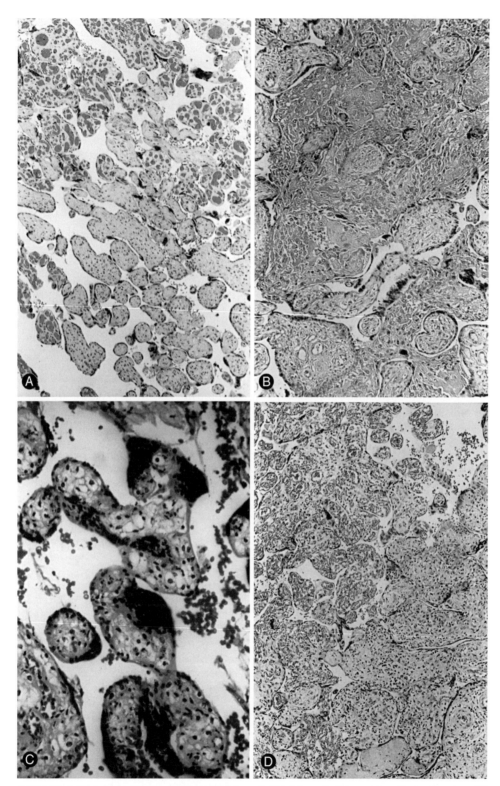

Figure 23–3. Histologic patterns of placental injury. *A,* Fetal thrombotic vasculopathy—avascular villi *(lower right)* due to upstream vascular occlusion. *B,* Massive perivillous fibrin deposition—fibrin with proliferating extravillous trophoblast encases terminal villi (especially *upper left*). *C,* Chronic uteroplacental underperfusion (increased syncytial knots)—aggregates of syncytiotrophoblast nuclei gather at one pole of the villus, leading to attenuation of the remaining syncytiotrophoblast cytoplasm, maximizing gas exchange. *D,* Villitis of unknown etiology—maternal T lymphocytes in the fetal villous stroma *(lower right)* lead to edema and fibrosis, which increase the diffusing distance between maternal and fetal circulations.

connective tissue diseases, diabetes mellitus, chronic hypertension, and chronic renal disease and in patients with an underlying thrombophilic condition.[1, 26, 27, 49, 50, 114]

FETAL VASCULAR PATHOLOGY

Fetal vessels within the umbilical cord are protected from compression by the cord matrix, a hydrated gel known as Wharton's jelly. Several processes lessen this protection: decreased hydration of the matrix, which can occur with *chronic uteroplacental underperfusion*,[54] torsion-related kinking of the cord to excessive coiling,[23] and insertion of the cord vessels into the membranes, which leaves them unprotected from trauma.[53] The critical parameters for deciding whether a putative cord lesion can be confirmed pathologically are thrombosis, necrosis, or hemorrhage at the proposed site of occlusion and histologic differences in cord structures located proximal and distal to the lesion.

Large vessels in the chorionic plate and stem villi may occasionally rupture, leading to *massive subchorial thrombosis*, a rare and often fatal lesion.[107] A more common process affecting these vessels is thrombotic occlusion *(fetal thrombotic vasculopathy)*.[87, 94] Factors predisposing to thrombosis are similar to those reported for thrombi in other organs: severe inflammation (villitis or chorioamnionitis), stasis and irritation (nuchal cords with meconium-stained fluid), inherited predispositions to clotting (protein C and S deficiencies, maternal antiphospholipid antibodies, factor V Leiden), and specific maternal disease states (diabetes mellitus).[3, 65, 92] Villi downstream of occlusive thrombi are avascular and hyalinized. Adverse sequelae of thrombotic vasculopathy include a decrease in the size of the fetal vascular bed available for gas exchange, coexistent thromboembolic disease in the fetus, or, in rare cases, a fetal consumptive coagulopathy with disseminated intravascular coagulation or thrombocytopenia.

Tertiary stem villous arterioles regulate placental resistance to fetal blood flow, the parameter evaluated in clinical pulsed-flow Doppler studies. These arterioles have been found to be numerically decreased in autosomal trisomies[97] and either obliterated or stenosed in patients with severe IUGR.[31, 35] A large proportion of placentas with *fetal arteriolar vasculopathy* also show clinical and pathologic evidence of *chronic uteroplacental underperfusion*.[112] Finally, it remains unclear whether fetal arteriolar vasculopathy is the cause or the result of IUGR. Placental arteriolar occlusion could cause placental hypoperfusion and growth retardation or alternatively might simply be the result of hypoperfusion by a sick, volume-depleted infant (see Chapter 13).

As described earlier, placental capillaries can leak fluid (villous edema) or blood (villous stromal hemorrhage), and both lesions have been shown to be associated with adverse outcome in very premature infants.[33, 76, 95] Frank rupture of capillaries is the cause of placental intervillous thrombi and may be associ-

ated with hypovolemia, fetal anemia, and a compensatory increase in circulating nucleated red blood cells.[48] Proliferation of villous capillaries (chorangiosis) is defined by a significant proportion of terminal villi having 10 or more capillary cross sections and has been associated with chronic villitis, meconium staining, diabetes, and congenital anomalies.[4]

INFECTION/INFLAMMATION

Acute chorioamnionitis is caused by cervicovaginal bacteria that either overwhelm normal cervical host defense systems or gain access to the amnionic cavity after rupture of membranes[15, 77] (see Chapter 22). The inflammatory response to bacterial infection is overwhelmingly neutrophilic and generally involves the membranes and chorionic plate but not the chorionic villi. Acute chorioamnionitis is by far the most common cause of preterm labor.[41, 94, 99] However, few delivered infants are septic at birth, attesting to the effectiveness of the placenta as a protective barrier.

Features indicating the duration of infection in chorioamnionitis can sometimes be helpful. In the initial stages (1 to 2 hours), maternal neutrophils marginate in the fibrin just below the chorionic plate (early chorionitis). Later, neutrophils, predominantly maternal, infiltrate the entire chorionic plate and the full thickness of the membranes (2 to 24 hours). A fetal neutrophilic response as manifest by transmigration across the umbilical vessel walls begins in the vein and later involves all three vessels (panvasculitis). This pattern, particularly when seen in a preterm birth, indicates an infection of 24 to 48 hours' duration. Later changes such as fetal neutrophils in the umbilical cord stroma (perivasculitis) and necrosis of the amnion (necrotizing chorioamnionitis) suggest more than 48 hours of infection. Finally, perivascular umbilical arcs of calcific debris, glycoprotein, and neovascularization (halo lesion) or a chronic mononuclear component (chronic chorioamnionitis) suggests prolonged infection of days' to weeks' duration.[34] Infants with placental halo lesions or chronic chorioamnionitis often have had occult membrane rupture and are at risk for pulmonary hypoplasia from secondary chronic oligohydramnios.[15, 77, 89] Data suggest that the fetal inflammatory response in chorioamnionitis is especially deleterious and may be a risk factor for severe neonatal morbidity (bronchopulmonary dysplasia, necrotizing enterocolitis, cranial ultrasound abnormalities, and long-term neurologic impairment).[37, 95] The patterns described earlier are typical for most bacteria. Unusual patterns that can suggest specific organisms are neutrophilic exudates involving the villi and intervillous space (suggestive of *Listeria monocytogenes* or *Campylobacter fetus*)[29] and microabscesses on the external surface of the umbilical cord (suggestive of *Candida albicans*).[42, 84]

Chronic placentitis is caused by organisms that enter the intervillous space by means of either the maternal bloodstream or the adjacent uterus. The hallmark of chronic placentitis is a destructive diffuse villitis with fibrosis, calcification, or both.[5] Although villous inflammation is generally emphasized, these infections also involve chorion, decidua, and other placental regions. This pattern of panplacentitis is typical of fetal infection by organisms of the TORCH group (*Toxoplasma gondii*, rubella virus, cytomegalovirus, and herpes simplex virus), *Treponema pallidum*, other herpesviruses (Epstein-Barr virus, varicella), and a host of other parasitic and protozoan infections rarely seen in the United States. Specific histopathologic features can indicate specific etiologic agents (e.g., increased Hofbauer cells, periarteritis, and necrotizing umbilical phlebitis in syphilis,[51, 83, 103] villous plasma cells in cytomegalovirus,[71] stromal necrosis and calcification in herpes simplex [personal observation], and umbilical cord pseudocysts in toxoplasmosis).[30]

Two other categories of neonatal infection that cannot be evaluated directly by placental pathology are transplacental and intrapartum infection. Transplacental infections spread to the fetus without affecting the placenta, presumably through breaks in the interhemal barrier (maternofetal transfusion). Important organisms in this category include human immunodeficiency virus,[57] hepatitis B virus,[60] human parvovirus B19,[20] and the enteroviruses.[70] Intrapartum infections, on the other hand, are acquired by the fetus during passage down a contaminated birth canal and hence also spare the placenta. Prominent in this category are venereal pathogens such as *Neisseria gonorrhoeae*, *Chlamydia trachomatis*, and human papillomavirus and some pathogens associated with neonatal sepsis (e.g., group B streptococci and *Escherichia coli*).[24]

Foci of chronic villous inflammation, *villitis of unknown etiology (VUE)*, are common in term placentas (5% of all placentas), whereas chronic placentitis attributable to the organisms listed earlier is rare (1 to 2 per 100 live births).[52, 102] For many years it was believed that some new organism would be discovered that could explain VUE, and indeed this may yet happen. However, certain features of VUE differ from chronic placentitis of infectious origin. First, VUE is confined to villi and generally involves only a fraction of the villous tree. Second, the predominant cells in VUE are CD4-positive T cells of maternal origin whereas the cells in chronic placentitis are predominantly macrophages, which are suspected, but not yet proven, to be of fetal origin.[39, 55] Third, VUE can be a recurrent disease associated with maternal autoimmunity whereas chronic placentitis due to infection rarely recurs because of acquired immunity.[91, 104] For all of these reasons many have argued that VUE represents a maternal antifetal immune response, a consequence of genetic differences between mother and fetus.[55, 92] Clinically, the relevance of VUE is its common association with IUGR, which can be attributed to its location in the villous stroma separating the maternal and fetal circulations.[52, 102]

DEVELOPMENTAL/STRUCTURAL LESIONS

The final group of lesions to be discussed are gross abnormalities in placental structure. As with structural abnormalities in the infant, these placental lesions can reflect either primary maldevelopment or secondary deformations and disruptions. Uterine abnormalities such as malformations, leiomyomas, or scars from previous surgical procedures are a major cause of abnormal placental development. These developmental abnormalities can be separated into two groups. First are abnormalities of lateral growth and membrane formation in which the placenta appears to migrate away from its original implantation site to optimize its blood supply, a process that has been termed *trophotropism*.[12] Trophotropism can lead to bilobation, accessory lobes, membranous cord insertions, and placenta previa, none of which is pathologic by itself. However, these placental anomalies can cause problems at delivery by placing fetal vessels at risk for rupture or, in some cases, predisposing to breech or transverse fetal presentations. The second abnormality is one of vertical growth. The uterine decidua is believed to regulate depth of uterine implantation. Prior surgery or other uterine abnormalities can interfere with normal decidualization, leading to uncontrolled placental growth into or through the uterine wall. This pattern, known as placenta acreta or percreta, most commonly causes postpartum hemorrhage but in selected cases can lead to uterine rupture.[88]

A second set of placental structural anomalies are those associated with deformations or disruptions in the fetus. Fetal deformation sequences attributable to *amniotic bands* (amputations) or prolonged oligohydramnios (clubfoot and pulmonary hypoplasia) are potential complications of early membrane rupture.[68, 115] Early membrane rupture and subsequent oligohydramnios are associated with a placental lesion known as *amnion nodosum*[56] (see Chapter 21). Amnion nodosum consists of white membrane excrescences that are the consequence of prolonged contact between fetal vernix and membrane amnion. Fetal disruptions are caused by in utero ischemia of either maternal or fetal origin. Transient interruption of maternal blood supply early in pregnancy has been correlated with limb and central nervous system anomalies.[17] Such episodes can present clinically as chronic abruption and pathologically as a *circumvallate placenta* (membranes arising inside the placenta perimeter with an associated fibrin rim due to peripheral accumulation of blood in a closed uterine environment).[14, 78]

A second cause of fetal vascular disruptions are vascular anastomoses in monochorionic twins[45] (see Chapter 18). Identical twins having a single monochorionic placenta and two separate amnionic sacs (monochorionic diamnionic) are at highest risk. Anastomoses can cause sudden circulatory shifts at the time of delivery or, if intrinsically unbalanced, chronic twin-to-twin transfusion. Dichorionic twin placentas, whether from identical or fraternal twins, are not affected. Interestingly, identical twins with only one amnionic cavity (monochorionic monoamnionic) rarely have twin-to-twin transfusion but commonly have another placental complication—entangled umbilical cords—which can lead to the death of one or both twins.

Although present for only a short time, tumors can develop in the placenta. The most common placental tumors are chorangiomas composed of proliferating fetal blood vessels (hemangiomas). Chorangiomas cause fetal pathologic conditions in two ways: by arteriovenous shunting, leading to hydrops fetalis, or by sequestering platelets, leading to disseminated intravascular coagulation.[11, 13] Choriocarcinomas (malignant trophoblastic tumors) can arise from the villi of second- and third-trimester placentas and metastasize to the fetus.[10, 18] The placenta also can be a metastatic site for malignant tumors of either the mother (most commonly acute myeloid leukemia, melanoma, and adenocarcinoma) or the fetus (e.g., congenital neuroblastoma).[101]

As mentioned earlier, it has recently become apparent that chromosomally normal infants do not always have chromosomally normal placentas. Placental aneuploidy or confined placental mosaicism, as this phenomenon has been called, can affect all or part of the placenta and is believed to explain some cases of idiopathic IUGR and intrauterine fetal demise.[44, 46, 47, 117] The morphologic sequelae of this phenomenon, if any, have not yet been established. Candidate lesions include dysmorphic villi of the type described in triploidy or monosomy X[81, 113] and delayed villous maturation, which has been described in the placentas of infants with congenital anomalies.[4]

CLINICAL CORRELATION

Finally, it is useful to put the various anatomic, physiologic, and pathologic reaction patterns discussed earlier in a clinical context by reviewing their involvement in a few common obstetric and neonatal disease syndromes (Box 23–2). Clearly such generalizations may be misleading in considering individual patients, but they can be useful in considering the range of possible diagnoses and causes in a particular case.

Preterm labor is most commonly associated with pathologic evidence of *acute chorioamnionitis*.[41, 58, 100, 105] The proportion of cases attributable to prior membrane rupture versus infection with intact membranes is difficult to specify. Five to ten percent of such cases will have pathologic evidence of prolonged infection. Because chorioamnionitis generally triggers preterm labor relatively rapidly, the majority of these cases probably represent membrane rupture with subsequent development of chorioamnionitis and preterm labor.

Most of the remaining cases of preterm birth fall into three groups: *placental abruption*, either acute or chronic, chronic maternal underperfusion with increased syncytial knotting, and uterine structural anomalies without associated placental abnormalities (e.g., cervical incompetence).[36, 73] Less commonly, preterm birth may be associated with *idiopathic chronic inflammation* (lymphoplasmacytic deciduitis, decidual perivasculitis, or eosinophilic chorionitis).[58, 100, 105]

■ **BOX 23–2**

CLINICOPATHOLOGIC CORRELATION

Preterm Labor
- Acute chorioamnionitis
- Abruption (acute or chronic)
- Chronic uteroplacental underperfusion
- Idiopathic chronic uterine inflammation

Intrauterine Growth Retardation
- Chronic uteroplacental underperfusion
- Villitis of unknown etiology
- Abruption (chronic)
- Fetal thrombotic vasculopathy
- Perivillous fibrin

Intrauterine Fetal Demise
- Large placenta with delayed villous maturation
- Massive fetomaternal hemorrhage/intervillous thrombi
- Hydrops fetalis (any cause)
- Multiple placental lesions

Neonatal Encephalopathy
- Abruption (acute)
- Umbilical cord accident
- Rupture of fetal vessels

Cerebral Palsy (Preterm)
- Severe villous edema
- Chorionic vessel thrombi
- Multiple placental lesions

Cerebral Palsy (Term)
- Fetal thrombotic vasculopathy
- Severe fetal chorioamnionitis
- Abruption (chronic)
- Multiple placental lesions

IUGR may be primarily constitutional, relating to small maternal size, malnutrition, or an anomalous fetus. When caused by uteroplacental disease, two clinicopathologic pictures predominate: *chronic uteroplacental underperfusion*, with or without associated hypertension, and *VUE*, generally in the absence of hypertension.[90, 93] Other less frequent uteroplacental causes of IUGR are *fetal thrombotic vasculopathy, chronic peripheral separation*, and *massive perivillous fibrin deposition* ("maternal floor infarction").

Intrauterine fetal demise, particularly at or near term, is often difficult to explain pathologically. One group at increased risk is that of large fetuses with histologically immature placentas, long umbilical cords, and reduced amniotic fluid.[8, 59, 67] A distinct subgroup in this category is infants of diabetic mothers who have long been known to be at increased risk for stillbirth. Two factors that may play a role in these gestations are susceptibility to cord accidents due to spatial constraints and *delayed villous maturation* due to continuing placental growth. This latter phenomenon could operate by decreasing adaptive mechanisms, such as syncytial knotting, that are available to mature placentas. A second common cause of stillbirth is *massive fetomaternal hemorrhage,* which is manifest in the placenta by intervillous thrombi and increased circulating nucleated red blood cells.[25] Fetomaternal hemorrhage and its accompanying anemia can cause congestive heart failure and *hydrops fetalis.* Clearly, hydrops of any cause can lead to stillbirth. Other causes of hydrops identifiable by placental examination include chronic infections such as human parvovirus B19, toxoplasmosis, and syphilis.[63] Finally, a third, smaller group of stillbirths show evidence of more than one of the following lesions: *chronic uteroplacental underperfusion, fetal thrombotic vasculopathy, VUE,* and *massive perivillous fibrin deposition.*[28]

Neonatal encephalopathy and cerebral palsy can be related to acute birth asphyxia, chronic intermittent hypoxia, chronic uteroplacental disease, or various combinations of these problems.[62] Placental findings associated with acute asphyxia include acute abruption, umbilical cord accidents, and *rupture of fetal vessels* (i.e., tears in villous parenchyma or umbilical or chorionic vessels).[5, 69, 98] Subacute or chronic intermittent stress is often accompanied by an increase in nucleated red blood cells in the placental circulation.[109, 110] Placental findings that have been associated with long-term neurologic impairment in preterm infants are severe villous edema, chorionic vessel thrombi, and multiple placental lesions.[95] Based on our own recent data and previous studies, long-term neurologic impairment in term infants may be associated with *fetal thrombotic vasculopathy, long-standing severe chorioamnionitis, chronic abruption,* and, again, multiple placental lesions.[9, 38, 61, 80, 96a, 118]

CONCLUSION

The placenta is the link that connects the clinical status of the neonate with underlying maternal and fetal disease processes. Careful evaluation of this organ not only provides useful diagnostic, prognostic, and therapeutic information but also enhances our overall understanding of perinatal biology. Communication among neonatologists, obstetricians, and placental pathologists brings together distinct pieces of a puzzle that none can fully solve alone. Through this process meaningful explanations of the reasons for adverse perinatal outcomes and their chances of recurrence can be provided for concerned physicians and family members.

■ REFERENCES

1. Abramowsky CR, et al: Decidual vasculopathy of the placenta in lupus erythematosus. N Engl J Med 303:668, 1980.

2. Acker D, et al: Abruptio placentae associated with cocaine use. Am J Obstet Gynecol 146:218, 1983.
3. Alles AJ, et al: The incidence of Factor V Leiden in fetal thrombotic events. Mod Pathol 10:1P, 1997.
4. Altshuler G: The placenta. In Sternberg SS (ed): Diagnostic Surgical Pathology. New York, Raven Press, 1989.
5. Altshuler G, et al: The human placental villitides: A review of chronic intrauterine infection. In Grundmann K (ed): Current Topics in Pathology. Berlin, Springer-Verlag, 1975.
6. Altshuler G, et al: Meconium-induced vasocontraction: A potential cause of cerebral and other fetal hypoperfusion and of poor pregnancy outcome. J Child Neurol 4:137, 1989.
7. Altshuler G, et al: Meconium-induced umbilical cord vascular necrosis and ulceration: A potential link between the placenta and poor pregnancy outcome. Obstet Gynecol 79:760, 1992.
8. Becker MJ, et al: The placenta. In: Pathology of Late Fetal Stillbirth. New York, Churchill Livingstone, 1989.
9. Bejar R, et al: Antenatal origin of neurologic damage in newborn infants: I. Preterm infants. Am J Obstet Gynecol 159:357, 1988.
10. Belchis DA, et al: Infantile choriocarcinoma: Reexamination of a potentially cureable entity. Cancer 72:2028, 1993.
11. Benirschke K: Recent trends in chorangiomas, especially those of multiple and recurrent chorangiomas. Pediatr Devel Pathol 2:264, 1999.
12. Benirschke K, et al: The Pathology of the Human Placenta. New York, Springer-Verlag, 1967.
13. Benirschke K, et al: Pathology of the Human Placenta, 4th ed. New York, Springer-Verlag, 2000.
14. Bey M, et al: The sonographic diagnosis of circumvallate placenta. Obstet Gynecol 78:515, 1991.
15. Blanc WA: Pathology of the placenta and cord in ascending and in haematogenous infection. In: Perinatal Infections (CIBA Foundation Symposium 77). London, Excerpta Medica, 1977.
16. Brace RA: Progress toward understanding the regulation of amniotic fluid volume: Water and solute fluxes in and through the fetal membranes. Placenta 16:1, 1995.
17. Brent RL: What is the relationship between birth defects and pregnancy bleeding? Teratology 48:93, 1993.
18. Brewer JI, et al: Gestational choriocarcinoma: Its origin in the placenta during seemingly normal pregnancy. Am J Surg Pathol 5:267, 1981.
19. Brosens IA, et al: The role of the spiral arteries in the pathogenesis of pre-eclampsia. In Wynn R (ed): Obstetrics and Gynecology Annual. New York, Appleton Century Crofts, 1972.
20. Caul EO, et al: Intrauterine infection with human parvovirus B19: A light and electron microscopy study. J Med Virol 24:55, 1988.
21. Chasnoff IJ, et al: Cocaine use in pregnancy. N Engl J Med 313:666, 1985.
22. College of American Pathologists Conference XIX on the Examination of the Placenta: Report of the working group on indications for placental examination. Arch Pathol Lab Med 115:701, 1991.
23. Collins JC, et al: Prenatal observation of umbilical cord abnormalities: A triple knot and torsion of the umbilical cord. Am J Obstet Gynecol 169:102, 1993.
24. Current concepts of infections of the fetus and newborn infant. In Remington JS, et al (eds): Infectious Diseases of the Fetus and Newborn Infant, 2nd ed. Philadelphia, WB Saunders Co, 1983.
25. de Almeida V, et al: Massive fetomaternal hemorrhage: Manitoba experience. Obstet Gynecol 83:323, 1994.
26. DeWolf F, et al: Fetal growth retardation and the maternal arterial supply of the human placenta in the absence of sustained hypertension. Br J Obstet Gynaecol 87:678, 1980.
27. DeWolf F, et al: Decidual vasculopathy and extensive placental infarction in a patient with repeated thromboembolic accidents, recurrent fetal loss, and a lupus anticoagulant. Am J Obstet Gynecol 142:829, 1982.
28. Driscoll SG: Autopsy following stillbirth: A challenge neglected. In Ryder OA, et al (eds): One Medicine. Berlin, Springer-Verlag, 1984.
29. Driscoll SG, et al: Congenital listeriosis: Diagnosis from placental studies. Obstet Gynecol 20:216, 1962.

30. Elliott WG: Placental toxoplasmosis: Report of a case. Am J Clin Pathol 53:413, 1970.

31. Fok RY, et al: The correlation of arterial lesions with umbilical artery Doppler velocimetry in the placentas of small-for-dates pregnancies. Obstet Gynecol 75:578, 1990.

32. Fox H: Pathology of the Placenta. London, WB Saunders Co, 1978.

33. Genest D, et al: Placental findings correlate with neonatal death in extremely premature infants (24–32 weeks): A study of 150 cases. Lab Invest 68:126A, 1993.

34. Gersell DJ, et al: Chronic chorioamnionitis: A clinicopathologic study of 17 cases. Int J Gynecol Pathol 10:217, 1991.

35. Giles WB, et al: Fetal umbilical artery flow velocity waveforms and placental resistance: Pathological correlation. Br J Obstet Gynaecol 92:31, 1985.

36. Golan A, et al: Incompetence of the uterine cervix. Obstet Gynecol Surv 44:96, 1989.

37. Gomez R, et al: The fetal inflammatory response syndrome. Am J Obstet Gynecol 179:194, 1998.

38. Grafe MR: The correlation of prenatal brain damage with placental pathology. J Neuropathol Exp Neurol 53:407, 1994.

39. Greco MA, et al: Phenotype of villous stromal cells in placentas with cytomegalovirus, syphilis, and nonspecific villitis. Am J Pathol 141:835, 1992.

40. Harris BA: Peripheral placental separation: A review. Obstet Gynecol Surv 43:577, 1988.

41. Hillier SL, et al: A case-control study of chorioamniotic infection and histologic chorioamnionitis in prematurity. N Engl J Med 319:972, 1988.

42. Hood IC, et al: The inflammatory response in candidal chorioamnionitis. Hum Pathol 14:984, 1983.

43. Hyde S, et al: A model of bacterially induced umbilical vein spasm, relevant to fetal hypoperfusion. Obstet Gynecol 73:966, 1989.

44. Johnson A, et al: Mosaicism in chorionic villus sampling: An association with poor perinatal outcome. Obstet Gynecol 75:573, 1990.

45. Johnson SF, et al: Twin placentation and its complications. Semin Perinatal 10:9, 1986.

46. Kalousek D, et al: Chromosomal mosaicism in term placentas and its association with high incidence of abnormal intrauterine development. Lab Invest 66:6P, 1991.

47. Kalousek DK, et al: Chromosomal mosaicism confined to the placenta in human conceptions. Science 221:665, 1983.

48. Kaplan C, et al: Identification of erythrocytes in intervillous thrombi: A study using immunoperoxidase identification of hemoglobins. Hum Pathol 13:554, 1982.

49. Khong TY: Acute atherosis in pregnancies complicated by hypertension, small-for-gestational age infants and diabetes mellitus. Arch Pathol Lab Med 115:722, 1991.

50. Kitzmiller JL, et al: Decidual arteriopathy in hypertension and diabetes in pregnancy: Immunofluorescent studies. Am J Obstet Gynecol 141:773, 1981.

51. Knowles S, et al: Umbilical cord sclerosis as an indicator of congenital syphilis. J Clin Pathol 42:1157, 1989.

52. Knox WF, et al: Villitis of unknown aetiology: Its incidence and significance in placentae from a British population. Placenta 5:395, 1984.

53. Kouyoumdijian A: Velamentous insertion of the umbilical cord. Obstet Gynecol 56:737, 1980.

54. Labarrere C, et al: Absence of Wharton's jelly around the umbilical cord: An unusual cause of perinatal mortality. Placenta 6:555, 1985.

55. Labarrere CA, et al: Immunohistologic evidence that villitis in human normal term placentas is an immunologic lesion. Am J Obstet Gynecol 162:515, 1990.

56. Landing BH: Amnion nodosum: A lesion of the placenta associated with deficient secretion of fetal urine. Am J Obstet Gynecol 60:1339, 1950.

57. Lapointe N, et al: Transplacental transmission of HTLV-III virus. N Engl J Med 312:1325, 1985.

58. Lettieri L, et al: Does "idiopathic" preterm labor resulting in preterm birth exist? Am J Obstet Gynecol 168:1480, 1993.

59. Leveno KJ, et al: Prolonged pregnancy: I. Observations concerning the causes of fetal distress. Am J Obstet Gynecol 150:465, 1984.

60. Lin HH, et al: Transplacental leakage of HBeAg-positive maternal blood as the most likely route in causing intrauterine infection with hepatitis B virus. J Pediatr 111:877, 1987.

61. Lipitz S, et al: Midtrimester bleeding: Variables which affect the outcome of pregnancy. Gynecol Obstet Invest 32:24, 1991.

62. Low JA, et al: The clinical diagnosis of asphyxia responsible for brain damage in the human fetus. Am J Obstet Gynecol 167:11, 1992.

63. Machin GA: Hydrops revisited: Literature review of 1,414 cases published in the 1980's. Am J Med Genet 34:366, 1989.

64. MacLennan AH: The ultrastructure of human trophoblast in spontaneous and induced hypoxia using a system of organ culture: A comparison and ultrastructural changes in preeclampsia and placental insufficiency. Br J Obstet Gynecol 72:113, 1972.

65. Manco-Johnson MJ, et al: Severe neonatal protein-C deficiency: Prevalence and thrombotic risk. J Pediatr 119:793, 1991.

66. Mandsager NT, et al: Maternal floor infarction of placenta: Prenatal diagnosis and clinical significance. Obstet Gynecol 83:750, 1994.

67. McLean FH, et al: Postterm infants: Too big or too small? Am J Obstet Gynecol 164:619, 1991.

68. Miller ME, et al: Compression-related defects from early amnion rupture: Evidence for mechanical teratogenesis. J Pediatr 98:292, 1981.

69. Miller PW, et al: Dating the time interval from meconium passage to birth. Obstet Gynecol 66:459, 1985.

70. Moustofi-Zadeh M, et al: Postmortem manifestations of echovirus 11 sepsis in five newborn infants. Hum Pathol 14:818, 1983.

71. Moustofi-Zadeh M, et al: Placental evidence of cytomegalovirus infection of the fetus and neonate. Arch Pathol Lab Med 108:403, 1984.

72. Naeye RL: Do placental weights have clinical significance? Hum Pathol 18:387, 1987.

73. Naeye RL: Pregnancy hypertension, placental evidences of low utero-placental blood flow and spontaneous premature delivery. Hum Pathol 20:441, 1989.

74. Naeye RL: Disorders of the Placenta, Fetus, and Neonate. St. Louis, Mosby–Year Book, 1992.

75. Naeye RL, et al: Abruptio placentae and perinatal death: A prospective study. Am J Obstet Gynecol 128:740, 1977.

76. Naeye RL, et al: The clinical significance of placental villous edema. Pediatrics 71:588, 1983.

77. Naeye RL, et al: Antenatal infections. In: Risk Factors in Pregnancy and Diseases of the Fetus and Newborn. Baltimore, Williams & Wilkins, 1983.

78. Naftolin F, et al: The syndrome of chronic abruptio placentae, hydrorrhea, and circumvallate placenta. Am J Obstet Gynecol 116:347, 1973.

79. Nelson DM, et al: Trophoblast interaction with fibrin matrix: Epithelialization of perivillous fibrin deposits as a mechanism for villous repair in the human placenta. Am J Pathol 136:855, 1990.

80. Nelson KB, et al: Antecedents of cerebral palsy: Multivariate analysis of risk. N Engl J Med 315:81, 1986.

81. Novak R, et al: Histologic analysis of placental tissue in first trimester abortions. Pediatr Pathol 8:477, 1988.

82. Page Faulk W, et al: Immunology of coagulation control in human placentae [abstract]. Am J Reprod Immunol Microbiol 16:113, 1988.

83. Qureshi F, et al: Placental histopathology in syphilis. Hum Pathol 24:779, 1993.

84. Qureshi F, et al: *Candida* funisitis: A clinicopathologic study of 32 cases. Pediatr Dev Pathol 1:118, 1998.

85. Ramsey EM, et al: Placental Vasculature and Circulation. Philadelphia, WB Saunders Co, 1980.

86. Rand JH, Wu X-X: Antiphospholipid-mediated disruption of the Annexin-V antithrombotic shield: A new mechanism for thrombosis in the antiphospholipid syndrome. Thromb Haemost 82:649, 1999.

87. Rayne SC, et al: Placental thrombi and other vascular lesions: Classification, morphology, and clinical correlations. Pathol Res Pract 189:2, 1993.

88. Read JA, et al: Placenta accreta: Changing clinical aspects and outcome. Obstet Gynecol 56:31, 1980.

89. Redline RW: Placenta and adnexa in late pregnancy. In Reed GB, et al (eds): Diseases of the Fetus and Newborn, 2nd ed. London, Chapman & Hall Medical, 1995.

90. Redline RW: Placental pathology: The neglected link between basic disease mechanisms and untoward pregnancy outcome. Curr Opin Obstet Gynecol 7:10, 1995.

91. Redline RW, et al: Clinical and pathological aspects of recurrent placental villitis. Hum Pathol 16:727, 1985.

92. Redline RW, et al: Villitis of unknown etiology is associated with major infiltration of fetal tissue by maternal inflammatory cells, Am J Pathol 143:473, 1993.

93. Redline RW, et al: Patterns of placental injury: Correlations with gestational age, placental weight, and clinical diagnosis. Arch Pathol Lab Med 118:698, 1994.

94. Redline RW, et al: Fetal thrombotic vasculopathy: The clinical significance of extensive avascular villi. Hum Pathol 26:80, 1995.

95. Redline RW, et al: Placental lesions associated with neurologic impairment and cerebral palsy in very low birth weight infants. Arch Pathol Lab Med 122:1091, 1998.

96. Redline RW, Wilson-Costello D: Chronic peripheral separation of placenta: The significance of diffuse chorioamnionic hemosiderosis. Am J Clin Pathol 111:804, 1999.

96a Redline RW, O'Riordan MA: Placental lesions associated with cerebral palsy and neurologic impairment following term birth. Arch Pathol Lab Med 124:1785, 2000.

97. Rochelson B, et al: A quantitative analysis of placental vasculature in the third-trimester fetus with autosomal trisomy. Obstet Gynecol 75:59, 1990.

98. Rogers BB, et al: Fetal acidosis and placental pathology. Lab Invest 62:85A, 1990.

99. Romero R, et al: Infection and preterm labor. Clin Obstet Gynecol 31:553, 1988.

100. Romero R, et al: The preterm labor syndrome: Biochemical, cytologic, immunologic, pathologic, microbiologic, and clinical evidence that preterm labor is a heterogeneous disease. Am J Obstet Gynecol 168:288, 1993.

101. Rothman LA, et al: Placental and fetal involvement by maternal malignancy: A report of rectal carcinoma and review of the literature. Am J Obstet Gynecol 116:1023, 1973.

102. Russell P: Inflammatory lesions of the human placenta. Placenta 1:227, 1980.

103. Russell P, et al: Placental abnormalities of congenital syphilis. Am J Dis Child 128:160, 1974.

104. Russell P, et al: Recurrent reproductive failure due to severe villitis of unknown etiology. J Reprod Med 24:93, 1980.

105. Salafia CM, et al: Placental pathologic findings in preterm birth. Am J Obstet Gynecol 165:934, 1991.

106. Seemayer TA: The graft-versus-host reaction: A pathogenetic mechanism of experimental and human disease. In Rosenberg HS, et al (eds): Perspectives in Pediatric Pathology. New York, Masson, 1980.

107. Shanklin DR, et al: Massive subchorial thrombohaematoma (Breus' mole). Br J Obstet Gynaecol 82:476, 1975.

108. Smith DW: Recognizable Patterns of Human Deformation. Philadelphia, WB Saunders Co, 1987.

109. Soothill PW, et al: Prenatal asphyxia, hyperlacticaemia, hypoglycaemia, and erythroblastosis in growth retarded fetuses. BMJ 294:1051, 1987.

110. Thilaganathan B, et al: Umbilical cord blood erythroblast count as an index of intrauterine hypoxia. Arch Dis Child 70:F192, 1994.

111. Tominaga T, et al: Accommodation of the human placenta to hypoxia. Am J Obstet Gynecol 94:679, 1966.

112. Trudinger BJ, et al: Flow velocity waveforms in the maternal uteroplacental and fetal umbilical placental circulations. Am J Obstet Gynecol 152:155, 1985.

113. Vanlijnschoten G, et al: Intra-observer and inter-observer variation in the interpretation of histological features suggesting chromosomal abnormality in early abortion specimens. Histopathology 22:25, 1993.

114. Van Pampus MG, et al: High prevalence of hemostatic abnormalities in women with a history of severe preeclampsia. Am J Obstet Gynecol 180:1146, 1999.

115. Vergani P, et al: Risk factors for pulmonary hypoplasia in second-trimester premature rupture of membranes. Am J Obstet Gynecol 170:1359, 1994.

116. Wallenburg HCS, et al: The pathogenesis of placental infarction: I. A morphologic study in the human placenta. Am J Obstet Gynecol 116:835, 1973.

117. Wilkins-Haug L, et al: Frequency of confined placental mosaicism in pregnancies with IUGR. Am J Obstet Gynecol 166:350, 1992.

118. Williams MA, et al: Adverse infant outcomes associated with first-trimester vaginal bleeding. Obstet Gynecol 78:14, 1991.

IV The Delivery Room

24 Anesthesia for Labor and Delivery

John S. McDonald

Jay J. Jacoby

Health care consumers clearly understand and expect that current regional anesthesia techniques are safe for the mother and not injurious to the fetus or neonate. At no other time in the history of medicine has it been more important for the specialists of neonatology, perinatology, and anesthesiology to cooperate and deliver a truly team-directed care continuum. One slip of communication or one disregard for fully informing the other colleague in this closely knit health care team can spell disaster for a good outcome. The team concept in labor and delivery is the key element in successful outcomes in high-risk obstetrics management. We see examples during high-risk gestations, in which obstetricians coordinate efforts with their trusted and skilled colleagues in the fields of neonatal medicine and anesthesiology.[3] The end result is and will continue to be favorable outcomes in situations in which a decade ago there was slim hope for such results.

A team concept for delivery of information to expectant mothers is also important. Many expectant mothers can come away from such discussions better informed and armed with knowledge that can dispel many of the "stories of childbirth" that haunt them so often. Psychological well-being can be promoted also by talking with patients to dispel many unfounded fears. At the same time, knowledge can also strengthen and empower the pregnant patient who is educated on understanding the physiology of pregnancy and expected changes of pregnancy by the anesthesiologist, obstetrician, and neonatologist together as a team.

The purpose of this chapter is to discuss specific contributions of the anesthesiologist member of the team and current methods of management of obstetric anesthesia. We also hope that the information presented may serve to enlighten our obstetric and pediatric colleagues in regard to many newer aspects of anesthesia management and allow them to develop both an understanding and an appreciation of the importance of the role of the anesthesiologist in this valuable team effort.

ANALGESIA FOR NORMAL LABOR AND DELIVERY

In the past three decades, the most popular intrapartum analgesic method today—lumbar epidural—made a clean sweep over all other challengers, including systemic analgesics and paracervical, pudendal, and subarachnoid blocks. Recent popularized methods also include patient-controlled analgesia by means of the systemic method and patient-controlled epidural anesthesia for labor pain control.

NATURAL CHILDBIRTH

Natural childbirth has relieved some labor pain in some patients for many years. It was introduced at a time that it was accepted as a godsend because of its contribution toward pain relief in lieu of other quasi-effective pain relief methods. Confusion about the exact nature of labor pain and its specific treatment is often due to lack of experience and many times to rank ignorance. This is because of inadequate dissemination of information about the other commonly available and newer modalities of treatment. Vociferous proponents of natural childbirth may have added to, rather than cleared up, many misconceptions. For example, one of these misconceptions is the insistence that pain need not occur during normal labor and that when it does it is due to modern cultural and environmental factors.

The natural childbirth method was popularized by Dick-Read[6] and others in the 1930s. An important contribution made by this method is it did emphasize the importance of physical training, health, and stamina in withstanding the rigors of labor and delivery.[13] Participants are schooled in the skills of conditioning and the concept that the birth process is a contest between themselves and the forces of parturition. In many patients this is an effective tool to combat pain and a sense of loss of control by the patient. Furthermore, the mother who is conditioned and in optimal physical shape fares better during the labor and delivery process than her unconditioned counterpart who is in poor physical condition.

SYSTEMIC METHODS

Opioids are potent individual narcotics that serve as primary agents for systemic pain relief in labor. Systemic analgesics are important to stem first-stage labor pain, because patients generally fear they will not be able to handle the severity of pain they believe they may encounter. What is different now as compared with a decade ago is that patients often believe strongly that it is their right to experience either a pain-free or nearly pain-free labor and delivery. Part of this latter feeling has developed from the current knowledge base that lumbar epidural anesthesia is now safe for both the mother and infant and it provides excellent pain relief at the same time. Some pregnant mothers have read or heard sordid stories about labor from others and secretly have become terrified of the prospect of labor pain or, worse, the possibility of inadequately managed labor pain. An open discussion should be held with the patient about the planned use of drugs for early first-stage labor, the type of anesthesia for later second-stage labor and delivery, and other medications such as oxytocics and Rh(D) immune globulin and their purposes, advantages, and disadvantages.

It is prudent to assure the patient and her family that the planned techniques and agents will be used to give the optimal benefit for both the mother and infant throughout the entire course of labor and delivery. The patient should be advised that in the early portion of labor the uterine musculature is more susceptible to systemically administered opioid type of medications and elevated levels of local anesthetics. After such instruction the patient and her family will be more understanding when the administration of these drugs is postponed until the labor curve is well developed (e.g., at 4 to 5 cm cervical dilation in primigravidas and 3 to 4 cm in multiparas). Centers with fewer than adequate personnel to provide anesthesia coverage in the evenings and nighttime hours can use either intravenous or intramuscular analgesia for systemic analgesia. In this way advantage is taken of the fact that this technique requires less knowledge of anatomy and less technical skill than regional methods.

The 1990s have provided us with a new level of maternal pain relief that supersedes the methods of earlier days. For example, first-stage labor pain in prior days was often alleviated by either intramuscular administration of meperidine (Demerol) or intermittent inhalation of trichloroethylene, methoxyflurane, or nitrous oxide; these methods are described in more detail by Bonica and coworkers.[1] The new methods of pain relief have attained a level of sophistication that affords excellent pain relief with concomitant safety for the infant and mother. This has been due largely to the development of the lumbar epidural technique far beyond its original single-dose bolus of anesthetic for local pain relief to the present

continuous microapplication of combined anesthetics and opioids for local effect. In addition, the first stage can also be managed by use of the patient-controlled analgesia technique, in which the patient administers her own medication on an ongoing basis as circumstances require.

The most important change in opioid administration in the past decade has been the advent of patient-controlled intravenous analgesia. In addition, small amounts of opioids do not have an adverse effect on the intrauterine fetus. Large amounts have a respiratory depressant effect on the neonate in the early minutes and hours after delivery. There are still some centers in the United States that do not have a sophisticated obstetric-anesthesiology service; in these centers, systemic pain relief provided by the intramuscular or intravenous administration of analgesics can help considerably to alleviate pain for parturients in the first stage of labor. The following is a brief description of some of the agents used in systemic relief of labor pain.

Sedatives

The agents currently in vogue in obstetrics include the barbiturates, the benzodiazepines, and the phenothiazines. Barbiturates are not analgesic agents at all. They once were popular for stand-alone use in the early latent phase of labor, when 100 to 200 mg would be given intramuscularly to determine whether patients really were in labor.[28] Today they rarely are used in these large doses because of their disorienting properties, and they are less frequently used in combination with narcotics because of the known late and lasting effects on the neonate in the first few days of life.

In the benzodiazepine group the only agent frequently used in obstetrics is diazepam, which has been studied intensively for the past 20 years. The benzodiazepines are not analgesics; their only beneficial effect is from their tranquilizing properties. In addition, there are adverse effects on the neonate. Diazepam may cause temperature-regulation problems in the neonate that last for nearly a week. The drug competes with bilirubin for albumin-binding sites, possibly resulting in elevated levels of free bilirubin and thus increasing the possibility of development of kernicterus. The newest of the benzodiazepines, midazolam, has not been used extensively in obstetrics. It is more potent than diazepam and is the most popular tranquilizing agent used in general anesthesiology today.

The phenothiazines are potent tranquilizers that block the uptake of dopamine by brain receptors.[16] They are metabolized in the liver by oxidation and are excreted in the urine as generally inactive metabolites. They also have several untoward side effects, which are more maternal than fetal or neonatal. These side effects include some extrapyramidal reactions, instability of blood pressure as a result of effects on vasomotor reflexes and direct myocardial depression, and a reduction in seizure threshold. In addition, approximately 1% of patients given a phenothiazine intravenously will experience an allergic reaction typified as obstructive jaundice. Another serious but rare complication is the neuroleptic malignant syndrome. This condition develops in 2 to 3 days and is characterized by hyperthermia, hypertonicity of skeletal muscles, and instability of the autonomic nervous system, manifested by alterations in blood pressure, tachycardia, or cardiac arrhythmia. This severe complication is very rare, occurring in only 0.1% of patients treated with phenothiazines. The most popular drugs for use in women in labor are promethazine (Phenergan), propiomazine (Largon), and hydroxyzine pamoate (Vistaril).[25] Currently, as in past years, they are most commonly used in small doses in combination with narcotics. Given in this way they have not been found to produce more neonatal depression than narcotics alone.

Narcotics

One of the most exciting events in the 1970s was the discovery of opioid receptors. The highest concentrations of these receptors apparently are in the limbic system, the thalamus, the hypothalamus, and the substantia gelatinosa of the spinal cord; they also have been found in peripheral tissues.[7, 15] Generally, the receptors have been divided into the five classes of mu, delta, kappa, sigma, and epsilon.[14] The primary disadvantage of narcotics is that the sharp pain of labor is not completely obtunded. They also cause drowsiness and mental clouding, which are not desirable during childbirth. Narcotics often cause nausea and vomiting and sometimes itching, and in large doses they cause respiratory depression.

Morphine sulfate is the old standby in obstetrics and was the primary agent used for pain relief for decades. Meperidine replaced morphine when it was discovered that it does not penetrate the blood-brain barrier of the fetus as completely as morphine. After intramuscular injection, the effect of meperidine develops in 15 minutes, with a peak effect in 40 to 60 minutes, a half-life of 7 minutes, and total duration of 2 to 4 hours.[18] The majority of the drug is bound to maternal protein, with only 28% of it in the fetus and neonate. Meperidine has attained its prominence in obstetric analgesia by virtue of its relatively short duration of action in the mother and relatively low central nervous system penetration in the fetus and neonate as compared with morphine.[25] Nonetheless, neonatal depression can occur and apparently is related to the amount of unmetabolized meperidine that has been transferred from mother to fetus rather than to the presence of the active metabolite normeperidine.[27] Neonatal depression correlates best with the injection-delivery interval; it occurs most often when meperidine is administered 2 to 3 hours before delivery, whereas intervals of less than 1 hour are associated with essentially no ill effects. Alphaprodine (Nisentil) is structurally similar to meperidine, with a shorter duration of action, although fewer

pharmacologic data are available for this drug than for meperidine.

Butorphanol (Stadol) is a popular synthetic parenteral analgesic in obstetrics. It is approved by the Food and Drug Administration and the manufacturer for use as an obstetric analgesic by the intramuscular or the intravenous route. Its potency is 5 times that of morphine and 40 times that of meperidine. Butorphanol is 80% protein bound in the mother. The onset of action occurs 10 minutes after intravenous injection, and its duration is as long as 3 to 4 hours, with a half-life of 2.7 hours.[17] Butorphanol metabolism takes place in the liver by dealkylation and hydroxylation; excretion is through the kidney. Respiratory depression resulting from 2 mg of butorphanol is the same as that resulting from administration of 10 mg of morphine. The respiratory and narcotic effects of butorphanol can be reversed with naloxone. Studies concluded that butorphanol is superior to meperidine as an analgesic and has no neonatal neurobehavioral effects.[9] For these reasons, this drug is rapidly gaining in popularity.

Pentazocine (Talwin) is another synthetic analgesic with both opioid agonist and weak antagonist properties. Analgesia occurs 2 to 3 minutes after intravenous injection, yet the elimination half-life of the drug is 2 hours. Higher dosages have been associated with certain psychomimetic effects, such as hallucinations. There is less nausea and vomiting with pentazocine than with other drugs and less placental transfer. Studies comparing it with meperidine, however, have revealed similar levels of neonatal depression with equipotent dosages. This drug has not become popular because it lacks any clear advantage over other analgesics commonly used for labor.

Fentanyl (Sublimaze) became one of the most popular narcotic drugs used in anesthesiology operating room environs, and it has begun to gain some acceptance in certain obstetric anesthesia circles. Generally it is used more as an adjunctive agent with a local anesthetic in the epidural space rather than as a solitary agent for systemic pain relief.

In summary, drugs used for systemic pain relief in the first stage of labor should be injected intravenously in small increments to minimize total fetal drug exposure and to adjust the dose more effectively to counteract maternal discomfort as cervical dilation progresses. The intramuscular route may be used also, but larger doses are necessary to obtain similar relief. The most frequently used analgesic drugs are meperidine, fentanyl, and alphaprodine; hydroxyzine (Atarax) or promethazine (Phenergan) often is administered as a tranquilizer.

One of the most significant advances in recent years is the discovery of antibody-specific pain receptors. This paves the way for possible development of pain blockers that are devoid of some of the side effects of currently used pain medications. The developments in this field will be worthy of close scrutiny over the next decade. There may well be a time in the future when we will be able to describe pain relief medication that is so specific it will carry few if any untoward side effects.

LABOR MECHANICS IN RELATION TO ANESTHESIA

The practitioner of obstetric anesthesia demands considerable knowledge that encompasses both the understanding of the pharmacology of drugs that are used for sedation and analgesia for the first stage of labor and the understanding of the basic obstetric labor mechanics. Included among these mechanics of labor are attitude, lie, presentation, and position. *Attitude* refers to the posture of the fetus in relation to itself only. The normal attitude is with the fetal back arched, the cervical spine in flexion with the chin in contact with the chest, and the arms, thighs, knees, and feet in complete flexion. *Lie* refers to the long-axis relationship between the fetus and mother. The most common is longitudinal, with fetal and maternal spines parallel. Less common are the oblique, with the fetal spine at an angle with the mother's axis, and the transverse, in which the fetal spine is actually at a right angle to the maternal spinal axis. *Presentation* is the anatomic part of the fetus that descends first into the birth canal. Cephalic, or vertex, presentation is the most common, followed by breech and shoulder presentations. *Position* refers to a predetermined anatomic point on the child (the occiput, chin, or sacrum) in reference to the right or left side of the mother.

Understanding the mechanisms of labor with the most common occipitoanterior presentation provides a working general understanding of normal progress and aids decision making in regard to optimal anesthetic management. Labor progress results from two important opposing forces: (1) the positive labor forces, which include the activity of the uterus and other positive muscle groups, and (2) the negative labor forces, which include the resistant force from the pelvic musculature and the bony pelvis.

The classic descriptive cardinal movements of labor are descent, flexion, internal rotation, extension, external rotation, restitution, and expulsion. They occur in concert with each other. Engagement of the fetal presenting part occurs as it enters the superior plane of the pelvis. This usually occurs during the last weeks of pregnancy in primigravidas and often not until at the onset of labor in multigravidas. Early in the first stage of labor, uterine contractions dilate and efface the cervix.

Descent is the first downward movement for the birth of the child, and it is constant throughout the mechanisms of flexion, internal rotation, extension, restitution, and external rotation. Descent can be delayed by many factors, such as failure in dilation, pelvic disproportion, ineffective uterine activity, and overtly resistant pelvic soft tissues. Descent naturally occurs more slowly in primigravidas than in multigravidas. It is always estimated by the station of the presenting part in its position relative to the transverse plane of the ischial spines.

Flexion occurs as soon as the vertex meets with substantial resistance, and it continues until the chin becomes completely flexed on the chest. This is perhaps the most important of the cardinal movements of labor because it allows the smaller suboccipitobregmatic diameter of 9.5 cm to be the leading part of the fetus instead of the larger occipitofrontal diameter of approximately 11.5 cm. Thus, flexion is vital to descent because it impressively substitutes a smaller negotiating diameter for a larger one and this allows for passage through the narrowest part of the pelvis, the midpelvis.

Internal rotation refers to the forward rotational movement of the head with continued movement downward through the birth canal. Internal rotation is affected by the bony pelvis and the pelvic floor musculature, which are amazingly complex. A successful rotation indicates that the fetal part endures a spiraling motion because of the funnel shape of the pelvic muscles. In the final phase of internal rotation, the vertex negotiates this muscular sling and ends in the anteroposterior position. Furthermore, the larger aspect of the fetal head, the occiput, comes to occupy the larger space of the maternal forepelvis. This aspect of the cardinal movements of labor must be understood. It explains why the incidence of persistent posterior position may be increased in some mothers in whom the pelvic muscles are partially paralyzed by regional techniques such as epidural, caudal, or subarachnoid block.

Extension, external rotation, and *expulsion* are the final three movements. They do not play a major role with regard to analgesia and anesthesia and more properly are the concern of the obstetrician instead of the anesthesiologist.

Labor is continuous and is divided into three stages: the first stage is from the onset of labor through complete dilation of the cervix; the second stage starts with complete cervical dilation and terminates at delivery; and the third stage begins with delivery and ends with either spontaneous placental expulsion or manual extraction of the placenta. The progress of labor is deemed abnormal when the obstetrician decides that labor is not moving along in accordance with the expectations for a particular patient. Various factors that may be responsible for the abnormal progress are a prolonged latent phase, protracted active phase, and secondary arrest of cervical dilation. When abnormal progress occurs, augmentation of labor usually begins with administration of oxytocin, which is a synthetic chemical stimulant for the uterus. Labor augmented with oxytocin is not dissimilar to normal spontaneous labor.

NERVE BLOCK METHODS

The technique of paracervical block has belonged to the obstetrician since its inception and is a procedure still exclusively performed by the obstetrician. It is mentioned here to round out and to include all past utilized analgesic methods. The reason for paracervical block being relegated to this status is the many documented reports of adverse fetal-neonatal effects due to paracervical injection. These vary, with a full spectrum of problems from minor neonatal depression to full-blown severe cerebral insult and even death. This technique still is performed in certain parts of the country even today, yet it continues to decline in popularity and is now being replaced by heavier reliance on lumbar epidural analgesia at centers where anesthesiologists practice pain relief for labor and delivery. Its use continues in those areas where such anesthesia coverage by anesthesiologists is not possible and serves as a good method of pain relief for the mother—it is the danger posed to the fetus that is still worrisome. Attention to use of dilute rather than concentrated local anesthetics and use of slow delivery should help to reduce the complications just mentioned.

The pudendal block is another technique the obstetrician performs for second-stage pain relief. It is accomplished by the careful deposition of local anesthetic in a narrowly circumscribed area of the pudendal nerve where it closely approaches the ischial spines in its course through the pelvis and out to the perineum. It produces complete pain relief for the perineum during the second stage of labor. Usually 10 mL of 2% lidocaine or 10 mL of 0.25% bupivacaine is injected by the obstetrician on each side to obtain an adequate block. Although this technique usually is very safe, there have been reports of maternal toxic reactions and even maternal infection and abscess formation. Because the pudendal nerve is the major peripheral nerve supplying the lower vagina and perineum, this technique is sufficient to produce perineal anesthesia for spontaneous delivery, low forceps delivery, episiotomy, and repair. It is not necessary to block adjacent nerves such as the ilioinguinal, the genital branch of the genitofemoral, and the perineal branch of the posterior femoral cutaneous, thus simplifying the technique and adding to its popularity. Because the pudendal nerve is peripheral, satisfactory analgesia can be obtained with use of even dilute solutions of local anesthetics such as 1.0% lidocaine or 0.125% bupivacaine.

Alterations of any of the maternal major physiologic systems (e.g., respiratory and cardiovascular) are not a consequence, unless a mistake in injection occurs and the anesthetic is deposited intravenously. Maternal complications that have been reported include systemic toxic reaction, local nerve trauma, vaginal hematoma, and, in the worst scenario, infection through the greater sciatic foramen into the joint capsule of the ipsilateral femur. Inadvertent injection of an epinephrine solution instead of a local anesthetic has resulted in maternal or fetal death or both. Because the pudendal block is administered at the very end of the first stage of labor, its effect on labor is of little or no consequence. Although it does not alter the intensity, frequency, or duration of uterine activity, it may interrupt the afferent limb of the perineal reflex; thus, it may somewhat reduce the urge to use the Valsalva maneuver effectively.

Performance of the pudendal nerve block by the transvaginal approach is certainly the most common

and preferred method of achieving pudendal block. With this method the operator uses the second and third finger of the hand opposite from the side he or she is blocking to position the needle guide into place at the ischial spine. The needle guide is referred to as the "Iowa trumpet" and is vital to the success of the block, because otherwise the needle catches repeatedly in the vaginal folds. After the guide is in place, the operator inserts the needle until the mucosa is contacted. Then the needle is inserted a few millimeters, and the entire 10 mL is injected slowly over 20 to 30 seconds, with aspiration before beginning and after each 2 mL. The needle must not be inserted as deeply as possible, because the local anesthetic could be deposited behind the nerve as it sweeps behind the ischial spine on its course down the vagina to the perineum.

The local infiltration block is accomplished by subcutaneous injection of a local anesthetic. Its primary use is for episiotomy pain. The block typically is administered just before maximal perineal distention by injection of 5 to 10 mL of 1% lidocaine without epinephrine. The principal advantage is that small amounts of local anesthetic can be injected into the subcutaneous compartment in which small nerve endings innervate peripheral tissues without seeking a specific nerve. The action is swift because the nerves are small and extremely sensitive even to dilute concentrations of local anesthetic.

One of the first uses of local infiltration or field block was by Greenhill, an obstetrician. Although it is a most simple technique to master, its practical application is not always satisfactory, because it does not produce complete pain relief. Although local relief may be adequate for the actual episiotomy, it is not sufficient to obliterate pain from perineal distention. It has no effect on labor, no detrimental maternal effects when properly applied, and no untoward fetal or neonatal effects.

The best method of infiltrating the subcutaneous tissues is to use a small-bore long needle (25 gauge), which can be the length of a spinal needle. This choice allows point penetration and subcutaneous infiltration of local anesthetic along the path the needle follows. In this fashion a solid line or block of analgesia can be created for the subsequent incision. Only a few minutes is required to ensure that adequate analgesia is obtained through the action of the local anesthetic.

REGIONAL METHODS

In the late 1950s papers were published that noted infants born of mothers who received regional anesthesia instead of general anesthesia were more active and vigorous at delivery. This was a fair comparison at the time, because general anesthesia meant deep levels of depression with agents such as cyclopropane, ether, and halothane. These older anesthetic agents are no longer used. Currently, general anesthesia for cesarean section is accomplished with short-acting muscle relaxants and mental obtundation with minuscule amounts of thiopental and only a 50% concentration of nitrous oxide. Because the mother has minimal drug exposure, the fetus also is exposed minimally whether administered through the intravenous, epidural, or pulmonary route.[8]

The superiority of epidural analgesia over narcotics and other systemic drugs in decreasing maternal work and oxygen consumption and maternal and fetal metabolic acidosis has been demonstrated impressively by many investigators.[19, 20] The continuous technique carries the added benefit of providing uninterrupted pain relief during the painful part of the first stage and the entire second and third stages. The continued reduction of concentration of local anesthetics used in labor also provides a safer environment for the fetus and neonate now as compared with even 5 to 10 years ago. This reduction has been promoted by the realization that we were using too highly concentrated anesthetics in the past. It also is a testimonial to the concerns for better childbirth methods whether they include obstetric or anesthesia issues. The overall tendency has been to provide safer, less painful, and more logical concern for the welfare of both the mother and her child.

SUBARACHNOID BLOCK

The subarachnoid block is a long-trusted, long-honored technique for terminal second-stage pain relief. Its use is very popular for primiparas; early on when 0.2 mg to 0.4 mg of tetracaine was administered with the patient in the sitting position, it usually produced a very low lumbar or sacral block. The latter was referred to as a saddle block, and it became extremely useful because of its effectiveness in providing perineal pain relief and its low incidence of complications. It is difficult to identify a more rapidly acting, dependable, or safe technique. The only difference today is that most saddle blocks are performed using the local anesthetic bupivacaine.

Subarachnoid block is safe and effective for cesarean section delivery if certain hazards are avoided. First, it is necessary to reduce the possibility of hypotension by providing rapid intravenous hydration just before maternal sympathetic blockade. Second, it is necessary to displace the uterus off the vena cava by lateral tilt. Third, maternal blood pressure must be monitored every 30 seconds for the first 5 minutes for early detection of a fall in maternal blood pressure so that immediate and effective countermeasures can be instituted.

Presently, the procedure is performed by anesthesiologists at most larger centers. The most popular drugs are tetracaine in a 0.5% concentration, lidocaine in a 5% concentration, or bupivacaine. Although the procedure often is deemed simple and safe, it has lethal consequences if attention to detail is not maintained, including control of the level of the anesthetic, alveolar ventilation, and maternal blood pressure.

LUMBAR EPIDURAL BLOCK

The pioneer work of one man, Dr. John G. P. Cleland, who dedicated a portion of his life to identifying the pain pathways of labor, stands as a monumental memorial to him. He worked with minimal equipment and spent extra hours and evenings during his training in surgery because he was sensitive to the anguish and cries of pain from the obstetric floors. His data, published in 1933, formed the foundation on which pain relief through lumbar epidural and caudal epidural blocks began.

Over the years the lumbar epidural method of pain relief for labor and cesarean section has undergone modifications.[5] Currently, the segmental lumbar epidural block is the single most useful and popular technique for providing first-stage analgesia with later second-stage pain relief.[26] It also minimizes the complications that formerly were associated with the larger spread of sympathetic block.[9] An alternative approach is the use of the lumbar epidural block for the first stage. The caudal epidural block for the second stage of labor is now infrequently used and when it is used it is mostly at medical teaching centers. This difficult technique allows the physician to insert the epidural catheters when the patient is not so uncomfortable and subsequently to administer less medication when the patient's discomfort demands pain relief. Even though the effects of the epidural block are complex, the incidence of hypotension is low compared with that with subarachnoid block. Spinal anesthesia predictably produces greater depression of heart rate, cardiac output, and mean arterial pressure than the lumbar epidural method.

Instances may occur when the aforementioned regional blocks are not fully effective in relieving pain during the second stage. In such an instance inhalation analgesia with nitrous oxide–oxygen (50% concentration) or subanesthetic concentrations of enflurane or isoflurane may be used to manage an otherwise extremely uncomfortable or uncooperative patient. A subanesthetic dose of ketamine is also very effective.

Psychoprophylaxis, with a competent staff dedicated to the technique and a suitably motivated patient, also may be effective in relieving the discomfort of the second stage. Ideally, the combination of psychoprophylaxis for early labor and the lumbar epidural or caudal epidural technique for added relief and later comfort during the bearing down efforts of the second stage provides optimal management of the normal patient.

INHALATION METHODS

Inhalation analgesia refers to the pain relief achieved for a brief period of time during the expulsion phase of the second stage of labor. This method of obtaining second-stage pain relief is quite old and was used primarily in the 1940s, 1950s, and 1960s to provide brief periods of pain relief for the mother when no regional technique was available. For the most part it was administered by either nurse anesthetists or nurses who were schooled simply in the technique of applying a mask to a patient and administering nitrous oxide–oxygen (the favorite combination of inhalation drugs) for a brief period during expulsion of the child.

There is a major difference between anesthesia with loss of consciousness and analgesia only, associated with full awareness. The latter technique provides for patient cooperation and alertness because of the small concentration of the drug administered, yet it offers the benefits of pain relief. Primary concerns in use of the inhalation technique include careful maintenance of the airway, prevention of aspiration, and maintenance of a light plane of analgesia. This technique also can be used to supplement inadequate blocks for perineal discomfort during second-stage expulsion. This method still has a role to play in brief delivery periods for patients who have inadequate analgesia.

One of the greatest concerns about using this technique is to make sure the patient does not enter the second stage and develop delirium and unwanted reflexes such as vomiting. All obstetric patients are asked to maintain a nothing-by-mouth status when they go into labor. The first concern of anyone working in the area of obstetric anesthesia is to prevent vomiting and aspiration, which can be done only when it is anticipated constantly. Inhalation techniques, when used in skilled hands, can provide an important adjunct for pain relief for the mother while presenting little or no threat to the fetus.

ANESTHESIA FOR SPECIAL CIRCUMSTANCES

DIABETES MELLITUS

One of the most significant endocrine disease states that impacts pregnancy and obstetric and anesthesia management is diabetes mellitus (see Chapter 15). This endocrine abnormality is unique in its effect on the health and welfare of both the mother and the infant. It can, for example, endanger the fetus because of large fetal size, it can result in placental deterioration, and it can cause both hyperglycemic and hypoglycemic threats that negatively impact both the fetus and the neonate. Thus, providing anesthesia for the diabetic obstetric patient demands close cooperation and coordination between the obstetrics team and anesthesiologist. Again, a prime example of this is a situation in which a preload administration of an intravenous bolus of 5% dextrose solution by an anesthesiologist could cause serious rebound hypoglycemia in the newborn and could initiate problems subsequently for the neonatologist. The alternative would be for the diabetic patient to receive the aforementioned preload with a solution that does not contain glucose.

Because oxygen supply to and carbon dioxide removal from the fetus are the primary determinants of fetal safety in utero, they must be protected at all costs for a diabetic's fetus, who, because of the mother's diabetes and the placental vascular disease, already has only a small margin of placental reserve. Because gas exchange depends on blood supply to the intervillous space, which in turn depends on maternal blood pressure, the latter must be maintained regardless of the analgesic technique chosen. The primary concern or complication of regional techniques has been maternal hypotension and the attendant reduction in blood flow to the intervillous space. We already noted that in the diabetic patient such an event can jeopardize the fetus already placed at risk. An important point here is to understand that no mother wants pain relief at the cost of risk to her unborn baby. Therefore, the specialty of obstetric anesthesiology always must have as its primary concern safety for the mother and fetus, followed by the secondary concern for pain relief of the mother.

DYSMATURITY

Dysmaturity refers to more than just a postmature fetus (see Chapter 13). It refers to an aging of the placenta and thus presents a notable risk to the fetus. Thus, the dysmature fetus is at risk similar to the fetus of a diabetic mother as noted earlier. The organ causing the direct risk is once again the placenta or lifeline organ, which, instead of enhancing gas exchange, undergoes degenerative change that creates greater and greater threats of hypoxia. Yet, although the fetus' continued life in utero is progressively threatened, it may do quite well in extrauterine life. Because of diminished placental perfusion, the anesthesiologist must be careful to maintain maximal blood flow to the fetus, who may have no placental reserve. Therefore, again, any method of analgesia that lowers maternal pressure may result in fetal embarrassment. The end result will be determined by the duration of the embarrassment. For example, a brief period of hypotension that is quickly diagnosed and successfully treated may not be of any consequence to the fetus but a longer period may cause dire consequences.

A secondary concern in dysmaturity is excessive fetal entrapment of drugs administered to the mother when that fetus is acidotic in utero. The neonatologist must be alerted to this possibility, because an initially vigorous infant may give a false sense of security to the medical team. Later, that very newborn may be diagnosed with hypotonia, hypotension, and respiratory depression that develop only as the drugs are flushed out into the system. The latter situation again underlines the importance of close communication and coordination between the neonatologist and anesthesiologist.

Providing labor and delivery analgesia is now not difficult for these cases but used to tax the ability of the obstetric anesthesiologist. Use of first-stage psychoprophylaxis with a carefully administered segmental epidural agent may be logical, because it allows the placement of an epidural catheter early in labor before the mother gets too uncomfortable. This can then be activated with a small continuous administration of local anesthetic and narcotic during cervical dilation.[19] Administering 4 to 6 mL of either 0.125% bupivacaine or 0.0625% bupivacaine with sufentanil by continuous infusion in the epidural space presents no threat of maternal hypotension.[29]

For the second stage several possibilities can be considered. Either 5 to 10 mL of 2% lidocaine can be administered through the epidural catheter, or a "saddle block spinal" or even analgesic concentrations of nitrous oxide in oxygen can be administered during the expulsion phase.

Cesarean section probably is done best with the patient under general anesthesia if there is definite evidence of fetal compromise identified by the obstetrician. This usually obviates any possible threat of hypotension to the already embarrassed fetus during the induction or subsequent delivery process. On the other hand, if the fetus is dysmature but otherwise healthy and not compromised, and if the mother insists on being awake for delivery, a modified epidural method can be considered. Naturally this entire scenario with all of its attendant risks is carefully spelled out to the parents for their complete understanding and agreement. Such a procedure can be carried out with minimal risk to the fetus, but it must be understood that in some rare situations of extensive preexisting fetal compromise the risk indeed may still be too great.

PREMATURITY

The premature infant has always been considered at an increased risk of central nervous system depression from anesthesia and analgesia (see Chapter 16). Therefore, the use of narcotic analgesics for discomfort in the first stage of labor should be restricted severely, specifically in centers with limited neonatal care. Relief of pain during the first stage of labor can be effected by use of selective regional analgesia while maternal and fetal homeostasis is maintained. Continuous segmental lumbar epidural analgesia is recommended for use with a minimal amount of longer-lasting local anesthetic and narcotic to reduce maternal and fetal drug accumulation. Lumbar epidural analgesia for first-stage labor and caudal epidural analgesia for second-stage labor also may be used. This is the same as described in the section on dysmaturity. The use of a paracervical block in premature labors should be avoided because of the hazard of inadvertently elevating fetal anesthetic drug levels as a result of fetal injection or even inadvertent intravascular injection. This may result in fetal arrhythmias secondary to the high local anesthetic blood levels that can lead to cardiac arrest in utero.

Several alternative forms of analgesia are available for the second stage of labor. A subarachnoid block may be restricted to the sacral area by manipulating the patient's position and using a hyperbaric solution to effect a true saddle block; this involves sacral nerves of S2 to S4. A bilateral pudendal block or local infiltration also may be used for restricted perineal analgesia because an effective bilateral block involves the identical S2 to S4 nerves. Alternatively, nitrous oxide can be administered during the pushing stages to offset the pain associated with maximal perineal distention. This can be given either intermittently or continuously, but either way it demands the full-time care of the anesthesiologist.

Psychoprophylaxis also may be an important adjunct to the management of the premature patient, chiefly because of high maternal motivation. The combination of psychoprophylaxis for the early first stage of labor followed by segmental lumbar epidural analgesia alone or with segmental caudal epidural analgesia may be one of the optimal choices in such premature labors.

TOXEMIA

Toxemia of pregnancy is also referred to as the syndrome of preeclampsia (see Chapter 14). The syndrome is manifested by three salient features: hypertension, edema, and proteinuria. For purposes of classification it is subdivided into mild, moderate, and severe categories. As in the previously discussed disease processes (i.e., diabetes and dysmaturity), the placenta is the affected end target organ, because generalized arterial disease is the primary problem. Once again, in the disease entity of toxemia blood supply to the growing fetus is the special consideration. Careful plans must be made for analgesia and anesthesia, because the use of regional blockade, as noted earlier, may result in serious sequelae for both mother and fetus. Management of toxemic patients must include a careful evaluation by the anesthesiologist. Special attention should be given to fluid balance, electrolyte stability, and urinary output. For the purpose of discussion, management of anesthesia for the patient with toxemia is divided into two categories: (1) the patient with mild toxemia, and (2) the patient with either moderate or severe toxemia.

The blood pressures of patients with mild toxemia are 140 to 160 mm Hg systolic and 90 mm Hg diastolic. The patients have a trace amount of proteinuria and only a slight amount of edema. They usually do not have fetal embarrassment before delivery or during the intrapartum period unless it is precipitated by some event such as severe hypotension or excessive uterine stimulation. These patients may obtain some relief of discomfort for the early first stage of labor through the use of psychoprophylaxis or a mild narcotic analgesic. However, if a patient wishes regional anesthesia, use of a segmental lumbar epidural block for the first stage of labor and a sacral block for the second stage should be considered. This technique is preferred in patients with preeclampsia, not only because there is a minimal effect on blood pressure after adequate fluid replacement but also because it can be instituted with minimal agitation to the patient and, once given, provides stable controlled blood pressure during contractions. An ineffective block at the time of delivery may also be supplemented by use of nitrous oxide and oxygen, a spinal block, or even an infiltration local anesthetic.

Now, on to the more significant challenge. Moderate and severe toxemia are considered together because fetal compromise often may be associated with more seriously elevated blood pressure (more than 160 mm Hg systolic and 100 mm Hg diastolic) and a greater degree of placental dysfunction. The primary problems are hypertension and associated cerebral complications, including hemorrhage, hypotension after regional block caused by reduced intravascular volume, muscle fatigue, and a tendency for muscle relaxant effects to be prolonged because of high doses of magnesium sulfate.

In patients with severe toxemia, physiologic changes are exaggerated and regional blockade in the presence of a reduced intravascular volume may result in considerable depression of blood pressure. Profound reductions in maternal systemic pressure may occur when standard epidural or low subarachnoid blocks are given. Restricted segmental lumbar epidural block has been used safely in patients with toxemia when careful attention has been paid to management of intravascular blood volume and small doses of local anesthetics have been used (not greater than 5 mL of drug at a time, with restriction of the analgesic block to the T10 to L2 levels). All patients are kept on their sides to offset the effect of the vena caval syndrome. For the second stage of labor, modified caudal analgesia, again with only S2 to S5 block, or a true saddle block may be the anesthetic technique of choice.

Practically speaking, when the obstetrician notifies the anesthesiologist that there is fetal compromise and a significantly elevated maternal blood pressure, providing general anesthesia really is the best choice for what most often is an anticipated cesarean section delivery. One maternal problem of concern is marked elevation of the mother's blood pressure during light anesthesia for delivery of the neonate. Ablation of significant overshoots in pressure can be managed by use of a potent vasodepressor by immediate and continuous intravenous delivery. This is not a complication to be taken lightly because some patients with eclampsia die as a result of cerebral hemorrhage.

FORCEPS AND VACUUM-ASSISTED DELIVERY

Continued critical appraisal of fetal and maternal trauma subsequent to midforceps deliveries has stringently curbed the use of such operative vaginal procedures. During midforceps maneuvers the operator must use an additional space-occupying instrument in a restricted pelvic area. Therefore, providing both profound vaginal tract and perineal analgesia and muscular relaxation are the key desirable requirements before starting the procedure. Because timing and specific requirements for rotation may be necessary, the obstetrician should determine these factors and, with the anesthesiologist, choose the most suitable technique and agent for each patient. During the induction of anesthesia the patient should not be stimulated by application of the forceps or attempted rotation until the anesthesiologist is ready for the obstetrician to proceed.

Regional anesthesia is the preferred method of pain relief because it provides complete analgesia and pro-

found relaxation without significant maternal or fetal depression. The subarachnoid block is the ideal choice because of minimal drug dose, rapid onset, and intense muscular relaxation. Lumbar epidural block or combined lumbar epidural block and caudal analgesia also will provide sensory analgesia and motor relaxation adequate for these procedures. Pudendal block is not adequate for midforceps rotational maneuvers; even when combined with light inhalation analgesia, it usually will not provide sufficient relaxation to protect the mother and fetus during these maneuvers. Inhalation analgesia with intubation and administration of a muscle relaxant could be used, but to do so is highly unusual; it is done only as a last resort if a suitable regional anesthetic has not been effective.

Elective or prophylactic low forceps deliveries require minimal analgesia restricted to the perineum and lower portion of the vagina. In addition, relaxation is not always necessary; a cooperative patient often may aid the descent and delivery with moderate Valsalva maneuvers. The duration of perineal analgesia needed is very short, because no manipulation is required and the time of traction is minimal. Local analgesia by infiltration and supplemental nitrous oxide, oxygen inhalation analgesia, or pudendal block may be all that is required in a cooperative patient. Saddle block, low caudal epidural, and lumbar epidural analgesia also may be used in low forceps delivery with good results.

Vacuum extraction is becoming much more popular and may be useful when the fetal position is not easily ascertainable or there is the need to avoid using a space-occupying instrument in tight pelvic conditions. It occasionally has been associated with reports of scalp lacerations, cephalohematomas, and intracranial hemorrhage (see Chapter 27). Analgesic requirements for vacuum extraction are not demanding. Some relief of discomfort and adequate vaginal relaxation during the introduction of the examiner's hand and manipulation of the extraction cup are all that is necessary. If the patient is cooperative and has a sufficiently relaxed vagina, this procedure may be performed without analgesia or anesthetic. When the parturient is not cooperative and the obstetrician has difficulty in actual placement of the vacuum cup, a saddle block may be performed to provide the needed vaginal analgesia and relaxation. This block denervates only sacral fibers and is compatible with continued uterine contractions and good Valsalva maneuvers, when they are required for descent and rotation of the fetal head. Lumbar epidural, caudal epidural, and pudendal analgesia also suffice to reduce pelvic diaphragmatic muscle tension and may be used successfully to aid in ease of application.

BREECH DELIVERY

Breech presentations (frank, complete, incomplete, and footling) occur in 3% to 5% of all mothers in labor. The perinatal morbidity and mortality rate in breech delivery is significantly greater than that associated with vertex delivery. In many centers all breech presentations except frank breech are considered managed best by cesarean section. Frank breech presentation may provide a wedge to the cervix of sufficient diameter to produce cervical dilation and simultaneously to protect the fetal umbilical cord from prolapse during dilation, descent, and rotation. In the frank breech subjected to vaginal delivery, the obstetrician and anesthesiologist should be prepared to provide immediate inhalation anesthesia and profound uterine relaxation during delivery of an entrapped head.

The primary life-threatening situation to the fetus is entrapment of the fetal head after delivery of the smaller-diameter pelvic girdle and shoulders. This is a special threat in a premature infant, whose head size is proportionately greater than the shoulder or pelvic girdle size. The midpelvis may also present a secondary threat to delivery of the fetal head; the cervix cannot be relaxed and dilated by means of drugs because its lower portion is primarily connective tissue. Normally, it takes 1 hour for each 2 cm of cervical dilation; this process cannot be accelerated even when there is profound myometrial relaxation caused by deep inhalation anesthesia. Persistent forceful attempts at dilation will produce maternal trauma, possible rupture of the lower uterine segment, and fetal injury. In contrast, many cases of breech delivery involve only increased tone of the lower uterine segment, which traps the fetal head, and the levator ani and coccygeal muscles, which hinder manipulation. The use of the inhalation anesthetic technique for emergency vaginal delivery may be the indicated treatment under these circumstances. The two phases of general anesthesia for emergency vaginal delivery include the preparatory phase, which may be performed during the preparation and draping of the patient for delivery, and the induction phase (Box 24-1).

BOX 24-1

GENERAL ANESTHESIA FOR EMERGENCY VAGINAL DELIVERY

Preparatory Phase
- Antacid, 30 mL PO
- Denitrogenation
- Glycopyrrolate, 0.2 mg IV
- d-Tubocurarine chloride, 3 mg IV

Induction Phase
- Thiopental sodium, 2.5 mg/kg IV
- Cricoid pressure
- Succinylcholine chloride, 80–100 mg IV
- Avoidance of positive pressure
- Endotracheal intubation
- Halothane, 2%–3%

A pudendal block may be used during the descent of the breech to the introitus. When descent is adequate, as shown by delivery of the umbilicus to the perineum, induction of general anesthesia is started. This gives the anesthesiologist adequate time to place an endotracheal tube and begin administration of an inhalation agent while the obstetrician is delivering the lower extremities and then the upper extremities and thorax of the fetus. By this time, both lower uterine segment and pelvic relaxation should be adequate for manipulation of the fetal head with the Piper forceps or by the Mauriceau maneuver. In situations in which a potent inhalation agent is administered and the anesthesiologist increases alveolar ventilation to effect rapid myometrial relaxation, endotracheal intubation and blood pressure monitoring to safeguard against possible hypotension are essential. If an anesthesiologist is called only at the time an obstetrician encounters difficulty with entrapment of the fetal head, it will be practically impossible to anesthetize the mother safely and effectively and provide optimal conditions for an atraumatic delivery.

Many times in the past, regional techniques such as subarachnoid, caudal, and epidural blocks were considered contraindicated for use in breech delivery, because they may decrease uterine contractions and prolong the first and second stages of labor. They were also considered to eliminate auxiliary forces and make spontaneous delivery impossible.

There was also a belief that regional procedures increased uterine contractility and were contraindicated in breech extractions. Today these are not valid arguments. If these procedures are not begun prematurely, uterine contractions are not diminished. Occasionally, there is diminished uterine contractility for a few minutes after the anesthetic is started, but then the uterus soon resumes contractions with the same intensity and duration. In some patients, contractions are enhanced by the relief of pain and elimination of the effects of anxiety and fear. Moreover, the perineal relaxation provided by the block can aid rather than impede the progress of labor by eliminating the resisting forces of the perineum.

The argument that epidural and subarachnoid blocks eliminate the auxiliary forces of labor is also not valid. It is true, of course, that these techniques eliminate the afferent limb of the reflex mechanism, which creates the patient's urge to bear down. It is also true that the auxiliary forces are necessary for spontaneous breech delivery and partial breech extraction. However, if the patient is not oversedated and is cooperative, she can be coached to bear down effectively. If analgesia does not extend above the T10 dermatome, the diaphragm and intercostal and abdominal muscles are not affected. For the patient to use these forces effectively, it is necessary that she be able to cooperate and that the obstetric nurse, anesthesiologist, or obstetrician coach her so she will bring the forces into action at the optimal time.

Certain benefits are derived by the fetus, the newborn, and the mother from caudal, epidural, and subarachnoid blocks. This is supported by reports from those medical centers where these techniques are used for breech delivery.[2, 4, 21–24] Perinatal mortality of infants born with regional anesthesia was consistently lower than that of those born with general anesthesia, especially among premature infants. Finally, neonatal depression and morbidity were significantly lower because of avoidance of direct depressant action and because of better obstetric conditions.[11, 12] For those same reasons, maternal complications were fewer and the length of labor was often decreased.[10] Especially today, with the minimal concentrations and amounts of drugs used, there is little if any effect on the mother or the fetus.

TWIN GESTATION

Internal podalic version and extraction are principally of historical significance. They have been associated with uterine rupture, cervical and perineal laceration, hemorrhage, and puerperal sepsis. A very high incidence of maternal death has been associated with the procedure. Nevertheless, under optimal conditions of uterine relaxation and full cervical dilation, internal podalic version and extraction may be useful in management of a second twin with fetal distress immediately after delivery of the first twin. Maternal and fetal safety depend on an experienced obstetrician working with a competent obstetric anesthesiologist. Unless conditions are optimum, cesarean delivery is the procedure of choice (see Chapter 18).

Success with version and extraction depends on adequate uterine relaxation. Before version and extraction the patient is prepared for general anesthesia in the routine fashion. In emergency circumstances some of the steps may be abbreviated (e.g., eliminating the prefasciculation curare and reducing the preoxygenation period to 15 seconds of hyperventilation). A rapid sequence induction is carried out with cricoid pressure. Once the endotracheal tube is inserted, halothane and oxygen are administered in an appropriate concentration and duration to achieve rapidly the uterine relaxation necessary for complete version and extraction, without excess residual postpartum atony. This requires close communication and interaction between the obstetrician and anesthesiologist during delivery. If at any time the obstetrician believes that manipulation is too difficult, a cesarean section should be performed.

For twin gestations with no contraindications for vaginal delivery after a trial labor, anesthesia can be by the epidural method. It is the most versatile method. In one large series of 130 women with twins who received epidural analgesia, an interesting disadvantage was found: the duration of the second stage was increased threefold when compared with women without epidural analgesia. This study was completed before 1987, however, and there have been substantial changes in practice since then. The most notable change has been the use of the continuous, low-concentration local anesthetic with minute levels of opioid and epinephrine. This provides excellent pain relief without the hazard of hypotension and allows the mother to advance through the first stage of labor in comfort. The second stage is managed with no additional anesthetic for nearly 80% of the patients, who have adequate perineal analgesia for delivery if the administration time is over 3 hours. For the remainder, a small, more concentrated dose of local anesthetic is administered for the purpose of blocking the sacral fibers just before vaginal delivery. Another method that can also provide suitable analgesia is the administration of small aliquots of opioid intravenously during labor for first-stage analgesia and the addition of a pudendal block with nitrous oxide supplementation as needed for the actual delivery. The nitrous oxide can be given either intermittently or continuously with changes in concentration from 20% to 30% to 50%, as needed.

CESAREAN SECTION DELIVERY

Ideally, use of general anesthesia for cesarean section should permit the mother to be unconscious and analgesic without jeopardizing the fetus and neonate. The nitrous oxide relaxant technique for cesarean section has gained popularity in the United States because nitrous oxide is not explosive, it reduces the need for more potent inhalation anesthetics that cause myometrial and neonatal depression, and it involves no risk of maternal hypotension. Thiopental is used to produce unconsciousness and amnesia, followed by muscle relaxants, nitrous oxide, and oxygen during the interval between induction and delivery. The analgesic effect of nitrous oxide is often less than optimal until after delivery. This approach is unlikely to produce hypotension; in skilled hands it should produce ideal fetal and neonatal conditions even in cases of known maternal, fetal, or uteroplacental compromise (Box 24–2).

The antacid regimen before induction is intended to elevate the gastric pH. The d-tubocurarine prevents fasciculations from succinylcholine and subsequent increased intragastric pressure that may expel gastric air and acid fluid into the esophagus. Misdirected positive pressure of oxygen in the esophagus could worsen this problem. Cricoid pressure against the vertebral body of the upper cervical spine effectively closes the esophagus and reduces the incidence of

---

■ **BOX 24–2**

NITROUS OXIDE RELAXANT TECHNIQUE FOR CESAREAN SECTION

Antacid, 30 mL PO
Glycopyrrolate, 0.2 mg IV
d-Tubocurarine chloride, 3 mg IV
Thiopental sodium, 2.5 mg/kg IV
No positive airway pressure
Cricoid pressure
Succinylcholine chloride, 80–100 mg IV for intubation
Nitrous oxide and oxygen, 50% mixture

gastric fluid escape into the upper airway. If there is fetal distress, increased maternal ventilation with oxygen only is indicated, in spite of the greater possibility of maternal recall. All patients should have left uterine displacement. Unless there is fetal distress, 50% oxygen is adequate for the inhalation technique; there is no significant improvement in fetal oxygenation when maternal arterial oxygen tension values rise above 300 mm Hg.

MANAGEMENT OF THE POSTPARTUM MOTHER

Postpartum recovery areas must be staffed by nurses who are fully trained in diagnosis and management of the multiple problems that can develop during the postpartum period in recovery from all types of delivery processes. Serious complications include inadequate ventilation, hypotension, hemorrhage, and convulsions. Unrecognized postpartum hemorrhage can also be life threatening. Most of the ventilation problems are those that relate to recovery from anesthetics and if detected promptly can be managed with little difficulty. If any problem develops, prompt response is imperative. There is no substitute for a thorough and complete evaluation of the patient. It must also be noted that whenever delirium, excitement, or restlessness occurs in the recovery period, oxygenation problems must first be ruled out before any assumptions are entertained that it simply may be due to inadequate pain relief or confusion on awakening.

Both hypertension and hypotension are problems that are noted in the postpartum period. Undetected postpartum hemorrhage may be fatal. Hypotension may first be noted when the patient arrives in the recovery room because her legs are then flat in bed. Before then, legs in stirrups helped to increase cardiac output owing to passive transfusion from the lower extremities. A quick way to check for this is to lift the patient's legs to the straight position and retake the blood pressure in 30 seconds. By this time the pressure should be back to near normal if there is a minimal or moderate amount of blood loss. Unless there is extensive blood volume loss the leg elevation method should be capable of producing the desired effect. Rarely have we found this maneuver to fail in such circumstances. If this maneuver does not result in an increase in the systolic pressure almost immediately, then one must further evaluate the cause. Interim treatment is rapid intravenous administration of fluid and small (10 mg) doses of ephedrine.

■ REFERENCES

1. Bonica JJ, McDonald JS: Principles and Practices of Obstetric Analgesia and Anesthesia, 2nd ed. Malvern, PA. Williams & Wilkins, 1995.
2. Chada YC, et al: Breech delivery and epidural analgesia. Br J Obstet Gynaecol 99:96, 1992.
3. Cohen SE: Walking with labor epidural analgesia: The impact of bupivacaine concentration and a lidocaine-epinephrine test dose. Anesthesiology 92:387, 2000.
4. Confine E, et al: Extradural analgesia in the management of singleton breech delivery. Br J Anaesth 57:892, 1985.
5. Crews JC: New developments in epidural anesthesia and analgesia. Anesthesiol Clin North Am 18:251, 2000.
6. Dick-Read G: Natural Childbirth. London, William Heinemann, 1933.
7. Goodman RR, et al: Multiple opiate receptors. In Kuhar MJ, et al (eds): Analgesics: Pharmacologic and Clinical Perspectives. New York, Raven Press, 1984.
8. Hodgkinson R, et al: Double-blind comparison of maternal analgesia and neonatal neurobehavior following intravenous butorphanol and meperidine. J Int Med Res 7:224, 1979.
9. Jouppila R, et al: The effect of segmental epidural analgesia on maternal and foetal acid-base balance, lactate, serum potassium and creatine phosphokinase during labour. J Acta Anaesth Scand 20:259, 1976.
10. Klufio CA, et al: Breech presentation and delivery. P N G Med J 34:289, 1991.
11. Mahomed K, et al: Outcome of term breech presentation. East Afr Med J 66:819, 1989.
12. Malik SJ, et al: Perinatal mortality in high risk pregnancy: A prospective study of preventable factors. Asia Oceania J Obstet Gynaecol 18:45, 1992.
13. Mandy AJ, et al: Is natural childbirth natural? Psychosom Med 14:431, 1952.
14. Pasternak GW: Multiple morphine and enkephalin receptors and the relief of pain. JAMA 259:1362, 1988.
15. Pert CG, et al: Opiate receptor: Demonstration in nervous tissue. Science 179:1011, 1973.
16. Powe CG, et al: Propiomazine hydrochloride in obstetrical analgesia. JAMA 181:290, 1962.
17. Quilligan EF, et al: Double-blind analgesic comparison of intravenous butorphanol and meperidine in obstetrical patients. J Obstet Gynecol 18:363, 1980.
18. Refstad SO, et al: Ventilatory depression of the newborn of women receiving pethidine or pentazocine. Br J Anaesth 52:265, 1980.
19. Richardson MG: Regional anesthesia for obstetrics. Anesthesiol Clin North Am 18:383, 2000.
20. Sangoul F, et al: Effect of regional analgesia on maternal oxygen consumption during the first stage of labor. Am J Obstet Gynecol 121:1080, 1975.
21. Schiff E, et al: Progression of labor in twin versus singleton gestations. Am J Obstet Gynecol 179:1181, 1998.
22. Schiff E, et al: Maternal and neonatal outcome of 846 term singleton breech deliveries: Seven-year experience at a single center. Am J Obstet Gynecol 175:18, 1996.
23. Songane FF, et al: Balancing the risks of planned cesarean section and trial of vaginal delivery for the mature, selected, singleton breech presentation. J Perinat Med 15:531, 1987.
24. Steinberg ES: Successful regional anesthesia for cesarean section for sextuplets. Anesth Analg 86:1236, 1998.
25. Stephens MB: Obstetric analgesia. Prim Care Mar 27:203, 2000.
26. Thalme B, et al: Lumbar epidural analgesia in labour: II. Effects on glucose, lactate, sodium chloride, total protein, haematocrit, and haemoglobin. Acta Obstet Gynaecol Scand 53:113, 1974.
27. Way WL, et al: Respiratory sensitivity of the newborn infant to meperidine and morphine. Clin Pharmacol Ther 6:454, 1965.
28. Yaksh TL, et al: Physiology and pharmacology of neuropathic pain. Anesthesiol Clin North Am 15:335, 1997.
29. Zador G, et al: Low-dose intermittent epidural anesthesia with lidocaine for vaginal delivery: II. Influence on labour and foetal acid-base status. Acta Obstet Gynaecol Scand Suppl 34:17, 1974.

25

Delivery Room Resuscitation of the Newborn

Ronald S. Bloom

In the human, the transition from fetus to neonate represents a series of rapid and dramatic physiologic changes. This transition goes smoothly most of the time; however, approximately 10% of the time the active intervention of a skilled individual or team is necessary to assist in that transition to ensure that it occurs with the least possible damage.

Although certain episodes of fetal asphyxia cannot be prevented, there are many circumstances in which, in the immediate neonatal period, a prompt and skilled resuscitation may prevent lifelong adverse sequelae. This, along with the fact that the need for intervention cannot always be predicted, has prompted the Guidelines for Neonatal Resuscitation to state: "At least one person skilled in initiating neonatal resuscitation should be present at every delivery. An additional person capable of performing a complete resuscitation should be immediately available."[33]

Although many elements of a resuscitation sequence have been agreed on, debate and discussion regarding the process continue. Research has yet to answer many questions. For the present, guidelines such as those published by the American Academy of Pediatrics and the American Heart Association[3] as well as those of the International Liaison Committee on Resuscitation (ILCOR)[33, 36] represent a middle ground for various contending views.

In this chapter I present an approach to neonatal resuscitation and at the same time attempt to provide an appreciation of the more common and controversial questions and a basis for understanding conflicting views.

THE FETUS

In utero the fetus depends on the placenta for gas exchange. Remarkably, the fetus thrives despite a Pao_2 in the 20s and, in terms of fuel metabolism, is not hypoxic. The tissues receive adequate amounts of oxygen, and anaerobic metabolic pathways are not ordinarily required. Adequate oxygen delivery is accomplished with an adaptive process primarily involving the architecture of the circulatory system, the charac-teristics of fetal hemoglobin, and the rate of perfusion of fetal organs.

The placenta, having the lowest resistance in the circulatory system of the fetus, preferentially receives blood from the systemic circulation. Approximately 40% of the total cardiac output of the fetus flows through the placenta.[73] Blood in the umbilical artery en route to the placenta has a Po_2 of 15 to 25 mm Hg.[44] In the human, umbilical venous blood returning from the placenta to the fetus, obtained by percutaneous umbilical vein sampling, has a Po_2 as high as 55 mm Hg.[50] However, when the umbilical venous blood is mixed with venous return from the body, the result is a lower Po_2. Although the oxygen tension of the fetus is low in postnatal terms, because of fetal hemoglobin's high affinity for oxygen, the oxygen content is only mildly diminished.

When the umbilical vein enters the abdomen of the fetus, the stream splits, with slightly more than half of the blood flowing through the ductus venosus into the inferior vena cava. The remaining blood perfuses portions of the liver. The umbilical venous return entering the inferior vena cava tends to stream and does not completely mix with less oxygenated blood entering the inferior vena cava from below. In the right atrium the crista dividens splits the inferior vena cava stream so that oxygenated blood from the umbilical vein flows through the foramen ovale into the left side of the heart. The less oxygenated blood returning from the body flows into the right ventricle (Fig. 25–1). (See also Chapter 43.)

In the fetus, blood flow through the lungs is diminished because of the high resistance of the fetal pulmonary circuit, the open ductus arteriosus, and the lower resistance of the systemic circuit. About 87% of the right ventricular output crosses the ductus and enters the aorta, bypassing the lungs. With little return from the pulmonary veins, oxygen in the umbilical venous blood crossing the foramen into the left atrium is only slightly diluted. Thus the most highly oxygenated blood perfuses the head and heart via the carotid and coronary arteries before its oxygen concentration is decreased by blood entering the aorta from the ductus arteriosus.

Another adaptive mechanism keeping the tissues oxygenated is the rate of perfusion of fetal tissues.

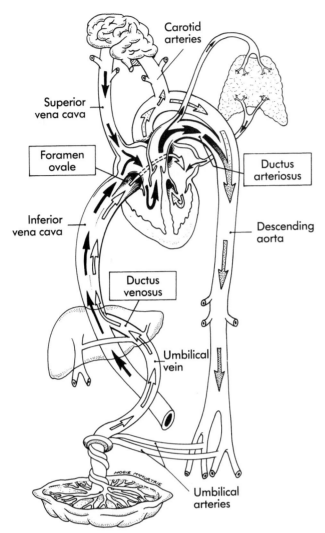

FIGURE 25–1. Fetal circulation.

Fetal tissues are perfused with blood at a higher rate than in the adult. The increased delivery of blood compensates for the low oxygen saturation in the fetus and the higher oxygen affinity of fetal hemoglobin.

Finally, the fetus has less of an oxygen demand than the newborn. With thermoregulation unnecessary in the fetus and respiratory effort limited, two significant consumers of oxygen in the newborn are either eliminated or markedly diminished in the fetus.

The P_{CO_2} of the fetus is slightly higher than adult levels, with an umbilical venous P_{CO_2} from 35 to 45 mm Hg. Elimination of carbon dioxide from the fetus is enhanced by maternal hyperventilation during pregnancy. Because of the lower P_{CO_2} of maternal blood, a gradient is created favoring the transfer of carbon dioxide across the placenta from fetal to maternal blood.

The low fetal P_{O_2} contributes to the architecture of the fetal circulation by helping to keep the pulmonary vascular resistance high. The low P_{O_2} and prostaglandin production by the fetus also play a significant role in keeping the ductus arteriosus patent. Thus the

low P_{O_2} is physiologically acceptable to the fetus. However, any compromise of fetal gas exchange or lack of effective transition at birth quickly results in asphyxia consisting of hypoxia, an elevated P_{CO_2}, and metabolic acidosis.

TRANSITION AT BIRTH

(See also Chapter 42, Part Two.)

The labor process is, to some extent, mildly asphyxiating. With each contraction, uterine blood flow decreases, with a resulting decrease in placental perfusion and a temporary impairment of transplacental gas exchange. This is accompanied by transient hypoxia and hypercapnia. The intermittent nature of labor permits the fetus to "recover" between each contraction; however, the effect is cumulative. Throughout a normal labor the fetus undergoes a progressive reduction in P_{O_2}, some increase in P_{CO_2}, a decrease in pH, and the accumulation of a base deficit (Table 25–1).[10]

With birth the neonate must establish the lungs as the site of gas exchange; the circulation, which in the fetus shunted blood away from the lungs, must now fully perfuse the pulmonary vasculature. Postnatal breathing is a continuum of in utero breathing movements that are well established but intermittent in the term fetus.[55] The events of birth stimulate peripheral and central chemoreceptors, cause tactile and thermal stimulation, and increase systemic blood pressure as a result of clamping of the cord. This combination is usually enough stimulation for the infant to pursue breathing vigorously.

Traditionally, it was thought that passage through the vaginal canal and the resulting "thoracic squeeze" resulted in clearance of a significant amount of lung fluid. We now know that during spontaneous birth with preceding labor the thoracic squeeze may have only a minor effect on clearance of lung fluid. A few days before a normal vaginal delivery the fetal production of lung fluid slows and alveolar fluid volume decreases. The process of labor is a powerful stimulus for the clearance of lung fluid, and that transfer of fluid from the air spaces is predominantly

TABLE 25–1   FETAL SCALP BLOOD VALUES DURING LABOR*

	EARLY FIRST STAGE	**LATE FIRST STAGE**	**SECOND STAGE**
pH	7.33 ± 0.03	7.32 ± 0.02	7.29 ± 0.04
P_{CO_2} (mm Hg)	44 ± 4.05	42 ± 5.1	46.3 ± 4.2
P_{O_2} (mm Hg)	21.8 ± 2.6	21.3 ± 2.1	16.5 ± 1.4
Bicarbonate (mmol/L)	20.1 ± 1.2	19.1 ± 2.1	17 ± 2
Base deficit (mmol/L)	3.9 ± 1.0	4.1 ± 2.5	6.4 ± 1.8

*Mean ± standard deviation.

From Boylan PC, et al: Fetal acid-base balance. In Creasy RK, et al (eds): Maternal-Fetal Medicine. Philadelphia, WB Saunders, 1989.

a process of active transport into the interstitium and drainage through the pulmonary circulation, with some fluid exiting through lymphatic drainage.[34] Although started before labor and influenced by the increasing levels of endogenous catecholamines, the process accelerates immediately after birth.[8]

The first few breaths must facilitate clearance of fluid from the lungs and establish a functional residual capacity (FRC).[77] The first breath of a spontaneously breathing infant has some unique characteristics. Although the peak inspiratory pressure is usually between −20 and −40 cm H₂O, the opening pressures are very low. That is, gas begins to enter the lungs at very low pressures, usually less than −5 cm H₂O pressure. Very high expiratory pressures are also generated, pressures that generally exceed the inspiratory pressure. This expiratory pressure, probably generated against a closed glottis, aids in clearing lung fluid and leads to a more even distribution of air throughout the lung. Thus, spontaneously breathing, vaginally delivered infants develop a significant FRC at the end of the first breath (Fig. 25–2).[46]

Expansion of the lungs is a stimulus for surfactant release,[38] which reduces alveolar surface tension, increases compliance, and helps develop a stable FRC. Simultaneously the act of ventilation alone will lower pulmonary vascular resistance.[15] Ventilation with air leads to a fall in P_{CO_2} and a rise in pH and P_{O_2}, also causing a fall in pulmonary vascular resistance. The relationships among pH, P_{O_2}, and pulmonary vascular resistance are illustrated in (Fig. 25–3).[67] Clearance of lung fluid and establishment of an FRC (along with an increase in pulmonary blood flow) facilitate ventilation.

With the onset of ventilation the fetal circulatory system assumes the adult pattern (Fig. 25–4). Coincident with clamping of the cord, the low-resistance placenta is removed from the systemic circuit and systemic blood pressure rises. This rise in systemic pressure, coupled with the fall in pulmonary vascular resistance and in pulmonary artery pressure, de-

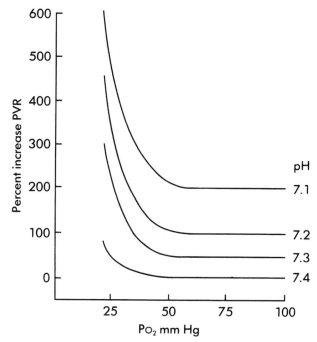

FIGURE 25–3. Pulmonary vascular resistance (PVR) in the calf. (From Rudolph AM, et al: Response of the pulmonary vasculature to hypoxia and H⁺ ion concentration changes. J Clin Invest 45:339, 1966.)

creases the right-to-left shunt through the ductus arteriosus. The increase in PaO_2 further stimulates closure of the ductus. With ductal shunting diminished, pulmonary artery blood flow increases, resulting in increased pulmonary venous return to the left atrium and increased pressure in the left atrium. Once the left atrial pressure exceeds right atrial pressure, the foramen ovale closes.[72]

Thus an uncomplicated transition from fetal to newborn status is characterized by loss of fetal lung fluid, secretion of surfactant, establishment of FRC, a fall in pulmonary vascular resistance, increased systemic pressure after removal of the low-resistance placenta from the systemic circuit, closure of two shunts (the ductus arteriosus and the foramen ovale), and an increase in pulmonary artery blood flow. In most circumstances the mild degree of asphyxia associated with labor is not enough to interfere with this process. However, the transition may be significantly altered by a variety of antepartum or intrapartum events, resulting in cardiorespiratory depression, asphyxia, or both.

CAUSES OF DEPRESSION AND ASPHYXIA

A newborn may be compromised because of problems initiated in utero with either the mother, the placenta, or the fetus itself (Box 25–1). A process initiated in utero may extend into the neonatal period, preventing a normal transition. An asphyxial process also may be neonatal in origin; that is, the infant appears well until required to breathe on his or her own.

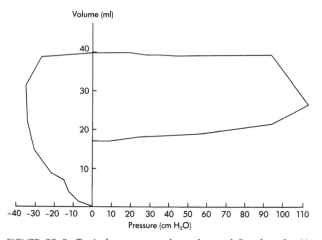

FIGURE 25–2. Typical pressure volume loop of first breath. Air enters the lung as soon as intrathoracic pressure falls. Expiratory pressure greatly exceeds inspiratory pressure. (From Milner AD, et al: Lung expansion at birth. J Pediatr 101:879, 1982.)

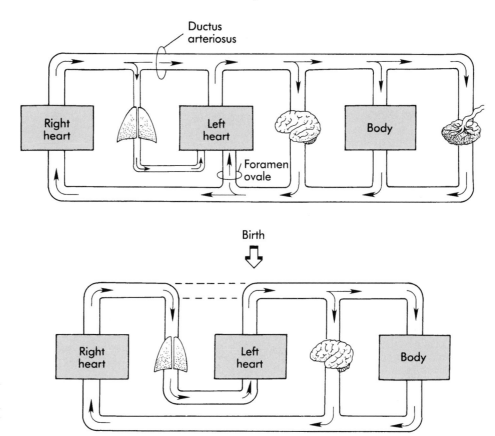

FIGURE 25–4. Comparison of fetal with adult circulatory system. (Modified from Dawes GS: Fetal and Neonatal Physiology. Chicago, Year Book Medical, 1968.)

Maternal causes of fetal compromise may be related to decreased uterine blood flow, which decreases the amount of oxygen transported to the placenta. Diminished uterine blood flow may result from maternal hypotension (as a result of drugs used to treat hypertension), regional anesthesia, eclampsia, or abnormal uterine contractions. Problems with the placenta, such as infarcts, premature separation, edema, or inflammatory changes, may impair gas exchange. The fetus also may be compromised because of fetal problems related to cord compression, for example, nuchal cord, prolapse, or a breech presentation with cord compression by the aftercoming head. A neonate may not breathe after delivery because of a number of problems, including drug-induced central nervous system depression, central nervous system anomalies or injury, spinal cord injury, mechanical obstruction of the airways, deformities, immaturity, pneumonia, or congenital anomalies.

Finally, there are some circumstances in which the infant may initiate breathing only to markedly diminish or stop breathing soon after birth. Examples include drug-induced depression in which the stimuli surrounding birth initially overcome the depression, diaphragmatic hernia, and spontaneous pneumothorax.

RESPONSE TO ASPHYXIA

The goal with any depressed or asphyxiated infant, whether the process is initiated in the fetal or the neonatal period, is to reverse the ongoing events as soon as possible and avoid permanent damage. An understanding of the response of the fetus or neonate to asphyxia aids in understanding the sequences of a resuscitative process.

When a fetus or neonate is subjected to asphyxia, the classic "diving" reflex takes place. This is simply an attempt to either accentuate or restore a fetal type of circulation. Hypoxia and acidosis increase vasoconstriction of the pulmonary vasculature (see Fig. 25–3).[64] The rise in pulmonary vascular resistance decreases pulmonary blood flow, decreasing left atrial return, which, in turn, lowers left atrial pressure. The drop in left atrial pressure increases right-to-left shunting across the foramen ovale. In the fetus, this directs the most highly oxygenated blood coming from the placenta to the left side of the heart. In the neonate, with no placenta, this shunting merely bypasses the lungs, making matters worse (Fig. 25–5).

In both the fetus and the neonate, the increase in noncerebral peripheral resistance during asphyxia results in a redistribution of blood flow, with increased flow to the head and heart and decreased flow to nonvital organs. Even though the oxygen content of the blood is low, during the early stages of asphyxia the amount of oxygen brought to the head and heart is maximized by the maintenance of cardiac output and the increased flow to these organs.[47, 65]

The increased peripheral resistance increases blood pressure early in the asphyxial period. The blood pressure will remain at reasonable levels as long as the myocardium is able to sustain cardiac output. As the asphyxia is not corrected, the infant again begins to gasp irregularly and the respirations cease (secondary apnea) unless positive pressure ventilation and successful resuscitation take place (Fig. 25–6).[21]

The longer the asphyxia has gone on, the longer it will take for the onset of spontaneous ventilation to occur after positive pressure ventilation is started (Fig. 25–7).[1] Asphyxia may begin before birth, and the infant may pass through any or all of these stages of the asphyxial response in utero. It may be difficult to determine at birth how far the asphyxial episode has progressed. Thus, with any depressed infant it is essential that resuscitation be initiated without delay.

Our goal, although we recognize that it is not always attainable, is to initiate resuscitation in a timely and effective manner so that the insults of hypoxia, ischemia, hypercapnia, and acidosis are reversed before they cause permanent injury (Box 25–2).

PREPARATION FOR RESUSCITATION

The key elements in preparing for resuscitation are anticipation of the problem, provision of adequate equipment, and presence of trained personnel. The chaos that, at times, occurs with resuscitation of an infant, especially an unexpected resuscitation, is primarily caused by either inadequate or unavailable equipment or staff members who are unskilled or have difficulty coordinating their activities. With some effort, both problems are avoidable.

the asphyxia progresses and hypoxia and acidosis worsen, the myocardium fails and both cardiac output and blood pressure fall.[22]

Superimposed on these circulatory and hemodynamic changes is a characteristic change in respiratory pattern. Initially there are gasping respirations (which may occur in utero). With continuing asphyxia, respirations cease in what is known as primary apnea. If

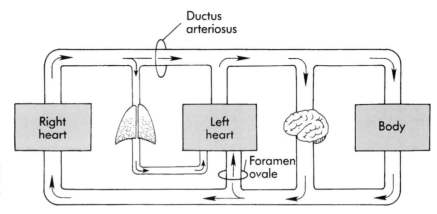

FIGURE 25–5. Neonatal circulatory response to asphyxia. (Modified from Dawes GS: Fetal and Neonatal Physiology. Chicago, Year Book Medical, 1968.)

ANTICIPATION

A careful review of the antepartum and intrapartum history can identify a number of problems that put a mother at risk of being delivered of a depressed or asphyxiated infant (see Box 25–1). Identifying a high-risk situation before delivery of the infant provides time for adequate preparation. Traditionally, a cesarean section of any type has been listed as a high-risk delivery. There is now enough available information to feel confident that an uncomplicated second cesarean section carries no greater risk for the infant than a vaginal delivery.[58] Thus, only if the cesarean section involves fetal distress or other complications is there any cause for added concern. It is important to stress that we are not able to identify every infant who may need assistance. Thus, at every delivery, equipment and personnel should be available in case of unanticipated respiratory depression.

ADEQUATE EQUIPMENT

Whenever an infant is delivered, appropriate equipment must be close at hand and in good working order. It is not acceptable for someone to need to leave the delivery room during a resuscitation to obtain an

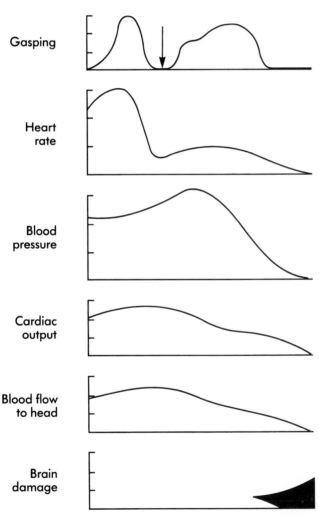

FIGURE 25–6. Schematic diagram of changes associated with asphyxia. Arrow indicates the point of primary apnea. (Modified from Dawes GS: Fetal and Neonatal Physiology. Chicago, Year Book Medical, 1968; and Phibbs RH: Delivery room management of the newborn. In Avery G [ed]: Neonatology, 3rd ed. Philadelphia, Lippincott, 1987.)

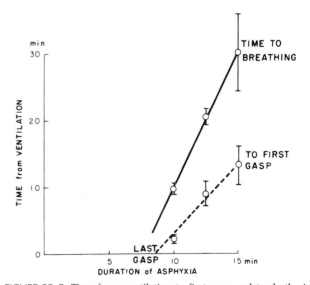

FIGURE 25–7. Time from ventilation to first gasp and to rhythmic breathing in newborn monkeys asphyxiated for 10, 12.5, and 15 minutes at 30°C. (From Adamsons K, et al: Resuscitation by positive pressure ventilation and *tris*-hydroxymethyl-aminomethane of rhesus monkeys asphyxiated at birth. J Pediatr 65:807, 1964.)

■ **BOX 25–3**

NEONATAL RESUSCITATION SUPPLIES AND EQUIPMENT

Suction Equipment

Bulb syringe
Mechanical suction
Suction catheter: Size 5 (or 6), 8, 10, or 12 Fr
Size 8 Fr feeding tube and 20 mL syringe
Meconium aspirator

Bag-and-Mask Equipment

Neonatal resuscitation bag with a pressure-release valve or pressure gauge; the bag must be capable of delivering 90% to 100% oxygen
Face masks—newborn and premature sizes (cushioned-rim masks preferred)
Oral airways—newborn (size 0) and premature sizes (size 00)
Oxygen source with intact flowmeter and tubing

Intubation Equipment

Laryngoscope with straight blades—No. 0 (premature) and No. 1 (term newborn)
Extra bulbs and batteries for laryngoscope
Endotracheal tubes—sizes 2.0, 2.5, 3.0, 3.5, 4.0 mm ID
Stylet (optional)
Scissors
Gloves
Tape or securing device for endotracheal tube

Medications

Epinephrine 1:10,000 (0.1 mg/mL) 3-mL or 10-mL ampules
Naloxone hydrochloride, 0.4 mg/mL in 1-mL ampules or 1.0 mg/mL in 2-mL ampules
Isotonic crystalloid (normal saline or Ringer's lactate) for volume expansion—100 or 250 mL
Sodium bicarbonate 4.2% (5 mEq/10 mL) in 10-mL ampules
Dextrose 5% and 10%, 250 mL
Sterile water

Other Equipment and Supplies

Radiant warmer
Stethoscope
Blood pressure monitor with transducer (desirable)
Adhesive tape—½-inch or ¾-inch wide
Syringes—1, 3, 5, 10, 20, 50 mL
Needles—25, 21, 18 gauge
Alcohol sponges
Umbilical artery catheterization tray
Umbilical tape
Umbilical catheters size 3.5, 5 Fr
Three-way stopcocks
Size 5 Fr feeding tube
Cardiotachometer with electrocardiographic oscilloscope (desirable)
Pressure transducer and monitor (desirable)
Pulse oximeter

Modified from American Heart Association/American Academy of Pediatrics: Textbook of Neonatal Resuscitation, 4th ed. Dallas, American Heart Association, 2000.

---

essential piece of equipment. Equipment that should be available at every delivery is listed in Box 25–3.

ADEQUATE PERSONNEL

Individuals vested with the responsibility of resuscitating infants should be adequately trained, readily available, and capable of working together as a team. Having trained personnel readily available means having someone present at every delivery who has the skill required to perform a complete resuscitation, with other available staff close at hand in case they are needed. At least two, if not three, people are needed to carry out a full resuscitation. Adequate training involves more than simply going through a course and receiving a certificate of completion. The neonatal resuscitation program of the American Heart Association/American Academy of Pediatrics and similar courses are simply starting points. They do not qualify one to assume independent responsibility. Before being given independent responsibility, an individual must work under the tutelage of experienced personnel in the delivery room.

Finally, the personnel available to the delivery room should be capable of working together as a team. If staff are skilled at carrying out their responsi-bilities and can anticipate each other's needs, the tension inherent in any resuscitation can be reduced and the process will go much more smoothly. In those institutions in which resuscitations are not frequent events, holding mock code drills on an ongoing basis will help to maintain skills and develop coordination among staff.

ROLE OF THE APGAR SCORE

The Apgar score is a tool that can be used objectively to define the state of an infant at given times after birth, traditionally at 1 minute and 5 minutes (Table 25–2).[4] Clearly, if the 1-minute Apgar score is very low, a resuscitation is necessary and in most circumstances should have already been started by 1 minute. The Apgar score should not be used as the primary indicator for resuscitation because it is not normally assigned until 1 minute of age. As noted earlier, an asphyxial process may begin in utero and continue into the neonatal period. Thus, to minimize the chances of brain damage, one should begin resuscitation as soon as there is evidence that the infant is not able to establish ventilation sufficient to maintain an adequate heart rate. Waiting until a 1-minute Apgar

TABLE 25–2 APGAR SCORE

SIGN	0	1	2
Heart rate	Absent	Less than 100 beats per minute	More than 100 beats per minute
Respiratory effort	Absent	Slow, irregular	Good, crying
Muscle tone	Flaccid	Some flexion of extremities	Active motion
Reflex irritability	No response	Grimace	Vigorous cry
Color	Pale	Cyanotic	Completely pink

score is assigned before initiating resuscitation only increases the chance of permanent damage in a severely asphyxiated infant.

ELEMENTS OF A RESUSCITATION

A resuscitation can be viewed as a series of elements (Box 25–4). The process is not a linear set of steps in which one marches inexorably from one point to another. Rather, it involves an evaluation of the infant's condition, a decision based on that evaluation, and action(s). These steps are repeated until the process is concluded. Figure 25–8 is an overview of the resuscitation process.

Virtually all infants undergo the initial steps. The vast majority of those requiring active resuscitation will respond to positive pressure ventilation: in a large series, only 0.12% of infants required chest compressions and medication. Of note is the fact that it was believed that in three fourths of these infants ineffective or improper ventilatory support was the presumed mechanism for the continued neonatal depression.[56] However, all infants, whether they require only the initial steps or a complete resuscitation, are entitled to a skilled and timely response, regardless of who is performing the resuscitation.

AN INITIAL QUICK OVERVIEW

Most infants are vigorous, cry upon birth, and breathe easily thereafter. There are many times when delivery room staff and the parents prefer that the infant go to the mother immediately after birth rather than be placed on a warmer and put through the "initial steps" in resuscitation. In most circumstances, a healthy and vigorous infant does not even require suctioning after delivery. With appropriate triaging and oversight many, if not most, infants can be directly given to the mother after birth without compromising the infant. It requires a rapid initial overview that will provide the information necessary to appropriately triage the infant. If the infant has not passed meconium in utero, is term, is breathing easily, is not cyanotic or pale, has good tone, and appears normal and vigorous, it may be appropriate to hand the child to the mother immediately after birth. As the mother holds the infant, it is probably a good idea to provide a light blanket to prevent rapid evaporative heat loss while covering the infant in such a way as to be able to observe the infant for signs of increasing distress. If, however, the infant has passed meconium in utero, is preterm, is not breathing easily, is cyanotic or pale, has diminished tone, or does not appear normal and vigorous, then the infant should be placed on a radiant warmer until a more thorough assessment of the infant can be done. The following steps apply to any infant who is not term, healthy, and vigorous at birth.

INITIAL STEPS

THERMAL MANAGEMENT

(See also Chapter 29.)

Delivery rooms are kept at a level of thermal comfort for the adults working in them. This leaves the neonate, with a very large surface area/mass ratio, susceptible to cold stress. Immediately after birth the infant should be placed in the microenvironment of a preheated radiant warmer. The infant should be thoroughly dried and the wet blankets promptly removed to avoid evaporative heat loss. These simple measures can minimize the drop in core temperature that the infant experiences at birth (Fig. 25–9).[45] Preventing excessive heat loss can become especially important with a preterm infant or an infant who is asphyxiated and hypoxic. Because hypoxia blunts the normal response to cold, a hypoxic infant will undergo a greater than normal drop in core temperature if not thermally protected.[12] Recovery from acidosis also is delayed by hypothermia.[2]

CLEARING THE AIRWAY

Normally the airway is cleared with the use of a bulb syringe or a suction catheter. The mouth is suctioned

---

BOX 25–4

ELEMENTS OF A RESUSCITATION

Initial steps
 Thermal management
 Clearing the airway
 Tactile stimulation
Establishment of ventilation
Chest compression
Medication

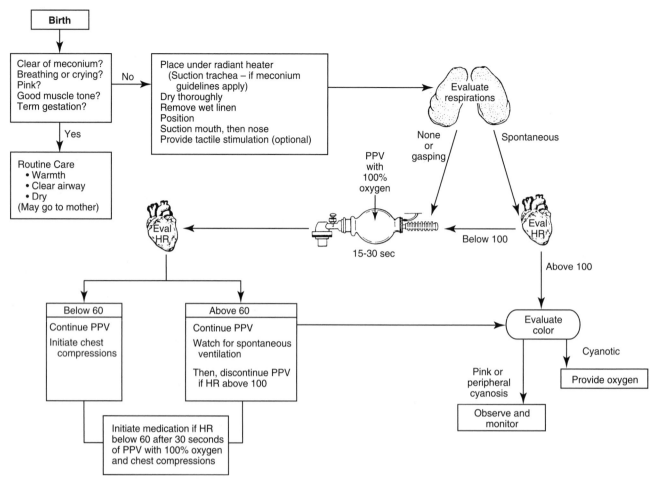

FIGURE 25–8. Overview of resuscitation in the delivery room. Note: Although many recommendations use a fixed heart rate (HR) number and take no account of a rising HR, I have retained the above recommendations (60 to 100) for reasons stated in the text. (Modified from American Heart Association/American Academy of Pediatrics: Textbook of Neonatal Resuscitation, 4th ed. Dallas, American Heart Association, 2000.)

first in case the infant gasps when the nose is suctioned. Care should be exercised to suction the infant gently because vigorous suctioning and stimulation of the posterior portion of the pharynx may induce bradycardia.[17] If a suction catheter is to be used, it is recommended that in the term infant the catheter be inserted no more than 5 cm from the lips and that the duration of suctioning be no more than 5 seconds.[36] The infant exposed to meconium in the amniotic fluid represents a special circumstance, to be discussed later.

TACTILE STIMULATION

Generally, the act of drying and suctioning the infant is enough tactile stimulation to initiate respiration. However, if the infant does not breathe after these efforts, slapping or flicking the soles of the feet or rubbing the infant's back may be enough additional stimulation to elicit regular respirations. If there is no immediate response to this additional stimulation, positive pressure ventilation should be quickly initiated. Continued tactile stimulation is not useful and may be harmful because the asphyxial process will

be permitted to persist that much longer. The decisions from this point revolve around the response of the infant—primarily heart rate, respirations, and color.

FREE FLOW OXYGEN

Considerable discussion has surrounded the decision to use either 100% oxygen or room air in the postasphyxial infant requiring positive pressure ventilation.[66, 71] However, if the infant is spontaneously breathing and the heart rate is more than 100 beats per minute, and yet the infant remains cyanotic, oxygen should be administered through a free flow system until it can be shown that the oxygen concentration can be lowered (SaO_2 greater than 85%) or that lowering the concentration makes no difference (cyanotic heart disease). A high concentration of oxygen can be obtained with an oxygen mask (with escape holes) held firmly over the face or an oxygen tube cupped in the hand. A flow-inflating bag also is capable of delivering high concentrations of oxygen. Caution should be exercised to be sure the mask is held

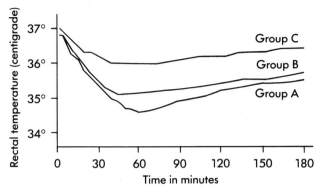

FIGURE 25–9. Mean core temperatures in three groups of infants, showing effect of drying and thermal protection immediately after birth. Group A: open crib, bathed within 1 hour; group B: open crib, no bath; group C: preheated incubator, dried immediately after birth, no bath. (From Miller DL, et al: Body temperature in the immediate neonatal period: The effect of reducing thermal losses. Am J Obstet Gynecol 94:964, 1966.)

lightly over the face to prevent positive pressure to the lungs.

It is best to heat and humidify the oxygen. During an emergency, cold, dry oxygen can be given; however, if free flow oxygen is to be continued for any period, it should be heated and humidified and given through wide-bore tubing. An oxygen blender and oximeter are useful in determining the amount of oxygen the infant requires. This is especially pertinent to the preterm infant.

If, after suctioning and tactile stimulation, the respirations are gasping or are insufficient to sustain the heart rate at greater than 100 beats per minute, positive pressure ventilation must be initiated.

POSITIVE PRESSURE VENTILATION

Under most circumstances, positive pressure ventilation can be provided quickly and effectively with a bag and mask. Some individuals who are skilled at inserting an endotracheal tube prefer to use this route for ventilation de novo.

RESUSCITATION BAGS

Regardless of the type of bag used, it should be specifically designed for use with neonates and hold between 200 and 750 mL. Whether a flow-inflating (anesthesia bag) or a self-inflating bag is used is mainly a matter of preference. Those who are experienced in the use of an anesthesia bag prefer it because they believe that it is more responsive and gives the individual greater control. However, an anesthesia bag takes more practice to use correctly than does a self-inflating bag.[35] Unless the entire staff is trained and comfortable using an anesthesia bag, it is wise to have self-inflating bags available.

Any bag, whether it be an anesthesia or a self-inflating bag, should be equipped with a pressure-relief (pop-off) valve or a pressure gauge or both.

Pressure-relief valves are built into most self-inflating bags and are set to vent pressures greater than 30 to 40 cm H_2O. However, the point at which the pressure-relief valve pops off may be highly variable.[25] If greater pressures are needed, the pop-off valve can be temporarily occluded with a finger. Adjustable pop-off valves are made to attach to an anesthesia bag. Any bag without a pop-off valve should have a pressure gauge attached. Pressure gauges with adjustable pop-off valves are also available.

It is important to check for faults in the bag-and-mask assembly before use in the delivery room. If the bags are reusable, cracks may appear with time, or a part may have been left out or improperly placed when the bag was reassembled after cleaning. One can check for faults by occluding the outlet with the palm of the hand and squeezing the bag. A pressure should be generated and/or the pop-off valve should open. It takes only a second or two to check a bag before use. It is much better to identify a faulty bag before use than to determine later that the infant's lungs are being inadequately ventilated because the bag does not work properly.

BAG AND MASK

With bag-and-mask ventilation, a mask with a cushioned rim is usually preferable to one with a noncushioned rim. The cushioned-rim masks tend to conform to the contour of the face more easily and generally require less pressure to obtain a seal. Masks come in more than one size, so the delivery room must have a selection of masks to accommodate infants from 500 gm or less to infants who are large for gestational age—4500 gm or more.

If a bag and mask are to be used for a prolonged period, a size 8 French feeding tube should be inserted through the mouth into the stomach to vent air going into the stomach. This also permits removal of any stomach contents, reducing the chance of aspiration.

BAG AND ENDOTRACHEAL TUBE

Insertion of an endotracheal tube is best accomplished by two people: one to insert the tube and ventilate the infant's lungs and the other to assist with the intubation and, after placement of the tube, to listen to the chest to ensure that proper placement of the tube has resulted in equal breath sounds on both sides of the chest. Tube sizes ranging from 2.0 to 4.0 should be available. Although intubation can be accomplished in most preterm infants with a No. 2.5 French tube or larger, there is the occasional infant with very low birth weight of 500 to 600 gm or less who may initially need a size 2.0 French tube (Table 25–3). If a soft, flexible wire stylet is to be used, it should be secured so that it stops about 0.5 to 1 cm from the end of the tube. A protruding stylet can cause damage to the larynx or the trachea. If the endotracheal tube is long, it is easier to manage if it is cut to about 13 cm and the adapter reconnected.

TABLE 25–3 ENDOTRACHEAL TUBE SIZES

TUBE SIZE (MM ID)	WEIGHT (gm)	GESTATIONAL AGE (wks)
2.0*	500–600 or less	25–26 or less
2.5	<1000	<28
3.0	1000–2000	28 to 34
3.5	2000–3000	34 to 38
3.5–4.0	>3000	>38

*May be needed if a size 2.5 Fr tube does not fit.
ID, internal diameter.

The correct position of the infant for intubation is with the head slightly extended. Inexperienced people sometimes hang the head over the edge of the warmer. This hyperextends the neck, moving the trachea anterior and making the glottis hard to visualize. Flexion of the neck also makes the glottis hard to visualize (Fig. 25–10).

Although much has been written about the intricacies of visualizing the glottis, to a large extent this depends on recognizing the place where the blade has been initially inserted and then moving it to the proper position. In general, the blade is either not inserted far enough, is off to the side, or is inserted too far and is in the esophagus (Fig. 25–11). The ability to recognize the position of the blade and then move to the proper position and recognize the landmarks of the glottis facilitates an efficient intubation (Fig. 25–12). In the larger infant the blade should be inserted into the vallecula and lifted to visualize the glottis. If the vallecula is too small in the smaller premature infant, the blade should be used to lift the epiglottis. If the glottis is too far anterior, gentle pressure over the larynx will bring it into view. This

pressure can be applied by either the assistant or the person doing the intubation (Fig. 25–13).

The tube should not be inserted down the center of the laryngoscope blade, which provides the line of sight, but alongside the blade. The intubator should always keep the tube in sight and insert the tube until the vocal cord guide (black line near the tip of the endotracheal tube) is at the level of the cords. This should place the tip of the tube at a point slightly above the carina. A tip-to-lip distance can be used to check the placement of the tube. Adding 6 to the weight of the infant (in kilograms) is a reasonable estimate of the centimeter marking that should occur at the lips when the tube is properly positioned (Table 25–4).

When the tube is placed in the airway, a bag should be attached and the infant's lungs ventilated while an assistant listens to both lungs. If the tube is properly positioned, there should be bilateral and equal breath sounds, a slight rise of the chest with each ventilation, no air heard entering the stomach, and no gastric distention. Another way of checking for an in-place endotracheal tube is to use a CO_2 detector. Recognize, however, that these may be inaccurate in the infant with very low birth weight.

Table 25–5 outlines some of the complications of the intubation procedure and their causes. Insertion of an endotracheal tube must be done quickly. Prolonged attempts to insert a tube simply extend the asphyxial period and increase the chance of permanent damage. If a tube has not been successfully inserted within approximately 20 seconds and the infant has bradycardia, the attempt should stop and the infant's lungs should be ventilated with a bag and mask. Another attempt at intubation can be made after a minute or so of bag-and-mask ventilation. In a severely asphyxiated infant requiring prolonged

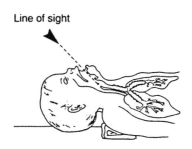

Infant in Correct Position

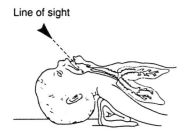

Neck Hyperextended

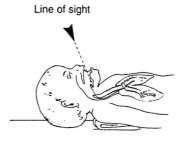

Neck Underextended

FIGURE 25–10. Effects of flexion and hyperextension on ability to visualize the glottis. (From American Heart Association/American Academy of Pediatrics: Textbook of Neonatal Resuscitation. Dallas, American Heart Association, 1994.)

Position	**Landmarks**	**Corrective Action**
Not inserted far enough	You see the tongue surrounding the blade	Advance the blade farther

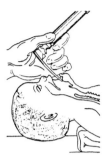 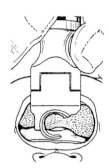 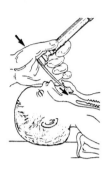

Position	**Landmarks**	**Corrective Action**
Inserted too far	You see the wall of the esophagus surrounding the blade	Withdraw the blade slowly until the epiglottis and glottis come into view

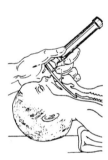 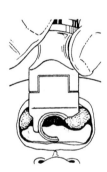 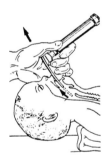

Position	**Landmarks**	**Corrective Action**
Inserted off to the side	In the posterior pharynx, you see part of the trachea to the side of the blade	Gently move the blade back to the midline, then advance or retreat according to the landmarks seen

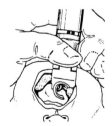 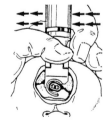

FIGURE 25–11. Examples of incorrect positioning of laryngoscope blade and how to take corrective action. (From American Heart Association/American Academy of Pediatrics: Textbook of Neonatal Resuscitation. Dallas, American Heart Association, 1994.)

Correct Position of Laryngoscope

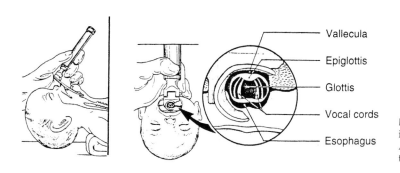

— Vallecula

— Epiglottis

— Glottis

— Vocal cords

— Esophagus

FIGURE 25–12. Correct view of glottis in preparation for intubation (From American Heart Association/American Academy of Pediatrics: Textbook of Neonatal Resuscitation. Dallas, American Heart Association, 1994.)

resuscitation, intubation is helpful at some point because it is easier to use a bag and tube for a prolonged period than a bag and mask.

LARYNGEAL MASK AIRWAY

Although the use of a bag and either a mask or an endotracheal tube is the most common method of providing positive pressure ventilation, another method that may have merit is the use of a laryngeal mask airway. A version is available for neonates weighing as little as 2.5 kg. Recent studies have supported the use of the laryngeal mask airway in neonatal resuscitation. However, at a pressure of approximately 23 cm an audible air leak develops. This will limit the use of the laryngeal mask airway in infants with poor compliance or in those who require higher

pressures for the first or subsequent breath. Larger studies are required to determine the training required, the usefulness of the device, its failure rate, and complications that may occur.[11, 28, 54]

POSITIVE PRESSURE VENTILATION

Positive pressure ventilation must accomplish much of what a spontaneous first breath accomplishes: it must establish a tidal volume and FRC. In some early work looking at the pulmonary response to positive pressure ventilation in the newborn, there was evidence that the inspiratory phase of the first breath should be somewhat prolonged. When the lungs of asphyxiated infants were ventilated at a rate of 30 to 40 breaths per minute, with an inspiratory time of only 1 second and pressures limited to 30 cm H_2O, an FRC was not established after the first breath in a majority of the cases. When it was, it was much smaller than that generated by a spontaneously breathing infant. However, if the inspiratory phase of the first assisted ventilation is prolonged to a mean of 5 seconds, an FRC is usually established on the first breath, and its volume approaches that of a spontaneously breathing infant (Table 25–6).[9, 66, 77, 78] Thus an argument was made for prolonging the inspiratory phase of the first breath and then continuing ventilation at ordinary inspiratory times.

However, further work, in which asphyxiated neonates were resuscitated with a median rate of inflation of 48 breaths per minute, a median inspiratory time of 0.51 second, and as much pressure as necessary

Before

After

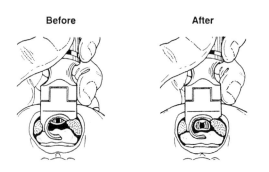

Pressure Applied by Operator

Pressure Applied by Assistant

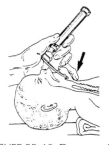

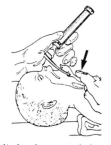

FIGURE 25–13. Downward pressure applied to larynx to help visualize the glottis. (From American Heart Association/American Academy of Pediatrics: Textbook of Neonatal Resuscitation. Dallas, American Heart Association, 1994.)

TABLE 25–4 ENDOTRACHEAL TUBE PLACEMENT

WEIGHT	DEPTH OF INSERTION (CM FROM UPPER LIP)
1 kg	7*
2 kg	8
3 kg	9
4 kg	10

*Infants weighing less than 750 gm may require only 6-cm insertion.
From American Heart Association/American Academy of Pediatrics: Textbook of Neonatal Resuscitation. Dallas, American Heart Association, 1994.

TABLE 25–5   COMPLICATIONS OF ENDOTRACHEAL INTUBATION

COMPLICATION	CAUSE
Hypoxia	Procedure taking too long; incorrect placement of tube
Bradycardia/apnea	Hypoxia
Vagal response	Stimulation of posterior pharynx by laryngoscope blade, endotracheal tube, or suction catheter
Pneumothorax	Overventilation of one lung caused by placement of tube in main bronchus (usually the right)
Contusions or lacerations of tongue, gums, pharynx, epiglottis, trachea, vocal cords, or esophagus	Rough handling of laryngoscope or endotracheal tube; laryngoscope blade that is too long or too short
Perforation of trachea or esophagus	Insertion of tube or stylet was too vigorous, or stylet protrudes beyond end of tube
Infection	Introduction of organisms by equipment or hands

From American Heart Association/American Academy of Pediatrics: Textbook of Neonatal Resuscitation. Dallas, American Heart Association, 1994.

until inflation of the lungs was observed, indicated that (1) we may need higher pressures than conventionally recommended and (2) with higher pressures an FRC can be established within four breaths (Fig. 25–14). In this study the initial pressures needed ranged from 28 to 60 cm H_2O, with a median of 40 cm H_2O. As positive pressure ventilation progressed, the median pressure needed to inflate the chest decreased to 29 cm H_2O, with a range of 18 to 42 cm H_2O.[76]

The conventional recommendations have indicated inspiratory pressures for the first breath of 30 to 40 cm H_2O; however, these may not be high enough. A better guide may be to ventilate with enough pressure

TABLE 25–6   ESTABLISHMENT OF AN FRC AFTER POSITIVE PRESSURE VENTILATION

	MEAN FRC (mL)	
	1-Second Inspiration	**Prolonged Inspiration (5 seconds)**
After first breath	7.5*	15.9
After 30 seconds	36.9	54.1

*Only 5 of 20 infants had a positive FRC.
Modified from Boon AW, et al: Lung expansion, tidal exchange and formation of the functional residual capacity during resuscitation of asphyxiated neonates. J Pediatr 95:1031, 1979; and from Vyas AD, et al: Physiologic responses to prolonged and slow-rise inflation in the resuscitation of the asphyxiated newborn infant. J Pediatr 99:635, 1981.

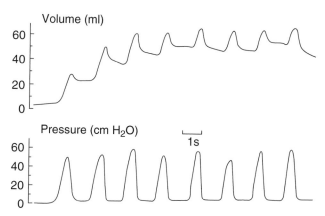

FIGURE 25–14. Resuscitation trace from an infant. Inspiration is upward on the volume trace. Note formation of functional residual capacity during first four inflations. (From Upton CJ, et al: Endotracheal resuscitation of neonates using a rebreathing bag. Arch Dis Child 66:39, 1991.)

to cause a gentle rise and fall of the chest (using higher pressures if necessary) than to adhere to the pressure settings on a manometer as the final determinant of adequate ventilation. There also appears to be advantages to a longer inspiratory time of the first breath.

There is now experimental evidence that one of the principal mechanisms causing lung injury is volutrauma from excessive tidal volumes.[13] This may be even more important than barotrauma from high airway pressures.[32] Thus, if overventilation is to be avoided, it is important to recognize that subsequent breaths will require less pressure than the initial breaths: from as low as 15 cm H_2O to as high as 42 cm H_2O. This becomes especially true in the preterm infant who can be quite easy to overventilate, adding the insult of volutrauma to that of a low $PaCO_2$ with subsequent risk of neurodevelopmental deficits.[29]

Table 25–7 outlines the most common problems associated with inadequate chest expansion. As soon as positive pressure ventilation begins, a second person should be summoned if he or she is not already present. This second individual should auscultate the chest to ensure equal air entry bilaterally and should listen to the heart rate.

CONTINUOUS POSITIVE AIRWAY PRESSURE VERSUS INTERMITTENT MANDATORY VENTILATION

In North America it is common to intubate preterm infants as part of the resuscitation process and continue with intermittent mandatory ventilation (IMV). In parts of Europe, however, the initial management of preterm infants may consist of using positive pressure to establish an initial FRC and then the use of continuous positive airway pressure (CPAP) in a spontaneously breathing infant in place of IMV. Intubation and IMV are used only with the failure of CPAP.[40, 43] In one study of infants with weights of less than 1000 gm and a gestational age of 24 weeks or more, 25% of the infants were never intubated. With

TABLE 27–7   PROBLEMS ASSOCIATED WITH INADEQUATE CHEST EXPANSION

PROBLEM	CORRECTION
Inadequate face mask seal	Reapply mask to face. Alter position of hand that holds mask.
Blocked airway	Bag and mask: Check infant's position. Suction mouth, oropharynx, and nose. Insert oral airway if indicated (Pierre Robin, macroglossia). Bag and endotracheal tube: Suction the tube.
Misplaced endotracheal tube	Remove endotracheal tube, ventilate with bag and mask, replace tube.
Inadequate pressure	Increase pressure, taking care not to overexpand the chest; may require adjusting or overriding the pop-off valve.

the use of a historical control, the overall incidence of intubation and IMV in the delivery room fell from 84% to 40%. Thirty-five percent of the infants were later intubated and put on IMV for a variety of reasons. Compared with the historical control, those managed with CPAP exhibited no increase in mortality or morbidity.[40] Although appealing, this strategy must be subject to a randomized controlled study before it can be recommended for widespread use in delivery room resuscitations.

ROOM AIR VERSUS 100% OXYGEN

There is now an accumulating body of knowledge with regard to the use and potential advantages of room air as opposed to 100% oxygen in the resuscitation of the asphyxiated infant. Because some of the damage to the asphyxiated infant may be caused by excess oxygen radical production during the reoxygenation period,[57, 62, 68] several investigators have examined the use of room air in place of 100% oxygen during resuscitation.

After a preliminary study indicating that room air is as effective as 100% oxygen in resuscitating newborns in need of positive pressure ventilation,[61] a large multicenter, controlled study involving data from 609 infants was conducted. The time to first breath and first cry was significantly shorter, and the 1-minute Apgar scores were significantly higher in infants resuscitated with room air as opposed to oxygen. There were no significant changes in mortality, presence of hypoxic-ischemic encephalopathy (HIE), acid-base balance, SaO_2, or PaO_2.[67]

Although most continue to recommend that all resuscitative efforts be made with 100% oxygen, this recommendation is undergoing increasing scrutiny and will likely undergo some modification as more

information becomes available regarding the specific types of infants who will tolerate (or may potentially benefit from) resuscitation with less than 100% oxygen.

In the vast majority of cases, ventilation alone will be sufficient to resuscitate the newborn. If ventilation is provided early in the asphyxial process, most often oxygenation will quickly occur and bradycardia will be reversed. If, however, asphyxia has progressed to the point where bradycardia is associated with a failing myocardium, chest compression will be necessary. Thus, if after 30 seconds of positive pressure ventilation with 100% oxygen the heart rate remains low, chest compression may be needed to assist a hypoxic and failing myocardium.

CHEST COMPRESSION

If after effective ventilation with 100% oxygen the heart rate remains low, chest compression should be initiated to help maintain cardiac output. The heart rate at which one begins chest compression varies with the source of the recommendations. ILCOR recommends initiating chest compressions at heart rates of 60 beats per minute or less.[36] The previous recommendations of the American Heart Association/ American Academy of Pediatrics started chest compressions if the heart rate is below 60 beats per minute or between 60 and 80 beats per minute and not rising. The new recommendations suggest starting chest compressions at a heart rate of 60 beats per minute or less because of the ease of teaching this value. To date there is little evidence to suggest one number over another.

Compression of the chest should occur over the lower third of the sternum, just below an imaginary line drawn between the nipples. Care should be taken not to apply pressure to the xyphoid process at the lower end of the sternum. The sternum can be compressed by using the thumbs with the fingers encircling the chest or by placing two fingers perpendicular to the sternum (Fig. 25–15). On the basis of very limited data, it has been suggested that a greater mean arterial pressure can be obtained with the thumb method.[19, 75] Regardless of which position is used, the persons providing ventilation and chest compression must position themselves so that they do not interfere with each other.

Each compression should depress the sternum about one third of the anterior-posterior diameter of the chest or until a palpable pulse is generated. A pulse should be palpable with each compression. Having a third person available to check the pulse is helpful. It is currently recommended that the chest be compressed 90 times a minute, with a ventilation interposed between each third compression. This provides 30 ventilations per minute. Thus, within a 2-second period, three chest compressions and a ventilation would occur.[3] Periodically, chest compression should be stopped briefly to see whether the spontaneous heart rate has risen. Once the heart rate has

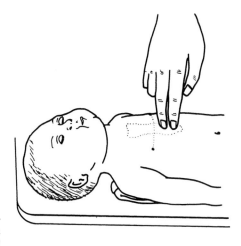

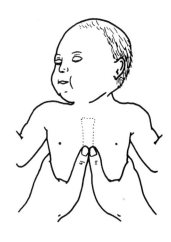

**Two finger
method**

**Thumb
method**

FIGURE 25–15. Two methods of applying chest compression. (From American Heart Association/American Academy of Pediatrics: Textbook of Neonatal Resuscitation. Dallas, American Heart Association, 1994.)

risen to 60 beats per minute, chest compressions can be stopped. The best way to monitor the effectiveness of chest compression is by means of arterial blood pressures obtained from a transducer attached to an umbilical artery catheter or a peripheral arterial line. These are not commonly available in delivery rooms.

An infant undergoing chest compression may receive ventilation by either a mask or an endotracheal tube. However, a tube has advantages over a mask in these situations. A tube provides more stability and prevents gas from entering the stomach should a compression overlap with a ventilation. If a bag and mask are used, an orogastric tube must be inserted into the stomach to ensure decompression of the stomach.

It is now recommended that ventilations be interposed between compressions.[36] The reason for coordination and not simultaneous ventilation and compression is based on a reconsideration of the data supporting simultaneous ventilation and compression/cardiopulmonary resuscitation (SVC/CPR) in the human adult, as well as on some laboratory evidence in infant animals.

In the adult there is clear evidence that it is not direct compression of the heart but a "thoracic pump" that plays a significant role in moving blood forward.[63] It was shown that in the adult SVC/CPR increased aortic pressure and improved cerebral circulation.[16] However, further work demonstrated that although cerebral circulation increased, myocardial blood flow diminished with SVC/CPR.[70] In a controlled clinical trial looking at SVC/CPR versus conventional ventilation in a prehospital setting, it became clear that SVC/CPR offered no advantages and the authors concluded that SVC/CPR should not be used in the clinical setting.[37] There also are some laboratory data showing no advantage to SVC/CPR in the newborn piglet.[6]

In addition to the fact that simultaneous ventilation and compression offered no advantage in the adult human or the newborn piglet, there are some poten-

tial limitations to simultaneous chest compression and ventilation in the newborn. These include a compromised tidal volume; in the patient without an endotracheal tube in place, high airway pressures necessary to effect a ventilation will increase the amount of gas diverted into the stomach. A pressure-monitor on the bag and mask would have limited value because it would be impossible to differentiate airway pressure associated with an adequate tidal volume from pressure associated with chest compression. Furthermore, because ventilation is frequently administered with a self-inflating bag and mask, it would be necessary to override the pressure pop-off valve (usually set at 35 to 40 mm Hg), or the pressure generated would not be enough to deliver an adequate tidal volume.[49]

For all of these reasons, interposition of ventilation and compression is recommended: one ventilation interposed between every three compressions. Until more data are generated, a definitive statement cannot be made regarding the two-finger versus the thumb method. Regardless of the method used, if chest compressions and ventilations do not raise the heart rate above 60 beats per minute within 30 seconds of well-coordinated chest compressions and ventilation, support of the cardiovascular system with medications is indicated.

MEDICATIONS

The use of medications is required when, despite ventilation and chest compression, the infant continues to have bradycardia or when the infant is born with no detectable heartbeat. In the latter circumstance, medications are started along with ventilation and chest compression. Medications can be given through either an umbilical catheter or an endotracheal tube. If an umbilical catheter is used, it should be inserted into the umbilical vein just beneath the skin.

If the catheter is inserted too high and becomes wedged in the liver, it can be dangerous because infusing solutions into the liver may cause liver necrosis. If there is any doubt regarding the placement of the catheter, it should be reinserted to the level of the skin so that direct infusion into the liver does not occur. Table 25–8 presents an overview of the various medications, their concentration, dosage, route, and precautions.

EPINEPHRINE

If positive pressure ventilation with 100% oxygen and chest compression are not successful in increasing the heart rate, use of medications is indicated. The first drug used should be epinephrine 1:10,000 (0.1 to 0.3 mL/kg). If necessary, the dose can be repeated every 3 to 5 minutes. Epinephrine not only has a beta-1 effect, which stimulates the heart, but, what is possi-

TABLE 25–8 MEDICATIONS FOR NEONATAL RESUSCITATION

MEDICATION	CONCENTRATION TO ADMINISTER	PREPARATION	DOSAGE/ ROUTE	TOTAL DOSE/INFANT			RATE/ PRECAUTIONS
Epinephrine	1:10,000	1 mL	0.1–0.3 mL/kg IV or ET	**Weight** 1 kg 2 kg 3 kg 4 kg		**Total mL** 0.1–0.3 mL 0.2–0.6 mL 0.3–0.9 mL 0.4–1.2 mL	Give rapidly May dilute with normal saline solution to 1–2 mL if giving ET
Volume expanders	Normal saline solution Ringer's lactate solution Whole blood 5% Albumin–saline solution	40 mL	10 mL/kg IV	**Weight** 1 kg 2 kg 3 kg 4 kg		**Total mL** 10 mL 20 mL 30 mL 40 mL	Give over 5–10 minutes
Sodium bicarbonate	0.5 mEq/mL (4.2% solution)	20 mL or two 10-mL prefilled syringes	2 mEq/kg IV	**Weight** 1 kg 2 kg 3 kg 4 kg	**Total Dose** 2 mEq 4 mEq 6 mEq 8 mEq	**Total mL** 4 mL 8 mL 12 mL 16 mL	Give *slowly*, over at least 2 minutes Give only if infant is being effectively ventilated
Naloxone hydrochloride	0.4 mg/mL	1 mL	0.1 mg/kg (0.25 mL/kg) IV, ET IM, SQ	**Weight** 1 kg 2 kg 3 kg 4 kg	**Total Dose** 0.1 mg 0.2 mg 0.3 mg 0.4 mg	**Total mL** 0.25 mL 0.50 mL 0.75 mL 1.00 mL	Give rapidly IV, ET preferred. IM, SQ acceptable Do not give if mother is suspected of narcotic addiction or on methadone maintenance (may result in severe seizures)
	1.0 mg/mL	1 mL	0.1 mg/kg (0.1 mL/kg) IV, ET IM, SQ	1 kg 2 kg 3 kg 4 kg	0.1 mg 0.2 mg 0.3 mg 0.4 mg	0.1 mL 0.2 mL 0.3 mL 0.4 mL	
Dopamine $$6 \times \frac{\text{Weight (kg)} \times \text{Desired dose } (\mu g/kg/min)}{\text{Desired fluid (mL/hr)}} = \frac{\text{mg of dopamine}}{\text{per 100 mL of solution}}$$			Begin at 5 μg/ kg/min (may increase to 20 μg/kg/min if necessary) IV	**Weight** 1 kg 2 kg 3 kg 4 kg		**Total μg/min** 5–20 μg/min 10–40 μg/min 15–60 μg/min 20–80 μg/min	Give as a continuous infusion, using an infusion pump Monitor heart rate and blood pressure closely Seek consultation

IM, intramuscular; ET, endotracheal; IV, intravenous; SQ, subcutaneous.
From American Heart Association/American Academy of Pediatrics: Textbook of Neonatal Resuscitation. Dallas, American Heart Association, 1987, 1990, 1994.

bly of more importance, also has an alpha effect that increases noncerebral peripheral resistance. By selective vasoconstriction of peripheral vascular beds, epinephrine increased cerebral and myocardial blood flow.[5] Although in pediatric[30] and adult cases[53] larger than recommended doses of epinephrine have been used, there is no information indicating an advantage of larger doses in neonates. On the contrary, there is concern about complications in adults given higher than recommended doses of epinephrine. Thus, high-dose epinephrine administration is not recommended.

Epinephrine can be given intravenously or through the endotracheal tube.[41] Although there is evidence that low pulmonary blood flow associated with a resuscitation does not decrease plasma levels after endotracheal instillation of epinephrine,[42] there is still uncertainty as to whether the dose of epinephrine should be increased when the drug is given through the endotracheal tube.[51, 60]

There is animal evidence that during a neonatal resuscitation a metabolic acidosis significantly attenuates the hemodynamic responses to epinephrine.[59] When epinephrine alone is not effective, consideration should be given to correction of acidosis and the possibility of hypovolemic shock—but only after establishing adequate ventilation.

VOLUME EXPANDERS

Although an asphyxiated infant may be in shock, this is usually not caused by hypovolemia but by decreased myocardial function and decreased cardiac output. In fact, most infants who have undergone intrauterine asphyxia are not hypovolemic. In some circumstances, however, hypovolemic shock is a real possibility (Box 25–5).

It must be recognized that both asphyxia and hypovolemia can result in shock, the former as a result of decreased myocardial function and decreased cardiac output. In addition, most of the causes of hypovolemic shock result in asphyxia in the infant. Thus, most hypovolemic infants are asphyxiated, but most asphyxiated infants are not hypovolemic. The problem is in distinguishing hypovolemic shock from asphyxial shock that does not involve hypovolemia.

■ **BOX 25–5**

CAUSES OF HYPOVOLEMIA

Decreased blood return from placenta
Cord compression resulting in venous but not arterial occlusion
Placental separation compromising placental blood return to the fetus
Maternal hypotension
Loss of blood from fetal-placental circulation
Hemorrhage from the fetal side of the placenta
Fetal-fetal transfusion
Incision of placenta during cesarean section

Because volume expanders may be detrimental in an infant who is not hypovolemic, how does one determine when they are needed? In the acute circumstance when, after adequate ventilation and oxygenation have been established, poor capillary filling persists and there is evidence or suspicion of blood loss with signs of hypovolemia, volume expanders should be given. If a pressure monitor and transducer are available in the delivery room, an umbilical arterial catheter may be used to obtain aortic blood pressure (Fig. 25–16). The use and placement of a central venous line have been debated; however, a low central venous pressure in the presence of poor capillary filling and a low aortic pressure is good evidence of hypovolemic shock and requires volume expansion.

To compound the problem in a hypovolemic infant, shock may not be evident at first in the asphyxial process. Early, there may be marked peripheral vasoconstriction, which will maintain blood pressure. With an effective resuscitation, peripheral vasodilation takes place. At this point a hypovolemic infant will begin to manifest shock.

In an acute situation the volume expander of choice is normal saline. Five percent albumin has been used and previously recommended but appears to offer no advantage over normal saline. In a randomized study of infants with low birth weight with hypotension, saline was compared to 5% albumin. No differences were noted in the number of infants who went on to receive pressor support. However, those given albumin had significantly more weight gain in the first 48 hours than those given normal saline.[69] This increase in weight may well be because albumin easily crosses capillary walls into the extravascular space, reducing the oncotic pressure difference between the vascular space and the interstitium and making fluid retention more likely.[26]

If time permits, fresh frozen plasma can be used. The best volume expander, although rarely available, is whole O-negative blood crossmatched against the mother's blood. This provides volume, oxygen-carrying capacity, and colloid.

Some have suggested that, in an emergency, blood be withdrawn from the fetal side of the placenta and infused into the infant. Although this should very rarely be necessary, if it must be done, it should be carried out in a sterile manner as soon as possible after the placenta is delivered. The syringe used to withdraw the blood should be heparinized and a filter attached to the syringe so that microclots can be filtered out before entering the syringe. Before the blood is infused into the infant, the filter should be changed and blood passed through the filter a second time during the infusion.

Infusion of volume expanders should consist of a volume of 10 mL/kg given over 5 to 10 minutes. If necessary, the infusion can be repeated. Delay in clamping of the cord is desirable in certain circumstances.

SODIUM BICARBONATE

The use of sodium bicarbonate should be discouraged during the acute phase of a neonatal resuscitation in

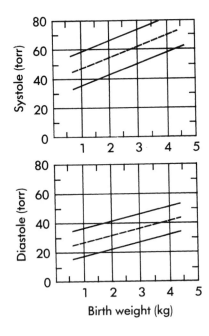

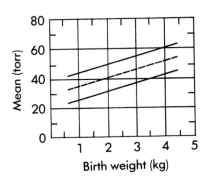

FIGURE 25–16. Systolic, diastolic, and mean aortic blood pressure as function of birth weight. (From Versmold H, et al: Aortic blood pressure during the first 12 hours of life in infants with birth weight 610–4220 grams. Pediatrics 67:607, 1981. Used with permission of the American Academy of Pediatrics.) (See also Appendix B.)

a delivery room. An asphyxiated infant may have both respiratory and metabolic acidosis. Adequate ventilation will correct the respiratory acidosis. The establishment of adequate circulation and oxygenation, along with sufficient carbohydrates for fuel, will stop progression of the acidosis, result in metabolism of lactic acid, and clear the remaining acidosis. (See also Chapter 34, Part Two.) There may be instances in a prolonged resuscitation when it is reasonable to use sodium bicarbonate. However, this should only be done after adequate ventilation is established.

In the absence of adequate ventilation, the administration of bicarbonate may be harmful. Bicarbonate administration results in an acute increase in carbon dioxide. The carbon dioxide crosses cell membranes quickly and will lower the pH of all major organs, including the heart and brain.[7] This can be attenuated with adequate ventilation. Therefore, before bicarbonate is administered, one must be certain that adequate ventilation is established. Another potential danger associated with the use of acute doses of bicarbonate is intracranial hemorrhage, especially in the preterm infant.[52]

If sodium bicarbonate is required, the recommended dose is 2 mEq/kg. To avoid a sudden increase in osmolality, with the risk of intracerebral hemorrhage, the concentration of bicarbonate should be 0.5 mEq/mL, infused at a rate of no more than 1 mEq/kg per minute; thus, it should take 2 minutes to infuse the entire dose. In the midst of a resuscitation this will seem like an impossibly long time.

DOPAMINE

There are times when the infant will have suffered enough myocardial compromise so that, despite resuscitative measures, poor cardiac output and hypotension remain. In these circumstances dopamine should be used. At doses up to 10 μg/kg per minute, dopamine has both an inotropic effect as well as an alpha-adrenergic effect. At these doses, however, the increased cardiac output will antagonize the alpha-adrenergic effect, resulting in increased cardiac output with only mild peripheral vasoconstriction. In higher doses the alpha-adrenergic effect predominates with generalized peripheral vasoconstriction. Moreover, in low doses of up to 5 μg/kg dopamine binds to dopaminergic receptors in the renal, mesenteric, and cerebral arteries, producing vasodilation.

Traditionally dopamine is started at 5 μg/kg per minute and the dose increased as necessary. However, there is some evidence that the neonate may respond to initial doses that are much smaller than those commonly recommended. If the dose reaches 20 μg/kg per minute of dopamine without adequate response, it is unlikely that raising the dose further will make a difference.

THE DRUG-DEPRESSED INFANT

Respiratory depression is not uncommon if a mother has been given a narcotic analgesic within 4 hours of delivery or an inhalation anesthetic before a cesarean section. If the depression is solely related to the drug, with no overlying asphyxia, the infant usually has a good heart rate and simply needs ventilation. If the problem is caused by an inhalation anesthetic, ventilation of the infant will usually remove the anesthetic from the infant's circulation. However, if the cause of the respiratory depression is due to administration of a narcotic to the mother within 4 hours of delivery, naloxone (Narcan) may be useful in antagonizing the respiratory depressant effect. The dose is 0.1 mg/kg. The preferred routes of administration of naloxone are through an endotracheal tube or an umbilical catheter. Naloxone can be given intramuscularly or subcutaneously, although when given using these routes there is a delayed onset of action because the drug needs to be absorbed from the injection site.

The duration of action of the narcotic may be longer than the duration of action of naloxone. Thus, the naloxone may wear off before the narcotic and the infant may slip back into respiratory depression. Repeated doses of naloxone may be necessary. It also is important to understand that naloxone should never be given to an infant of a narcotic-addicted mother because the infant may have acute withdrawal symptoms, including seizures.

IMMEDIATE CARE AFTER ESTABLISHING ADEQUATE VENTILATION AND CIRCULATION

Once an infant is stabilized after resuscitation, the next steps require deliberate consideration. The future course of the infant's resuscitation is related to how well the lungs function and to the presence or absence of a good respiratory drive. Many infants improve rapidly, quickly attaining good lung compliance, adequate pulmonary blood flow, and spontaneous respiration. In these infants, resuscitative efforts can be withdrawn within a matter of minutes. Attention must be paid to the amount of assisted ventilation needed as the infant is improving. As compliance improves there is a tendency to overventilate the infant's lungs. In addition, although 100% oxygen was needed initially, the amount of oxygen can often be lowered to avoid hyperoxygenation. The latter is especially important in the preterm infant.

PROLONGED ASSISTED VENTILATION

(See also Chapter 42, Part Four.)

Some infants will need a ventilator after the immediate resuscitation. In the severely asphyxiated infant, central nervous system depression may inhibit spontaneous ventilation (see Fig. 25–7). As pointed out earlier, the longer the asphyxial process lasts, the longer it takes for resumption of spontaneous ventilation. Most of the infants in this category also will have some degree of pulmonary compromise related to the asphyxial process. Some infants with primary lung disease will initially breathe spontaneously; however, these infants subsequently may need assisted ventilation, either IMV or CPAP, to attain adequate blood gases. Whenever an infant is in need of ventilation for more than the immediate resuscitative period, evaluation of blood gases obtained from an umbilical arterial line should guide the ventilatory support.

GLUCOSE

As soon as the hypoxia is corrected, an infusion of glucose at about 8 mg/kg per minute should be started. Adjustment of the glucose infusion rate will depend on follow-up of blood sugars. The purpose of the glucose is twofold: to provide fuel and to help eliminate the metabolic acidosis. A steady infusion of glucose will provide fuel to an infant who will have depleted much of his or her glycogen, especially myocardial glycogen, during the asphyxial episode. This infusion will thus help prevent the hypoglycemia that frequently accompanies asphyxia. It is important to recognize that glucose should not be started until the infant is adequately oxygenated. Anaerobic metabolism of carbohydrate leads to the formation of additional lactic acid, worsening the acidosis.

FLUIDS

The urine output of any infant undergoing an asphyxial episode should be carefully monitored. Oliguria is a common complication of asphyxia, and an infant can easily be overloaded with fluid. Fluid should be restricted until there is evidence of adequate urine output. The need to restrict fluid and yet give glucose emphasizes the importance of considering glucose infusion in terms of milligrams of glucose per kilogram of body weight per minute, rather than the amount of 10% glucose to be given. The concentration of infused glucose will depend on how much fluid can be given to the infant. (See also Chapter 34.)

FEEDING

During the asphyxial process, ischemia of the intestine occurs as a result of vasoconstriction of the mesenteric vessels. Because of the suggested relationship between ischemia of the intestine and necrotizing enterocolitis, it may be prudent to withhold enteral feedings for a few days in the asphyxiated infant. (See also Chapters 33 and 45, Part Five.)

OTHER PROBLEMS

Other complications of asphyxia that are of concern include hypocalcemia, disseminated intravascular coagulation, seizures, cerebral edema, and intracerebral hemorrhage, as discussed elsewhere in this text.

SPECIAL PROBLEMS DURING RESUSCITATION

PREVENTION OF MECONIUM ASPIRATION

(See also Chapter 42, Part Five.)

If meconium is present in the amniotic fluid, there is a chance that meconium will enter the mouth of the fetus and be aspirated into the lungs. Aspiration of meconium can result in a ball valve obstruction of the airways, causing gas trapping and pneumothorax. It can also cause a reactive inflammatory process. Because meconium-stained amniotic fluid is frequently associated with asphyxia in the newborn, the inability to effect adequate ventilation combined with the initial asphyxia may result in enough hypoxia and acidosis to maintain the increased resistance of the pulmonary vasculature and a persistence of fetal circulation.

The management of the infant born through meconium has represented a controversial area, with varying recommendations. The work of Carson and colleagues[14] in 1976 set in place a virtually universal agreement on the need to suction the hypopharynx after delivery of the head and before delivery of the shoulders. This should be done with a size 10 Fr or larger suction catheter. It is the management of the infant after birth that has generated controversy.

The hallmark study of Gregory and associates[31] in 1974, done before suctioning on the perineum was common, recommended that "all infants born through thick, particulate, or pea soup meconium should have the trachea aspirated immediately after birth." This was reinforced in a retrospective, uncontrolled study by Ting and coworkers[74] in 1975, in which vigorous infants with slight meconium were excluded. Ting and coworkers recommended immediate tracheal suction for infants born through meconium-stained amniotic fluid.

As a result of the Gregory and Ting studies and a 1977 statement by the American Academy of Pediatrics Committee on Fetus and Newborn, which said nothing about suctioning the hypopharynx on the perineum, intubation and tracheal suctioning became routine in many nurseries.

In the early and mid-1980s there were reports in the obstetrics literature that, even with "appropriate" management of the infant, meconium aspiration syndrome continued to occur.[20, 24] In the neonatal resuscitation guidelines of 1986,[48] it was suggested that all infants with thick meconium undergo intubation and tracheal suction. No distinction was made with regard to the depressed versus the vigorous infant. In 1988, Linder and colleagues[39] published a controlled, randomized trial examining the value of endotracheal intubation and suction in *vigorous* infants. They noted that in vigorous infants the morbidity, including complications of intubation, was 2% greater in infants who had undergone intubation and suctioning. In 1990, Cunningham and associates[18] proposed a standard of care that reserved intubation largely for infants who were depressed and who required positive pressure ventilation.

In 1992 the American Academy of Pediatrics/American College of Obstetricians and Gynecologists *Guidelines for Perinatal Care*[27] recommended that, in the presence of thick meconium *and* respiratory depression, the larynx be visualized, and if meconium is seen, the trachea be intubated and suctioned. It was noted that if the infant is vigorous, the indication for visualization of the cords and endotracheal suction is "less clear." In an article reporting a retrospective chart review in 1992, Wiswell and coworkers[79] argued that endotracheal intubation should not be limited to depressed infants because 54% of their study infants with meconium aspiration syndrome did not need positive pressure ventilation and were presumed vigorous at birth, including one infant with only thin meconium. Wiswell and coworkers also noted no significant adverse sequelae associated with intubation.

In 2000, a multicenter study looked at vigorous infants with a gestational age of more than 37 weeks

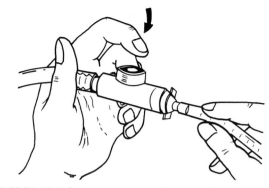

FIGURE 25–17. Adapter to connect endotracheal tube to mechanical suction. (From American Heart Association/American Academy of Pediatrics: Textbook of Neonatal Resuscitation. Dallas, American Heart Association, 1994.)

who were born through meconium-stained amniotic fluid of any consistency. In these vigorous infants intubation and tracheal suctioning did not offer any advantage over expectant management.[80]

All depressed infants, with either thick or thin meconium, should undergo direct tracheal suctioning. However, it now appears that vigorous infants, regardless of the thickness of the meconium in the amniotic fluid, need not be handled in a special way. Although some may still recommend that the vigorous infant with thick meconium undergo endotracheal suctioning, clinical judgment should be used to determine whether the difficulty in intubation of a vigorous infant outweighs the advantages of intubation and suctioning.

If intubation is to be done and meconium removed from the trachea, the best method is to attach an adapter to the endotracheal tube so that suction can be directly applied using regulated wall suction at approximately 100 mm Hg as the tube is withdrawn (Fig. 25–17). The trachea can then be reintubated and suctioned again if necessary. Because some infants with thick meconium are severely asphyxiated, it may not be possible to clear the trachea completely before beginning positive pressure ventilation. Clinical judgment determines the number of reintubations needed.

PNEUMOTHORAX

(See also Chapter 42, Part Five.)

A pneumothorax is a potential problem whenever positive pressure ventilation is used. A pneumothorax should be suspected in any infant who is improving during a resuscitative effort and then suddenly decompensates. Listening to the infant, one may hear unequal breath sounds and distant heart sounds, which may be shifted from the normal position in the left side of the chest. The affected side of the chest will be hyperinflated compared with the nonaffected side and will have less movement during ventilation. If the pneumothorax is large enough to obstruct venous return, cardiac output will fall and the infant will become hypotensive. When these events occur in an infant who is otherwise stable, a pneumothorax is easy to suspect. However, when a pneumothorax occurs early during resuscitation of a severely compromised infant, the signs and symptoms are not as obvious and a high index of suspicion is needed. When immediate intervention in the delivery room is needed, it may be necessary to insert a needle into the thorax before radiographic confirmation.

DIAPHRAGMATIC HERNIA

(See also Chapters 11, Part Two, 42, Part Five, and 45, Part Four.)

An infant with a diaphragmatic hernia whose bowel suddenly fills with air as a consequence of spontaneous or mask ventilation may appear much the same as an infant with a pneumothorax.

To prevent gas from entering the intestines, one should always use an endotracheal tube when ventilating the lungs of an infant with a suspected diaphragmatic hernia. An orogastric tube should be inserted as soon as possible to remove air before it passes into the portion of intestine located in the chest. Forcing air into the intestine with bag-and-mask ventilation increases the chances of inflating intrathoracic stomach or bowel, further compromising pulmonary function.

ERYTHROBLASTOSIS/HYDROPS

(See also Chapters 20, 21, and 44.)

Successful resuscitation of an infant with hydrops demands preparation of a coordinated team with preassigned responsibilities. The team should be prepared at delivery to perform a partial (or, rarely, complete) exchange transfusion with O-negative packed cells crossmatched against the mother. In addition, they should be prepared to perform a thoracentesis, paracentesis, and complete resuscitation.

The infant with hydrops may not only be severely anemic but also is likely to have ascites, a pleural effusion, and pulmonary edema. Furthermore, such infants frequently have had chronic intrauterine and intrapartum asphyxia. Because they are usually premature, respiratory distress syndrome may be an overlying confounding complication. On delivery, the infant should immediately undergo intubation because of poor lung compliance and the risk of pulmonary edema. High ventilator pressures are typically needed. If adequate ventilation cannot be attained and there is evidence of fluid in the abdomen or pleural space, consideration should be given to performing a paracentesis as well as a thoracentesis. Ultrasonography done before delivery may be helpful in determining the amount of fluid present. If the abdomen is markedly distended, the paracentesis should be performed first to relieve pressure on the diaphragm; this may need to be followed with a thoracentesis. Although most of these infants will initially have a normal blood volume, after a large amount of ascitic and pleural fluid has been removed, some of this fluid may reaccumulate, lowering vascular volume. Therefore, careful attention should be paid to maintenance of intravascular volume and the prevention of shock after resuscitation.

A hematocrit obtained immediately at birth will determine the need for an exchange transfusion (usually partial) in the delivery room. If the infant is extremely anemic and in need of oxygen-carrying capacity, catheters should be inserted into both the umbilical vein and artery to permit a slow isovolemic exchange with packed cells, which will result in minimal impact on the already borderline hemodynamic status of the infant. These lines also can be used to monitor central venous pressure and aortic pressure to determine the volume needs of the infant. This is especially important when large amounts of fluid are removed from the thorax or abdomen.

SCREENING FOR CONGENITAL DEFECTS

(See also Chapters 26 and 28.)

Two percent to three percent of infants are born with a congenital anomaly that will require intervention soon after birth. If undetected, some of the anomalies may result in life-threatening problems. Immediately after birth, choanal atresia or diaphragmatic hernia may result in respiratory distress. Other problems may appear later, such as aspiration caused by esophageal atresia (with esophageal fistula) or a high intestinal obstruction. A rapid screening test for congenital defects that can easily be performed by the delivery room staff can help identify many of these defects, along with others that are not life-threatening but require prompt recognition and intervention.

EXTERNAL PHYSICAL EXAMINATION

A rapid external physical examination will identify obvious abnormalities such as abnormal facies, and limb, abdominal wall, or spinal column defects. A close look at the abdomen may reveal a scaphoid abdomen, which is a clue to a diaphragmatic hernia. If an umbilical vessel count reveals only two vessels, there is a possibility of other defects, especially involving the genitourinary tract.

INTERNAL PHYSICAL EXAMINATION

Because infants are preferential nasal breathers, bilateral *choanal atresia* will result in respiratory difficulty and require an airway at birth (see also Chapter 42, Parts Five and Six). Bilateral choanal atresia can be ruled out quickly if the infant is able to breathe while the mouth is held closed. Some infants with unilateral choanal obstruction appear normal until an examiner closes the mouth and then sequentially obstructs the nostrils with a finger. When the patent nostril is obstructed, such infants will have difficulty breathing. Confirmation of choanal atresia results from the insertion of a soft nasogastric tube into each nostril. If an obstruction is reached within 3 to 4 cm, choanal atresia is a possibility.

An examination of the mouth will identify a cleft

palate. Inserting a nasogastric tube through the mouth may help identify an *esophageal atresia* or a high intestinal obstruction. If the tube does not reach the stomach, an esophageal atresia, most often associated with a tracheoesophageal fistula, is a likely possibility. A few cubic centimeters of air forced through the tube, while listening over the stomach, will confirm that the tube is in the stomach. Once the tube is in the stomach, the contents of the stomach can be suctioned. If more than 15 to 20 mL of gastric contents is obtained, the chances of a high intestinal obstruction are increased. The same tube can then be removed and gently inserted into the anal opening. Easy passage of the catheter for 3 cm into the anus makes atresia unlikely. A minute or so spent screening for congenital defects in this way may help to avert many future problems.

■ REFERENCES

1. Adamsons K, et al: Resuscitation by positive pressure ventilation and *tris*-hydroxymethyl-aminomethane of rhesus monkeys asphyxiated at birth. J Pediatr 65:807, 1964.
2. Adamsons K, et al: The influence of thermal factors upon oxygen consumption of the newborn human infant. J Pediatr 66:45, 1965.
3. American Heart Association/American Academy of Pediatrics: Textbook of Neonatal Resuscitation, 4th ed. Dallas, American Heart Association National Center, 2000.
4. Apgar V: A proposal for a new method of evaluation of the newborn infant. Anesth Analg 32:260, 1953.
5. Berkowitz ID: Epinephrine dosage effects on cerebral and myocardial blood flow in an infant swine model of cardiopulmonary resuscitation. Anesthesiology 75:1041, 1991.
6. Berkowitz ID, et al: Blood flow during cardiopulmonary resuscitation with simultaneous compression and ventilation in infant pigs. Pediatr Res 26:558, 1989.
7. Bersin RM: Effects of sodium bicarbonate on myocardial metabolism and circulatory function during hypoxia. In Arieff AI (ed): Hypoxia, Metabolic Acidosis, and the Circulation. Oxford, England, Oxford University Press, 1992.
8. Bland R: Formation of fetal lung liquid and its removal near birth. In Polin RA, et al (ed): Fetal and Neonatal Physiology, Philadelphia, WB Saunders Co, 1992, p 782.
9. Boon AW, et al: Lung expansion, tidal exchange and formation of the functional residual capacity during resuscitation of asphyxiated neonates. J Pediatr 95:1301, 1979.
10. Boylan PC, et al: Acid-base physiology in the fetus. In Creasy RK, et al (eds): Maternal-Fetal Medicine. Philadelphia, WB Saunders Co, 1989.
11. Brimacombe J: The laryngeal mask airway for neonatal resuscitation. Pediatrics 93:874, 1994.
12. Bruck K: Temperature regulation in the newborn infant. Biol Neonate 3:65, 1961.
13. Carlton DP, et al: Lung overexpansion increases pulmonary microvascular protein permeability in lambs. J Appl Physiol 69:577, 1990.
14. Carson BE, et al: Combined obstetric and pediatric approach to prevent meconium aspiration syndrome. Am J Obstet Gynecol 126:712, 1976.
15. Cassin S, et al: The vascular resistance of the foetal and newly ventilated lung of the lamb. J Physiol 171:61, 1964.
16. Chandra N, et al: Augmentation of carotid flow during cardiopulmonary resuscitation by ventilation at high airway pressure simultaneous with chest compression. Am J Cardiol 48:1053, 1981.
17. Cordero L Jr, et al: Neonatal bradycardia following nasopharyngeal stimulation. J Pediatr 78:441, 1971.
18. Cunningham AS, et al: Tracheal suction and meconium: A proposed standard of care. J Pediatr 116:153, 1990.
19. David R: Closed chest massage in the newborn infant. Pediatrics 81:552, 1988.
20. Davis RO, et al: Fetal meconium aspiration syndrome occurring despite airway management considered appropriate. Am J Obstet Gynecol 151:731, 1985.
21. Dawes GS: Birth asphyxia, resuscitation, brain damage. In Foetal and Neonatal Physiology. Chicago, Year Book Medical, 1968, p 141.
22. Downing SE, et al: Influences of arterial oxygen tension and pH on cardiac function in the newborn lamb. Am J Physiol 211:1203, 1966.
23. Dunn PM: Localization of the umbilical catheter by postmortem measurements. Arch Dis Child 41:69, 1966.
24. Falciglia HS: Failure to prevent meconium aspiration syndrome. Obstet Gynecol 71:349, 1983.
25. Finer NN, et al: Limitations of self-inflating resuscitators. Pediatrics 77:417, 1986.
26. Fleck A, et al: Increased vascular permeability: A major cause of hypoalbuminemia in disease and injury. Lancet 1:781, 1985.
27. Freeman RK, et al (eds): American Academy of Pediatrics American College of Obstetricians and Gynecologists Guidelines for Perinatal Care, 3rd ed. Elk Grove Village, Ill, American Academy of Pediatrics, 1992.
28. Gandini D, Brimacombe JR: Neonatal resuscitation with the laryngeal mask airway in normal and low birth weight infants. Anesth Analg 89:642, 1999.
29. Gannon CM: Volutrauma, $PaCO_2$ levels and neurodevelopmental sequelae following assisted ventilation. Clin Perinatol 25:159, 1998.
30. Goetting MG, et al: High-dose epinephrine improves outcome from pediatric cardiac arrest. Ann Emerg Med 20:22, 1991.
31. Gregory GA, et al: Meconium aspiration in infants: A prospective study. J Pediatr 85:848, 1974.
32. Hernandez LA, et al: Chest wall restriction limits high airway pressure-induced lung injury in young rabbits. J Appl Physiol 66:2364, 1989.
33. International Guidelines for Neonatal Resuscitation: An excerpt from the Guidelines 2000 for cardiopulmonary resuscitation and emergency cardiovascular care: International Consensus on Science. Pediatrics 106, 2000. Available at: http://www.pediatrics.org/cgi/content/full/106/3/e29.
34. Jain L: Alveolar fluid clearance in developing lungs and its role in neonatal transition. Clin Perinatol 26:585, 1999.
35. Kanter RK: Evaluation of mask-bag-ventilation in resuscitation of infants. Am J Dis Child 141:761, 1987.
36. Kattwinkel J, et al: ILCOR advisory statement: Resuscitation of the newly born infant. Pediatrics 103(4):e56, 1999. Available at:http://www.pediatrics.org/cgi/content/full/103/4/e56.
37. Krisher JP, et al: Comparison of pre-hospital conventional and simultaneous compression-ventilation cardiopulmonary resuscitation. Crit Care Med 17:1263, 1989.
38. Lawson EE, et al: Augmentation of pulmonary surfactant by lung expansion at birth. Pediatr Res 13:611, 1979.
39. Linder N, et al: Need for endotracheal intubation and suction in meconium-stained neonates. J Pediatr 112:6135, 1988.
40. Linder W, et al: Delivery room management of extremely low birth weight infants: Spontaneous breathing or intubation? Pediatrics 103:961, 1999.
41. Lindermann R: Resuscitation of the newborn with endotracheal administration of epinephrine. Acta Pediatr Scand 73:210, 1984.
42. Lucus VW Jr, et al: Epinephrine absorption following endotracheal administration: Effects of hypoxia-induced low pulmonary blood flow. Resuscitation 27:31, 1994.
43. Lundstrom KE: Initial treatment of preterm infants-continuous positive airway pressure or ventilation? Eur J Pediatr 155(Suppl 2):S25, 1996.
44. Meschia G: Placental respiratory gas exchange and fetal oxygenation. In Creasy RK, et al (eds): Maternal-Fetal Medicine: Principles and Practice. Philadelphia, WB Saunders Co, 1989.
45. Miller DL, et al: Body temperature in the immediate neonatal period: The effect of reducing thermal losses. Am J Obstet Gynecol 94:964, 1966.
46. Milner AD, et al: Lung expansion at birth. J Pediatr 101:879, 1982.
47. Morin CM, et al: Response of the fetal circulation to stress. In

Polin RA, et al (eds): Fetal and Neonatal Physiology. Philadelphia, WB Saunders Co, 1992, p 620.

48. Neonatal Resuscitation in American Heart Association: Standards and guidelines for cardiopulmonary resuscitation and emergency care. JAMA 255:2969, 1986.

49. Neonatal Resuscitation Steering Committee—AHA/AAP: Why change the compression and ventilation rates during CPR in neonates? Pediatrics 93:1026, 1994.

50. Nicolaides KH, et al: Ultrasound-guided sampling of umbilical cord and placental blood to assess fetal well-being. Lancet 1:1065, 1986.

51. Orlowski JP, et al: Endotracheal epinephrine is unreliable. Resuscitation 19:103, 1990.

52. Papile LA, et al: Relationship of intravenous sodium bicarbonate infusion and cerebral intraventricular hemorrhage. J Pediatr 93:834, 1978.

53. Paradis NA, et al: The effect of standard and high-dose epinephrine on coronary perfusion pressure during prolonged cardiopulmonary resuscitation. JAMA 265:1139, 1991.

54. Paterson SJ, et al: Neonatal resuscitation using the laryngeal mask airway. Anesthesiology 80:1248, 1994.

55. Patrick J, et al: Patterns of human fetal breathing during the last 10 weeks of pregnancy. Obstet Gynecol 56:24, 1980.

56. Perlman JM, et al: Cardiopulmonary resuscitation in the delivery room: Associated clinical events. Arch Pediatr Adolesc Med 149:20, 1995.

57. Poulsen JP, et al: Hypoxanthine, xanthine, and uric acid in newborn pigs during hypoxia followed by resuscitation with room air or 100% oxygen. Crit Care Med 21:1058, 1993.

58. Press S, et al: Cesarean delivery of full-term infants: Identification of those at high risk for requiring resuscitation. J Pediatr 106:477, 1985.

59. Preziosi MP, et al: Metabolic acidemia with hypoxia attenuates the hemodynamic responses to epinephrine during resuscitation in lambs. Crit Care Med 21:1901, 1993.

60. Quinton DN, et al: Comparison of endotracheal and peripheral intravenous adrenaline in cardiac arrest: Is the endotracheal route reliable? Lancet 1:828, 1987.

61. Ramji S, et al: Resuscitation of asphyxic newborn infants with room air or 100% oxygen. Pediatr Res 34:809, 1993.

62. Rootwelt T, et al: Hypoxemia and reoxygenation with 21% or 100% oxygen in newborn pigs: Changes in blood pressure, base deficit, and hypoxanthine and brain morphology. Pediatr Res 32:107, 1992.

63. Rudikoff MT, et al: Mechanisms of blood flow during cardiopulmonary "thoracic pump supported" resuscitation. Circulation 61:345, 1980.

64. Rudolph AM, et al: Response of the pulmonary vasculature to hypoxia and H^+ ion concentration changes. J Clin Invest 45:339, 1966.

65. Rudolph AM, et al: Fetal cardiovascular response to stress. In Wiknjosastro WH, et al (eds): Perinatology. New York, Elsevier Science, 1988.

66. Saugstad OD: Resuscitation of newborn infants: Do we need new guidelines? Prenat Neonat Med 1:26, 1996.

67. Saugstad OD, et al: Resuscitation of asphyxiated newborn infants with room air or oxygen: An international controlled trial: The Resair 2 Study. Pediatrics 102:e1, 1998. Available at: http://www.pediatrics.org/cgi/content/full/102/1/e1.

68. Saugstad OD: Oxygen toxicity in the neonatal period. Acta Paediatr 79:881, 1990.

69. So KW, et al: Randomized controlled trial of colloid or crystalloid in hypotensive preterm infants. Arch Dis Child 76:F43, 1997.

70. Swenson RD, et al: Hemodynamics in humans during conventional and experimental methods of cardiopulmonary resuscitation. Circulation 78:630, 1988.

71. Tarnow-Mordi WO: Room air or oxygen for asphyxiated babies? Lancet 352:341, 1998.

72. Teitel DF: Circulatory adjustments to postnatal life. Semin Perinatol 12:96, 1988.

73. Teitel DF: Physiologic development of the cardiovascular system in the fetus. In Polin RA, et al (eds): Fetal and Neonatal Physiology. Philadelphia, WB Saunders, 1992, p 615.

74. Ting P, et al: Tracheal suction in meconium aspiration. Am J Obstet Gynecol 122:767, 1975.

75. Todres ID, et al: Methods of external cardiac massage in the newborn infant. J Pediatr 86:781, 1975.

76. Upton CJ, et al: Endotracheal resuscitation of neonates using a rebreathing bag. Arch Dis Child 66:39, 1991.

77. Vyas H, et al: Intrathoracic pressure and volume changes during the spontaneous onset of respiration in babies born by cesarean section and by vaginal delivery. J Pediatr 99:787, 1981.

78. Vyas H, et al: Physiologic responses to prolonged and slow-rise inflation in the resuscitation of the asphyxiated newborn infant. J Pediatr 99:635, 1981.

79. Wiswell TC, et al: Intratracheal suctioning, systemic infection, and the meconium aspiration syndrome. Pediatrics 89:203, 1992.

80. Wiswell TC, et al: Delivery room management of the apparently vigorous meconium-stained neonate: Results of the multicenter, international collaborative trial. Pediatrics 105:1, 2000.

26

Physical Examination and Care of the Newborn

part one

PHYSICAL EXAMINATION OF THE NEWBORN

Tom Lissauer

Immediately after a baby is born, all parents want to know "Is my baby all right?" A quick, initial physical examination of all newborns should be performed in the delivery room to check that there are no major anomalies or birth injuries, that the newborn's tongue and body appear pink, and that breathing is normal. The whole of the newborn's body must be checked. This will usually allow the health care provider to reassure the parents that their infant looks well and appears normal.

Many serious congenital anomalies will have been identified prenatally, their presence anticipated, and a management plan made before delivery. If the newborn is sufficiently preterm or small for gestational age, has a significant problem diagnosed prenatally, or is unwell (e.g., with respiratory distress), the newborn will need to be admitted to an intermediate or intensive care nursery in accordance with hospital guidelines (see Part Two). If the mother had hydramnios, a feeding tube should be passed into the stomach to exclude esophageal atresia. When the infant is born, the parents will have been informed if it is a boy or girl. If there is any doubt about the infant's gender, it is important not to guess but to inform the parents that further evaluation is required before a definite decision is made.

During the first few hours after birth, healthy newborns are usually alert and reactive and will suck at the breast. This will provide an initial opportunity for the mother to form a close attachment with her infant and to establish breast milk feeding. Medical interference during this time should be kept to a minimum if the infant is well.

ROUTINE EXAMINATION OF THE NEWBORN

Every newborn infant should have a "routine examination of the newborn."[1, 18] This is a detailed examination performed by an experienced health care provider within 24 hours of birth. Its purpose is to

- Detect congenital abnormalities not already identified at birth (e.g., congenital heart disease and congenital dislocation of the hip)
- Identify common neonatal problems and initiate their management or reassure the parents
- Check for potential problems arising from maternal disease, familial disorders, or those detected during pregnancy
- Provide an opportunity for the parents to discuss any questions about their infant
- Initiate health promotion for the newborn

Before approaching the mother and infant, the mother and infant's medical and nursing notes should be checked (see Chapter 2). Items of particular relevance are

- The mother's age, occupation, and social background
- Family history
- History of maternal drug or alcohol abuse
- Details of previous pregnancies and any medical problems encountered by her children
- History of maternal disease and drugs taken during pregnancy
- Results of pregnancy screening tests (e.g., blood tests, prenatal ultrasound scans)
- Special diagnostic procedures (e.g., amniocentesis, chorionic villous sampling)
- Problems during labor and delivery
- Infant's condition at birth and if resuscitation was required
- Any concerns about the infant from nursing staff or parents
- The infant's birth weight
- The gestational age and if there is any uncertainty about it
- The infant's gender

INTRODUCTION TO THE MOTHER

The health care provider should introduce himself or herself to the mother or preferably to both parents and explain the purpose of the examination. It is usually best at this stage to inquire if there are any problems with feeding and if there are any other worries about the infant. Before starting the examination, the health care professional must perform a thorough hand washing and ensure that the newborn can be examined in a warm, private area with good lighting.

ORDER OF THE EXAMINATION

The exact sequence in which the newborn is examined is not important. What is important is that all aspects of the newborn are examined at some stage and that the whole of the infant is observed. Indeed, if the newborn is quiet, one may well take the opportunity to listen to the heart and examine the eyes directly. It is convenient to make one's general observations of the newborn's appearance, posture, and movements while undressing him or her, to conduct the examination from head to foot, to examine the hips, and then to pick the newborn up and turn him or her over to examine the back (Fig. 26–1). A checklist is helpful to record the findings of the examination and to ensure that nothing has been omitted.

MEASUREMENTS

The infant's birth weight, gender, and gestational age should be noted. The 10th to 90th centile for weight at 40 weeks' gestation for a male infant is 2.9 to 4.2 kg (mean, 3.6 kg), and for a female infant it is 2.8 to 4 kg (mean 3.5 kg) (see Appendix). The birth weight centile can be ascertained from the growth chart. If the infant's gestational age is uncertain, it can be determined (± 2 weeks' gestational age) using a standardized scoring scheme. The head circumference should be measured at its maximum to identify microcephaly or macrocephaly and to serve as a reference for future measurements. However, it can change markedly in the first few days because of molding of the head during delivery. The 10th to 90th centile is 33 to 37 cm at 40 weeks. The infant's length is measured routinely in the United States but not in the United Kingdom (48 to 53 cm at 40 weeks). Because the hips and lower legs need to be held extended by an assistant, the length is rarely measured accurately enough to identify short stature or serve as a reliable reference value when measured routinely.[18] The length of the arms and legs relative to that of the trunk is observed, although short limbs from skeletal dysplasias can be difficult to appreciate in the immediate newborn period.

GENERAL OBSERVATION OF THE NEWBORN'S APPEARANCE, POSTURE, AND MOVEMENTS

Much valuable information can be gleaned by simply observing the newborn. The skin of a newborn looks reddish pink. He or she may appear plethoric from polycythemia or unduly pale from anemia or shock. If polycythemia or anemia is suggested, the hemoglobin concentration or hematocrit should be checked. Jaundice within the first 24 hours of birth, unless mild, is most likely to be hemolytic and requires investigation and treatment.

Central cyanosis is best observed on the tongue. If present, this requires urgent investigation. If there is any doubt, the newborn's oxygen saturation should be checked with a pulse oximeter. Polycythemic infants may appear cyanosed because they have more than 5 gm of reduced hemoglobin per 100 mL even though they are adequately oxygenated.

The facial appearance is observed. If abnormal, does the newborn have a syndrome?

Part of the overall examination is to observe the newborn's posture and tone. Is he or she moving all four limbs fully and are they held in a normal, flexed position?

HEAD

The fontanelle and sutures are palpated. The size of the anterior fontanelle is very variable. After delivery, the sagittal sutures are often separated whereas the coronal sutures are overriding. The posterior fontanelle is often open, but small. If the fontanelle is tense when the newborn is not crying, this may be from raised intracranial pressure and cranial ultrasonography should be performed. A tense fontanelle is also a late sign of meningitis.

EYES

The eyes should be checked both by inspection and with an ophthalmoscope. The red reflex should be elicited using an ophthalmoscope. The red retinal reflex can be seen if the lens is clear but not if it is opaque from a congenital cataract or glaucoma. If the red reflex is abnormal, an ophthalmologist should be consulted urgently. Congenital cataract is the most common form of preventable childhood blindness.

EARS

The shape, size, and position of the ears are checked. Low-set ears are those where the top of the pinna falls below a line drawn from the outer canthus of the eye at right angles to the face. Low-set or abnormal ears are a characteristic of a number of syndromes.

PALATE

The palate needs to be inspected, including posteriorly, to exclude a posterior cleft palate. It should also be palpated to detect an indentation of the posterior palate from a submucous cleft or a posterior cleft palate.

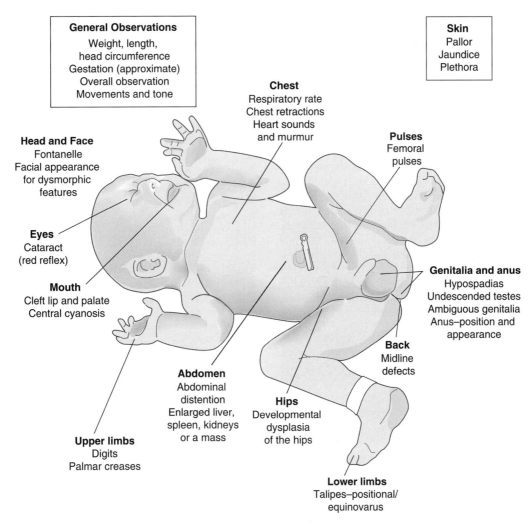

FIGURE 26–1. Main features of routine examination of the newborn.

BREATHING

Breathing and chest wall movement are observed. The respiratory rate should be less than 60 breaths per minute without chest retraction or flaring of the alae nasi or grunting. If the breathing is normal, it is very rare for any significant abnormalities to be detected on auscultation. If respiratory distress is present, further evaluation is required immediately.

EXAMINATION OF THE HEART

The normal heart rate is 110 to 150 beats per minute in term infants but may drop to 85 beats per minute during sleep. The heart sounds should be loudest on the left side of the chest and no murmurs should be present.

PALPATION OF THE ABDOMEN

Observation will readily reveal abdominal distention. For palpation, the infant needs to be relaxed. The abdomen is palpated to identify any masses. The liver is normally palpable 1 to 2 cm below the costal mar-

gin. The spleen tip may be palpable, as may the kidney on the left side.

FEMORAL PULSES

These can be palpated when the infant is quiet. Their pulse pressure is reduced if there is coarctation of the aorta. If suggested clinically, it can be confirmed by comparing the blood pressure in the arms and legs. The pulse pressure is increased if there is a patent ductus arteriosus.

GENITALIA

In boys, the penis is checked for length and the position of the urethral orifice. The presence of testes in the scrotum is confirmed, especially if the scrotum is poorly developed. In girls, the clitoris and labia minora are prominent if preterm but are covered by the labia majora at full term. The position and appearance of the anus is also inspected. Passage of urine and meconium should be checked.

EXTREMITIES

The hands and arms and feet and legs are examined to identify an abnormality, such as extra digits. Infants who were in an extended breech position in utero may maintain this posture for some days after birth.

HIPS

The hips are checked for developmental dysplasia of the hips. It is best left toward the end of the examination because the procedure is uncomfortable. To successfully perform this examination, the infant needs to lie supine on a flat, firm surface and be relaxed, because crying or kicking will result in tightening of the muscles around the hip. The pelvis is stabilized with one hand. With the other hand the examiner's middle finger is placed over the greater trochanter and the thumb over the lesser trochanter. The Barlow test is performed to dislocate posteriorly an unstable hip that is lying in the joint (see Chapter 52, Part Three).[6] The hip is flexed and adducted, and the femoral head is gently pushed downward. If the hip can be dislocated, the femoral head will be pushed posteriorly out of the acetabulum and will move with a "clunk."

Next, the hip is checked to see if it can be returned from a dislocated position back into the acetabulum (the Ortolani test) (see Chapter 52, Part Three). With the hip abducted, upward leverage is applied. A dislocated hip will return with a "clunk" into the acetabulum. This is best felt but can sometimes also be observed. It should also be possible to abduct the hips fully, but this may be restricted if the hip is dislocated and may be the only abnormal sign of developmental dysplasia of the hips. Any newborn with developmental dysplasia of the hips should be checked for a neuromuscular disorder, and the spine should be examined to exclude spina bifida.

THE BACK AND SPINE AND MUSCLE TONE

The newborn is picked up under the arms, while supporting the head. If hypotonic, the newborn will feel as though he or she is slipping through one's hands. Most newborns will support their weight with their feet. On turning the infant prone, they can lift the head to the horizontal and straighten the back. Hypotonic newborns flop down like a rag doll. The whole of the back and spine are checked for midline and other defects and for any curvature of the spine.

A detailed neurologic examination is only required if an abnormality has been detected. Some pediatricians routinely perform a Moro reflex, when sudden head extension causes symmetric extension followed by flexion of all limbs. However, if normal movement of all four limbs has been observed, no further information will be elicited from this procedure. Because infants appear to find it unpleasant and parents are often alarmed and upset by it, it is best omitted from the routine examination.

Most newborns will be found to be normal on their routine examination. The parents should be strongly reassured that the examination was normal, and any concerns they have about their newborn should be answered fully.

LESIONS THAT RESOLVE SPONTANEOUSLY

There are a number of conditions that may be observed during the routine examination and may alarm parents but that resolve spontaneously.

PERIPHERAL AND TRAUMATIC CYANOSIS

Peripheral cyanosis confined to the hands and feet is common during the first day of life and is of no clinical significance.

Traumatic cyanosis is blue discoloration of the skin, often with petechiae. It may affect the presenting part in a face or breech presentation of the head and neck if the umbilical cord was wrapped around the infant's neck. However, the tongue remains pink.

BRUISING OF THE HEAD

There may be marked molding from the head having to squeeze through the birth canal. Newborns who have been in the breech position in utero often have a prominent occipital shelf. A *caput succedaneum* is when there is bruising and edema of the presenting part of the head. It extends beyond the margins of the skull bones. A *cephalhematoma* is from bleeding between the periosteum and the skull bone. It is confined within the margins of the skull sutures, usually affecting the parietal bone. Bruising and abrasions after forceps deliveries, from scalp electrodes, or from fetal blood sampling are relatively common (see Chapter 27).

SWOLLEN EYELIDS

Swelling of the eyelids is common in newborns and resolves over the first few days of life. There may also be a mucoid discharge, often called a "sticky eye." When present on the first day of life it usually resolves spontaneously. The eyelids can be cleansed with sterile water. This needs to be contrasted to the erythematous, swollen eyelids with purulent eye discharge seen in conjunctivitis in the first day of life from gonococcal infection, although this is extremely rare in developed countries irrespective of whether newborns are given prophylactic eye drops.

SUBCONJUNCTIVAL HEMORRHAGES

Subconjunctival hemorrhages are common. They occur during delivery and resolve in 1 to 2 weeks.

PEELING DRY SKIN

Dry skin is common, especially in post-term infants.

CAPILLARY HEMANGIOMA OR STORK BITES

These pink macules appear on the upper eyelids, the mid forehead, and the nape of the neck from distention of dermal capillaries. Those on the eyelids and forehead fade over the first year, whereas those on the neck become covered with hair.

NEONATAL URTICARIA (ERYTHEMA TOXICUM)

This common rash usually starts on the second or third day of life. There are white pinpoint papules at the center of an erythematous base. Eosinophils are present on microscopy. The lesions migrate to different sites (see Chapter 50).

MILIA

Benign white cysts may be present on the nose and cheeks from retention of keratin and sebaceous material in the pilaceous follicles.

EPSTEIN PEARLS AND CYSTS OF THE GUMS

Small white pearls may be visible along the midline of the palate (Epstein pearls).

Cysts of the gums (epulis) and on the floor of the mouth (ranula) are mucus retention cysts and do not need any treatment.

HARLEQUIN COLOR CHANGE

There is longitudinal reddening down one half of the body with a sharply demarcated blanching down the other side. This lasts for a few minutes. It is thought to be due to vasomotor instability.

PROMINENCE OF THE CLAVICLE

Clavicular fractures most often occur during difficult delivery of the shoulders. A lump on the clavicle may be palpated or observed or identified because the infant keeps the arm immobile. It results from callus around a fracture and will heal without treatment.

BREAST ENLARGEMENT

This may occur in newborns of either gender. A small amount of milk ("witches' milk") may be discharged.

HYDROCELES

These are not uncommon in boys and usually resolve spontaneously.

VAGINAL DISCHARGE

There may be a white vaginal discharge or small amount of bleeding from maternal hormonal withdrawal. There may also be prolapse of a ring of vaginal mucosa.

MONGOLIAN BLUE SPOTS

These are blue-black macular discolorations at the base of the spine or on the buttocks. They occasionally also occur on the legs and other parts of the body. They occur most often in African-American or Asian infants and fade slowly over the first few years of life. They are of no clinical significance but are occasionally misdiagnosed as bruises.

UMBILICAL HERNIA

These hernias are common especially in African-American infants. No treatment is indicated because they usually resolve within the first few years of life.

SIGNIFICANT ABNORMALITIES DETECTED ON ROUTINE EXAMINATION

The prevalence of the most common significant congenital abnormalities is shown in Table 26–1. Some of them will be detected prenatally, but many are first noted in the delivery room or during the routine examination of the newborn. These lesions are described briefly here but are considered in more detail elsewhere in the book.

SYNDROMES

Identification of abnormal facies and other abnormalities may lead one to suspect that the newborn has a syndrome. Down syndrome is by far the most common. The characteristic facies is often more difficult to recognize in the immediate neonatal period than in later life, but other abnormalities, such as the flat occiput, hypotonia, bilateral single palmar creases, and a pronounced "sandal gap" and abnormal skin crease between the big and first toe are helpful additional signs. In practice, the parents will usually need to be informed of the diagnosis before the results of

TABLE 26–1 PREVALENCE OF SERIOUS CONGENITAL ANOMALIES (PER 1000 LIVE BIRTHS)

ANOMALY	PREVALENCE
Congenital heart disease	6–8 (0.8 identified in the first day of life)
Congenital dislocation of the hip	0.8 (about 7/1000 have an abnormal initial examination)
Talipes equinovarus	1.5
Down syndrome	1.5
Cleft lip and palate	0.8
Urogenital (hypospadias, undescended testes)	1.2
Spina bifida/anencephalopathy	0.5

the chromosome analysis are available. An experienced pediatrician should always confirm the diagnosis clinically before the parents are informed.

Many hundreds of syndromes have been described. When the diagnosis is uncertain, a book or computer database should be consulted and advice sought from a pediatrician or clinical geneticist.

PORT-WINE STAIN (NEVUS FLAMMEUS)

These lesions are due to a vascular malformation of the capillaries in the dermis. They are usually present at birth. When disfiguring, the appearance of these lesions can now be improved using laser therapy. When affecting the distribution of the trigeminal nerve it may be associated with intracranial vascular anomalies (Sturge-Weber syndrome). Severe lesions on the limbs are associated with bone hypertrophy (Klippel-Trénaunay syndrome). Port-wine stains need to be differentiated from strawberry nevi (cavernous hemangioma), which are not present at birth but appear during the first month or two of life.

BRACHIAL PLEXUS LESIONS

These cause lack of active movement of the affected limb; passive movement is not painful or restricted. The most common is an Erb palsy from an upper root palsy (C5, C6, and sometimes C7). The arm is held internally rotated and pronated in the "waiter's tip" position. Although most brachial plexus injuries resolve, those that do not recover steadily over the first 2 months of life or are severe should be referred to a specialist because surgical repair may then be indicated. Accompanying respiratory symptoms may be secondary to damage of phrenic nerve roots (see Chapter 27).

EYE ABNORMALITIES

On checking the eyes with an ophthalmoscope, the cornea may be opaque from a congenital cataract or enlarged and hazy from congenital glaucoma. A coloboma is a defect in the iris, resulting in a keyhole-shaped pupil. It may be associated with a defect in the retina. Newborns with these eye abnormalities should be referred immediately to an ophthalmologist.

CLEFT LIP AND PALATE

If cleft lip and palate are recognized prenatally, the parents will be forewarned and counseled about the likely appearance and management. When diagnosed at birth, the parents will need to be reassured about the good cosmetic results after surgical repair. Before and after photographs of other children are often helpful. Assistance in establishing feeding may be required. The infant will need to be referred to a multidisciplinary craniofacial service.

MICROGNATHIA

Micrognathia may be associated with glossoptosis and a posterior cleft palate (Pierre Robin syndrome) and may result in upper airway obstruction.

NECK ABNORMALITIES

Redundant skin over the posterior neck together with a flat occiput are features of Down syndrome. A webbed neck is a feature of Turner syndrome, which may also be associated with lymphedema of the feet. A short webbed neck may indicate abnormalities of the cervical spine (Klippel-Feil syndrome). Cystic hygromas are soft, fluctuant swellings that transilluminate.

EAR ABNORMALITIES

Malformations of the ear may be associated with hearing loss. Affected infants should have their hearing checked. Skin tags anterior to the ear and accessory auricles should be removed by a plastic surgeon. Accessory auricles are associated with an increased risk of renal anomalies.

EXTRA DIGITS

These are usually connected by a thin skin tag but can be completely attached containing bone. They should then be removed by a plastic surgeon. If tied off with a silk thread, a stump of skin may remain. Polydactyly may be familial, but it also may be from a dysmorphic syndrome.

HEART MURMURS

Most murmurs audible in the first few days of life are innocent and originate from the acute angle at the pulmonary artery bifurcation or are from a patent ductus arteriosus or tricuspid regurgitation.[3] Features of an innocent murmur are

- Soft (grade 1–2/6) murmur at left sternal edge
- No clicks audible
- Normal pulses
- Otherwise normal clinical examination

However, some murmurs are caused by congenital heart disease. Features suggesting that a murmur is significant are[24]

- Pansystolic
- Loud (grade 3/6) or more
- Harsh quality
- Best heard in the upper left sternal edge
- Abnormal second heart sound
- Femoral pulses difficult to feel or other abnormality on clinical examination

With the use of these clinical criteria, clinical examination was correct in identifying significant heart lesions in almost all cases examined by general pediatricians[11, 19] as well as by pediatric cardiologists.[24, 29] If a heart murmur is detected, an experienced pediatrician or pediatric cardiologist should be consulted. If the murmur is thought to be significant or cannot confidently be diagnosed as innocent, the infant should be referred for echocardiography promptly. With wide availability of echocardiography and increasing fear of missing a significant heart lesion, the referral rate of newborns with heart murmurs continues to rise.

The usefulness of electrocardiography and chest radiography in assisting to distinguish innocent from significant murmurs is controversial. The neonatal ECG and chest radiograph are difficult to interpret, and these tests have been found to rarely change decisions based on the clinical examination.[29, 30] An ECG and chest radiograph are usually performed as a baseline for those with an abnormality on echocardiography.

If the murmur has the features of an innocent murmur and an echocardiogram is not performed, a follow-up examination should be arranged for 2 to 6 weeks and the parents warned to seek medical assistance if their infant becomes symptomatic with poor feeding, labored breathing, or cyanosis. Most innocent murmurs will disappear in the first year of life, the majority in the first 3 months. However, any mention of a heart murmur will create considerable parental anxiety, which may continue for years. Attention needs to be paid to this to avoid parents continuing to worry about their child's heart although the murmur has disappeared.[32]

MIDLINE ABNORMALITY OVER THE SPINE OR SKULL

Spina bifida is often diagnosed prenatally. Affected infants will need to be referred to a neurosurgical service. A nevus, swelling, or tuft of hair along the spine or middle of the skull requires further evaluation because it may indicate an underlying abnormality of the vertebrae, spinal cord, or brain. An ultrasound or magnetic resonance image will delineate the anatomy. Sacrococcygeal pits are common and harmless, whereas a dermal sinus above the natal clefts should be investigated, because it may extend into the intraspinal space and place the infant at increased risk of meningitis.[16]

SINGLE UMBILICAL ARTERY

This occurs in about 0.3% of newborns. About 40% of infants with a single umbilical artery have other major congenital malformations, particularly of the genitourinary system, and have a significant mortality.[15, 22] A single umbilical artery in an otherwise normal infant is associated with asymptomatic renal anomalies in 7% in one series.[7] The yield from performing ultrasound screening of the kidneys and urinary tract when this is an isolated finding is low and is further reduced by routine prenatal ultrasound screening for congenital anomalies. It is probably best reserved for those who also have other anomalies.

ENLARGED KIDNEYS/BLADDER

If on palpation of the abdomen abnormally large renal masses or an enlarged bladder in a male infant is detected, ultrasonography is required urgently to identify urinary outflow obstruction. Most, but not all, infants with urinary outflow obstruction are now detected on prenatal ultrasound screening, as are other major abnormalities of the kidneys and urinary tract. Siblings of children with vesicoureteric reflux should be screened for this condition because up to 40% will also be affected.[28]

GENITALIA

In the male, the position of the urethral meatus is abnormal in hypospadias; it may be glandular, coronal, in the middle of the shaft, or perineal. Glandular hypospadias without chordee does not usually require any treatment, but more severe forms will require corrective surgery and a specialist's opinion should be sought and circumcision withheld. If a testis is undescended, it should be rechecked at several months of age. If still undescended, referral to a pediatric surgeon or urologist is indicated. Neonatal *testicular torsion* usually occurs at some time before birth. A pediatric surgeon should be consulted urgently, although the testis is rarely salvageable because it has usually already undergone infarction.

TALIPES

Positional talipes is quite common and is from the position of the fetus *in utero,* especially if there was oligohydramnios. If held in the equinovarus position, the newborn should be able to fully abduct and dorsiflex the foot and ankle. If this maneuver can be performed, no treatment is required; if not, the infant is likely to have talipes equinovarus and needs to be referred directly to a pediatric orthopedic surgeon. When the feet are held in calcaneus valgus position, this is usually from the position of the feet in utero. It should be possible to dorsiflex the foot to bring its dorsal surface into contact with the anterior lower leg and to achieve normal plantarflexion. If this can be achieved, spontaneous resolution can be expected.

LIMITATIONS OF THE ROUTINE EXAMINATION OF THE NEWBORN

Examination of a newborn in the delivery room and at a routine examination will identify a number of problems, many of which are transient, though some are permanent and significant. However, some significant abnormalities will not be identified. Sometimes this is due to inexperience of the examiner or the difficulty of performing a satisfactory examination in an uncooperative newborn (e.g., getting a good view of the eyes and red reflex). However, some significant abnormalities will not be identified because of the limitations of the examination itself. Parents may become upset or angry when it becomes evident at a later stage that their child has a significant problem. They need to be made aware that not all abnormalities can be detected at this stage. It also stresses the importance of clear documentation of the routine examination for future reference. Some of the major limitations of the clinical examination are listed below:

1. *Identification of syndromes.* These can be difficult or impossible to identify in the immediate neonatal period but become apparent as the child grows older.
2. *Jaundice.* Jaundice usually develops after 24 hours of age, unless due to hemolysis. Significant jaundice may develop at several days of age, although the infant has been said to be normal only 1 or 2 days beforehand.
3. *Congenital heart disease.* Whereas 6 to 8 infants per 1000 live births have congenital heart disease, only 0.8 per 1000 are identified on the first day of life, many of whom are symptomatic. At the time of the newborn examination, the pressure in the right side of the heart is still relatively high and the ductus arteriosus may still be patent. Infants with a ventricular septal defect, the most common congenital heart lesion, may not have a heart murmur at the routine examination because the pressure difference between the left and right sides of the heart will be insufficient to generate turbulent flow at this stage. More worrying, ductal dependent lesions may present clinically with heart failure, shock, cyanosis, or death just days or weeks after a normal routine examination. In coarctation of the aorta, the femoral pulses may be palpable at the initial examination because of blood flow through the ductus arteriosus.
4. *Developmental dysplasia of the hip.* As a screening test, clinical examination for developmental dysplasia of the hip is problematic.[10] Ideally, all affected infants should be identified in the neonatal period, because early treatment prevents or reduces the need for surgery. In practice, a significant proportion of infants who subsequently require surgery are not identified in the neonatal period. A survey from the United Kingdom suggested that the operative rate had remained unchanged since screening was introduced, at 0.7/1000 live births,[17] although a more recent study from South Australia found a lower operative rate, at 0.45/1000 births, but still only 56% of these infants were identified at the initial clinical examination.[9] However, development dysplasia of the hip was diagnosed in 7.7/1000 live births highlighting that the hips of most infants with an abnormal neonatal hip examination are normal. Failure to identify developmental dysplasia of the hip at the initial examination may be because the examiner is inexperienced, but in some infants with a flat acetabular shelf the clinical examination may be

normal in the neonatal period but progresses with age.[27] Also, the irreducible dislocated hip is easily missed on examination. The role of ultrasound in the early recognition of development dysplasia of the hip is yet to be established. In many centers ultrasound screening is used for those at increased risk (i.e., if there is a positive family history, if the newborn was a breech presentation, or if the infant has a neuromuscular disorder), as well as if there is any abnormality detected on clinical examination.[8] In some centers, universal ultrasound screening is performed, but the false positive rate is high. If there is any doubt about the hip examination, a consultation should be obtained.

HEALTH PROMOTION

The routine examination is an opportunity to provide health promotion for parents. Some of the many issues that can be raised are listed below:

1. *Prevention of sudden infant death syndrome (SIDS).* All parents should be advised that infants should sleep on their backs and that overheating and parental smoking are risk factors. These measures appear to have markedly reduced the incidence of SIDS in many countries.
2. *Promotion of breast milk feeding.* Mothers should be encouraged and assisted with their breast milk feeding.
3. *Hearing and vision screening.* Children at increased risk of deafness (e.g., family history, malformations of the ear including skin tags and pits)[21] must be referred for early hearing testing. In the United States, universal neonatal hearing screening is close to reality. Similarly, infants at increased risk of visual loss should be referred to an ophthalmologist. The parents should be given advice about the early detection of hearing and vision loss.
4. *Safe vehicular transport.* The newborn period is a good opportunity to provide advice on the need for car seats for infants.

REPEAT EXAMINATION

With the early discharge of mothers and their newborns from a hospital, it is no longer practicable for infants to have two full "routine examinations" before discharge. It has also been found that two detailed examinations within such a short space of time is of limited value in the identification of additional abnormalities.[25] Infants should be checked within 24 hours of discharge from hospital, although in practice this may often be accomplished with one physical examination.[1] However, before an infant is discharged, the health care provider should check that the infant has fed satisfactorily, is not significantly jaundiced, and is breathing normally and that the mother is able to care adequately for her infant and that the infant is going to a suitable environment. Follow-up care for the infant should also be in place. Although early discharge is accompanied by an increased readmission rate to hospital, it is reassuringly low.[23]

ASSESSMENT OF GESTATIONAL AGE

Formal assessment of gestational age is unnecessary for the routine newborn examination. The best guide to an infant's gestational age is an early antenatal ultrasound evaluation combined with information about the mother's last menstrual period. An evaluation of the clinical methods of assessing gestational age showed that clinical methods had 95% confidence intervals of 17 days whereas the antenatal ultrasound had 95% confidence intervals of less than 7 days.[31] Clinical testing is most important for infants whose gestational age is unknown or discrepant with their growth.

Four methods can be employed to assess gestational age: physical criteria,[14, 26] neurologic examination,[2] combined physical and neurologic examination,[4, 12] and examination of the lens of the eye.[20] Table 26–2 lists some of the physical criteria used to

establish gestational age and shows how they progress in an orderly fashion with increasing gestation. The assessment of gestational age using neurologic criteria involves the assessment of posture, passive and active tone, reflexes, and righting reaction.[2]

Although the physical criteria can be used to establish gestational age immediately after delivery, the neurologic criteria require the infant to be in an alert, rested state, which may not occur until the second day of life. Infants who are asphyxiated at the time of delivery, who have a primary neurologic disorder, or who are affected by maternal medication cannot be assessed using neurologic criteria until they have recovered.

Gestational age can be assessed most accurately by combining the physical criteria and the neurologic assessment. Dubowitz described and developed such a combined scoring system.[13] Its disadvantage is that it involves the assessment of 11 physical criteria and 10 neurologic findings. Although the physical criteria allow clear distinction of infants with varying gestational ages greater than 34 weeks, neurologic criteria are essential to differentiate infants between 26 and 34 weeks when the physical changes are less evident. Ballard and her colleagues abbreviated the Dubowitz scoring system to include six neurologic and six physical criteria to shorten the time taken. The revised

TABLE 26–2 ESTIMATION OF GESTATIONAL AGE

EVALUATION	APPROXIMATE WEEK OF GESTATION WHEN FINDINGS APPEAR								
	24	28	30	32	34	36	38	40	
Head circumference in cm ± 2 SD		23–28.3	25–30.4	26.8–32.4	28.6–34	30.5–35.5	32–36.5	33–37	Based on 300 single live births—all white
Sole creases		Anterior transverse crease only →				Occasional creases anterior two thirds →		Sole covered with creases →	
Breast nodule diameter		Not palpable-absent →				2 mm →	4 mm →	7 mm →	If small may represent fetal malnutrition
Scalp hair		Fine and fuzzy / Hard to distinguish individual strands →					Thick and silky / Appears as individual strands →		
Earlobe		Pliable—no cartilage →				Some cartilage →		Stiffened by thick cartilage	
Testes and scrotum		Testes in lower canal Scrotum small—few rugae →				Intermediate →		Testes pendulous, scrotum full, extensive rugae →	

From Behrman RE, et al: In utero disease and the newborn infant. In Schulman I (ed): Advances in Pediatrics, vol 17. Chicago, Year Book Medical, 1970; modified from Amiel-Tison, Brett, Koenigsbergh, and Usher.

Ballard examination (Fig. 26–2) includes assessment for extremely premature infants.[5]

Regardless of the method used, the assessment of gestational age using physical and neurologic criteria is accurate only to ±2 weeks, with a tendency toward overestimation in extremely premature infants.

part two
CARE OF THE NEWBORN
Susan D. Izatt

Because newborns have differing needs based on gestation or illness, perinatal facilities and care must be tailored to provide a range of medical services appropriate to the delivery population. In this chapter, the physical facilities and environmental recommendations for newborn care are outlined. Basic care appropriate for all newborns is subsequently addressed. These suggestions are offered as minimal standards. The American Academy of Pediatrics (AAP) *Guidelines for Perinatal Care* should be used in conjunction with state regulations in the implementation and review of neonatal facilities and care.[38]

PHYSICAL FACILITIES

NORMAL NURSERY

A normal nursery provides routine care for well full-term infants of between 37 and 42 weeks' gestation. Care may also be provided for healthy near-term infants who weigh more than 2000 gm and are at least of 35 weeks' gestation.

The number of bassinets in the nursery should exceed the number of maternal beds to allow for situations including multiple births and extended neonatal hospitalizations. If combination labor/delivery rooms or infant rooming-in is utilized, fewer bassinets may be present in the nursery. Each bassinet should have 30 square feet of floor space, with the bassinets 3 feet apart in all directions.

One nursing staff member is recommended for each six to eight infants. One registered nurse per shift is required to supervise care in the newborn nursery but does not necessarily have to be in constant attendance and may share responsibilities in an adjacent obstetric area. All staff members caring for newborns should be trained in neonatal resuscitation and ideally should have successfully completed the American Academy of Pediatrics formal program on newborn resuscitation (see Chapter 25).

A specific pediatrician should be designated as the physician responsible for general, medical, and administrative policies affecting these infants and should regularly review all such matters. Each infant should have a particular physician responsible for medical care.

The newborn nursery should have foot-controlled sinks and soap dispensers to allow adequate hand washing before and between patient contact. The room should be well illuminated, allowing for examination and procedures. Resuscitation equipment, a functional wall clock with a second hand, and ready access for portable radiography is needed for unexpected neonatal emergencies. Cabinet and counter storage within the nursery is needed for routine newborn supplies. Current AAP guidelines recommend one pair of electrical outlets for each two neonatal positions and one oxygen, suction, and compressed air outlet for each four patient stations.

INTERMEDIATE OR TRANSITIONAL CARE

(See also Chapter 3.)

Intermediate care nurseries provide medical support for newborns requiring 6 to 12 hours of nursing care per day. Infants who require this care include premature infants of less than 35 weeks' gestation, infants who are small for gestational age (weighing less than 2000 gm), and term infants with medical conditions of moderate severity, including hypoglycemia and sepsis. These infants should not require ventilatory assistance for more than several hours.

Infants requiring intermediate care can be managed in an area either completely separated or contiguous to the well-baby nursery or the neonatal intensive care unit (NICU). This area may be located in the delivery suite. Care in this area generally requires 100 to 120 square feet per infant. There should be 4 feet on all sides between bassinets and/or incubators in this area. The aisles in this area should be 5 feet wide. Infants requiring intermediate care can be located in a single large room or in smaller rooms with sufficient space to house 3 to 4 infants, because this level of care requires a nurse for every 3 to 4 patients. Because 3 to 4.5 infants per 100 deliveries require the services of such a unit, the need for an intermediate care area should be based on annual delivery rate.

One nursing staff member is recommended for every 3 to 4 infants. At least one registered nurse must be in attendance on each shift and should be part of the pediatric nursing service and have no nursing responsibilities other than those related to care of these infants. All staff members caring for newborns in the intermediate care nursery should be trained in neonatal resuscitation and ideally should have successfully completed the American Academy of Pediatrics formal program on newborn resuscitation.

Nurses in the intermediate care nursery should be able to initiate intravenous therapy. They also must be trained to care for infants requiring assisted ventilation for 2 to 3 hours. Nurses in these units should be able to initiate or change therapy, even when a physician is not present, using established protocols. Neonatal nurse practitioners may provide primary

NEUROMUSCULAR MATURITY

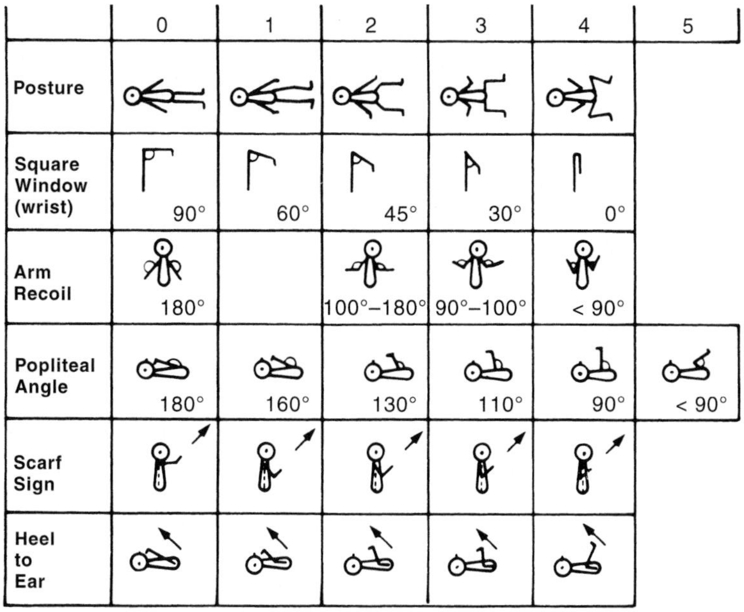

	0	1	2	3	4	5
Posture						
Square Window (wrist)	90°	60°	45°	30°	0°	
Arm Recoil	180°		100°–180°	90°–100°	< 90°	
Popliteal Angle	180°	160°	130°	110°	90°	< 90°
Scarf Sign						
Heel to Ear						

PHYSICAL MATURITY

Skin	gelatinous red. transparent	smooth pink. visible veins	superficial peeling &/or rash few veins	cracking pale area rare veins	parchment deep cracking no vessels	leathery cracked wrinkled
Lanugo	none	abundant	thinning	bald areas	mostly bald	
Plantar creases	no crease	faint red marks	anterior transverse crease only	creases ant. 2/3	creases cover entire sole	
Breast	barely percept.	flat areola no bud	stippled areola 1–2 mm bud	raised areola 3–4 mm bud	full areola 5–10 mm bud	
Ear	pinna flat. stays folded	sl. curved pinna; soft with slow recoil	well-curv. pinna; soft but ready recoil	formed & firm with instant recoil	thick cartilage ear stiff	
Genitals	scrotum empty no rugae		testes descending. few rugae	testes down good rugae	testes pendulous deep rugae	
Genitals	prominent clitoris & labia minora		majora & minora equally prominent	majora large minora small	clitoris & minora completely covered	

MATURITY RATING

Score	Wks
5	26
10	28
15	30
20	32
25	34
30	36
35	38
40	40
45	42
50	44

FIGURE 26–2. Assessment of gestational age using the revised Ballard method. (From Ballard JL, et al: New Ballard Score, expanded to include extremely premature infants. J Pediatr 119:417, 1991.)

care in these units, working with the assigned nurse and supervised by the medical director. In other units, nurse clinicians with expanded technical skills may be assigned to these nurseries.

Respiratory therapists with training in newborn care work collaboratively with the nursing staff and medical director to provide airway stabilization and subsequent ventilation therapy. Each unit should clearly define the role and responsibility of the respiratory therapist in its hierarchy to maximize the efficient and appropriate use of its staff.

Medical direction of the unit should be provided by a board-certified neonatologist or by a board-certified pediatrician with additional training in the management of infants at high risk. In coordination with the senior nursing staff, the pediatrician or neonatologist should establish guidelines for the admission, management, and/or transfer of infants with medical issues.

The intermediate care unit should have the basic design and equipment found in the normal nursery, with the addition of incubators and/or radiant heaters, monitoring equipment, and respirators. The resuscitation equipment must be readily available, ideally on an emergency cart. Infusion pumps should be used to control administration of fluids. As per the AAP guidelines, there should be eight electrical outlets, two oxygen outlets, two compressed air outlets, and two suction outlets per patient station. All electrical units should be connected to an auxiliary power source. The area also requires a special electrical outlet to power the portable x-ray unit.

The laboratory, radiology, and ultrasound technicians should either be in the hospital or on call 24 hours to guarantee their availability to the nursery. Respiratory therapists with expertise in the care of the newborn should be in the hospital at all times.

INTENSIVE CARE

(See also Chapter 3.)

Infants requiring continuous cardiorespiratory support and/or constant nursing care require admission to an NICU. Generally, infants admitted to NICUs have not been previously discharged to home. Occasionally, older infants who have issues related to prematurity may be readmitted to this area with appropriate isolation. Infants with sepsis, meningitis, pneumonia, or other infections may remain in this area at the discretion of the director of the nursery with the institution of appropriate isolation procedures.

The NICU must be in an area separated from the well-baby nursery, but it may be contiguous to the intermediate care nursery. In the design of new units, this area should be adjacent to the delivery suites if possible. Older hospitals may be unable to rearrange existing facilities to provide this access at reasonable costs. The unit should also be easily accessible from the hospital's emergency area. A minimum of 150 net square feet per infant is needed to provide this care. The unit should have at least 6 feet between patient care areas, and the aisles should be 8 feet wide. An

estimated 1 to 1.5 infants per 100 deliveries will need intensive care services. This, combined with the estimated number of neonatal transfers, should dictate the need and size of the NICU.

There should be a 1:2 nurse/patient ratio with a 1:1 ratio for infants requiring multisystem support and a ratio greater than 1:1 for unstable infants (e.g., an infant requiring extracorporeal membrane oxygenation). Nurses in this area should have no other assignments outside this nursery unless it is on regular rotation to an intermediate nursery. All nurses in this area should have a closely supervised, well-controlled orientation program with its duration suited to the needs of the particular nurse; nurses without this orientation should not work in this area. The nurses should also be trained in resuscitation of the newborn and ideally should have successfully completed the American Academy of Pediatrics formal program on newborn resuscitation. The unit should have a head nurse who is responsible for the overall nursing management and jointly responsible with the medical director for administration of the service.

Respiratory therapists with special expertise in newborn ventilation work collaboratively with the nursing staff and medical director to provide airway stabilization and subsequent ventilation therapy in the NICU.

The director of this unit should be a full-time, board-certified neonatologist. In-house coverage on a 24-hour basis by pediatric resident staff, neonatal fellows, neonatologists, or specially trained neonatal nurses is essential, and consultants must be available in all medical and surgical specialties. In NICUs without house staff or fellow coverage, the neonatologist provides 24-hour in-hospital coverage, often in combination with a staff of nurse practitioners, neonatal nurses, and respiratory therapists.

This area should have all the equipment required for intermediate care, as well as more extensive cardiorespiratory monitoring and supportive facilities. The area should also have sufficient space for desks and cabinets and adequate storage space to avoid clutter. As outlined in the AAP guidelines, there should be 12 to 16 electrical outlets, two to four oxygen and compressed air outlets, and two to four suction sources for each infant. All electrical outlets should be on both regular and emergency power. There should also be a special outlet for x-ray and ultrasound units.

The laboratory and radiology departments must provide 24-hour in-house service. Where delays in blood gas results are unavoidable because of the location of the laboratories or limitation of personnel, a unit to measure pH, Po_2, and Pco_2 should be available within the nursery. The laboratory or respiratory therapy department should be responsible for quality control of the blood gas machine, checking performance standards at least once a day or as required by state health code.

The infection control personnel of the hospital working with the designated nursery personnel must be responsible for surveillance of infection and implementation and maintenance of appropriate environmental controls. An isolation room should be available for infants with contagious disease, ideally within the NICU.

Provisions should be made to ensure admission for sick infants transferred from smaller services. To ensure accomplishment of this task, all normal nurseries and intermediate care units should have an ongoing relationship with a regional NICU. Ideally, infants at high risk should be delivered in institutions capable of providing intensive care from the moment of delivery. Nonetheless, it is estimated that 40% of neonatal problems are at present unpredictable. To provide for such emergencies, an effective transport system with specially trained nursing and medical personnel as described in Chapter 3 is essential.

GENERAL CONSIDERATIONS FOR NEWBORN CARE UNITS

LIGHTING

Ambient lighting should allow easy detection of both cyanosis and jaundice. Concerns have been raised regarding the intensive light environment in many nurseries, in particular the effect on infants with very low birth weight who spend weeks to months in this area. These issues suggest that nurseries be prudent until further data are available and attempt to control excessive illumination. Ambient lighting levels in intensive care should be adjustable through a range of 1 to 60 foot-candles (ft-c). The Illuminating Engineering Society (IES) recommends 10 to 20 ft-c, with diurnal variation with nighttime levels as low as 0.5 ft-c. All nurseries should have the capability for adjustable illumination. Separate procedure lighting should be available to each bed station, which provides no more than 100- to 500-ft-c illumination. Temporary increases in illumination should be possible without increasing light levels for all infants in the same room. Lighting should minimize shadows and glare.

Light reduction has not been shown to decrease the incidence of retinopathy of prematurity.[46] However, reduced light exposure does not appear deleterious to central visual development in the premature infant.[47] Because preliminary studies suggest diurnal cycling may enhance growth and development of the premature infant, the ability to reduce ambient lighting to levels as low as 0.5 ft-c as per IES guidelines is recommended.

WALLS, FLOORS, AND CEILINGS

True skin color is best seen in nurseries with walls that are pale beige or off-white; brighter tones of blue and yellow interfere with the ability to evaluate jaundice and cyanosis. The walls should be easily cleaned and protected at contact points with movable equipment.

Windows provide an important psychological benefit to staff and families. At least one source of daylight should be visible from newborn care areas. External windows in patient rooms should be glazed with insulating glass to minimize heat gain or loss, and they should be located at least 2 feet away from the bed. Outside awnings in parts of the country where radiant heat gain is a problem also reduce the chance of overheating. The windows must also have the ability to be shaded, with the units either self-contained or easily cleaned.

Floor surfaces should be easily cleaned and minimize the growth of microorganisms. The surface should be resilient to heavy use and frequent cleaning. Although carpet is acceptable for use in the NICU, it should not be used around sinks, in isolation areas, or in holding areas.

Acoustical ceiling systems are highly desirable in the NICU, but the construction must be nonfriable and prohibit the passage of particles above the ceiling into the room below.

TEMPERATURE CONTROL AND VENTILATION

For more information on temperature control, see Chapter 29. Present AAP guidelines recommend the air temperature in nurseries should be maintained between 75°F and 79°F (24°C and 26°C), with relative humidity between 30% and 60%. The AAP Section on Perinatal Pediatrics has recently suggested that the NICU provide an air temperature of between 72°F and 78°F (22°C and 26°C).[39] These temperature and humidity ranges prevent excessive heat loss or gain for the infant and ensure personnel comfort.

The AAP guidelines suggest a minimum of six changes of room air per hour, with a minimum of two changes being outside air, for control of infection. The fresh air intake should be located at least 25 feet from exhaust outlets of ventilation systems, combustion equipment stacks, medical/surgical vacuum systems, plumbing vents, or areas that may collect vehicular exhausts or other exhaust fumes. Air to the NICUs should be filtered with at least 90% efficiency. A slight positive pressure differential between the unit and adjacent hallways should exist within the ventilation system.

OXYGEN AND COMPRESSED AIR

Oxygen and compressed air are generally supplied to the NICU from a central source. The capability to provide mixtures of air and oxygen producing concentrations from 21% to 100% must be available. These mixtures should be available at atmospheric pressure and pressures up to 50 to 60 pounds per square inch in units where positive pressure ventilators are used. Warning devices to alert personnel to falls in pressure should be part of each system. Compressed air systems require detailed planning and meticulous care once they are operational. Air should be washed, filtered, and then dehumidified before delivery into the system. All intakes must be closely checked to minimize the introduction of contaminated air. Small compressor units should be operated pneumatically and not electrically because of an increasing number of power failures in some urban areas.

ACOUSTICS

The design of new or renovated intensive care units should include consideration of sound abatement (see Chapter 29). Monitors, respirators, ventilation systems, incubators, and staff all create noise. The AAP Committee on Environmental Health has recommended that sound should be monitored both in the NICU and within the incubators, with a noise level of greater than 45 dB to be avoided.[34] These recommendations are based on studies of premature infants treated with environmental interventions, including sound reduction, which demonstrated improved neurologic development and decreased duration of respiratory support.

Architectural sound reduction strategies include acoustical ceiling systems, sound-absorbing wall panels, and carpeting. Careful selection of monitoring equipment and communication systems combined with staff education can further enhance sound control in the NICU.

ELECTRICITY

The medical profession is often uninformed about electrical hazards related to the use of equipment (see Chapter 30). In an attempt to minimize electrical hazards, certain recommendations can be made. The use of a single ground of low-resistance wire is particularly effective when connected to all outlets in the nursery. Frequent checking of the integrity of this ground and all wiring will prevent the hazard of stray electrical currents. When more than one piece of electrical equipment is used, there must be enough outlets at each incubator to accommodate the equipment, with all units connected to a common ground. All electrical equipment should be tested and maintained by a qualified engineer to detect defective equipment and current leakage and to specify appropriate safety precautions both at installation and at regular subsequent intervals. Plugs on all equipment should be hospital grade, and extension cords, adapters, and junction boxes must not be used. The Joint Commission on the Accreditation of Healthcare Organizations provides standards for current leakage allowances, preventive maintenance, and quality of equipment that should be followed.

All electrical outlets in the NICU must be on the hospital's emergency circuit to maintain life support systems. A minimum of 16 to 20 simultaneously accessible electrical outlets should be provided at each patient care spot. In-service training programs should be maintained to educate all nursery personnel in the proper use of equipment and recognition of potential electrical hazards. All new equipment should be checked for proper insulation and approved by a qualified engineer before use in a clinical area, regardless of previous approvals by the manufacturer.

SINKS

There should be a sink adjacent to the door in each area, one basin for every six to eight patient positions within the regular nursery, one for every three to four patients in an intermediate care unit, and one for every one to two infants in the NICU. All basins should have foot, knee, or remote controls for hot and cold water and soap. Scrub brushes and paper towels should be conveniently placed near each basin. The basins should not be built into counters used for other purposes, and sinks should drain properly and avoid splashing. The scrub area should also contain facilities for storing clothing, cabinets for clean gowns, receptacles for soiled gowns, and a clock for timing of hand washing.

CONTROL OF ENVIRONMENT

The establishment of stringent microbiologic environmental control has been a significant factor in reduction of nosocomial infections in nurseries. Critical evaluation of these controls should be ongoing, because new studies may permit modification of previously established standards. Before altering existing procedures and techniques, personnel must compare the type of facility where the study was conducted with their own institution. Many smaller hospitals have continued their established environmental controls, acknowledging inherent differences between their own facilities and those where innovations have been initiated.

Studies have demonstrated that cover gowns are not necessary for regular nursery or NICU personnel as long as hand-washing standards are strictly enforced. If an infected or potentially infected neonate is to be handled outside the bassinet, a long-sleeved cover gown should be worn over clothing and discarded after use.

Thorough hand washing eliminates the most common route of cross infection within nurseries. It requires accessible antiseptic agents and a sufficient number and proper location of wash basins. Correct preparation for initial hand washing before entering the nursery includes removal of rings, watches, and bracelets. Sleeves need to be rolled above the elbow. The hands and arms should be washed for 3 minutes, followed by a thorough rinse and drying. A similar scrub should be done before procedures. After the initial 3-minute scrub, a 10-second wash should be subsequently used before and after handling each neonate. An unpublished study of a 30-second wash of the hands and arms using an antiseptic agent offers promising results, with fewer colony-forming units of bacteria found on the skin as compared with the 3-minute scrub and with less skin abrasion.[49]

An antiseptic agent should be used for washing before entering the nursery, before a procedure, and before and after handling an infant. Antiseptic agents should kill pathogenic bacteria, should not be sensitizing, should be easy to use, should be nonstaining, and should have lasting antibacterial action. The most commonly used agents are chlorhexidine gluconate (4%) or iodophors, both of which are effective against gram-positive and gram-negative bacteria. Hexachlorophene solutions may be used during nursery outbreaks of staphylococcal infections but should not be used routinely.

The cleaning of equipment requires establishment of specific, detailed guidelines that are well known to all personnel. The aim of cleaning most equipment is disinfection (killing or decreasing the number of organisms known to be the potential cause of infection), but sterilization (killing of all organisms) is mandatory for certain items, such as surgical instruments. Steam autoclaving remains the preferred method of sterilization because of cost and safety, but it is limited because of damage to certain equipment. Thus gas sterilization has been recommended as the ideal solution to the problems of cleaning and disinfection, but such a gas system is not always available.

The most commonly used disinfectants are iodophors, chlorine compounds, phenolic compounds, and glutaraldehyde. Caution must be exercised to follow directions with certain phenolic disinfectants. Excessive use of a phenolic disinfectant in greater concentrations than recommended or on surfaces with which neonates have direct contact has been associated with hyperbilirubinemia.

Before disinfection of equipment, thorough cleaning is necessary to remove dust particles and grease that may partially inactivate the disinfectant. Supervisory personnel should check the disinfectant procedure itself, as well as periodically culture recently disinfected equipment. Specific guidelines for cleaning various equipment used in NICUs are available in a manual of the American Academy of Pediatrics on hospital care of newborns. Stethoscopes are a particular source of infection that should require a specific policy for cleaning and care in obstetric and newborn units.[51]

Meticulous attention to details and supervision of the technique of all personnel are critical for safe, effective microbiologic controls.

SAFETY

The incidence of reported infant abduction in the United States (birth through 6 months) is three to four cases per year. This tragedy profoundly affects the family, the health care staff, and the health care facility.[40] Analysis has revealed that the best deterrents to infant abduction are education and cooperation, with the development of an institutional multidisciplinary plan being essential. Technology is allowing more sophisticated methods of infant monitoring, but it will not replace simple interventions such as newborn safety guidelines given to and reviewed with new mothers post partum and clear photographic identification of all medical care providers and support staff.

BASIC CARE OF THE NEWBORN

PRENATAL HISTORY AND MATERNAL INFORMATION

Clear communication between the obstetrician/midwife and pediatrician/nurse practitioner is needed around the time of delivery to allow optimal care of the newborn. If the pregnancy and delivery is uncomplicated, the maternal chart may be adequate. Prenatal screens, including blood type and antibody status, hepatitis B status, serologic screening, and sexually transmitted disease status should be readily available. A thorough history of the mother including occupation, drug exposure, past and present medical problems, past and present obstetrical problems, family history, and social issues is essential. Intrapartum events including maternal fever, prolonged or premature rupture of membranes, fetal heart rate abnormalities, preeclampsia, meconium-stained fluid, group B *Streptococcus* status, and maternal antibiotic treatment contribute to the postpartum care of the infant. This information allows the identification and timely intervention of medical and social issues potentially affecting the well-being of the newborn.

NEWBORN ASSESSMENT

The clinical status of the infant must be evaluated immediately after birth in the delivery room. Resuscitation and stabilization may be needed as outlined in Chapter 25. Premature infants, ill newborns, or infants with congenital abnormalities may require transfer to an intermediate care unit or NICU after initial assessment and stabilization. Before leaving the delivery room, identical bands that specify the mother's name, the mother's admission number, the infant's sex, and the date and time of birth should be placed on the infant and mother. If placement of the identification bands is not possible due to the clinical status of the patient, the bands should accompany the infant and be placed as soon as medically appropriate.

The gestation of the infant should be determined from the mother's last menstrual period or from an ultrasound performed at less than 20 weeks. A Ballard examination should be performed on all infants within 12 hours of birth to confirm the gestational age (see Part One). If the mother received late or no prenatal care, the Ballard examination can be used to establish the gestational age. Anthropometric measurements should be plotted to assess size for gestational age, allowing for identification of infants at risk because of being either small for gestation or large for gestation.

Within 2 hours of birth, healthy newborns should have a preliminary assessment, including vital signs, physical examination, and review of infant risk factors. Newborns should be closely monitored for respiratory distress, poor color, diaphoresis, jitteriness, or abnormal tone during the first 6 to 12 hours after birth during the transition phase.

If the infant's care provider was not at the delivery, he or she should be notified of the infant's birth following the guidelines established at the delivery facility. Examination of the newborn should be performed within 24 hours of birth and within 24 hours before discharge (see Part One). With shortened hospital stays, one newborn examination may be acceptable and has been found to be safe when prospectively studied.[41, 43]

FEEDING

Human milk is the preferred feeding for all infants, including sick and premature newborns, with rare exceptions. Breast milk feeding should be initiated shortly after birth in a well newborn, preferably within the first hour of life. Infants should be nursed whenever they show signs of hunger, approximately 8 to 12 times every 24 hours. No supplements should be given unless a medical indication such as dehydration exists. If supplementation is needed, methods that avoid bottle feeding, including a supplemental nursing system, cup feeding, and finger feeding, should be considered.

In-hospital lactation support for all breast-feeding mothers and infants is encouraged. Identification of potential breast-feeding problems before discharge allows teaching and follow-up support, optimizing successful breast milk feeding and minimizing medical complications, including dehydration and hyperbilirubinemia. First-time breast-feeding mothers should be seen by a health care provider knowledgeable in lactation within several days of discharge.

If a mother chooses to formula-feed her infant, the formula should be iron fortified. Soy protein–based formulas are not believed to be superior to cow's milk–based formulas in the prevention of atopic disease.[33] Because infants with cow's milk protein enteropathy are often sensitive to soy protein, a formula derived from hydrolyzed protein or synthetic amino acid should be used in these patients. Soy protein–based formulas are not recommended for premature infants who weigh less than 1800 gm.

Most term infants who are bottle feeding will rapidly progress from 15 to 30 mL every 3 to 4 hours to 75 to 90 mL by 4 to 5 days of life. Vigorous premature infants may require smaller (5 to 10 mL) feedings at more frequent intervals (every 2 hours) before progressing to larger, less frequent feedings (see Chapter 33, Part One).

SKIN CARE

Newborn skin differs significantly from adult skin (see Chapter 50). The dermal thickness of the term infant is 60% of that of an adult and declines further in thickness with decreasing gestation. Although the stratum corneum is similar to the adult at term, a marked decrease in the cell layer thickness is seen in premature infants of less than 32 weeks' gestation. These differences contribute to increased permeability to topically applied agents and increased risk of damage to skin integrity.

The American Academy of Pediatrics currently recommends dry skin care for the healthy term newborn. The benefits of this approach are reduction of heat loss by exposure, decrease in skin trauma, limitation of exposure to agents with unknown toxicity, and reduction in nursing time. With this technique, cleansing is delayed until an infant's temperature has stabilized. Then fresh water or nonmedicated soap is used to remove blood and meconium from the face and head. The rest of the infant's skin may be left untouched, leaving the vernix caseosa in place. For the duration of hospitalization, the buttocks and perianal region can be cleaned with fresh water or a mild soap at diaper changes or as often as necessary. Whatever agent is used on a newborn's skin, it should either be dispensed as a single unit container or be restricted to one infant's use to prevent spread of infection through the unit.

Care practices that impact skin must be closely monitored in the NICU.[45, 48] Adhesives including tape, electrodes, and skin bonding agents all damage the epidermal layer on removal. Chemical damage from alcohol and povidone-iodine (Betadine) affects the epidermal and dermal layers of skin. Intravenous extravasations can lead to tissue necrosis, requiring strict observation of infusion sites and prompt intervention if infiltration is suspected. With decreasing gestation, minimal intervention to the fragile skin surface can lead to significant disruption of the skin integrity. Alterations of skin integrity diminish the skin barrier function, leading to infection and alterations in fluid balance. Close attention must be paid to any topically applied substance in the nursery or intensive care unit.

Skin disinfection, prior to procedures, is predominantly with povidone-iodine. It should be allowed to dry for 30 seconds before the procedure and completely removed with sterile saline or water after the procedure to prevent further absorption because the iodine may affect thyroid function. Use of isopropyl alcohol is discouraged because it is less effective in reducing bacterial colonization and more damaging to the skin.

Efforts should be made to prevent skin trauma from adhesives by minimizing tape use, backing the adhesive with cotton or tape, and delaying tape removal until at least 24 hours after application. Pectin barriers under the adhesives mold and adhere well to body contours and help the adhesives to adhere in moist conditions. In premature infants routine application of emollients improves skin integrity and can prevent excessive skin drying, skin cracking, and fissures.

Skin breakdown may occur from infection, friction, pressure sores, trauma from adhesive removal, and diaper dermatitis. Areas of breakdown should be cleansed with warmed sterile water and covered with petrolatum-based emollients and ointments. These form a semi-occlusive layer that facilitates migration of the epithelial cell. The use of antibacterial ointments may be appropriate. Transparent adhesive dressings may be used on uninfected wounds because bacteria and fungi may proliferate under the dressing.

Cord care attempts to control outbreaks of streptococcal and staphylococcal disease. There is no single method of cord care that is recommended to prevent colonization and subsequent disease. Currently, acceptable agents include triple dye or bacitracin. Alcohol may be used to dry the cord, but it is ineffective in preventing cord colonization.

VITAMIN K THERAPY

The AAP guidelines state that every neonate should receive a single parenteral 0.5 to 1.0 mg dose of natural vitamin K1 oxide (phytonadione) within 1 hour of birth to aid in the prevention of vitamin K–dependent hemorrhagic disease of the newborn (HDN). Breastfed infants are at risk of late HDN if untreated due to the low concentrations of vitamin K in breast milk combined with preferential gut colonization with bacteria that cannot produce vitamin K. Additionally, infants with cholestatic liver disease are also at risk of late HDN believed to be due to decreased absorption of fat-soluble vitamin K from the bowel.

In 1992, several studies linked intramuscular vitamin K and childhood cancers.[52] Although subsequent evaluation did not confirm this finding, the efficacy of oral vitamin K prophylaxis was studied. Oral vitamin K has been found to be effective in the prevention of classic HDN. However, supplementation with repeat doses of oral vitamin K did not prevent all cases of late HDN. It is presently recommended to use intramuscular vitamin K for prevention of both classic and late HDN, with the alternative of oral vitamin K to be offered to families refusing the intramuscular form.

EYE PROPHYLAXIS

Prophylaxis against gonococcal ophthalmia neonatorum is mandatory for all newborns and should be instilled within 1 hour of birth. Two drops of 1% silver nitrate in a single-dose container or a 1- to 2-cm ribbon of sterile ophthalmic ointment containing erythromycin (0.5%) or tetracycline (1%) in a single-use tube are acceptable prophylactic regimens. The treatment needs to reach all parts of the conjunctival sac, and the eyes should not be irrigated after instillation.

CIRCUMCISION

Circumcision of the male newborn remains a controversial topic. The AAP Task Force on Circumcision has stated that although some potential benefits of neonatal circumcision exist, the data are not sufficient to recommend routine neonatal circumcision.[35] Parents need to be informed of the risks and benefits of neonatal circumcision and allowed to consider the information before giving consent for the procedure. Families should be encouraged to include cultural and religious traditions as well as medical information in decision making regarding circumcision.

If circumcision is elected, analgesia should be provided to the infant. Present methods for procedural analgesia include subcutaneous ring block, dorsal penile nerve block, and eutectic mixture of local anesthetics (EMLA).[44] Supplemental methods of pain control including sucrose on a pacifier, upper extremity swaddling, and acetaminophen should be incorporated into the protocol for newborn circumcision. Discharge should be delayed for 2 hours after the circumcision is performed to observe for bleeding. The caregivers should be instructed in the care and appearance of the circumcision.

NEWBORN SCREENING

Newborn screening protocols should be developed in every nursery based on existing state guidelines. As described in Chapter 48, newborn screening is a preventative public health strategy used for early identification of treatable disorders that significantly affect health and development. The disorders screened for using newborn testing vary from state to state, and health care providers should be knowledgeable regarding their specific state newborn screening protocols.

Multiple components form an effective newborn screening program. Foremost, families and health care providers must understand the goals of newborn screening. Health care providers obtaining the samples must be trained to draw appropriate samples, which are then expediently delivered to a central testing facility. The samples should be run promptly and reliably, with rapid follow-up of infants with abnormal screening results. Families with affected infants should have readily available sources for education, genetic counseling, and psychosocial support.

The authority or agency performing the screening test is responsible for transmitting the results to the physician. The health care provider caring for the infant should carefully document the results of the newborn screen in the patient's medical record.

HEARING SCREENING

Bilateral hearing loss is estimated at 1 to 3 per 1000 healthy newborns, with the average age of detection at 14 months.[36] The Joint Committee of Infant Hearing proposed in 1994 a goal of identifying hearing loss in infants before 3 months of life, with intervention begun by 6 months of age (see Chapter 40).[37]

Present systems of newborn hearing screening rely on questionnaires identifying infants at risk for hearing loss by screening criteria. It is estimated that only 50% of infants with congenital hearing loss are identified using this technique.

Universal hearing screening of all infants has been proposed and is actively being studied.[42, 50] No specific screening method has been proven to be superior, with criteria that included the ability to detect hearing loss of more than 35 dB in the better ear, a false positive rate of less than 3%, and a false negative rate of 0. If universal hearing screen is practiced, families and health care workers need to be educated regard-

---

■ **BOX 26–1**

SCHEDULE FOR IMMUNIZATION OF PRETERM INFANTS

- Vaccine doses should not be reduced for preterm infants.
- If an infant is still hospitalized at 60 days of life and weighs at least 1500 gm, the infant should be given diphtheria and tetanus toxoids and acellular pertussis (DTaP), *Haemophilus influenzae* type B (Hib) conjugate, inactivated poliovirus (IPV), and pneumococcal conjugate (PCV). These immunizations may be given over two or three days to minimize the number of injections given to these tiny babies at a single time.
- Infants with a birth weight of less than 2 kg and whose mothers are Hb$_S$Ag-negative should receive the first hepatitis B vaccine (Hep B):
  - just before hospital discharge, if the infant's weight is 2 kg or more, or
  - at 2 months of age when the other immunizations are given.
  The second dose should be given at least one month after the first dose.
  The third dose should be given at least 4 months after the first dose, at least 2 months after the second dose, and not before 6 months postnatal age.
- Preterm infants whose birth weight is less than 2 kg and whose mothers are Hb$_S$Ag-positive should be given Hepatitis B Immune Globulin (HBIG) within 12 hours of birth and a concurrent Hep B at a different site. This initial vaccine dose should not be counted in the required 3 doses to complete the immunization series.

- Preterm infants with birth weight less than 2 kg and whose mothers are Hb$_S$Ag-unknown should be given Hep B within 12 hours of birth. The maternal Hb$_S$Ag status should be determined and HBIG given to the infant if the mother is Hb$_S$Ag-positive. If the maternal status cannot be determined within 12 hours of birth, HBIG should be given. This initial vaccine dose should not be counted in the required 3 doses to complete the immunization series.
- Breast feeding of the infant by an Hb$_S$Ag-positive mother poses no additional risk for acquisition of HBV infection by the infant.
- Live virus vaccines should *never* be given during hospitalization.
  These include OPV, MMR, adenovirus, and BCG.
- Immunizations (other than live-virus vaccines that should *never* be given during hospitalization) may be given during corticosteroid administration.
- Infants with chronic respiratory tract disease should be given the influenza immunization annually in the fall once they are 6 months postnatal age and older. *Family and other caregivers should also receive influenza vaccine annually in the fall to protect the infant from exposure.*
- Palivizumab (Synagis) should be given in accordance with RSV policy.

BCG, bacille Calmette-Guérin; Hb$_S$Ag, hepatitis B surface antigen; MMR, measles-mumps-rubella; OPV, poliovirus vaccine live oral; RSV, respiratory syncytial virus.
Adapted by Jill E. Baley, MD, from the AAP Red Book 2000.

---

ing the implications of testing. Clearly defined pathways for follow-up of abnormal screening tests would be required that include both medical and social components. In a significant portion of children who have hearing loss, it develops after birth.

IMMUNIZATIONS

Preterm infants should generally be immunized at the usual chronologic age in most cases. However, modification of immunization schedules is needed to accommodate the unique immunologic characeristics of these infants. The schedule adopted at our institution is shown in Box 26–1, as modified from the 2000 Red Book of the AAP.

FAMILIES

The most important component in the care of the well or sick newborn is the family. An infant is not treated in isolation from those who are most attached and who have the most to offer. As described in Chapter 32, newborn care in any facility should be family

centered. From mother-infant care in the normal nursery to intensive care unit policies that actively encourage parental care and input, active effort needs to be continuously focused on enhancing the role families play in the care of their newborn. Respect should be given to cultural and religious beliefs that are important to each family.

ACKNOWLEDGMENTS

Drs. Lissauer and Izatt and the editors acknowledge the contributions of Drs. Susan Aucott and Michele Walsh-Sukys to the previous edition of the chapter, from which many sections remain largely unchanged.

■ REFERENCES

Part One: Physical Examination of the Newborn

1. American Academy of Pediatrics, American College of Obstetricians & Gynaecologists: Guidelines for Perinatal Care, 4th ed. Elk Grove Village, Ill, American Academy of Pediatrics, 1997.
2. Amiel-Tison C: Neurological evaluation of the maturity of newborn infants. Arch Dis Child 43:89, 1968.

3. Arlettaz R, Archer NJ, Wilkinson AR: Natural history of innocent heart murmurs in newborn babies: A controlled echocardiographic study. Arch Dis Child 78:F166, 1998.
4. Ballard JL, et al: A simplified score for assessment of fetal maturation of newly born infants. J Pediatr 95:769, 1979.
5. Ballard JL, et al: New Ballard Score, expanded to include extremely premature infants. J Pediatr 119:417, 1991.
6. Barlow TG: Early diagnosis and treatment of congenital dislocation of the hip. J Bone Joint Surg Br 44:B292, 1962.
7. Bourke WG, et al: Isolated single umbilical artery—the case for screening. Arch Dis Child 68:600, 1993.
8. Chan A, et al: Perinatal risk factors for developmental dysplasia of the hip. Arch Dis Child 76:F94, 1997.
9. Chan A, et al: Late diagnosis of congenital dislocation of the hip and the presence of a screening programme: South Australia population based study. Lancet 354:1514, 1999.
10. Clarke NMP: Diagnosing congenital dislocation of the hip. BMJ 305:435, 1992.
11. Du Z-D, Rougin N, Barak M: Clinical and echocardiographic evaluation of neonates with heart murmurs. Acta Paediatr 86:752, 1997.
12. Dubowitz L, et al: Clinical assessment of gestational age in the newborn infant. J Pediatr 77:1, 1970.
13. Dubowitz L, Dubowitz V: The neurological assessment of the preterm and full-term newborn infant. In: Clinics in Developmental Medicine, No. 79 SIMP. London, WH Heinemann, 1981.
14. Farr V, et al: The definition of some external characteristics used in the assessment of gestational age of the newborn infant. Dev Med Child Neurol 8:507, 1966.
15. Froelich L, et al: Follow up of infants with single umbilical artery. Pediatrics 52:6, 1973.
16. Gibson P, et al: Lumbosacral skin markers and identification of occult spinal dysraphism in neonates. Acta Paediatr 84:208, 1995.
17. Godward S, Dezateux C: Surgery for congenital dislocation of the hip in the UK as a measure of outcome of screening. Lancet 351:1149, 1998.
18. Hall DMB: Health for All Children, 3rd ed. Oxford, England, Oxford University Press, 1995, pp 90–108.
19. Hansen LK, Birkebaek NH, Oxhoj H: Initial evaluation of children with heart murmurs by the non-specialised paediatricians. Eur J Pediatr 154:15, 1995.
20. Hittner HM, et al: Assessment of gestational age by examination of anterior vascular capsule of lens. J Pediatr 91:455, 1977.
21. Kugelman A, et al: Preauricular tags and pits in the newborn: The role of hearing tests. Acta Paediatr 86:170, 1997.
22. Leung AKC, et al: Single umbilical artery: A report of 159 cases. Am J Dis Child 148:108, 1989.
23. Liu LL, et al: The safety of newborn early discharge. JAMA 278:293, 1997.
24. McCrindle BW, et al: Cardinal clinical signs in the differentiation of heart murmurs in children. Arch Paediatr Adolesc Med 150:169, 1996.
25. Moss GD, et al: Routine examination in the newborn period. BMJ 302:878, 1991.
26. Parkin JM, Hey EN, Clowes JS: Rapid assessment of gestational age at birth. Arch Dis Child 51:259, 1976.
27. Sanfridson J, Redland-Johnell I, Uden A: Why is congenital dislocation of the hip still missed? Analysis of 96,891 infants screened in Malmo, 1956–1987. Acta Orthop Scand 62:87, 1991.
28. Scott JES, et al: Screening newborn babies for familial ureteric reflux. Lancet 350:396, 1997.
29. Smythe JF, et al: Initial evaluation of heart murmurs: Are laboratory tests necessary? Pediatrics 86:497, 1990.
30. Temmerman AM, Mooyaart EL, Taverne PP: The value of the routine chest roentgenogram in the cardiological evaluation of infants and children: A prospective study. Eur J Pediatr 150:623, 1991.
31. Wariyar U, Tin W, Hey E: Gestational assessment assessed. Arch Dis Child 77:F216, 1997.
32. Young PC: The morbidity of cardiac nondisease revisited. Is there lingering concern associated with an innocent murmur? Am J Dis Child 147:975, 1993.

Part Two: Care of the Newborn

33. American Academy of Pediatrics, Committee on Nutrition: Soy protein-based formulas: Recommendations for use in infant feeding. Pediatrics 101:148, 1998.
34. American Academy of Pediatrics, Committee on Environmental Health. Noise: A hazard for the fetus and newborn. Pediatrics 100:724, 1997.
35. American Academy of Pediatrics, Task Force on Circumcision: Circumcision policy statement. Pediatrics 103:686, 1999.
36. American Academy of Pediatrics, Task Force on Newborn and Infant Hearing: Newborn and infant hearing loss. Pediatrics 103:527, 1999.
37. American Academy of Pediatrics, Joint Committee on Infant Hearing: Joint Committee on Infant Hearing 1994 position statement. Pediatrics 95:152, 1995.
38. American Academy of Pediatrics, American College of Obstetricians and Gynecologists: Guidelines for Perinatal Care, 4th ed. Elk Grove Village, Ill, AAP/ACOG, 1997.
39. American Academy of Pediatrics, Section on Perinatal Pediatrics, Committee to Establish Recommended Standards for Newborn ICU Design: Recommended standards for newborn ICU design. J Perinatol 19:S1, 1999.
40. Bellig L: Infant abduction safeguard program. Neonatal Network 17:52, 1998.
41. Glazener CMA, et al: Neonatal examination and screening trial (NEST): A randomized, controlled, switchback trial of alternative policies for low risk infants. BMJ 318:627, 1999.
42. Grote JJ: Neonatal screening for hearing impairment. Lancet 355:513, 2000.
43. Hall DMB: The role of the routine neonatal examination. BMJ 318:619, 1999.
44. Lander J, et al: Comparison of ring block, dorsal penile nerve block, and topical anesthesia for neonatal circumcision: A randomized controlled trial. JAMA 278:2157, 1997.
45. Lund C: Prevention and management of infant skin breakdown. Nurs Clin North Am 34:907, 1999.
46. Reynolds JD, et al: Lack of efficacy of light reduction in preventing retinopathy of prematurity. N Engl J Med 338:1572, 1998.
47. Roy M-S, et al: Effects of early reduced light exposure on central visual development in preterm infants. Acta Paediatr 88:459, 1999.
48. Siegfried EC: Neonatal skin and skin care. Dermatol Clin 16:437, 1998.
49. Walsh-Sukys MC: personal communication, March 17, 2000.
50. Wessex Universal Neonatal Hearing Screening Trial Group: Controlled trial of universal neonatal screening for early identification of permanent childhood hearing impairment. Lancet 352:1957, 1998.
51. Wright IM, et al: Stethoscope contamination in the neonatal intensive care unit. J Hosp Infect 29:65, 1995.
52. Zipursky A: Prevention of vitamin K deficiency bleeding in newborns. Br J Haematol 104:430, 1999.

27

Birth Injuries

Henry H. Mangurten

Birth injuries are those sustained during the birth process, which includes labor and delivery. They may be avoidable, or they may be unavoidable and occur despite skilled and competent obstetric care, as in an especially hard or prolonged labor or with an abnormal presentation. Fetal injuries related to amniocentesis and intrauterine transfusions and neonatal injuries after resuscitation procedures are not considered birth injuries. However, injuries related to the use of intrapartum monitoring of the fetal heart rate and collection of fetal scalp blood for acid-base assessment are included. Factors predisposing the infant to birth injury include macrosomia, prematurity, cephalopelvic disproportion, dystocia, prolonged labor, abnormal presentation, and certain operative deliveries, particularly vacuum extraction.

The significance of birth injuries may be assessed by review of mortality data. In 1981, birth injuries ranked sixth among major causes of neonatal death, resulting in 23.8 deaths per 100,000 live births.[66] During the ensuing decade, because of refinements in obstetric techniques and the increased use of cesarean deliveries over difficult vaginal deliveries, a dramatic decline occurred in birth injuries as a cause of neonatal death. Statistics for 1993 revealed a reduction to 3.7 deaths per 100,000 live births; because of the emergence of other conditions, birth injuries ranked 11th among major causes of neonatal death.[67] The most recent figures available (for 1998) identify only the 10 leading causes of infant death, with no mention of birth injuries.[24]

Despite a reduction in related mortality rates, birth injuries still represent an important source of neonatal morbidity[64] and neonatal intensive care unit admissions. Of particular concern are severe intracranial injuries after combined methods of vaginal delivery (vacuum-assisted and forceps delivery) and failed attempts at operative vaginal delivery.[64]

The clinician should consider the broad spectrum of birth injuries in the differential diagnosis of neonatal clinical disorders. Although many injuries are mild and self-limited, others are serious and potentially lethal. This chapter describes both conditions that can be managed by observation only and those that require more aggressive intervention.

INJURIES TO SOFT TISSUES

ERYTHEMA AND ABRASIONS

Erythema and abrasions frequently occur when dystocia has occurred during labor as a result of cephalopelvic disproportion or when forceps have been used during delivery. Injuries caused by dystocia occur over the presenting part; forceps injury occurs at the site of application of the instrument. Forceps injury frequently has a linear configuration across both sides of the face, outlining the position of the forceps. The affected areas should be kept clean to minimize the risk of secondary infection. These lesions usually resolve spontaneously within several days with no specific therapy.

PETECHIAE

Occasionally, petechiae are present on the head, neck, upper portion of the chest, and lower portion of the back at birth after a difficult delivery; they are observed more frequently after breech deliveries.

ETIOLOGY. Petechiae are probably caused by a sudden increase in intrathoracic and venous pressures during passage of the chest through the birth canal. An infant born with the cord tightly wound around the neck may have petechiae only above the neck.

DIFFERENTIAL DIAGNOSIS. Petechiae may be a manifestation of an underlying hemorrhagic disorder. The birth history, early appearance of the petechiae, and absence of bleeding from other sites help to differentiate petechiae caused by increased tissue pressure or trauma from petechiae caused by hemorrhagic disorders (see Chapter 44). The localized distribution of the petechiae, the absence of subsequent crops of new lesions, and a normal platelet count exclude neonatal thrombocytopenia. The platelet count also may be low because of infections or disseminated intravascular coagulation. Infections may be clinically distinguished from traumatic petechiae by the presence of other signs and symptoms. Disseminated intravascular coagulation usually is associated with excessive and persistent bleeding from a variety of sites. Petechiae usually are distributed over the entire body when associated with systemic disease.

TREATMENT. If the petechiae are caused by trauma, neither corticosteroids nor heparin should be used. No specific treatment is necessary.

PROGNOSIS. Traumatic petechiae usually fade within 2 or 3 days.

ECCHYMOSES

Ecchymoses may occur after traumatic or breech deliveries. The incidence is increased in premature infants, especially after a rapid labor and poorly controlled delivery. When extensive, ecchymoses may reflect blood loss severe enough to cause anemia and, rarely, shock. The reabsorption of blood from an ecchymotic area may result in significant hyperbilirubinemia (Fig. 27–1).

TREATMENT. No local therapy is necessary. The rise in serum bilirubin that follows severe bruising may be decreased by the use of phototherapy (see also Chapter 46). Ecchymoses rarely result in significant anemia.

PROGNOSIS. The ecchymoses usually resolve spontaneously within 1 week.

SUBCUTANEOUS FAT NECROSIS

(See also Chapter 47, Part Two.)

Subcutaneous fat necrosis is characterized by well-circumscribed indurated lesions of the skin and underlying tissue.

ETIOLOGY. The cause of subcutaneous fat necrosis is uncertain, although obstetric trauma is considered a

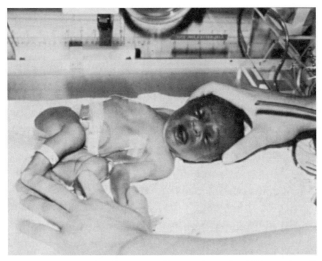

FIGURE 27–1. Marked bruising of entire face of a 1490-gm female infant born vaginally after face presentation. Less severe ecchymoses were present on extremities. Despite use of phototherapy from the first day, icterus was noted on the third day and exchange transfusions were required on the fifth and sixth days.

possibility. Many affected infants are large and have been delivered by forceps or after a prolonged, difficult labor involving vigorous fetal manipulation. The distribution of the lesions usually is related to the site of trauma, which explains the frequent involvement of shoulders and buttocks. Other etiologic factors that have been implicated include hypothermia, local ischemia, and intrauterine asphyxia. One suggested mechanism of pathogenesis proposes that diminished in utero circulation and mechanical pressure during labor and delivery result in vascular compromise to specific areas, which eventually causes localized fat necrosis.[11] This condition has also been described in an infant whose mother used cocaine during pregnancy. The authors postulate that cocaine may be a factor because of decreased placental perfusion with subsequent hypoxemia and alteration of the maternal and fetal pituitary-adrenal axes.[9]

PATHOLOGY. Initially, histopathologic studies reveal endothelial swelling and perivascular inflammation in the subcutaneous tissues. They are followed by necrosis of fat and a dense granulomatous inflammatory infiltrate containing foreign body type giant cells with needle-shaped crystals resembling cholesterol.

CLINICAL MANIFESTATIONS. Necrotic areas usually appear between 6 and 10 days of age but may be noted as early as the second day or as late as the sixth week. They occur on the cheeks, neck, back, shoulders, arms, buttocks, thighs, and feet, with relative sparing of the chest and abdomen. The lesions vary in size from 1 to 10 cm; rarely, they may be more extensive. They are irregularly shaped, hard, plaquelike, and nonpitting (Fig. 27–2). The overlying skin may be colorless, red, or purple. The affected areas may be slightly elevated above the adjacent skin; small lesions may be easily moveable in all directions. There is no local tenderness or increase in skin temperature.

Marked symptomatic hypercalcemia may develop in infants with subcutaneous fat necrosis at 3 to 4 weeks of age; this has been characterized by vomiting, weight loss, anorexia, fever, somnolence, and irritability, with serum calcium levels as high as 16.2 mg/ dL.[13, 35] Improvement generally has occurred after intravenous hydration, furosemide, and hydrocortisone therapy. Investigators have suggested extrarenal production of 1,25-dihydroxyvitamin D by the granulomatous cells of fat necrosis as a possible mechanism for the hypercalcemia.[13, 35]

DIFFERENTIAL DIAGNOSIS. The differential diagnosis includes lipogranulomatosis and sclerema neonatorum, which carry a serious prognosis, and nodular nonsuppurative panniculitis, which is usually associated with fever, hepatosplenomegaly, and tender skin nodules.

TREATMENT. These lesions require only observation. Surgical excision is not indicated.

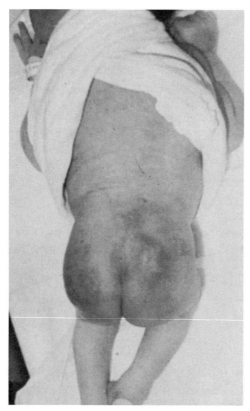

FIGURE 27–2. Subcutaneous fat necrosis in a 2900-gm term infant delivered vaginally; pregnancy, labor, and delivery were completely uncomplicated. Note nodular lesion located on right buttock and surrounded by erythema *(darkened area)*. (Courtesy of Dr. Rajam Ramamurthy, Cook County Hospital, Chicago.)

PROGNOSIS. The lesions slowly soften after 6 to 8 weeks and completely regress within several months. Occasionally, minimal residual atrophy, with or without small calcified areas, is observed. Affected infants should be followed closely during the first 6 weeks for potential development of hypercalcemia. It is important to treat this complication without delay to prevent central nervous system (CNS) and renal sequelae.[13]

LACERATIONS

Accidental lacerations may be inflicted with a scalpel during cesarean section. They usually occur on the scalp, buttocks, and thighs, but they may occur on any part of the body. If the wound is superficial, the edges may be held in apposition with butterfly adhesive strips. Deeper, more freely bleeding wounds should be sutured with the finest material available, preferably 7-0 nylon. Rarely, the amount of blood loss and depth of wound require suturing in the delivery room. After repair, the wound should be left uncovered unless it is in an area of potential soiling, such as the perineal area; in such locations the wound should be sprayed with protective plastic. Healing is usually rapid, and the sutures may be removed after 5 days.

INJURIES TO THE HEAD

SKULL

Caput Succedaneum

Caput succedaneum, a frequently observed lesion, is characterized by a vaguely demarcated area of edema over that portion of the scalp that was the presenting part during a vertex delivery.

ETIOLOGY. Serum or blood or both accumulate above the periosteum in the presenting part during labor. This extravasation results from the higher pressure of the uterus or vaginal wall on those areas of the fetal head that border the caput. Thus, in a left occiput transverse presentation, the caput succedaneum occurs over the upper and posterior aspect of the right parietal bone; in a right-sided presentation it occurs over the corresponding area of the left parietal bone.

CLINICAL MANIFESTATIONS. The soft swelling is usually a few millimeters thick and may be associated with overlying petechiae, purpura, or ecchymoses. Because of the location external to the periosteum, a caput succedaneum may extend across the midline of the skull and across suture lines. After an especially difficult labor, an extensive caput may obscure various sutures and fontanelles.

DIFFERENTIAL DIAGNOSIS. Occasionally, a caput succedaneum may be difficult to distinguish from a cephalhematoma, particularly when the latter occurs bilaterally. Careful palpation usually indicates whether the bleeding is external to the periosteum (a caput) or beneath the periosteum (a cephalhematoma).

TREATMENT. Usually no specific treatment is indicated. Rarely, a hemorrhagic caput may result in shock and require blood transfusion.

PROGNOSIS. A caput succedaneum usually resolves within several days.

Cephalhematoma

Cephalhematoma is an infrequently seen subperiosteal collection of blood overlying a cranial bone. The incidence is 0.4% to 2.5% of live births; the frequency is higher in male infants and in infants born to primiparous mothers.

ETIOLOGY. A cephalhematoma is caused during labor or delivery by a rupture of blood vessels that traverse from skull to periosteum. Repeated buffeting of the fetal skull against the maternal pelvis during a prolonged or difficult labor and mechanical trauma caused by use of forceps in delivery have been implicated. Recently, Petrikovsky and associates[47] have described seven infants in whom cephalhematoma or caput succedaneum was identified prenatally *prior to* onset of labor. Occurrence of premature rupture of membranes in five of the pregnancies suggests an etiology of fetal head compression by the uterine walls, resulting from oligohydramnios subsequent to the ruptured membranes.

CLINICAL MANIFESTATIONS. The bleeding is sharply limited by periosteal attachments to the surface of one cranial bone; there is no extension across suture lines. The bleeding usually occurs over one or both parietal bones. Less often it involves the occipital bones and, very rarely, the frontal bones. The overlying scalp is not discolored. Because subperiosteal bleeding is slow, the swelling may not be apparent for several hours or days after birth. The swelling is often larger on the second or third day, when sharply demarcated boundaries are palpable. The cephalhematoma may feel fluctuant and often is bordered by a slightly elevated ridge of organizing tissue that gives the false sensation of a central bony depression. In 1974, Zelson and coworkers[68] noted an underlying skull fracture in 5.4% of cephalhematomas. These fractures are almost always linear and nondepressed.

RADIOGRAPHIC MANIFESTATIONS. Radiographic manifestations vary with the age of the cephalhematoma. During the first 2 weeks, bloody fluid results in a shadow of water density. At the end of the second week, bone begins to form under the elevated pericranium at the margins of the hematoma; the entire lesion is progressively overlaid with a complete shell of bone.

DIFFERENTIAL DIAGNOSIS. A cephalhematoma may be differentiated from caput succedaneum by (1) its sharp periosteal limitations to one bone, (2) the absence of overlying discoloration, (3) the later initial appearance of the swelling, and (4) the longer time before resolution. Cranial meningocele is differentiated from cephalhematoma by pulsations, an increase in pressure during crying, and the demonstration of a bony defect on a radiograph. An occipital cephalhematoma may be confused initially with an occipital meningocele and with cranium bifidum because all occupy the midline position.

TREATMENT. Therapy is not indicated for the uncomplicated cephalhematoma. Rarely, a massive cephalhematoma may result in blood loss severe enough to require transfusion. Significant hyperbilirubinemia also may result, necessitating phototherapy or other treatment of jaundice (see also Chapter 46).

The most common associated complications are skull fracture and intracranial hemorrhage. Linear fractures do not require specific therapy, but radiographs should be taken at 4 to 6 weeks to ensure closure and to exclude formation of leptomeningeal cysts; depressed fractures require immediate neurosurgical consultation. Specific treatment of blood loss or hyperbilirubinemia or both may be indicated if there has been an intracranial hemorrhage. Routine incision or aspiration of a cephalhematoma is contraindicated because of the risk of introducing infection.

Rarely, bacterial infections of cephalhematomas occur, usually in association with septicemia and meningitis. Focal infection should be suspected when a sudden enlargement of a static cephalhematoma occurs during the course of a systemic infection, with a relapse of meningitis or sepsis after treatment with antibiotics, or with the development of local signs of infection over the cephalhematoma (Fig. 27–3). Diagnostic aspiration may be indicated. If a local infection is present, surgical drainage and specific antibiotic therapy should be instituted. Osteomyelitis of the underlying skull may be a rare concurrent problem.[42, 44] The diagnosis may be suggested by periosteal elevation and overlying soft tissue swelling on skull radiographs. A computed tomographic (CT) finding of permeative bone destruction confirms the diagnosis.

PROGNOSIS. Most cephalhematomas are resorbed within 2 weeks to 3 months, depending on their size; most of those are resorbed by 6 weeks. In a few patients, calcium is deposited (Fig. 27–4), causing a bony swelling that may persist for several months and, rarely, up to 1½ years.

Radiographic findings persist after the disappearance of clinical signs. The outer table remains thickened as a flat, irregular hyperostosis for several months. Widening of the space between the new shell of bone and the inner table may persist for years; the space originally occupied by the hematoma usually

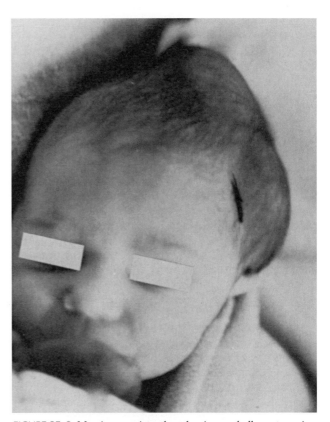

FIGURE 27–3. Massive, persistently enlarging cephalhematoma in a 13-day-old female infant delivered by midforceps after occiput-posterior presentation. Surgical drainage revealed 300 mL of yellowish material that cultured *Escherichia coli*.

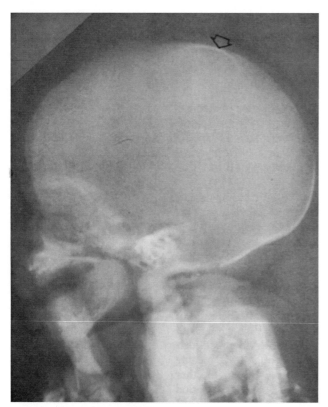

FIGURE 27–4. Calcified cephalhematoma in left parietal region of 5-week-old girl. Infant weighed 1410 gm at birth and was delivered rapidly because of prolapsed cord. Hard left parietal swelling was detected at 5 weeks by nurses during feeding.

develops into normal diploic bone, but cystlike defects may persist at the sites of the hematoma for months or years. Rarely, a neonatal cephalhematoma may persist into adult life as a symptomless mass, the cephalhematoma deformans of Schüller.

Subgaleal Hemorrhage

Subgaleal hemorrhage (SGH) is a collection of blood in the soft tissue space between the galea aponeurotica and the periosteum of the skull (Fig. 27–5). The incidence is approximately 4 per 10,000 deliveries, with an even higher incidence after instrumental deliveries. Ng and colleagues[45] have reported an incidence of 64 per 10,000 deliveries when vacuum extraction is performed!

ETIOLOGY. The most common predisposing factor is difficult instrumental delivery, particularly midforceps delivery and vacuum extraction.[22, 48] The risk of SGH may be reduced by use of softer silicone vacuum cups instead of the original rigid metallic ones.[6] Other factors include coagulopathies,[12, 54] prematurity, macrosomia, fetal dystocia, and precipitous labor.[31] The loose connective tissue of the subgaleal space can accommodate as much as 260 mL of blood.[48] SGH may result from an associated skull fracture or rupture of an interosseous synchondrosis (primarily between the parietal bones), in turn causing injury to

major intracranial veins or sinuses. Another possible mechanism results from distortion of or traction on emissary veins bridging the subdural and subgaleal spaces.[22]

CLINICAL MANIFESTATIONS. Early manifestations may be limited to pallor, hypotonia, and diffuse swelling of the scalp. The development of a fluctuating mass straddling cranial sutures, fontanelles, or both is highly suggestive of the diagnosis.[22] Because blood accumulates beneath the aponeurotic layer, ecchymotic discoloration of the scalp is a later finding.[48] This often is associated with pitting edema and progressive posterior spread toward the neck and lateral spread around the ears, frequently displacing the ears anteriorly (Fig. 27–6). Periorbital swelling and ecchymosis also are commonly observed.[48] Eventually, hypovolemic shock and signs of cerebral irritation develop. The clinician should be aware of occasional "silent presentation," in which a fluctuant mass is not apparent initially despite serial clinical examinations.[45] SGH should be considered in infants who show signs of hypoperfusion and falling hematocrit after attempted or successful vacuum delivery, even in the absence of a detectable fluctuant mass.

RADIOGRAPHIC MANIFESTATIONS. Standard radiographs of the skull may identify possible associated fractures. CT scanning may demonstrate abundant epicranial blood, parieto-occipital bone dehiscence, bone fragmentation, and posterior cerebral interhemispheric densities compatible with subarachnoid hemorrhage.[22]

DIFFERENTIAL DIAGNOSIS. In contrast to cephalhematoma, SGH is characterized by its more diffuse distribution, more rapid course, significant anemia, signs of CNS trauma (e.g., hypotonia, lethargy, seizures), and frequent lethal outcome.

TREATMENT. Prompt restoration of blood volume with fresh frozen plasma or blood is essential. If the bleeding continues, gentle compression wraps may be applied to the head; however, the value of this therapy is only anecdotal.[6] In the presence of continued deterioration, surgery may be considered as a last resort. A bicoronal incision allows for exposure of the subgaleal space. Bipolar cauterization of any bleeding points can then be accomplished, and a drain can be left in the subgaleal space.

PROGNOSIS. Nearly 25% of infants with SGH die.[31, 48]

Skull Fractures

Fracture of the neonatal skull is uncommon because the bones of the skull are less mineralized at birth and thus more compressible. In addition, the separation of the bones by membranous sutures usually permits enough alteration in the contour of the head to allow its passage through the birth canal without injury.

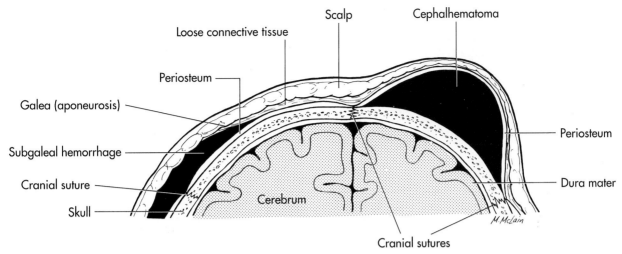

FIGURE 27–5. Subgaleal hemorrhage and cephalhematoma.

ETIOLOGY. Skull fractures usually follow a forceps delivery or a prolonged, difficult labor with repeated forceful contact of the fetal skull against the maternal symphysis pubis, sacral promontory, or ischial spine. Recently, this has been described following a vacuum extraction delivery.[29] Most of the fractures are linear. Depressed fractures almost always result from forceps application. However, they may occur spontaneously after cesarean section[18, 20] or vaginal delivery without forceps. Factors that have been implicated include pressure on the fetal skull by a maternal bony prominence (e.g., sacral promontory) or uterine fibroid, a fetal hand or foot, or the body part of a twin. Occipital bone fractures usually occur in breech deliveries as a consequence of traction on the hyperextended spine of the infant when the head is fixed in the maternal pelvis.

CLINICAL MANIFESTATIONS. Linear fractures over the convexity of the skull frequently are accompanied by soft tissue changes and cephalhematoma. Usually the infant's behavior is normal unless there is an associated concussion or hemorrhage into the subdural or subarachnoid space. Fractures at the base of the skull with separation of the basal and squamous portions of the occipital bone almost always result in severe hemorrhage caused by disruption of the underlying venous sinuses. The infant may then exhibit shock, neurologic abnormalities, and drainage of bloody cerebrospinal fluid from the ears or nose.

Depressed fractures are visible, palpable indentations in the smooth contour of the skull, similar to dents in a Ping-Pong ball (Fig. 27–7). The infant may be entirely free of symptoms unless there is an associated intracranial injury.

RADIOGRAPHIC MANIFESTATIONS. The diagnosis of a simple linear or fissure fracture is seldom made without radiographs in which fractures appear as lines and strips of decreased density. Depressed fractures appear as lines of increased density. On some views they are manifested by an inward buckling of bone with or without an actual break in continuity. Either type of fracture may be seen on only one view.

DIFFERENTIAL DIAGNOSIS. Occasionally, the fragments of a linear fracture may be widely separated and may simulate an open suture. Conversely, parietal foramina, the interparietal fontanelle, mendosal sutures, and innominate synchondroses may be mistaken for fractures. In addition, normal vascular grooves, "ripple lines" that represent soft tissue folds of the scalp, and lacunar skull may be mistaken for fractures.

TREATMENT. Uncomplicated linear fractures over the convexity of the skull usually do not require treat-

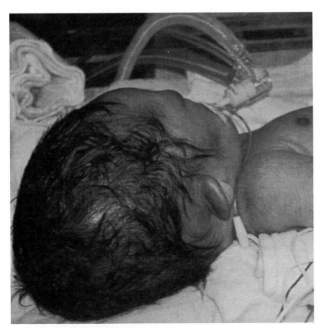

FIGURE 27–6. Clinical manifestations of subgaleal hemorrhage. Note anteriorly displaced ear.

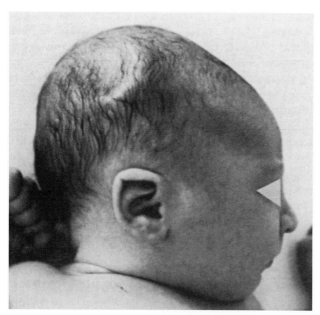

FIGURE 27–7. Depressed skull fracture in term male infant delivered after rapid (1 hour) labor. Infant was delivered by occiput-anterior presentation after rotation from occiput-posterior position.

ment. Fractures at the base of the skull often necessitate blood replacement for severe hemorrhage and shock in addition to other supportive measures. If cerebrospinal fluid rhinorrhea or otorrhea is present, antimicrobial coverage is indicated to prevent secondary infection of the meninges.

Small (less than 2 cm) "Ping-Pong" fractures may be observed without surgical treatment. Loeser and associates[38] reported on three infants with depressed skull fractures in whom spontaneous elevation of the fractures occurred within 1 day to 3½ months of age. Follow-up at 1 to 2½ years revealed normal neurologic development in all three.

Several nonsurgical methods have been described for elevation of depressed skull fractures in certain infants:

1. A thumb is placed on opposite margins of the depression and gentle, firm pressure exerted toward the middle. After several minutes of continuous pressure the area of depression gradually disappears.[52]
2. A hand breast pump is applied to the depressed area. Petroleum jelly placed on the pump edges ensures a tighter seal, and gentle suction for several minutes results in elevation of the depressed bone.[56]
3. A vacuum extractor is placed over the depression, and a negative pressure of 0.2 to 0.5 kg/cm^2 is maintained for approximately 4 minutes.[55, 62]

Because these methods are technically easier and less traumatic, they may be preferable to surgical intervention in a symptom-free infant with an isolated lesion.

Comminuted or large fractures associated with neurologic signs or symptoms should be treated by immediate surgical elevation of the indented segment to prevent underlying cortical injury from pressure. Other indications for surgical elevation include manifestations of cerebrospinal fluid beneath the galea and failure to elevate the fracture by nonsurgical manipulation.

PROGNOSIS. Simple linear fractures usually heal within several months without sequelae. Rarely, a leptomeningeal cyst may develop from an associated dural tear, and meninges or part of the brain may protrude through the fracture. The fracture line may widen rapidly within weeks, or a large defect in the skull may be noted many months later. If detected early, the cyst may be excised successfully and brain atrophy prevented. It is therefore advisable to repeat skull radiographs within 2 to 3 months to detect early widening of the fracture line. Color Doppler imaging has been demonstrated to enhance earlier diagnosis of leptomeningeal cyst during the second week of life.[65]

Basal fractures carry a poor prognosis. When separation of the basal and squamous portions of the occipital bone occurs, the outcome is almost always fatal; surviving infants have an extremely high incidence of neurologic sequelae.

The prognosis for a depressed fracture is usually good when treatment is early and adequate. When therapy is delayed, especially with a large depression, death may occur from pressure on vital areas of the brain. Because the natural history of depressed skull fractures in neonates has not been clearly elucidated, the outcome is uncertain for infants with smaller lesions managed either by simple observation or by surgery after significant delays. Despite the apparently normal outcome in the three infants reported by Loeser and associates,[38] one cannot completely exclude the possibility that subtle neurologic sequelae may develop years later.

Intracranial Hemorrhage

(See Chapter 38, Part Five.)

FACE

Facial Nerve Palsy

(See also Chapter 38.)

Facial nerve palsy in the neonate may follow birth injury or rarely may result from agenesis of the facial nerve nucleus. The latter condition occasionally is hereditary but usually is sporadic.

ETIOLOGY. Traumatic facial nerve palsy most often follows compression of the peripheral portion of the nerve, either near the stylomastoid foramen, through which it emerges, or where the nerve traverses the ramus of the mandible. The nerve may be compressed by forceps, especially when the fetal head has been grasped obliquely. The condition also occurs after spontaneous deliveries in which prolonged pressure was applied by the maternal sacral promontory. Less frequently, injury is sustained in utero, often in association with a mandibular deformity, by the persistent position of the fetal foot against the superior ramus of the mandible. An extremely rare cause is the pressure of a uterine tumor on the nerve.

This condition may occur rarely with a simultaneous ipsilateral brachial plexus palsy, most likely secondary to compressive forces during delivery.[16] Contributing factors include prolonged second stage of labor and midforceps delivery.

A traumatic facial nerve palsy may follow a contralateral injury to the CNS, such as a temporal bone fracture, or hemorrhage, tissue destruction, or both to structures within the posterior fossa. This CNS injury is less frequent than peripheral nerve injury.

CLINICAL MANIFESTATIONS. Paralysis is usually apparent on the first or second day but may be present at birth. It usually does not increase in severity unless considerable edema occurs over the area of nerve trauma. The type and distribution of paralysis are different in central facial paralysis compared with peripheral paralysis.

Central paralysis is a spastic paralysis limited to the lower half or two thirds of the contralateral side of the face. The paralyzed side is smooth and full and often appears swollen. The nasolabial fold is obliterated, and the corner of the mouth droops. When the infant cries, the mouth is drawn to the normal side, the wrinkles are deeper on the normal side, and movement of the forehead and eyelid is unaffected. Usually other manifestations of intracranial injury appear, most often a sixth cranial nerve palsy.

Peripheral paralysis is flaccid and, when complete, involves the entire side of the face. When the infant is at rest, the only sign may be a persistently open eye on the affected side, caused by paralysis of the orbicular muscle of the eye. With crying, the findings are the same as in a central facial nerve injury, with the addition of a smooth forehead on the involved side. Because the tongue is not involved, feeding is not affected.

A small branch of the nerve may be injured, with involvement of only one group of facial muscles. Paralysis is then limited to the forehead, eyelid, or mouth. Peripheral paralysis caused by nerve injury distal to the geniculate ganglion may be accompanied by a hematotympanum on the same side.

DIFFERENTIAL DIAGNOSIS. Central and peripheral facial nerve palsies must be distinguished from nuclear agenesis (Möbius syndrome). The latter frequently results in bilateral facial nerve palsy; the face is expressionless and immobile, suggesting muscle fibrosis. Other cranial nerve palsies and deformities of the ear, palate, tongue, mandible, and other bones may be associated with Möbius syndrome. Congenital absence or hypoplasia of the depressor muscle of the angle of the mouth also may simulate congenital facial palsy and has been associated with an increased incidence of other congenital anomalies.

TREATMENT. No specific therapy is indicated for most facial palsies. If the paralysis is peripheral and complete, initial treatment should be directed at protecting the cornea with an eye pad and instilling 1% methylcellulose drops every 4 hours. The functional state of the nerve should be followed closely. Falco and colleagues[19] proposed the following comprehensive approach:

1. Distinguish developmental from acquired lesions on the basis of the birth history and a detailed physical examination. Patients thought to have developmental palsy should be examined with radiologic and electrodiagnostic studies and brainstem-evoked response as appropriate.
2. Because of the expected 90% likelihood of complete spontaneous recovery, patients should be observed for 1 year before surgical intervention is considered. If recovery is suggested by physical examination or serial electromyography, observation without surgery may be delayed until the second birthday. Infants who require surgery are best treated with decompression or neuroplasty or both.

PROGNOSIS. Most facial palsies resolve spontaneously within several days; total recovery may require several weeks or months. Electrodiagnostic testing is beneficial in predicting recovery; repeatedly normal nerve excitability indicates a good prognosis, but decreased or absent excitability early in the course suggests a poor outlook. The subsequent appearance of muscle fibrillation potentials indicates nerve degeneration. The prognosis in surgically treated infants worsens with increasing age at treatment.

Fractures and Dislocations of Facial Bones

Facial bone fractures may occur during passage through the birth canal, during forceps application and delivery, and during obstetric manipulation (most often the Mauriceau maneuver for delivery of the fetal head in a breech presentation). Manipulation may result in mandibular fractures and mandibular joint damage but is rarely severe enough to cause separation of the symphysis of the mandible. Fracture of the nose may result in early respiratory distress and feeding difficulties. The most frequent nasal injury is dislocation of the cartilaginous part of the septum from the vomerine groove and columella. This may result from intrauterine factors such as a uterine tumor or persistent pressure on the nose by fetal small parts or during delivery from pressure on the nose by the symphysis pubis, sacral promontory, or perineum. The presence of nasal septal dislocation may be differentiated from the more common normal variant of a misshapen nose by a simple compression test, in which the tip of the nose is compressed[14] (Fig. 27–8). In the presence of septal dislocation, the nostrils collapse and the deviated septum becomes more apparent; in the normal nose, no nasal deviation occurs with compression.

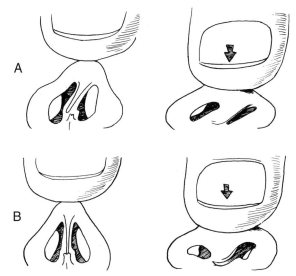

FIGURE 27–8. Result of finger compression *(A)* when nasal septum is dislocated. Normal septal relationship *(B)* results in no nasal deviation with pressure. (Modified from Daily W, et al: Nasal septal dislocation in the newborn. Mo Med 74:381, 1977.)

Infants who sustain nasal trauma during the birth process may demonstrate stridor and cyanosis, even in the absence of septal dislocation. Miller and co-workers[43] noted high nasal resistance in three such infants, of whom only one was found to have septal dislocation. The authors postulated the presence of edema and narrowed nasal passages from compression forces on the midface during delivery. The problem may be exaggerated by repeated nasal suctioning or transnasal bronchoscopy. These procedures and oral feeding should be avoided until the infant re-establishes normal nasal ventilation. Transcutaneous oxygen and carbon dioxide tensions and pulse oximetry measurements are useful in monitoring these infants.

TREATMENT. Fractures of the maxilla, lacrimal bones, and nose warrant immediate attention because they unite quickly, with fixation in 7 to 10 days. Nasal trauma frequently requires extensive surgery, so the pediatrician should request immediate consultation with a surgeon with expertise in nasal surgery. While waiting, the pediatrician should provide an oral airway to relieve respiratory distress. Often the surgeon can grasp the traumatized nose and elevate and re-mold it manually, relieving the respiratory distress. Fractures of the septal cartilage also may be reduced by simple manual remolding, but most are associated with hematomas that should be promptly incised and drained. The surgeon can visualize the deformity with an infant nasal speculum, place a septal elevator in the nose, and guide the septal cartilage into the vomerine groove; an audible and palpable click indicates return of the septum into position.[60]

Early reduction and immobilization also are advised for a displaced fracture of the mandible because rapid, firm union may occur as early as 10 to 14 days. Generally, adequate alignment can be achieved with an acrylic mandibular splint and circum-mandibular wires, which are maintained in place for 3 weeks. In more severe cases with canting of the mandibular alveolar ridge, perialveolar wires below the infraorbital rims have been used with excellent results. This procedure can prevent canted occlusion and possible facial asymmetry as the child grows, thus avoiding later extensive and costly reconstructive surgery.[50]

PROGNOSIS. If the fracture is reduced and fixated within a few days, rapid healing without complication is the usual course. If treatment is inadequate, missed, or delayed, subsequent developmental deformities are common. Ankylosis of the mandible in the second year of life is thought to result from birth trauma to the temporomandibular joint. A young child has been described with unilateral mandibular hypoplasia, which was thought to have resulted from fibrous ankylosis caused by perinatal trauma to the condylar cartilage of the ipsilateral temporomandibular joint.[7] Other deformities may not become apparent until adolescence or young adulthood.

EYES

(See also Chapter 51.)

Mechanical trauma to various regions of the neonatal eye usually occurs during abnormal presentation, in dystocia from cephalopelvic disproportion, or as a result of inappropriate forceps placement in normal deliveries. Most of the injuries are self-limited and mild and require no specific treatment.

Eyelids

Edema, suffusion, and ecchymoses of the eyelids are common, especially after face and brow presentations or forceps deliveries. Severely swollen lids should be forced open by an ophthalmologist for examination of the eyeball; retractors may be necessary. These findings usually resolve within a week without treatment, although an infant has been reported with totally everted upper eyelids that required suturing for 4 days before they would remain in the normal position.[51] Some believe that these injuries represent a possible cause of congenital ptosis.

A less common injury is laceration, including disruption of the lacrimal canaliculus. This has been associated with multiple upper-eyelid lacerations, including a full-thickness vertical wound lateral to the punctum and a full-thickness laceration through the lower eyelid with transection of the canaliculus after a low forceps delivery. Microsurgical repair of the lacrimal system and eyelids, including lacrimal intubation with a silicone stent, has been successful. Follow-up at 14 months revealed normal tear drainage with no amblyopia or residual deformity.[28]

An infant has been reported with superficial eyelid lacerations caused by an internal fetal monitoring spiral electrode.[37] At delivery the electrode was attached to the eyelid. Marked facial edema related to brow presentation apparently obscured the lacerations until 14 hours of age, when much of the edema had resolved. Periorbital edema was believed to have protected the infant from more serious injury to the eyelid and globe.

Lagophthalmos, the inability to close an eye, is an occasional finding thought to result from facial nerve injury by forceps pressure. It usually is unilateral. The exposed cornea should be protected by an eye pad and methylcellulose drops instilled every 4 hours. The condition usually resolves within a week.

Orbit

Orbital hemorrhage and fracture may follow direct pressure by the apex of one forceps blade, most often in high forceps extractions. In most instances, death occurs immediately. Surviving infants demonstrate traumatic eyelid changes, disturbances of extraocular muscle movements, and exophthalmos. The presence of the latter two findings warrants immediate ophthalmologic consultation. Subsequent management also may require neurosurgical and plastic surgery consultations.

Sympathetic Nervous System

Horner syndrome, resulting from cervical sympathetic nerve trauma, frequently accompanies lower brachial plexus injury (see later in this chapter). The syndrome consists of miosis, partial ptosis, slight enophthalmos, and anhidrosis of the ipsilateral side of the face. Although small, the pupil reacts to light. The presence of neurologic signs indicating brachial plexus injury helps distinguish this syndrome from intracranial hemorrhage as a cause of anisocoria. Pigmentation of the ipsilateral iris is frequently delayed to several months of age; occasionally, pigmentation never occurs. Resolution of other signs of the syndrome depends on whether the injury to the nerve is transient or permanent.

Subconjunctival Hemorrhage

Subconjunctival hemorrhage, characterized by bright red patches on the bulbar conjunctiva, is a relatively common finding in the neonate. It may be found after a difficult delivery but often is noted after easy, completely uncomplicated deliveries. This finding is considered to result from increased venous pressure in the infant's head and neck, produced by obstruction to venous return consequent to compression of the fetal thorax or abdomen by uterine contractions during labor.[34] If the infant is otherwise well, management consists of reassuring the parents. The blood is usually absorbed within 1 to 2 weeks. As the blood pigments break down and are absorbed, the color changes from bright red to orange and yellow.

External Ocular Muscles

Injury involving the external ocular muscles may result from direct trauma to the cranial nerve (in the form of compression or surrounding hemorrhages) or from hemorrhage into the muscle sheath, with subsequent fibrosis. The sixth cranial nerve (abducens) is the most frequently injured cranial nerve because of its long intracranial course; the result is paralysis of the lateral rectus muscle. This injury may follow a tentorial laceration with extravasation of a small amount of blood around the intracranial portion of the nerve. The involvement may be mild and transient; internal strabismus noted at birth may resolve gradually within 1 to 2 months. The seventh cranial nerve may be injured simultaneously with the sixth nerve by compression with forceps. Improvement in lateral gaze of the affected eye may appear within 1 to 2 months. Alternate patching of either eye in the severely affected infant maintains visual acuity until, with time, maximum improvement has occurred. At 6 months the degree of nerve regeneration may be evaluated. Some infants subsequently require surgical repair of their strabismus.

Fourth cranial nerve (trochlear) palsy occurs infrequently. It may follow small brainstem hemorrhages with nuclear damage. The affected muscle is the superior oblique, which mainly turns the eye inferiorly and medially. This condition is difficult to identify in the newborn infant. Surgical correction may be necessary later.

Third cranial nerve (oculomotor) palsy, when complete, causes paralysis of the inferior oblique and medial, superior, and inferior rectus muscles. This results in ptosis, a dilated fixed pupil, and outward and downward deviation of the eye, with inability to adduct or elevate up and in or up and out or to depress down and out. This palsy also may occur in partial form, with or without pupillary involvement. Partial palsies may recover function spontaneously within several months, whereas complete palsies usually require surgical intervention.

Optic Nerve

The optic nerve may be injured directly by a fracture in the region of the optic canal or from a shearing force on the nerve, with resultant hemorrhage into the nerve sheath. The latter injury seldom is recognized because of the more apparent and severe changes in the sensorium. Occasionally, a fracture through the optic foramen results in formation of callus, which slowly compresses the nerve. A difficult forceps delivery is a frequent preceding event. If optic nerve injury is not diagnosed within several hours with prompt surgical intervention, irreversible damage is likely. The result is optic atrophy and blindness. This is characterized by a blue-white optic disc, in contrast to the grayish disc of the normal neonate. In primary optic atrophy (e.g., that caused by birth trauma), the disc margin is well defined and fine vessels are rarely present in the disc tissue. In secondary atrophy the disc margin is blurred; a central gray area and evidence of intraocular disease are present.

Cornea

A diffuse or streaky haziness of the cornea is relatively common. This is usually caused by edema related to the birth process but also may follow use of a silver nitrate solution more concentrated than 1%. The haziness usually disappears in 7 to 10 days. When it persists, a rupture of the Descemet membrane has probably occurred, usually because of malpositioning of forceps at delivery. The consequence of a ruptured Descemet membrane is a leukoma or diffuse white opacity of the cornea. This results from interstitial damage of the substantia propria by fluids entering through the tear in the membrane. These leukomas are often permanent and, despite patching of the contralateral eye and use of glasses, are accompanied by a high incidence of amblyopia and strabismus.

A ruptured Descemet membrane has been reported after a prolonged delivery in which low forceps were used after unsuccessful attempts at vacuum extraction.[61] Because of significant corneal astigmatism at 2 months, a gas-permeable hard contact lens was applied. Patching of the contralateral eye was continued. Assessment of visual acuity at 13 months, with the use of spatial frequency sweep visual-evoked potentials, demonstrated an excellent visual result.

Intraocular Hemorrhage

Trauma at birth may result in retinal hemorrhage, hyphema, or vitreous hemorrhage, with retinal hemorrhage the most common. The cause is most likely compression of the fetal head, resulting in venous congestion. The fetal head is compressed two to four times more forcefully than other fetal parts during the second stage of labor. Retinal hemorrhage is more common in primiparous deliveries and after forceps or vacuum extraction; it is rare after cesarean section. It may occur in normal deliveries. The most common lesion is the flame-shaped or streak hemorrhage found mainly near the disc and sparing the macula and extreme periphery; it usually disappears within 1 to 3 days (occasionally 5 days) with no residual effects. Rarely, hemorrhages may take as long as 21 days to resolve. Retinal hemorrhages may reduce the resolving power of the macula, either bilaterally to produce nystagmus or unilaterally to produce amblyopia, which may not always respond to prolonged covering of the fixing eye with improvement of the amblyopic eye.

Hyphemas and vitreous hemorrhages usually result from misplacement of forceps and often are associated with ruptures of Descemet membrane. One infant has been described in whom a hyphema developed in one eye after spontaneous delivery.[49] The hyphema usually is clear of gross blood within 5 days; during this time the infant should be handled gently and fed frequently to minimize crying and agitation. If blood persists or secondary hemorrhage occurs, systemic administration of acetazolamide (Diamox) and surgical removal of blood may be necessary.

Vitreous hemorrhage is manifested by large vitreous floaters, blood pigment seen with the slit lamp, and an absent red reflex. The prognosis is guarded; if resolution does not occur in 6 to 12 months, surgical correction should be considered.

EARS

The proximity of ears to the site of application of forceps makes them susceptible to injury at birth. Most of the injuries are mild and self-limited, but serious injuries may occur because of slipping or misplacement of forceps (Fig. 27–9).

Abrasions and Ecchymoses

Abrasions must be cleansed gently to minimize the risk of secondary infection. Ecchymoses, if extensive and involving other areas of the body, may result in hyperbilirubinemia.

Hematomas

Hematomas of the external ear, if not treated promptly, liquefy slowly, followed by early organization and development of cauliflower ear. Wide incision and evacuation of the hematoma may be indicated.

Lacerations

Lacerations of the auricle may be repaired by the pediatrician if they are superficial and involve only

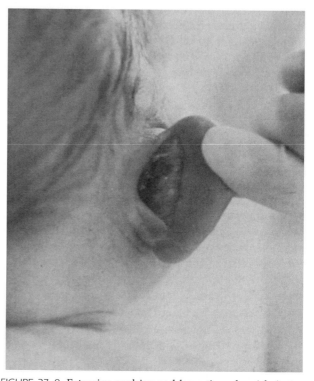

FIGURE 27–9. Extensive avulsion and laceration of auricle in term infant, resulting from forceful traction of misplaced forceps. (Courtesy of Dr. Bhagya Puppala, Lutheran General Children's Hospital, Park Ridge, Ill.)

skin. After thorough cleansing and draping, the wound edges are sutured with interrupted 6-0 or 7-0 nylon sutures, with exact edge-to-edge approximation. If the laceration involves cartilage, surgical consultation should be obtained because of the tendency toward postoperative perichondritis, which is refractory to treatment and leads to subsequent deformities. A sterile field and more meticulous presurgical preparation are essential. A contour pressure dressing is applied postoperatively.

VOCAL CORD PARALYSIS

Unilateral or bilateral paralysis of the vocal cords is uncommon in the neonate.

ETIOLOGY. Unilateral paralysis may be a consequence of excessive traction on the head during a breech delivery or lateral traction with forceps in a cephalic presentation. The recurrent laryngeal branch of the vagus nerve in the neck is injured. The left side is involved more often because of this nerve's lower origin and longer course in the neck. Bilateral paralysis may be caused by peripheral trauma involving both recurrent laryngeal nerves, but more frequently it is caused by a CNS insult such as hypoxia or hemorrhage involving the brainstem.

CLINICAL MANIFESTATIONS. An infant with a unilateral paralysis may be completely free of symptoms when resting quietly, but crying is usually accompanied by hoarseness and mild inspiratory stridor. When associated with difficulty in feeding and clearing secretions, concurrent involvement of the 12th (hypoglossal) cranial nerve should be suspected, particularly if the tongue on the ipsilateral side does not protrude and demonstrates fasciculations. Hypoglossal paralysis also has been described in association with ipsilateral upper brachial plexus injury.[25] Affected infants demonstrate difficulty in sucking, with swelling and immobility of the affected side of the tongue. This 12th cranial neuropathy can be confirmed by concentric needle electromyography of the tongue.[23] Bilateral paralysis results in more severe respiratory symptoms. At birth the infant may have difficulty in establishing and maintaining spontaneous respiration; later, dyspnea, retractions, stridor, cyanosis, or aphonia may develop.

DIFFERENTIAL DIAGNOSIS. Unilateral paralysis of the vocal cords must be distinguished from congenital laryngeal malformations that produce neonatal stridor. A history of difficult delivery, especially involving excessive traction on the fetus, may suggest laryngeal paralysis; previously the diagnosis was confirmed only by direct laryngoscopic examination. The availability of the flexible fiberoptic laryngoscope at the bedside has facilitated earlier diagnosis without disrupting the infant's environment. Serial examinations to monitor progress also can be conducted with ease because the infant need not be transported to the operating room.

Bilateral paralysis also must be distinguished from a number of causes of respiratory distress in the neonate (see Chapter 42, Part Five); stridor should suggest the larynx as the site of disturbance. Direct or flexible fiberoptic laryngoscopy is necessary to establish the diagnosis.

TREATMENT. Infants with unilateral paralysis should be observed closely until there is evidence of improvement. Gentle handling and frequent small feedings will aid in keeping the infant quiet and minimizing the risk of aspiration. Bilateral paralysis necessitates immediate tracheal intubation to establish an airway. Tracheostomy is required subsequently in most patients. Laryngoscopic examinations then should be performed at intervals to look for evidence of return of vocal cord function; early extubation may be attempted if complete return occurs within a short time.

PROGNOSIS. Unilateral paralysis usually resolves rapidly without treatment, and complete resolution occurs within 4 to 6 weeks. Birth injury–induced glossolaryngeal paralysis or paresis should resolve spontaneously by 6 months of age.[23] Recognition of this subtle condition is important for two reasons. First, its self-limited course is encouraging, thus avoiding needless alarm in the parents with concern about more ominous conditions such as Werdnig-Hoffmann disease. Second, unnecessary invasive and aggressive procedures can be avoided.

The prognosis for bilateral paralysis is more variable. If untreated, a funnel deformity may develop in the lower sternal area; this may appear as early as the 15th day of life. After tracheostomy a decrease in the severity of the deformity may occur within several weeks. Some of the affected infants subsequently regain normally shaped chests; others may have residual fixed depressions, occasionally severe enough to require surgical correction. The recovery of vocal cord function varies in time and degree. Some infants may show partial recovery within a few months, with several years elapsing before complete movement of the cords is restored. Other infants who have been followed for years show no improvement. Bilateral paralysis of central origin may improve completely if it is caused by cerebral edema or hemorrhage that rapidly resolves.

INJURIES TO THE NECK AND SHOULDER GIRDLE

FRACTURE OF THE CLAVICLE

(See also Chapter 52.)

The clavicle is the most frequently fractured bone during labor and delivery. Most clavicular fractures are of the greenstick type, but occasionally the fracture is complete.

ETIOLOGY. The major causes of clavicular fractures are difficult delivery of the shoulders in vertex presentations and extended arms in breech deliveries. Vigorous, forceful manipulation of the arm and shoulder usually has occurred. However, fracture of the clavicle may also occur in infants after apparently normal labor and delivery.[33, 46] It has been suggested that some fetuses may be more vulnerable to spontaneous birth trauma secondary to forces of labor, maternal pelvic anatomy, and in utero fetal position.[46]

CLINICAL MANIFESTATIONS. Most often a greenstick fracture is not associated with any signs or symptoms but is first detected after the appearance of an obvious callus at 7 to 10 days of life. Thus the majority of neonatal clavicular fractures will be diagnosed at discharge or at the first follow-up visit.[32] Complete fractures and some greenstick fractures may be apparent shortly after birth; movement of the arm on the affected side is decreased or absent. Deformity and, occasionally, discoloration may be visible over the fracture site with obliteration of the adjacent supraclavicular depression as a result of sternocleidomastoid muscle spasm. Passive movement of the arm elicits cries of pain from the infant. Palpation reveals tenderness, crepitus, and irregularity along the clavicle. Moro reflex on the involved side is characteristically absent. Radiographs confirm the diagnosis of fracture.

DIFFERENTIAL DIAGNOSIS. A similar clinical picture of impaired movement of an arm with an absent Moro reflex may follow fracture of the humerus or brachial palsy. The fracture is confirmed by radiographs; palsy is accompanied by additional clinical findings.

TREATMENT. Therapy is directed toward minimizing the infant's pain. The affected arm and shoulder should be immobilized with the arm abducted more than 60 degrees and the elbow flexed more than 90 degrees. A callus forms, and pain usually subsides by 7 to 10 days, when immobilization may be discontinued.

PROGNOSIS. Prognosis is excellent, with growth resulting in restoration of normal bone contour after several months.

FRACTURE OF RIBS

Rib fractures related to labor and delivery are exceedingly rare, with a total of seven reported cases since 1977.[41]

ETIOLOGY. Risk factors are similar to those related to fracture of the clavicle, including macrosomia, a primigravida mother, shoulder dystocia, and delivery by midforceps or vacuum extraction.

CLINICAL MANIFESTATIONS. Specific clinical manifestations are often absent, making diagnosis difficult, unless a chest radiograph is obtained for other reasons, including suspected clavicular fracture (Fig. 27–10), respiratory distress, or cyanosis.

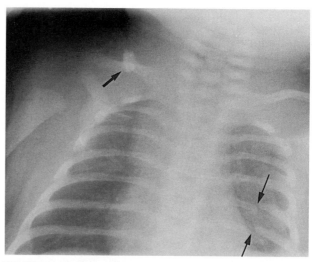

FIGURE 27–10. Chest radiograph of a 4905-gm female delivered by midforceps after right shoulder dystocia. On the 11th day, a prominent mass was noted in the right midclavicular region. Radiograph reveals a right midclavicular fracture (*thick arrow*) with slight superior angulation and incidental fractures of left fifth and sixth ribs (*thin arrows*). (From Mangurten HH, et al: Incidental rib fractures in a neonate. Neonat Intensive Care 12:15, 1999.)

MECHANISM OF INJURY. This injury is initiated when the anterior shoulder is impacted behind the symphysis pubis, with the other shoulder attempting to descend into the posterior compartment of the pelvis (Fig. 27–11). This results in compression forces on the fetal arms and thorax, leading to spontaneous rib fractures on the same side as the posterior shoulder (Fig. 27–12).

TREATMENT. No specific treatment is required. However, it is extremely important to document this injury immediately after birth to avoid later unwarranted

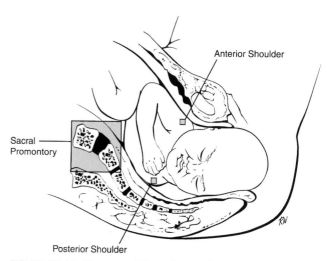

FIGURE 27–11. Diagram of fetus during delivery, illustrating impaction of anterior shoulder (*right*) behind the symphysis pubis, with left shoulder attempting to descend into posterior compartment of the pelvis. (From Mangurten HH, et al: Incidental rib fractures in a neonate. Neonat Intensive Care 12:15, 1999.)

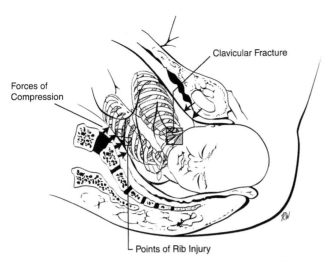

FIGURE 27–12. Diagram of fetus, illustrating compression forces on the fetal arms and thorax, which results in spontaneous fractures of right clavicle and left fifth and sixth ribs. (From Mangurten HH, et al: Incidental rib fractures in a neonate. Neonat Intensive Care 12:15, 1999.)

accusation of parents or other caretakers for suspicion of child abuse.

PROGNOSIS. Prognosis is excellent, with spontaneous healing within several months.

BRACHIAL PALSY

(See also Chapters 38 and 52.)

Brachial palsy is a paralysis involving the muscles of the upper extremity that follows mechanical trauma to the spinal roots of the fifth cervical through the first thoracic nerves (the brachial plexus) during birth. Three main forms occur, depending on the site of injury: (1) Duchenne-Erb, or upper arm, paralysis, which results from injury of the fifth and sixth cervical roots and is by far the most common; (2) Klumpke, or lower arm, paralysis, which results from injury of the eighth cervical and first thoracic roots and is extremely rare; and (3) paralysis of the entire arm, which occurs slightly more often than the Klumpke type.

ETIOLOGY. Most cases of brachial palsy follow a prolonged and difficult labor culminating in a traumatic delivery. The affected infant is frequently large, relaxed, and asphyxiated and thereby vulnerable to excessive separation of bony segments, overstretching, and injury to soft tissues. Injury of the fifth and sixth cervical roots may follow a breech presentation with the arms extended over the head; excessive traction on the shoulder in the delivery of the head may result in stretching of the plexus. The same injury may follow lateral traction of the head and neck away from one of the shoulders during an attempt to deliver the shoulders in a vertex presentation. More vigorous traction of the same nature will result in paralysis of the entire arm. The mechanism for iso-

lated lower arm paralysis is uncertain; it is thought to result from stretching of lower plexus nerves under and against the coracoid process of the scapula during forceful elevation and abduction of the arm. Excessive traction on the trunk during a breech delivery may result in avulsion of the lower roots from the cervical cord. In most patients the nerve sheath is torn and the nerve fibers are compressed by the resultant hemorrhage and edema. Less often the nerves are completely ruptured and the ends severed, or the roots are avulsed from the spinal cord with injury to the spinal gray matter.

An increasing number of reports have described "no shoulder" brachial plexus palsy unrelated to excessive traction during delivery.[21, 46] Some authorities have suggested an intrauterine insult *preceding* labor, such as compression by uterine tumors or maternal pelvic bony prominences.[21]

CLINICAL MANIFESTATIONS. The infant with upper arm paralysis holds the affected arm in a characteristic position, reflecting involvement of the shoulder abductors and external rotators, forearm flexors and supinators, and wrist extensors. The arm is adducted and internally rotated, with extension at the elbow, pronation of the forearm, and flexion of the wrist. When the arm is passively abducted, it falls limply to the side of the body. Moro, biceps, and radial reflexes are absent on the affected side. There may be some sensory deficit on the radial aspect of the arm, but this is difficult to evaluate in the neonate. The grasp reflex is intact. Any signs of respiratory distress may indicate an accompanying ipsilateral phrenic nerve root injury (see following section).

Lower arm paralysis involves the intrinsic muscles of the hand and the long flexors of the wrist and fingers. The hand is paralyzed, and voluntary movements of the wrist cannot be made. The grasp reflex is absent; the deep tendon reflexes are intact. Sensory impairment may be demonstrated along the ulnar side of the forearm and hand. Frequently, dependent edema and cyanosis of the hand and trophic changes in the fingernails develop. After some time there may be flattening and atrophy of the intrinsic hand muscles. Usually an ipsilateral Horner syndrome (ptosis, miosis, and enophthalmos) also is present because of injury involving the cervical sympathetic fibers of the first thoracic root. Often this is associated with delayed pigmentation of the iris, sometimes of more than 1 year's duration.

When the entire arm is paralyzed, it is usually completely motionless, flaccid, and powerless, hanging limply to the side. All reflexes are absent. The sensory deficit may extend almost to the shoulder.

DIFFERENTIAL DIAGNOSIS. The presence of a flail arm in a neonate may be caused by cerebral injury or by a number of injuries about the shoulder. Cerebral injury is usually associated with other manifestations of CNS injury. A careful radiographic study of the shoulder, including an examination of the lower cervical spine, clavicle, and upper humerus, should be made to exclude tearing of the joint capsule, fracture of the clavicle, and fracture, dislocation, or upper epiphyseal detachment of the humerus. Posterior dislocation of the humeral head may be difficult to identify with standard radiographs. Torode and Donnan have used CT scans to demonstrate that posterior dislocation is more common than previously believed.[63] Hunter and coworkers[30] reported an infant in whom a posterior dislocation was uncertain with standard radiographs. Ultrasound clearly revealed a posterior dislocation. Because posterior dislocation will complicate resolution of the palsy, ultrasound evaluation should be considered early in the management of these infants.

TREATMENT. The basic principle of treatment historically has been conservative, with initial emphasis on prevention of contractures while awaiting recovery of

the brachial plexus. This approach has recently been replaced by a more comprehensive program that combines initial conservative management with closer follow-up and earlier decision regarding surgical intervention. This new approach is best represented by the care plan developed by Shenaq and colleagues (Fig. 27–13).[59]

This approach is initiated with a thorough and complete physical examination that includes careful palpation of the sternocleidomastoid muscle for contracture or pseudotumor; inspection for fractures of the clavicle, humerus, or ribs; observation for abdominal asymmetry, which could indicate paralysis of the hemidiaphragm; and assessment for ocular asymmetry, which may indicate associated Horner syndrome.

Ancillary investigations, including computed tomography or myelography and magnetic resonance imaging, could be helpful in detecting possible avul-

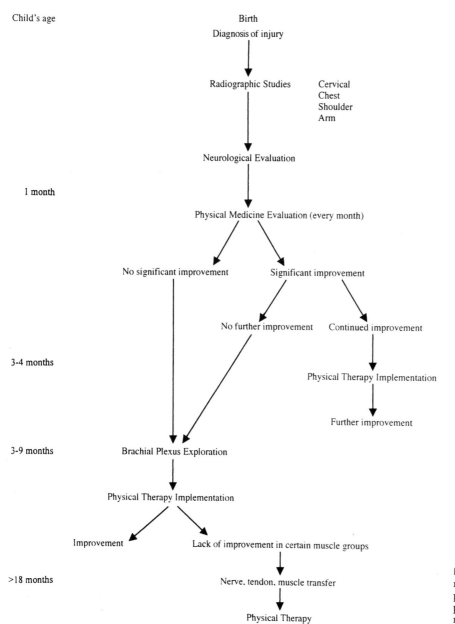

FIGURE 27–13. Treatment protocol for management of obstetric brachial plexus palsy. (From Shenaq SM, et al: Brachial plexus birth injuries and current management. Clin Plast Surg 25:527, 1998.)

sions. Electromyography has been unreliable in predicting extent of damage.

Some infants may demonstrate discomfort because of a painful traumatic neuritis affecting the brachial plexus. If no discomfort is apparent and other lesions as noted earlier are ruled out, early passive range of motion exercises, particularly involving the elbow and wrist, should be instituted. Because of shorter nursery stays, the mother should receive early demonstration and written instructions describing these exercises. She should then begin to work with the infant under the guidance of the therapy staff. Exercises include shoulder rotation, elbow flexion and extension, wrist flexion and extension, finger flexion and extension, and thumb abduction, adduction, and opposition. The infant should be re-evaluated every month. If improvement in deltoid, biceps, and triceps function has not occurred by the third month of life, functional outcome without surgery is unlikely. Consequently, a decision for surgery should be made by the end of the third month, followed by primary brachial plexus exploration during the fourth month.

Initial surgical intervention beyond 12 months of age at the level of the cervical root alone has resulted in disappointing outcomes. However, more recently infants referred at this age have been offered a combined cervical root and infraclavicular exploration with neurolysis, graph reconstruction, and nerve transfer of appropriate elements in both anatomic compartments, with evidence of improving outcomes.

The initial surgical therapy may include a team of neurosurgeons, plastic surgeons, and physiatrists who collaborate in the exploration, evaluation, and repair of the injury. This aggressive approach has resulted in up to 90% of patients demonstrating useful function of muscle groups above the elbow. Function below the elbow has resulted in 50% to 70% recovery due to the increased distance required for nerve regeneration.

PROGNOSIS. Continued close follow-up includes serial evaluation of shoulder, elbow, forearm, wrist, finger, and thumb function. Based on the child's progress over time, a decision is made regarding further treatment. Physical therapy is continued until there is no further progress or the deficit is debilitating. For the infant who continues to demonstrate lack of improvement in certain muscle groups, secondary surgical reconstruction is available, with a variety of options dependent on the individual deficit. In summary, the infant who does not improve spontaneously now has increased hope for recovery due to recent advances in microsurgery and nerve-transfer techniques.

Although the majority (93% to 95%) of infants achieve return of function with conservative management, the remainder with persistent deficits may go on to develop long-term severe handicaps of the affected extremity. Early treatment offers significant improvement for approximately 90% of these children. Later treatment reduces this number to 50% to 70%. To avoid missing the window of opportunity for time-

lier and more successful treatment, infants with brachial plexus palsy should be referred to centers that have an established comprehensive program for the broad spectrum of infants with this condition.

PHRENIC NERVE PARALYSIS

(See also Chapter 42, Part Five.)

Phrenic nerve paralysis results in diaphragmatic paralysis and rarely occurs as an isolated injury in the neonate. Most injuries are unilateral and are associated with an ipsilateral upper brachial plexus palsy.

ETIOLOGY. The most common cause is a difficult breech delivery. Lateral hyperextension of the neck results in overstretching or avulsion of the third, fourth, and fifth cervical roots, which supply the phrenic nerve.

CLINICAL MANIFESTATIONS. The first sign may be recurrent episodes of cyanosis, usually accompanied by irregular and labored respirations. The respiratory excursions of the involved side of the diaphragm are largely ineffectual, and the breathing is therefore almost completely thoracic, so that no bulging of the abdomen occurs with inspiration (Fig. 27–14A, B). The thrust of the diaphragm, which often may be felt just under the costal margin on the normal side, is absent on the affected side. Dullness to percussion and diminished breath sounds are found over the affected side. In a severe injury, tachypnea, weak cry, and apneic spells may occur.

RADIOGRAPHIC MANIFESTATIONS. Radiographs taken during the first few days may show only slight elevation of the affected diaphragm, occasionally so subtle that it may be considered normal. Additional films will show the more apparent elevation of the diaphragm, with displacement of the heart and mediastinum to the opposite side (see Fig. 27–14C). Frequently, areas of atelectasis appear bilaterally. Early diagnosis can be confirmed by real-time ultrasonographic examination of the diaphragm, which reveals abnormal motion of the affected hemidiaphragm. This procedure provides the added advantage of availability at the bedside. Fluoroscopy should be reserved for the equivocal case. In still questionable cases, diagnosis can be further enhanced by transvenous electrical stimulation of the phrenic nerve.

DIFFERENTIAL DIAGNOSIS. Careful physical examination should allow differentiation between CNS, cardiac, and pulmonary causes of neonatal respiratory distress. The diagnosis can be confirmed by fluoroscopy and electrical stimulation of the phrenic nerve.

TREATMENT. Most infants require only nonspecific medical treatment. The infant should be positioned on the involved side, and oxygen should be administered for cyanosis or hypoxemia. Intravenous fluids may be necessary for the first few days. If the infant begins to show improvement, progressive oral or ga-

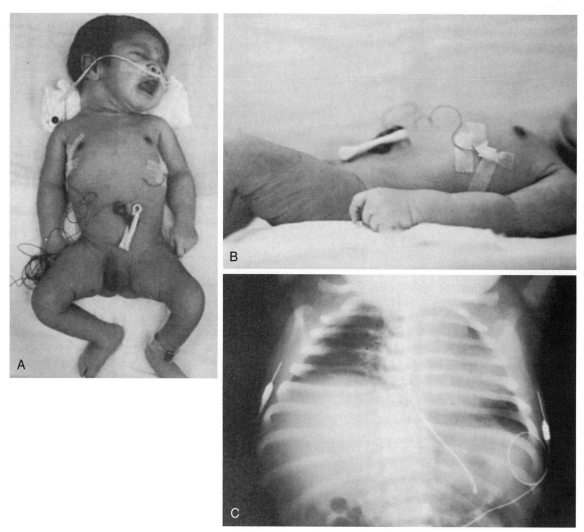

FIGURE 27–14. *A*, Nine-hour-old 3190-gm female infant born after difficult total breech extraction; during delivery, cervix clamped down on head, necessitating extensive tugging and pulling on both arms. Note markedly hyperexpanded chest and classic appearance of both upper extremities in Erb palsy positions. *B*, Lateral view of same infant, demonstrating increased anterior-posterior diameter of chest and close-up view of left upper extremity adducted at shoulder, extended at elbow, and pronated and flexed at wrist. *C*, Significant elevation of right hemidiaphragm to level of fifth thoracic vertebra in same infant, compatible with paralysis of right hemidiaphragm. Note significant shifting of heart and mediastinum to the left.

vage feedings may be started. Antibiotics are indicated if pneumonia occurs.

Infants with more severe respiratory distress, particularly those with bilateral phrenic nerve palsy, may require assisted ventilation shortly after delivery. de Vries Reilingh and associates[17] have reviewed their experience with 23 infants who incurred phrenic nerve injury as neonates. Infants who had not recovered diaphragmatic function after 30 days of conservative treatment did not demonstrate spontaneous recovery thereafter. Accordingly, these investigators recommend limiting conservative treatment to 1 month, assuming the infant is adequately oxygenated with conventional techniques. The absence of definite improvement after 1 month is considered evidence of disruption of the phrenic nerve, thereby minimizing chances of complete spontaneous recovery. Infants in this category should be considered candidates for plication of the diaphragm early in the second month of life.

PROGNOSIS. Many infants recover spontaneously. If avulsion of the cervical nerves has occurred, spontaneous recovery is not possible, and in the absence of surgery the infant is susceptible to pneumonia in the atelectatic lung. Infants treated surgically do well, with no recurrence of pneumonia and no late pulmonary or chest wall complications.

INJURY TO THE STERNOCLEIDOMASTOID MUSCLE

Injury to the sternocleidomastoid muscle is designated muscular torticollis, congenital torticollis, or sternocleidomastoid fibroma. Its cause and pathologic features have been controversial.

ETIOLOGY. The birth trauma theory suggests that the muscle or fascial sheath is ruptured during a breech or difficult delivery involving hyperextension of the muscle. A hematoma develops and is subsequently invaded by fibrin and fibroblasts with progressive formation of scar tissue and shortening of the muscle. The intrauterine theory postulates abnormal pressure, position, or trauma to the muscle during intrauterine life. Another theory suggests a hereditary defect in the development of the muscle. Others have noted pathologic findings resembling infectious myositis, suggesting an infection in utero or a muscle injured at delivery. Davids and coworkers,[15] using magnetic resonance imaging in visualizing live infants and cadaver dissections and injection studies, suggest that congenital muscular torticollis results from intrauterine or perinatal compartment syndrome. According to this investigation, the sternocleidomastoid muscle compartment, defined by the external investing fascia of the neck, contains only the sternocleidomastoid muscle. In utero or intrapartum positioning of the head and neck in forward flexion, lateral bending, and rotation can result in the ipsilateral sternocleidomastoid muscle kinking on itself. If the kinking continues for a prolonged period in utero, an ischemic injury at the site could develop, followed by subsequent edema and development of a compartment syndrome. Therefore, the mechanism of injury is localized kinking or crush, in contrast to the previously suspected mechanism of stretching or tearing (Fig. 27–15).

CLINICAL MANIFESTATIONS. A mass in the midportion of the sternocleidomastoid muscle may be evident at birth, although usually it is first noted 10 to 14 days after birth. It is 1 to 2 cm in diameter, hard, immobile, fusiform, and well circumscribed; there is no inflammation or overlying discoloration. The mass enlarges during the following 2 to 4 weeks and then gradually regresses and disappears by age 5 to 8 months.

A transient torticollis produced by contracture of the involved muscle appears soon after birth. The head tilts toward the involved side, and the chin is somewhat elevated and rotated toward the opposite shoulder. The head cannot be moved passively into normal position. If the deformity persists beyond 3 or 4 years, the skull becomes foreshortened. Flattening of the frontal bone and bulging of the occipital bone occur on the involved side, whereas the contralateral frontal bone bulges and the occiput is flattened. The ipsilateral eyebrow is slanted; the clavicle and shoulder become elevated compared with the opposite normal side, and the ipsilateral mastoid process becomes more prominent. If treatment is not instituted, a lower cervical, upper thoracic scoliosis subsequently develops. Rarely, calcification develops in the affected muscles.

DIFFERENTIAL DIAGNOSIS. Careful radiographic examination should be made of the cervical spine and shoulders to rule out Sprengel deformity or the Klippel-Feil syndrome, cervical myelodysplasia, and occipitalization of the atlas. In clinically equivocal cases, CT scans may differentiate classic muscular torticollis from other cervical soft tissue lesions that may cause torticollis (e.g., hemangioma, lymphangioma, and teratoma).

TREATMENT. Treatment should be instituted as early as possible. The involved muscle should be stretched to an overcorrected position by gentle, even, and persistent motion with the infant supine. The head is flexed forward and away from the affected side, and the chin is rotated toward the affected side. The mother can be instructed to repeat this maneuver

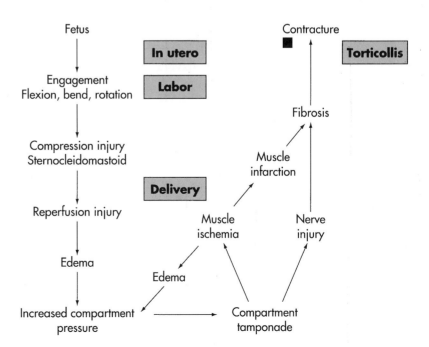

FIGURE 27–15. Algorithm illustrating the Davids study,[15] suggesting that congenital muscular torticollis results from intrauterine or perinatal compartment syndrome.

several times a day. The infant also should be stimulated to turn the head spontaneously toward the affected side; the crib may be positioned so that the infant must turn to the desired position of overcorrection in looking for window light or at a mobile or favorite rattle. During sleep the infant should be placed on the side of the torticollis; in this position, sandbags should be placed on each side of the infant's body for fixation. An alternative approach involves a helmet that is custom made for the infant. Rubber straps made of surgical drain tubing attached to the helmet are in turn fixed to the side rails of the crib at night, with appropriate adjustments made to force the infant to sleep on the prominent side of the head. This results in stretching of the shortened sternocleidomastoid muscle.

Conservative therapy should be continued for 6 months. If the deformity has not been fully corrected, surgery should be considered to prevent permanent skull and cervical spine deformities. Ultrasonography may be useful in defining the quantity of normal muscle remnant surrounding the lesion, thereby helping to determine whether the infant requires no treatment at all, conservative stretching, or surgery.[10]

Procedures that have been used include distal tenotomy, muscle lengthening, and excision of the affected muscle. All are followed by some problems. After tenotomy, contractures may recur. Lengthening is difficult because of imprecision in estimating how much elongation will be adequate for subsequent growth. Complete excision will deform the outline of the neck. Akazawa and associates[1] reported favorable results after partial resection. This was followed postoperatively with massive cotton bandaging of the neck in the neutral position for 3 weeks. Plaster casts, a brace, and physical therapy were not used. They recommend the period between 1 and 5 years of age as the optimum for surgery.

PROGNOSIS. Most infants treated conservatively show complete recovery within 2 to 3 months. If surgery is necessary and if it is performed early, the facial asymmetry will disappear almost entirely. Infants treated before their first birthday have a better outcome than those treated later, regardless of the type of treatment. Nonsurgical treatment after 1 year is rarely successful.

INJURIES TO THE SPINE AND SPINAL CORD

Birth injuries to the vertebral spine and spinal cord are rarely diagnosed. It is not certain whether the low incidence is real, reflecting improved obstetric techniques, or represents a tendency for postmortem examination to overlook spine and spinal cord lesions.

ETIOLOGY. These injuries almost always result from breech deliveries,[8] especially difficult ones in which version and extraction were used. Other predisposing factors include brow and face presentations, dystocia

(especially shoulder), prematurity, primiparity, and precipitous delivery.

The injuries are usually caused by stretching of the cord. However, Hankins[27] reported an infant with lower thoracic spinal cord injury following application of maternal fundal pressure to relieve shoulder dystocia. Magnetic resonance imaging revealed focal spinal cord swelling involving T9 through T12, thought to represent ischemia and/or infarction due to a compressive injury. The most common mechanism responsible is probably forceful longitudinal traction on the trunk while the head is still firmly engaged in the pelvis. When combined with flexion and torsion of the vertebral axis, this becomes a more significant problem. Occasionally, a snap is felt by the obstetrician while traction is exerted. Although cesarean delivery has been recommended as optimal for infants in breech presentation with a hyperextended head, Maekawa and colleagues[40] documented spinal cord injury after cesarean section. In fact, the mother had reported weak fetal movements during the third trimester, which suggests that injury was occurring before delivery. Difficulty in delivery of the shoulders in cephalic presentations may result in a similar mechanism of injury. The spinal cord is very delicate and inelastic. Its attachments are the cauda equina below and the roots of the brachial plexus and medulla above. Because the ligaments are elastic and the muscles delicate, the infant's vertebral column may be stretched easily. In addition, the dura is more elastic in the infant than in the adult. Consequently, strong longitudinal traction may be expected to cause elongation of the spinal column and to stretch the spinal cord and its membranes. The possible result is vertebral fracture or dislocation or both and cord transection. Most often, hemorrhage and edema produce a physiologic transection. The lower cervical and upper thoracic regions are most often involved, but occasionally the entire length of the spinal canal contains a heavy accumulation of blood.

CLINICAL MANIFESTATIONS. Affected infants may follow one of four clinical patterns. Those in the first group are either stillborn or in poor condition from birth, with respiratory depression, shock, and hypothermia. They deteriorate rapidly; death occurs within several hours, often before neurologic signs are obvious. These infants usually have a high cervical or brainstem lesion.

The second group consists of infants who at birth may appear normal or show signs similar to those of the first group; these infants die after several days. Cardiac function is usually relatively strong. Within hours or days the central type of respiratory depression that is initially present may be complicated by respiratory distress of pulmonary origin, usually pneumonia. The spinal lesion, usually in the upper or midcervical region, frequently is not recognized for several days, when flaccidity and immobility of the legs are noted. Occasionally, urinary retention may be the first symptom. Paralysis of the abdominal wall is manifested by a relaxation of the abdominal wall and bulging at the flanks when the infant is held upright. The intercostal muscles may be affected if the lesion is high enough. Sensation is absent over the lower half of the body. Deep tendon reflexes and spontaneous reflex movements are absent. The infant is constipated. The brachial plexus is involved in approximately 20% of all cases. The spinal column is usually clinically and radiographically normal.

The third group, with lesions at the seventh cervical to first thoracic vertebra or lower, comprises infants who survive for long periods, some for years. Paraplegia noted at birth may be transient. The lesion in the cord may be mild and reversible, or it may result in permanent neurologic sequelae with no return of function in the lower cord segments. The skin over the involved part of the body is dry and scaly, predisposing the infant to bedsores and ulcers. Muscle atrophy, severe contractures, and bony deformities follow. Bladder distention and constant dribbling persist, and recurring urinary tract infections and pneumonia are common. Within several weeks or months this clinical picture is replaced by a stage of reflex activity, or paraplegia-in-flexion. This is characterized by return of tone and rigid flexion of the involved extremities, improvement in skin condition with healing of decubiti, and periodic mass reflex responses consisting of tonic spasms of the extremities, spontaneous micturition, and profuse sweating over the involved part of the body.

Infants in the fourth group have subtle neurologic signs of spasticity thought to represent cerebral palsy. These patients have experienced partial spinal cord injuries and occasional cerebrovascular accidents.

DIFFERENTIAL DIAGNOSIS. During the first few weeks of life injuries to the spinal cord may be confused with amyotonia congenita or myelodysplasia associated with spina bifida occulta[53] (see also Chapter 38). The former may be differentiated by the generalized distribution of the weakness and hypotonia and by the presence of normal sensation and sphincter control. The latter is usually associated with some cutaneous lesions over the sacral region such as dimples, angiomas, or abnormal tufts of hair; it is always associated with defects in the spinal lamina. Other conditions less often considered include transverse myelitis and spinal cord tumors, particularly in infants who demonstrate paralysis after an apparently normal labor and delivery. Cerebral hypotonia should be considered in infants who also demonstrate cranial nerve abnormalities, persistent primitive reflexes, and a dull facial appearance, contrasting to the bright, alert facies of the infant with spinal cord trauma. However, the concomitant occurrence of cerebral damage in an infant with spinal cord injury may confound the diagnosis. A final consideration is the infant with bilateral brachial plexus palsy with associated motor and sensory loss, or Horner syndrome; the demonstration of normal lower extremity function should rule out spinal cord injury.

Although somatosensory-evoked potential has been used in establishing a diagnosis of spinal cord injury,[5] cervical responses are generally small and can be difficult to detect even in clinically normal infants; in addition, scalp potentials overlying the somatosensory cortex may be absent in normal term neonates.[36] Ultrasonography has been used to evaluate severe spinal cord injury in neonates.[3] The procedure is easily performed at the bedside with no disturbance of the patient. Initial cord edema, hematomyelia, and hemorrhage outside the cord can be assessed. Magnetic resonance imaging is the only procedure that provides a direct image of the spinal cord and clearly is the most reliable modality available to evaluate presumptive cervical spinal cord injury in the infant.[36] Previous limitations of ferromagnetic ventilators and monitors can now be circumvented by manual ventilation combined with nonferromagnetic monitors. Another option is the use of a nonferromagnetic ventilator.

TREATMENT. Treatment is supportive and usually unsatisfactory. The infant affected at birth requires basic resuscitative and supportive measures. Infants who survive present a therapeutic challenge that can be met only by the combined and interested efforts of the pediatrician, neurologist, neurosurgeon, urologist, psychiatrist, orthopedist, nurse, physical therapist, and occupational therapist.

While the infant is reasonably stable, cervical and thoracic spine radiographs should be obtained. In the rare occurrence of vertebral fracture or dislocation or both, immediate neurosurgical consultation is necessary for reduction of the deformity and relief of cord compression, followed by appropriate immobilization. Lumbar puncture in the acute period is of little practical value and may aggravate existing cord damage if the infant is excessively manipulated during the procedure. After several days, however, a persistent spinal fluid block may be demonstrated and may be an indication for exploratory laminectomy at the site of trauma. This possibility should be suspected in an infant with partial paraplegia and normal radiographs.

Prompt and meticulous attention must be given to skin, bladder, and bowel care. The position of paralyzed parts should be changed every 2 hours. Areas of anesthetic skin should be washed, dried, and gently massaged daily. Lamb's-wool covers are helpful in preventing pressure necrosis of skin. Benzoin tincture applications help protect the skin in pressure areas. A decubitus ulcer is treated by scrupulous cleansing and complete freedom from weight bearing and friction. An indwelling urethral catheter should be inserted within several hours after severe cord trauma at any level. In the smaller infant a size 3 feeding tube may be used. However, in the term infant a size 5 feeding tube can usually be inserted. Repeated instrumentation should be avoided. Cultures of urine should be obtained weekly and as clinically indicated. Antibiotic therapy should be used only in the presence of infection. After several weeks, the infant reaches the stage of paraplegia-in-flexion, and urinary retention usually is replaced by regular episodes of spontaneous voiding. The indwelling catheter may then be removed, and postvoid bladder residuals should be measured. A renal sonogram and a conventional fluoroscopically guided voiding cystourethrogram should be obtained. If there are large postvoid residuals (more than 10 to 15 mL), or if there is an abnormal renal sonogram or cystogram, urodynamic studies may be necessary. A high-pressure neurogenic bladder is treated with an anticholinergic agent such as oxybutynin chloride, 0.5 to 2.0 mg/kg per day in three or four divided doses, concurrently with clean intermittent bladder catheterization every 3 to 4 hours. Treatment of the low-pressure neurogenic bladder requires only clean intermittent catheterization.

The first infection should be treated with the appropriate antibiotic for 2 weeks. After the neonatal period this should be followed by suppressive therapy. During the first 2 months of life, this may include amoxicillin, 20 mg/kg PO in one daily dose, or ampicillin, 50 mg/kg IV daily. After 2 months, any of the following options is appropriate: trimethoprim and sulfamethoxazole (Bactrim, Septra), 2 mg/kg per day in one daily dose; nitrofurantoin (Furadantin), 1.5 to 2 mg/kg in one daily dose; or cefprozil, 15 mg/kg in one daily dose. This therapy should be continued for 6 to 12 months or longer, depending on the reversibility of the lesion. Cultures of urine should be obtained at 1 week, monthly for 3 months, and then every 3 months for 1 year or until recovery.

Fecal retention also is a common problem, especially after total cord transection. Appropriate dietary balance should aid in keeping the stools soft. Early use of glycerin suppositories at regular intervals will encourage automatic defecation. Digital manipulation may be necessary to relieve fecal impaction.

Finally, physical rehabilitation should be instituted early in an attempt to minimize deformity. After several years, orthopedic procedures may still be necessary to correct contractures and bony deformities.

PROGNOSIS. The prognosis varies with the severity of the injury. Most severe injuries result in death shortly after birth. Infants with cord compression from vertebral fractures or dislocations or both may recover with reasonable return of function if prompt neurosurgical removal of the compression is performed. Infants with mild injuries or partial transections may recover with minimal sequelae. Infants who exhibit complete physiologic cord transection shortly after birth without vertebral fracture or dislocation have an extremely poor outlook for recovery of function. Many die in infancy of ascending urinary tract infection and sepsis. Long-term survivors have been reported to live into their third decade. They are extremely rare, and although they may have normal intelligence and learn to walk with special appliances, these children face the late complications of pain, spasms, autonomic dysfunction, bony deformities, and genitourinary, psychiatric, and school problems.

MacKinnon and colleagues[39] have published an algorithm for predicting outcome in infants with upper cervical spinal cord injury; the algorithm is based on age at first breath and rate of recovery of breathing and limb movements in the first few weeks and months of life. For infants with rapid recovery, the prognosis was clarified by age 3 weeks. Infants who demonstrated very slow or no recovery of breathing or extremity movements by 3 months of age universally had a poor outcome. Patients with intermediate rates of recovery were thought to have an uncertain long-term prognosis at 3 months of age.

INJURIES TO INTRA-ABDOMINAL ORGANS

Although birth trauma involving intra-abdominal organs is uncommon, it frequently must be considered by the physician who cares for neonates because deterioration can be fulminant in an undetected lesion, and therapy can be very effective when a lesion is diagnosed early. Intra-abdominal trauma should be suspected in any newborn with shock and abdominal distention or pallor, anemia, and irritability without evidence of external blood loss.

RUPTURE OF THE LIVER

The liver is the most frequently injured abdominal organ during the birth process. The autopsy incidence of liver injury varies from 0.9% to 9.6%.[58]

ETIOLOGY. Birth trauma is the most significant factor contributing to liver injury. The condition usually occurs in large infants, infants with hepatomegaly (e.g., infants with erythroblastosis fetalis and infants of diabetic mothers), and infants who underwent breech delivery. Manual pressure on the liver during delivery of the head in a breech presentation is probably a typical mechanism of injury. Prematurity and postmaturity also are thought to predispose the infant to this injury. Other contributing factors include asphyxia and coagulation disorders. Trauma to the liver more often results in subcapsular hematoma than actual laceration of the liver.

CLINICAL MANIFESTATIONS. The infant usually appears normal the first 1 to 3 days, but rarely for as long as 7 days. Nonspecific signs related to loss of blood into the hematoma may appear early; they include poor feeding, listlessness, pallor, jaundice, tachypnea, and tachycardia. A mass may be palpable in the right upper quadrant of the abdomen. The hematocrit and hemoglobin values may be stable early in the course, but serial determinations will suggest blood loss. These manifestations are followed by sudden circulatory collapse, usually coincident with rupture of the hematoma through the capsule and extravasation of blood into the peritoneal cavity. The abdomen then may be distended, rigid, and dull to percussion, occasionally with a bluish discoloration of the overlying skin, which may extend over the scrotum in male infants. Abdominal radiographs may suggest the diagnosis by revealing liver enlargement, an abnormal course of a nasogastric tube or umbilical venous catheter, or uniform opacity of the abdomen, indicating free intraperitoneal fluid. Although paracentesis can confirm whether the latter indicates free blood in the peritoneal cavity, ultrasonography offers a noninvasive method of diagnosis.[58] Fresh intrahepatic hemorrhage will appear echogenic, with possible enlargement of the involved lobe; with involution of the hemorrhage, the lesion becomes more echolucent and may disappear. CT scan of the abdomen also may assist in establishing a diagnosis of subcapsular hemorrhage without rupture.

DIFFERENTIAL DIAGNOSIS. This lesion is one of several that can result in hemoperitoneum; others include trauma to the adrenal glands, kidneys, gastrointestinal tract, and spleen. Presence of a right upper quadrant mass suggests trauma to the liver, but absence of a mass does not rule it out. Abdominal radiography, ultrasonography, and intravenous pyelography may assist in pinpointing the site of trauma, but ultimately a definitive diagnosis can be made only by laparotomy.

TREATMENT. Immediate management consists of prompt transfusion with packed red blood cells, as well as recognition and correction of any coagulation disorder. This should be followed by laparotomy with evacuation of the hematoma and repair of any laceration with sutures placed over a hemostatic agent. Any fragmented, devitalized liver tissue should be removed to prevent subsequent fatal secondary hemorrhage. Occasionally, hemostasis may be difficult to achieve at surgery. Consequently, blood transfusion and the tamponade of intra-abdominal pressure might be adequate therapy in some infants.

PROGNOSIS. In unrecognized liver trauma with formation of a subcapsular hematoma, shock and death may result if the hematoma ruptures through the capsule, reducing the pressure tamponade and resulting in new bleeding from the liver. Recognition of the possibility of liver rupture in infants with a predisposing birth history, followed by early diagnosis and prompt therapy, should improve the prognosis. Early diagnosis and correction of any existing coagulation disorder also will improve the prognosis.

RUPTURE OF THE SPLEEN

Rupture of the spleen in the newborn occurs much less often than rupture of the liver. However, recognition of this condition is equally important because of its similar potential for fulminant shock and death if the diagnosis is delayed.

ETIOLOGY. The condition is most common in large infants, infants delivered in breech position, and infants with erythroblastosis fetalis or congenital syphilis in whom the spleen is enlarged and more friable and thereby susceptible to rupture either spontaneously or after minor trauma. An underlying clotting defect also has been implicated. Rupture of the spleen has occurred in normal-sized infants with uneventful deliveries and no underlying disease.

CLINICAL MANIFESTATIONS. Clinical signs indicating blood loss and hemoperitoneum are similar to those described for hepatic rupture. The hemoglobin and hematocrit values decrease, and abdominal paracentesis may reveal free blood. Several infants have been described in whom the blood was circumscribed within the leaves of the phrenicosplenic ligament and therefore was not clinically detectable. Occasionally, a left upper quadrant mass may be palpable, and radiographs of the abdomen may show medial displacement of the gastric air bubble.

DIFFERENTIAL DIAGNOSIS. Rupture of the liver and trauma to the adrenal glands, kidneys, and gastrointestinal tract must be distinguished.

TREATMENT. Packed red blood cells should be transfused promptly, and any coexisting clotting defect should be corrected. This should be followed by immediate exploratory laparotomy. Every attempt should be made to repair and preserve the spleen to prevent the subsequent increased risk of infection.[57]

PROGNOSIS. With early recognition and emergency surgery, survival rate should approach 100%.

ADRENAL HEMORRHAGE

Neonatal adrenal hemorrhage is more common than previously suspected; some autopsy studies have revealed a high incidence of subclinical hemorrhage. Massive hemorrhage is much less common, and the incidence is difficult to determine because the diagnosis is often unsuspected and considered retrospectively only years later, when calcified adrenal glands are unexpectedly found on radiographs or at autopsy.

ETIOLOGY. The most likely cause is birth trauma; risk factors include macrosomia, diabetes in the mother, breech presentation, congenital syphilis, and dystocia. Placental hemorrhage, anoxia, hemorrhagic disease of the newborn, prematurity, and, more recently, neuroblastoma have been implicated. Pathologic findings vary from unilateral minute areas of bleeding to massive bilateral hemorrhage. The increased size and vascularity of the adrenal gland at birth may predispose it to hemorrhage.

CLINICAL MANIFESTATIONS. Signs vary with the degree and extent of hemorrhage. The classic findings are fever, tachypnea out of proportion to the degree of fever, yellowish pallor, cyanosis of the lips and fingertips, a mass in either flank with overlying skin discoloration, and purpura. Findings suggesting adrenal insufficiency include poor feeding, vomiting, diarrhea, obstipation, dehydration, abdominal distention, irritability, hypoglycemia, uremia, rash, listlessness, coma, convulsions, and shock.

RADIOGRAPHIC MANIFESTATIONS. Initial radiographic manifestations may be limited to widening of the retroperitoneal space with forward displacement of the stomach and duodenum or downward displacement of the intestines or kidneys. In time, calcification may appear. Typically, this is rimlike and has been observed as early as the 12th day of life. After several weeks the calcification becomes denser and retracted and assumes the configuration of the adrenal gland (Fig. 27–16). Ultrasonographic examination of the neonate is an excellent adjunctive method of diagnosis. Abdominal ultrasonography performed during the first several days may reveal a solid lesion in the location of the adrenal hemorrhage; this is thought to represent either clot fragmentation or diffuse clotted blood throughout the adrenal gland. If adrenal hemorrhage is suspected, ultrasonographic examination should be repeated at 3- to 5-day intervals. If adrenal hemorrhage has occurred, the lesion will change from a solid to a cystic appearance, coincident with liquefaction, degeneration, and lysis of the clot (Fig. 27–17).

DIFFERENTIAL DIAGNOSIS. Adrenal hemorrhage must be distinguished from other causes of abdominal hemorrhage. In addition, when a mass is palpable, the differential diagnosis must include the multiple causes of flank masses in the newborn, such as genitourinary anomaly, Wilms tumor, and neuroblastoma. If the infant is large or the delivery is traumatic or breech, an adrenal hemorrhage is most likely. Neuroblastoma may be distinguished by persistent-demonstration of a solid lesion on serial ultrasound examinations and by increased excretion of vanillylmandelic acid and other urinary catecholamines in

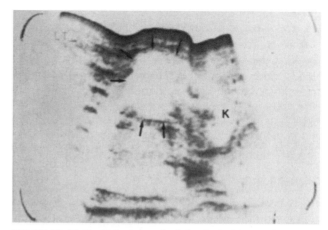

FIGURE 27–17. Sagittal gray-scale abdominal ultrasound examination of a 4564-gm male infant whose mother had gestational diabetes. Problems included fracture of right clavicle, hyperbilirubinemia requiring three exchange transfusions, and abdominal distention with large left flank mass. Ultrasound examination at 14 days demonstrated fluid-filled mass (arrows) superior to left kidney (K), representing adrenal hemorrhage. (Courtesy of Dr. John C. McFadden, Lutheran General Children's Hospital, Park Ridge, Ill.)

85% to 90% of affected infants. Blood pressure measurements and radiographs also may help to evaluate this possibility.

TREATMENT. Significant blood loss should be replaced with packed red blood cell transfusion. Suspicion of adrenal insufficiency may warrant the use of intravenous fluids and corticosteroids. The decision for surgical intervention is dictated by the location and degree of hemorrhage. If it appears to be retroperitoneal

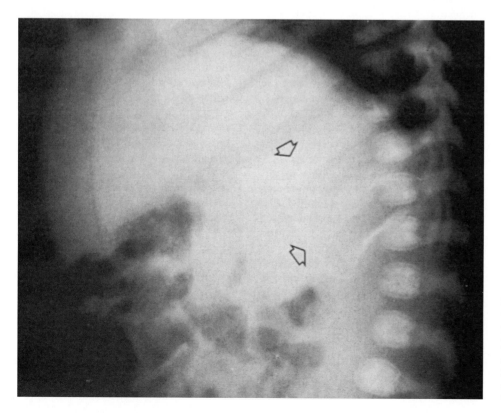

FIGURE 27–16. Lateral abdominal radiographs of a 5312-gm male infant delivered vaginally, with difficulty after shoulder dystocia. At 48 hours, fever, icterus, and slow feeding were noted and a mass was palpable above the left kidney. At 31 days there was dense, retracted calcification (arrows) that assumed the configuration of the adrenal gland.

and limited by the perinephric fascia, some recommend blood replacement and careful observation in the hope of spontaneous control by tamponade; often this approach is successful, and surgery is not necessary. If paracentesis reveals blood or if blood loss exceeds replacement, exploratory laparotomy is indicated. Surgery may involve evacuation of hematoma, vessel ligation, and adrenalectomy with or without nephrectomy. When the hemorrhagic process extends to the peritoneal cavity, peritoneal exploration and evacuation of clots are indicated.

PROGNOSIS. Small hemorrhages are probably often asymptomatic and have no associated significant morbidity, judging from the unexpected discovery of calcified adrenal glands on abdominal radiographs taken for other reasons later in infancy and childhood. If hemoperitoneum or adrenal insufficiency or both develop, the outlook depends on the speed with which diagnosis is made and appropriate therapy instituted. Surviving infants should be followed closely after discharge from the hospital. Adrenal function should be tested with adrenocorticotropic hormone stimulation at a later date to determine whether a normal response occurs in the urinary excretion of 17-hydroxycorticosterone.

RENAL INJURY

Birth-related injury to the kidneys occurs rarely and less often than injury involving the liver, spleen, or adrenal gland.

ETIOLOGY. Factors that predispose an infant to any form of intra-abdominal injury also may affect the kidneys. They include macrosomia, malpresentation (especially breech), and precipitous labor or delivery or both. The potential for renal injury is enhanced by a pre-existing anomaly (e.g., hydronephrosis).

CLINICAL MANIFESTATIONS. The infant may demonstrate the same signs of blood loss and hemoperitoneum noted in the other intra-abdominal lesions. More specific signs include ascites, flank mass, and gross hematuria. Radiographs may confirm the presence of ascites and flank mass. Ultrasonographic examination may further define the mass (e.g., presence of cysts) and reveal ascites and retroperitoneal hematoma. Application of a Doppler probe to the renal hilus and the region of the vessels can assist in assessing renal arterial and venous flow. In ambiguous cases CT scanning may help to clarify ultrasonographic findings.

DIFFERENTIAL DIAGNOSIS. Other lesions that cause hematuria must be considered. They include renal tumor with hemorrhage and renal vein thrombosis with infarction.

TREATMENT. After providing supportive measures similar to those used in other intra-abdominal injuries, one should consider laparotomy. Possible findings at surgery include kidney rupture or transection, renal pedicle avulsion, and kidney necrosis. Use of an intraoperative Doppler probe can determine the status of renal blood flow. If there is no flow, nephrectomy is indicated.

PROGNOSIS. Early recognition of possible renal vascular injury may lead to earlier intervention, with the potential for kidney salvage.

INJURIES TO THE EXTREMITIES

FRACTURE OF THE HUMERUS

After the clavicle, the humerus is the bone most often fractured during the birth process.

ETIOLOGY. The most common mechanisms responsible are difficult delivery of extended arms in breech presentations and of the shoulders in vertex presentations. Besides traction with simultaneous rotation of the arm, direct pressure on the humerus also is a factor. This may account for the occurrence of fracture of the humerus in spontaneous vertex deliveries. The fractures are usually in the diaphysis. They are often greenstick fractures, although complete fracture with overriding of the fragments occasionally occurs.

CLINICAL MANIFESTATIONS. A greenstick fracture may be overlooked until a callus is noted. A complete fracture with marked displacement of fragments presents an obvious deformity that calls attention to the injury. Often the initial manifestation of the fracture is immobility of the affected arm. Palpation reveals tenderness, crepitation, and hypermobility of the fragments. The ipsilateral Moro response is absent. Radiographs confirm the diagnosis.

DIFFERENTIAL DIAGNOSIS. The differential diagnosis includes all the previously noted lesions that cause immobility of the arm. An associated brachial plexus injury occasionally occurs.

TREATMENT. The affected arm should be immobilized in adduction for 2 to 4 weeks. This may be accomplished by maintaining the arm in a hand-on-hip position with a triangular splint and a Velpeau bandage, by strapping the arm to the chest, or by application of a cast.

PROGNOSIS. The prognosis is excellent. Healing is associated with marked formation of callus. Moderate overriding and angulation disappear with time because of the excellent remodeling power of infants. Complete union of the fracture fragments usually occurs by 3 weeks. Fair alignment and shortening of less than 1 inch indicate satisfactory closed reduction. Fractures of the long bones in infants always result in epiphyseal stimulation; the closer the fracture to the epiphyseal cartilage, the greater is the degree of subsequent overgrowth.

FRACTURE OF THE FEMUR

Although a relatively infrequent injury, fracture of the femur is by far the most common fracture of the lower extremity in the newborn.

ETIOLOGY. Fracture of the femur usually follows a breech delivery when the leg is pulled down after the breech is already partially fixed in the pelvic inlet or when the infant is improperly held by one thigh during delivery of the shoulders and arms. Femoral fracture even may occur during cesarean delivery.[2] Infants with congenital hypotonia may be more prone to this injury if their underlying disorder (e.g., severe Werdnig-Hoffmann disease) is associated with decreased muscle bulk at birth.

CLINICAL MANIFESTATIONS. Usually an obvious deformity of the thigh is seen (Fig. 27–18); as a rule the bone breaks transversely in the upper half or third, where it is relatively thin. Less often the injury may not be appreciated until several days after delivery, when swelling of the thigh is noted; this swelling may be caused by hemorrhage into adjacent muscle. The infant refuses to move the affected leg or cries in pain during passive movement or with palpation over the fracture site. Radiographs almost always show overriding of the fracture fragments.

TREATMENT. Optimal treatment is traction-suspension of both lower extremities, even if the fracture is unilateral. The legs are immobilized in a spica cast; with Bryant traction the infant is suspended by the legs from an overhead frame, with the buttocks and lower back just raised off the crib. The legs are extended and the thighs flexed on the abdomen. The weight of the infant's body is enough to overcome the pull of the thigh muscles and thereby reduce the deformity. The infant is maintained in this position for 3 to 4 weeks until adequate callus has formed and new bone growth has started. During the treatment period, special attention should be given to careful feeding of the infant and to protection of bandages and casts from soiling with urine and feces.

PROGNOSIS. The prognosis is excellent; complete union and restoration without shortening are expected. Extensive calcification may develop in the areas of surrounding hemorrhage but is resorbed subsequently.

DISLOCATIONS

Dislocations caused by birth trauma are rare. Often an apparent dislocation is actually a fracture displaced through an epiphyseal plate. Because the epiphyseal plate is radiolucent, a fracture occurring adjacent to an unmineralized epiphysis will give a radiographic picture simulating a dislocation of the neighboring joint. This type of injury has been termed *pseudodislocation.*[26] Because the humeral and proximal femoral epiphyses are usually not visible on radiographs at birth, a pseudodislocation can occur at the shoulder, elbow, or hip.

Of the true dislocations, those involving the hip and knee are probably not caused by the trauma of the birth process. Most likely they are either intrauterine positional deformities or true congenital malformations. A true dislocation resulting from birth trauma is that involving the radial head. This has been associated with traumatic breech delivery. Examination reveals adduction and internal rotation of the affected arm, with pronation of the forearm; Moro response is poor, and palpation reveals lateral and posterior displacement of the radial head. This is confirmed by radiographs. With supination and extension the radial head can be reduced readily. This should be done promptly, followed by immobilization of the arm in this position in a circular cast for 2 to 3 weeks. Early recognition and treatment should result in normal growth and function of the elbow.

Bayne and associates[4] illustrated the importance of establishing an early diagnosis when they described a term infant with a swollen, tender elbow after breech delivery. Movement produced obvious pain. Radiographs at that time and again at 8 months of age were misinterpreted as normal. At 1 year an orthopedist diagnosed anteromedial dislocation. Because of several unsuccessful attempts at closed reduction, future osteotomy was required to treat this now permanent deformity.

EPIPHYSEAL SEPARATIONS

As with dislocations, epiphyseal separations are rare. They occur mostly in primiparity, dystocic deliveries, and breech presentations, especially those requiring manual extraction or version and extraction. Any de-

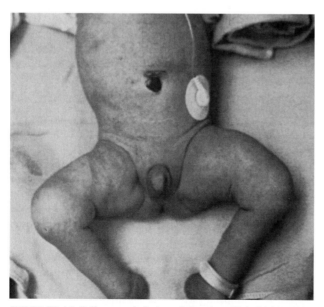

FIGURE 27–18. Fullness and obvious deformity of left thigh in 4020-gm male with Werdnig-Hoffmann disease. Muscle wasting of both lower extremities also is apparent. Radiograph confirmed fracture of proximal third of left femur.

livery associated with vigorous pulling may predispose the infant to this injury. The upper femoral and humeral epiphyses are most often involved. Usually on the second day the soft tissue over the affected epiphysis develops a firm swelling with reddening, crepitus, and tenderness. Active motion is limited, and passive motion is painful. If the injury is in the upper femoral epiphysis, the infant assumes the frog-leg position with external rotation of the leg.

Early radiographs will show only soft tissue swelling, with occasional superolateral displacement of the proximal femoral metaphysis. Because the neonatal femoral capital epiphysis is not ossified, this can be interpreted mistakenly as congenital hip dislocation. However, the presence of pain and tenderness would make dislocation unlikely. Besides plain radiographs of the hips, an infant with a history and physical examination compatible with traumatic epiphysiolysis should also be studied by ultrasonography before manipulation is attempted. This examination would demonstrate a normal femoroacetabular relationship, in contrast to the abnormal findings in an infant with septic arthritis and congenital hip dislocation. In addition, in the presence of traumatic epiphysiolysis the femoral head and neck would not be continuous, in contrast to the findings of septic arthritis and congenital hip dislocation. Further differentiation between traumatic epiphysiolysis and septic arthritis can be provided by arthrocentesis; in epiphysiolysis the joint does not contain excess fluid, and what is obtained may be serosanguineous, whereas in septic arthritis, purulent fluid is obtained. After 1 to 2 weeks, extensive callus appears, confirming the nature of the injury; during the third week, subperiosteal calcification appears.

If possible, treatment should be conservative. Closed reduction and immobilization are indicated within the first few days before rapidly forming fibrous callus prevents mobilization of the epiphysis. The hip is immobilized in the frog-leg position as in congenital dislocation. Poorly immobilized fragments may require temporary fixation with a Kirschner wire. Union usually occurs within 10 to 15 days. Untreated or poorly treated epiphyseal injuries may result in subsequent growth distortion and permanent deformities such as coxa vara. Mild injuries carry a good prognosis.

OTHER PERIPHERAL NERVE INJURIES

In contrast to the brachial plexus and phrenic and facial nerves, other peripheral nerves are injured less often at birth and usually in association with trauma to the extremity. Radial palsy has occurred after difficult forceps extractions, both from pressure of incorrectly applied forceps and in association with fracture of the arm. Occasionally, the palsy occurs later, when the radial nerve is enmeshed within the callus of the healing fracture. Frequently, associated subcutaneous fat necrosis overlies the course of the radial nerve along the lateral aspects of the upper arm. The presence of isolated wristdrop with weakness of the wrist,

finger, and thumb extensors, skin changes overlying the course of the nerve, and absence of weakness above the elbow distinguish this condition from brachial plexus injury. Palsies of the femoral and sciatic nerves have occurred after breech extractions; sciatic palsy has followed extraction by the foot. Passive range-of-motion exercises are usually the only therapy required. Complete recovery usually occurs within several weeks or months.

TRAUMA TO THE GENITALIA

Soft tissue injuries involving the external genitalia sometimes occur, especially after breech deliveries and in large infants.

SCROTUM AND LABIA MAJORA

Edema, ecchymoses, and hematomas can occur in the scrotum and labia majora, especially when they are the presenting parts in a breech presentation. Because the male newborn has a pendulous urethra that is vulnerable to compression or injury, it is possible for significant trauma to occur after a protracted labor in the breech position; the mechanism is believed to be compression of the urethra against a firm structure in the maternal bony pelvis. Rarely this may cause marked temporary hydronephrosis after delivery. The hydronephrosis usually resolves within 3 days. Because of laxity of the tissues, the degree of swelling and of discoloration occasionally is extreme enough (Fig. 27–19) to evoke considerable concern among the medical and nursing staff, especially regarding deeper involvement (e.g., periurethral hemorrhage and edema), which might hinder normal micturition. However, this has not generally been a problem, and

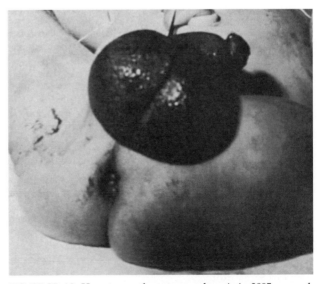

FIGURE 27–19. Hematoma of scrotum and penis in 3895-gm male infant delivered vaginally after frank breech presentation. Infant voided at 22 hours and regularly thereafter. Swelling diminished appreciably within 5 hours and was gone by third day. Discoloration was greatly diminished by second day.

frequently these infants void shortly after arriving in the nursery. Spontaneous resolution of edema occurs within 24 to 48 hours, and resolution of discoloration occurs within 4 to 5 days. Treatment is not necessary. Secondary ulceration, necrosis, or eschar formation is rare unless an associated underlying condition such as herpes simplex infection is present.

DEEPER STRUCTURES

Much less often, birth trauma may involve the deeper structures of the genitalia. If the tunica vaginalis testis is injured and blood fills its cavity, a hematocele is formed. Absence of transillumination distinguishes this from a hydrocele. If the infant appears in pain, the scrotum may be elevated and cold packs applied. Spontaneous resolution is the usual course.

The testes may be injured, often in association with injury to the epididymis. Usually the involvement is bilateral. The testes may be enlarged, smoothly rounded, and insensitive. The infant may be irritable, with vomiting and poor feeding. Urologic consultation is indicated; occasionally, exploration and evacuation of blood are necessary, especially with increasing size of the testes. Severe trauma may result in atrophy or failure of the testes to grow. The occasional finding in older children of a circumscribed fibrous area within the testicular tissue is thought to represent past birth trauma to the gland.

INJURIES RELATED TO INTRAPARTUM FETAL MONITORING

Continuous monitoring of the fetal heart rate and the intermittent sampling of fetal scalp blood for determination of acid-base status often are used to monitor the fetus during labor. Thousands of patients have been monitored by these methods (see also Chapters 9 and 30). The relative infrequency of complications indicates that in experienced hands these procedures are generally safe. However, certain specific complications have occurred.

INJURIES RELATED TO DIRECT FETAL HEART RATE MONITORING

Direct monitoring of the fetal heart rate during labor depends on application of an electrode to the fetal scalp or other presenting part. Superficial abrasions, lacerations, and hematomas can occur rarely at the site of application of the electrode. These complications require no specific therapy beyond local treatment.

Rarely, abscesses of the scalp may follow application of scalp electrodes. These abscesses usually have been sterile and have required only local treatment. Systemic signs or symptoms require evaluation for possible septicemia.

Lauer and Rimmer[37] reported a potentially more serious complication related to use of a spiral fetal scalp electrode, as noted earlier in this chapter. At delivery the electrode was noted to be attached to the infant's eyelid, resulting in a superficial laceration. Marked surrounding edema was considered to have protected the infant from more severe injury.

INJURIES RELATED TO FETAL SCALP BLOOD SAMPLING

Fetal biochemical monitoring requires puncture of the presenting part, usually the scalp, with a 2-mm blade and the collection of blood under direct visualization in a heparinized tube. Major complications that may occur rarely are excessive bleeding and accidental breakage of the blades. The bleeding can be stopped by pressure, but on occasion this may require sutures. Rarely blood replacement may be required. It is important to obtain a detailed family history of bleeding disorders before initiation of this procedure.

The second major complication has been breakage of the blade within the fetal scalp. Removal soon after delivery has been recommended to prevent secondary infection. This has been accomplished by use of a magnet attached to a small forceps that probes the puncture site and elicits a click as the blade is attracted to the magnet. On occasion, radiographic localization followed by a small incision is necessary for withdrawal of the blade.

■ REFERENCES

1. Akazawa H, et al: Congenital muscular torticollis: Long-term follow-up of thirty-eight partial resections of the sternocleidomastoid muscle. Arch Orthop Trauma Surg 112:205, 1993.
2. Alexander J, et al: Femoral fractures at caesarean section: Case reports. Br J Obstet Gynaecol 94:273, 1987.
3. Babyn PS, et al: Sonographic evaluation of spinal cord birth trauma with pathologic correlation. AJR Am J Roentgenol 151:763, 1988.
4. Bayne O, et al: Medial dislocation of the radial head following breech delivery: A case report and review of the literature. J Pediatr Orthop 4:485, 1984.
5. Bell HJ, et al: Somatosensory evoked potentials as an adjunct to diagnosis of neonatal spinal cord injury. J Pediatr 106:298, 1985.
6. Benaron DA: Subgaleal hematoma causing hypovolemic shock during delivery after failed vacuum extraction: A case report. J Perinatol 13:228, 1993.
7. Berger SS, et al: Mandibular hypoplasia secondary to perinatal trauma: Report of case. J Oral Surg 35:578, 1977.
8. Brans YW, et al: Neonatal spinal cord injuries. Am J Obstet Gynecol 123:918, 1975.
9. Carraccio C, et al: Subcutaneous fat necrosis of the newborn: Link to maternal use of cocaine during pregnancy. Clin Pediatr 33:317, 1994.
10. Chan YL, et al: Ultrasonography of congenital muscular torticollis. Pediatr Radiol 22:356, 1992.
11. Chen TH, et al: Subcutaneous fat necrosis of the newborn. Arch Dermatol 117:36, 1981.
12. Cohen DL: Neonatal subgaleal hemorrhage in hemophilia. J Pediatr 93:1022, 1978.
13. Cook JS, et al: Hypercalcemia in association with subcutaneous fat necrosis of the newborn: Studies of calcium-regulating hormones. Pediatrics 90:93, 1992.
14. Daily W, et al: Nasal septal dislocation in the newborn. Mo Med 74:381, 1977.
15. Davids JR, et al: Congenital muscular torticollis: Sequela of intrauterine or perinatal compartment syndrome. J Pediatr Orthop 13:141, 1993.
16. de Chalain TM, et al: Case report: Unilateral combined facial nerve and brachial plexus palsies in a neonate following a midlevel forceps delivery. Ann Plast Surg 38:187, 1997.
17. de Vries Reilingh TS, et al: Surgical treatment of diaphragmatic

eventration caused by phrenic nerve injury in the newborn. J Pediatr Surg 33:602, 1998.

18. Eisenberg D, et al: Neonatal skull depression unassociated with birth trauma. AJR Am J Roentgenol 143:1063, 1984.

19. Falco NA, et al: Facial nerve palsy in the newborn: Incidence and outcome. Plast Reconstr Surg 85:1, 1990.

20. Garza-Mercado R: Intrauterine depressed skull fractures of the newborn. Neurosurgery 10:694, 1982.

21. Gherman RB, et al: Brachial plexus palsy: An in utero injury? Am J Obstet Gynecol 180:1303, 1999.

22. Govaert P, et al: Vacuum extraction, bone injury and neonatal subgaleal bleeding. Eur J Pediatr 151:532, 1992.

23. Greenberg SJ, et al: Birth injury induced glossolaryngeal paresis. Neurology 37:533, 1987.

24. Guyer B, et al: Annual summary of vital statistics—1998. Pediatrics 104:1229, 1999.

25. Haenggeli CA, et al: Brachial plexus injury and hypoglossal paralysis. Pediatr Neurol 5:197, 1989.

26. Haliburton RA, et al: Pseudodislocation: An unusual birth injury. Can J Surg 10:455, 1967.

27. Hankins GDV: Lower thoracic spinal cord injury—a severe complication of shoulder dystocia. Am J Perinatol 15:443, 1998.

28. Harris GJ: Canalicular laceration at birth. Am J Ophthalmol 105:322, 1988.

29. Hickey K, McKenna P: Skull fracture caused by vacuum extraction. Obstet Gynecol 88:671, 1996.

30. Hunter JD, et al: The ultrasound diagnosis of posterior shoulder dislocation associated with Erb's palsy. Pediatr Radiol 28:510, 1998.

31. Ilagan NB, et al: Radiological case of the month. Arch Pediatr Adolesc Med 148:65, 1994.

32. Joseph PR, et al: Clavicular fractures in neonates. Am J Dis Child 144:165, 1990.

33. Kaplan B, et al: Fracture of the clavicle in the newborn following normal labor and delivery. Int J Gynecol Obstet 63:15, 1998.

34. Katzman GH: Pathophysiology of neonatal subconjunctival hemorrhage. Clin Pediatr 31:149, 1992.

35. Kruse K, et al: Elevated 1,25-dihydroxyvitamin D serum concentrations in infants with subcutaneous fat necrosis. J Pediatr 122:460, 1993.

36. Lanska MJ, et al: Magnetic resonance imaging in cervical cord birth injury. Pediatrics 85:760, 1990.

37. Lauer AK, Rimmer SO: Eyelid laceration in a neonate by fetal monitoring spiral electrode. Am J Ophthalmol 125:715, 1998.

38. Loeser JD, et al: Management of depressed skull fracture in the newborn. J Neurosurg 44:62, 1976.

39. MacKinnon JA, et al: Spinal cord injury at birth: Diagnostic and prognostic data in twenty-two patients. J Pediatr 122:431, 1993.

40. Maekawa K, et al: Fetal spinal-cord injury secondary to hyperextension of the neck: No effect of cesarean section. Dev Med Child Neurol 18: 229, 1976.

41. Mangurten HH, et al: Incidental rib fractures in a neonate. Neonat Intensive Care 12:15, 1999.

42. Miedema CJ, et al: Primarily infected cephalhematoma and osteomyelitis in a newborn. Eur J Med Res 4:8, 1999.

43. Miller MJ, et al: Oral breathing in response to nasal trauma in term infants. J Pediatr 111:899, 1987.

44. Mohon RT, et al: Infected cephalhematoma and neonatal osteomyelitis of the skull. Pediatr Infect Dis J 5:253, 1986.

45. Ng PC, et al: Subaponeurotic haemorrhage in the 1990s: A 3-year surveillance. Acta Paediatr 84:1065, 1995.

46. Peleg D, et al: Fractured clavicle and Erb's palsy unrelated to birth trauma. Am J Obstet Gynecol 177:1038, 1997.

47. Petrikovsky BM, et al: Cephalhematoma and caput succedaneum: Do they always occur in labor? Am J Obstet Gynecol 179:906, 1998.

48. Plauche WC: Subgaleal hematoma: A complication of instrumental delivery. JAMA 244:1597, 1980.

49. Pohjanpelto P, et al: Anterior chamber hemorrhage in the newborn after spontaneous delivery: A case report. Acta Ophthalmol 57:443, 1979.

50. Priest JH: Treatment of a mandibular fracture in a neonate. J Oral Maxillofac Surg 47:77, 1989.

51. Rainin EA: Eversion of upper lids secondary to birth trauma. Arch Ophthalmol 94:330, 1976.

52. Raynor R, et al: Nonsurgical elevation of depressed skull fracture in an infant. J Pediatr 72:262, 1968.

53. Rossitch E, et al: Perinatal spinal cord injury: Clinical, radiographic and pathologic features. Pediatr Neurosurg 18:149, 1992.

54. Ryan CA, et al: Vitamin K deficiency, intracranial hemorrhage, and a subgaleal hematoma: A fatal combination. Pediatr Emerg Care 8:143, 1992.

55. Saunders BS, et al: Depressed skull fracture in the neonate: Report of three cases. J Neurosurg 50:512, 1979.

56. Schrager GO: Elevation of depressed skull fracture with a breast pump. J Pediatr 77:300, 1970.

57. Schullinger JN: Birth trauma. Pediatr Clin North Am 40:1351, 1993.

58. Share JC, et al: Unsuspected hepatic injury in the neonate: Diagnosis by ultrasonography. Pediatr Radiol 20:320, 1990.

59. Shenaq SM, et al: Brachial plexus birth injuries and current management. Clin Plast Surg 25:527, 1998.

60. Silverman SH, et al: Dislocation of the triangular cartilage of the nasal septum. J Pediatr 87:456, 1975.

61. Stein RM, et al: Corneal birth trauma managed with a contact lens. Am J Ophthalmol 103:596, 1987.

62. Tan KL: Elevation of congenital depressed fracture of the skull by the vacuum extractor. Acta Paediatr Scand 63:562, 1974.

63. Torode I, Donnan L: Posterior dislocation of the humeral head in association with obstetric paralysis. J Pediatr Orthop 18:611, 1998.

64. Towner D, et al: Effect of mode of delivery in nulliparous women on neonatal intracranial injury. N Engl J Med 341:1709, 1999.

65. Voet D, et al: Leptomeningeal cyst: Early diagnosis by color Doppler imaging. Pediatr Radiol 22:417, 1992.

66. Wegman ME: Annual summary of vital statistics—1981. Pediatrics 70:835, 1982.

67. Wegman ME: Annual summary of vital statistics—1993. Pediatrics 94:792, 1994.

68. Zelson C, et al: The incidence of skull fractures underlying cephalhematomas in newborn infants. J Pediatr 85:371, 1974.

28

Congenital Anomalies

Louanne Hudgins

Suzanne B. Cassidy

Congenital anomalies, whether they are isolated (single) or part of syndromes, are a common cause of medical intervention, long-term illness, and death. The neonatologist or perinatologist often is the first person to identify necessary evaluations and management and to explain the cause of the anomalies and the prognosis for the child to the parents. This chapter reviews some of the significant etiologic and epidemiologic aspects of congenital anomalies. It provides an approach to and a framework for the evaluation of the infant with congenital anomalies, with emphasis on conditions that are apparent in the delivery room.

TERMINOLOGY

It is important to distinguish between "congenital" and "genetic," terms that are often confused. *Congenital* means present at birth, but it does not denote etiology, which may or may not be *genetic* (i.e., determined by genes). An *anomaly* is a structural defect, a deviation from the norm. A major anomaly is an anomaly that requires significant surgical or cosmetic intervention, whereas a minor anomaly has no significant surgical or cosmetic importance. Minor anomalies overlap with normal phenotypic variations and are discussed later in this chapter. It is important to classify congenital anomalies as major anomalies, minor anomalies, or normal variations, because their implications are different for both the infant and the family.

A useful approach to determining the etiology of a congenital anomaly is to consider whether it represents a malformation, deformation, or disruption.[33] A *malformation* is a primary structural defect in tissue formation, usually owing to abnormal development (morphogenesis) of the tissue for genetic or teratogenic reasons, such as a neural tube defect or a congenital heart defect. A *deformation* results from abnormal mechanical forces, often related to intrauterine constraint, acting on normally developed tissues.[12] Clubfoot and altered head shape often are due to deformation. Deformations occurring late in gestation often are reversible with removal of the force or with

positioning. Breech or other abnormal positioning in utero, oligohydramnios, and uterine anomalies are the most common causes of deformations. Observation of the position of comfort of the infant combined with a careful history of fetal movement, position, and fluid volume can be very helpful in identifying an anomaly as a deformation. A *disruption* represents interruption of development of intrinsically normal tissue, and it usually affects a body part rather than a specific organ. Vascular occlusion and amniotic bands are common causes of disruptions. Monozygotic twinning and prenatal cocaine exposure are common predisposing factors for disruptions on the basis of vascular interruption.

Disruptions and isolated deformations are generally sporadic, with negligible or low recurrence risks. Malformations, however, may predispose a fetus to deformations, such as renal agenesis (a malformation) causing *Potter sequence,* in which facial and limb deformations and pulmonary hypoplasia result from oligohydramnios. A neural tube defect, also a malformation, predisposes a fetus to hip dislocation and clubfoot, owing to lack of movement below the level of the lesion.

Many congenital malformations can have more than one cause, often with different possible associated anomalies and different recurrence risks. Cleft lip and palate, for example, can be isolated or can be part of dozens of different syndromes and can be multifactorial, autosomal dominant, autosomal recessive, X-linked, chromosomal, or teratogenic in etiology.[10]

If more than one anomaly is present in an individual, one should consider whether it is part of a sequence, association, or syndrome, which have different implications for prognosis and recurrence risk. *Sequence* refers to a pattern of multiple anomalies derived from a single known or presumed cause. An example is the oligohydramnios sequence, often referred to as *Potter syndrome,* which consists of limb deformations; simple ears, a beaked nose, and infraorbital creases (Potter facies); and pulmonary hypoplasia. These features are present when there is a lack of amniotic fluid, be it secondary to chronic leakage of amniotic fluid or lack of fetal urine (renal agenesis). *Association* refers to a nonrandom occurrence of multiple malformations for which no specific or common etiology has been identified. An example is the *VATER (or VACTERL) association,* an acronym for a pattern of anomalies consisting of *v*ertebral abnormalities, *a*nal atresia, (*c*ardiac anomalies,) *t*racheo*e*sophageal fistula, and *r*enal and *r*adial (*l*imb) dysplasia.[29] *Syndrome* refers to a recognized pattern of anomalies with a single, specific cause, such as Holt-Oram syndrome, in which radial dysplasia and cardiac defects occur as a consequence of an autosomal dominant gene.[15] As is the case of many syndromes, the etiology is unknown.

Phenotype is the observable manifestation of *genotype,* which is the genetic constitution of an individual; therefore, when one speaks of the phenotypic features, reference is being made to the observable physical features present in that individual.

EPIDEMIOLOGY AND ETIOLOGY

MAJOR MALFORMATIONS

Approximately 2% of newborn infants have a serious anomaly that has surgical or cosmetic importance (Tables 28–1[13] and 28–2[14]). This proportion is a minimum estimate because it is based only on the examination of newborn infants; additional anomalies are detected with increasing age. The etiology of malformations can be divided into broad categories: genetic (multifactorial, single gene [mendelian], or chromosomal), teratogenic, and unknown.

Genetic

MULTIFACTORIAL. The largest number (86%) of congenital malformations are isolated,[13] and most isolated malformations are believed to be the consequence of multifactorial inheritance involving the interaction of multiple genetic and environmental factors. The most common and familiar birth defects fall into this category, including congenital heart defects, neural tube defects, cleft lip and palate, clubfoot, and

TABLE 28–2   TYPE AND ETIOLOGY OF MAJOR MALFORMATIONS IN 18,155 NEWBORNS

MALFORMATION		NUMBER
Multifactorial Inheritance		128 (0.7%)
Anencephaly-myelomeningocele-encephalocele	25	
Cardiac anomalies	45	
Cleft lip and/or palate	14	
Clubfoot	21	
Congenital hip dislocation	12	
Hypospadias	8	
Omphalocele	2	
Bilateral renal agenesis	1	
Mendelian Inheritance		67 (0.4%)
Autosomal dominant disorders (excluding polydactyly)	57	
Autosomal recessive disorders	9	
X-linked recessive disorders	1	
Chromosomal Abnormalities		27 (0.2%)
Down syndrome	21	
Trisomy 13	3	
Other	3	
Teratogenic Conditions		15 (0.1%)
Infants of diabetic mothers	14	
Effects of warfarin	1	
Unknown		107 (0.6%)
Total Number Affected		**344 (2%)**

Data from Holmes LB: Current concepts in genetics: Congenital malformations. N Engl J Med 295:204, 1976.

congenital hip dysplasia. The genetic contribution to such complex disorders is being unraveled with techniques developed as a consequence of the Human Genome Project. In most cases, multiple genetic components are involved, some with large effects and some with small contributions.

SINGLE GENE (MENDELIAN). Single major genes are responsible for causing 0.4% of newborns to have major malformations (see Table 28–2). The most common mode of mendelian inheritance for major malfor-

TABLE 28–1   MALFORMATIONS IN 12,000 CONSECUTIVE NEWBORNS

MALFORMATION	NUMBER OF NEWBORNS	TOTAL MALFORMATIONS (%)	TOTAL NEWBORNS (%)
Localized	**161**	**85.6**	**1.34**
Multifactorial inheritance	70	37.2	0.58
Mendelian inheritance	41	21.8	0.34
Unknown	50	26.6	0.42
Multiple	**27**	**14.4**	**0.22**
Chromosomal	11	5.9	0.09
Mendelian inheritance	6	3.2	0.05
Unknown	10	5.3	0.08
Totals	**188**	**100**	**1.56**

Data from Holmes LB: Inborn errors of morphogenesis: A review of localized hereditary malformations. N Engl J Med 291:763, 1974.

mations is autosomal dominant, with a minority of major malformations owing to autosomal recessive or, rarely, X-linked genes (see Table 28–2). Limb anomalies, including postaxial polydactyly, syndactyly, and brachydactyly, constitute the most prevalent major localized malformations, and they are frequently the result of a dominant gene. Any type of malformation, however, may be under the control of a single gene, including multiple anomalies arising in different structures or organ systems. Relatively little is understood about the biochemical defects underlying the production of malformations by mutant genes, although advances are being made. For example, *Smith-Lemli-Opitz syndrome*, characterized by genital abnormalities, syndactyly of the second and third toes, ptosis, and wide alveolar ridges, has been found to be associated with a defect in cholesterol biosynthesis.[18] Although a biochemical or molecular basis increasingly is being recognized, specific diagnosis still relies heavily on the family history and clinical evaluation.

An excellent reference for all single gene conditions is *Mendelian Inheritance in Man*,[24] which now has an excellent on-line version (www.ncbi.nlm.nih.gov/omim).

CHROMOSOMAL (see also Chapter 7). About 0.2% of newborns have a major malformation as a result of a chromosomal disorder, amounting to 10% of all the major congenital malformations (see Table 28–2). It is important to note, however, that approximately 0.6% of newborns have noteworthy chromosomal anomalies, but that the abnormalities are not detectable by physical examination at birth in 66% of these infants.[16] Included among these early phenotypically undetectable chromosomal anomalies are common disorders of the sex chromosomes, such as 47,XXY, 47,XYY, and 47,XXX. The most prevalent malformation syndrome owing to an abnormal chromosomal constitution in newborns is *Down syndrome*, or *trisomy 21*, which occurs in approximately 1 in 660 births.[16] The other common trisomies are *trisomy 18* and *trisomy 13*, each occurring in approximately 1 in 10,000 births. All three trisomies occur more frequently with increased maternal age. Other well-known chromosomal syndromes are *Klinefelter syndrome* (47,XXY), occurring in 1 in 1000 male births, and *Turner syndrome* (45,X), present in 1 in 5000 female births. Many other types of chromosomal aberrations have been identified using chromosome banding techniques, including translocations, inversions, ring chromosomes, marker chromosomes, and deletions.[30] Not all deletions are detectable by routine cytogenetic analysis, however. Fluorescence in situ hybridization (FISH) is a technique that uses fluorescently labeled DNA probes and chromosome metaphase spreads to identify microdeletions associated with such conditions as *Prader-Willi syndrome* (long arm of chromosome 15),[6] *Miller-Dieker* syndrome (short arm of chromosome 17), *Williams syndrome* (long arm of chromosome 7),[22] and *velocardiofacial/DiGeorge syndrome* (long arm of chromosome 22).[7] FISH continues to contribute to better definitive

diagnosis for conditions involving multiple congenital anomalies.

Teratogenic

(See also Chapter 12.)

A *teratogen* is anything external to the fetus that causes a structural or functional disability postnatally. Teratogens can be drugs and chemicals, altered metabolic states in the mother, infectious agents, or mechanical forces.[17] Known teratogenic factors cause only 5% to 10% of congenital anomalies despite the ever-expanding list of potential teratogens in our increasingly chemical environment (Table 28–3).[2] Before one can attribute malformations to a teratogenic agent, there must be one anomaly, only a few specific anomalies, or a recognizable pattern of anomalies found to occur at increased incidence over the background risk in infants exposed at the appropriate developmental stage (usually 2 to 12 weeks' gestation). With only a few exceptions, teratogenic agents do not affect every exposed infant, which is probably related to genetic susceptibility factors. Dose and timing of exposure also affect teratogenic potential.

Although many drugs have teratogenic potential, several commonly used drugs are worthy of some discussion. Alcohol is thought to be the most common teratogen to which a fetus may be exposed.[17] Chronic maternal alcohol use during pregnancy is associated

TABLE 28–3 ETIOLOGY OF HUMAN MALFORMATIONS

ETIOLOGY	MALFORMED LIVE BIRTHS (%)
Environmental	**10**
Maternal conditions	4
Alcoholism, diabetes, endocrinopathies, phenylketonuria, smoking, nutritional problems	
Infectious agents	3
Rubella, toxoplasmosis, syphilis, herpes simplex, cytomegalic inclusion disease, varicella, Venezuelan equine encephalitis	
Mechanical problems (deformations)	2
Amniotic band constrictions, umbilical cord constraint, disparity in uterine size and uterine contents	
Chemicals, drugs, radiation, hyperthermia	1
Genetic	**20–25**
Single gene disorders	
Chromosomal abnormalities	
Unknown	**65–70**
Polygenic/multifactorial (gene-environment interactions)	
"Spontaneous" errors of development	
Other unknowns	

Modified from Brent RL: Evaluating the alleged teratogenicity of environmental agents. Colin Perinatol 13:609, 1986.

with increased perinatal mortality and intrauterine growth restriction, as well as congenital anomalies such as cardiac defects, microcephaly, short palpebral fissures, and other anomalies (Fig. 28–1). Long-term effects include mental retardation and behavioral problems. Alcohol carries serious risks when it is used almost at any time during pregnancy in sufficient quantities, because the central nervous system continues to develop throughout pregnancy. For this reason, it is recommended that women avoid alcohol, even in small amounts, throughout their pregnancy.[17] (See Chapter 36.)

Some altered metabolic states in the mother also are known to have teratogenic potential. One of the most common is maternal diabetes mellitus. Infants of diabetic mothers are at increased risk for congenital heart defects, sacral dysgenesis, and central nervous system abnormalities such as holoprosencephaly and others.[25] In this population, there is an approximately threefold increase in congenital anomalies over those in the general population. The risk for congenital anomalies seems to be lower in offspring of diabetic mothers with better control of blood glucose, but this is not absolute, and factors other than blood glucose levels are thought to play a role in teratogenesis. (See Chapter 15 and Chapter 47, Part One.)

Anticonvulsants are a common category of teratogens to which a fetus is likely to be exposed. Although the medical literature is somewhat contro-versial, clinical geneticists, dysmorphologists, and clinical teratologists generally identify a variable but recognizable pattern of anomalies and developmental defects that occur at significantly increased frequency among fetuses exposed to all currently used anticonvulsants.[31]

Congenital anomalies also may be associated with certain infections during pregnancy. The most common and best understood infections are represented by the acronym TORCH, which stands for *t*oxoplasmosis, *o*ther agents (including syphilis), *r*ubella, *c*ytomegalovirus, and *h*erpes simplex. Although the sequelae of these infections may not be apparent until later, one should consider these congenital infections in neonates with intrauterine growth retardation, microcephaly, chorioretinitis, intracranial calcification, microphthalmia, or cataracts. Confirmation of the specific diagnosis should be made by antibody studies and other evaluations such as ophthalmologic examination and imaging studies. (See Chapters 22 and 37.)

Mechanical forces also may be categorized as teratogens. Deformations, such as clubfoot, may be from intrauterine constraint secondary to mechanical forces such as uterine fibroids. Disruption of the amnion also may be associated with deformations and other limb anomalies.

Unknown

Approximately 66% of major malformations have no recognized etiology if one includes those of presumed polygenic and multifactorial etiology.[2] As our understanding of congenital anomalies increases, it is likely that specific genetic and environmental causes will be identified. For example, in recent years, folic acid has been recognized to decrease the risk of neural tube defects, thus implicating folic acid deficiency in the etiology of the anomalies.[35] Specific genes have been identified as causing the multifactorial disorder Hirschsprung disease.[1]

ANOMALIES IN ABORTED FETUSES

Spontaneously aborted fetuses have a higher incidence of malformations than do newborns (Table 28–4),[14, 28] which presumably represents a natural selection process. The common major malformations present in newborns that are of presumed multifactorial inheritance, such as neural tube defects and cleft lip or palate, are also frequent in aborted fetuses and may be more severe. Other malformations, such as cloacal exstrophy, are relatively rare in newborns but are comparatively common in aborted fetuses.

In addition to these rather localized anomalies, multiple congenital anomalies commonly occur, including well-recognized syndromes that are caused by single genes and chromosomal abnormalities (Table 28–5).[5] It is estimated that approximately half of all fetuses aborted by 20 weeks' gestation, including those whose existence was not yet known to the mothers, have a chromosome abnormality. The most common single chromosome abnormality is 45,X, fol-

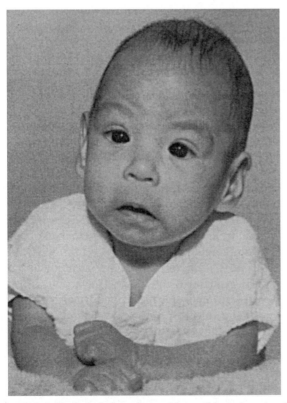

FIGURE 28–1. Fetal alcohol syndrome. Note mild ptosis, epicanthal folds, flat nasal bridge, short nose, smooth philtrum, and thin upper vermilion border. (From Dworkin PH [ed]: Pediatrics, 2nd ed. Malvern, Pa, Lea & Febiger, 1992, p 168.)

TABLE 28-4 PREVALENCE OF LOCALIZED MALFORMATIONS IN SPONTANEOUSLY ABORTED FETUSES AND NEWBORNS (per 1000)

MALFORMATION	SPONTANEOUS ABORTIONS*			NEWBORNS†
	2 to 8 Weeks	9 to 18 Weeks	19 Weeks	
Anencephaly-myelomeningocele-encephalocele	31	10	116	1.4
Cleft lip/palate	3	14.5	0	0.8
Cloacal exstrophy	0	7.3	10.6	0.1
Polydactyly	0	7.3	0	0.1

*Data from Nelson T, et al: Collection of human embryos and fetuses. In Hook EB, et al (eds): Monitoring Birth Defects and Environment: The Problem of Surveillance. New York, Academic Press, 1971.

†Data from Holmes LB: Current concepts in genetics: Congenital malformations. N Engl J Med 295:204, 1976.

lowed by triploidy. Both conditions are more common in aborted fetuses than in newborns. The trisomies, as a group, account for over 50% of all chromosomally abnormal pregnancy losses. The most frequent trisomy, accounting for almost 33% of all trisomies, is trisomy 16, which does not occur in newborns.[20] Trisomy 21, the most common trisomy in newborns, occurs in less than 10% of all recognized trisomic conceptions. Unbalanced products of translocations account for 2% to 4% of all chromosomally abnormal fetuses and are three to six times more frequent in aborted fetuses than in newborns.

MINOR ANOMALIES AND PHENOTYPIC VARIANTS

Although major malformations often are easy to identify, minor anomalies, by their nature, are more subtle

TABLE 28-5 DIAGNOSES IN 375 CONSECUTIVE CASES OF PREGNANCY LOSS

DIAGNOSIS	≤20 wks (%)	>20 wks (%)
Chromosomal abnormalities	19.4	15.7
Trisomies	54	47
Triploidy/tetraploidy	18	5.2
45,X	16	15.8
45,X mosaic	6	0
Deletion/duplication	0	15.8
Other	6	15.8
Placental abnormalities	12	5.8
Infection	7	6.6
Cord problems	7	5
Neural tube defects	6	10
Central nervous system abnormalities	1.2	5
Twins	7.4	3.3
Skeletal dysplasias	2	2.5
Recognizable syndromes	1.2	5.8
Hemoglobinopathies	0	4
Early amnion rupture sequence	3.5	5
Abdominal wall defects	1.2	0
Renal abnormalities	1.2	3.3
Cardiac abnormalities	0.7	4
Other	6.5	9
Total cases with diagnoses	76	85
Diagnoses unknown	24	15

Modified from Curry CJR: Pregnancy loss, stillbirth, and neonatal death: A guide for the pediatrician. Pediatr Clin North Am 39(1):157, 1992.

and may not be appreciated unless they are specifically sought. Minor anomalies, however, are significant. They may be part of a characteristic pattern of malformations and thus may provide clues to a diagnosis. Also, their occurrence may be an indication of the presence of a more serious anomaly. In one large study of 4305 newborns, 19.6% of the 162 babies with major malformations had three or more minor anomalies.[21] A single minor anomaly, however, was associated with a major malformation in only 3.7% of cases.[21]

Minor anomalies are most frequent in areas of complex and variable features, such as the face and distal extremities (Table 28-6).[23] Among the most common features are lack of a helical fold of the pinna and complete or incomplete single transverse palmar crease patterns.[23] Typical single transverse palmar crease (simian crease) occurs in almost 3% of normal newborns, but it appears in 45% of individuals with trisomy 21.[19]

Among the most frequent phenotypic variants, those present in 4% or more of the population, are a folded-over helix of the pinna and mongolian spots in blacks and Asians (Table 28-7).[23] Before attributing medical significance to an apparent minor anomaly or phenotypic variation, it is useful to determine whether the anomaly is present in other family members or whether it is frequent in the patient's ethnic group. It is common for isolated minor anomalies such as syndactyly of the second and third toes to be familial.

RACIAL DIFFERENCES

The prevalence of congenital malformations varies significantly among racial groups. This variation is most likely the consequence of differing genetic predispositions and variable environmental factors operating in diverse areas. Table 28-8[8, 9] shows the prevalence of common major congenital malformations in white Americans, African Americans, and the Chinese. It is of interest that certain anomalies are especially common in a particular race, such as polydactyly in African Americans and hypospadias and clubfoot in white Americans. Minor malformations may show an equally striking racial predisposition. Brushfield spots are common in white Americans but

TABLE 28–6 COMMON MINOR MALFORMATIONS IN NEWBORNS (FREQUENCY GREATER THAN 1:1000)

MINOR MALFORMATION	NEWBORNS (%)
Craniofacial	
Borderline micrognathia	0.32
Eye	
Inner epicanthal folds	0.42
Ear	
Lack of helical fold	3.52
Posteriorly rotated pinna	0.25
Preauricular and/or auricular skin tags	0.23
Small pinna	0.14
Auricular sinus	0.12
Skin	
Capillary hemangioma other than on face or posterior aspect of neck	1.06
Pigmented nevi	0.49
Mongoloid spots in white infants	0.21
Hand	
Simian creases	2.74
Bridged upper palmar creases	1.04
Bilateral combinations	0.51
Other unusual crease patterns	0.28
Clinodactyly of fifth finger	0.99
Foot	
Partial syndactyly of second and third toes	0.016
Total	12.34

Data from Marden PM, et al: Congenital anomalies in the newborn infant, including minor variations: A study of 4142 babies by surface examination for anomalies and buccal smear for sex chromatin. J Pediatr 64:357, 1964.

are rare in African Americans. Umbilical hernias, however, are common in African American infants but are relatively infrequent in white American infants. The widely varying frequencies of various traits in different races demonstrate that whether any given characteristic is considered to be a minor anomaly or a phenotypic variant may be strongly dependent on the race of the patient being studied. One of the best examples is mongolian spots, which occur in almost 50% of black or Asian infants but in only 0.2% of white infants.[23]

EVALUATION

Every infant with a congenital anomaly should receive a thorough diagnostic evaluation; without one, accurate information about the natural history of the condition and the recurrence risk for similarly affected future children cannot be provided. Therefore, an accurate diagnosis and etiology are needed.

When a child is born with one or more anomalies, a number of considerations should guide the physician in the evaluation. The most critical factors to be considered are the detailed prenatal and family history, the dysmorphic physical examination (including

careful observation and measurements of individual features), and the use of appropriate diagnostic tests and evaluations, particularly if there is more than one anomaly. It is essential to identify whether the malformation is isolated or part of a constellation of anomalies. It is also essential to identify whether there are other major or minor anomalies, including perhaps inapparent internal malformations, and to recognize well-described patterns of malformations. Practice in such recognition or consultation with others who have such expertise may be required. The severity of an anomaly can sometimes be helpful in identifying whether it may be associated with other anomalies and in predicting the prognosis for the infant.

HISTORY

The evaluation of an infant with congenital anomalies begins with a detailed history. The important goal is to identify a possible genetic predisposition, environmental factor, or other clue to the cause of the anomalies. It is useful to begin with the pregnancy to document fetal movement and vigor, complications, illnesses, maternal use of any medications, or possible exposure to teratogens, as well as the timing of all complications and exposures (see Chapter 12). The extent of smoking and alcohol consumption should be determined, and every mother should be asked about illicit drug use. A careful three- to four-generation family history, charted in a concise manner in the form of a pedigree, should be constructed, using squares for males and circles for females. Horizontal lines indicate genetic union, and vertical lines indicate genetic descent. All abortions and stillbirths should be noted. A question always should be specifically asked about possible consanguinity. A simple way to inquire is to ask if the families of the affected child's

TABLE 28–7 COMMON PHENOTYPIC VARIANTS

PHENOTYPIC VARIANT	NEWBORNS (%)
Craniofacial	
Flat nasal bridge	7.3
Ear	
Folded-over upper helix	43.0
Darwinian tubercle	11.0
Skin	
Capillary hemangioma on face and/or posterior aspect of neck	14.3
Mongolian spots in blacks and Asians	45.8
Hand	
Hyperextensibility of thumbs	12.3
Foot	
Mild calcaneovalgus	4.7
Genital	
Hydrocele	4.4

Data from Marden PM, et al: Congenital anomalies in the newborn infant, including minor variations: A study of 4142 babies by surface examination for anomalies and buccal smear for sex chromatin. J Pediatr 64:357, 1964.

TABLE 28–8 FREQUENCY OF COMMON CONGENITAL MALFORMATIONS IN VARIOUS RACIAL GROUPS (per 1000)

MALFORMATION	WHITE AMERICANS*	AFRICAN AMERICANS*	CHINESE†
Anencephaly-myelomeningocele-encephalocele	2.4	0.9	1.5
Cleft lip and palate	1.1	0.6	1.3
Cleft palate	0.6	0.4	
Clubfoot (talipes equinovarus)	3.9	2.3	0.1
Polydactyly	1.2	11.0	1.5
Hypospadias	2.4	1.2	0.6

*Data from Erickson JD: Racial variations in the incidence of congenital malformations. Ann Hum Genet 39:315, 1976.

†Data from Emanuel I, et al: The incidence of congenital malformations in a Chinese population: The Taipei collaborative study. Teratology 5:159, 1972.

parents are related in any way. If so, then the charting should indicate the exact relationships. The presence of other relatives with congenital anomalies of any type or with growth or developmental abnormalities should be recorded along with other pertinent information, such as the maternal and paternal ages and the nature of the anomaly. Family photographs are often very useful in clarifying questions of possible unusual facial features. The pedigree should, at a minimum, include all siblings and parents of the proband as well as aunts, uncles, cousins, and grandparents. In the case of possible dominant or X-linked disorders, a more extensive pedigree may be needed.

PHYSICAL EXAMINATION

(See also Chapter 26.)

The goal of the physical examination of an infant with congenital anomalies is to determine if an anomaly is isolated or to detect a recognizable pattern of malformations so that a specific etiologic determination can be made. In addition, careful attention must be directed not only to an exact description of the major anomalies but also to apparent minor anomalies or variations. Distinctive physical features may become clues in figuring out the cause of multiple congenital anomalies; therefore, a detailed inspection of various features of external anatomy and measurement of them where appropriate should be performed. Objective description of anomalous features allows for accurate use of resources or consultants. In this section, an outline of this external examination is presented by region or structure, and certain helpful points, as well as aspects of the differential diagnosis, are discussed. Greater detail in regard to examination and abnormalities of various organ systems is given in other relevant chapters in this book. The authors also refer the reader to various resources in which the anomalies and syndromes mentioned in this section are discussed at length.[3, 11, 19, 34]

Skin

(See also Chapter 50.)

Normal infant skin, particularly when exposed to cold temperatures, shows a marbling pattern termed *cutis marmorata* or *livedo reticularis*. In rare instances, this pattern may be unusually prominent and familial, inherited as an autosomal dominant trait. A similar prominent pattern may occur in those with trisomy 21, hypothyroidism, or Cornelia de Lange syndrome.

A variety of lesions with altered pigmentation may provide useful clues to a diagnosis. Café-au-lait spots are characteristic of *neurofibromatosis*, but they also occur in other conditions and may be isolated, especially in darkly pigmented babies. Hypopigmented macules may be the earliest manifestation of tuberous sclerosis in the young infant. Multiple irregular pigmented lesions arranged in whorls are very suggestive of incontinentia pigmenti, but this disorder usually presents initially with a vesicular rash. An angiomatous patch over one side of the face may be an isolated anomaly or part of the *Sturge-Weber syndrome*. More than one skin hemangioma should raise suspicion of internal vascular lesions.

Generalized edema may obscure many minor anomalies, making diagnosis difficult. Turner syndrome, trisomy 21, and Noonan syndrome should be considered in newborns with generalized edema.

Hair

The relative sparseness or prominence of body hair should be noted. Sparse hair is characteristic of an ectodermal dysplasia, but it does occur in other syndromes, such as cartilage-hair hypoplasia and oculodentodigital syndrome. Generalized hirsutism is typical of Cornelia de Lange syndrome, fetal hydantoin syndrome, and fetal alcohol syndrome, but it also may occur in those with trisomy 18. It also may be a racial (Hispanic, American Indian) or familial characteristic.

Abnormal scalp hair patterns may reflect underlying brain abnormalities. In microcephaly, there may be a lack of the normal parietal whorl, or the whorl may be displaced more centrally or posteriorly. In addition, the frontal hair may show a prominent upsweep. A low posterior hairline occurs with a short or webbed neck, as in Turner syndrome and Noonan syndrome. Punched-out scalp lesions in the parietal

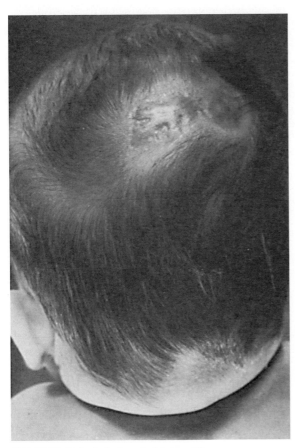

FIGURE 28–2. Scalp lesions in trisomy 13.

aly) to a decrease in this dimension (brachycephaly). Premature infants and those with trisomy 18 characteristically have dolichocephaly (Fig. 28–3), but either type of head shape may be of familial or racial origin. Many Asian and American Indian infants, for example, have strikingly brachycephalic heads.

Premature fusion of cranial sutures (craniosynostosis) results in an abnormal configuration in head shape. Various types occur depending on the sutures involved (see Chapter 38, Part Eight). Torticollis or abnormal mechanical forces in utero can cause asymmetric head shape (plagiocephaly).

A common anomaly in head shape is frontal bossing, which is frequent in some skeletal dysplasias such as achondroplasia and in some cases of hydrocephaly.

Face

The face is composed of a series of structures, each demonstrating considerable normal variation and providing a distinctive and particularly unique appearance to every human being. Because examination of the face is both complex and important, a systematic approach is necessary. It is never sufficient to describe the face merely as "funny looking" or unusual. Specific abnormalities must be analyzed and quantified, when appropriate, even though an overall gestalt impression may suggest a diagnosis in some cases.

Eyes

Hypotelorism occurs when the eyes are unusually close together; *hypertelorism* occurs when the eyes are too far apart. Clinically, hypotelorism and hypertelorism are defined by the interpupillary distance, which may be estimated in a relaxed patient by measuring between the midpoints of the pupils. It is usually impossible to measure the interpupillary distance of a newborn; therefore, two other relevant and useful measurements that are easier to obtain are the inner canthal distance and the outer canthal distance. *Telecanthus* is an increase in the inner canthal distance, and it may occur in the absence of hypertelorism, such as in Waardenburg syndrome type I. There are other factors that may create an illusion of hypertelorism, such as epicanthal folds and a flat nasal bridge; therefore, a subjective impression should always be confirmed by measurement of all three distances, if possible. From the prognostic and diagnostic points of view, it is important to identify hypotelorism, because often it is associated with *holoprosencephaly*, a major malformation of the central nervous system that usually is associated with severe disturbance of brain function and early death. Holoprosencephaly can be isolated or can be part of trisomy 13 (Fig. 28–4). Hypertelorism, however, occurs in a number of syndromes, such as frontonasal dysplasia, and even when it is severe, it is less likely to be related to an underlying brain malformation. Figures 28–5 and

occipital area (aplasia cutis congenita) are typical of trisomy 13 or may be seen in isolation and may be familial (Fig. 28–2).

Head

(See also Chapter 38, Part Eight.)

The size of the head, measured by the maximum head circumference, and the sizes of the anterior and other fontanels should be compared with those of appropriate standards. Head size varies with age, sex, and racial group and correlates with body size. Macrocephaly as an isolated anomaly often is familial and inherited in an autosomal dominant fashion; therefore, determining the head circumferences of the parents is helpful. However, macrocephaly may be a manifestation of several disorders, including hydrocephaly and various conditions affecting the skeletal system, such as achondroplasia. Microcephaly can also be familial, either autosomal dominant or recessive, but it is more commonly a manifestation of many syndromes that result in mental retardation. Large fontanels occur in hypothyroidism; in trisomies 21, 18, and 13; and in many bone disorders, such as hypophosphatasia and cleidocranial dysostosis. A small anterior fontanel may be a sign of failure of normal brain growth.

The normal shape of the head may vary from an increase in the anteroposterior diameter (dolichoceph-

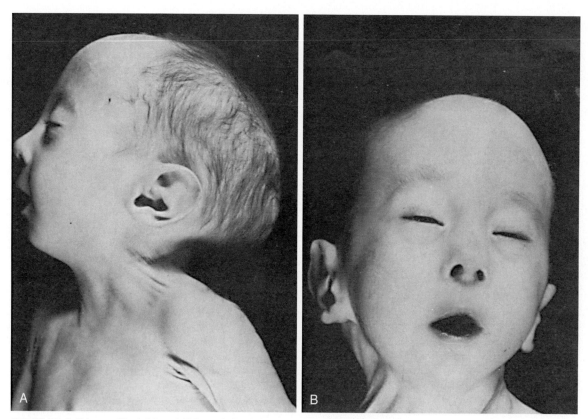

FIGURE 28–3. Trisomy 18. *A,* Note dolichocephaly. *B,* Note small mouth and anomalous ears.

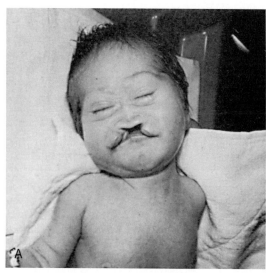

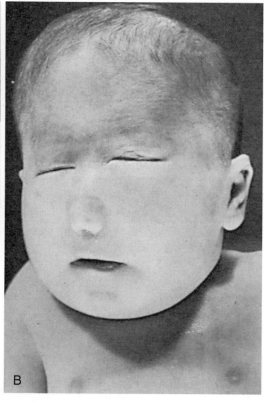

FIGURE 28–4. Trisomy 13. *A,* Note anomalous midline facial development with hypotelorism, midline cleft lip, and lack of a nose. *B,* Note hypotelorism and abnormal nose.

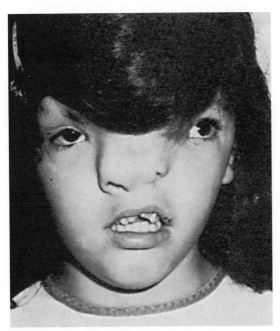

FIGURE 28–5. Frontonasal dysplasia with hypertelorism and bifid nose.

28–6 illustrate hypertelorism with midline facial anomalies.

Epicanthal folds are a feature of normal fetal development, and they may be present in normal infants. They are characteristic in trisomy 21 (Fig. 28–7A, B), but they occur in many other malformation syndromes, especially in those that include a flat nasal bridge.

Normally, an imaginary line through the inner and outer canthi should be perpendicular to the sagittal plane of the face. An upward slant to the palpebral fissure is seen in trisomy 21 (see Fig. 28–7), and a downward slant is seen in mandibulofacial dysostosis

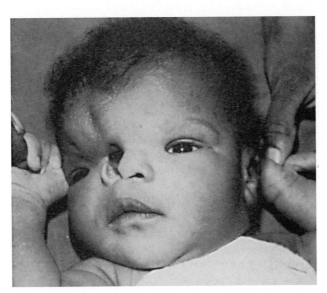

FIGURE 28–6. Frontonasal dysplasia with nasal cleft.

(see Fig. 28–7C). Both types of slant can be part of a number of other syndromes.

Palpebral fissure length is measured from the inner canthus to the outer canthus. Short palpebral fissures may occur in association with other ocular anomalies, such as microphthalmia, and they are characteristic of syndromes such as *fetal alcohol syndrome* (see Fig. 28–1) and *trisomy 18* (see Fig. 28–3B).

A *coloboma* is a developmental defect in the normal continuity of a structure, and it often is used in reference to the eye. Colobomas may involve the eyelid margin, as those seen in *Treacher Collins syndrome* (see Fig. 28–7C), or the iris and retina, as those seen in *CHARGE association* (coloboma, heart disease, atresia choanae, retardation of growth development, genital hypoplasia, ear anomalies and/or deafness). Identification of a coloboma should lead to a formal eye evaluation.

Synophrys, or fusion of the eyebrows in the midline, is common in hirsute infants, and it usually occurs in Cornelia de Lange syndrome. It also may be familial.

Other types of anomalies involving the internal structure of the eyes are discussed in Chapter 51.

Ears

The external ear, or pinna, commonly shows great variation, but a number of anatomic landmarks can be identified and should be described when evaluating the anomalous ear. These landmarks include the helix, antihelix, tragus, antitragus, external meatus, and lobule (Fig. 28–8). If the ears appear to be large or small, they should be measured by obtaining the maximum length of the pinna from the lobule to the superior margin of the helix. Preauricular tags or pits may be isolated or associated with other abnormalities of the pinna (Fig. 28–9).

Low-set ears are designated when the helix joins the head below a horizontal plane passing through the outer canthus perpendicular to the vertical axis of the head (Fig. 28–10). It is critical that this condition be assessed with the head in vertical alignment with the body, because any posterior rotation of the head can create an illusion of low-set ears. The relative placement of the ears is more a function of head shape and jaw size than of an intrinsic anomaly of the ear.

When the vertical axis of the ear deviates more than 10 degrees from the vertical axis of the head, the ears are posteriorly rotated. This anomaly often is associated with low-set ears and represents a lag in the normal ascent of the ear during development (Figs. 28–11 and 28–12).

It is important to note that any significant abnormality of the external ear may be an indication of additional anomalies of the middle or inner ear and associated hearing loss; therefore, an early hearing assessment is indicated in such cases (see Chapter 40). Figure 28–13 illustrates a patient with hemifacial microsomia, whose findings include a severely malformed pinna and an absent ear canal. This condition

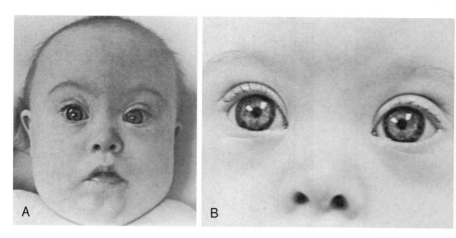
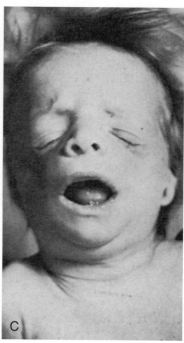

FIGURE 28–7. *A*, Trisomy 21. Note epicanthal folds and mongoloid slant of eyes. *B*, Enlargement of eyes of patient in *A*. Note Brushfield spots on irides. *C*, Mandibulofacial dysostosis (Treacher Collins syndrome) with antimongoloid slant of eyes. Note coloboma, or notch, in left eyelid.

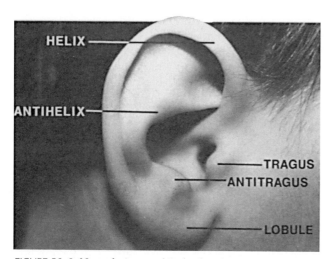

FIGURE 28–8. Normal pinna and its landmarks.

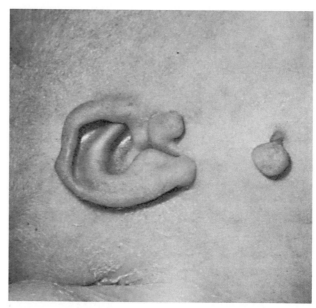

FIGURE 28–9. Preauricular tags with malformed pinna.

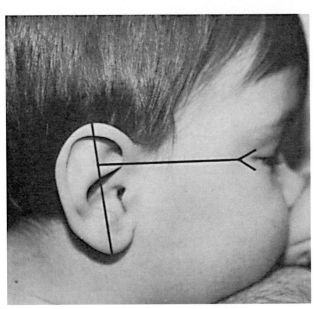

FIGURE 28–10. Normal pinna and its orientation with respect to eyes.

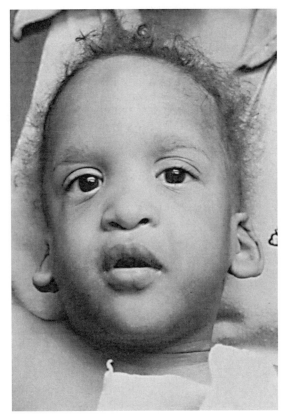

FIGURE 28–12. Facial view of patient in Figure 28–11.

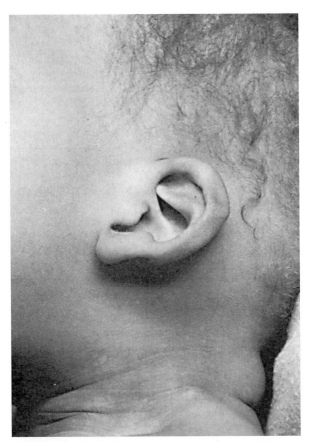

FIGURE 28–11. Abnormal pinna that is low set and posteriorly rotated in patient with Smith-Lemli-Opitz syndrome.

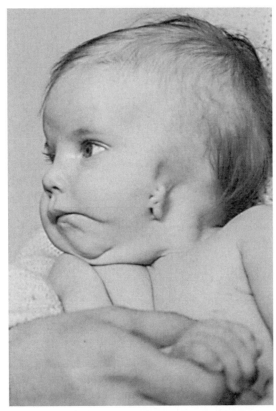

FIGURE 28–13. Hemifacial microsomia showing mandibular hypoplasia, severely malformed pinna, and absent ear canal.

is an example in which an early hearing assessment is essential, because hearing loss is likely.

Nose

The nose, like the external ear, shows great individual variation, but certain alterations in shape are frequent in malformation syndromes involving the face. The nose may be unusually thin with hypoplastic alae nasi, as in *Hallerman-Streiff syndrome*, or it may be unusually broad, as in *frontonasal dysplasia* (see Fig. 28–5). A depressed nasal bridge with an upturned nose occurs in many skeletal dysplasias, such as achondroplasia. When the depression is severe, the nostrils may appear to be anteverted and the nose may appear to be shortened. A hypoplastic nose is often syndromic, and a nose with a single nostril is highly suggestive of holoprosencephaly (see Fig. 28–4).

Mouth

(See also Chapter 42, Part Six.)

The mouth is a complex structure with component parts that each require separate evaluation. The size and shape of the mouth may be altered. A small mouth, or microstomia, should be noted; it occurs in trisomy 18 (see Fig. 28–3). Macrostomia, a large mouth, should be noted as well; it may be present in such conditions as mandibulofacial dysostosis (see Fig. 28–7C). Severe macrostomia may result in association with a lateral facial cleft. The corners of the mouth may be downturned, as in Prader-Willi syndrome and other conditions with hypotonia. An asymmetric face during crying occurs with congenital deficiency in the depressor anguli oris muscle on one side, and this may be associated with other abnormalities, such as hemifacial microsomia and velocardiofacial syndrome.

Prominent, full lips occur in various syndromes, including Williams syndrome. A thin upper lip may be seen in Cornelia de Lange syndrome and in fetal alcohol syndrome (see Fig. 28–1).

A cleft upper lip is usually lateral, as in the common multifactorial *cleft lip* (and/or palate) anomaly. The presence of pits in the lower lip associated with a cleft lip or palate, however, is suggestive of Van der Woude syndrome, which is inherited in an autosomal dominant manner. A median cleft lip is very suggestive of holoprosencephaly (see Fig. 28–4A). In fact, there are many diverse syndromes with cleft lip and/or palate that are important to identify, because they may have other associated malformations and relatively high genetic risks of recurrence. Therefore, it is important to evaluate the infant with cleft lip and/or palate carefully for evidence of other malformations in order to give accurate recurrence risk and prognostic information to the family.

Isolated *cleft palate* is different genetically than cleft lip. Mild forms of cleft palate are represented by submucosal clefts, pharyngeal incompetence with nasal speech (velopharyngeal insufficiency), and bifid

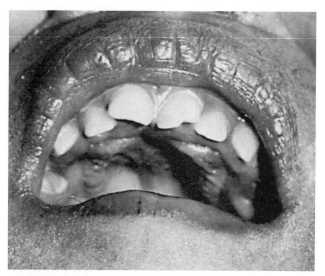

FIGURE 28–14. Prominent alveolar ridges in patient with Smith-Lemli-Opitz syndrome.

uvula. A high arched palate may occur normally, but it is also a feature of many syndromes, especially if hypotonia or another long-standing neurologic abnormality is present. Hypertrophied alveolar ridges are apparent in the palate along the inner margin of the teeth, and they are suggestive of *Smith-Lemli-Opitz syndrome* (Fig. 28–14) if seen in an infant.

Macroglossia may be relative, as in the Pierre Robin malformation complex, in which the primary abnormality is mandibular hypoplasia. In other cases, such as hypothyroidism, Beckwith-Wiedemann syndrome, and Down syndrome, the tongue protrudes and is enlarged. A cleft or irregular tongue or oral frenula occur in various syndromes such as the orofaciodigital syndromes.

The lower portion of the mouth is formed by the mandible, which in young infants is relatively small. An excessively small mandible is termed *micrognathia,*

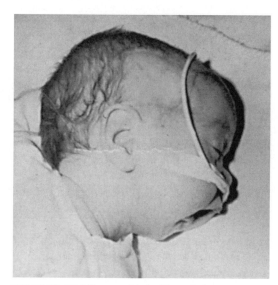

FIGURE 28–15. Micrognathia in Pierre Robin sequence.

which is a feature of many syndromes. It is characteristic in the Pierre Robin sequence, which consists of the triad of micrognathia, glossoptosis, and a U-shaped cleft palate, as opposed to the common V-shaped cleft. A typical patient is shown in Figure 28–15. The Pierre Robin sequence may be part of a syndrome, such as Stickler syndrome (hereditary arthro-ophthalmopathy), and thus other anomalies and a family history must be sought. In other syndromes, the maxilla likewise may be hypoplastic, decreasing the prominence of the upper cheeks (malar hypoplasia).

Neck

The neck may be short, and limitation of rotation should raise the suspicion of fusion of cervical vertebrae, as in a Klippel-Feil anomaly. Excessive skinfolds are characteristic of Turner syndrome (Fig. 28–16), Noonan syndrome, and Down syndrome. In these examples, the excess nuchal skin often represents resolution of a cystic hygroma that was present prenatally.

Chest

The thoracic cage may be unusually small as part of a skeletal dysplasia, such as *thanatophoric dysplasia*

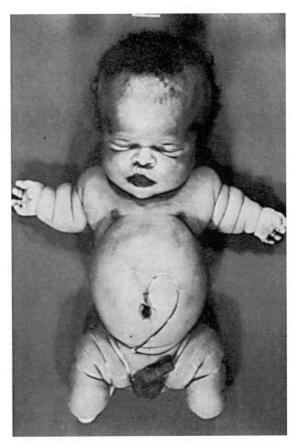

FIGURE 28–17. Thanatophoric dwarf. Note short limbs and narrow thoracic cage.

(Fig. 28–17) or *Jeune asphyxiating thoracic dystrophy*. The sternum itself may be unusually short, which is typical in trisomy 18, or it may be altered in shape, as is seen in pectus excavatum or pectus carinatum. The latter anomalies are commonly seen in a variety of skeletal dysplasias and connective tissue disorders (see Chapter 42, Part Five).

Abdomen

(See also Chapter 45.)

Hypoplasia of the abdominal musculature may occur in association with intrauterine bladder outlet obstruction and other anomalies of the urogenital system. It results in a characteristic prune-belly appearance (see Chapter 49). An omphalocele, in which abdominal contents protrude through the umbilical opening, may be part of the Beckwith-Wiedemann syndrome (see Chapter 47, Part One) or chromosomal abnormalities such as trisomy 13. Gastroschisis, however, is usually an isolated disruption in which the abdominal contents protrude through the periumbilical abdominal wall. Anomalies of a more minor nature, such as inguinal or umbilical hernias, occur in normal infants, but they are more frequent in various syndromes, particularly in connective tissue disorders.

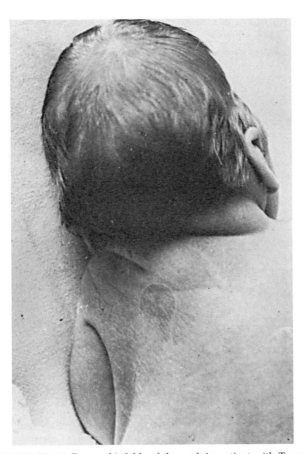

FIGURE 28–16. Excess skinfolds of the neck in patient with Turner syndrome.

Anus

(See also Chapter 45.)

Imperforate anus may be isolated or may occur as the mildest expression of a caudal regression sequence, in which other anomalies such as sacral dysgenesis are seen. It is most commonly part of a constellation of anomalies, such as the VATER association. It also can be seen in a number of chromosomal abnormalities.

Genitalia

(See also Chapter 47, Part Four.)

Hypogenitalism can be seen in association with hypotonia in Prader-Willi syndrome or with low-set dysplastic ears, syndactyly of the toes, and thickened alveolar ridges in Smith-Lemli-Opitz syndrome. Genital ambiguity is associated with renal anomalies and an increased risk for Wilms tumor in Denys-Drash syndrome.

Spine

(See also Chapter 38.)

Among the most common congenital anomalies are the neural tube defects, which involve abnormalities of the central nervous system along with defects in the associated bony structures. Minor external anomalies, particularly of the lower spine, include unusual pigmentary lesions, hair tufts, dimples, and sinuses. Some of these changes, such as hair tufts and sinuses above the gluteal cleft, may be an indication of a more significant deeper anomaly and require further evaluation, such as magnetic resonance imaging (MRI).

Extremities

Extremities may be relatively long, as occur in Marfan syndrome or homocystinuria, or unusually short, as occur in a diverse group of skeletal dysplasias, the most common being achondroplasia. A simple guide to evaluating relative extremity length is to determine where the fingertips are in relation to the thighs when the upper extremities are adducted alongside the body. In the normal infant, the fingertips fall below the hip joint in the midthigh region. When the upper extremities are short, they align with the hip joint or above (see Fig. 28–17); when they are relatively long, they may reach the knees. A more precise and useful measurement is to determine the upper segment–to–lower segment ratio. The distance from the pubis to the heel constitutes the lower segment. By subtracting the lower segment measurement from the length, one obtains the upper segment. In normal newborns this upper segment–to–lower segment ratio is about 1.7 and decreases with age to approximately 1.0 in the adult. A high ratio suggests relative shortening of the extremities, and a low ratio implies either unusually long extremities or a foreshortened trunk, as may occur in spondyloepiphyseal dysplasia.

Paired extremities may be asymmetric in either length or overall size, suggesting either atrophy of one or hypertrophy of the other. The distinction may be difficult to make at times, although it is often evident if an extremity is unusually large or excessively small. Hypertrophy of limbs may be a manifestation of Beckwith-Wiedemann syndrome or Klippel-Trénaunay-Weber syndrome. Isolated hemiatrophy may occur with long-standing corticospinal tract damage as well, as in Russell-Silver syndrome. It is important to identify hemihypertrophy because individuals with this finding are at increased risk for intra-abdominal tumors, such as Wilms tumor, and thus require close monitoring.

Foreshortening of long bones leads to various limb abnormalities, depending on the segments involved. A number of terms have been used to describe such anomalies. *Rhizomelia* denotes proximal shortening of the limbs, such as those in achondroplasia. *Mesomelia* refers to shortening of the middle segment, and *acromelia* refers to relative shortening of the hands and/or feet. A shortened forearm with secondary prominence of skinfolds in a newborn with thanatophoric dysplasia is shown in Figure 28–18.

The hands and feet have epidermal ridges and creases forming a variety of configurations. Normally, there are two deep transverse palmar creases that do not completely cross the palm. In various conditions, such as trisomy 21, there may instead be a single transverse palmar crease (a simian crease). Single palmar creases may be completely transverse across the palm or may be bridged or incomplete (Fig. 28–19*A*,

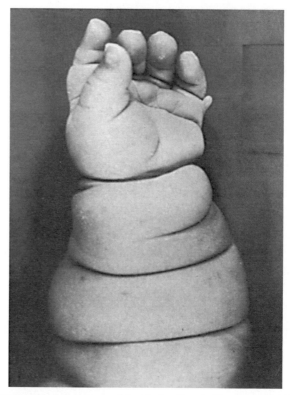

FIGURE 28–18. Forearm and hand of patient in Figure 28–17. Note rudimentary postaxial polydactyly.

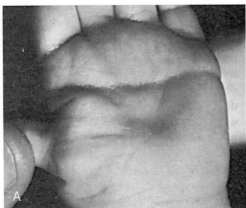
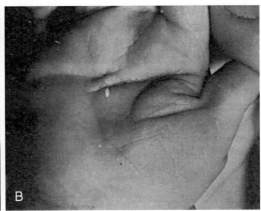

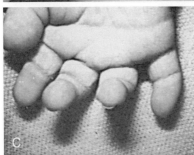

FIGURE 28–19. *A,* Simian crease. *B,* Incomplete bridged simian crease. *C,* Hand of patient with trisomy 21 showing simian crease, brachydactyly, and clinodactyly of fifth finger with single phalangeal crease.

B). They may become more apparent when the palm is slightly flexed. A single phalangeal crease on the fifth finger, instead of the normal two, occurs as a consequence of a hypoplastic middle phalanx and results in clinodactyly (incurving of the digit). This is frequently seen in trisomy 21 (see Fig. 28–19*C*) and in a number of other conditions.

The foot also has ridge patterns. A sandal pattern of deep furrows is typical of mosaic trisomy 8 (Fig. 28–20). Figure 28–21 illustrates the increased separation of the first and second toes and a prominent interdigital furrow in trisomy 21.

Dermatoglyphics, the study of configurations of the characteristic ridge patterns of the volar surfaces

of the skin, can sometimes aid in the diagnosis of the newborn with congenital anomalies. The scope of this subject is beyond that of this chapter and the reader is referred to other sources.[26]

The hands and feet may be enlarged as a result of lymphedema. This is characteristic of infants with Turner or Noonan syndrome, in which the dorsum of the hands and feet may have a puffy appearance (Fig. 28–22). Congenital lymphedema can also be an

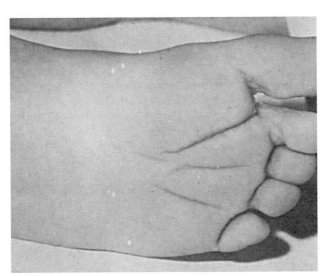

FIGURE 28–20. Sandal line furrows in trisomy 8.

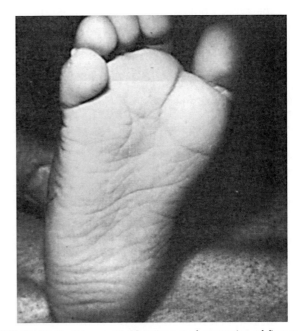

FIGURE 28–21. Trisomy 21. Note increased separation of first and second toes.

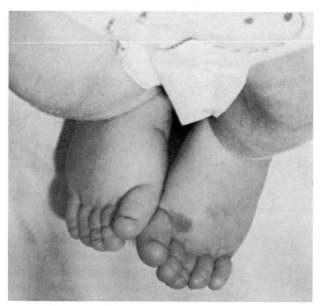

FIGURE 28–22. Dorsal edema of feet in patient with Turner syndrome.

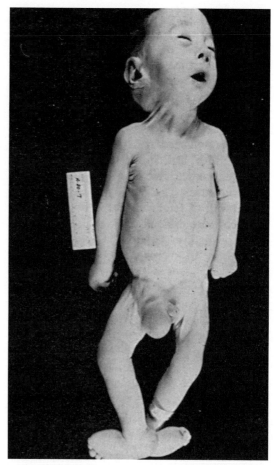

FIGURE 28–23. Trisomy 18. Note right hydrocele and rocker-bottom feet.

autosomal dominantly inherited condition with variable expressivity.

Rocker-bottom feet (Fig. 28–23) are manifested by a prominent heel and a loss of the normal concave longitudinal arch of the sole. They are common in trisomy 18 and other syndromes.

Significant anomalies of the underlying structure produce alterations in the normal form of the hands and feet. Such abnormalities may be classified into the following categories: absence deformities, polydactyly, syndactyly, brachydactyly, arachnodactyly, and contracture deformities (see Chapter 52).

Absence anomalies are of various types, and the etiology and possible associated malformations vary with the type. Congenital absence of an entire hand is termed *acheiria*, and absence of both hands and feet is *acheiropodia*. *Ectrodactyly* refers to a partial or total absence of the distal segments of a hand or foot with the proximal segments of the limbs more or less normal. All such anomalies are examples of terminal transverse defects and may occur sporadically or as part of a syndrome. The term ectrodactyly is frequently misused for the lobster-claw anomaly, which is best described as split hand/split foot. In this anomaly, the central rays are deficient, and there is often fusion of the remaining digits. Split hand/split foot may be seen in isolation, when it is of autosomal dominant origin, or it may be seen with other anomalies.

It is useful to determine whether the defects involve primarily the radial, or preaxial, side of the limb or the ulnar, or postaxial, side. For example, blood dyscrasias such as the Fanconi pancytopenia syndrome and the thrombocytopenia-absent radius (TAR) syndrome commonly involve radial deficiency (see Chapter 44).

Polydactyly refers to partial or complete supernumerary digits and is one of the most common hand malformations. Postaxial polydactyly is more frequent than preaxial, particularly in blacks (Fig. 28–24). As an isolated anomaly, polydactyly may be inherited as an autosomal dominant trait. It also may be a manifestation of a multiple malformation syndrome. Postaxial polydactyly may occur in a variety of syn-

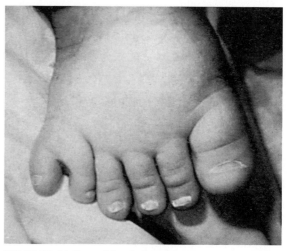

FIGURE 28–24. Postaxial polydactyly.

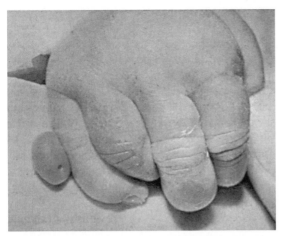

FIGURE 28–25. Postaxial polydactyly in trisomy 13.

dromes, including trisomy 13 (Fig. 28–25), chondroectodermal dysplasia, Meckel-Gruber syndrome, and Bardet-Biedl syndrome. Preaxial polydactyly is characteristic of Carpenter syndrome and Majewski short rib–polydactyly syndrome.

Syndactyly refers to fusion of digits; it is usually cutaneous, but it may involve bone. Minimal syndactyly of the second and third toes is common in normal newborns. More extensive syndactyly is shown in Figure 28–26 and can be seen in trisomy 21 and Smith-Lemli-Opitz syndrome. As an isolated anomaly, different clinical types may be distinguished, but each of them is inherited as an autosomal dominant trait with variable expressivity and incomplete penetrance. Extensive syndactyly often is part of a syndrome, and typical examples include some of the craniosynostosis conditions, such as Apert and Pfeiffer syndromes.

Brachydactyly refers to shortening of one or more digits owing to anomalous development of any of the phalanges, metacarpals, or metatarsals. Various clinical types may be distinguished, but most isolated forms of brachydactyly are inherited in an autosomal dominant fashion. Brachydactyly is also a component of numerous disorders, including skeletal dysplasias such as achondroplasia, and syndromes such as Albright hereditary osteodystrophy and Down syndrome (see Fig. 28–19C).

Arachnodactyly refers to unusually long, spider-like digits, and it is characteristic but not invariable in Marfan syndrome and homocystinuria. The appearance of brachydactyly and arachnodactyly can be confirmed by measuring and determining a middle finger–to–total hand length ratio, which is normally approximately 0.43 in the newborn.

A variety of congenital joint deformities involving the limbs may occur. *Arthrogryposis*, multiple congenital contractures, is most often sporadic and may be associated with oligohydramnios or may be the result of some underlying neuromuscular abnormality. Talipes equinovarus or calcaneovalgus deformities of the ankle are common isolated joint contractures (see Chapter 52). Contractures also may occur in numerous syndromes. Joint hypermobility is frequent in various connective tissue disorders, such as Marfan and Ehlers-Danlos syndromes.

Clinodactyly, as discussed previously, designates an incurving of a digit, most commonly of the fifth finger. This condition is common in trisomy 21 and other syndromes (see Fig. 28–19C). A characteristic clinodactyly involving the fourth and fifth fingers radially and second finger in an ulnar direction occurs in trisomy 18 (Fig. 28–27) or, less often, in trisomy 13.

Camptodactyly is irreducible flexion of the digits. In the hand it usually involves the fifth finger, but it may affect other fingers as well. Isolated camptodactyly may be inherited as an autosomal dominant trait. Camptodactyly also may be part of a syndrome such as trisomy 8, trisomy 10q, and Freeman-Sheldon syndrome.

EVALUATION OF THE STILLBORN

Evaluation of the stillborn is essential and is very similar to that of the live-born infant. A thorough

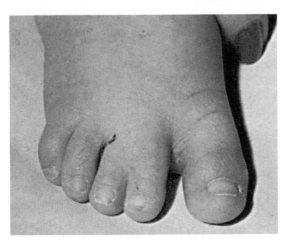

FIGURE 28–26. Syndactyly between second and third toes.

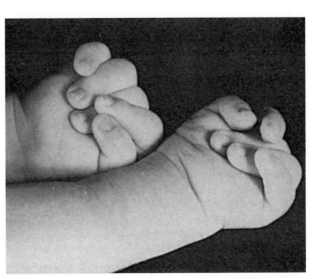

FIGURE 28–27. Trisomy 18. Note characteristic clinodactyly of second, fourth, and fifth fingers.

surface examination by the clinician is useful to identify minor anomalies that may not be apparent to the pathologist as rigor mortis sets in. If indicated, a sample of blood and/or skin should be obtained as soon as possible under sterile conditions for chromosome analysis. Skin can be placed in viral culture media or sterile saline and sent to the laboratory for fibroblast culture. Cells from the fetal side of the placenta may grow when macerated fetal tissue may not. Examination of the stillborn and the placenta by the pathologist may identify internal anomalies that lead to a definitive diagnosis.

There has been controversy over whether it is the responsibility of the perinatologist or the neonatologist to evaluate pregnancy loss.[36] As a result, this important function often has been inadequately performed, leaving the family with little understanding of the nature and etiology of the anomaly, the recurrence risk, and methods of preventing future occurrences. The grieving process, a natural and constant result of fetal loss, is left unaddressed and is made much more difficult without an understanding of the cause of the loss. In addition to the obvious role of the pathologist to learn as much as possible from the examination of the aborted fetus, the clinician is essential in encouraging the family to allow fetal evaluation and to allow the pathologist to conduct it. The clinician also should direct additional testing and meet with the family when the evaluation is complete to ensure that the family receives medical and genetic counseling. Given the decreasing gestational age at fetal viability, it seems reasonable to assume that before 20 weeks' gestation, responsibility of pregnancy loss evaluation rests with the perinatologist, and after this date it falls to the neonatologist. Pregnancy loss before 20 weeks occurs in at least 12% to 15% of all pregnancies[32] and in 1% to 2% of pregnancies after 20 weeks, when it is usually called stillbirth.[4, 27] It is optimal for each hospital to develop a protocol for evaluating fetal loss, including which fetuses to study and which evaluations are appropriate.[4]

DIAGNOSTIC TESTING AND INDICATIONS

Once the history and clinical findings are noted, various laboratory studies may be indicated to aid in making an accurate diagnosis.

In a newborn with one or more obvious major malformations or with multiple minor anomalies, imaging studies are often indicated to identify other anomalies. Ultrasound of the head and abdomen are useful to screen for major structural anomalies of the brain and kidneys. Head ultrasound is a crude study for brain abnormalities, and if brain abnormalities are suspected, more definitive testing such as computed tomography (CT) or MRI is indicated. Echocardiography also is helpful, because congenital heart defects are among the most common major malformations. Detection of major anomalies involving the brain, heart, and kidneys is useful for diagnostic purposes, and it also may allow for more accurate prognostication.

Routine chromosome analysis is indicated in newborns with ambiguous genitalia, two or more major anomalies, multiple minor anomalies, or growth restriction in association with anomalies. Because a routine karyotype on peripheral blood allows for better resolution than a karyotype from amniocentesis and thus will allow detection of small deletions or duplications, such a study should be performed even if a prenatal chromosome analysis had normal findings.

FISH will allow for identification of microdeletions not detectable by routine cytogenetic analysis (Table 28–9). In fact, it has been shown that a significant number of neonates with conotruncal heart defects will have a 22q microdeletion such that this testing is justified in patients with truncus arteriosus, interrupted aortic arch, and tetralogy of Fallot.

Molecular genetic analysis is an increasingly useful tool in diagnosing the newborn with congenital anomalies. For example, in those babies with unexplained hypotonia and contractures, DNA testing may identify an expansion in the myotonic dystrophy gene. As more disease-causing genes are identified, molecular analysis will undoubtedly become a cost-effective aid in diagnosis.

Another area of burgeoning research that is likely to result in useful diagnostic testing is that of metabolic disorders. These conditions were traditionally thought of as not being associated with congenital anomalies, but this notion is changing. A definitive diagnosis of Smith-Lemli-Opitz syndrome, which is associated with syndactyly of the second and third toes, genital abnormalities, ptosis, thick alveolar ridges, malformations of the heart, and other anomalies, can be made by obtaining a low serum choles-

---

TABLE 28–9 COMMON MICRODELETION SYNDROMES IDENTIFIABLE BY FLUORESCENCE IN SITU HYBRIDIZATION (FISH)

SYNDROME	CLINICAL FEATURES IN NEWBORN PERIOD	CHROMOSOMAL LOCATION
Prader-Willi syndrome	Hypotonia, hypogenitalism	15q
Velocardiofacial/DiGeorge syndrome	Conotruncal heart defects, palatal abnormalities, ear anomalies, hypocalcemia	22q
Williams syndrome	Supravalvular aortic stenosis, hypercalcemia, full lips, periorbital fullness	7q
Miller-Dieker syndrome	Lissencephaly (smooth brain)	17p

terol level and an elevated 7-dehydrocholesterol level. Presumably, many other conditions with congenital anomalies will be found to have a biochemical basis, which will allow for more definitive diagnoses.

The neonate with ambiguous genitalia requires a battery of tests, including chromosome analysis to determine genotypic sex, pelvic ultrasound to identify internal genitalia, and endocrine testing (17-OH progesterone, testosterone, luteinizing hormone, follicle-stimulating hormone). It is best to defer assignment of sex until many of these tests have been performed and a urologist has evaluated the newborn. A psychologist can be very useful in helping the family deal with the uncertainty.

Ophthalmology evaluation also can be useful in diagnosing the neonate with congenital anomalies, especially if brain malformations or neurologic abnormalities are present. This evaluation also should be performed if small genitalia are present in a male (septo-optic dysplasia) or if features of CHARGE association are present.

The value of the postmortem examination cannot be overemphasized. A thorough evaluation by an experienced pathologist can yield findings that would not be identified otherwise and that may lead to a definitive diagnosis and thus information about recurrence risk and possible prenatal testing in future pregnancies. The role of the clinician is to educate the family on the importance of such an evaluation.

Once a thorough history has been taken, a physical examination has been performed, and appropriate testing is under way, the clinician should identify those features that are most unique (Fig. 28–28). Sometimes a pattern is readily recognized, such as Down syndrome in a child with an atrioventricular canal, hypotonia, palpebral fissures that slant up, small squared ears, and fifth finger clinodactyly. However, a review of reference texts often is required to determine whether the findings represent a previously described condition. A clinical geneticist/dysmorphologist may be especially helpful at this point. Other evaluations also may be indicated (see "Diagnostic Testing and Indications," earlier).

Sometimes a diagnosis does not become apparent until later in life as the physical features change and other structural or functional abnormalities become apparent. Parents should be counseled about this possibility and that even though a diagnosis may not be apparent, the findings may very well have a genetic basis and recurrence in future pregnancies is possible.

GENETIC COUNSELING

Genetic counseling is a communication process during which families are informed about the abnormalities present in the affected individual, with medical and genetic knowledge discussed in practical language. A description of the abnormality, the natural history, associated abnormalities, and prognosis for the disorder are provided. The etiology of the abnormality (if known), whether genetic or nongenetic, is

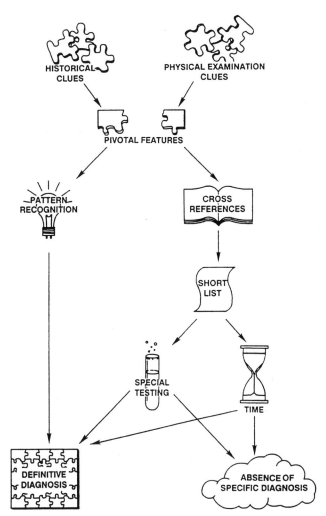

FIGURE 28–28. Diagnostic strategies: the Sherlock Holmes model. (From Aase JM: Diagnostic Dysmorphology. New York, Plenum Publishing Corp, 1990.)

explained in such a manner that the family can understand. The family also is given reassurance that the condition in the affected individual is not the fault of any individual, and information about recurrence risk is provided.

Those family members who are at increased risk of being affected or having affected offspring, as determined by pedigree analysis and etiology, are identified, and prenatal diagnostic testing, if possible, is described, including the complications and accuracy. Assistance in reaching a decision about prenatal testing and in accessing it is offered. Genetic counselors provide supportive counseling to families, assist families in coping with a lifelong condition, and serve as patient advocates. Information about appropriate community services and family support organizations also is offered.

Genetic counseling can be given by anyone willing to take the time and to make the effort. Genetic counselors, sometimes called genetic associates, are individuals with a master's degree who have been specifically trained to understand genetic disorders and congenital anomalies and to help families with the psychological and emotional adaptation to having a family member with a serious and chronic problem. Medical geneticists are physicians (or sometimes doctors of philosophy) who have received special training in genetic counseling and in the diagnosis and management of genetic disorders and birth defects.

EDUCATIONAL RESOURCES AND SUPPORT ORGANIZATIONS

With almost universal access to the Internet, the number of education resources in the genetics arena has increased greatly. In addition to more general references for the medical community, which can be helpful to families, most individual conditions now have their own websites.

Because most congenital anomalies and genetic disorders are relatively rare, usually occurring with a frequency of 1 in 1000 or less, family support organizations have been developed to help combat the isolation and grief felt by families who have or have had an affected child. These groups usually offer support and empathy and serve as a clearinghouse for information about the disorder and its management. Often they have a newsletter for members that describes helpful coping mechanisms and keeps families updated on relevant resources and research. Many have their own website and chatroom.

Such organizations often have been started by and are usually staffed by parents of affected individuals or by affected individuals themselves. As a result, they vary greatly both in the format and content of what they offer and in the accuracy of the information they distribute. Organizations for more frequent disorders, such as Down syndrome and Prader-Willi syndrome, are generally large and professionally run; offer educational forums, such as an annual conference and lay literature; keep listings of resources locally and nationally; and may even offer grant funding for research on the disorder. Smaller organizations for less common conditions may serve primarily a social and support function. Because of this variability in the knowledge of support organizations and the resultant uncertainty concerning the accuracy of information provided, it is advisable for the physician to become familiar with an organization and its functions before referring a family.

A national organization, the Alliance of Genetic Support Groups, serves as a resource to identify whether a designated organization exists for a specific condition and also lists more general organizations. The Alliance supplies contact information and data about the organizations. It prints a directory of national genetic voluntary organizations and related resources, which it updates regularly. The Alliance can be reached by calling 1-800-336-GENE. Another group, the National Organization for Rare Disorders (NORD), functions as a clearinghouse for information on genetic disorders; it will send a summary of this information written for lay individuals for a small fee, will match families, and will make medical referrals, if appropriate. NORD can be reached at 1-800-999-NORD.

SUMMARY

It is the role of the neonatologist to direct the evaluation of the newborn or stillborn with congenital anomalies. Diagnostic testing and evaluations along with consultation of references and specialists in the field, such as clinical geneticists and dysmorphologists, may be helpful. The goal is to identify the etiology so that accurate information on prognosis and recurrence risk can be shared with the family.

■ REFERENCES

1. Bolk S, et al: A human model for multigenic inheritance: Phenotypic expression in Hirschsprung disease requires both the RET gene and a new 9q31 locus. Proc Natl Acad Sci U S A 97:268, 2000.
2. Brent RL: Evaluating the alleged teratogenicity of environmental agents. Clin Perinatol 13:609, 1986.
3. Buyse ML (ed): Birth Defects Encyclopedia. Dover, Blackwell Scientific Publications, 1990.
4. Curry CJR, et al: A protocol for the investigation of pregnancy loss. Clin Perinatol 17:723, 1990.
5. Curry CJR: Pregnancy loss, stillbirth, and neonatal death: A guide for the pediatrician. Pediatr Clin North Am 39:157, 1992.
6. Delach JA, et al: Comparison of high resolution chromosome banding and fluorescence in situ hybridization (FISH) for the laboratory evaluation of Prader-Willi syndrome and Angelman syndrome. Am J Med Genet 52:85, 1994.
7. Driscoll DA, et al: Prevalence of 22q11 microdeletions in DiGeorge and velocardiofacial syndrome: Implications for genetic counseling and prenatal diagnosis. J Med Genet 30:813, 1993.
8. Emanual I, et al: The incidence of congenital malformations in a Chinese population: The Taipei collaborative study. Teratology 5:159, 1972.
9. Erickson JD: Racial variations in the incidence of congenital malformations. Ann Hum Genet 34:315, 1976.
10. Gorlin RJ, et al: Orofacial clefting syndromes: General aspects. In Gorlin RJ, et al (eds): Syndromes of the Head and Neck. New York, Oxford University Press, 1990.
11. Gorlin RJ, et al (eds): Syndromes of the Head and Neck. New York, Oxford University Press, 1990.
12. Graham JM: Smith's Recognizable Patterns of Human Deformation. Philadelphia, WB Saunders, 1988.
13. Holmes LB: Inborn errors of morphogenesis: A review of localized hereditary malformations. N Engl J Med 291:763, 1974.
14. Holmes LB: Current concepts in genetics: Congenital malformations. N Engl J Med 295:204, 1976.
15. Holt M, et al: Familial heart disease with skeletal malformations. Br Heart J 22:236, 1960.
16. Hook EB: Contribution of chromosome abnormalities to human morbidity and mortality. Cytogenet Cell Genet 33:101, 1982.
17. Hoyme HE: Teratogenically induced fetal anomalies. Clin Perinatol 17:547, 1990.
18. Irons M, et al: Defective cholesterol biosynthesis in Smith-Lemli-Opitz syndrome. Lancet 341:1414, 1993.
19. Jones KL (ed): Smith's Recognizable Patterns of Human Malformation. Philadelphia, WB Saunders, 1997.
20. Kaji T, et al: Anatomic and chromosomal anomalies in 639 spontaneous abortuses. Hum Genet 55:87, 1980.
21. Leppig KA, et al: Predictive value of minor anomalies. I. Association with major malformations. J Pediatr 110:530, 1987.
22. Lowery MC, et al: Strong correlation of elastin deletions, de-

tected by FISH, with Williams syndrome: Evaluation of 235 patients. Am J Hum Genet 57:49, 1995.

23. Marden PM, et al: Congenital anomalies in the newborn infant, including minor variations: A study of 4142 babies by surface examination for anomalies and buccal smear for sex chromatin. J Pediatr 64:357, 1964.

24. McKusick VA, et al (eds): Mendelian Inheritance in Man: A Catalog of Human Genes and Genetic Disorders. Baltimore, The Johns Hopkins University Press, 1998.

25. Mills JL: Malformations in infants of diabetic mothers. Teratology 25:385, 1982.

26. Mulvihill JJ, et al: The genesis of dermatoglyphics. J Pediatr 75:579, 1969.

27. Nelson K, et al: Malformations due to presumed spontaneous mutations in newborn infants. New Engl J Med 320:19, 1989.

28. Nelson T, et al: Collection of human embryos and fetuses. In Hook EB, et al (eds): Monitoring Birth Defects and Environ-ment: The Problem of Surveillance. New York, Academic Press, 1971.

29. Quan L, et al: The VATER association. J Pediatr 82:104, 1973.

30. Schinzel A: Catalog of Unbalanced Chromosome Aberrations in Man. Berlin, Walter de Gruyter & Co, 1983.

31. Seaver L, et al: Teratology in pediatric practice. Pediatr Clin North Am 39:111, 1992.

32. Simpson JL: Genetic causes of spontaneous abortion. Contemp Obstet Gynecol 35:25, 1990.

33. Spranger J, et al: Errors of morphogenesis: Concepts and terms. J Pediatr 100:160, 1982.

34. Stevenson RE, et al (eds): Human Malformations and Related Anomalies. New York, Oxford University Press, 1993.

35. Werler MM, et al: Periconceptional folic acid exposure and risk of occurrent neural tube defects. JAMA 269:1257, 1993.

36. Winter RM: The malformed fetus and stillbirth: Whose patient? Br J Obstet Gynaecol 90:499, 1983.

V Provisions for Neonatal Care

29 The Physical Environment

Michael H. LeBlanc*

THE THERMAL ENVIRONMENT

Protecting infants against excessive heat loss improves their chances for survival,† reduces their bodies' need to perform heat-producing metabolic work,[1, 3, 15, 37, 89] and eliminates the problems associated with rewarming of cold infants.‡

TEMPERATURE, SURVIVAL, AND DEVELOPMENT OF INCUBATORS

Although incubators can be traced back to ancient Egypt, where they were used for the hatching of chicken eggs, incubators used for human infant care did not exist until the late 1870s. The incubator was part of the primal technology in Professor Tarnier's method for enhancing the survival of prematurely born babies. The history of incubators is the history of neonatal medicine, which includes the bizarre but critically important use of incubators to display human infants in side show exhibits. Other sources provide excellent reviews of this colorful period (see also Chapter 1).[21, 101]

This chapter summarizes only the more current history of incubators, dating from 1957. It was in 1957 that Silverman and Blanc reported that premature infants who were housed in incubators humidified to more than 80% had higher survival rates than babies in incubators humidified to less than 60%.[102] The investigators speculated that these results were related to thermal differences. This belief was reinforced in 1958 when babies who were housed in humidified, convectively heated incubators survived at a greater rate when the air temperature was controlled to 32°C than when it was 29°C.[103] It must be noted that premature sick infants largely contributed to the significant differences in mortality noted in these and subsequent studies. There has been no systematic study of the effect of thermal conditions on survival of full-term infants.

In 1963, Agate and Silverman, in an attempt to

separate the salutary effect of environmental humidity from that of temperature, designed an enclosed air-temperature–controlled incubator with supplemental warmth provided by a radiant heater controlled in response to skin temperature.[2] The incubator control ensured that the infant had normal and stable body temperatures and reflected an appreciation of the specific importance of radiant heat losses in simple convectively heated incubators.

The new incubator was used to compare survival rates of premature infants of similar skin temperatures housed in an incubator of one humidity setting with those housed in an incubator of a contrasting humidity setting.[104] The results indicated that enhanced survival could not be credited to the nonthermal use of high humidity in an enclosed, radiantly heated incubator. The results do not negate other evidence that humidity control remains extremely important when warming some infants in convectively heated incubators.[6, 102]

Subsequent survival studies demonstrated a significant thermal advantage for neonates housed in radiantly heated, skin-temperature–controlled, enclosed incubators than those housed in much colder air-temperature–controlled incubators.[16, 29, 56] However, because of difficulties encountered in fabrication, the radiant heater design was replaced by the convective systems that are commercially available today.[63]

A convective heater controlled using simple or proportional control logic produces an environment markedly different from that produced in a radiantly heated incubator.[2] In a radiantly heated, enclosed incubator, the air temperature is stable because it is controlled separately; in a convectively heated skin-temperature–controlled incubator, air temperatures can vary over short periods by 3°C to 4°C and after severe disruptions by as much as 5°C to 10°C (Fig. 29–1).[2, 83] These rapid excursions in temperature have been associated with apneic spells in some premature infants.[83] The excursions in temperature are initiated by errors in the measurement of skin temperature, caused by laying the baby on the skin probe, the skin probe coming loose, or by procedures that cool the infant. The excursions are sustained in convectively heated, skin-temperature–controlled incubators by the

---

*Much of the text and all of the illustrations were taken from the previous edition of this chapter, written by Paul H. Perlstein.

†References 16, 29, 56, 86, 102–104.

‡References 17, 19, 57, 68, 83, 114.

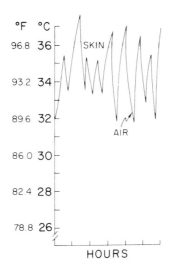

FIGURE 29–1. Typical air temperatures in a convectively heated incubator servocontrolled to maintain an infant's skin temperature at 36°C.

long delay between turning the heater on and getting the skin temperature to rise. The radiant incubator has a more rapid heating response time and thus a more stable environment. However, the controlled trials of the radiant incubator did not test a stable environment versus an unstable environment; they tested a stable warm environment versus a cold stable environment. Warm was better.[16, 29]

After observing that temperature instability caused apnea, Perlstein and coworkers designed a computer-controlled incubator to provide a more stable environment.[87] In 1976, improved survival was reported when babies were housed in computer-controlled, convectively heated incubators constrained to prevent wide thermal environmental changes.[86] The computer-controlled incubator achieved stability by controlling the average of the skin and environmental temperatures rather than just the skin temperature and, like a good nurse, adjusting the environmental temperature control point slowly (0.01°C per min) until the skin temperature was in the accepted range of 35.5°C to 36°C. This process reduced the rapid response of the system to errors in measurement of skin temperature and controlled, through the environmental temperature equation, the rapidly responsive air temperature. Although documented to enhance survival, the radiantly heated and the computer-controlled convective incubator systems are not commercially available, and the commercial incubator systems now available have not been documented to improve infant survival. The skin-temperature–servo-controlled, convectively heated incubator was not tested in clinical trials against the radiantly heated incubator. We found the skin-temperature–servo-controlled, convectively heated incubator wanting in clinical trials against the computer-controlled incubator. It is reassuring, however, that in response to available data, some manufacturers have modified their incubators and control algorithms to emulate the environmental stability of the studied devices.[18, 63]

TEMPERATURE AND HOMEOTHERMY

Babies are homeotherms who increase and decrease their heat production to maintain their internal body temperatures within a narrow range.[15, 49, 52] The consequences of prolonged and maximum heat production include the loss of life-sustaining substrates and their conversion to acidic metabolic by-products (Fig. 29–2).* Infants with apparently similar characteristics can vary significantly in their competence as homeotherms. Developmental characteristics,[49, 84, 85] sleep state,[28] normal adaptation,† central nervous system damage,[25] sedation,[23] shock, hypoxia,[24] and drugs[23, 97] all may reduce or eliminate the metabolic response to cold. After prolonged cold stress, depletion of hormonal and energy stores also may reduce homeostatic responsiveness and produce the classic signs of severe cold injury.[19, 68]

The concept of an optimum thermal environment for newborn infants evolved during the 1960s.[1, 15] This idealized setting, called the *neutral thermal environment,* is characterized as "the range of environmental temperature within which the metabolic rate is at a minimum and within which temperature regulation is achieved by non-evaporative physical processes alone."[12] Because these simple conditions can be met even by infants with low body temperatures,[1, 15] the definition, for clinical purposes, has been expanded to include a requirement that the environment must

---

*References 15, 22, 37, 89, 107, 116.
†References 38, 39, 43, 47, 85, 111.

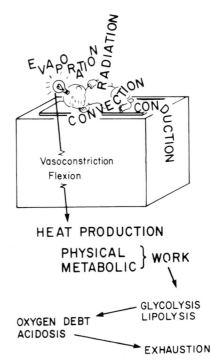

FIGURE 29–2. Homeothermy in newborns. On sensing loss of body heat, the infant minimizes heat loss from the skin and increases metabolic rate. The increase in metabolism can produce acidosis and substrate depletion.

also ensure a normal body temperature when applied to newborns.

The necessity of maintaining neutral thermal conditions has never been proved; in fact, there are physiologic arguments against the use of these conditions in generating thermal control strategies for use in newborn care.[27, 38, 43] An infant not exposed to periodic cold stress may adapt to the protective environment and lose the ability to respond by activation of brown fat when exposed to an unfamiliar cold stimulus.[38, 39, 85] However, because current technology does not provide reliable methods for creating continuous neutral thermal conditions for sustained periods of care,[61, 75, 106] this argument is not of practical importance. Additionally, in very premature infants who require the most intense care, the concept of thermoneutrality loses specific meaning, because very premature infants often cannot generate additional heat in a heat-losing environment.[53, 122]

Premature infants of less than 29 weeks' gestation may behave like poikilotherms.[122] A poikilotherm, instead of increasing heat production like a homeotherm, has a proportional decrease in metabolic rate and body temperature when in a cool environment.[12] However, very premature infants are not expected to have the elaborate mechanism that land-dwelling poikilotherms have developed to maintain enzymatic balance and membrane fluidity over a range of temperatures. In addition, vertebrate poikilotherms regulate their body temperature, but they do so solely by behavioral mechanisms. The optimum environment for very premature infants who behave like poikilotherms is not known, but it is assumed that one should at least ensure that the infant has a normal body temperature.

THE PHYSICS OF HEAT EXCHANGE

The temperature of an object is a measure of the balance between heat leaving and entering the object. Heat can be lost only from a substance that is warmer to one that is cooler; therefore, an infant loses heat only when the surrounding environment is colder than the infant.

Homeothermic infants are alerted to cold stress when thermal receptors throughout the body,[15] especially in the skin[1, 74, 88] or airways,[93] are stimulated. The face is particularly sensitive; and even when the infant's body is warm, cooling of the face causes a responsive rise in metabolic rate.[73, 100] Conversely, warming of the facial skin when the body is cold suppresses homeothermically induced hypermetabolism.[15, 73] Because the brain accounts for a large proportion of a newborn's basal heat production,[91] the skin of the head is always warm and the heat losses from the head are disproportionately large.[8, 110] Thus, the responsiveness of the thermal control system of the infant to facial temperature is appropriate.

In spite of common perceptions, body temperature alone does not predict the metabolic state of an infant[1, 15] unless the infant's temperature and the environmental temperature are stable. It is well documented that an infant with any body temperature can become hypermetabolic if the environmental temperature drops sufficiently below the skin temperature to cause a rate of heat loss exceeding the rate of heat generated by the infant's basal metabolic activity (Fig. 29–3).[1, 15] Even with a low body temperature, however, if the environmental temperature is rising or is close enough to the skin temperature to limit heat loss to a rate not exceeding the rate of basal heat production, an infant does not become hypermetabolic.[15] High body temperatures also activate distress mechanisms that produce an increase in metabolic work.[42]

An infant can limit heat loss by flexing his limbs to reduce the skin surface area exposed to the environment.[15, 120] An infant can increase the exposed body surface area by extending his limbs. This capability is compromised in premature, unconscious, sedated, or physically restrained babies. Infants also can reduce shunting of internal heat to body surfaces by vasoconstricting peripheral vessels.[54, 127] This mechanism can be defeated by shock or some autonomic drugs. An infant may generate heat by crying and becoming hyperactive when cold stressed to the point of jitteriness or shivering.[3, 15]

A cold-stressed infant primarily depends on mechanisms that cause chemical thermogenesis.[15] When an infant is stimulated by cold, norepinephrine[95, 108] is released, inducing lipolysis in brown fat stores principally found in the interscapular, paraspinal, and perirenal areas.[80] Because of the protein thermogenin, brown fat can decouple oxidative phosphorylation and break down fats to produce heat,[80] without the inhibitory feedback loop of ATP (adenosine triphosphate) production. Triglycerides in the fat are broken down to fatty acids and glycerol. The fatty acids enter thermogenic metabolic paths that end in the common pool of metabolic acids. Brown fat is turned on in response to skin thermoreceptors prior to a decrease in core temperature, and shivering is initiated by a decrease in core temperature.[15]

Glycolysis also may be stimulated during severe stress when epinephrine released from the adrenals activates glycogen stores, which may result in transient hyperglycemia.[89] Lowered blood sugars in cold-stressed infants also have been reported,[22] possibly caused by inhibition of glycolysis by lipolysis or by exhaustion of glycogen stores.

The absolute maximum or "summit" amount of heat production is affected by gestational and postnatal age and is demonstrably less during the first days of life.[15, 44, 52, 98] Both basal and maximal heat production increase dramatically in the first week of life in the term infant to adjust for the infant's high surface area–to–mass ratio (four times that of his mother). The rate of heat loss is directly proportional to the magnitude of the difference between the infant's skin temperature (TS) and the temperature of the environment (TE).[1, 62] This proportion can be expressed mathematically by introducing a constant called the thermal transfer coefficient (h), the value of which depends on the material of the substance transferring the heat. The thermal transfer coefficient describes the

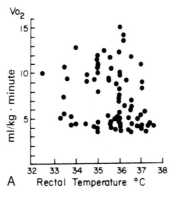
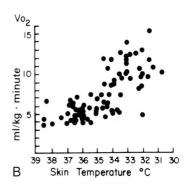

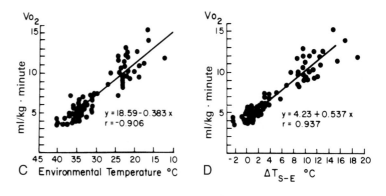

FIGURE 29–3. The relationship between oxygen consumption (VO₂) and (A) rectal temperature in various environments, (B) skin temperature in various environments, (C) environmental temperature when incubator walls and air are within ±2°C of each other, (D) the difference between skin and environmental temperatures (ΔT_{S-E}) when incubator walls and air are within ±2°C of each other. The poor correlation of skin temperature with oxygen consumption was accounted for by measurements in which environmental temperature was either rising or falling. (Modified from Adamson K Jr, et al: The influence of thermal factors upon oxygen consumption of the human infant. J Pediatr 66:495, 1965.)

rate at which heat leaves the body surface, and it is related to body shape and thickness, the thickness of the boundary layer of air surrounding the body, and the characteristic way in which tissue absorbs or reflects radiant energy.

$$\text{Heat loss} = h \times (TS - TE) \times (\text{Surface area})$$

The exposed surface area of the infant is critical in the equation used to calculate heat loss.[120] An infant who is diapered or swaddled has less exposed surface and different heat exchange characteristics than an infant who is unclothed.[17, 75] Quantitatively, the most important reason term babies have trouble staying warm is that they are born with four times the surface area–to–mass ratio of their mothers and only 1.5 times the basal metabolic heat production rate. Infants double their basal metabolic rate at a week of age. Until that time, they require a warmer temperature or more clothing than their mothers. In addition, an infant's maximal heat production increases from twice his basal metabolic rate to the adult value of four times the basal rate in the first week.[15, 44] Thus, a term baby's maximal heat production per m² (i.e., per unit of heat loss) increases from 20% of adult levels to 75% of adult levels in the first week. Premature babies make the same adjustment, but it occurs much more slowly. In places in which term newborns are exposed to cooler temperatures, severe hypothermia in infants is common.[114] The basic evolutionary response to this problem is behavioral. Babies are quite sensitive to cold. They respond behaviorally by crying and thereby elicit a holding response from their mother that places them against their mother's warm body.

Heat loss is also modified by the thermal conductance of an infant. The thermal conductance is computed using the difference between the infant's core and skin temperatures multiplied by a thermal coefficient describing the speed with which heat is transferred from the interior to the exterior of the body. This variable coefficient depends on body size, tissue composition and thickness, skin blood flow, and vascular shunting. The differences between body shapes and sizes and tissue thickness result in infants having thermal conduction and transfer coefficients that are higher than those in adults. Because of this difference in coefficients, infants lose more heat per m² than do adults in identical heat-losing environments[15, 51]; however, this is quantitatively much less important than their larger surface area–to–mass ratio.

DEFINITION OF NORMAL BODY TEMPERATURE

In 1964, Silverman and Agate defined body temperature as a weighted value in which a colonic measurement contributed 60% and a skin measurement contributed 40%.[106] For practical purposes, however, it is traditional to rely on a single-site measurement. There is no reason to believe that infants have a different normal temperature than do adults. If an infant's internal temperature is within the range of 36.5°C to 37.5°C (with a ±0.5°C diurnal variation), the infant's temperature is probably normal. Because body temperature is a measure of only the balance between heat production and net heat loss, a normal body temperature should not be confused with a "normal" metabolic rate (Fig. 29–4).[1]

INTERNAL BODY TEMPERATURE MEASUREMENTS

Although esophageal and tympanic membrane temperatures have been used in some physiologic studies,[85] rectal temperature is easier to take in a clinical setting and more traditionally equated with the infant's internal body temperature.

In measuring the rectal temperatures of newborn babies, the depth of insertion of the thermometer is very important. The difference between rectal temperature measured by a thermistor inserted 1 cm and one inserted 5 cm into the rectum can exceed 1.5°C.[58] As a corollary, serial readings should be taken at a common depth. Ideally, thermometers used for temperature transduction in babies should be accurate to ±0.1°C and have a range that spans 33°C to 40°C.

Over the years, some concern has been expressed about the danger of perforation or other injury when using rigid thermometers to transduce rectal temperatures. Measurement of axillary temperature has been suggested as a safer alternative.[14] Although axillary temperatures have been found only variably comparable to simultaneous measurement of rectal temperature, if care is taken to place the thermometer firmly in the axilla with the infant's arm held against the body of the infant, accurate and comparable temperature readings can be obtained if a sufficient period of time is allowed for the transducer to reach its maximum reading.[59] Some electronic thermometers extrapolate temperature based on the expected thermal characteristics of the patient population for which they were designed rather than directly measure the maximum reading. With this type of device, using a transducer designed for an adult on infants can result in large errors.[81]

Electronic devices using infrared sensors for measuring heat in the ear canal also are available for estimating core temperatures. As yet, the study results using these devices do not generate a level of confidence sufficient to recommend their use in neonates.[126]

The placement of a temperature-sensing device between the bare skin of an infant and the underlying mattress surface has been studied, and it appears to

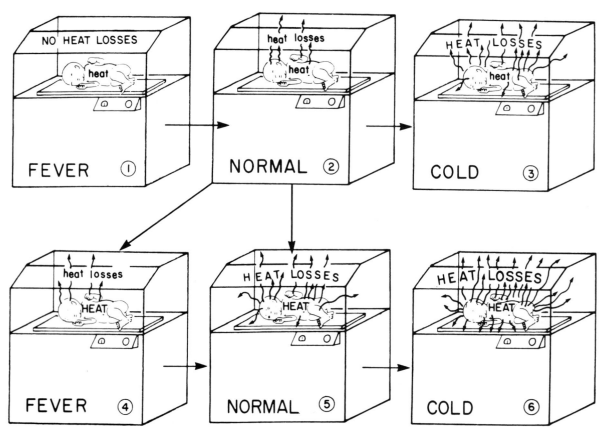

FIGURE 29–4. *1,* Fever caused by total elimination of heat losses from a minimally metabolic infant. *2,* Normal temperature when heat losses are minimized and equal to heat produced by a minimally metabolic infant (neutral thermal conditions). *3,* Hypothermia caused by large heat losses from an infant who is temporarily poikilothermic. *4,* "Fever" when heat losses are less than the heat produced by a hypermetabolic infant. *5,* Normal temperature when heat losses are large but equal to heat produced by a hypermetabolic infant. *6,* Hypothermia caused by very large heat losses that exceed the heat produced by a hypermetabolic infant. Heat, minimum heat production; HEAT, maximum heat production; FEVER, internal temperature > 37.5°C; NORMAL, internal temperature of 35.5°C to 37.5°C; COLD, internal temperature < 35.5°C.

provide another alternative for estimating core temperatures.[69] Thus, rolling the baby over so that he or she is lying on his skin temperature probe in a skin-temperature–controlled incubator or radiant warmer causes the sensor to read a core rather than a skin temperature and inappropriately causes the temperature to plummet.

SKIN TEMPERATURE MEASUREMENTS

Skin temperatures are usually measured with thermocouples or thermistors attached to the skin. These three-dimensional transducers sense the environment surrounding their tops, sides, and bottoms, and they are prone to multiple influences that can result in factitious temperature readings.[6, 30, 64] The larger the temperature difference between the infant and his environment, the greater are the artifacts. Use of a well-designed flat probe with a surface of a thermal conductor and a back of a thermal insulator generally results in adequate accuracy for clinical use. Even with poorly designed cylindrical probes, placing an insulated foam pad over the sensor in the more moderate environment of an incubator usually results in adequate accuracy.

Attachment of the skin sensor reduces evaporative water loss of the skin surrounding the probe and artificially raises the measured skin temperature in infants with large insensible water loss.[6] If the very premature infant's core temperature remains below her skin temperature after achieving thermal stability, raising the local humidity often fixes the problem.

Additionally, there is a very wide distribution of different temperatures over varying skin surface sites.[55, 84] These variations make interpretation of a single skin temperature difficult. These differences can be quite significant in a clinical setting because attachment sites sometimes must be changed to prevent skin irritation. Also, the rotation of infants into various positions requires changing attachment sites so that the infant's body does not cover the probe and cause a measurement that reflects the core temperature rather than the skin temperature.[31, 69]

In practice, it is common to move single skin probes freely so that they are always on a skin surface exposed to the environment. In search of a mean surface temperature, the transducers usually are not attached over the least and most vasoreactive body regions. Body prominences and the extremities, therefore, are the least favored attachment sites. It also is sensible to avoid placing probes on the skin over the metabolically reactive brown fat collections in the intrascapular region (Fig. 29–5).[84, 105] Additionally, attachment near heat-producing transcutaneous gas-monitoring transducers or over areas of bruised or burned skin results in false temperature measurements.[99]

ENVIRONMENTAL TEMPERATURE MEASUREMENTS

The environment in which an object resides is defined as everything that surrounds the object. For discus-

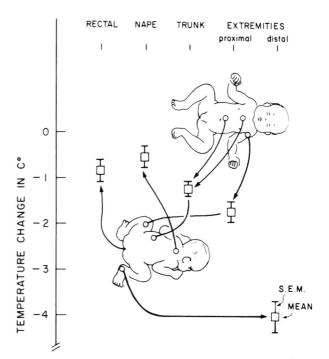

FIGURE 29–5. Cooling of skin over different body surfaces after naked infants were exposed for 1 hour to room temperatures ranging between 23°C and 29°C. Note how the nape of the neck that sits over a collection of brown fat stays much warmer than other sites. (Modified from Silverman WA, et al: Warm nape of the neonate. Pediatrics 33:984, 1964. Copyright American Academy of Pediatrics 1964.)

sion purposes, the environment can be separated into four mechanisms by which heat is lost from the body: conduction, convection, radiation, and evaporation.[62, 102]

Conductive and Convective Heat Losses

Conduction is the transfer of heat between contacting solid objects of different temperatures. Conductive heat flow is linearly proportional to the difference in temperature, the area of contact, and the thermal conductivity of the material. Thermal conductivity of common materials varies by more than 1000. Good thermal conductors are metals and water. Good thermal insulators are foam rubber, ceramic, wood, or wool. On a cold day, metal feels colder than wood because of its higher conductivity. In ordinary circumstances, heat losses by conduction can be kept to a minimum by ensuring that an infant is lying on a warm mattress of very low conductivity or that the swaddled infant is wrapped in prewarmed materials. If the mattress and swaddling materials are at the same temperature as the infant's skin, no heat loss or gain occurs by conduction. If the infant is placed on a cold table or is wrapped in a blanket at room temperature, heat losses can be large. Conversely, if an infant is placed close to a hot water bottle or heating pad that is warmer than the infant, the infant gains heat at a rate directly proportional to the temperature difference between the conductive heat source and the infant's skin. Hot, thermally conductive objects placed close to an infant's skin should not exceed 40°C to avoid skin burns.[109]

Convection can be thought of as a special subset of conduction, referring to heat exchange between a solid object and the liquid or gaseous material in the environment. When heated, air expands and rises, creating the air flow of natural convection.[65] Convective heat losses are proportional to the difference between skin and air temperatures and the area of exposed skin. Convective heat losses also are higher with higher rates of air flow.[65, 82] The effect of the air temperature is modified by an associated wind chill factor.[124] The measured air temperature should be that perceived by the infant; thus, the air temperature 5 to 10 cm from the infant's skin surface should be the temperature measured. The measurement should be close enough to reflect the air around the infant yet far enough away to measure air rather than skin temperature. Measurement of air temperatures elsewhere in an incubator vary by up to 10°C in older incubators. Current manufacturing standards allow no more than 2°C variation when the temperature is measured 10 cm above the mattress. Sometimes it is necessary to monitor multiple air temperatures that influence heat exchange over different body surfaces. When an infant is in a head hood flushed by air or oxygen, head hood temperature may be different from that in the incubator chamber.[73, 88, 100] Convective losses also include heat exchanges that occur between the respiratory system and cooler gases delivered by respirators.[113] Thus, warming and humidifying inspired gas is important to prevent convective heat loss (see Chapter 42, Part Four).

Radiant Heat Losses

Heat loss by radiation is heat loss at the speed of light from a warmer object to a cooler one with which the warmer object is not in contact. Objects can be characterized by their ability to absorb or emit energy in the infrared range of the electromagnetic spectrum. The degree to which infrared rays are absorbed or emitted is called the emissivity of an object, and emissivity can range from near 0 for a perfectly reflecting substance such as shiny silver to the value of almost 1 for a substance that, like carbon black, absorbs and emits all infrared energy received. Human skin is more like carbon than silver and is considered to have an emissivity of 1 for most purposes. When measuring the temperature of the skin by its infrared emissions, the 2% to 10% of radiant energy reflected by the skin from a very hot object like a radiant warmer heater contaminates the measurement; otherwise, assuming a skin emissivity of 1 works well. Emissivity is related more to the tissue's moisture content, texture, and porosity than to its color.

The walls of the incubator or room, the heater of the warmer, and the mattress on which the infant is lying are examples of surfaces with which babies exchange radiant heat. These routes of heat exchange are essentially independent of all other routes. An infant can get cold in a room containing air warmer than the infant's skin if the walls and windows are sufficiently cold. An infant in the warm air of an incubator can get cold if the incubator walls are cold, and an infant in an incubator with cold air can get overheated if the walls are too hot. Because of the radiant "greenhouse" effect, an infant in an incubator also can get too hot even if the incubator walls are not subjected to any obvious heating. Because the acrylic plastic walls of most incubators are opaque to infrared waves, they behave like the glass in a greenhouse through which visible short-wave light rays pass easily. On absorption of the short electromagnetic waves by the house plants, the short waves are converted into heat energy and re-emitted as long infrared rays that, upon reaching the glass inner surface, are absorbed and not transmitted. The glass is heated by the infrared energy, and this energy is re-emitted toward the plants. In this way visible light can be used to generate heat, which is trapped in the greenhouse whose contents become warmer.

It is not uncommon to find infants in incubators near windows become cold in the evening when incubator walls radiate their heat to the night-chilled glass panes. The same infants can be found overheated in the morning when the bright sun streams through glass and plastic to warm the incubator occupant. Such environmental changes can occur without causing changes in incubator air temperature. To define environmental temperature requires at least a measurement of surrounding wall temperatures with which the infant lives in radiant harmony. Because radiant exchanges are quantitatively related not only to absolute temperature gradients but also to the distance between the surfaces exchanging heat, to the solid angles of the surfaces relative to the each other, and to the emissivity of each of the radiant surfaces, no single measurement can provide anything but an approximation of an infant's radiant world.[62] When an infant is within the chamber of an enclosed incubator, however, the measurements are greatly simplified and the approximations are more believable than those made when an infant is in an open crib.[121]

Evaporative Heat Losses

With every milliliter of water that evaporates, approximately 580 calories of body heat are lost[48]; therefore, it is theoretically possible to use insensible weight loss measurements to estimate the amount of heat that an infant has lost by this mechanism. Because accurate and continuous insensible weight loss measurements are somewhat difficult to obtain, this form of monitoring is reserved for research purposes. (See also Chapter 34.)

To understand heat loss by evaporation is to appreciate the distinction that exists between humidity and vapor pressure.[112] The vapor pressure of water is the specific atmospheric pressure of water vapor at any given temperature at which water can exist in both its liquid and vaporous states. The partial pressure of water vapor is the actual pressure exerted by water vapor at any given temperature. If the partial pressure equals the vapor pressure, the vapor is saturated. If the partial pressure is less than the vapor pressure, the vapor is unsaturated. Relative humidity (RH) is a percentage expression of this degree of saturation and is computed using the following equation:

$$RH (\%) = \frac{100 \times \text{Partial pressure of water vapor}}{\text{Vapor pressure at same temperature}}$$

Although relative humidity is easy to quantitate, it is not the relative humidity that actually sets up the driving force causing evaporative water losses; it is the difference between the partial pressure of the water vapor in the boundary layers around the infant's body and the vapor pressure of water in the environment outside this boundary layer. The vapor pressure rises with higher temperature; therefore, as long as the infant's skin is warmer than the environment, evaporative losses can occur even when the humidity is 100%. Evaporative losses also can be increased by turbulent convective air currents introduced using resuscitation bags and head hoods during care.[65, 82] Quantitatively, evaporative heat loss accounts for the largest part of the difference in thermal requirements between a term infant and a preterm infant. Evaporative heat losses increase exponentially as gestational age is reduced and as the stratum corneum gets thinner.[63] Evaporative heat loss decreases exponentially as a premature infant ages.[62]

In a hot environment, adults can increase their evaporative water loss by a factor of 10, drenching their bodies with sweat. Term infants can increase their evaporative water loss by a factor of four, producing visible sweat on their brow. Preterm infants, depending on gestation, can double their evaporative water loss, but they do not produce visible sweat.[15]

HOW TO KEEP A BABY WARM

Prevention of heat loss is often best achieved by simple methods applied with common sense. Because heat loss requires the presence of a thermal gradient, the prevention of heat loss is achieved by either warming the environment or covering the baby.

The Delivery Room

An in utero fetus is warmer than the mother.[119, 123] Born wet, warm, and naked into the usual environment of a delivery room, the newborn infant loses heat rapidly. Even if the oxygen consumption of a homeothermic infant increases to the maximum possible, the heat produced is still two or three times less than the heat loss. The consequences of this heat loss depend on many factors, including the general condition of the infant at birth. Poorly protected infants tend to develop metabolic acidosis mixed with variably successful compensatory respiratory alkalosis.[37, 76, 107] Based on various methods used to protect infants, elimination of heat loss in a clinical setting can be effective, but it is seldom complete.[4, 8, 37] If no decrease in temperature occurs at delivery, babies are admitted to the nursery with a core temperature of 37.8°C.[1a] Typically, babies lose 2°C in their first half hour.

In the delivery room a large proportion of heat loss is caused by evaporation.[41, 44] The skin should be dried with warm towels and evaporative losses should be limited by using plastic bags or other swaddling materials to insulate the skin from the dry room air.[8, 63] Even with the most careful drying of the newborn, it is almost impossible to dry the hair completely. To keep the head warm, it is necessary to use caps or hooded blankets (Table 29–1).[8, 120]

To keep the resuscitation of a newborn from interfering with thermal protection, the child should be placed on a preheated radiant warmer at full heater power at the start of the resuscitation. If the child requires more than 10 minutes of resuscitation, the temperature probe should be secured to the infant to control the skin temperature.

The control of heat loss must not be loosened during the transfer of an infant from the delivery room to another care area. Even within the delivery room, the infant should remain swaddled for display to the parents. If the mother desires skin-to-skin contact with her infant, they should be swaddled together under warm blankets (see Chapter 32). The use of another person as a heat source for keeping a newborn warm has been popularly termed *kangaroo care* and seems to be effective when it is applied appropriately.[20, 78] In transferring a sick baby to the neonatal intensive care unit, the caretaker should be sure that the transport incubator is prewarmed and that the hot air in the transport incubator is not allowed to escape by widely opening the incubator to place the baby inside.

The Nursery

Swaddling may be an ancient practice, but it is not archaic. In fact, it is a simple and effective method for keeping larger babies warm who do not need to be unclothed for procedures or observation.[4, 39, 50] Infants who are swaddled can be maintained in cooler ambient environments and can tolerate wider variations in environmental temperatures than infants who are naked.[50] Nonetheless, swaddling alone does not keep small preterm infants warm at room temperature, and even term babies require additional heat if they must be exposed for observation. The alternatives when more heat is needed can be reduced to three common choices:

1. Warm the room.
2. Place the infant in a warm, enclosed incubator.
3. Place the infant under an open radiant heater.

THE WARM ROOM.   Heating a room to 36°C or 37°C to keep some small and sick infants warm may distress personnel working in the nursery. These conditions also may be unfavorable for larger and healthier in-

TABLE 29–1   POSTNATAL TEMPERATURE DECREASE WITHIN 30 MINUTES WITH VARIOUS METHODS FOR LIMITING HEAT LOSS

METHOD	SOURCE OF DATA	30-MINUTE TEMPERATURE (°C)*	30-MINUTE FALL IN TEMPERATURE (°C)†
Infant placed in crib 30–40 cm under 60 W bulb covered with warm blanket; later dressed and put in incubator	Miller et al[76]	35.5 ± 2.6	2.6
Infant placed in preheated crib, covered loosely with warm blanket, and then bathed, dressed, and swaddled	Miller et al[76]	35.6 ± 0.14	2.5
Infant swaddled in warm dry towel	Baum et al[4]	36.1 ± 0.59	2.0
Infant dried, placed in incubator (procedures through portholes)	Miller et al[76]	36.2 ± 0.15	1.9
Naked infant, 80 cm under 750 W radiant heater	Besch et al[8]	36.2 ± 0.10	1.9
Transparent swaddler without head shield	Besch et al[8]	36.2 ± 0.11	1.9
Naked infant, 64 cm under 400 W radiant heater	Du et al[31]	36.4 ± 0.16	1.7
Silver swaddler	Baum et al[4]	36.6 ± 0.61	1.5
Transparent swaddler with head shield	Besch et al[8]	36.9 ± 0.09	1.2
Transparent swaddler with head shield and 750 W radiant heater at 80 cm	Besch et al[8]	37.3 ± 0.11	0.8

Modified from Besch NJ, et al: The transparent baby bag: A shield against heat loss. N Engl J Med 284:125, 1971.
*Mean ± standard error of the mean.
†From fetal intrauterine temperature of 38.1°C.

fants in the same area. For long-term care, heating and humidifying nurseries to appropriate temperatures is probably the least desirable method for limiting heat losses from infants, although in short-term situations such as in radiology departments, operating rooms, and treatment rooms, this method of protection can be the most applicable and effective. Raising the room temperature to meet the needs of a small infant is an important responsibility of those who deliver infants at home. Ambulances used for transportation between institutions should always be warmed before initiating the transfer. Wrapping a small swaddled infant in a heated water pad controlled to a temperature of 40°C or less and adjusted with continuous measurement of skin and core temperatures can be used for brief periods, whereas warming the room or using a radiant heater are impractical.

CONVECTIVELY HEATED INCUBATORS. Convectively heated incubators create a microclimate in which to care for an individual infant.[18] They provide a single- or double-layer plastic-walled chamber in which an infant is placed on an insulating mattress. The plastic walls of the chamber can be opened or have portholes in various places to provide hand access to the enclosed infant. All convectively heated incubators use fans to force filtered room air at various rates of flow over relatively large heaters and, in some devices, pans that can be filled with water to increase environmental humidity. The heating of incubator air can be controlled by a feedback loop mechanism referenced to the temperature within the chamber itself or elsewhere in the air stream that heats the chamber. The heating also can be controlled in a feedback loop that

references the heater-on or heater-off decision to a narrow band of infant skin temperatures. Proportional control is when the heater output is proportional to the difference between the set and the measured skin temperature within this band. Some incubators use more complicated digital or analog control schemes.[63] All incubators should have an upper limit of air temperature beyond which an alarm will sound and the heater will turn off. This prevents overheating the infant if the temperature probe becomes dislodged. Only a few studies of the differences between various convectively heated incubators have been published, but they all confirm that general statements assuming homogeneity in the environments produced are somewhat naive.[63]

The differences become very clear when comparing how different incubators react when their control systems and environmental chambers are subjected to influences that potentially disrupt their integrity. It is important to know how far an incubator can be opened without lowering the environmental temperature. Care should be provided in a way that does not cool the incubator, which usually means opening only the portholes and not the front wall of the incubator. In maintaining incubator air temperatures, positioning of the sensing thermistor may make it vulnerable to situations that might cause false temperature recordings. For example, a poorly placed air temperature probe may be warmed by a covering of diapers and blankets lying in the incubator or artificially cooled by a stream of cold oxygen from a resuscitation bag placed carelessly next to the infant.

In general, although incubator chambers can be cooled rapidly, they take a relatively long time to reach a stable thermal equilibrium during warming;

therefore, the incubator should be warmed before placing an infant within the chamber. A prewarmed incubator should always be ready and available in anticipation of the arrival of a sick infant. Prewarming an incubator so that the air is at 36°C produces a thermal environment of approximately 35°C, which is sufficient to reduce heat loss from most infants. Very premature infants, however, may require chamber temperatures in excess of 38°C to remain warm. If oxygen is to be administered by head hood or respirator, the gas humidification chambers also should be prewarmed.

Because the initial care provided a sick infant ordinarily requires multiple entries into the incubator chamber, it is reasonable, especially when caring for very small infants, to provide the infant with some form of additional thermal protection. This protection can be provided by increasing the incubator humidity to maximum levels,[46] keeping the infant partially swaddled with the head covered with a cap,[8, 110] or using a supplementary portable radiant heat source over the incubator top (Fig. 29–6). Heating the mattress area also can be used to provide the infant with additional warmth.[115] Overprotection must be avoided,[17, 42] and the initial focus of thermal control should simply be the prevention of heat loss without excessive concern about optimizing the environment for long-term care.

After stabilizing the infant, various guidelines can be used when adjusting incubator temperatures for infants of various sizes and ages.[18, 44, 94] No available guidelines, however, negate the need to measure and record the infant's core and skin temperatures along with incubator air temperatures periodically, if not

continuously. Orders should specify the desired ranges for both incubator and infant temperatures and for the site of air temperature measurement, which should be that perceived by the infant. If not already incorporated as part of the incubator control equipment, many types of relatively inexpensive electronic thermometers can be purchased to make these measurements. The incubator temperature should be increased and decreased about 0.5°C per hour as needed to maintain the infant's temperature within the specified normal range either by the nurses or by the incubator control algorithm. Because of the possible induction of apnea, rapid and large changes in temperature[83] and humidity[86] should be prevented, especially when the incubator houses a small, sick premature infant. If a simple proportion control incubator is used, air control produces a more stable and predictable environment than does skin control.[7]

Controlling a convective heater by a simple or proportional control algorithm to maintain an infant's skin temperature at a specified level is best reserved for healthier, more mature infants. Because body warming is offset by environmental cooling in a skin-temperature–controlled incubator, an infant who becomes hypermetabolic[13] because of sepsis may not become febrile, thus disguising the infant's problem. It is therefore imperative that careful records of skin and environmental temperatures be maintained to diagnose when an infant becomes infected. When using skin control, the thermistor probe must be firmly attached to the skin and carefully protected against artifacts that might interfere with the accurate transduction of the infant's true temperature.[64, 70, 99] For most babies a skin temperature in the range of 36.0°C

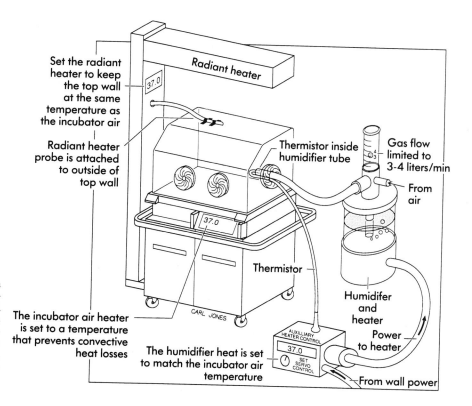

FIGURE 29–6. The method for using a radiant heater and an auxiliary humidification source to augment the thermal protection of very small and cold infants in an enclosed convectively heated incubator. This enhanced system provides independent control over the radiant, evaporative, and convective environmental components.

to 36.5°C provides a suitable environment. In one study, more apneic spells were observed in premature infants whose skin temperatures were controlled to 36.8°C than those whose skin temperatures were controlled to 36°C.[26]

During the ongoing monitoring of incubators in a busy intensive care nursery, incubators were found to be out of predictable control more than 10% of the time because of unrecognized events that interfered with equipment's proper functioning.[87] Alarm systems can and have been designed to warn of such disruptions, but only an understanding of incubator frailty, constant awareness, and unflagging attentiveness can reduce the occurrence of these alarm conditions and the exposure of incubated infants to unintended hazards. In addition, enclosed incubators can be protective only when they are kept closed. If the limits of skill and requirements of care preclude keeping the incubator closed during care procedures, use of open radiantly heated beds should be considered.

CONVECTIVE HEATING AND THERMONEUTRALITY. The only way to certify that an infant with a normal body temperature is in a neutral thermal environment is to continuously monitor the infant's metabolic rate. This monitoring is usually performed by measuring the infant's oxygen consumption, which requires techniques not suited for ongoing clinical care.[98] To approximate thermoneutrality, the caretaker should set an infant's incubator temperature to the estimated thermoneutral temperature based on published charts, then adjust the air temperature to maintain the infant's skin temperature and core temperature in the acceptable ranges. Based on data available, it is probable that an infant is in a minimum metabolic state if the incubator environment is stable and the baby's skin temperature is between 36°C and 36.5°C. Given the individual variation in neutral thermal skin temperatures[67] and artifacts in the measurement of surface temperature,[6, 64] a baby's physiologic responses to the environmental temperature should also be considered. A baby who is lying spread-eagle and has warm, flushed hands and feet and sweat on his brow perceives his environment as too hot regardless of what his temperature is. A baby who appears hunched, is fully flexed with cold and blue hands and feet, and is shivering and crying perceives his environment as too cold regardless of what his temperature is. As the infant ages, his basal heat production increases (Fig. 29–7)[92, 98] and his evaporative heat losses decrease.[62] Evaporative heat loss can change dramatically in the first two weeks of life. For infants of more than 1000 gm at birth, Scopes has provided the most complete data for helping resolve this problem of changing requirements with age and has reduced his observations to guidelines for incubator temperature settings. These guidelines include expected temperature ranges for infants who are undressed and infants who are swaddled (cot nursed) during care[96] (Fig. 29–8). Other guidelines exist for very small premature infants who may require envi-

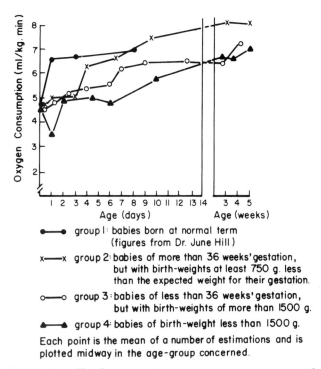

FIGURE 29–7. The change in minimum oxygen consumption with age. (From Scopes JW: Metabolic rate and temperature control in the human body. Br Med Bull 22:88, 1966.)

ronmental temperatures higher than their skin and core temperatures to remain warm[92] (Table 29–2).

OVERHEAD (OPEN) RADIANTLY HEATED BEDS. The use of overhead radiant heaters to keep infants warm has become popular because they provide unimpeded access to infants receiving intensive care. Overhead radiant heaters are usually high-energy heat sources that require the use of skin servocontrol to ensure that infants do not become overheated when under their influence. The only exception to this requirement is when radiant heaters are used to protect infants for short periods immediately after birth. The heat loss from the wet body of a freshly delivered newborn is sufficiently great to balance even the heat provided by the 60 mW/cm² potential in the most powerful radiant heaters. It is good that this balance exists, because the attachment of a skin servocontrol probe to the amniotic fluid–covered skin of a baby can be very difficult, and temperatures recorded may be unreliable.

Because of the known risk of causing hyperthermia when using a radiant heater, manufacturers have been improving the alarm logic in heater control designs. There also are provisions for silencing alarms. Failure to reactivate silenced alarms may expose infants under radiant heaters to a subsequent risk of severe hyperthermia; thus, the safe use of a radiant heater requires an informed awareness of the specific way that the alarms operate when the heater is used. Most radiant warmers sound an alarm if the probe is more than 0.5°C above or below the desired control temperature (a broken wire in a probe is read as off scale

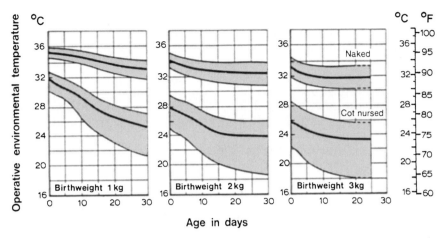

Age in days

FIGURE 29–8. The usual ranges of environmental temperatures needed to provide warmth for infants weighing 1 to 3 kg at birth in draft-free, uniform-temperature surroundings at 50% relative humidity; upper curves represent naked infants, lower curves represent swaddled, "cot-nursed" babies. *Thick lines,* Usual "optimum" temperature; *shaded area,* range within which to maintain normal temperature without increasing heat production or evaporative water loss by more than 25%. The operative environmental temperature inside a single-walled incubator is less than the internal air temperature recorded by the thermometer; the effective environmental temperature provided by the incubator can, however, be estimated by subtracting 1°C from the air temperature for each 7°C the incubator air temperature exceeds room temperature. (From Hey EN: The care of babies in incubators. In Gairdner D, et al (eds): Recent Advances in Paediatrics, 4th ed. London, Churchill Livingstone, 1971.)

low), which means that an alarm sounds for the common event of displacement of the skin probe from the skin. If the skin probe comes off the skin slowly, the heater output gradually increases and the baby is overheated by the time the alarm sounds and the condition is corrected. After the probe is reattached the alarm sounds because now the skin is too warm. A well-designed warmer allows the alarm to be silenced but rearms it within 15 minutes. Because rare events like total malfunction of the control system of the warmer can occur with the heater on, the caretaker must understand the cause of the alarm and correct it before silencing the alarm. To help decide if the warmer is functioning properly, one must ask

what should the heater be doing at this skin temperature. You should then place your hand beneath the heater to verify that the heater is doing what it is supposed to be doing. The proper attachment of a thermistor probe to the skin of an infant under a radiant heater remains undefined. Various authoritative opinions have been expressed that support techniques of attachment that both maximally and minimally shield the probe from the infrared energy emitted by the heater element. Because insulated probes do provide different information than do exposed probes, a technique consistent with the manufacturer's instructions is recommended during the care of any infant.

TABLE 29–2   APPROXIMATE INCUBATOR AIR TEMPERATURES (°C) FOR VERY PREMATURE INFANTS IN INCUBATORS HUMIDIFIED TO AT LEAST 30%

GESTATIONAL AGE (wks)	POSTNATAL AGE (wks)						
	1	**2**	**3**	**4**	**5**	**6**	**7**
25	38.0	37.7	37.5	37.2	36.9	36.6	36.3
26	37.7	37.4	37.1	36.8	36.6	36.3	36.0
27	37.3	37.1	36.8	36.5	36.2	35.9	35.7
28	37.0	36.7	36.4	36.2	35.9	35.6	35.3
29	36.7	36.4	36.1	35.8	35.5	35.3	35.0
30	36.3	36.0	35.8	35.5	35.2	34.9	34.6
31	36.0	35.7	35.4	35.1	34.9	34.6	34.3
32	35.6	35.4	35.1	34.8	34.5	34.2	34.0
33	35.3	35.0	34.7	34.5	34.2	33.9	33.6
34	35.0	34.7	34.4	34.1	33.8	33.6	33.3
35	34.6	34.3	34.1	33.8	33.5	33.2	32.9
36	34.3	34.0	33.7	33.4	33.2	32.9	32.6

The radiantly heated open bed is unquestionably convenient and allows superior access to the infant compared with the enclosed convectively heated incubator. Data exist, however, to suggest some special problems to consider when using a radiant heat source. Infants under radiant heaters have higher insensible losses of water than do infants housed in enclosed incubators (see Chapter 34, Part One).[121, 125] The fluid and electrolyte management of infants under radiant heaters must be modified from that provided to infants housed in enclosed incubators. Because the fluid losses immediately after birth vary widely from infant to infant and change more gradually as the infant ages, the specific replacement requirements can be determined only by carefully and frequently assessing the needs of each infant. Either frequent body weights or frequent serum sodium levels should be assessed in the first few days in infants of less than 28 weeks' gestation who are nursed under radiant warmers. Using the simplifying assumption that in the first few days total body sodium stays constant and thus changes in serum sodium reflect changes in total body water, a ratio of approximately 6 mL total body water change per kg body weight per mEq change in sodium concentration can be derived. Some improvement of the fluid loss problem is possible by using polyurethane membranes or lotions to cover the baby's skin.[60, 63, 117] Alternatively, a plastic heat shield can reduce insensible water loss under a radiant heater.[34] Either a small chamber around the baby is created that the evaporation from the infant humidifies or a larger chamber is created to contain external humidity.[125] For the warmer to work as designed, the top wall of the constructed chamber should be transparent to the emitted energy of the warmer.[61] Although most plastic films provide adequate transparency, pure polyethylene (GLAD wrap) is the most transparent. If a very immature infant cannot be kept warm under a radiant warmer, raising the humidity around the infant or otherwise reducing his evaporative water losses is usually the answer. When plastic sheeting is used as a barrier to evaporation, hyperthermia can occur if the skin probe gradually becomes dislodged from the skin and attaches to the plastic.[70] The plastic sheeting should not be placed close enough to the skin probe to allow this to happen. A good practical approach is to swaddle the child in plastic wrap until the initial procedures are competed, exposing only the needed body parts. Thereafter, a humidified box should be made by lifting the plastic off the skin.

The introduction of radiant heating has provided a valuable alternative way to keep infants warm. In some settings this is the only controllable way to protect them against heat loss.

RADIANT HEATING AND THERMONEUTRALITY. A meta-analysis of studies comparing oxygen consumption of premature babies in incubators and radiant warmers,[61] both controlled to provide the same abdominal skin temperature, show a slightly higher metabolic requirement in the radiant warmers. The babies nursed in the radiant warmers also had cooler foot temperatures, which may reflect differences in the relationship of abdominal skin temperature to mean skin temperature; that is, babies nursed in radiant warmers may have a lower mean skin temperature than babies nursed in incubators if they both have the same abdominal skin temperature. Consistent with this, there is evidence that a skin temperature of 36.5°C ± 0.5°C rather than 36.0°C ± 0.5°C is needed for minimal metabolic rate in a radiant warmer.[6] Particular infants may have a neutral thermal skin temperature at or beyond either of these extremes in either device. Errors in skin temperature measurement are more important in infants in radiant warmers because the thermal gradients between the infant's skin and various parts of his environment are much larger with a radiant warmer.[5, 64]

THE COLD INFANT

Simply stated, infants get cold when heat losses exceed heat production. Defining a specific temperature beneath which an infant can be declared to be cold is less simple. An infant with homeothermic responses may become hypermetabolic and acidotic if the body temperature cools from 37°C to 36°C. Because such an infant is responding to cooling, it would be justifiable to believe that this infant with a body temperature of 36°C is cold. Assume that the same infant is now cooled further to 35°C and then rewarmed to 36°C. The infant at this same body temperature of 36°C is no longer hypermetabolic.[1] Is the 36°C body temperature in this warming infant still to be considered cold? Because of such dilemmas, it is better to define hypothermia using dynamic rather than static criteria. In general, an infant is cold only if the baby senses the heat loss as a stress and responds with a metabolic increase in heat production. As the normal rise in temperature that occurs because of the specific dynamic action of food is not considered to be fever, the normal drop in body temperature that occurs when an infant falls asleep should not be considered hypothermia. The use of the word "cold" implies that the condition is potentially or actually harmful. When cold is used as a sign of infant condition, it requires further study to determine if the sign reflects a true symptom from the infant's perspective. One infant with a body temperature of 35.5°C may be hyperactive, vasoconstricted, tachypneic, tachycardic, hypermetabolic, and acidotic. Another with the same temperature may be sleeping and content. It is difficult to believe that similar meaning is contained when cold is applied as a description of their conditions.

In spite of a common perception, there is no clear basis for including hypothermia as a subtle sign of sepsis. This idea has never been proved, although an infant may not become hypermetabolic and febrile when septic because of reduced responsiveness to bacterial pyrogens. Profound sepsis, however, that produces shock and vasodilatation can increase heat loss while suppressing an infant's normal homeothermic reactions. Such an infant, although previously able to maintain a warm body temperature in a cool environment, may get colder in the same environment. To decipher the meaning of each of these situations when examining an infant with a lower-than-usual body temperature requires more investigation than is possible using only a thermometer. Although the lower limit of normal temperature is frequently cited as being 36°C, individual variation beyond this value does exist.

Helping a Cold Infant Rewarm

Debates about the comparative virtues of rapid versus slow rewarming procedures notwithstanding, there is no convincing argument available to certify any method as better than another. Published arguments are based on evidence from uncontrolled studies.[57, 79] The only controlled study showed no difference in outcome for slow or rapid rewarming.[114] Because rewarming some infants may induce apnea, an infant should be constantly observed and the environment carefully analyzed and controlled during the rewarming process.[83] As a first step in rewarming, a heat-gaining environment should be produced to eliminate any further significant heat losses from the infant. In a radiant warmer, set the skin temperature to 36.5°C to produce rapid rewarming and to 1°C above the core temperature to produce slow rewarming. The existence of a heat-gaining environment can be certified only if the infant begins to get warmer. In an incubator, simply warming the air temperature to a level that is higher than the infant's temperature is inadequate. The actual environmental temperature in a convectively heated, single-walled incubator is probably 1° to 2°C less than the measured air temperature.[44, 45]

Evaporative losses should be minimized by raising the incubator's humidity.[46] In small infants in radiant warmers, raise the humidity around the infant or otherwise reduce his evaporative heat loss. Radiant losses in incubators should be minimized by protecting the incubator walls from excessive cooling or by use of an inner heat shield.[45] If evaporative and radiant losses are minimized, the absolute air temperature becomes more meaningful.

A temperature-monitoring thermistor or thermometer should be suspended directly in the air over the infant's body to measure actual incubator air temperature. Air temperature of 36°C usually provides a sufficient heat-gaining gradient for any infant with a skin temperature below 35°C. The gradient also should be sufficiently narrow to prevent too rapid transfer of heat from the environment to the infant. The goal is to produce an environment in which the infant is rewarmed by the heat actually generated by the infant. Excessive external warming of an infant tends to cause vasodilation of the skin vessels,[42, 54, 72, 127] which can result in shunting and pooling of blood to a degree that produces decreases in blood pressure. Continual monitoring of the rewarming infant's core temperature can be used to certify that heating of the skin temperature has not become excessive. The rate of warming should be such that the skin temperature is never more than 1°C warmer than the coexisting core temperature.

If in this initial environment the infant's temperature ceases to decrease or slowly begins to increase, maintain the settings at that level and continue monitoring all temperatures. If the temperature of the infant continues to decrease, raise the incubator temperature 1°C to 37°C, and look for any previously undiscovered source of heat loss (Fig. 29–9). If within 15 minutes the body temperature has not stabilized when the air temperature is 37°C, raise the air temper-

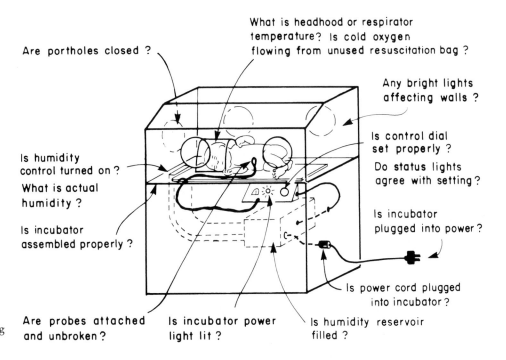

What is headhood or respirator temperature? Is cold oxygen flowing from unused resuscitation bag?

Are portholes closed ?

Any bright lights affecting walls ?

Is humidity control turned on ? What is actual humidity ?

Is incubator assembled properly ?

Is control dial set properly ? Do status lights agree with setting?

Is incubator plugged into power ?

Is power cord plugged into incubator ?

Are probes attached and unbroken ?

Is incubator power light lit ?

Is humidity reservoir filled ?

FIGURE 29–9. Troubleshooting an incubator.

ature to 38°C and, assuming that a heat sink still exists, look again for any further potential causes of the heat loss. In these searches, incubator humidity should be measured and certified to be at a level of more than 70%.

Heating an incubator to an air temperature of more than 38°C is sometimes difficult because of overriding safety thermostats built into most incubators. If the source of heat loss escapes discovery when the air temperature is at 38°C, this failure does not provide reason to allow an infant to continue to cool. The infant can be swaddled, or a radiant heater can be suspended over the incubator and, with the probe attached to the outside of the top wall of the plastic chamber, controlled to raise the incubator wall temperature slowly by 1°C increments until heat losses are completely offset. If an infant becomes apneic during rewarming, the rate of warming should be slowed. On occasion, it may be necessary to halt the warming process completely for a period to allow the infant to adjust to the new conditions, even though the infant may still be hypothermic (see Fig. 29–6).

THE BABY WHO IS TOO HOT

There are many important studies on the physiologic significance of fever.[3, 13, 17, 42, 95] Most neonatal thermoregulatory studies have focused on the effects, prevention, and amelioration of hypothermia. Hyperthermia has been noted primarily as a sign of hypermetabolism when an infant is septic or otherwise stimulated. It is probably beneficial to cool an infant who has become febrile because of exposure to an overheated environment. Whether it is good to cool infants who are febrile because they are septic or otherwise stressed by internal conditions is less clear, although it is usually attempted.

An infant with a body temperature higher than 37.5°C often is considered to be abnormally warm. To determine whether the elevated temperature is caused by an increase in heat production, which might occur if the infant is septic, or by a decrease in heat loss, some simple presumptive clinical measures can be made.

A physiologically competent infant responds to overheating from a hot environment by incorporating heat-losing mechanisms.[42] The infant's skin vessels dilate, the infant may appear flushed, the infant's hands and feet are suffused and warm, and the infant assumes a spread-eagle posture. Evaporative losses increase and, though they are uncommonly observed in premature infants, active sweating may be noted in the full-term infant.[35] If the heat stress is severe, the infant may begin to protest and complain, becoming hyperactive and irritable.[17, 42] During rapid warming the skin of the infant is warmer than the infant's core temperature.[54, 72]

An infant who is febrile because of an increase in endogenous heat production reflects a state of stress. The febrile infant, during the phase of rising temperature, perceives his environment to be too cold. The infant is vasoconstricted, and compared with the skin

on the trunk, the extremities appear pale and blue and feel cold. Unlike the gradients expected in overheated infants, the core temperature of the hypermetabolic infant is warmer than the skin temperature.

Simultaneous measurements of rectal, abdominal skin, and foot temperatures often help to distinguish the term infant who is febrile because of iatrogenic overheating from the infant who is hypermetabolic because of sepsis or stimulating drugs. In the afebrile and minimally metabolic infant, the abdominal skin temperature is usually no more than 1°C to 2°C cooler than the infant's rectal temperature. The term infant's foot temperature is no more than 2°C to 3°C colder than the abdominal skin temperature. In the febrile and hypermetabolic infant, the rectal temperature is warmer than the skin temperature, and the foot temperature is more than 3°C colder than the abdominal skin temperature. In the overheated infant, the rectal temperature is the same or colder than the skin temperature, and the foot temperature is less than 3°C cooler than the abdominal skin temperature.[72] Because a baby responds rapidly to environmental temperature, for this analysis to work, one must look at the infant at the time the hyperthermia is discovered, not 30 minutes later. Babies younger than 24 hours of age who are hyperthermic are almost always overheated rather than hypermetabolic.

WEANING FROM AN INCUBATOR TO AN OPEN CRIB

When the processes of care no longer require an infant to be naked, the infant can be swaddled.[96] If the neutral thermal environment of a swaddled infant of the infant's age, weight, and maturity includes room temperature, the infant can be weaned to a crib.[71, 96] When the infant is mature and healthy enough to compensate for the increased metabolic rate by increasing caloric intake,[39, 75] it is acceptable to allow the infant to be slightly hypermetabolic provided the core temperature is normal.

THE NONTHERMAL ENVIRONMENT

SOUND

Infants in incubators are exposed to continuous noise levels of 50 to 86 dB, with frequent peaks that can reach levels of 90 to 100 dB and beyond.[9] The sounds associated with routine care, paging systems, radios and the addition of each new piece of life-support equipment can add 15 to 20 dB to the background noise.[36, 66] The American Academy of Pediatrics (AAP) has recommended that efforts be directed toward reducing the known high levels of noise in nurseries.[2a] The industrial standard that allows the exposure of workers to 90 dB for an 8-hour day is probably too generous when establishing criteria for infants. Young animals, including humans, suffer auditory damage at much lower sound levels than do adults of their species.[11, 32, 36, 66, 77] From animal studies, drugs commonly used in the nursery, such as diuretics and antibiotics, are known to potentiate noise-induced hearing loss.[10] Whether noise can potentiate the effects of other suspected or known causes of hearing loss, including that associated with hypoxic-ischemic encephalopathy, hyperbilirubinemia, and infectious agents such as cytomegalovirus, is still undocumented.[9]

Sounds, especially impact sounds, can cause some infants to become hypoxic as part of a startle response.[66] These sounds can be produced as part of normal care processes such as opening and closing incubator doors or as by-products of hospital paging systems or can result when equipment alarms are activated. Nurseries are too noisy, and the recommendation by the AAP committee to reduce these noise levels to less than 70 dB is sensible.[77] Both background sound levels and impact noises can be reduced by asking personnel to care for the infants more quietly. Respirator alarms are especially loud and can be silenced during airway suctioning and other care by temporarily using a plug to seal the open patient connector that produces the alarm. (See also Chapter 40.)

LIGHT

With rare exception, the lighting, the colors, the decorations, and the windows with a view in nurseries are examples of environmental factors designed to suit the observational and psychological needs of adults who provide infants with care. Daylight-simulating illumination enhances the ability to observe color and other changes that occur in sick infants. It is, however, unclear whether the illumination is otherwise beneficial or harmful to the infants, although the high-level illumination of most special care nurseries almost certainly is perceived by the infants. However, early data suggesting that a link exists between background nursery light levels and the occurrence of retinopathy of prematurity in premature human infants[33, 40] has been disproved.[90] Optimal illumination in the nursery is discussed elsewhere in the book (see Chapter 26, Part Two).

MERCURY TOXICITY

(See also Chapter 12.)

Because thermometer breakage may cause toxic mercury levels in incubator air, mercury thermometers should not be used in incubators.[118]

■ REFERENCES

1. Adamsons K Jr, et al: The influence of thermal factors upon oxygen consumption of newborn human infants. J Pediatr 66:495, 1965.
1a. Adamsons K Jr, Towell ME: Thermal homeostasis in the fetus and newborn. Anesthesiology 26:531, 1965.
2. Agate FJ, Silverman WA: The control of body temperature in the human premature infant by low energy infrared radiation. Anat Rec 136:152, 1963.
2a. American Academy of Pediatrics and the American College of Obstetricians: Guidelines for Perinatal Care, 4th ed. Elk Grove Village, IL, 1997.
3. Bach V, et al: Regulation of sleep and body temperature in response to cool and warm environments in neonates. Pediatrics 93:789, 1994.
4. Baum JD, et al: The silver swaddler: Device for preventing hypothermia in the newborn. Lancet 1:672, 1968.
5. Baumgart S: Radiant heat loss versus radiant heat gain in premature neonates under radiant warmers. Biol Neonate 57:10, 1990.
6. Belgaumkar TK, et al: Effects of low humidity on small premature infants in servocontrol incubators. I. Decrease in rectal temperatures. Biol Neonate 26:337, 1975.
7. Bell EF, et al: Air versus skin temperature servo control of infant incubators. J Pediatr 103:954, 1983. (See also: Reply to editorial correspondence. J Pediatr 104:958, 1984.)
8. Besch NJ, et al: The transparent baby bag: A shield against heat loss. N Engl J Med 284:121, 1971.
9. Bess FH, et al: Further observations on noise levels in infant incubators. Pediatrics 63:100, 1979.
10. Bhattacharyya JK, et al: Ototoxicity and noise-drug interaction. J Otolaryngol 13:361, 1984.
11. Bhattacharyya JK, et al: Age related cochlear toxicity from noise and antibiotics: A review. J Otolaryngol 15:15, 1985.
12. Bligh J, et al: Glossary of terms for thermal physiology. J Appl Physiol 35:941, 1973.
13. Bonadio WA, et al: Relationship of fever magnitude to rate of serious bacterial infections in neonates. J Pediatr 116:733, 1990.
14. Brown PJ, et al: Taking an infant's temperature: Axillary or rectal thermometer? N Z Med J 105:309, 1992.
15. Bruck K: Heat production and temperature regulation. In Stave U (ed): Perinatal Physiology. New York, Plenum Publishing Corp, 1978.
16. Buetow KC, et al: Effect of maintenance of "normal" skin temperature on survival of infants of low birth weight. Pediatrics 34:163, 1964.
17. Cheng TL, et al: Effect of bundling and high environmental temperature on neonatal body temperature. Pediatrics 92:238, 1993.
18. Chessex P, et al: Environmental temperature control in very low birth weight infants cared for in double-walled incubators. J Pediatr 113:373, 1988.
19. Cohen IJ, et al: Thrombocytopenia of neonatal cold injury. J Pediatr 104:620, 1984.
20. Colonna F, et al: The "kangaroo-mother" method: Evaluation of an alternative model for the care of low birth weight newborns in developing countries. Int J Gynaecol Obstet 31:335, 1990.
21. Cone TE: History of the care and feeding of the premature infant. Boston, Little, Brown & Co, 1985.
22. Cornblath J, Schwartz R: Disorders of carbohydrate metabolism in infancy. In Cornblath J, Schwartz R (eds): Major Problems in Clinical Pediatrics, vol 3, Philadelphia, WB Saunders, 1966.
23. Cree JE, et al: Diazepam in labour: Its metabolism and effect on the clinical condition and thermogenesis of the newborn. Br Med J 3:251, 1973.
24. Cross K, et al: The gaseous metabolism of the newborn infant breathing 15 percent oxygen. Acta Paediatr Scand 47:217, 1958.
25. Cross K, et al: Lack of temperature control in infants with abnormalities of the central nervous system. Arch Dis Child 46:437, 1971.
26. Daily WJ, et al: Apnea in premature infants: Monitoring incidence, heart rate changes, and an effect of environmental temperature. Pediatrics 43:510, 1969.
27. Daniel SS, et al: Hypothermia and the resuscitation of asphyxiated fetal rhesus monkeys. J Pediatr 68:45, 1966.
28. Darnall RA Jr, et al: The effect of sleep state on active thermoregulation in the premature infant. Pediatr Res 16:512, 1982.
29. Day RL, et al: Body temperature and survival of premature infants. Pediatrics 34:171, 1964.
30. Dollberg S, et al: Effect of insulated skin probes to increase skin-to-environmental temperature gradients of preterm infants cared for in convective incubators. J Pediatr 124:799, 1994.
31. Du JNH, et al: The baby in the delivery room: A suitable microenvironment. JAMA 207:1502, 1969.

32. Falk SA, et al: Noise-induced inner ear damage in newborn and adult guinea pigs. Laryngoscope 84:444, 1974.
33. Fisher DA, et al: Neonatal thyroidal hyperactivity. Am J Dis Child 107:574, 1964.
34. Fitch CW, et al: Heat shield reduces water loss. Arch Dis Child 59:886, 1984.
35. Foster KG, et al: The response of the sweat glands of the newborn baby to thermal stimuli and to intradermal acetylcholine. J Physiol (Lond) 203:13, 1969.
36. Gadeke R, et al: The noise level in a children's hospital and the wake-up threshold in infants. Acta Paediatr Scand 58:164, 1969.
37. Gandy GM, et al: Thermal environment and acid-base homeostasis on human infants during the first few hours of life. J Clin Invest 43:751, 1964.
38. Glass L, et al: Effect of the thermal environment on cold resistance and growth of small infants after the first week of life. Pediatrics 41:1033, 1968.
39. Glass L, et al: Relationship of thermal environment and caloric intake to growth and resting metabolism in the late neonatal period. Biol Neonate 14:324, 1969.
40. Glass P, et al: Effect of bright light in the hospital nursery on the incidence of retinopathy of prematurity. N Engl J Med 313:401, 1985.
41. Hammarlund K, et al: Transepidermal water loss in newborn infants. Acta Paediatr Scand 72:721, 1983.
42. Harpin VA, et al: Responses of the newborn infant to overheating. Biol Neonate 44:65, 1983.
43. Heath M, et al: Thermoregulatory heat production in cold-reared and warm-reared pigs. Am J Physiol 233:R273, 1983.
44. Hey EN: The care of babies in incubators. In Gairdner D, et al (eds): Recent Advances in Paediatrics, 4th ed. London, Churchill Livingstone, 1971.
45. Hey EN, et al: Heat losses from babies in incubators. Arch Dis Child 42:57, 1967.
46. Hey EN, et al: Effect of humidity on production and loss of heat in the newborn baby. Arch Dis Child 43:166, 1968.
47. Hey EN, et al: Temporary loss of a metabolic response to cold stress in infants of low birthweight. Arch Dis Child 44:323, 1969.
48. Hey EN, et al: Evaporative water loss in the newborn baby. J Physiol 200:605, 1969.
49. Hey EN, et al: The optimum thermal environment for naked babies. Arch Dis Child 45:328, 1970.
50. Hey EN, et al: Oxygen consumption and heat balance in the cot-nursed baby. Arch Dis Child 45:335, 1970.
51. Hey EN, et al: The total thermal insulation of the newborn baby. J Physiol (Lond) 207:683, 1970.
52. Hill JR, et al: Heat balance and the metabolic rate of newborn babies in relation to environmental temperature; and the effect of age and of weight on basal metabolic rate. J Physiol (Lond) 180:239, 1965.
53. Hull D: Thermal control in very immature infants. Br Med Bull 44:971, 1988.
54. Jahnukainen T, et al: Dynamics of vasomotor thermoregulation of the skin in term and preterm neonates. Early Hum Dev 33:133, 1993.
55. Johnson KJ, et al: Infrared thermometry of newborn infants. Pediatrics 87:34, 1991.
56. Jolly H, et al: A controlled study of the effect of temperature on premature babies. J Pediatr 60:889, 1962.
57. Kaplan M, et al: Improved prognosis in severely hypothermic newborn infants treated by rapid rewarming. J Pediatr 105:470, 1984.
58. Karlberg P: The significance of depth of insertion of the thermometer for recording rectal temperatures. Acta Paediatr Scand 38:359, 1949.
59. Keeling EB: Thermoregulation and axillary temperature measurements in neonates: A review of the literature. Matern Child Nurs J 20:124, 1992.
60. Knauth A, et al: Semipermeable polyurethane membrane as an artificial skin for the premature neonate. Pediatrics 83:945, 1989.
61. LeBlanc MH: Relative efficacy of an incubator and an open warmer in producing thermoneutrality for the small premature infant. Pediatrics 69:439, 1982.
62. LeBlanc MH: The physics of thermal exchange between infants and their environment. Medical Instrumentation 21:11, 1987.
63. LeBlanc MH: Thermoregulation: Incubators, radiant warmers, artificial skins, and body hoods. Clin Perinatol 18:403, 1991.
64. LeBlanc MH, et al: Artifacts in the measurement of skin temperature under infant radiant warmers. Ann Biomed Eng 13:443, 1985.
65. Lewis HE, et al: Aerodynamics of the human microenvironment. Lancet 50:1273, 1969.
66. Long JG, et al: Noise and hypoxemia in the intensive care nursery. Pediatrics 65:143, 1980.
67. Malin SW, et al: Optimal thermal management for low birth weight infants nursed under high-powered radiant warmers. Pediatrics 79:47, 1987.
68. Mann TP, et al: Neonatal cold injury. Lancet 1:229, 1957.
69. Mayfield SR, et al: Temperature measurement in term and preterm neonates. J Pediatr 104:271, 1984.
70. Mayock D, et al: Neonatal hyperthermia secondary to a plastic thermal blanket. Crit Care Med 14:817, 1986.
71. Medoff-Cooper B: Transition of the preterm infant to an open crib. J Obstet Gynecol Neonatal Nurs 23:329, 1994.
72. Messaritakis J, et al: Rectal-skin temperature difference in septicaemic newborn infants. Arch Dis Child 65:380, 1990.
73. Mestyan J, et al: The significance of facial skin temperature in the chemical heat regulation of premature infants. Biol Neonate 7:243, 1964.
74. Mestyan J, et al: Surface temperatures versus deep body temperature and the metabolic response to cold of hypothermic premature infants. Biol Neonate 7:230, 1964.
75. Mestyan J, et al: The total energy expenditure and its components in premature infants maintained under different nursing and environmental conditions. Pediatr Res 2:161, 1968.
76. Miller DL, et al: Body temperature in the immediate neonatal period: The effect of reducing thermal losses. Am J Obstet Gynecol 94:964, 1966.
77. Miller RW, et al: Noise pollution: Neonatal aspects. Committee on Environmental Hazards, American Academy of Pediatrics. Pediatrics 54:476, 1974.
78. Mondlane RP, et al: Skin-to-skin contact as a method of body warmth for infants of low birth weight. J Trop Pediatr 35:321, 1989.
79. Motil KJ, et al: The effects of four different radiant warmer temperature set points used for rewarming neonates. J Pediatr 85:546, 1974.
80. Nedergaard J, Cannon B: Brown adipose tissue: Development and function. In Polin RA, Fox WW (eds): Fetal and Neonatal Physiology. Philadelphia, WB Saunders, 1992, p 314.
81. Ogren JM: The inaccuracy of axillary temperatures measured with an electronic thermometer. Am J Dis Child 144:109, 1990.
82. Okken A, et al: Effects of forced convection of heated air on insensible water loss and heat loss in preterm infants in incubators. J Pediatr 101:108, 1982.
83. Perlstein PH, et al: Apnea in premature infants and incubator air temperature changes. N Engl J Med 282:461, 1970.
84. Perlstein PH, et al: Age relationship to thermal patterns on the backs of cold stressed infants. Biol Neonate 20:127, 1972.
85. Perlstein PH, et al: Adaptation to cold in the first three days of life. Pediatrics 54:411, 1974.
86. Perlstein PH, et al: Computer-assisted newborn intensive care. Pediatrics 57:494, 1976.
87. Perlstein PH, et al: Incubator control with computer assistance. Perinatology Neonatology 1:16, 1977.
88. Pribylova H: The importance of thermoreceptive regions for the chemical thermoregulation of the newborn. Biol Neonate 12:13, 1968.
89. Pribylova H, et al: The effect of body temperature on the level of carbohydrate metabolites and oxygen consumption in the newborn. Pediatrics 37:743, 1966.
90. Reynolds JD, et al: Lack of efficacy of light reduction in preventing retinopathy of prematurity. N Engl J Med 338:1572, 1998.
91. Rojas RD, et al: A mathematical model of premature baby thermoregulation and incubator dynamics. In Cerroloza, et al (eds): Simulation Modeling in Bioengineering. Boston, Computational Mechanics Publications, 1996, p 23.

92. Rutter N, et al: Variations in the resting oxygen consumption of small babies. Arch Dis Child 53:850, 1978.
93. Sant'ambrogio G, et al: Laryngeal cold receptors. Respir Physiol 59:35, 1985.
94. Sauer PJJ, et al: New standards for neutral thermal environment of healthy very low birthweight infants in week one of life. Arch Dis Child 59:18, 1984.
95. Schmitt BD: Fever in childhood. Pediatrics 74:929, 1984.
96. Scopes JW: Metabolic rate and temperature control in the human body. Br Med Bull 22:88, 1966.
97. Scopes JW, et al: The effect of intravenous noradrenaline on the oxygen consumption of newborn animals. J Physiol (Lond) 165:305, 1963.
98. Scopes JW, et al: Minimal rates of oxygen consumption in sick and premature newborn infants. Arch Dis Child 41:407, 1966.
99. Seguin JH, et al: Local skin hyperthermia due to transcutaneous electrode heat. J Perinatol 8:393, 1988.
100. Shvartz E: Effect of a cooling hood on physiological responses to work in a hot environment. J Appl Physiol 29:36, 1970.
101. Silverman WA: Incubator-baby side shows. Pediatrics 64:127, 1979.
102. Silverman WA, Blanc WA: The effect of humidity on survival of newly born premature infants. Pediatrics 20:477, 1957.
103. Silverman WA, et al: The influence of the thermal environment upon the survival of newly born premature infants. Pediatrics 22:876, 1958.
104. Silverman WA, et al: A sequential trial of the nonthermal effect of atmospheric humidity on survival of newborn infants of low birth weight. Pediatrics 31:719, 1963.
105. Silverman WA, et al: Warm nape of the newborn. Pediatrics 33:984, 1964.
106. Silverman WA, Agate FJ: The oxygen cost of minor changes in heat balance of small newborn infants. Acta Paediatr Scand 55:294, 1966.
107. Stephenson JM, et al: The effect of cooling on blood gas tensions in newborn infants. J Pediatr 76:848, 1970.
108. Stern L, et al: Environmental temperature, oxygen consumption and catecholamine excretion in newborn infants. Pediatrics 36:367, 1965.
109. Stoll AM, Green LC: Relationship between pain and tissue damage due to thermal radiation. J Appl Physiol 14:373, 1959.
110. Stothers JK: Head insulation and heat loss in the newborn. Arch Dis Child 56:530, 1981.
111. Stothers JK, et al: The effect of feeding on neonatal oxygen consumption. Arch Dis Child 54:415, 1979.
112. Sulyok E, et al: Effect of relative humidity on thermal balance of the newborn infant. Biol Neonate 21:210, 1972.
113. Sulyok E, et al: Respiratory contribution to the thermal balance of the newborn infant under various ambient conditions. Pediatrics 51:641, 1973.
114. Tafari N, et al: Aspects on rewarming newborn infants with severe accidental hypothermia. Acta Paediatr Scand 63:595, 1974.
115. Topper WH, et al: Thermal support for the very-low-birthweight infant: Role of supplemental conductive heat. J Pediatr 105:810, 1984.
116. Turnell R: The influence of different environmental temperatures on pulmonary gas exchange and blood gas changes after birth. Acta Paediatr Scand 64:57, 1975.
117. Vernon H, et al: Semipermeable dressing and transepidermal water loss in premature infants. Pediatrics 86:357, 1990.
118. Waffarn F, et al: Mercury vapor contamination of infant incubators: A potential hazard. Pediatrics 64:640, 1979.
119. Walker D, et al: Temperature of the human fetus. Br J Obstet Gynaecol 76:503, 1969.
120. Wheldon AE: Energy balance in the newborn baby: Use of a manikin to estimate radiant and convective heat loss. Phys Med Biol 27:285, 1982.
121. Wheldon AE, et al: The heat balance of small babies nursed in incubators and under radiant warmers. Early Hum Dev 6:131, 1982.
122. Wheldon AE, et al: Incubation of very immature infants. Arch Dis Child 58:504, 1983.
123. Wood C, et al: Temperature of the human fetus. Br J Obstet Gynaecol 71:768, 1964.
124. Yamaguchi T, et al: An application of computational fluid mechanics to the air flow in an infant incubator. Ann Biomed Engineering 20:497, 1992.
125. Yeh TF, et al: Reduction of insensible water loss in premature infants under the radiant warmer. J Pediatr 94:651, 1979.
126. Yetman RJ, et al: Comparison of temperature measurements by an aural infrared thermometer with measurements by traditional rectal and axillary techniques. J Pediatr 122:769, 1993.
127. Young IM: Vasomotor tone in the skin blood vessels of the newborn infant. Clin Sci 22:325, 1962.

30 Biomedical Engineering Aspects of Neonatal Monitoring

Susan R. Hintz

David A. Benaron

David K. Stevenson

Monitoring in the neonatal intensive care unit (NICU) has improved dramatically since the inception of neonatology as a specialty. Many devices are relied on increasingly to alert the physician to developing problems and even to direct care as technologic advances make the management of infants in the NICU more complex. Although currently employed monitoring systems are diverse, they should all meet a few basic requirements. The system should be reliable, a requirement that applies to both the sensitivity and the specificity of the information relayed by the system and to long-term equipment integrity. It should be relatively simple to operate and should provide information in an easy-to-interpret manner. The system must be safe for patient use, which is especially important in the neonatal population because the sensors or probes, the portion of the system that comes in contact with the patient, must be appropriately sized and nonirritating to sensitive skin. The ideal system should be noninvasive, or at least not require invasive procedures beyond which will be needed for optimal patient care. The system should provide continuous or near-continuous, real-time information, such that personnel may respond to an event occurring at the time the information is relayed. It should be relatively small and portable. The system must be safe for personnel, and must not interfere with other vital equipment required for the care of the patient.

To meet those requirements, a system must be engineered appropriately and dependably. Monitoring systems have afforded enormous benefits to the patient and to the clinician, but they have become such an integral part of the NICU environment that a basic understanding of the shortfalls of such equipment has been overlooked. Although the technical aspects of monitoring systems may not appear to be important when caring for patients, the clinician should be aware of the basic instrumentation of each system and the system's potential limitations. This chapter reviews cardiac, respiratory, blood pressure, transcutaneous, and pulse oximetry monitoring and the emerging technology of near-infrared spectroscopy. An excellent examination of several of these systems also can be found in the previous edition of this text.[53]

CARDIAC MONITORING

In the modern NICU, heart rate and rhythm strip monitoring are considered to be the standard of care. This information, which may report the first warning signal of patient decompensation, is usually taken for granted. However, the electrocardiogram (EKG) is an indispensable tool that delivers vital information simply and noninvasively to the physician regarding molecular and cellular events of the heart.

BIOLOGIC BASIS

Electrocardiographic recording provides a one-dimensional view of the heart, based on time-dependent, electrical potential changes between two points on the body.[42] The origin of this electrical signal lies in the transmembrane potential, the result of differences in concentration of ions inside compared to that outside the cells; in a resting cell, this electrical difference is approximately -90 mV. When a cardiac cell is activated, a cardiac action potential occurs, consisting of rapid depolarization followed by a period of repolarization (Fig. 30–1). The rapidity of the depolarization phase, the slope of repolarization, and the shape of this action potential are different depending on cardiac cell type; for instance, the initial depolarization phase in cells of the His-Purkinje system is extremely rapid, but it is much slower in nodal cells. These electrical changes in cardiac cells are the result

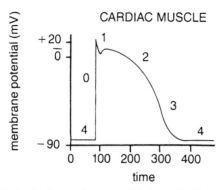

FIGURE 30–1. Cardiac action potential for a Purkinje fiber with phases 0 to 4 as marked. (From Katz AM: Physiology of the Heart, 2nd ed, New York, Raven Press, 1992.)

of the opening and closing of complex ion channels in the cell membrane, first postulated by Hodgkin and Huxley in the 1950s,[35] and they are now known to be regulated not only by electrical impulses but by selective gene expression. In the normal heart, an electrical impulse arising in the sinoatrial (SA) node is propagated through the atria, then the ventricles, ending with the area around the outflow tracts. It is more difficult to explain how the spreading depolarization and repolarization of cardiac cells are translated into an EKG. The theory most often cited to explain this phenomenon is referred to as the *dipole* theory.[27]

A dipole is an electrical source that is asymmetric with respect to charge. As discussed earlier, the outside of a myocardial cell at rest is positively charged when compared with the cytosol, whereas during excitation, depolarization occurs within the cell and the outside then is negatively charged in comparison. The heart during excitation, when viewed from the surface, may therefore be considered to be a dipole because excited myocardium is negatively charged with respect to myocardium at rest. Clinical application of this principle is made possible because the heart is surrounded by tissues of the body that act as a conductor for the electrical current. Therefore, the potentials generated by the dipole, in this case the heart, may be measured at the body surface by a recording electrode, or lead. From this background, it can be understood that a surface lead placed facing an approaching wave of excitation would record a positive potential, represented on the EKG as an upward deflection (Fig. 30–2). Although the dipole theory is useful for understanding how cardiac electrical activity is detectable on the body surface, it is an oversimplified explanation because the tissues surrounding the heart are inconsistent conductors and the heart is not truly a single dipole, but rather multiple dipoles.

LEADS AND LEAD PLACEMENT

It is not obvious how a lead placed on the surface of the body transmits information regarding electrical activity of the heart. Simply stated, a lead is an elec-

trode consisting of metal that forms the communication connection from the heart, which is a system involving electrical conduction, to the instrumentation.[12] In order for this process to occur, a *redox*, or oxidation-reduction reaction, must occur at the electrode surface, allowing for energy conversion, which is made possible by the reversible transfer of ions from a metal into an electrolyte solution. Theoretically, this completely reversible system describes an electrode in which the change in *equilibrium potential* is zero; however, in reality, there are several problems that can cause an electrode to operate irreversibly, at which point it is said to be *polarized*. Polarization can result in practical difficulties in using electrodes for biologic monitoring. One cause of polarization is referred to as *charge-transfer overvoltage*, which results when the transfer of ions from the metal into solution does not balance the deposition of ions on the metal surface. This imbalance is caused by differences in how much energy is required to deposit ions onto a metal surface, and thus varies with different metal types. Another potential cause of polarization is *resistance polarization*, which describes changes in the potential of the electrode system owing to films that have accumulated, or changes in the concentration of electrolytes in the diffusion layer. These changes could be caused by production and deposition of electrolytes or other ionic species by the body.

The type of electrode used for clinical application has been a matter of intense study and research over many years.[26] The hydrogen electrode, which is a platinized electrode in an acid solution with hydrogen gas bubbled through it, is the most reproducible. It is used as the zero potential standard against which all other electrodes are measured, but clearly it is not appropriate for clinical use. In his early studies, Einthoven's approach was to immerse the arms and feet of his human subjects into buckets filled with saline, using the arms and feet as electrodes. However, of primary importance in the development of clinically useful electrodes was the investigation of metals in which electrode-electrolyte interfaces resulted in the smallest and most stable voltage potential, because this potential and its variations can be responsible for

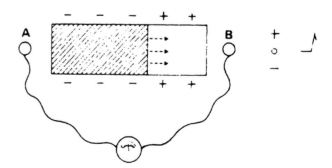

FIGURE 30–2. Wave of depolarization in a strip of myocardium after stimulation on the left side. Electrode B is facing a greater positivity than is electrode A, thus an upward deflection is observed in the chart recorder at right. (From Katz AM: Physiology of the Heart, 2nd ed, New York, Raven Press, 1992.)

significant artifact. Researchers made a number of other observations, including that a uniform film of electrolyte-containing material on the electrode when applied electrolytically serves to decrease this noise or artifact. For this reason, silver–silver chloride electrodes are extremely useful for noninvasive measurements in the clinical arena because they have been found to be extremely stable, and they have been suggested to be the most reliable electrodes next to hydrogen electrodes. Silver–silver chloride electrodes can be prepared in a variety of forms, and they have been developed for special use in the NICU setting.

The most popular type of electrode used for EKG monitoring in the NICU is a silver–silver chloride, foil-based, recessed or floating electrode. When using this type of electrode, the metal does not come into contact with the subject directly; contact with the patient is instead made through an electrolyte solution. In the past, the metal electrodes were placed on the patient after separate application of an electrolyte paste or gel. Numerous companies now market very flexible, prewired neonatal and pediatric EKG monitoring electrodes in which cloth surrounds a small silver–silver chloride electrode with the lead already attached to a safety socket. This type of unit is backed by a sticky adhesive electrolyte gel, referred to as *hydrogel,* of which the precise composition varies with manufacturer. The hydrogel serves as both the required electrolyte interface solution and the reversible adhesive. These electrodes are generally packaged in sets of three, are relatively inexpensive, and are designed for one-time use.

Neonatal probe placement is a unique area of concern that requires special consideration. Improper lead placement is a particular problem in premature infants, because the shape of the thorax yields a limited flat surface for electrode placement. In addition, the premature infant's small size markedly restricts the space available for lead placement, occasionally resulting in electrodes placed too close to each other or that are at right angles to the main P and QRS vectors. Additional problems are encountered when many noninvasive surface monitors and other equipment prevent proper placement of electrodes, leading to worrisome artifacts caused by patient movement or manipulations. Tremulousness and myoclonic seizures have been reported to simulate atrial flutter in the newborn, and EKGs performed during chest percussion have been mistaken to represent tachyarrythmias.[57] The most common causes of EKG artifacts are related to poor skin contact with the electrodes: 1) poor adhesiveness resulting from multiple probe replacement, 2) poor positioning on a nonflat thoracic surface, such as a bony prominence, and 3) poor contact resulting from excessive lotion or gel on the skin surface. Few studies have investigated optimal EKG probe location on the neonate body surface. Lead placement for the patient in the NICU is, in practice, frequently dictated by issues such as the position of other necessary equipment or probes on a small patient. Baird and colleagues, however, did study the best positioning of leads for both respira-

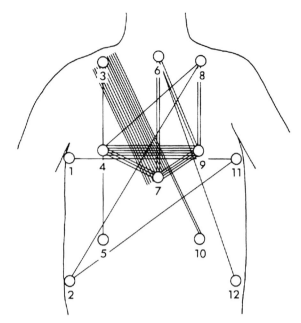

FIGURE 30–3. Optimal locations for cardiopulmonary monitoring electrodes on preterm and term infants. Electrodes between positions 3 and 7 generally have the best results.[4]

tory and EKG signal in both term and preterm infants.[4] They found that the best EKG signal was found with one lead at the right midclavicular line at the level of T4 and the other at the xyphoid in term infants, whereas lead placement in a line parallel but shifted to the left was best in premature infants (Fig. 30–3).

Also of great importance in the consideration of EKG probe placement is the fragility of the skin of the patient, especially in the case of a premature infant. Previous reports have emphasized the possibility of skin damage with adhesive-based probes in premature infants, specifically EKG probes. In extremely premature infants, removal of adhesive probes has been associated with stripping of the stratum corneum layer, which may be associated with increased permeability to toxic chemicals, as well as leading to a site of entry for infectious agents.[31] Furthermore, transepidermal water losses (measured using an evaporimeter technique) have been shown to be extremely high in areas of the skin of preterm infants on which traditional adhesive probes were placed then removed.[10] This water loss may result in substantial clinical complications, especially in the most premature infants whose epidermal barrier is already weak and whose water losses are significant. Other types of skin injury, such as anetoderma, have been identified in association with EKG probe placement in preterm infants and those with extremely low birth weight, and they may be linked to cleansers or irritants trapped under the adhesive or to local hypoxemia.[14]

EKG DEVICE AND SAFETY

Most nurseries now use computer-based cardiac monitoring systems. These systems have obvious advan-

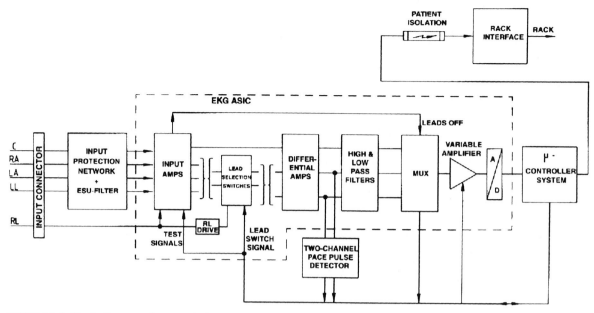

FIGURE 30–4. Block diagram of a typical electrocardiogram (EKG) module monitoring system. (Courtesy of Hewlett-Packard Corporation and Agilent Technologies.)

tages over older devices: they can store information in memory, thereby providing the opportunity for trend analysis and review; they frequently possess the capability to assess more complex EKG parameters, allowing for recognition of specific rate and rhythm disturbances; they usually have more sophisticated filtering components in order to reduce noise and artifacts; and they allow for multiple patient parameters to be viewed on a single display, with the availability of blood pressure, pulse oximetry, and other computer modules.

A typical, simplified EKG module diagram is shown in Figure 30–4. As the EKG signals pass from the patient to the monitor via the electrode leads, an input protection network provides electrical isolation, preventing electrical shock to the patient, and filters extraneous high frequency signals from the rest of the system. The signal is next selected with respect to lead, then amplified. In many systems, the common mode signal from behind the lead selectors is used to drive the right leg amplifier in order to prevent interference from 60 Hz power lines, a common source of artifact. High-pass and low-pass filters usually are employed, allowing for independent selection of diagnostic, monitoring, or filter bandwidths for each channel. Finally, an analog-to-digital (A/D) circuit converts the signal to one that can be presented to and understood by the microprocessor. The microprocessor then presents the signal to other ancillary modules for further processing by specialized evaluation modules.

Troubleshooting problems with EKG monitoring should be approached in a systematic fashion, and with knowledge of one's particular monitoring device. However, the most important causes of artifact are often fairly simple to correct, including poor contact between skin and electrode or improper place-

ment of leads. Problems with the EKG equipment, including cables and cable connections, or, less likely, internal hardware or software failure within the EKG module, also may be contributory. Finally, electrical interference from other equipment may lead to artifacts (Table 30–1).

Recommendations for safe current limits for electrocardiographs have been set by the American Heart Association (AHA).[46] These recommendations address two aspects of electrical safety. First, the level of current allowable to flow through any patient-connected lead has been established at 10 μA. This recommendation is based on studies by Watson and associates,[61] which showed that the smallest current needed to produce ventricular fibrillation through an endocardial electrode in humans is 15 μA, and it was considered to be unrealistic from an engineering standpoint to establish a limit lower than 10 μA. Second, the recommended allowable chassis leakage current, or the unintentional current that flows from the electrocardiograph to ground, has been established at 100 μA. A limit of 10 μA is the optimal goal because of the small potential for the patient to contact the case either directly or indirectly while being

TABLE 30–1 POTENTIAL CAUSES OF EKG ARTIFACTS

Improper electrode placement
Poor skin contact
Patient movement: hiccups, myotonic jerks, seizures, tremors
Improper lead selection
60 Hz interference
Electrical interference from other equipment or appliances
Internal EKG module hardware or software failure

simultaneously grounded through another pathway; however, with the increasing technical complexity of monitoring systems, design challenges meeting this standard are prohibitive.

RESPIRATORY MONITORING

Respiratory assessment and monitoring are essential in the NICU. Although physical examination can provide information regarding the quality of an infant's pulmonary effort, it is a noncontinuous evaluation. Continuous monitoring is critical in the ill patient, but the quantity of information varies greatly with the method used. Surface monitoring techniques are used routinely in the NICU to monitor respiratory rate, but they are unable to provide detailed information regarding further pulmonary parameters and are often subject to artifact. Methods of sensing ventilation requiring tight connections with the patient airway often provide the most data, but they are more invasive and until recently were impractical for continuous use. It is important for all care providers to understand the benefits and limitations of the respiratory monitoring systems used in the care of their patients (see Chapter 42, Part Two).

SURFACE AND NONINVASIVE MONITORING

The most frequently employed method of indirect monitoring in infants is *transthoracic electrical impedance*. This method measures electrical impedance changes between two electrodes on the thorax during respiration. The signal obtained could potentially be dominated by the signal generated by the polarization layer in the electrodes, so a high frequency current (greater than 25 kHz) is passed though the electrodes to minimize this possibility. By using this modulation technique, the same electrodes that are used for EKG measurement can be used for respiration detection in many devices. The impedance change caused by breathing activity is extracted from the baseline impedance of the thorax, amplified, and converted to digital form for presentation to the microprocessor. Depending on the device being used, the microprocessor then performs a number of functions, including analyzing the signal for apnea, high respiratory rate, low respiratory rate, alarm triggering and presenting the analyzed rate for display on the monitor. Unfortunately, the change in impedance with breathing can be very small with respect to the baseline thoracic impedance. Therefore, introduction of artifact, commonly seen with improper lead placement, poor skin contact, or patient movement, is a frequent problem with this approach to respiratory monitoring. In the case of obstructive apnea, a breathing movement may be detected when no breath truly has been taken. In addition, transthoracic changes in electrical impedance are caused by other physical changes not related to respiration, and these changes also may lead to incorrect signal display or false alarms. Although impedance changes related to EKG signals are filtered

out by special signal-processing algorithms in most currently used microprocessor-based monitors, other changes in thoracic blood volume may result in transthoracic impedance changes. These changes may be detected, processed, and reported as a breath when no breath has been taken, or they may lead to a missed breath when one has actually occurred. Alarms may be triggered falsely as a result; conversely, no alarm may sound when an apneic event has occurred.

Inductance plethysmography is another indirect method for monitoring respiration. This instrument places a one-turn electrical wire coil around the chest and abdomen of the infant. The coil is incorporated into an elastic strap that conforms to the curvature of the infant. An electromagnetic property of each coil, known as the inductance, varies with the area outlined by the coil. This property is measured and yields signals that are proportional to the changes in area of the thorax and abdomen as the infant breathes. This signal can be used to detect apnea and to report breath rate. Theoretically, this method could provide a signal proportional to tidal volume, thus giving an indirect estimate of this parameter.

Carbon dioxide detection also has been used to detect patterns of ventilation, based on the concentration of carbon dioxide in expired air being higher than that of inspired air. A small tube is placed at the nares and/or mouth and a small amount of suction is applied to the tube, causing expired air to flow into the tube.[59] The gas is directed to an instrument that has a rapid carbon dioxide sensor, and changes are processed and displayed as respiratory rate. This system allows free head movement and is less likely to have direct interference from patient movements. However, the gas transport tubes must remain in position, thus requiring close observation. Moisture accumulation in the tubing, if not noted and corrected by an observer, may limit reliability.

OTHER MONITORING TECHNIQUES

Available for the adult patient population for many years, highly sophisticated ventilatory techniques and continuous monitoring systems are now integral to the NICU. With increasing interest and concern regarding the influence of differing ventilatory strategies on long-term pulmonary outcomes and significant recent technologic advances, continuous *pneumotachography* now is frequently encountered in NICUs.

Sensors, or transducers, that have been developed to detect signals such as airflow and pressure are placed in series with the airway.[16] These signals are converted to an electrical analog, then amplified and filtered. The signals are processed by an A/D converter, then presented to the microprocessor, which further processes the data with respect to computational tasks, alarm triggering, and other factors (Fig. 30–5). The processed information is displayed on a monitor. The two basic categories of sensors most commonly used for neonatal pulmonary monitoring are *flow sensors* and *pressure sensors*.

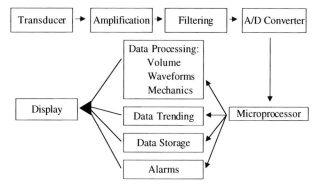

FIGURE 30–5. Simplified block diagram of a respiratory monitoring system.

Flow sensors are classified with respect to how the transducer obtains information as *differential pressure type* or *thermal type*. The most common type of differential pressure sensor is one based on a fixed orifice within a tubular attachment placed in series with the airway. Pneumatic transmission lines are placed upstream and downstream of the fixed orifice, and a differential pressure is detected between them by the transducer. The flow rate can be calculated because it is known that the differential pressure signal is proportional to the square of the flow rate. Volume calculations can then be undertaken by the microprocessor.[18] Another type of differential pressure sensor is the Fleisch, or laminar flow type, in which many capillary tubes, or in some cases a screen, are between the pneumatic transmission lines. The differential pressure across these tubes is approximately linearly proportional to the flow rate. Because of the mathematical relationships used to solve for flow, the Fleisch differential pressure sensors may be accurate over a wider range than the fixed orifice type. However, capillary tubes are more likely to have problems with moisture or secretions. Another category of flow transducer, based on the properties of heat convection, is the thermal anemometer. In these transducers, an element secured within a tube placed in line with the airway is heated continuously. As air flows past the heated wire or film, the element cools. Electrical current is delivered to the element to again attain the elevated temperature. The amount of current required is proportional, however nonlinear, to the gas flow. A second heated element is added to the system if bidirectional flow measurement is needed. These devices are accurate over a wide range, but they may be prone to difficulties stemming from particulate matter or secretions. Pressure transducers are constructed so that a thin diaphragm is flexed in response to pressure. A sensing element associated with the diaphragm then transmits the information regarding the amount of displacement sensed. The material used for the sensing element changes its electrical characteristics proportional to the strain applied. This same basic technology is used for both airway pressure transducers and esophageal pressure transducers.

BLOOD PRESSURE MONITORING

Blood pressure monitoring of the newborn can be undertaken using a variety of methods and technologies.[45] Depending on the clinical requirements, blood pressure may be measured continuously and directly through the use of electrical transducers and catheters or indirectly through the use of occlusive devices (cuffs) and manual or automatic methods of detecting pulsations.

DIRECT MONITORING

Most direct blood pressure monitoring devices used in the NICU are the "catheter-type" transducer. In these devices, fluid exerts a force against a diaphragm, and the sensed deflection of the diaphragm is relayed as an electrical signal. The early versions of these instruments were relatively cumbersome, extremely expensive, and because they were reusable had to be sterilized between each use. However, the advent of solid-state construction has allowed for smaller, less expensive, and disposable transducers.

A pressure transducer is simple in concept, but it is a complicated system. It is well known, according to Pascal's law, that a pressure transducer will detect the same pressure as that seen at the distal tip of a fluid-filled tube (such as a catheter) as long as the two are at the same level. However, this is true only for static pressures, and because blood pressure represents a complex oscillating pattern, other factors influence the response of the catheter-transducer unit. These factors include the *mass* of all components; the *stiffness* or compliance of the "elastic" component of the transducer, which is described by the number of cubic millimeters of fluid required for the application of 100 mm Hg; and the *viscous drag*, also referred to as *damping*, which represents a retarding force that is proportional to the velocity of movement of the fluid in the transducer-catheter system. These factors are related to pressure by the following equation:

$$(M)\frac{d^2x}{dt^2} + (R)\frac{dx}{dt} + Kx = P(t)$$

where:

$$
\begin{aligned}
M &= \text{effective mass} \\
x &= \text{distance moved} \\
R &= \text{viscous drag factor} \\
K &= \text{stiffness} \\
P(t) &= \text{pressure applied}
\end{aligned}
$$

Although seemingly complicated in this form, it is simple when compared with the actual case in which the viscous drag of the fluid in the transducer must be considered separately from that of the fluid in the catheter, which in turn is influenced by resistance of the catheter. Distortions could exist in the system so that additional undulations not truly relayed at the tip of the catheter could be detected at the level of the transducer. This artificial detection could lead to a problem known as *overshoot*, which causes the transducer to read a pressure higher than that which exists at the catheter tip. The degree to which this potential problem exists is influenced by the viscous drag or damping factor, which is proportional to the viscosity of the fluid, the square of the catheter length, and volume displacement and is inversely proportional to the catheter diameter cubed and the square of the density of the fluid. If the damping factor is 1.0 there would be no overshoot, but the rise time would be unacceptably long. A damping factor of zero is not possible and not desirable; the amplitude of the wave at the transducer in this case would become larger and larger. In practice, systems with damping factors of approximately 0.7 are used.[12]

Clinically, it is well known that air bubbles in the system also can significantly influence the performance of the device, owing to air being compressible and that an air bubble would therefore increase the volume displacement and lead to an increased damping factor and prolonged rise time. This problem may be of particular concern when, as in most cases, using the same catheter for infusion of fluids and medications. In addition to artifact, introduced bubbles could cause significant, potentially life-threatening patient complications, especially if air is introduced to the arterial side or to the venous side, in the case of central venous pressure monitoring. Distortion may be caused by movement of the catheter. Although actual pressure is the same at the catheter tip, low frequency oscillations may be produced by movement of the catheter tip within the vessel. This type of artifact often is easily detected and usually addressed simply with stabilization of the catheter.

Arterial and venous pressures can be measured by catheter-transducer systems. In the neonate, these measurements are usually accomplished by accessing the umbilical vessels, introducing flushed catheters into the appropriate vessels, then placing a transducer at the proximal end of the catheter. Care should be taken so that the transducer is at the level of the distal tip of the catheter. For most transducer sets, establishing a "zero" pressure reading before obtaining meaningful patient data is necessary. As with all transducers, a signal is passed through isolation before analysis by the remainder of the system. In the case of pressure monitors, mean blood pressure is calculated, which is not the simple arithmetic average of systolic and diastolic pressures but is the area under a single pulse wave divided by the width of the pulse. Alarm systems are also incorporated into typical modular blood pressure monitors, allowing for selection of systolic, diastolic, or mean pressure alarm points.

INDIRECT MONITORING

Indirect blood pressure monitoring is accomplished through use of an occlusive device, usually the familiar "cuff" that contains an inflatable bladder with a tube for entrance and exit of air. The cuff is placed around an extremity and is inflated to an adequately high pressure to cause occlusion of arterial flow distal to the cuff. The placement of the cuff on either upper arm or calf, two popular sites in the preterm infant, has not been shown to result in significant differences in pressure readings in this population.[45] During the deflation of the cuff, measurements may be obtained regarding systolic and diastolic pressure levels. Selecting the proper cuff size is of great importance and cannot be overemphasized.[2] The AHA recommends that a cuff width approximately 40% of the member circumference be used; using a cuff that is too narrow may result in blood pressure measurements that are falsely high because the pressure in the cuff could be high compared with the underlying tissue. In addition, the cuff should be applied snugly because a loose cuff may provide falsely high values, and it should be at the same level as the heart when making measurements. A number of cuff sizes are now available for the neonatal population making correct size selection easier.

The most commonly taught method of indirect pressure monitoring is the *auscultatory method*, in which the examiner rapidly inflates then slowly deflates the cuff while listening for distal Korotkoff sounds with a stethoscope. Unfortunately, this method is not useful in neonates because the frequency spectrum of arterial sounds in this age group cannot be routinely heard. The most frequently used method to assess blood pressure noninvasively in the newborn is the *oscillometric method* (Fig. 30–6). In this method, cuff pressure is raised quickly to above the systolic blood pressure. As pressure is slowly released from the cuff, the cuff pressure approaches the systolic pressure and the artery begins to pulsate; the small pulsations or oscillations are communicated to the arterial pressure sensor through the edge of the cuff. A pressure sensor also exists in these systems to monitor the true pressure of the cuff. When the cuff pressure drops below the systolic pressure, blood rushes into the artery, causing oscillations to be larger. With continued deflation, the oscillations become larger as more blood flows into the tissue until a

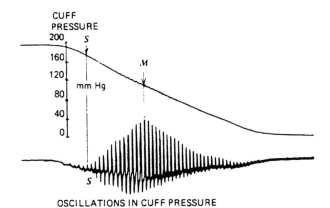

FIGURE 30–6. The oscillometric method of blood pressure monitoring. S, systolic pressure; M, mean pressure. (From Geddes LA: Cardiovascular Devices and Their Applications, New York, John Wiley and Sons, 1984. Reprinted by permission of John Wiley & Sons, Inc.)

maximum point very close to the true mean arterial pressure of oscillation is reached.[25] Oscillations continue to decrease as cuff pressure is slowly decreased.

In addition to pressure sensors, these devices have pressure pumps and deflation systems that are controlled by microprocessor technology. The oscillatory signals are extracted then converted to a digital signal and analyzed by the microprocessor. It is important to note that systolic and diastolic blood pressure is deduced through extrapolation, using attenuation rate of signal on both sides of the maximum oscillatory readings and often internal reference measurements. Each system has a slightly different algorithm, and differences in readings among devices and between the oscillometric and direct methods have been shown in the newborn population.[28, 54] Many systems have timing modes that allow for frequent automatic readings to be taken, and many systems now offer multiple patient modes, allowing for selection of adult, pediatric, or neonatal parameters. Mode selection is most important in terms of cuff inflation and overpressure maximum safety limits controlled by the microprocessor.

Indirect blood pressure monitoring may be ideal in certain clinical situations in the newborn nursery, but there are important issues to consider. First, although indirect blood pressure monitoring is noninvasive, it is a noncontinuous method. In specific instances of critically ill infants, direct and continuous monitoring may be required. Second, this method is extremely sensitive to patient movement; therefore, gentle restraint often is needed to obtain a reliable reading. Finally, a full range of cuff sizes should be available to ensure accuracy of readings.

TRANSCUTANEOUS OXYGEN AND CARBON DIOXIDE MONITORING

Transcutaneous blood gas monitoring is a concept that has been considered and studied for hundreds of years.[11] After the development of clinically useful sensors in the late 1960s, patient investigations followed, focused especially on the newborn population, owing to skin permeability to gas and to the need for noninvasive monitoring devices.[40] Although subsequent technical advances have made their use for long-term monitoring less widespread, these systems are still used routinely in many nurseries (see Chapter 42, Part Three).

OXYGEN MONITORING

Transcutaneous oxygen tension ($P_{tc}O_2$) measurement is based on the principle of extracellular oxygen diffusion across the skin. These systems use electrodes, separated from skin and isolated from room air by an adhesive, semipermeable membrane. The oxygen from the skin reacts with the platinum/silver-chloride sensor to create an electrical current proportional to the concentration of oxygen. This signal is relayed by cable to the device where further analysis and display functions are carried out. Because measurements are made transcutaneously, electrodes are best placed on an area of the body where the epidermis is thin and capillary network is dense. Even with this proviso, $P_{tc}O_2$ will not approach correlation with PaO_2 unless the capillary bed is arterialized through heating; therefore, systems provide for electrode heating to 43°C to 44°C before placement. These systems require calibration before each use and recalibration every 2 to 6 hours depending on the system and clinical circumstances. Studies have demonstrated a linear relationship between $P_{tc}O_2$ measurements and PaO_2, although values may be discrepant in neonates at high or low PaO_2 levels, and accuracy differs between different instruments.[9, 19]

Several factors may be associated with inaccurate $P_{tc}O_2$ readings. The sensor must be placed on well-perfused skin, which may be exceedingly difficult with an infant suffering from septic or cardiac shock because local hypoperfusion may be present. The skin site chosen also may not be maximally permeable to gas if scarring or edema is present or if the site chosen is covered with thickened skin. The sensor and device must be properly prepared, placed, and calibrated before making measurements. Air bubbles under the sensor, insecure seal with the skin, or faulty calibration may be responsible for inaccuracies. Because of these potential problems, clinical correlation of $P_{tc}O_2$ readings with arterial blood gases should be undertaken. $P_{tc}O_2$ monitoring has been associated with some dermatologic complications[8, 29]; therefore, care must be taken to move sensor position and inspect underlying skin frequently and to avoid placement of sensors on infants with gelatinous or fragile skin.

CARBON DIOXIDE MONITORING

Transcutaneous carbon dioxide ($P_{tc}CO_2$) monitoring is possible through the use of a pH-sensitive glass electrode with a silver–silver chloride reference electrode. Carbon dioxide, which diffuses through the skin and semipermeable membrane attaching the sensor to the skin, causes analyte pH changes that result in an electrical signal, which is relayed through a cable to a device for further analysis and display. Heating the skin is not as crucial for $P_{tc}CO_2$ determination, but heated electrodes have been shown to provide better correlation of $P_{tc}CO_2$ with $PaCO_2$, although transcutaneous measurements are consistently greater than arterial values. Calibration for these systems is required, and calibration time and response time are improved when heated electrodes are used. Combined $P_{tc}CO_2$ and $P_{tc}O_2$ sensors now are used routinely, although some debate exists regarding the possibility that single electrodes may perform slightly better.[22] $P_{tc}CO_2$ monitoring systems have demonstrated better sensitivity and specificity in the detection of hypercarbia than hypocarbia in term and premature infants, and different systems have slightly different levels of accuracy.[9, 22, 44] This form of monitoring has proven useful clinically in the continuous, noninvasive evaluation of recently extubated infants.[44] Conversely to the $P_{tc}O_2$ readings that may be falsely low in scenarios of poor perfusion, $P_{tc}CO_2$ will likely be falsely high. Concerns regarding sensor placement and $P_{tc}co_2$ system calibration are similar to those of $P_{tc}O_2$ devices. In addition, the potential for skin injury also exists with these systems.

PULSE OXIMETRY

Pulse oximetry has become an invaluable aspect of monitoring in the NICU. This technology is advantageous because it is continuous and noninvasive, it may act as a complement to other monitoring techniques, and in some cases, it can lead to a reduction in more invasive monitoring or testing. Its widespread introduction has changed the way medicine is practiced. The simplicity of this tool, however, may be deceptive, and the assumptions made may not be apparent. It is therefore crucial to understand the underlying principles and potential limitations of this technology.

PRINCIPLES

Pulse oximetry is an optical method for estimating arterial oxygen saturation (SaO_2) by measuring the color of arterial blood at two or more wavelengths of light.[6] Hemoglobin absorbs light differently after it has bound oxygen, reflecting a change in color (Fig. 30–7). The amount of light absorbed by hemoglobin in vitro is dictated by Beer's law:

$$A = \epsilon CL$$

where A is absorbance, ϵ is a constant, C is hemoglobin concentration, and L is the optical path length or the distance light has traveled through the solution. Numerous methods for estimating hemoglobin oxygen saturation have been developed, but most rely on measuring total absorbance at two different wavelengths, one in which there is a large difference in

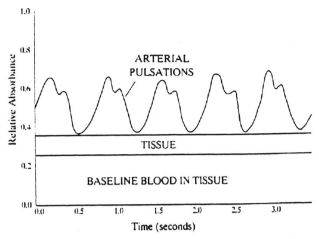

FIGURE 30–8. Influence of arterial pulsations on relative absorbance in vivo. (From Benaron DA, et al: Noninvasive methods for estimating in vivo oxygenation. Clin Pediatr 5:258, 1992.)

absorbance between deoxyhemoglobin (Hb) and oxyhemoglobin (HbO_2) and another above the isobestic point where Hb and HbO_2 absorbance are not different. Two equations can then be constructed and solved simultaneously, with saturation ultimately derived from percentage HbO_2 to Hb.[49] Unfortunately, the situation in vivo is highly complicated compared with that of the ideal in vitro system. There are absorbers in the body apart from hemoglobin, and light itself is reflected and scattered, making reliable calculations difficult with Beer's law alone. Early ear oximeters attempted to circumvent these complications by subtracting the light attenuated by bloodless tissue, accomplished by measuring light transmission after vigorously squeezing the pinna, from the total amount of light transmitted through the ear.[63] Hewlett-Packard developed the first widely used oximeter, which used a broad spectrum of light, measuring absorbance at eight different wavelengths.[50] This device was highly accurate, but it was cumbersome, expensive, and unsuitable for neonates because of the large size of the ear probe (10 cm x 10 cm).

Development of modern pulse oximetry occurred after variation in ear lobe absorbance was noted with each heartbeat, from a minimum during diastole to a maximum during systole.[1] During diastole, the volume of venous and arterial blood is constant, with the sum of diastolic absorbance from tissue and from blood forming a baseline. During systole, tissues swell with incoming arterial blood. Subtracting the diastolic baseline from the total noted at systole yields a signal because of arterial blood (Fig. 30–8). This signal is analyzed at two wavelengths, and saturation is determined.

The instrumentation of pulse oximeters is easily understood from this background. Light transmission is accomplished by a probe placed on a well-perfused capillary bed, such as a finger or toe in larger infants, or across a palm or foot in smaller infants. Adhesive-backed bandage material is used for neonatal probes. Two light-emitting diodes (LEDs) generate red (i.e.,

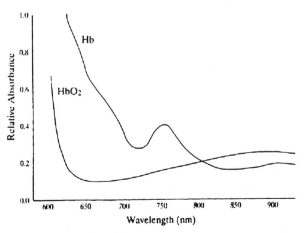

FIGURE 30–7. Relative absorption of light by hemoglobin (Hb) and oxyhemoglobin (HbO_2). (From Benaron DA, et al: Noninvasive methods for estimating in vivo oxygenation. Clin Pediatr 5:258, 1992.)

660 nm) or near-infrared (i.e., 940 nm) light. The LEDs are generally supplied with a chopped current at a high frequency to allow it to be distinguished from ambient light, which is accomplished in different ways by different manufacturers. A photodiode is opposite the LEDs and detects ambient light, as well as the red and near-infrared light, and a current is generated that represents the intensity of light detected at each wavelength. The current then passes through an isolation network and converted to voltage, which in turn is presented to a high pass filter that rejects ambient light. Before presentation to the microprocessor, the signal passes through an A/D converter. Depending on the pulse oximeter model or module, the microprocessor then derives the oxygen saturation value (SpO_2), a plethysmogram waveform, and a pulse value calculated from the plethysmographic signal.

LIMITATIONS

Many assumptions are made in order to derive an estimate of SaO_2 noninvasively, but these assumptions can lead to serious errors if they are not met (Table 30–2). Perhaps the most important is the assumption of adequate pulse pressure. Because the technology of pulse oximetry is dependent on subtraction of a baseline absorbance from that measured at systole, pulse oximetry may be unreliable in low perfusion states. Clinically, infants in septic shock or in significant cardiac failure, those who most require oxygenation monitoring, may have unreliable or undetectable SpO_2 measurements. Low light transmission may result in a signal too weak to measure adequately. Even with optimal probe placement, this phenomenon may be observed in edematous infants. Skin pigmentation, however, does not appear to have significant effects on SpO_2 accuracy.[20] It also is crucial for neonatologists to recognize that the accuracy of pulse oximetry is approximately $\pm 3\%$ (when saturation is 80% to 95%)[21] and does not allow for precise estimation of PaO_2 at saturations greater than 95%.[33] This understanding is particularly important in monitoring extremely premature infants at risk for retinopathy of prematurity. Inaccuracy is also inherent in the case of poorly saturated patients. In these situations, SpO_2 may be an inaccurate or insensitive reflection of actual SaO_2,[43] or it may appear clinically acceptable owing in part to the presence of high fetal hemoglobin (HbF) levels in the newborn circulation, but PaO_2 may

be unacceptably low. Although HbF does not affect oximeter accuracy itself in any clinically significant way, other hemoglobin forms, such as methemoglobin and carboxyhemoglobin, can significantly affect accuracy of the saturation reading owing to their relative absorbance at the wavelengths used by pulse oximeters.[64] Although this problem is rarely clinically relevant, it can greatly complicate and delay diagnosis if not recognized. Electrical or optical interference can lead to incorrect saturation estimates by burying the absorbance signal in noise. The signal from an oximeter may be extremely small compared with other signals,[15] and it may be obscured if power sources are not shielded properly. Interference by light sources alone is generally easy to remedy by placing an opaque cover over the pulse oximeter site. Movement is also a significant source of error or artifact in pulse oximetry, caused by the inability of most devices to consistently detect a pulse change and alterations in baseline patient blood volume during motion.[34] This problem can lead to substantial difficulties in optimal management during air or ground transports of critically ill infants.

POTENTIAL SOLUTIONS

There is no doubt that pulse oximetry is a rapid, noninvasive, and generally reliable monitoring system; many of the problems encountered in the clinical arena that affect pulse oximetry can be remedied or improved so that consistent readings can be obtained. However, the assumptions underlying conventional pulse oximetry cannot be altered, and, especially in the case of motion, solutions are difficult to achieve.

Several companies have attempted to circumvent the problems presented by motion by designing pulse oximetry systems with complex filtering algorithms. After extensive benchtop and clinical research, Masimo Corporation developed a system employing a unique recessed sensor design (low noise optical probe [LNOP®]), minimizing (though not eradicating) the effects of venous blood movement during motion, and a software algorithm referred to as the Discrete Saturation Transform™ (DST) (Fig. 30–9). In this algorithm, a noise reference is built for incoming red and infrared signals for all saturations from 1% to 100%. An adaptive filter is used to remove correlated frequencies between the noise signal and incoming red and infrared signals, and the remaining output is measured and plotted for all possible saturations. If several peaks are generated, as with motion, that considered to be most consistent with arterial pulsation is reported. This algorithm is different from conventional pulse oximetry in that it calculates SpO_2 without first having to reference the pulse rate. This system has been studied in adult volunteers in scenarios of motion and low perfusion and was found to be superior to other traditional or advanced pulse oximeters tested.[5, 62] Initial studies in the neonatal population indicate co-oximetry validation of the method, improved sensitivity and specificity, and dramatically improved reliability on transport and dur-

---

TABLE 30–2 CLINICAL ISSUES THAT MAY
AFFECT PULSE OXIMETRY

> Poor pulse pressure
> Significant hyperoxia
> Severe hypoxia
> Presence of other hemoglobin forms
> Electrical interference
> Optical interference
> Motion

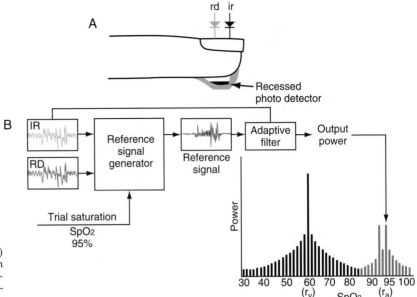

FIGURE 30–9. *A,* Low noise optical probe (LNOP®) design. *B,* Schematic of the Discrete Saturation Transform™ for pulse oximetry analysis. ir, infrared; r_a, aterial optical density ratio; rd, red; r_v, venous optical density ratio. (Courtesy of Masimo Corporation.)

ing extracorporeal membrane oxygenation (ECMO) therapy compared with traditional pulse oximetry.[24, 30, 32, 36] Other companies also have developed signal processing algorithms, such as Oxismart™, which is incorporated into many of the newer Nellcor pulse oximeters (Mallinkrodt, Inc.), to attempt to address the problems encountered with motion and frequent false alarms.[56]

Pulse oximetry systems with this type of technology may be more expensive than traditional pulse oximetry systems, specifically as a result of the cost of the probes or sensors; the increased cost may outweigh the potential benefits for many newborn nurseries. In addition, this technology is currently limited to separate unit systems and thus could not be incorporated into the monitoring module systems already in place in many newborn nurseries. However, in situations in which movement is expected, such as during ground or air transport or transport within a facility, this technology may be beneficial. Further studies in the neonatal population should be undertaken.

CONTINUOUS BLOOD GAS MONITORING

Intravascular sensors for blood gas analysis offer the benefit of continuous or near-continuous measurements of pH, PaO_2, $PaCO_2$, and in some cases certain electrolytes, without patient blood loss or need to wait for results. These devices have been used and studied in the adult population for applications such as intra- and postoperative monitoring and have been found to provide good agreement with traditional in vitro blood gas measurements.[60, 65] In addition, retrospective studies have revealed that these types of catheters can be used in the term and premature

neonatal population with complication rates consistent with umbilical catheterization alone.[13, 55] There are several types of "in-line" monitoring systems, each of which having a slightly different theory of operation.

One such type of monitoring system, of which the Neotrend™ system is representative, can report a number of parameters, including pH, $PaCO_2$, PaO_2, and temperature, owing to a sensor that is placed within a 4 F umbilical artery catheter (Fig. 30–10). The Neotrend™ sensor consists of three optical sensors and mirror within 0.5 mm diameter sheath, and a thermocouple for temperature measurements. The pH sensor uses the principle that phenol red dye changes color reversibly in response to hydrogen ions. Hydrogen ions permeate through a microporous hollow fiber containing the dye; absorption is measured at 555 nm; and pH is calculated. The $PaCO_2$ sensor uses this same principle; however, the membrane surrounding a phenol red–bicarbonate solution is surrounded by a gas-permeable but not an ion-permeable membrane. The PaO_2 sensor is based on the principle of fluorescence quenching. An oxygen-sensitive ruthenium-based dye is immobilized in a gas-permeable complex, and an excitation beam at 460 nm is transmitted. The excitation light is absorbed by the indicator dye and fluorescent light is emitted; when oxygen is present the fluorescent light is quenched, allowing for calculation of PaO_2. A dedicated screen displays results continuously, and data trends are recorded for 10 minutes to 24 hours. This system has the advantage of allowing for continuous multiparameter assessment of the critically ill newborn, reducing blood sampling, and potentially reducing the chance of infection owing to multiple line access events. Currently, a special catheter must be used in conjunction with the sensor, and calibration is required before insertion, in vivo, and occasionally throughout the period of use. Initial

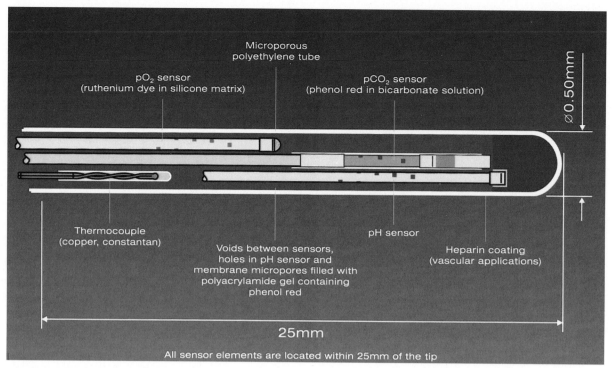

Microporous
polyethylene tube

pO$_2$ sensor
(ruthenium dye in silicone matrix)

pCO$_2$ sensor
(phenol red in bicarbonate solution)

Ø0.50mm

Thermocouple
(copper, constantan)

Voids between sensors,
holes in pH sensor and
membrane micropores filled with
polyacrylamide gel containing
phenol red

pH sensor

Heparin coating
(vascular applications)

25mm

All sensor elements are located within 25mm of the tip

FIGURE 30–10. Cross section through multiparameter Neotrend™ continuous in-line monitoring system. (Courtesy of Diametrics Medical Ltd.)

studies in the neonatal population revealed bias and precision data that would suggest that this type of system could be of potential clinical benefit, although the need for traditionally obtained arterial blood gases will not be completely eliminated.[51]

Another approach to blood gas monitoring has been used in the VIA-LVM (low volume mode) Monitor (VIA® Medical Corporation, San Diego, Calif). In this system, the monitor is a microprocessor-based instrument that integrates the functions of a volumetric infusion pump with an electrolyte and blood gas parameter measurement system (Fig. 30–11). The sen-

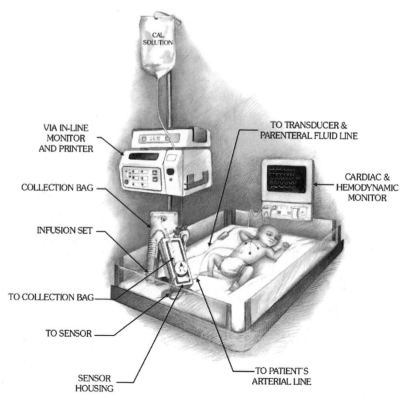

CAL
SOLUTION

VIA IN-LINE
MONITOR
AND PRINTER

COLLECTION BAG

INFUSION SET

TO COLLECTION BAG

TO SENSOR

SENSOR
HOUSING

TO PATIENT'S
ARTERIAL LINE

TO TRANSDUCER &
PARENTERAL FLUID LINE

CARDIAC &
HEMODYNAMIC
MONITOR

FIGURE 30–11. VIA-LVM blood gas and chemistry monitoring system. (Courtesy of VIA® Medical Corporation.)

sor set consists of two flow cells, a sensor cell and a reference cell connected in series. The sensor cell is connected to the IV cannula and contains ion selective electrodes (ISE) to measure pH, Na, K, and $PaCO_2$. A Clark electrode and electrical conductance technology are used to measure $PaO2$ and hematocrit, respectively. This system employs a closed-loop system whereby a reversible pump withdraws 1.5 cc of blood from any arterial line to the sensor set, analysis is performed, and the blood is returned to the patient followed by a 0.5 mL post-sample flush from an in-line heparinized solution, which is also the calibration fluid. Results are displayed approximately 70 seconds after sampling and may be printed out. The system has a 40-sample memory so that trends may be noted. An initial two-point calibration is required, after which one-point self-calibrations are performed after each sample and every 30 minutes. Studies in the adult population using this system have reported performance criteria acceptable by the current Medicare Clinical Laboratory Improvement Amendments (CLIA) proficiency standards.[3] Initial results from a multicenter evaluation of this system in the neonatal intensive care population[7] suggest that data obtained from this monitoring system agree with results from laboratory-based analyzers within CLIA limits.

NEAR-INFRARED SPECTROSCOPY

TECHNOLOGY DEVELOPMENT

Despite the enormous advances in neonatal monitoring technologies in recent years, current methods have failed to reliably and prospectively identify infants at risk for poor neurodevelopmental outcome. Although some clinical indicators and interventional factors have been examined, no powerful associations have been detected. A method for early identification of infants at risk for poor neurodevelopmental outcome is needed so that future neuroprotective techniques and therapies can be appropriately employed. On the brink of emerging from the research and development phase, near-infrared spectroscopy may offer possibilities for the future of neonatal diagnostic monitoring technology.

Transillumination, or the passage of light through the body, is a concept that has been in development since the early 1800s. Transillumination of the head, first described in 1831 by Richard Bright, was later recognized as the first light-based diagnosis of hydrocephalus. The technique was modified, and although still crude, was used to diagnose intracranial hemorrhage in the neonate at a time when head ultrasound was not yet available.[17] Jobsis showed that if near-infrared light with a wavelength of 700 to 1000 nm was used instead of visible light, absorption by tissue was low enough for spectral measurements to be made across the head of an animal with a diameter of 5 to 6 cm. Light within these wavelengths could then be used to measure total hemoglobin and oxygenation noninvasively within the tissue (see Fig. 30–

7).[41] These developments have led to a proliferation of near-infrared spectroscopy (NIRS) research.

All near-infrared devices to study the brain have a few basic principles in common. Light within the near-infrared wavelengths is emitted from fiberoptic cables placed on the head. Near-infrared light is a nonionizing and safe form of radiation, and it is known to penetrate the scalp and skull to reach the brain. There the photons are scattered and absorbed to varying degrees based on the physical and chemical properties of the brain. The depth of the penetration is in part a function of the emitter-detector separation; the greater the distance between the two, the deeper the penetration. The photons are therefore transmitted through a portion of the brain to the detector bearing "information" about the function of the brain. Mathematical derivations of Beer's law that take the scattering properties of tissues into account are used to calculate oxy-, deoxy-, and total hemoglobin. Numerous devices have been developed in multiple laboratories including University of Illinois, Urbana; University of Pennsylvania; Stanford University; University College, London; Phillips Corporation; ISS, Inc.; Siemens; and Hamamatsu. Because of their noninvasive nature, these devices can be used at the bedside of critically ill patients and can make continuous, often real-time measurements.

CLINICAL APPLICATION

An important aspect of obtaining data by a noninvasive method is ensuring that measurements are reflective of the site of interest. In addition to benchtop phantom and pathologic sample studies, a clinically useful headband[37] has allowed in vivo studies, which revealed site specificity with regard to intraventricular hemorrhage in the neonatal population (Fig. 30–12).[39] The creation of bedside, noninvasive NIRS functional imaging systems also has led to studies revealing real-time activation of sensorimotor cortex during passive movements in the premature infant.[38] Further studies with NIRS have demonstrated changes in cerebral blood volume during exchange transfusions and during the induction of extracorporeal membrane oxygenation (ECMO), leading to speculation over loss of cerebral autoregulation in the sick newborn population.[47, 52] Studies using NIRS to investigate cerebral oxygenation in the newborn have underscored the fact that present clinical indicators and monitoring systems may not reflect potentially important changes in the brain. Presumably "simple" procedures, such as endotracheal suctioning of term and preterm infants, can result in significant changes in cerebral oxygenation and blood volume that cannot necessarily be anticipated or compensated for using traditional parameters such as pulse oximetry.[23] Similarly, NIRS methods have demonstrated that in a particular subset of the ill preterm population, a strong correlation between systemic blood pressure and cerebral oxygenation parameters may be predictive of later neurologic injury, suggesting that impaired cerebrovascular autoregulation could be identifiable

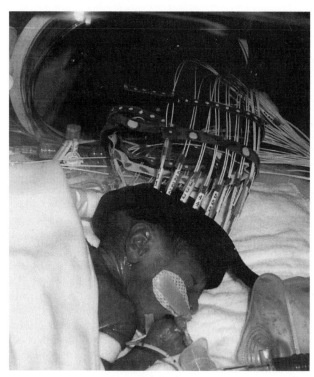

FIGURE 30–12. Fiberoptic headband for near-infrared spectroscopy measurements by the time-of-flight and absorbance method in place on a premature infant.

by NIRS techniques.[58] In addition, and perhaps most important for the clinician, small preliminary outcome studies have indicated that NIRS-obtained measures of cerebral blood flow and volume may be highly sensitive in the prediction of death or disability in the asphyxiated neonatal population.[48] Cerebral hemodynamic abnormalities could be witnessed in evolution by NIRS yet be clinically silent using current monitoring techniques. In the future, continuous, bedside cerebral monitoring by NIRS could potentially identify infants at risk for permanent neurodevelopmental damage, allowing for proper application of rapidly developing neuroprotective interventions.

■ REFERENCES

1. Aoyagi T, et al: Improvement of the earpiece oximeter. In Abstracts of the 13th Conference of the Japanese Society of Medical Electronics and Biological Engineering 90–91. Osaka, Japan, 1974.
2. Arafat M, Mattoo TK: Measurement of blood pressure in children: Recommendations and perceptions of cuff selection. Pediatrics 104:e30, 1999.
3. Bailey PL, et al: Evaluation in volunteers of the VIA V-ABG automated bedside blood gas, chemistry, and hematocrit monitor. J Clin Monit Comput 14:339, 1998.
4. Baird TM, et al: Optimal lead placement for monitoring the ECG and breathing in infants. Pediatr Pulmonol 7:276, 1989.
5. Barker SJ, Shah NK: The effects of motion on the performance of pulse oximeters in volunteers. Anesthesiology 86:101, 1997.
6. Benaron DA, et al: Noninvasive methods for estimating in vivo oxygenation. Clin Pediatr 5:258, 1992.
7. Billman G, et al: Multicenter evaluation of a novel low volume blood gas and chemistry monitor for neonates. Pediatr Res 45:37A, 1999.
8. Boyle RJ, Oh W: Erythema following transcutaneous PO_2 monitoring. Pediatrics 65:333, 1980.
9. Carter B, et al: A comparison of two transcutaneous monitors for the measurement of arterial PO_2 and PCO_2 in neonates. Anaesth Intensive Care 23:708, 1995.
10. Cartlidge PHT, Rutter N: Karaya gum electrocardiographic electrodes for preterm infants. Arch Dis Child 62:1281, 1987.
11. Cassady G: Transcutaneous monitoring in the newborn infant. J Pediatr 103:837, 1983.
12. Cobbold RSC: Transducers for Biomedical Measurements. New York, Wiley-Interscience, 1974.
13. Cohen RS, et al: Retrospective analysis of risks associated with an umbilical artery catheter system for continuous monitoring of arterial oxygen tension. J Perinatol 15:195, 1995.
14. Colditz PB, et al: Anetoderma of prematurity in association with electrocardiographic electrodes. J Am Acad Dermatol 41:479, 1999.
15. Costarino AT, et al: Falsely normal saturation reading with the pulse oximeter. Anesthesiology 67:830, 1987.
16. Donn SM: Neonatal and Pediatric Pulmonary Graphics: Principles and Clinical Applications. Armonk, New York, Futura Publishing Company, 1998.
17. Donn SM, et al: Rapid detection of neonatal intracranial hemorrhage by transillumination. Pediatrics 64:843, 1979.
18. Dransfield DA, Philip AGS: Respiratory airflow measurement in the newborn. Clin Perinatol 12:21, 1985.
19. Duc G, et al: Reliability of continuous transcutaneous PO_2 in respiratory distress syndrome of the newborn. Birth Defects 15:305, 1979.
20. Emery JL: Skin pigmentation as an influence on the accuracy of pulse oximetry. J Perinatol 7:329, 1990.
21. Fanconi S: Pulse oximetry for hypoxemia: A warning to users and manufacturers. Intensive Care Med 15:540, 1989.
22. Fanconi S, Sigrist H: Transcutaneous carbon dioxide and oxygen tension in newborn infants: Reliability of a combined monitor of oxygen tension and carbon dioxide tension. J Clin Monit 4:103, 1988.
23. Gagnon RE, et al: Variations in regional cerebral blood volume in neonates associated with nursery care events. Am J Perinatol 16:7, 1999.
24. Gangitano ES, et al: Near continuous pulse oximetry during newborn ECLS. ASAIO J 45:125, 1999.
25. Geddes LA: The Direct and Indirect Measurement of Blood Pressure. Chicago, Year Book Publishers, 1970.
26. Geddes LA: Electrodes and the Measurement of Bioelectric Events. New York, Wiley-Interscience, 1972.
27. Geddes LA: Cardiovascular Devices and Their Applications. New York, Wiley-Interscience, John Wiley and Sons, 1984.
28. Gevers M, et al: Accuracy of oscillometric blood pressure measurement in critically ill neonates with reference to the arterial pressure wave shape. Intensive Care Med 22:242, 1996.
29. Golden SM: Skin craters—a complication of transcutaneous oxygen monitoring. Pediatrics 67:514,1981.
30. Goldstein MR, et al: Pulse oximetry in transport of poorly-perfused babies. Pediatrics 102:818, 1998.
31. Harpin VA, Rutter N: Barrier properties of the newborn infant's skin. J Pediatr 102:419, 1983.
32. Hay WW, et al: Pulse oximetry in the NICU: Conventional vs. Masimo SET. Pediatr Res 45:304A, 1999.
33. Hay WW Jr, et al: Neonatal pulse oximetry: Accuracy and reliability. Pediatrics 83:717, 1989.
34. Hay WW Jr, et al: Pulse oximetry in neonatal medicine. Clin Perinatol 18:441, 1991.
35. Hodgkin AL, Huxley AF: A quantitative description of membrane current and its application to conduction and excitation in nerve. J Physiol (Lond) 117:500, 1952.
36. Holmes M, et al: Co-oximetry validation of a new pulse oximeter in sick newborns. Resp Care 43:860, 1998.
37. Hintz SR, et al: Stationary headband for clinical time-of-flight optical imaging at the bedside. Photochem Photobiol 68:361, 1998.
38. Hintz SR, et al: Bedside functional imaging of the premature infant brain during passive motor activation. SPIE 3597:221, 1999.
39. Hintz SR, et al: Bedside imaging of intracranial hemorrhage in

the neonate using light: Comparison with ultrasound, CT and MRI. Pediatr Res 45:54, 1999.

40. Huch R, et al: Transcutaneous measurement of blood PO_2 ($tcPO_2$)—Method and application in perinatal medicine. J Perinat Med 1:183, 1973.

41. Jobsis FF: Non-invasive infra-red monitoring of circulatory parameters. Science 198:1264, 1977.

42. Katz AM: Physiology of the Heart, 2nd ed, ch 20, The Electrocardiogram. Raven Press, New York, 1992.

43. Kelleher JF: Pulse oximetry. J Clin Monit 5:37, 1989.

44. Kost GJ, et al: Monitoring of transcutaneous carbon dioxide tension. AJCP 80:832, 1983.

45. Kunk R, McCain GC: Comparison of upper arm and calf oscillometric blood pressure measurement in preterm infants. J Perinatol 16:89, 1996.

46. Laks MM, et al: Recommendations for safe current limits for electrocardiographs: A statement for healthcare professionals from the Committee on Electrocardiography, American Heart Association. Circulation 93:837, 1996.

47. Liem KD, et al: Cerebral oxygenation and hemodynamics during induction of ECMO as investigated by NIRS. Pediatrics 95:555, 1995.

48. Meek JH, et al: Abnormal cerebral haemodynamics in perinatally asphyxiated neonates related to outcome. Arch Dis Child Fetal Neonatal Ed 81:F110, 1999.

49. Mendelson Y: Pulse oximetry: Theory and applications for non-invasive monitoring. Clin Chem 38:1601, 1992.

50. Merrick EB, Hayes TJ: Continuous, non-invasive measurements of arterial blood oxygen levels. Hewlett-Packard Journal 28:2, 1976.

51. Morgan C, et al: Continuous neonatal blood gas monitoring using a multiparameter intra-arterial sensor. Arch Dis Child 80:F93, 1999.

52. Murakami Y, et al: Changes in cerebral hemodynamics and oxygenation in unstable septic newborns during exchange transfusion. Kurume Med J 45:321, 1997.

53. Neuman M: Biomedical engineering aspects of neonatal monitoring. In Fanaroff AA, Martin RJ (eds): Neonatal-Perinatal Medicine, 6th ed, St. Louis, Mosby, 1997.

54. Pichler G, et al: Non-invasive oscillometric blood pressure measurement in very-low birthweight infants: A comparison of two different monitor systems. Acta Paediatr 88:1044, 1999.

55. Pollitzer MJ, et al: Continuous monitoring of arterial oxygen tension in infants: Four years of experience with an intravascular oxygen electrode. Pediatrics 66:31, 1980.

56. Rheineck-Leyssius AT, Kalkman CJ: Advanced pulse oximeter signal processing technology compared to simple averaging. II. Effect on frequency of alarms in the postanethesia care unit. J Clin Anesth 11:196, 1999.

57. Stranger P, et al: Electrocardiograph monitor artifacts in a neonatal intensive care unit. Pediatrics 60:689, 1977.

58. Soul JS, du Plessis AJ: Near-infrared spectroscopy. Sem Ped Neurol 6:101, 1999.

59. Thach BT, Stark AR: Spontaneous neck flexion and airway obstruction during apneic spells in preterm infants. J Pediatr 94:275, 1979.

60. Venkatesh B, et al: Continuous measurements of blood gases using a combined electrochemical and spectrophotometric sensor. J Med Eng Tech 18:165, 1994.

61. Watson AB, et al: Electrical thresholds for ventricular fibrillation in man. Med J Aust 1:1179, 1973.

62. Weber W, et al: Low perfusion-resistant pulse oximetry. J Clin Monit 11:284, 1995.

63. Wood EH, Geraci JE: Photoelectric determination of arterial oxygen saturation in man. J Lab Clin Med 34:387, 1949.

64. Wukitsch MW, et al: Pulse oximetry: Analysis of theory, technology and practice. J Clin Monit 4:290, 1988.

65. Zollinger A, et al: Accuracy and clinical performance of a continuous intra-arterial blood-gas monitoring system during thoracoscopic surgery. Br J Anaesth 79:47, 1997.

31 Anesthesia in the Neonate

John E. Stork

The last decade has seen such major advances in neonatology that meaningful survival of infants weighing as little as 1000 gm has become almost routine. Pediatric anesthesia also has developed as a specialty, showing clear differences between adults and children with respect to medical needs and the patients' reactions to anesthesia and surgery. Nowhere are these differences more profound than in the neonate, particularly the premature infant. Immaturity of organ systems, homeostatic control mechanisms, and metabolic pathways are major complicating factors. Meticulous attention to detail, as well as a thorough understanding of neonatal physiology, pharmacology, and pathophysiology are prerequisites for the successful use of anesthesia in the preterm neonate. Consequently, there are obvious benefits from having personnel with experience and training specifically in the care of neonates. Studies have demonstrated decreased anesthesia-related morbidity in children anesthetized by pediatric anesthesiologists compared with those anesthetized by nonpediatric anesthesiologists.[18] The operating room (OR) environment also must be specifically adapted for neonatal care. The same degree of intensive care provided to the neonate in the neonatal intensive care unit (NICU) must continue in the OR, with the goal of maintaining or perhaps improving the overall medical condition of the infant. Inadequate ventilation, lack of careful temperature control, and other problems typical of trying to adapt adult anesthesia equipment to the neonate are not acceptable.

Anesthesia consists of three components:

1. Analgesia (pain relief)
2. Amnesia (absence of awareness or recall of surgical events)
3. Akinesia (lack of movement)

COMPONENTS OF ANESTHESIA

ANALGESIA

It has been suggested that the neonate's perception of pain is blunted or nonexistent. Because it was felt that anesthesia itself could induce or augment instability in the sick infant, minimal anesthesia to neonates was considered to be the safest approach. In some cases, this has included the performance of surgical procedures using only neuromuscular blockade. It has become increasingly clear that minimal anesthesia is an untenable position. Ethical treatment requires caregivers to do all that is possible to alleviate pain. With neonates and children, it has become a parental expectation that all possible measures be taken to minimize any pain. Although it is true that anesthetizing the infant requires careful attention to specific factors peculiar to neonatal physiology and metabolism, it can be performed safely.

There is clear evidence that although the infant does not self-report pain, neonates do experience discomfort and stress in response to painful stimuli as encountered during procedures and surgery.[3, 11, 15] By late gestation, the fetus is neuroanatomically and physiologically capable of transmitting pain.[2] Term and preterm neonates exhibit physiologic and hormonal responses to painful stimuli, which may even be exaggerated, compared with older children and adults.[2, 4] This stress response is characterized by overall sympathetic stimulation, with increased catecholamine production, a hyperdynamic circulation, increased oxygen demand, insulin resistance, increased gluconeogenesis, and a catabolic state, and can be inhibited by anesthesia, as shown in Figure 31–1.[5] Blunting the stress response to pain and surgery with appropriate anesthesia may improve outcome, even in the premature neonate, as shown in Table 31–1 from a study by Anand and colleagues in which fentanyl anesthesia markedly decreased the incidence of postoperative complications in a group of premature neonates.[5]

Pain experienced early in life may influence the individual's response to pain later. Behavioral and physiologic studies suggest an enhanced response to pain in former premature infants who experienced multiple noxious stimuli as neonates.[4] A very recent animal study may provide a basis for this effect. An inflammatory lesion lasting 5 to 7 days was induced in the hind paw of newborn rat pups. When examined as adults, these animals demonstrated neuroanatomic changes, with increased nociceptive dorsal horn primary afferents. These neurons exhibited increased

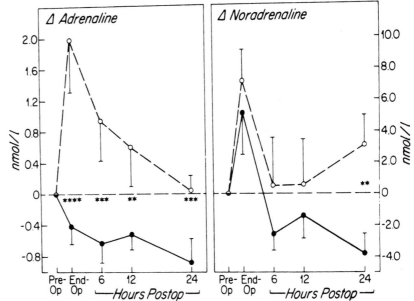

FIGURE 31-1. The change from baseline of adrenaline and noradrenaline in nmol/L preoperatively to the end of the operation and for the first 24 hours thereafter. The two groups reflect nitrous oxide–fentanyl anesthesia (*closed circles*) and nitrous oxide anesthesia (*open circles*). In the fentanyl-anesthetized patients there was no increase in adrenaline or noradrenaline, not only intraoperatively but also for the first 24 hours postoperatively, indicating a significantly blunted stress response.

spontaneous and evoked firing rates. Behaviorally, the adult animals also demonstrated heightened response to pain.[30]

More recent surveys of doctors and nurses demonstrate that an awareness of the problem of pain in neonates has replaced a previous lack of recognition of the problem. In a survey by Porter and associates, 60% of doctors and nurses believed that infants can feel the same amount of pain as can adults, whereas 27% believed infants feel more pain. About 10% continue to believe infants feel less pain than do adults.[28, 29] Although the need for intraoperative anesthesia and postoperative pain management is essentially universally accepted, pain associated with procedures in the NICU, such as invasive lines and chest tube insertions, is in many cases inadequately managed. A recent statement by the American Academy of Pediatrics and Canadian Pediatric Society highlights the problems of pain and stress in the neonate and makes recommendations for reduced exposure to pain and treatment interventions.[1]

AMNESIA

The need for analgesia during surgery of the neonate is accepted, but the benefits of amnesia are less clear.

TABLE 31-1   PERIOPERATIVE COMPLICATIONS

COMPLICATION	CONTROL	FENTANYL
Frequent bradycardia	4	1
Hypotension, poor circulation	4	0
Glycosuria	1	0
Acidosis	2	0
Increased ventilatory requirements	4	1
Intraventricular hemorrhage	2	0
Total complications	17	2

From Anand KJS, et al: Randomized trial of fentanyl anaesthesia in preterm babies undergoing surgery: Effects on the stress response. Lancet 1:243, 1987.

Whether awareness during surgery has any longstanding developmental consequences remains an open question. If adequate analgesia is provided, does awareness alone in the absence of pain cause stress in the neonate? What level of awareness does a preterm neonate possess? Parental expectations are generally clear—a sick child should not suffer—and it is important for the anesthesiologist to consider the question of awareness in the neonate.

AKINESIA

Muscle relaxants have been used commonly in neonates, and in the recent past they were often (sadly) the primary component of anesthesia. Neonatal surgery is a delicate procedure, so ideal operative conditions for most procedures require muscular paralysis. Paralyzing without adequate analgesia and sedation, however, is as inappropriate in the neonate as it is in the adult.

HOMEOSTASIS

Although not generally considered to be a component of anesthesia, maintenance of homeostasis is an important aspect of anesthesia care. Temperature regulation, fluid and electrolyte balance, cardiorespiratory function, nutritional balance, and maintenance of circulating red cell volume are several aspects of homeostasis, which can be adversely affected during surgery. Meticulous monitoring and care are necessary in the OR to ensure the best surgical outcome.

NEONATAL PHYSIOLOGY AND DEVELOPMENT

There are specific anatomic and physiologic differences among neonates, older children, and adults, many of which directly impact anesthetic administration and management. Maturation of organ systems and metabolic processes also vary significantly between preterm and term neonates. Major changes, primarily in cardiac and respiratory function, take place at birth, and an understanding of this transition phase is a prerequisite for the pediatric anesthesiologist. (See also Chapters 42 and 43.)

THE TRANSITION PHASE

Prior to birth, the pulmonary circulation is a high resistance circuit, the lungs receive little blood flow, and oxygenation is a placental function. At birth, approximately 35 mL of amniotic fluid is expelled from the lungs, the lungs re-expand, and respiration begins. Compliance of the lung is initially very low, and the first breath may require negative forces of 70 cm H_2O or more. With oxygenation and lung distention, pulmonary vascular resistance (PVR) decreases and pulmonary blood flow and cardiac output increase. Increasing pulmonary flow, coupled with decreased venous return from the inferior vena cava with clamping of the placenta leads to an increase in left atrial pressure higher than the right arterial pressure and closure of the foramen ovale. In normal situations the ductus arteriosus closes somewhere between 1 and 15 hours after birth. Although PVR decreases, the pulmonary arterioles possess abundant smooth muscle, and the pulmonary vascular bed remains very reactive. In this setting, hypoxia, hypercarbia, or acidosis can cause a sudden increase in PVR and a return to a fetal circulatory pattern, a condition known as persistent fetal circulation (PFC) or persistent pulmonary hypertension of the neonate (PPHN). This is an acute, life-threatening condition, as shunt fraction increases to 70% to 80% and profound cyanosis results. In addition to providing adequate anesthesia, careful attention intraoperatively to factors that increase PVR in the neonate is critical. (See also Chapter 43.)

RESPIRATORY PHYSIOLOGY

(See also Chapter 42, Part Two.)

Anesthetic agents are respiratory depressants. Central regulation of breathing is obtunded under anesthesia, with a significant decrease in the ventilatory response to increased CO_2. Lung volume and functional residual capacity (FRC) are small related to body size in the neonate compared with those of older children and adults. Alveolar ventilation per unit lung volume is very high, because the neonate's metabolic rate is about twice that of an adult. Most of this alveolar ventilation is provided by a rapid respiratory rate of 35 to 40 per minute because tidal volume is limited due to the structure of the chest wall. One consequence of the small FRC and high metabolic rate in the neonate is a diminished reserve. Changes in FiO_2 are rapidly seen as changes in PO_2, and the neonate quickly desaturates if ventilation is interrupted. This occurrence limits time for intuba-

tion, and airway management can be difficult. The high alveolar ventilation also accounts for a very rapid uptake of inhalational anesthetic agents, especially in premature infants, which can contribute to a tendency to overdose with these agents. Closing volume, which is the lung volume at which smaller airways tend to collapse, is very close to FRC in neonates. It is well known that anesthesia causes decreases in FRC.[17] In the neonate this decrease can result in airway closure at end-expiration, with resultant atelectasis, $\dot{V}/\dot{Q}$ mismatch, and increased intrapulmonary shunting. The awake infant uses laryngeal braking to provide some degree of auto–positive end-expiratory pressure (auto-PEEP) and to maintain FRC, but laryngeal braking is diminished by anesthesia. In the premature neonate the immature alveoli are thick walled and saccular. Surfactant production begins at 23 to 24 weeks' gestation, but it may remain inadequate until 36 weeks. Lung volumes and compliance are therefore further decreased in the very premature infant. Whereas the lung is less compliant in the infant than in older children, the chest wall in the infant is very compliant. This combination accounts for about 75% of an increased work of breathing, with the remainder attributed to airway resistance. Because resistance to airflow is inversely proportional to the fourth power of the radius of the airway, the work of breathing is markedly increased in the small premature infant. Changes in airway resistance are common during anesthesia, often due to small endotracheal tubes and equipment factors such as valves in the breathing circuit. Kinking of the tube or the presence of secretions also can adversely affect resistance. Respiratory failure from fatigue can occur easily. The low FRC, increased closing volume and increased work, along with changes induced by anesthetics combine to essentially require controlled positive pressure ventilation during operative procedures. Infants already being ventilated require some increase in their ventilator settings after induction of anesthesia, and postoperatively infants usually require increased ventilatory support.

Tracheomalacia is common in premature infants, and if low in the airway, it may not be obviated by intubation. Bronchomalacia may result in airway collapse on expiration. Continuous positive airway pressure (CPAP) or PEEP increases FRC and decreases closing volume and helps to stent open the airway during anesthesia. Somewhat slower respiratory rates should be used with positive pressure ventilation to allow time for passive exhalation and to prevent air trapping. The premature lung is very susceptible to barotrauma and oxygen toxicity. Pneumothorax and interstitial emphysema may develop if high-peak inspiratory pressures are used. Airway anatomy in the infant also differs from older children. The infant's head is much larger when compared with body size than that of older children, although the infant's neck is short. The infant's tongue is large, but the larynx is higher and anterior, with the cords located at C4 in the infant compared with that at C5 or C6 in the adult. The epiglottis of the infant is soft and folded.

In an adult, the larynx is cylindrical in shape, with the narrowest point at the glottis. The neonate's larynx is conical, with the narrowest point in the subglottic area at the cricoid ring. Endotracheal tube size must be carefully considered to prevent airway trauma. Subglottic stenosis is a common complication especially with longer-term intubation. Even modest airway edema can be serious. At the cricoid ring, as little as 1 mm of edema results in a 60% reduction in the cross-sectional area of the airway, resulting in increased airway resistance and increased work of breathing. Laryngomalacia is common in the premature infant and can result in obstruction. Periodic breathing with intermittent apneic spells is common in neonates up to 3 months of age. Small premature infants have a biphasic ventilatory response to hypoxia, with an initial increase in ventilation, followed by a progressive decrease, and apnea. The ventilatory response to CO_2 also is decreased, and as noted, is further decreased by anesthesia. Postoperative apneic spells are common in premature infants, although incidence decreases with advancing postconceptional age. These episodes can be secondary to the immature respiratory control system (central), a floppy airway (obstructive), or both (mixed or combined).

CARDIAC PHYSIOLOGY

(See also Chapter 43, Part Three.)

The transitional cardiac changes were discussed earlier. Immediately after birth, with an open ductus arteriosus most of the cardiac output is from the left ventricle, and left ventricular end-diastolic volume is very high. Consequently, the neonatal heart functions at the high end of the Starling curve. As PVR decreases, output from the two ventricles becomes balanced at 150 to 200 mL/kg per minute. Heart rate is rapid at 130 to 160. Because end-diastolic volumes are already high, the infant heart is not able to increase stroke volume to a significant degree, and increases in cardiac output are entirely dependent on increases in heart rate. Baseline blood pressure is lower in infants than in older children, particularly in preterm infants; because cardiac output is increased, this is due to a low systemic vascular resistance. All anesthetic agents have significant effects on the cardiovascular system to varying degrees. Inhalational agents tend to be cardiovascular depressants,[25] and they can result in decreased myocardial contractility and bradycardia and subsequent decreased cardiac output. Most anesthetic agents cause decreased autonomic tone and peripheral vasodilation, decreasing both afterload and preload. Because baroreceptor reflexes also are blunted by anesthesia, these decreases may make it impossible for the infant to compensate for pre-existing volume contraction or volume losses during anesthesia. In the sick neonate, inotropic support may be necessary, and almost all infants require some degree of volume loading during anesthesia. This belief may be at odds with current thoughts on respiratory management, which emphasize diuresis, and volume therapy needs to be carefully balanced

to support tissue perfusion, urine output, and metabolic needs.

FETAL HEMOGLOBIN

(See also Chapter 44.)

The infant has about 80% fetal hemoglobin at birth. Hemoglobin F (HbF) has a P50 of 20 mm Hg, compared with a P50 of 27 mm Hg for hemoglobin A, which means that HbF has a higher affinity for oxygen and that the hemoglobin dissociation curve is shifted to the left. In utero this favors transport of oxygen from the maternal to the fetal circulation. Another way to express this is that for any given oxygen saturation, the infant has a lower Po_2. Unloading of oxygen at the tissue level also is diminished, although this is compensated for by an increased hemoglobin level of about 17.5 gm/dL at birth. The decreased unloading, however, can result in tissue hypoxia if Po_2, hemoglobin, or cardiac output decrease intraoperatively, with secondary development of metabolic acidosis. The hemoglobin rises slightly just after birth, then it decreases progressively to a level of 9.5 to 11 gm/dL by 7 to 9 weeks of life, owing to decreased red cell life span, increasing blood volume, and immature hematopoiesis. Fetal hemoglobin synthesis begins to decrease after 35 weeks' gestation, and HbF is completely replaced by HbA by 8 to 12 weeks of life, paralleling the decrease in hemoglobin and helping to maintain tissue oxygenation.

RENAL PHYSIOLOGY

(See also Chapter 49.)

The fetus has as many nephrons as do adults from 34 weeks' gestation on, although the nephrons are immature, and the glomerular filtration rate (GFR) is about 30% of the adult at birth. With increasing cardiac output and decreasing renal vascular resistance, renal blood flow and GFR increase rapidly over the first few weeks of life, and reach adult levels by about one year of life. The diminished function over the first year is actually well balanced to the infant's needs, because much of the neonate's solute load is incorporated into body growth and excretory load is smaller. Several aspects of renal physiology are pertinent to anesthesia care. First, the neonatal kidney has only limited concentrating ability, seemingly owing to a diminished osmotic gradient in the renal interstitium, whereas antidiuretic hormone secretion and activity are normal. Coupled with an increased insensible loss owing to a "thin" skin and increased ratio of surface area to volume, the limited concentrating ability of the kidney implies a tendency to become water depleted if intake or administration is not adequate. The neonatal kidney also is not able to efficiently excrete dilute urine and therefore cannot handle a large free water load. In addition, primarily owing to a short, immature proximal tubule, infants are obligate sodium wasters. There is then a tendency toward hyponatremia, especially if too much free water is administered intraoperatively, which can easily happen with continuous infusions from invasive pressure transducers, especially if adult transducers are used. Again, owing to the lower GFR, the neonate also cannot handle a large sodium load and can easily develop volume overload and congestive heart failure. One final aspect concerns acid-base status; the neonatal kidney wastes small amounts of bicarbonate, owing to an immature proximal tubule; thus, infants are born with a mild proximal renal tubular acidosis, with serum bicarbonate about 20 mmol/L. These changes are all greater in the preterm infant, particularly before nephrogenesis is complete at 34 weeks.

TEMPERATURE REGULATION

(See also Chapter 29.)

Given a large surface area, small body volume, and minimal insulation, neonates are extremely prone to heat loss. Any degree of cold stress is detrimental and increases metabolic demands in the neonate. Infants are unable to shiver effectively, and cold stress causes catecholamine release, which stimulates nonshivering thermogenesis by brown fat. The increased catechols can be detrimental, causing increased pulmonary and systemic vascular resistance, increased cardiac stress, and increased O_2 consumption. Anesthesia blunts thermoregulatory sensitivity[7, 34, 35] and interferes with nonshivering thermogenesis and brown fat metabolism.[10] Anesthesia also increases heat loss by inducing cutaneous vasodilation. At all times, including during transport and in the OR, the infant must be subjected to a neutral thermal environment. An overly warm environment of course can be equally detrimental. Core temperature must be carefully monitored at all times in the OR.

CARBOHYDRATE METABOLISM

(See also Chapter 47, Part One.)

The neonate has a high glucose demand related to the high brain mass of 12% compared with that of 2% in the adult. Carbohydrate reserves in the normal newborn are relatively low, and even lower in the infant with low birth weight. Immediately after birth, glucose is only available from glycogen stores in the liver, although gluconeogenesis is activated within 8 hours of birth. Hypoglycemia can readily occur if the infant is deprived of a glucose source, but hyperglycemia can also be a problem in the perioperative period. Insulin response is deficient in preterm babies, and high catecholamines owing to intraoperative stress can result in hyperglycemia. Usually, IV glucose (D10) or IV hyperalimentation should be continued intraoperatively, especially in infants of low birth weight without adequate glycogen or fat stores. However, in the sicker infants it is important to monitor serum glucose, because hyperglycemia may intervene.

PREOPERATIVE EVALUATION AND PREPARATION

The preoperative evaluation is extremely important in the neonate, and it should encompass the infant's physical condition, including any disease states, degree of transition from fetal to newborn physiology, and presence of any congenital anomalies. Particular attention should be paid to cardiorespiratory status, any required ventilatory or hemodynamic support, blood chemistries, and nutritional support. The courses of pregnancy, labor, and delivery and a full maternal history are important details. As is the case with older children, a family history of anesthetic difficulties may be important. Maternal diseases such as diabetes, systemic lupus erythematosus, and preeclampsia are clearly reflected in the neonate. Potential congenital infections, oligohydramnios, intrauterine growth restriction, and maternal drug and alcohol use are also important considerations. Gestational age, as well as birth weight and postnatal age obviously impact anesthetic care. Birth weight does not necessarily accurately reflect maturity unless the infant is appropriate for gestational age (AGA), defined as being within two standard deviations of the mean for the gestational age. Infants who are small for gestational age (SGA) are more mature than their birth weight would indicate. Infants who are large for gestational age (LGA) are often children of diabetic mothers, and they are at increased risk of hypoglycemia in the first 48 hours after birth. Newborns are characterized by birth weight as *low birth weight* (LBW, 2.5 kg or less), *very low birth weight* (VLBW, 1.5 kg or less) and *extremely low birth weight* (ELBW, less than 1000 gm). *Term* is gestational age from 37 to 42 weeks; *preterm* is younger than 37 weeks; and *postterm* is older than 42 weeks. A history of birth asphyxia or neonatal resuscitation and Apgar scores are important. History should include complete details of present illness and treatment. Medications and administration times, details of vascular access, and respiratory parameters including ventilator type and settings are all critical details especially in the sicker infants. Infants on high-frequency oscillatory ventilation (HFOV) may need to be switched to conventional ventilation and observed for several hours to facilitate movement to an OR. If the infant is on some other modality, such as inhaled nitric oxide or extracorporeal membrane oxygenation, arrangements may also need to be made, and transport to the OR will require more resources and assistance.

The time of the last oral feed should be ascertained, especially in elective surgery in healthier infants. Attenuation of airway reflexes with induction of anesthesia places the infant at risk of aspiration of acidic gastric contents, and it can lead to serious inflammatory pneumonitis. NPO guidelines are summarized in Table 31–2,[32] and they are somewhat more liberal for newborns than adults. In part this reflects more rapid

TABLE 31–2 NPO GUIDELINES

INTAKE	TIME
Clear liquids	2 hrs
Breast milk	4 hrs
Formula	6 hrs

gastric emptying, although in an infant, dehydration occurs much more quickly than in an adult, and this is a concern in the infant without an IV. As in adults, gastric emptying is delayed with stress, anxiety, and illness. Infants with diseases such as pyloric stenosis, duodenal atresia, malrotation, or other obstructive lesions are considered NPO before surgery, and they will need an IV to maintain appropriate hydration. Despite the NPO status, there generally will be significant gastric contents and rapid sequence or awake intubation are required. Emptying the stomach via nasogastric drainage is not dependable and usually not adequate. Nasogastric feeds in intubated infants also should be discontinued at an appropriate time, because the infant may need to be reintubated perioperatively and a full stomach would increase the risk for aspiration. Physical exam includes vital signs, including temperature. Volume status needs to be carefully assessed, because major shifts can occur easily during surgery. Many infants requiring surgery are ill. Infants with congenital anomalies often have multiple defects, which may well have an impact on anesthetic care. Often a group of defects suggest a well-recognized and characterized syndrome. Some of the more common syndromes with their anesthetic implications are listed in Table 31–3, although this list is by no means complete.

Difficult intubation is a common problem in infants with congenital defects, and the airway needs to be carefully assessed. Given the tendency of rapid desaturation in infants, difficulties with intubation can be extremely serious. In infants who are already intubated, tube size and position should be evaluated. The pressure at which a leak occurs around the tube should be documented. Nurses should be questioned about the quantity and consistency of secretions and need for frequent suctioning. The small tubes required in premature infants can easily be blocked by tenacious secretions and are easily dislodged. If there is any question about adequacy of intubation, the infant should be electively reintubated before surgery; emergently replacing an endotracheal tube under the drapes after beginning an operation is not a benign procedure. A complete clinical physical exam should be performed, with particular attention paid to cardiorespiratory status. Laboratory studies and x-ray films need to be reviewed, if applicable. Hemoglobin level usually should be greater than 13 gm/dL to ensure adequate oxygen delivery to the tissues, given the decreased unloading at the tissue level by fetal hemoglobin. Metabolic acidosis should be corrected, preferably by reversal of the cause of the acidosis. Electrolyte levels help to guide fluid management; hypocalcemia should be corrected. For most operations, it is important to check that blood for transfusion is available; for major procedures, fresh frozen plasma and platelets for transfusion also may be required.

There are several specific areas that should be explored by the anesthesiologist. As previously dis-

TABLE 31–3   ANESTHETIC IMPLICATIONS OF SOME NEONATAL SYNDROMES

SYNDROME	CLINICAL MANIFESTATIONS	ANESTHETIC IMPLICATIONS
Adrenogenital syndrome	Defective cortisol synthesis Electrolyte abnormalities Virilization of females	Supplement cortisol
Analbuminemia	Almost absent albumin	Sensitive to protein-bound drugs (thiopental, curare, bupivacaine)
Andersen syndrome	Midface hypoplasia Kyphoscoliosis	Difficult airway Impaired respiratory function
Apert syndrome	Craniosynostosis Hypertelorism Congenital heart disease possible	Difficult airway Increased ICP Cardiac evaluation, prophylactic antibiotics
Chiari malformation	Hydrocephalus Cranial nerve palsies Other CNS lesions	Aspiration precautions Vocal cord paralysis Latex allergy precautions
Arthrogryposis multiplex congenita	Contractures Restrictive pulmonary disease	Care in positioning Difficult airway Postoperative ventilation
Beckwith-Wiedemann	High birth weight Macroglossia Neonatal hypoglycemia	Difficult airway Monitor blood glucose, continuous glucose infusion, avoid boluses
CHARGE syndrome	Coloboma Heart defects Atresia choanae Retardation Genital hypoplasia Ear deformities	Bilateral choanal atresia may require oral airway Cardiac evaluation, prophylactic antibiotics
Cherubism	Intraoral masses Mandibular, maxillary tumors	Difficult airway Possible cor pulmonale

Table continued on following page

TABLE 31–3 ANESTHETIC IMPLICATIONS OF SOME NEONATAL SYNDROMES *Continued*

SYNDROME	CLINICAL MANIFESTATIONS	ANESTHETIC IMPLICATIONS
Cornelia de Lange syndrome	Micrognathia, macroglossia Upper airway obstruction Microcephaly Congenital heart disease	Difficult airway Cardiac evaluation, prophylactic antibiotics
Cretinism	Macroglossia Goiter Decreased metabolic rate Myxedema Adrenal insufficiency	Difficult airway Delayed gastric emptying Fluid and electrolyte imbalance Sensitivity to cardiac and respiratory depressants Stress steroids
Cri du chat syndrome	Abnormal larynx, odd cry Microcephaly Hypertelorism, cleft palate Cardiac abnormalities	Difficult airway Cardiac evaluation, prophylactic antibiotics
Crouzon disease	Craniosynostosis Hypertelorism	Difficult airway Increased ICP
Dandy-Walker syndrome	Hydrocephalus Other CNS lesions	Increased ICP Latex allergy precautions
DiGeorge syndrome	Absent thymus, parathyroids Immunodeficiency Stridor Cardiac anomalies	Monitor calcium Exaggerated response to muscle relaxants Blood for transfusion irradiated Cardiac evaluation, prophylactic antibiotics
Down syndrome (trisomy 21)	Atlantoaxial instability Macroglossia Congenital subglottic stenosis Duodenal atresia Cardiac defects (AV canal) Mental retardation	Difficult airway, use smaller tube Care with neck manipulation Cardiac evaluation, prophylactic antibiotics
Dwarfism	Odontoid hypoplasia, atlantoaxial instability Micrognathia, cleft palate	Care with neck manipulation Cardiac evaluation, prophylactic antibiotics
Ellis–van Creveld syndrome	Ectodermal defects, short extremities Congenital heart defects Chest abnormalities Abnormal maxilla	Difficult airway Impaired respiratory function Cardiac evaluation, prophylactic antibiotics
Goldenhar syndrome	Maxillary hypoplasia, micrognathia Cleft or high arched palate Eye and ear abnormalities Hemivertebra or vertebral fusion Congenital heart defects Spina bifida	Difficult airway Cervical spine evaluation Cardiac evaluation, prophylactic antibiotics
Holoprosencephaly	Midline deformities of face, brain Dextrocardia, VSD Incomplete rotation of colon Hepatic malfunction, hypoglycemia Mental retardation, seizures	Difficult airway Postoperative apneas Cardiac evaluation, prophylactic antibiotics
Holt-Oram syndrome (heart-hand syndrome)	Radial dysplasia Congenital heart defects	Cardiac evaluation, prophylactic antibiotics
Jeune syndrome	Chest malformations Pulmonary hypoplasia and cysts Renal disease	Respiratory insufficiency, high risk of barotrauma Renal failure
Klippel-Feil syndrome	Fusion of cervical vertebrae Congenital heart defects	Difficult intubation Cardiac evaluation, prophylactic antibiotics
Möbius syndrome	Paralysis of CN VI and VII Micrognathia Recurrent aspiration Muscle weakness	Difficult airway Aspiration precautions
Mucopolysaccharidoses (Hurler and Hunter syndromes)	Macroglossia Hepatosplenomegaly Hydrocephalus Odontoid hypoplasia and atlantoaxial subluxation Valvular heart disease and cardiomyopathy	Difficult airway Coagulation abnormal Cervical spine Cardiac evaluation Increased ICP

TABLE 31–3 ANESTHETIC IMPLICATIONS OF SOME NEONATAL SYNDROMES *Continued*

SYNDROME	CLINICAL MANIFESTATIONS	ANESTHETIC IMPLICATIONS
Noonan syndrome	Micrognathia Webbed neck, short stature Congenital heart defects Hydronephrosis or hypoplastic kidneys	Difficult airway Cardiorespiratory evaluation Renal dysfunction
Oral-facial-digital syndrome	Cleft lip and palate Mandibular, maxillary hypoplasia Hydrocephalus Polycystic kidneys Digital abnormalities	Difficult airway Increased ICP Renal dysfunction
Osteogenesis imperfecta	Blue sclera, pathologic fractures, deafness Congenital heart defects Increased metabolism and hyperpyrexia	Difficult airway Careful positioning and padding Hyperpyrexia with anesthesia (not MH)
Pierre Robin	Micrognathia Cleft palate Glossoptosis Congenital heart defects Cor pulmonale	Difficult airway, LMA may be useful Cardiac evaluation, prophylactic antibiotics
Potter syndrome	Renal agenesis Low-set ears Pulmonary hypoplasia	Spontaneous pneumothorax Respiratory insufficiency Renal failure
Prune-belly syndrome	Absent abdominal musculature Renal dysplasia Pulmonary hypoplasia	Respiratory insufficiency Renal failure
Sturge-Weber syndrome	Vascular malformations and hemangiomas (intracranial)	Possible blood loss
Treacher Collins syndrome	Facial, pharyngeal hypoplasia Micrognathia, choanal atresia Congenital heart defects	Extremely difficult airway Cardiac evaluation, prophylactic antibiotics
Trisomy 18	Congenital heart disease common Micrognathia	Difficult airway Cardiac evaluation, prophylactic antibiotics
Turner syndrome	Micrognathia Webbed neck, short stature Congenital heart defects Renal anomalies	Difficult airway Cardiac evaluation, prophylactic antibiotics Renal insufficiency
VATER syndrome	*V*ertebral anomalies Imperforate *a*nus *T*racheo*e*sophageal fistula *R*adial dysplasia *R*enal anomalies Ventricular septal defect	Cardiac evaluation, prophylactic antibiotics TEF management
Williams syndrome	Elfin facies Infantile hypercalcemia Supravalvular aortic stenosis	Cardiac failure
Zellweger syndrome	Craniofacial dysmorphism Glaucoma Peroxisomal abnormalities in kidney and liver	Difficult airway Impaired renal drug excretion Electrolyte imbalance Abnormal coagulation

AV, atrioventricular; CN, cranial nerve; CNS, central nervous system; ICP, intracranial pressure; LMA, laryngeal mask airway; MH, malignant hyperpyrexia; TEF, tracheoesophageal fistula; VSD, ventricular septal defect.

cussed, the pulmonary circulation in the neonate is hyperreactive, and in the near term infant lung disease, asphyxia, and surgical stress can initiate episodes of pulmonary hypertension, resulting in decreased cardiac output and desaturation. Any history of such spells requires increased vigilance to avoid hypoxia, hypercarbia, and acidosis, which tend to increase pulmonary resistance. Congenital anomalies of the heart also must be carefully evaluated. Right-to-left shunts affect the oxygenation of the infant, but left-to-right shunts typically result in volume over-

load. The infant should be carefully evaluated for signs of congestive heart failure such as hepatic congestion, enlarged heart, and edema. The presence of single ventricle physiology is particularly important because the anesthesiologist needs to take great care to maintain balance between the pulmonary and systemic circulations. Abnormal pulses may indicate coarctation of the aorta. Intrinsic arrhythmias are unusual in the neonate, although congenital heart block may occur in infants of mothers with systemic lupus erythematosus. Neurologic function also should be carefully assessed. Hemodynamic changes during surgery may affect cerebral blood flow. A history of seizures should increase the anesthesiologist's level of suspicion for intraoperative seizure if there are unexplained tachycardias or blood pressure elevations. The presence of intraventricular hemorrhage requires increased care with hemodynamic stability and is a contraindication to procedures requiring anticoagulation. A history of hydrocephalus mandates avoidance of factors that increase intracranial pressure.

TRANSPORT, MONITORING, AND OPERATING ROOM EQUIPMENT

Where to perform surgery is an important question to ask. Initially, it seems obvious—surgery is performed in the OR; however, with neonates, particularly the very premature infant, the answer is less clear-cut. Transport of the infant may be as great a risk as the surgery itself. Great care needs to be taken to avoid cold stress. In some situations, if the surgical procedure is appropriate, if the surgeon is cooperative, and if a suitable locale is available, it may be preferable to perform some procedures in the NICU. Obvious basic requirements for a suitable locale include a clean area that can be closed off from traffic and adequate equipment including lights, surgical equipment and supplies, appropriate monitors, and anesthesia equipment. In our institution, we routinely perform patent ductus arteriosus (PDA) ligations in infants as small as 450 gm in a treatment room area of our NICU, which can be closed off and converted to a mini-OR. In most situations however, transport to the OR is necessary.

For all but the healthiest neonates, a physician experienced in neonatal resuscitation and who has the ability to manage critically ill neonates should accompany the transport. In most situations, this person should be the anesthesiologist. Heat loss during transport must be addressed because the hospital corridors are rarely neutral thermal environments. If the infant is in an isolette, the isolette should be used for transport, as heat is retained even when it is unplugged. A child on an open radiant warmer should be covered, including the head. In some institutions plastic wrap is used to retain heat and to reduce evaporative losses. Disposable chemical warmer packs are available and can be used under the infant in either an isolette or on the radiant warmer. Monitoring during transport varies depending on the condition of the infant. As a minimum, a pulse oximeter provides pulse rate and SaO_2. In most ill neonates electrocardiogram (EKG) and blood pressure should also be monitored, especially if the child has an indwelling arterial line. Any pumps providing infusions to the infant should have adequate battery power to operate throughout the transport, especially if vasoactive drips are running. For our infants dependent on vasoactive infusions, such as postoperative cardiac patients, we use a system with five syringe pumps and one IV infusion pump on a free-rolling IV pole. The syringe pumps provide a very stable rate and have a long battery life, and the entire system is compact, thereby minimizing the equipment needing transport. These pumps also run accurately at a low (0.5 mL per hour) rate so that concentrated infusions can be used, minimizing fluid delivered to the neonate.

The intubated infant requires hand bagging during transport. Particular care must be taken not to dislodge the endotracheal tube; small changes can result in either extubation or endobronchial intubation, particularly in the very premature infant. A self-inflating bag can be used to ventilate with room air, which may be necessary in infants with congenital heart disease and single ventricle physiology, whereas 100% oxygen can be delivered using an anesthesia bag and oxygen tank. Intermediate levels of FiO_2 require the use of a portable blender; for most neonates this is rarely needed during transfer. The anesthesia bag always should include a manometer, because it is easy to reach pressures that can result in acute barotrauma, such as pneumothorax. A laryngoscope, endotracheal tubes, and a face mask should be taken on transport, in case the endotracheal tube is dislodged. A complete round of resuscitative medications also should accompany any infant being transported to or from the NICU. Some transports require multiple personnel. It is not unusual in our ORs to transport infants on extracorporeal membrane oxygenation, or those receiving inhaled nitric oxide. With planning and an adequate number of personnel, this situation can be accomplished with minimal risk to the infant.

OPERATING ROOM EQUIPMENT AND MONITORING

The OR should not merely replicate NICU capabilities, it should surpass them, because the neonate will be subjected to the additional stress and destabilization of surgery. It is helpful if the room itself has adequate temperature control, because it may be necessary to increase room temperature to obtain a neutral thermal environment. Prior to draping, radiant heat lamps can be used, although care must be taken to not place the lamps too close to the infant because overheating can occur. The operating tables for neonates should use a heating pad. For longer cases, forced air heaters such as the Bair Hugger® can be used, with a "full access" disposable air blanket that is placed under the child. Maintenance fluids, because they are given at a relatively slow rate, can usually be given at room temperature, but fluid warmers must be available for blood or faster fluid administration. Cooling is rarely necessary, but it is possible to overheat an infant if care is not taken. Temperature must be monitored (see also Chapter 29). Core temperature is best temperature to monitor. It can be measured with a rectal, nasopharyngeal, or an esophageal probe. Bladder and tympanic membrane probes are rarely used in neonates because of size. Skin temperature is a poor second choice to core measurements.

TABLE 31–4 ROUTINE MONITORING REQUIREMENTS

ROUTINE	OPTIONAL

Precordial or esophageal stethoscope
Pulse oximeter
Electrocardiogram
Blood pressure
   Noninvasive
   Arterial line—UAC, radial, femoral
Temperature
   Core—rectal, esophageal, nasopharyngeal
   Skin
End-tidal CO_2
Peak inspiratory pressure, tidal volume, PEEP
FiO_2
Blood glucose
	Central venous pressure
	Blood gases—pH, PCO_2, PO_2
	Urine output
	Electrolytes

Routine monitoring requirements for neonates are shown in Table 31–4. Continuous pulse oximetry has revolutionized anesthesia, and it is a standard of care in the neonate as in the adult. In some situations, particularly with congenital heart disease or persistent pulmonary hypertension of the neonate (PPHN), two pulse oximeters may be used to monitor both preductal and postductal saturations. Heart rate is monitored from both the pulse oximeter and the EKG. Disposable neonatal EKG pads are needed, both from a size standard and because they may adhere better to the vernix caseosa–covered skin of the neonate. Noninvasive blood pressure can be measured, and most currently available machines have neonatal cuffs and a neonatal mode, which uses a smaller air volume for cuff inflation and is accurate in the neonate.

Invasive arterial pressure measurements from an indwelling line should be routine in the majority of sicker or more premature infants. Common sites are the umbilical artery, either radial artery, and the femoral artery (as a last resort). Dorsalis pedis is rarely useful, but an axillary or posterior tibial line may be used on some occasions. The arterial line site needs to be considered in relation to the clinical condition of the neonate; for example, if a coarctation is present, a right radial line should be used. Similarly, if a right Blalock-Taussig shunt is planned, a left radial line is appropriate. Arterial lines in the neonate must be treated with the greatest delicacy. If blood is drawn from the line a small syringe should be used, and suction should never be applied, because the artery easily can go into spasm. The line always should be flushed gently, again with a syringe, and not with a pressure bag attached to the transducer. For the smaller neonates, an IV infusion pump (not a pressure bag) should be used to keep a continuous flow through the transducer, both to prevent inadvertent flushing and to limit the rate of fluid administration through the transducer (3 mL per hour with the pressure bag versus 0.5 mL per hour with the pump). End-tidal CO_2 measurements also have become a standard of care, and they can be very helpful, but obtaining accurate numbers in a small neonate can be difficult. With a typical aspirating capnograph, the accuracy depends on the actual site of sampling, the type of anesthesia circuit used, and the volume of fresh gas flow through the circuit. Patient factors such as right-to-left shunt also may alter the values. The most accurate measurements are obtained using a low dead space circuit, with the sampling site in the endotracheal tube, not on the circuit. This location is accomplished by passing a small catheter into the endotracheal tube; recently we have used an endotracheal tube connector with a side port molded into it (Respiratory Support Products, Inc.) to which the capnograph sampling tubing can be attached. Blood glucose should be monitored intermittently during anesthesia; the importance of central venous pressure, urine output, and blood gases depends on the situation.

The standard anesthesia machine in most ORs is equipped with a relatively rudimentary volume-limited, time-cycled ventilator, which even with a pediatric bellows is poorly suited for neonatal ventilation. Small tidal volumes are very difficult to set, and tidal volume and pressure vary tremendously depending on the fresh gas flow. In the best of hands, these ventilators are impossible to use with premature neonates. Several methods have been used to get around this limitation. The simplest is to use hand ventilation throughout the case, thereby avoiding the ventilator. Although this method does allow some manual "feel" for pulmonary compliance, in many ways it limits the ability of the anesthesiologist to carry out other duties in caring for the patient. It also is very difficult to reproducibly apply PEEP when hand ventilating. A second method is to bring an NICU ventilator to the OR. The typical neonatal ventilator is pressure-limited and time-cycled. Because this ventilator is pressure-limited, it has an additional safety margin over a volume-limited ventilator in preventing barotrauma, and it can be used to ventilate the smallest neonates. PEEP also is easy to add. A disadvantage of pressure-limited ventilation is that tidal volume varies with changes in compliance, and care must be taken during surgery to monitor tidal volume as well as blood gases and end-tidal CO_2 to ensure adequacy of ventilation. Using a neonatal ventilator usually prevents the use of inhalation anesthetic agents, and it requires an intravenous anesthetic technique. As a third choice, in some centers, ventilators have been retrofitted with vaporizers to allow for the use of inhalational agents. More recently, newer anesthesia machines incorporate significantly more sophisticated ventilators, capable of either volume-limited or pressure-limited ventilation. Our ORs are currently equipped with either Ohmeda Excel® or Aestiva® machines, each incorporating the 7200 SmartVent. These ventilators can be used in pressure-limited, time-cycled mode, and they incorporate a spirometer that can measure expired tidal volumes as small as 10 mL. Fresh gas flow is uncoupled from tidal volume, and changes in flows do not affect ventilation materially. PEEP can easily be added, without the external valves used in older machines. These machines have now been used routinely in our institution in infants as small as 500 gm. Similar machines are possibly available from other manufacturers.

The circle breathing system, with inspiratory and expiratory valves, and incorporating a CO_2 absorber have become standard in adult anesthesia. A major advantage is that a semiclosed technique with very low gas flows can be used, thereby conserving anesthetic agent. Similar circle systems, appropriately sized for infants, with lower compliance tubing and smaller bags are commonly used in neonates. Many centers continue to use variants of the Mapleson D circuit, which has no valves and does not use an absorber, depending on higher fresh gas flows to prevent rebreathing. This circuit does have several advantages, particularly for smaller infants. The compliance of the tubing and the dead space is less; this can be critical in the smallest infants with very small tidal volumes, allowing adequate ventilation with lower pressures. In the rare situation in which the infant is allowed to breath spontaneously, the absence of valves markedly decreases the work of breathing. The Bain circuit is a variant of the Mapleson D circuit in which the fresh gas flow passes through a tube that is concentric with the expiratory tube. This makes a compact circuit and helps to minimize heat loss. We have found that the Mapleson D–type circuit is easily adapted to allow ventilation with subambient FiO_2 and nitric oxide, but a discussion is beyond the scope of this chapter.

Obviously, the OR must be equipped with appropriately sized airway equipment, including Miller size 0 and 1 blades, Macintosh size 2 and 3 blades, uncuffed endotracheal tubes, and nasopharyngeal and oropharyngeal airways. An assortment of special blades should be available for difficult airway cases. The laryngeal mask airway (LMA) is a relatively new device that fits in the pharynx, covering both the glottis and the esophageal opening. A cuff seals against the walls of the pharynx. The LMA is very useful for maintaining an airway in adults who develop upper airway obstruction under anesthesia. Positive pressure ventilation should be avoided with LMAs because it does not occlude the esophagus and may notably increase the risk of aspiration. LMAs are available in small sizes (1, 1½), but are not commonly used in the neonate. The LMA can be very helpful in intubating some infants with congenital anomalies, such as Pierre Robin. Essentially, the LMA is positioned and a fiberoptic bronchoscope is passed through the LMA and into the trachea. An endotracheal tube can then be passed through the LMA over the bronchoscope. The neonatal fiberoptic bronchoscope is essential for difficult airway cases. This scope is limited by extreme flexibility, and it does not have a suction channel, but it will pass through a 2.5 tube.

GENERAL ANESTHESIA

Although there continues to be some interest in regional anesthesia for some specific procedures in the neonate, most infants receive general anesthesia. Successful delivery of general anesthesia in neonates requires knowledge of developmental pharmacology to predict and to understand the responses of premature infants to anesthetic drugs. Size has an effect on response to anesthetics, and developmental age has a profound impact on the dose response, distribution, and metabolism of these drugs. Anesthetic agents can be classified in several ways. If we consider the components of anesthesia, we can classify drugs according to their analgesic, amnesic, and akinetic effects. A complete anesthetic agent would have potency in all three areas. We also can consider the mode of delivery, that is, inhalational agents versus intravenous agents.

INHALATIONAL AGENTS

Although common in older children, inhalational anesthesia has not been extensively used in premature infants. Use of inhalational agents was felt to be extremely dangerous, and based on reports of hemodynamic instability and cardiovascular collapse, it was believed that neonates would not tolerate these drugs.[24] In reality, these agents can be used safely, although very careful administration is required. The anesthetic effect of inhalational agents depends on the partial pressure of the anesthetic in the brain and on the potency of the agent. For several reasons, neonates develop very high partial pressures of the inhalational agents in the brain much more rapidly than do older children and adults. First, as already discussed, the ratio of alveolar ventilation to FRC in neonates is 5:1 compared with 1.5:1 in adults, and as a consequence, alveolar anesthetic concentration equilibrates with inspired concentration very quickly. Secondly, a greater fraction of the cardiac output in the neonate is distributed to the vessel-rich group and consequently the brain, and finally, the solubility of the inhaled anesthetics in blood is less in neonates than in adults.[21] Brain tissue equilibrates very quickly with the alveolar concentration of anesthetic and increases the risk of overdose in the neonate. The po-

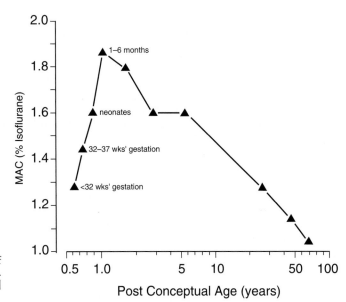

FIGURE 31–2. The minimum alveolar concentration (MAC) of isoflurane and postconceptual age on a semilogarithmic scale. (From LeDez KM: The minimum alveolar concentration [MAC] of isoflurane in preterm neonates. Anesthesiology 67:301, 1987.)

tency of inhalational anesthetics is expressed using the minimal alveolar concentration (MAC). The MAC is the concentration at which 50% of patients exhibit no response to stimulation such as skin incision. MAC is related to postconceptual age and is lowest in very premature neonates, rising to a peak at a postconceptual age of about 1 year, then decreasing progressively from childhood through adulthood. Figure 31–2 shows this relationship for isoflurane.[20] As shown, isoflurane is more potent (lower MAC) in premature neonates than in older infants, but this is not markedly different from that of adults, and difficulties using inhalational anesthetics are related more to the rapid uptake and equilibration.

Common inhalational anesthetics are halothane, isoflurane, sevoflurane, and nitrous oxide. Desflurane and enflurane are rarely used in the neonate. The inhalational anesthetics are complete anesthetics, with both analgesic and amnesic properties. In previous years halothane probably was the most commonly used, because it is minimally irritating to the airway, and it can be used for a very smooth mask induction of anesthesia. It is unfortunate that halothane was used so commonly; it is a significant myocardial depressant and sensitizes the heart to catecholamine-induced arrhythmias. Isoflurane, in contrast, is very pungent and cannot be used for mask induction, but it has less effect on cardiac output than does halothane. Systemic vascular resistance is decreased by isoflurane, and hypotension can result, especially if preload is diminished. Moderate volume loading helps to minimize any decrease in blood pressure. Isoflurane also causes cerebral vasodilation, and in the absence of hypotension, cerebral blood flow increases. In adults, isoflurane decreases cerebral metabolism and is cerebral protective. Sevoflurane recently has become very popular in pediatric anesthesia for mask induction. It is not irritating to the airway, and it is almost insoluble in blood, so that equilibration between brain and alveolus occurs rap-

idly. Thus onset of anesthesia during mask induction is very fast. Cardiovascular effects are more similar to isoflurane than to halothane. There is little published experience with sevoflurane in preterm infants, although it is certainly being used, primarily for mask inductions in healthier neonates. Nitrous oxide is an inhalational anesthetic, but it is not in the same class as the halogenated agents. It is a weak anesthetic, with a MAC of 104% in adults, so that to reach MAC, nitrous oxide would have to be provided at hyperbaric pressures. Obviously, the need for oxygen as part of our inspired gases prevents achievement of these levels. Nitrous oxide also is almost insoluble, and onset of effect is therefore fast. Unfortunately, insolubility and the high concentrations that are necessary for any meaningful effect cause nitrous oxide to enter progressively and to expand any gas-filled space in contact with the circulation, which rapidly leads to bowel distension or expansion of pneumothorax. If ventilation is interrupted for any reason, nitrous oxide also rapidly fills the alveoli, leading to dilution of the alveolar oxygen, producing a hypoxic mixture and rapid desaturation. Nitrous oxide is for these reasons best limited to an adjunct used during mask induction, switching to an air-oxygen mixture during maintenance anesthesia.

INTRAVENOUS AGENTS

Intravenous agents include sodium thiopental, propofol, ketamine, various narcotics, and the benzodiazepines. Other intravenous agents are rarely or never used in neonates. Sodium thiopental is an ultrashort-acting barbiturate used primarily as an induction agent. There is some evidence that premature neonates are more sensitive to thiopental than are older infants, possibly because of decreased binding by serum proteins.[46] Thiopental is primarily a hypnotic, with little analgesic activity. Usage is limited in smaller and sicker neonates because it has negative inotropic activity, and it is a peripheral vasodilator. Hypotension is therefore common, particularly in volume-depleted patients.

Propofol is a phenol derivative supplied as an emulsion in lipid, which in older children and adults is used as an induction agent, and it maintains anesthesia when given as a continuous infusion. Propofol is increasingly used for long-term sedation in adult and pediatric intensive care units, although there have been case reports of complications with long-term usage in children.[27] Recovery from the drug is rapid in adults due to redistribution and metabolism by liver and tissues. Propofol has less negative inotropic action compared with thiopental, but it is a powerful peripheral vasodilator, and hypotension is a common problem. The drug is designed as a complete anesthetic, but it does not have powerful analgesic effects, and for painful operations it should be used with narcotics. Propofol has been used in older infants, but there is little experience with the drug in premature infants, although some authors claim good results.[37] One would expect a slower recovery with less fat and muscle to which to redistribute and possibly slower hepatic metabolism owing to immaturity.

Ketamine, a phencyclidine derivative, provides good hypnosis and amnesia and excellent analgesia. It is used rarely in adults and older children because it can cause a dissociative state with confusion, hallucinations, and other severe psychological side effects. Ketamine stimulates the sympathetic nervous system and therefore causes minimal respiratory and cardiovascular depression. Blood pressure may rise, and increased intracranial pressure (ICP) is a concern in infants with hydrocephalus or those at risk for intraventricular hemorrhage. Ketamine can be useful in breaking hypercyanotic spells in the infant with congenital heart disease and right-to-left shunt because it will both anesthetize and increase systemic vascular resistance.

Fentanyl, a synthetic opioid, is widely used in neonatal anesthesia, and it is the most commonly used anesthetic for the premature infant. It has a wide safety margin and beneficial effects on hemodynamic stability. Fentanyl can block pulmonary hypertensive crises, and it is useful in infants with pulmonary hypertension, such as congenital diaphragmatic hernia, PPHN, and some cardiac defects.[41] Dosing has varied widely in the literature from as much as 50 to 60 μg per minute to as low as 10 to 12.5 μg per minute.[47] The pharmacokinetics of fentanyl in the early neonatal period are widely variable, depending on gestational and postnatal age and the type of surgery and medical problems of the infant.[31] Fentanyl is primarily metabolized in the liver, with only a small amount excreted unchanged by the kidneys. Clearance is lowest in the most premature infants, and it increases with gestational age and with age after birth, probably reflecting increasing hepatic maturation. Volume of distribution of fentanyl also seems to vary depending on gestational age and disease state.[31] Neonates with increased intra-abdominal pressure appear to have slower clearance of fentanyl.

Slower clearance is likely due to decreased hepatic blood flow resulting from the increased intra-abdominal pressure. Such a relationship has been demonstrated in neonatal lambs.[14, 23] Given the highly variable pharmacodynamics, fentanyl dosing needs to be individualized and titrated to effect. There is a fairly wide therapeutic range, and even with high doses, hemodynamic stability is maintained. All narcotics, however, are respiratory depressants, and with higher doses of fentanyl, prolonged respiratory depression occurs, necessitating postoperative assisted ventilation.

Fentanyl in combination with a muscle relaxant has become the standard for anesthesia in the premature neonate. It should be noted, however, that although fentanyl is a potent analgesic, it is not necessarily a complete anesthetic, and in occasional adults, awareness has occurred with high-dose fentanyl alone. In the past, it was suggested that this was of minimal importance because neonates are not "aware," especially if pain was adequately treated. This belief is less well accepted today, and benzodiazepines or inhalation agents such as isoflurane are more commonly added to fentanyl anesthesia. Other synthetic narcotics, such as alfentanil and sufentanil, rarely have been used in neonates. In adults, alfentanil is less potent than is fentanyl, but it has a shorter half-life, whereas sufentanil is more potent than fentanyl. Pharmacokinetics in infants are probably similar to those of fentanyl, and there does not appear to be any significant advantage when compared with fentanyl.[24] Remifentanil is a new opioid whose duration of action is terminated by hydrolysis by tissue esterases. Consequently, remifentanil does not accumulate or have prolonged duration of action. A half-life of 4.4 minutes and a clearance of 80 mL/kg per minute have been reported in the neonate,[9] but there is very little experience with this drug.

Morphine is the principal opium alkaloid, and it is the standard against which analgesics are measured. Morphine is less potent than fentanyl, but it has a longer duration of action and is more commonly used for postoperative pain. As with fentanyl, duration of action is further increased in the premature infant. As with all narcotics, respiratory depression is a major side effect. Unlike fentanyl, morphine causes histamine release, which limits its use as an anesthetic agent.

The benzodiazepines are agents that produce sedation, anxiolysis, and amnesia, but little analgesia. As such, they are not complete anesthetic agents, although in adults they have been very useful in combination with an opioid. Experience in neonates is very limited. Midazolam is a very short-acting benzodiazepine, and it has been the most commonly used in anesthesia. Metabolism is almost entirely hepatic, and it should be expected that duration would be prolonged by immature hepatic function in the preterm neonate. Midazolam vasodilates and can cause hypotension. In high doses it can cause respiratory depression, although this is more common in conjunction with opioids. Midazolam and the longer acting benzodiazepine lorazepam have been used for sedation in the NICU with mixed results. The Cochrane Neonatal Collaborative Review Group recently subjected several studies on sedation in the NICU using midazolam to a meta-analysis. In the two studies analyzed, infants treated with midazolam were more sedated (as judged by varying scoring systems) compared with infants treated with placebo. There were no differences in the incidence of intraventricular hemorrhage, pulmonary outcome, length of NICU stay, or mortality. The incidence of poor neurologic outcome was higher in the midazolam group, which at least raises questions as to the safety of midazolam infusion in these infants.[26]

Muscle relaxants, though not anesthetic agents, are commonly used in anesthesia for neonates. They are often grouped according to mechanism of action, that is, depolarizing versus nondepolarizing, but it is more important to consider rapidity of onset and duration of action. Succinylcholine chloride is the only depolarizing agent currently used, and it remains the standard for rapid onset and rapid disappearance. As such, it is primarily used in one situation—for rapid sequence intubation. In adults it also frequently is used when a difficult airway is feared. Given the limited reserve and rapid desaturation in infants, the difficult airway problem is probably better handled with awake intubation, so that spontaneous ventilation can be maintained. The ED_{95} (effective dose in 95 percent of the population receiving the dose) in neonates for succinylcholine is twice that of adults at 1.5 to 2 mg/kg. Action is terminated by metabolism by plasma pseudocholinesterase. Succinylcholine is not routinely used in children because of several rare but serious adverse reactions. In patients with some myopathies or neurologic diseases, succinylcholine can cause overwhelming hyperkalemia, muscle necrosis, and cardiac arrest, which is refractory to resuscitation. Bradycardia also occasionally occurs during intubation in the infant using succinylcholine. For this reason, some routinely administer atropine during a rapid sequence intubation. Despite these reactions, succinylcholine at this point remains the choice for rapid sequence.

Nondepolarizing relaxants competitively inhibit acetylcholine at the neuromuscular junction. Pancuronium bromide is a long-acting relaxant, and it is probably the most commonly used relaxant in neonates when early extubation is not a problem. Onset occurs over several minutes, and it cannot be used for rapid sequence. Pancuronium has some vagolytic action and increases the heart rate. Vecuronium bromide is an intermediate-acting relaxant occasionally used in neonates. It has little effect on the cardiac system, although it may cause bradycardia in combination with narcotics. Cis-atracurium undergoes spontaneous degradation by a chemical process (Hoffman elimination), and duration is not affected by liver or kidney function. Atracurium, its parent compound, is rarely used today because it causes histamine release. Rocuronium bromide is a newer agent with a rapid onset of action; however, it has not replaced succinyl-

choline for rapid sequence. Rapacuronium bromide also has a fast onset, but it is a very new agent and there is no information regarding use in neonates. Most relaxants probably have a prolonged duration of action in premature neonates, and frequency of dosing should be determined using a nerve stimulator to measure response to four spaced stimuli (train-of-four response). At the completion of surgery muscle relaxation with nondepolarizing agents should be reversed with an anticholinesterase, typically neostigmine, and an anticholinergic, usually atropine in the neonate.

INDUCTION OF GENERAL ANESTHESIA

Most sick infants have IV access, and an IV induction can be performed. Premedication rarely is given to neonates, although some would recommend atropine prior to laryngoscopy and intubation. Healthier infants without IV access can undergo mask induction, typically with 50% nitrous oxide and sevoflurane, after which IV access is rapidly obtained. Infants with a full stomach, most commonly those with intra-abdominal pathology, must have an IV rapid sequence induction or an awake intubation. In rapid sequence intubation, the infant is first preoxygenated with 100% FiO_2. Thiopental and succinylcholine, with or without atropine, are then rapidly pushed while an assistant performs the Sellick maneuver, pressure applied to the cricoid cartilage to prevent regurgitation of gastric contents. Positive pressure ventilation is not performed, and the infant is intubated expertly as soon as conditions are appropriate, usually after 45 to 90 seconds. There is little room for error with rapid sequence, and it should be performed only by individuals with significant expertise. Awake intubation with continued spontaneous ventilation is an alternative, and it may be most appropriate for infants with difficult airways, such as Pierre Robin and Goldenhar syndromes. Minimal sedation can be given, but protective airway reflexes should not be obtunded. Once the airway is secured, induction can continue by intravenous or inhalational route. Management of the difficult airway requires careful planning and the availability of additional "trained hands." A pediatric fiberoptic bronchoscope and a range of special purpose laryngoscope blades may be useful. Pediatric ear, nose, and throat consultation may also be of value. An LMA may assist with ventilation, but it does not protect the airway. The pediatric bronchoscope also can be used to intubate through the LMA.

MAINTENANCE OF ANESTHESIA

Maintenance of anesthesia requires monitoring as previously discussed. Temperature must be carefully controlled and adjustments in heating or cooling must be appropriately made. Fluid and metabolic requirements also must be carefully assessed throughout the course of the surgery. Fluids should be administered with an infusion pump to prevent inadvertent overload. It is generally easiest to calculate and administer maintenance fluids separately from replacement. Maintenance fluids should include glucose, unless the infant is known to be hyperglycemic. Intravenous hyperalimentation, or a dextrose-electrolyte solution can be used, depending on the size, age, and clinical condition of the neonate. Third space losses should be initially replaced with a balanced crystalloid solution such as Ringer's irrigation. Blood loss can also initially be replaced with crystalloid. Third space losses can be impressive, ranging from 2 to 15 mL/kg per hour especially during procedures with large amounts of bowel exposed, such as gastroschisis and omphalocele. Many infants, especially if they are hypoalbuminemic, should receive some of their replacement as colloid, usually 5% albumin. In the sickest neonates, transfusion with packed red cells, fresh frozen plasma, and platelets may be required. Urine output should be followed as one sign of adequate fluid replacement.

RECOVERY FROM ANESTHESIA

Emergence from anesthesia in the smallest and sickest premature infants is generally a prolonged event, because these neonates are not typical candidates for extubation at the conclusion of surgery; instead, they require continued intensive care in the NICU. Immaturity of drug clearance systems also prolongs recovery from the effects of most anesthetic agents in this group of infants. Transport from the OR involves the same considerations of temperature maintenance and airway management that have previously been discussed. Older and healthier infants usually can be extubated following surgery. Neuromuscular blockade should be reversed, as previously discussed. Hypothermia is a block to extubation if temperature control has not been adequate, and infants with hypothermia may need to be actively warmed. The infant should have resumed regular rhythmic respiration; to achieve this, ventilation may need to be decreased toward the end of the anesthetic to allow the PCO_2 to rise to mildly hypercapnic levels. Volume status must be adequate, and plasma hemoglobin should be close to normal. Flexion of the hip and contraction of the rectus abdominis muscle have been used as signs of adequate motor strength, and the infant usually begins to gag on the tube.[24] Laryngospasm can occur on extubation, and the anesthesia personnel need to be ready to treat and reintubate if necessary.

As previously discussed, premature infants often experience periodic breathing, and there is a risk of postoperative apnea in this population. Cote and coworkers have done a meta-analysis of data from eight separate studies and have found wide variability between institutions.[8] It was clear, however, that the risk of apnea was strongly inversely related to gestational age and postconceptual age. Anemia appears to be a significant risk factor for apnea. In one study the incidence of apneas was 80% in infants with hematocrits less than 30, and only 21% in those with normal hematocrits.[45] Prolonged postoperative apnea (defined as apnea > 15 seconds) occurs in approximately

70% of preterm infants less than 43 weeks' postconceptual age and decreases to less than 5% by postconceptual age 50 to 60 weeks.[8, 22] Most episodes occur within 2 hours of anesthesia, but they may start as late as 12 hours and recur for as long as 48 hours. IV caffeine (10 mg/kg) has been used to reduce the risk of apnea, although it does not reduce this risk to zero.[24, 43] A conservative approach is to avoid elective surgery and anesthesia until the former preterm infant reaches 60 weeks' postconceptual age, at which time the risk of postoperative apnea appears small. If surgery cannot be delayed, it is probably prudent to admit the child after surgery and monitor the child for 12 to 24 hours after surgery or after the last apneic episode.

REGIONAL ANESTHESIA

Although most neonates receive general anesthesia, a regional anesthetic is a viable option for certain procedures. Spinal and epidural (caudal) anesthesia is most common, although local infiltration or nerve block also is useful in certain specific procedures, such as circumcision, where a dorsal penile nerve block has been shown to be safe and effective. In most cases, regional anesthesia is an adjunct to general anesthesia, although a regional technique without general anesthesia can be used in some neonates considered to be high risk, for example, the infant with bronchopulmonary dysplasia. Spinal anesthesia without general anesthesia for inguinal hernia repair has been suggested as an alternative in infants at risk for postoperative apneas, although data are somewhat conflicting. Although several studies show a decrease in the incidence of apnea with spinal anesthesia,[13, 44] others see no difference,[19] but the infants receiving spinal anesthesia did have higher postoperative minimum oxygen saturations and heart rates. Supplemental sedation during the spinal anesthetic does increase the incidence of apneas. Spinal anesthesia can be induced using a 25-gauge Quincke needle at the L4 or L5 level (below the cauda equina). Either tetracaine or lidocaine can be used depending on the length of procedure. Caudal anesthesia also is a useful option. The epidural space can be entered via the caudal route through the sacrococcygeal membrane. Caudal anesthesia can be given as a single shot, using a 22-gauge short bevel needle, or a catheter can be threaded into the epidural space for continuous caudal anesthesia. With the continuous technique, the catheter can be threaded up into the epidural space, often high enough to give midthoracic anesthesia.[16] This technique seems to be well tolerated without significant hemodynamic effect. In the infant at high risk, caudal or spinal anesthesia can be used without additional sedation for appropriate procedures such as inguinal hernia repair. In this situation, simple nonpharmacologic comfort measures such as a pacifier are useful, and the technique seems to be well tolerated. More commonly, a single-shot caudal is used in combination with general anesthesia, which not only allows a "lighter" general anesthetic but also is very effective for postoperative pain relief. After a caudal anesthesia with bupivacaine, most infants are free of pain immediately after inguinal hernia repair, with relief continuing for at least 3 to 4 hours. Spinal and caudal anesthesia are quite safe. The most significant but thankfully rare complication of spinal or caudal anesthesia is inadvertent intravascular injection of local anesthesia that results in seizures, arrhythmias, and cardiac arrest.[12, 42]

Local nerve blocks are rarely used in neonates. An exception is dorsal penile nerve block (DPNB) for *neonatal circumcision*. Safety and efficacy have been well documented, and in one prospective report of short-term complications, no significant problems were noted after DPNB in more than 7000 infants over an 8-year period.[36] Other simple methods, such as a sucrose-dipped pacifier, or a padded and physiologic restraint chair further decrease objective signs of distress during circumcision performed with DPNB.[38] Eutectic mixture of local anesthetics (EMLA) cream also has been used for neonatal circumcision. Although absorption of prilocaine, a component of EMLA, has the potential for causing methemoglobinemia, EMLA did not lead to measurable changes in methemoglobin levels in several studies and appears safe for both premature and term infants.[39] Care should, however, be taken. When used for circumcision, EMLA is more effective than no anesthesia, but it is not as effective as DPNB.[6, 40] There are additional scattered reports of other uses for EMLA, including venous and arterial puncture, lumbar puncture, suprapubic puncture, and minor surgical procedures.[33]

■ REFERENCES

1. American Academy of Pediatrics, Committee on Fetus and Newborn, Committee on Drugs, Section on Anesthesiology, Section on Surgery, Canadian Pediatric Society, Fetus and Newborn Committee: Prevention and management of pain and stress in the neonate. Pediatrics 105:454, 2000.
2. Anand KJS, Hickey PR: Pain and its effects in the human neonate and fetus. N Engl J Med 217:1321, 1987.
3. Anand KJS: Neonatal stress responses to anesthesia and surgery. Clin Perinatol 17:207, 1990.
4. Anand KJS: Clinical importance of pain and stress in preterm neonates. Biol Neonate 73:1, 1998.
5. Anand KJS, et al: Randomized trial of fentanyl anaesthesia in preterm babies undergoing surgery: Effects on the stress response. Lancet 1:243, 1987.
6. Butler-O'Hara M, et al: Analgesia for neonatal circumcision: A randomized controlled trial of EMLA cream versus dorsal penile nerve block. Pediatrics 101(4):E5, 1998.
7. Bissonnette B, et al: The thermoregulatory threshold in infants and children anesthetized with isoflurane and caudal bupivacaine. Anesthesiology 73:1114, 1990.
8. Cote CJ, et al: Postoperative apnea in former preterm infants after inguinal herniorrhaphy: A combined analysis. Anesthesiology 82:809, 1995.
9. Davis PJ, et al: Remifentanil pharmacokinetics in neonates [abstract]. Anesth Analg 87:A1064, 1997.
10. Dicker A, et al: Halothane selectively inhibits non-shivering thermogenesis: Possible implications for thermoregulation during anesthesia of infants. Anesthesiology 82:491, 1995.
11. Fitzgerald M, Anand KJS: Developmental neuroanatomy and neurophysiology of pain. In Schecter NL, et al (eds): Pain in

Infants, Children and Adolescents. Baltimore, Williams and Wilkins, 1993, p 11.
12. Fried E, et al: Electrocardiographic and hemodynamic changes associated with unintentional intravascular injection of bupivacaine with epinephrine in infants. Anesthesiology 79:394, 1994.
13. Frumiento C, et al: Spinal anesthesia for preterm infants undergoing inguinal hernia repair. Arch Surg 135:445, 2000.
14. Gauntlett IS, et al: Pharmacokinetics of fentanyl in neonatal humans and lambs: Effects of age. Anesthesiology 69:683, 1988.
15. Gunnar MR, et al: Neonatal stress reactivity: Predictions to later emotional temperament. Child Dev 66:1, 1995.
16. Gunter JB, Eng C: Thoracic epidural anesthesia via the caudal approach in children. Anesthesiology 76:935, 1992.
17. Hatch D, et al: Anaesthesia and the ventilatory system in infants and young children. Br J Anaesth 68:398, 1992.
18. Holman RS: Pediatric morbidity and mortality in anesthesia. Pediatr Clin North Am 41:239, 1994.
19. Krane EJ, et al: Postoperative apnea, bradycardia and oxygen desaturation in formerly premature infants: Prospective comparison of spinal and general anesthesia. Anesth Analg 80:7, 1995.
20. LeDez KM, Lerman J: The minimum alveolar concentration of isoflurane in preterm neonates. Anesthesiology 67:301, 1987.
21. Lerman J, et al: Age and the solubility of volatile anesthetics in blood. Anesthesiology 61:139, 1984.
22. Malviya S, et al: Are all preterm infants younger than 60 weeks postconceptual age at risk for postanesthetic apnea? Anesthesiology 78:1076, 1993.
23. Masey SA, et al: Effect of abdominal distension on central and regional hemodynamics in neonatal lambs. Pediatr Res 19:124, 1985.
24. Mellor DJ, Lerman J: Anesthesia for neonatal surgical emergencies. Semin Perinatol 22:363, 1998.
25. Murray DJ, et al: Comparative hemodynamic depression of halothane versus isoflurane in neonates and infants: An echocardiographic study. Anesth Analg 74:329, 1992.
26. Ng E, et al: Intravenous midazolam infusion for sedation of infants in the neonatal intensive care unit [review]. Cochrane Database Syst Rev 2:CD002052, 2000.
27. Parke TJ, et al: Metabolic acidosis and fatal myocardial failure after propofol infusion in children: Five case reports. BMJ 305:613, 1992.
28. Porter F: Pain assessment in children: Infants. In Schecter NL, et al (eds): Pain in Infants, Children and Adolescents. Baltimore, Williams and Wilkins, 1993, p 87.
29. Porter FL, et al: Pain and pain management in newborn infants: A survey of physicians and nurses. Pediatrics 100:626, 1997.
30. Ruda MA, et al: Altered nociceptive neuronal circuits after neonatal peripheral inflammation. Science 289:628, 2000.
31. Saarenmaa E, et al: Gestational age and birth weight effects on plasma clearance of fentanyl in newborn infants. J Pediatr 136:767, 2000.
32. Schreiner MS: Preoperative and postoperative fasting in children. Pediatr Clin North Am 41:111, 1994.
33. Sethna, N: Regional anesthesia and analgesia. Semin Perinatol 22:380, 1998.
34. Sessler DI, et al: The thermoregulatory threshold in humans during halothane anesthesia. Anesthesiology 68:836, 1988.
35. Sessler DI, et al: Isoflurane-induced vasodilation minimally increases cutaneous loss. Anesthesiology 74:226, 1991.
36. Snellman LW, Stang HJ: Prospective evaluation of complications of dorsal penile nerve block for neonatal circumcision. Pediatrics 95:705, 1995.
37. Spaeth JP, et al: Anesthesia for the micropremie. Semin Perinatol 22:390, 1998.
38. Stang HJ, et al: Beyond dorsal penile nerve block: A more humane circumcision. Pediatrics 100(2):E3, 1997.
39. Taddio A, et al: Safety of lidocaine-prilocaine cream in the treatment of preterm neonates. J Pediatr 127:1002, 1994.
40. Taddio A, et al: Efficacy and safety of lidocaine-prilocaine cream for pain during circumcision. N Engl J Med 336:1197, 1997.
41. Vacanti JP, et al: The pulmonary hemodynamic response to perioperative anesthesia in the treatment of high-risk infants

with congenital diaphragmatic hernia. J Pediatr Surg 19:672, 1984.

42. Ved S, et al: Ventricular tachycardia and brief cardiovascular collapse in two infants after caudal anesthesia using a bupivacaine-epinephrine solution. Anesthesiology 79:1121, 1993.

43. Wellborn LG, et al: High-dose caffeine suppresses postoperative apnea in former preterm infants. Anesthesiology 71:347, 1989.

44. Wellborn LG, et al: Postoperative apnea in former preterm infants: Prospective comparison of spinal and general anesthesia. Anesthesiology 72:838, 1990.

45. Wellborn LG, et al: Anemia and postoperative apnea in former preterm infants. Anesthesiology 74:1003, 1991.

46. Westrin P, et al: Thiopental requirements for induction of anesthesia in neonates and infants one to six months of age. Anesthesiology 71:344, 1989.

47. Yaster M: The dose response of fentanyl in neonatal anesthesia. Anesthesiology 66:433, 1987.

32 | Care of the Mother, Father, and Infant

Marshall H. Klaus

John H. Kennell

PROVISION FOR CARE

The struggles of parents of premature infants who are learning to cope with their babies provided the stimulus to explore how parents develop a close attachment to their healthy, full-term infants. Initially, research on parent-infant attachment focused mainly on the parents of full-term infants. As investigators began to study the ways in which the parent of a premature infant manages to meet the needs of the immature, sleepy, fragile baby, they noted many common adaptations and problems. In recent years, many investigators have looked closely at the complex and confusing ecology that parents encounter when the birth of a premature, sick, or malformed infant brings them into an intensive care nursery.

Research in these intensive care units is not easy or straightforward; it is frequently confounded by harassed, overworked nurses and physicians, overwhelmed parents, and critically sick infants. Observations based on the completed studies suggest several interventions that appear to have merit and deserve further investigation in the traditional hospital environment. Some investigators have been refreshingly innovative and have broken down the walls of the intensive care unit to create a new and more positive environment for parents of sick infants.

In an attempt to determine what triggers, fosters, or disturbs a mother's attachment to her infant, information has been gathered from clinical observations during medical care procedures, naturalistic observations of mothering, long-term, in-depth interviews of mothers, and results from closely controlled studies on the parents of full-term and premature infants. This chapter attempts to integrate these studies into a general framework from which to develop some clinical recommendations.

Events that are important to the formation of a mother's attachment to her infant include the following:

A. Before pregnancy
　1. Planning the pregnancy
B. During pregnancy

　1. Confirming the pregnancy
　2. Accepting the pregnancy
　3. Becoming aware of fetal movement
　4. Perceiving the fetus as a separate individual
　5. Labor
C. Birth and after
　1. Birth
　2. Touching and smelling the baby
　3. Seeing the baby
　4. Breast feeding the baby
　5. Caring for the baby
　6. Accepting the infant as a separate individual and welcoming the infant into the family

By observing and studying the human mother according to these events, we can begin to describe how the parents of a normal, healthy infant build a bond with their baby.

BEFORE PREGNANCY

The literature on child development suggests that children are socialized by the powerful process of imitation or modeling. Their behavior is influenced by how they are mothered or what they observe. Long before a woman becomes a mother, she has obtained a repertoire of mothering behaviors through observation, play, and practice. She already has learned whether infants should be picked up when they cry, when and how much they are carried, and whether they should be chubby or thin. It is an interesting phenomenon that these modes of conduct, absorbed when children are very young, become unquestioned imperatives for them throughout life.[6] Unless adults consciously and painstakingly reexamine these learned behaviors, they will probably unconsciously repeat them when they become parents.

PREGNANCY

Pregnancy appears to be a developmental crisis involving two particular adaptive tasks: the acceptance of pregnancy and the perception of the fetus as a separate individual.

ACCEPTANCE OF PREGNANCY

During the first stage of pregnancy a woman must come to terms with the knowledge that she is going to be a mother. When she first realizes that she is pregnant, a mother often has mixed feelings. Many considerations, ranging from a change in her familiar patterns to more serious matters, such as economic and housing hardships or interpersonal difficulties, influence her acceptance of the pregnancy. This initial stage, as outlined by Bibring,[5] is the mother's identification of the growing fetus as an "integral part of herself."

PERCEPTION OF THE FETUS AS A SEPARATE INDIVIDUAL

The second stage of pregnancy involves a growing awareness of the baby in the uterus as a separate individual. It usually starts with the remarkably powerful event of *quickening*, the sensation of fetal movement. This perception occurs earlier for mothers who see their baby's movements on the screen during ultrasonography. During this period, the woman must begin to change her concept of the fetus from a being that is part of herself to a living baby who will soon be a separate individual. Bibring believes that this realization prepares the woman for birth and physical separation from her child.[5] In turn, this preparedness lays the foundation for a relationship with the child.

After quickening, a woman usually has fantasies about what the baby will be like, attributing some personality characteristics to the child and developing feelings of attachment.[5] At this time, she may further accept her pregnancy and show significant changes in attitude toward the fetus. Objectively there usually is some outward evidence of the mother's preparation. She may purchase clothes or a crib, select a name, or rearrange her home to accommodate a baby, a type of human "nesting."

The production of a normal child is a major goal of most women, yet most pregnant women have hidden fears that the infant may be abnormal or reveal some of their own secret inner weaknesses. Brazelton has clarified the importance of these changes and turmoil that occur during pregnancy for the subsequent development of attachment to the new infant:

> The prenatal interviews with normal primiparas, in a psychoanalytic interview setting, uncovered anxiety which often seemed to be of pathological proportions. The unconscious material was so loaded and distorted, so near the surface, that before delivery one felt an ominous direction for making a prediction about the woman's capacity to adjust to the role of mothering. And yet, when we saw her in action as a mother, this very anxiety and the distorted unconscious material could become a force for reorganization, for readjustment to her important new role. I began to feel that much of the prena-

> tal anxiety and distortion of fantasy could be a healthy mechanism for bringing her out of the old homeostasis which she had achieved to a new level of adjustment. . . . I now see the shakeup in pregnancy as readying the circuits for new attachments, as preparation for the many choices which they must be ready to make in a very short critical period, as a method of freeing her circuits for a kind of sensitivity to the infant and his individual requirements which might not have been easily or otherwise available from her earlier adjustment. Thus, this very emotional turmoil of pregnancy and that in the neonatal period can be seen as a positive force for the mother's adjustment and for the possibility of providing a more individualized environment for the infant.[7]*

The caregiver's ability to help parents during this emotional turmoil probably has a strong influence on determining whether the pregnancy will be a positive or negative experience in the woman's life.[8]

Cohen, however, emphasizes that any stress, such as moving to a new geographic area, marital infidelity, death of a close friend or relative, previous abortions, or loss of previous children, that leaves the mother feeling unloved or unsupported or that precipitates concern for the health and survival of either her infant or herself may delay preparation for the infant and retard bond formation.[11] After the first trimester, behaviors that are a reaction to stress and suggest rejection of pregnancy include a preoccupation with physical appearance or negative self-perception, excessive emotional withdrawal or mood swings, excessive physical complaints, absence of any response to quickening, or lack of any preparatory behavior during the last trimester.

A mother's and father's behavior toward their infant is derived from a complex combination of their own genetic endowments, the infant's responses to the parents, a long history of interpersonal relationships with their own families and with each other, experiences with this or previous pregnancies, the practices and values of their cultures, their socioeconomic status, and probably most important, the way they were raised by their own parents. The mothering or fathering behavior of each woman and man, the ability of each parent to tolerate stresses, and the needs each parent has for special attention differ greatly and depend on a mixture of these factors.

A remarkable illustration of how early caretaking of an infant, understood by the child through a complex mental process, becomes a template for the child's own parenting in later life is the case of Monica, who was born with esophageal atresia. Monica required gastrostomy feedings and was never held in anyone's arms during feeding. At 21 months of age, surgery established continuity between Monica's mouth and stomach. Systematic filming by George Engel over the next 30 years of her life showed that she repeated her own early feeding experience[15]; in

---

*From Brazelton TB: Early Child Dev Care 2:259, 1973. Copyright © Gordon and Breach Science Publishers, Inc. Reprinted by permission of the author and the publisher.

every feeding situation Monica never held in her arms a doll as a little girl, infants for which she was responsible as an adolescent baby sitter, or infants as a mother. She fed each of her four babies with the baby's back on her knees. Monica also played with her babies in the same fashion that she was played with, that is, only when they were flat on their backs for diapering or a bath. Thus, in spite of other examples and recommendations, her own experience in infancy became the persistent model for her caretaking as a baby sitter and mother.

Figure 32–1 is a schematic diagram of the major influences on parental behavior and the resulting disturbances that may arise from them. At the time the infant is conceived, some of these determinants, such as the mothering the father and mother received when they were infants, the practices of their culture, their endowments, and their relationships with their own families, are contributed by the parents. We originally believed these determinants were fixed and unchangeable. However, other investigators have argued that the influence of some of these may be changed during the crisis of birth. Other determinants relate to the hospital culture. For example, the attitudes, statements, and practices of the nurses and physicians in the hospital; whether there is early suckling and rooming-in or separation from the infant in the first days of life; the infant's temperament; and whether the infant is healthy, sick, or malformed obviously also affect the relationship. Most mothers and fathers develop warm and close attachments with their infants. However, a series of mothering disorders ranging from mild anxiety, such as persistent concerns about a baby after a minor problem that has been completely resolved in the nursery, to the most severe manifestation, the battered child syndrome, occurs with a few parents. Some problems result in part from separation and other unusual circumstances that occur in the early newborn period as a conse-

quence of present hospital care policies. Experiences during labor, parent-infant separation, and hospital practices during the first hours and days of life are the most easily manipulated variables in this scheme. Recent studies have partly clarified some of the steps in mother-infant attachment during this early period.

To minimize the number of unknowns for a mother while she is in the hospital, she and the father (or other supportive companion who will stay with her throughout labor and delivery) should visit the maternity unit to see where labor and delivery will take place. They should learn about delivery routines and all the procedures and medication the mother will receive before, during, and after delivery (see Chapter 24). Reducing the possibility of surprise increases confidence during labor and delivery. For an adult, just as for a child entering the hospital for surgery, the more meticulously detailed every step and event is in advance, the less the subsequent anxiety. The less anxiety the mother experiences while delivering and becoming attached to her baby, the better will be her immediate relationship with the infant.

LABOR

Before childbirth moved from the home to the hospital, the practice in industrialized nations was for women in the community to support the mother in labor, often with the assistance of a trained or untrained midwife. In all but 1 of the 128 cultures studied by anthropologists, a family member or friend, usually a woman, remained with the mother during labor and delivery. Although more fathers, relatives, and friends have been allowed into labor and delivery rooms in the past 10 years, a significant number of mothers still labor and deliver in some hospitals without continuous emotional and physical support.

The clinical value of continuous emotional and physical care during childbirth is clearly supported by the results of the 15 randomized clinical trials conducted over the past two decades. Beneficial findings are consistent across the studies despite different cultural, medical, and social practices.[22]

A meta-analysis by Scott and colleagues revealed that continuous social support during labor and delivery has a significantly greater beneficial impact on childbirth outcomes than does intermittent support.[51] The presence of a doula with mothers on an intermittent basis in six studies when compared to control mothers without doula support was not significantly associated with any improved outcomes. In contrast, continuous support for mothers in five studies was significantly associated with a 36% reduction in the need for analgesia, a 71% decrease in the need for oxytocin augmentation, a 57% reduction in the use of forceps, a 51% decrease in cesarean sections, and an average shortening of the duration of labor by 98 minutes.[27, 31, 54] Thus, some of the original studies may have underestimated the positive effects of social support during childbirth by not requiring support to be provided continuously to experimental subjects.

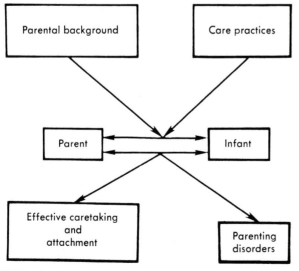

FIGURE 32–1. Major influences on parent-infant attachment and outcomes.

In the South African study (the only study continuing for 6 weeks after delivery), the results revealed favorable effects of continuous support during labor on the subsequent psychological health of the women and infants in the group of women with support from a doula. At 24 hours, the mothers with a doula had significantly less anxiety compared with the mothers without doulas, and fewer doula-supported mothers considered the labor and delivery to have been difficult. At 6 weeks postpartum, there was a significantly greater proportion of women breast feeding in the doula group (51% versus 29%), and feeding problems were significantly fewer in the doula group (16% versus 63%).[32]

The doula-supported mothers noted that it took an average of 2.9 days for them to develop a relationship with their baby compared with 9.8 days for the mothers without doulas. These results suggest that support during labor expedited the doula-supported mothers' readiness to bond with their babies. Using other measures, mothers in the doula group were again significantly less anxious, had scores on the depression scale that were significantly lower than those of the control group, and had higher levels of self-esteem at 6 weeks postpartum. They also felt significantly more satisfied with their partner 6 weeks postterm (71% versus 30%) and felt their baby was better than the standard baby, more beautiful, more clever, and easier to manage, whereas the control mothers perceived that their baby was slightly less attractive than a standard infant.

We concur with the Cochrane database that "given the clear benefits and no known risks associated with intra-partum support, every effort should be made to ensure that all laboring women receive support, not only from those close to them but also from specially trained caregivers (nurses, midwives, or lay women)."[22]

AFTER BIRTH

Immediately after the birth parents enter a unique period in which the parents' attachment to their infant usually begins to blossom and in which events may have many effects on the family. The first feelings of love for the infant are not necessarily instantaneous with the initial contact.[45] Many mothers have shared with us their distress and disappointment when they did not experience feelings of love for their baby in the first minutes or hours after birth. It should be reassuring for them and similar mothers to learn about two studies of normal, healthy mothers in England.

MacFarlane and associates asked 97 mothers from Oxford, "When did you first feel love for your baby?"[35] The replies were as follows: during pregnancy, 41%; at birth, 24%; first week, 27%; and after the first weeks, 8%.

In a study of two groups of primiparous mothers,[47] 40% recalled that their predominant emotional reaction when holding their babies for the first time was

indifference. The same response was reported by 25% of 40 multiparous mothers. Another 40% of both groups felt immediate affection. Most mothers in both groups had developed affection for their babies within the first week. The onset of this maternal affection after childbirth was more likely to be delayed if the membranes were ruptured artificially, if the labor was painful, or if the mothers had been given meperidine (Demerol).

The mother has an intense interest in her newborn baby's open eyes. When left alone with her infant in the first hour of life, 85% of what a mother says is related to the infant's eyes. "Please look at me." "If you look at me, I know you love me."[29] In the first 45 minutes of life the infant is awake and alert and in the quiet alert state.[14]

Information in closely related fields has greatly augmented our understanding of the beginning of parent-infant interactions. Detailed studies of the amazing behavioral capacities of the normal neonate in the quiet alert state have shown that the infant sees, hears, imitates facial gestures, and moves in rhythm to the mother's voice in the first minutes and hour of life, resulting in a beautiful linking of the reactions of the two and a synchronized "dance" between the mother and infant (see the importance of "state," Chapter 41).[33] The infant's appearance coupled with this broad array of sensory and motor abilities evokes responses from the mother and father and provides several channels of communication that are most helpful in the initiation of a series of reciprocal interactions and in the process of attachment.

With the mother's strong desire to touch and see her child, nature has provided for the immediate and essential union of the two. The alert newborn rewards the mother for her efforts by following her with his or her eyes, thus maintaining their interaction and kindling the tired mother's fascination with her baby.

Lind and coworkers in Stockholm have shown that a surprising increase in blood flow to the breast occurs when a mother hears the cries of her infant.[34] In addition, when the infant sucks the nipple, it induces a marked increase in both prolactin secretion in the mother, as well as oxytocin, to contract the uterus and decrease bleeding.

A renewed interest in the first minutes, hours, and days of life has been stimulated by several provocative behavioral and physiologic observations in both mother and infant. These assessments and measurements have been made during labor, birth, and the immediate postnatal period, and at the beginning breast feedings. They provide a compelling rationale for major changes in care in the perinatal period for both mother and infant. These findings fit together to form a new way to view the mother-infant dyad.

A SENSITIVE PERIOD

It is necessary to appreciate that the time period of labor, birth, and for the next several days can probably best be defined as a *sensitive period*. During this time, the mother and probably the father are strongly influenced by the quality of care they receive during the perinatal period. The more appropriately and humanely the mother is cared for, the more sensitive she is 6 weeks later in the care of her own infant.

Winnicott also described this period.[61] He reported a special mental state of the mother in the perinatal period that involves a greatly increased sensitivity to and focus on the needs of the baby. He indicated that this state of "primary maternal preoccupation" starts near the end of pregnancy and continues for a few weeks after the birth of the baby. A mother needs nurturing support and a protected environment to develop and maintain this state. This special preoccupation and the openness of the mother to her baby are probably related to the bonding process. Winnicott wrote that "only if a mother is sensitized in the way I am describing, can she feel herself into her infant's place, and so meet the infant's needs." In the state of "primary maternal preoccupation," the mother is better able to sense and provide what her new infant has signaled, which is her primary task. If she senses the needs and responds to them in a sensitive and timely manner, mother and infant will establish a pattern of synchronized and mutually rewarding interactions. It is our hypothesis that as the mother-infant pair continues this dance pattern day after day, the infant will develop a secure attachment.

This heightened sensitivity might explain observations by Kaitz and colleagues.[23, 24] In an innovative and well-designed series of studies, they investigated whether normal mothers were able to discriminate their own babies from other infants on the basis of smell, touch, face recognition, or cry recognition after several hours with their infants. They tested each sense separately and noted that smell was the most salient. After 5 hours of contact, nearly 100% of mothers were able to recognize the smell of their own infant. Parturient women know their infant's distinctive features after minimal exposure using olfactory and tactile cues, whereas discrimination based on sight and sound takes longer to develop. Kaitz and colleagues suggested that this order may reflect a fundamental property we share with subhuman species.

The clinical observations of Rose and associates[49] and Kennell and coworkers[26] suggested that affectional ties can be easily disturbed and may be permanently altered during the immediate postpartum period. Relatively mild illness in the newborn such as slight elevations of bilirubin levels, slow feeding, additional oxygen for 1 to 2 hours, and the need for incubator care in the first 24 hours for mild respiratory distress appears to affect the relationship between mother and infant. The mother's behavior is often disturbed during the first year or more of the infant's life, even though the infant's problems are completely resolved before discharge and often within a few hours. That early events have long-lasting effects is a principle of the attachment process. A mother's anxieties about her baby in the first few days after birth, even about a problem that is easily resolved, may affect her relationship with the child

long afterward. This has been described by Green and Solnit as the "vulnerable child syndrome."[20a]

In the past 30 years, multiple studies have focused on whether additional time for close contact of the mother and infant alters the quality of attachment. These studies have addressed the question of whether there is a sensitive period for parent-infant contact in the first minutes, hours, and days of life that may alter parents' later behavior with their infant. In many biologic disciplines, these moments have been called sensitive periods. However, in most examples of a sensitive period in biology, the observations are made of the young of the species rather than of the adult. Evidence for a sensitive period comes from the following series of studies. Note that in each study increasing mother-infant time together or increased suckling improves caretaking by the mother.[29]

In six out of nine randomized trials of early contact with suckling (during the first hour of life), both the number of women breast feeding and the length of their lactation were significantly increased for mothers who had early contact compared with the women in the control group who had their first contact with suckling at 3 hours.

In addition, studies of Brazelton and others have shown that if nurses spend as few as 10 minutes helping mothers discover some of their newborn infants' abilities, such as turning to the mother's voice and following the mother's face or imitation and assisting mothers with suggestions about ways to quiet their infants, the mothers became more appropriately interactive with their infants face to face and during feedings at 3 and 4 months of age.

O'Connor and colleagues carried out a randomized trial with 277 mothers in a hospital that had a high incidence of parenting disorders.[42] One group of mothers had their infants with them for 6 additional hours on the first and second day, but they had no early contact. The routine care group began to see their babies at the same age but only for 20-minute feedings every 4 hours, which was the custom throughout the United States at that time. In the follow-up studies, 10 children in the routine care group experienced parenting disorders, including child abuse, failure to thrive, abandonment, and neglect during the first 17 months of life compared with two cases in the experimental group, who had 12 additional hours of mother-infant contact. A similar study in North Carolina that included 202 mothers during the first year of life did not find a statistically significant difference in the frequency of parenting disorders[52]; 10 infants failed to thrive or were neglected or abused in the control group compared with seven in the group that had extended contact. When the results of these two studies are combined in a meta-analysis ($P = .054$), it appears that simple techniques, such as adding additional early time for each mother and infant to be together and closing the newborn nursery, may lead to a significant reduction in child abuse. However, a much larger study is necessary to confirm and validate these relatively small studies.

Evidence suggests that many of these early interactions also take place between the father and his newborn child. Parke in particular demonstrated that when fathers are given the opportunity to be alone with their newborns, they spend almost exactly the same amount of time as mothers do holding, touching, and looking at them.[44]

In the triadic situation the father tends to hold the infant nearly twice as much as the mother, vocalizes more, touches the infant slightly more, but smiles at the infant significantly less than the mother. The father clearly plays the more active role when both parents are present, in contrast to the cultural stereotype of the father as a passive participant. In fact, in this triadic interaction the mother's overall interaction declines. All but one of the fathers whom Parke studied had attended labor and birth, and this could be expected to produce an unusual degree of father-infant attachment. However, he conducted another study using a similar design but in which the fathers rarely participated in labor and birth. Despite these social and institutional differences, the fathers again played the more active and dominant role with increased holding, vocalizing, and touching.

In an interesting and significant observation of fathers, Rödholm noted that paternal caregiving greatly increased when the father was allowed to interact and establish eye-to-eye contact with his infant for 1 hour during the first hours of life.[48] Keller and associates have reported that the group of fathers who received extended postpartum hospital contact with their infants, compared with a traditional contact group, engaged in more *en face* behavior and vocalization with their infants and were more involved in infant caretaking responsibilities 6 weeks after the baby's birth.[25] They also had higher self-esteem scores than did fathers in the other group.

Parke believed that the father must have an extensive early exposure to the infant in the hospital and home, where the parent-infant bond is initially formed.[44] Parke indicated that the father is much more interested in and responsive toward his infant than U.S. culture has acknowledged.

Though there continues to be debate on the interpretation and significance of the many research studies with regard to the effects of early and extended contact for mothers and fathers with their infants on their ability to bond,[30] all sides agree that all parents should be offered early and extended time with their infants.[3, 29] An extensive review of this subject is summarized as follows.[16]

The restriction of early postnatal mother-infant interaction that has been such a common feature of the care of women giving birth in hospitals has undesirable effects.[16] Disruption of mother-infant interaction in the immediate postnatal period may set some women on the road to breast feeding failure and altered subsequent behavior toward their children.

Pediatricians, psychologists, and others have indeed debated this issue. This skepticism does not, however, constitute grounds for acquiescing in hospital routines that lead to unwanted separation of mothers from their babies. Because such policies may actually do harm, they should be changed forthwith.

PRACTICAL CONSIDERATIONS

The newborn should be thoroughly dried with warm towels after birth to avoid the loss of heat, and once it is clear that the infant has good color and is active and normal (usually within 1 to 5 minutes), the baby can be given to his mother. At this time, the warm and dry infant can be placed between the mother's breasts, on her abdomen, or if she desires, next to her.

When newborns are kept close to their mother's body or on their mother, the transition from life in the womb to existence outside the uterus is made much easier for them. The newborn recognizes his mother's voice and smell,[12, 57] and her body warms him to just the right temperature.[10] In this way, the infant can experience sensations somewhat similar to what he felt during the last several weeks of uterine life (Fig. 32–2).

Often, the baby's lips are placed near or on the mother's nipple immediately after birth. Some babies do start to suckle, but the majority just lick the nipple or peer up at the mother. They appear to be much more interested in the mother's face, especially in her eyes. When left on their own, babies most commonly begin to suckle 30 to 40 minutes after birth.[59]

One of the most exciting observations made in the modern era is the discovery that the newborn has the ability to find the mother's breast and to decide when to take the first feeding. In order not to remove the taste and smell of the mother's amniotic fluid, it is necessary to delay washing the baby's hands and the mother's breasts. The baby uses the taste and smell of the amniotic fluid on his hands to make a connection with a certain lipid substance on the nipple related to the amniotic fluid.[57]

The infant usually begins with a time of rest and

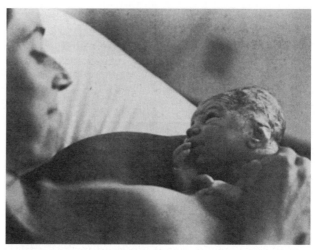

FIGURE 32–2. A mother and her infant shortly after birth. (From Klaus MH, et al: Amazing Newborn. Perseus, Cambridge, Mass, 1985, p 137, with permission. Copyright Suzanne Arms Wimberley.)

quiet alertness, rarely crying and often appearing to take pleasure in looking at the mother's face. Around 30 to 40 minutes after birth (sometimes longer), the newborn begins making mouthing movements, sometimes with lip smacking, and shortly after, saliva begins to pour down the infant's chin. When placed on the mother's abdomen, babies maneuver in their own ways to reach the nipple. They often use stepping motions of their legs to move ahead, and to move horizontally toward the nipple, they use small push-ups, lowering one arm first in the direction they wish to go. These efforts are interspersed with short rest periods. Sometimes babies change direction mid-course. These actions take effort and time. Parents find patience well worthwhile if they wait and observe their infant's first journey.

In the photos in Figure 32–3, one newborn is seen successfully navigating. At ten minutes of age, the newborn first begins to move toward the left breast. Repeated mouthing and sucking of the hands and fingers is commonly observed (see Fig. 32–3A). With a series of pushups and rest periods, the infant gets to the right breast completely unassisted (see Fig. 32–3B). The infant, with lips on the areola, now begins to suckle effectively while closely observing the mother's face (see Fig. 32–3C).

This sequence is helpful to the mother as well as the baby, because the massaging and suckling of the breast induces an oxytocin surge into her blood stream, which possibly helps contract the uterus, expelling the placenta and closing off many blood vessels in the uterus, thus reducing bleeding. In addition, the stimulation and suckling help in the manufacture of prolactin in the mother but also oxytocin in the brain in both the mother and the baby. Oxytocin, the "love hormone," in the dyad probably begins to enhance their early ties together. Mother and baby appear to be carefully adapted for these first moments together.

To allow this first intimate encounter, injection of vitamin K, application of eye ointment, washing, and any measuring of the infant's weight, height, and head circumference should be delayed for at least an hour. Over 95% of full-term infants are normal at birth. In a few moments they easily can be evaluated to ensure that they are healthy. After thorough drying, they can be placed safely on their mother's chest if their parents wish it.

The odor of the nipple appears to guide a newborn to the breast.[57] If the right breast is washed with soap and water, the infant will crawl to the left breast, and vice versa. If both breasts are washed, the infant will

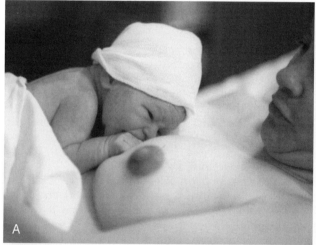

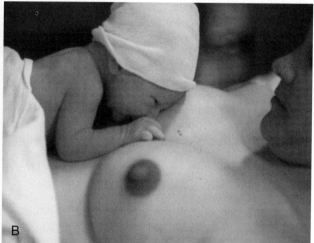

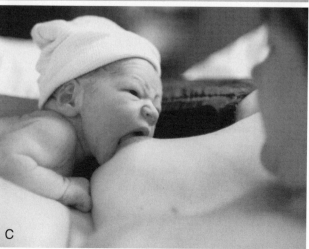

FIGURE 32–3. *A*, Infant about 15 minutes after birth, sucking on his unwashed hand and possibly looking at mother's left nipple. *B*, An arm pushup, which helps the infant to move to mother's right side. *C*, At 45 minutes of age the infant moved to the right breast without assistance and began sucking on the areola of the breast. The infant has been looking at the mother's face for 5 to 8 minutes. (Photographed by Elaine Siegel.) (From Klaus MH, et al: Your Amazing Newborn. Perseus, Cambridge, Mass, 1998, p 12.)

go to the breast that has been rubbed with the amniotic fluid of the mother. The special attraction of the newborn to the odor of his mother's amniotic fluid may reflect the time in utero when, as a fetus, it swallowed the liquid. It appears that amniotic fluid contains some substance that is similar to some secretion of the breast, though not the milk. Amniotic fluid on the infant's hands probably also explains part of the interest in sucking the hands and fingers seen in the photographs in Figure 32–3. This early hand-sucking behavior is markedly reduced when the infant is bathed before the crawl. With all these innate programs, it almost seems as if the infant comes into life carrying a small computer chip with instructions.

At childbirth we possibly can observe developmental stages of our own evolution. Many separate abilities enable a baby to do these tasks. Stepping reflexes help the newborn push against his mother's abdomen to propel him toward the breast. Pressure of the infant's feet on the abdomen may help the expulsion of the placenta and the reduction of uterine bleeding. The ability to move a hand in a reaching motion enables the baby to claim the nipple. Taste, smell, and vision all help the newborn detect and find the breast.[33] Muscular strength in neck, shoulders, and arms helps newborns bob their heads and do small pushups to inch forward and from side to side. This whole scenario may take place in a matter of minutes, most often occurring within 30 to 60 minutes, but it is all within the capacity of the newborn. It appears that our young, like other baby mammals, know how to find their mother's breast.

Swedish researchers have shown that the normal infant who is dried and placed naked on the mother's chest and then covered with a blanket maintains his or her body temperature as well as the infant who is warmed with an elaborate, high-tech heating device that usually separates the mother and baby. The same researchers found that when the infants have skin-to-skin contact with their mothers for 90 minutes after birth, they cry hardly at all compared with infants who were dried, wrapped in a towel, and placed in a bassinet.[10] In one group of mothers who did not receive pain medication, whose babies were not taken away during the first hour of life for a bath, and whose babies who did not receive vitamin K or application of eye ointment, 15 of 16 babies placed on their mother's abdomen were observed to make the trip all on their own to their mother's breast, latch on, and begin to suckle effectively.[46] It seems likely that each of these features—the crawling ability of the infant, the decreased crying when close to the mother, and the warming capabilities of the mother's chest—are adaptive and evolved genetically to help preserve the infant's life.

Suckling of the breast by the infant stimulates the production of oxytocin in both the mother's and infant's brain, and this oxytocin in turn stimulates the vagal motor nucleus, releasing 19 different gastrointestinal hormones, including insulin, cholecystokinin, and gastrin. Five of the 19 hormones stimulate growth of the baby's and mother's intestinal villi and increase the surface area and the absorption of calories with each feeding. The stimuli for this release are touch on the mother's nipple and the inside of the infant's mouth. These responses were essential for survival ten thousand years ago when periods of famine were more common before the development of modern agriculture and the storage of grain. The increased gut motility with each suckling also may help remove meconium with its large load of bilirubin.

These research findings may explain some of the underlying physiologic and behavioral processes and provide additional support for the importance of 2 of the 10 caregiving procedures that the United Nations International Children's Emergency Fund (UNICEF) is promoting as part of its Baby-Friendly Hospital Initiative to increase breast feeding, which involves early mother-infant contact, with an opportunity for the baby to suckle in the first hour, and mother-infant rooming-in throughout the hospital stay.

Following the introduction of the Baby-Friendly Hospital Initiative in maternity units in several countries throughout the world, an unexpected observation was made. In Thailand, in a hospital in which a disturbing number of babies were abandoned by their mothers, the use of rooming-in and early contact with suckling significantly reduced the frequency of abandonment from 33 out of 10,000 births to 1 out of 10,000 births a year.[9] Similar observations have been made in Russia, the Philippines, and Costa Rica when early contact and rooming-in were introduced. These reports are additional evidence that the first hours and days of life are a sensitive period for the human mother,[29] which may be due in part to the special interest that a mother has shortly after birth in hoping her infant will look at her and the infant's ability to interact in the first hour of life during the prolonged period of the quiet alert state. There is a beautiful interlocking at this early time of the mother's interest in the infant's eyes and the baby's ability to interact and to look eye-to-eye.

A possible key to understanding what is happening physiologically in these first minutes and hours comes from investigators who noted that if the lips of the infant touch the mother's nipple in the first hour of life, a mother will decide to keep her baby in her room 100 minutes longer on the second and third day during her hospital stay than another mother who does not have contact until later.[60] This decision may be explained in part by small infusions of oxytocin (the love hormone) occurring in both the infant's and mother's brains when breast feeding occurs. It is of interest that in sheep, dilatation of the cervical os during birth releases oxytocin within the brain that, acting on receptor sites, appears to be important for the initiation of maternal behavior and for the facilitation of bonding between mother and baby.[28] In humans, there is a blood-brain barrier for oxytocin, and only small amounts reach the brain via the blood stream. However, multiple oxytocin receptors in the brain are supplied by production from the brain. Increased levels of brain oxytocin result in slight sleepiness, euphoria, a raised pain threshold, and feelings of increased love for the infant. It appears that during breast feeding, raised blood levels of oxytocin are associated with increased brain levels; women who exhibit the largest plasma oxytocin concentrations are the most sleepy.

Measurements of plasma oxytocin levels in 18 healthy women who had their babies on their chests with skin-to-skin contact immediately after birth showed significant elevations compared with the antepartum levels, and a return to antepartum levels at 60 minutes. For most women, a significant and spontaneous peak concentration was recorded about 15 minutes after delivery, with expulsion of the placenta.[41] Most mothers had several peaks of oxytocin up to 1 hour after delivery. The vigorous oxytocin release after delivery and with breast feeding not only may help contract the uterine muscle to prevent bleeding, but it may enhance bonding of the mother to her infant. These findings may explain an observation made in France in the 19th century when many poor mothers were giving up their babies. Nurses recorded that mothers who breast fed for at least 8 days rarely abandoned their infants.

We hypothesize that a cascade of interactions between the mother and the baby occurs during this early period, locking them together and ensuring further development of attachment. The remarkable change in maternal behavior with just the touch of the infant's lips on the mother's nipple; the effects of additional time for mother-infant contact; the reduction in abandonment with early contact, suckling, and rooming-in; and the increased maternal oxytocin levels shortly after birth in conjunction with known sensory, physiologic, immunologic, and behavioral mechanisms all contribute to the attachment of the mother to the infant.

PREMATURE OR SICK INFANTS

In the years since parental visiting has been permitted in the intensive care nursery, studies have revealed that most parents continue to suffer severe emotional stress. Harper and coworkers noted that emotional stress occurred even when parents had close contact with their infants.[21] However, despite the anxiety, parents believed the opportunity to have this contact was helpful, and over 90% of parents questioned were opposed to restricting their contact with their infants. Most parents thought that holding their infant made the infant feel more loved. Benfield and colleagues noted that when infants are transported to a neonatal intensive care unit, most parents experienced grief reactions.[4] It is interesting that the level of their response was unrelated to the severity of the baby's problems.

From interviews and observations, researchers suggested that early parental reactions predicted how the mother would manage with her infant in the early weeks at home. From interviews Mason found that if the mother expressed a fairly high level of anxiety, actively sought information about the condition of her baby, showed strong maternal feelings for the baby, and had strong support from the father, there usually was a favorable outcome.[37] If the mother showed a low level of anxiety and activity, her relationship with her child probably would be poor.

Minde and associates noted that the most important variables are the mother's relationship with her mother, the mother's relationship with her father, and whether the mother had a previous abortion.[38] Highly interacting mothers in the nursery visited and telephoned the nursery more frequently while the infants were hospitalized and stimulated their infants more at home. Moreover, the authors noted that mothers who touched and fondled their infants more in the nursery had infants who opened their eyes more. Minde noted the contingency between the infant's eyes being open and the mother's touching and also between gross motor stretches and the mother's smiling. He and his colleagues could not determine to what extent the sequence of touching and eye opening reflected the primary contribution of the mother or the infant. Thus, from interviews and observations these researchers noted that mothers who become involved, interested, and anxious about their infants have an easier time when the infant is taken home.[38, 39]

In the last 20 years, numerous studies have revealed that if small, premature infants are touched, rocked, fondled, or cuddled daily during the stay in the nursery, they may have significantly fewer apneic periods, increased weight gain, fewer stools, and in some studies even advances in certain areas of higher central nervous system functioning that persist for a short time after discharge from the hospital.[20]

Fondling the premature infant for 5 minutes every hour for 2 weeks alters bowel motility, crying, activity, and growth. Gentle massage of preterm infants also results in less stress behavior, superior performance on the Brazelton neonatal assessment, and, more important, better performance on a developmental assessment at 8 months.[19] Several students of young premature infants, including Brazelton,[8] have perceptively noted that when some infants' visual attention is captured by an adult, the baby is so captivated by the experience that the infant may forget to breathe and often become quite blue. Until we have defined more closely the sensory needs and tolerances of these infants, it is wise to observe how the immature infant manages these exciting experiences. It is hoped that in the future infants will be able to regulate their own environment, just as Als has adapted the environment of each infant to meet individual needs.[1] As an example, Thoman and coworkers demonstrated that premature infants in an isolette would move and spend more time in contact with a small, breathing teddy bear than with a nonmoving teddy bear.[55] It is interesting that the infants with breathing teddy bears had a greater increase in quiet sleep 8 weeks after leaving the hospital. The long-term effects of altering the early environment of premature infants was emphasized when researchers turned the light out at night in a growing nursery in England for the last 2 weeks of a hospital stay for one group of infants but left it on for another group.[36] The two groups of infants appeared to be similar until 5 to 6 weeks after discharge. At 6 weeks after discharge, infants whose nursery had day and night cycles for the 2 weeks of hospital stay slept 2 hours longer per 24 hours and spent 1 hour less each day feeding, but 3 months after discharge they were 1 lb heavier than infants who did not have the light out at night.

Based on his observations of many normal mothers and their full-term infants, Winnicott noted that what the baby observes in the caretaker's face in the early months of life helps the baby develop a concept of self.[62] He noted that some infants have mothers who do not imitate the baby, and thus the babies do not see themselves. In these situations he postulated that the infant's own creative capacity may be atrophied and that such infants would look for other ways of getting to know themselves from the environment. The important observation that Winnicott noted was that in normal mother-infant dyads the mother often followed or imitated the infant.

Trevarthen confirmed these observations in mothers and infants using fast-film technique and noted that mothers imitate their babies during spontaneous play.[56] He also noted that the mother's imitation of the infant's behavior, rather than the reverse, sustained their interaction and communication. Detailed analysis revealed that mothers were studiously imitating the infant's expression with a lag of a few tenths of a second; therefore, the infant was choosing the rhythm.

In a series of creative experimental manipulations of infant-mother face-to-face interactions, Field noted that the mother and the normal full-term infant were interacting about 70% of the time in their spontaneous play.[18] However, when the mother was asked to increase her attention-getting behavior (stimulation), her activity increased to 80% of the time, and strikingly, the infant's gaze decreased to 50%. When the mother imitated the movements of the infant, which greatly reduced her activity, the infant's gaze time greatly increased.

Field noted that in the spontaneous situation the mothers of preterm infants considered to be high risk were interacting up to 90% of the time, whereas the infant was looking only 30% of the time. If the mother was told to use attention-getting gestures, her activity increased to more than 90% of the time and the infant's gaze decreased further. If her interactions were decreased by asking her to imitate the baby's movements, the infant's gaze increased greatly. Although generally the mother's activity was aimed at encouraging more activity or responsiveness from the premature infant, the approach appeared to be counterproductive, leading to less instead of more infant responsiveness. Thus, by three separate and different techniques it appears that mothers of normal infants follow or mirror their infant's behavior for significant periods.

INTERVENTIONS FOR PARENTS OF PREMATURE INFANTS

To help parents deal with the stressful situation of having a sick or small infant, several interventions have been introduced. In some cases these behaviors have involved the parents and infants together, whereas others have focused on either the parent or the infant.[23] The following interventions have been adopted in many intensive care units:

- Opening the intensive care nursery to parents
- Transporting the mother to be near her infant
- Maternal day care for premature infants
- Rooming-in for the parent of a premature infant
- Individualized nursing care plans (Als method)
- Early discharge
- Listening to parents (interviewing) during the infant's hospitalization and after discharge
- Parent groups
- Programmed contact and reciprocal interaction
- Transporting the healthy premature infant to the mother[29]
- Home-based intervention for young parents[29]
- Discussion with the parents after discharge[29]
- Kangaroo baby care (holding the infant skin to skin)
- Nurse home visitation

Individualized nursing care plans, kangaroo baby care, and rooming-in deserve special mention.

INDIVIDUALIZED NURSING CARE PLANS (ALS METHOD)

(See also Chapter 41.)

To reduce the disruptive effects of the nursery environment, Als and colleagues have developed a method of individualized care of the premature infant that takes into account what each infant finds soothing or disruptive during a formal observation.[1] This detailed examination is performed in the first days after birth and becomes the basis for each infant's nursing care plan. Their requirements for light, sound, position, and detailed nursing are developed only after the meticulous behavioral assessment.

They demonstrated that for infants at high risk and those who have low birth weight, the individualized nursing care plans involving their behavioral and environmental needs remarkably altered the infants' outcome.

In three randomized trials using the preceding procedure, infants receiving individualized behavioral management required many fewer days on a respirator and fewer days on supplemental oxygen; their average daily waking time increased; they were discharged many days earlier; and they also had a lower incidence of intraventricular hemorrhage. In addition, following discharge their behavioral development progressed more normally, and their parents more easily developed ways of sensing their needs and responding and interacting with them in a pleasurable fashion. Parents have an easier time adapting to premature infants who are more responsive. As the infant develops, the parents gain much by assisting with the observations and helping the nurse develop the care plan.

KANGAROO BABY CARE

In South America, the United States, and Europe, mothers and fathers have found that holding the infant skin to skin is uniquely helpful as they develop a tie to their infant.[58] At the first skin-to-skin experience the mother is usually tense, so it is best for the nurse to stay with her to answer questions and make any necessary adjustments in position and measures to maintain warmth such as blankets. A few mothers find that one experience is enough for them. However, most mothers discover that the experience is especially pleasurable. After the "kangaroo" contact some mothers have mentioned timidly that they began for the first time to feel close to their baby and feel that the baby was theirs. Without prompting, one mother said that she was feeling much better because she was now doing something for her baby that no one else could do.

It is our belief that skin-to-skin care is useful in helping parents develop a closer tie to their infant. Properly detailed observations have noted that the infant's heart rate, temperature, and respiratory rate are stable with kangaroo care, and there is no increase in pauses in breathing during the daily 1- to 1½-hour experience. Additionally, significant increases in milk output and an increase in the success of lactation have been documented with skin-to-skin care.

ROOMING-IN

One approach to helping parents adapt to a sick or premature infant has been developed by Donald Garrow at a district general hospital in High Wycombe, England. The 20-bed special infant care unit accommodates 8 mothers at a time and has 250 admissions each year. No matter how seriously ill they may be, 70% of the babies have their mothers with them from the first few hours of life. Fathers may stay at night, and young siblings may visit as frequently as desired each day. Six of the mothers' rooms open directly into the infant special care unit so the parents can easily see or care for their infants. Infection has not resulted from allowing free entry to fathers, siblings, and grandparents. However, parents are advised that children with diarrhea, fever, an upper respiratory tract infection, or any exposure to a contagious disease should stay home. Many mothers come to this special unit immediately after giving birth, and the nursery staff cares for both the mother and infant. Generally the mothers eat together, which allows time for sharing experiences and mutual support. When an infant death occurs, the mother involved usually remains on the unit for a day or so and the nurses, together with one or two other mothers, are often able to help her begin her grief work.

It was the impression of the staff when we visited the High Wycombe unit that the parents move more quickly to assume caregiving tasks, are less jealous of the staff, are more chatty, and adapt more readily to the birth of a sick infant than previously, when mothers could not room in. Plans are being made to develop units like this in the United States.

In several countries throughout the world, including Argentina, Chile, Brazil, South Africa, Ethiopia, and Estonia, mothers of premature infants live in a room adjoining the premature nursery or they room in. This arrangement was made because of a shortage of nurses; however, the solution appears to have multiple benefits. It allows the mother to continue producing milk, permits her to take on the care of the infant more easily, greatly reduces the caregiving time required for these infants, and allows a group of mothers of premature infants to talk over their situation and to gain from mutual discussion and support.

We recommend the following procedures:

- It is useful and safe for the mother to have the baby placed in her bed in the first hour of life with a heat panel above them when a premature baby weighing 1.5 to 2.5 kg is delivered and appears to be doing well without grunting and retractions. We do not recommend this approach unless the physician is sure the infant is healthy. We recommend that a skilled neonatal nurse be available in the room for the visits of the immature infant.

- A mother and her infant should be kept near each other in the same hospital, ideally on the same floor. When the long-term significance of early mother-infant contact is kept in mind, a modification of restrictions and territorial traditions usually can be arranged.[2, 29]

- If the baby does have to be moved to a hospital with an intensive care unit, the mother should be given a chance to see and touch her infant, even if the baby has respiratory distress and is in an oxygen hood or on a respirator. The house officer or the attending physician stops in the mother's room with the transport incubator and encourages her to touch and look at her baby. A comment about the baby's strength and healthy features may be long remembered and appreciated.

- In such a transfer we encourage the father to follow the transport team to the hospital so he can see what is happening with his baby. He uses his own transportation so that he can stay in the premature unit for a few hours. This extra time allows him to get to know the nurses and physicians in the unit, to find out how the infant is being treated, and to talk with the physician about what is expected to happen to the baby in the succeeding days. We allow him to come into the nursery, and we explain in detail everything that is going on with his infant. We ask him to help act as a link between us and his family by relaying information to the baby's mother, and we request that he come to our unit before he visits the baby's mother so that he can let her know how the baby is doing. We suggest that he take an instant photograph, even if the infant is on a respirator, so that he can describe the baby's care in detail to the baby's mother.

- In many communities the mother is transported from the community hospital before delivery to the maternity division of the medical center so she will be with her baby after birth. More often the mother is being transported with the baby after delivery.

- A mother should be permitted to enter the premature nursery as soon as she is able to maneuver easily. When she makes her first visit, it is important to anticipate that she may become faint or dizzy when she looks at her infant. We always have a stool nearby so that she can sit down, and a nurse stays at her side during most of the visit, describing in detail the procedures being carried out, such as respiration and heart rate monitoring, the umbilical catheter and endotracheal tube placement, feeding through the various infusion lines, and the functioning of the incubator and ventilator.

- We encourage grandparents, brothers, sisters, and other relatives to view the infant through the glass window of the nursery so they will begin to know and to feel attached to the infant. We believe it is important to arrange for the grandparents and special close friends or relatives to enter the nursery and visit the baby, particularly when the baby is very ill or expected to die, so that they can provide firsthand support and understanding to the parents. We selectively allow siblings to enter the nursery when we believe it will truly relieve (and not aggravate) a child's confusion and anxiety.

- It is necessary to find out what the mother believes is going to happen or what she has read about any problem that may have developed. We try to move at her pace during any discussion to ensure her understanding.

- In discussing the infant's condition by telephone with the mother who is still in the referring hospital, we ask the father to stand nearby so that we can talk to them both at the same time and they can hear the same message. This group communication reduces misunderstanding and usually is helpful in assuring the mother that we are telling her the whole story.

- If the sick infant has a reasonable chance of survival, we are cautiously optimistic with the parents from the beginning. No evidence has shown that the parents will be harmed by early optimism if a favorable prediction proves to be incorrect and the baby expires. Parents can almost always be prepared before the baby actually dies. If the infant lives and the physician has been pessimistic, it is more difficult for parents to become closely attached. We recognize that this recommendation is contrary to many past customs and places a heavy burden on the physician. It is our belief that if the infant does expire, we must

continue to work with the mother and father and to help them with their mourning reactions.

- Once the possibility that a baby has brain damage has been mentioned, the parents will not forget it. Therefore, unless we are convinced that the baby is damaged, we do not mention the possibility of any brain damage or retardation to the parents.

- It is important to emphasize that if there is a clear objective finding such as a cardiac abnormality or a specific congenital malformation, there is no reason to hide it from the parents.

- It is important to remember that feelings of love for the baby are often elicited through eye-to-eye contact. Therefore, if an infant is under bilirubin lights, we turn them off and remove the eye patches so the mother and her infant can see each other.

- From our previous observations, we have found that keeping a book in which to record parental phone calls and visits is useful in determining which mothers are likely to require additional help from a social worker or extra discussions about the health of their infant.[17] If a mother visits the nursery fewer than three times in 2 weeks, the chance of her developing a mothering disorder increases. Therefore, if her visiting pattern is less than that of most other mothers, she is given extra help in adapting to the hospitalization.

- Mothers should look to nurses for guidance, support, and encouragement when they first handle the child. The nurse's guidance in showing the mother how to hold, dress, and feed the infant can be extremely valuable. Often mothers need special reassurance and permission before they can enjoy caring for their baby. In a sense, the nurse assumes the role of the mother's own mother, teaching her the basic techniques of mothering.

- In recent years a number of neonatal intensive care units have formed groups of parents of premature babies who meet once a week or more often for 1- to 2-hour discussions.[39]

In a controlled study of a self-help group, Minde and associates reported that parents who participated in the group visited their infants in the hospital significantly more often than did parents in the control group.[38] The self-help parents also touched, talked to, and looked at their infants in the en face position more and rated themselves as more competent on infant care measures. These mothers continued to show more involvement with their babies during feedings and were more concerned about their general development 3 months after their discharge from the nursery.

INFANTS WITH CONGENITAL MALFORMATIONS

The birth of an infant with a congenital malformation presents complex challenges to the physician in charge and to the infant's family. Despite the relatively large number of infants with congenital anomalies, our understanding of how parents develop an attachment to a malformed child remains incomplete. Although previous investigators agree that the child's birth often precipitates major family stress, relatively few have described the process of family adaptation during the infant's first year of life. A major advance was Solnit and coworkers' conceptualization of parental reactions.[53] They emphasized that a significant aspect of adaptation is the necessity for parents to mourn the loss of the normal child they had expected. Other observers have noted the pathologic aspects of family reactions. Less attention has been given to the more adaptive aspects of parental attachments to children with malformations.

Parental reactions to the birth of a child with a congenital malformation appear to follow a predictable course. For most parents initial shock, disbelief, and a period of intense emotional upset, including sadness, anger, and anxiety, are followed by gradual adaptation marked by a lessening of intense anxiety and emotional reactions (Fig. 32–4). This adaptation is characterized by an increased satisfaction with and ability to care for the baby. These stages in parental reactions are similar to those reported in other crisis situations, such as with terminally ill children. The shock, disbelief, and denial reported by many parents seem to form an understandable attempt to escape the traumatic news of the baby's malformation, so discrepant with usual parental expectations for a normal newborn.[13]

As stated, Solnit and coworkers have likened the crisis of the birth of a child with a malformation to the emotional crisis after the death of a child, in that the mother must mourn the loss of her expected, normal infant. In addition, she must become attached to her living, damaged child. However, the sequence of parental reactions to the birth of a baby with a malformation differs from that after the death of a child in yet another respect. The mourning or grief work apparently does not occur in the usual manner because of the complex issues raised by continuation of the child's life and the demands of physical care. The parents' sadness, which is important initially in their relationship with their child, diminishes in most instances once the parents take over the physical care.[50] Most parents reach a point at which they are able to care adequately for their children and cope effectively with disrupting feelings of sadness and anger. Sadly not all parents reach the point of complete resolution, and Olshansky has described chronic sorrow that envelops the family of a mentally defective infant.[43] The mother's initiation of the relationship with her child is a major step in the reduction of anxiety and emotional upset associated with the trauma of the birth. As happens with normal children, the mother's initial experience with her infant seems to release positive feelings that aid the mother-child relationship after the stresses associated with the news of the child's anomaly and, in many instances, the separation of mother and child in the hospital.

INTERVENTIONS FOR PARENTS OF MALFORMED INFANTS

To help parents deal with the situation of having an infant with a congenital malformation, we offer the following interventions:

- The infant should be left with the mother for the first 2 or 3 days, if medically feasible. If the child is rushed to the hospital where special surgery will eventually be performed, the mother will not have enough opportunity to become attached to the infant. Even if the surgery is required immediately, as for bowel obstruction, it is best to bring the baby to the mother first, allowing her to touch and handle the infant and to point out to her how normal he or she is in all other respects.
- The parents' mental picture of the anomaly is often far more alarming than the actual problem. Any delay during which the parents suspect that a problem may exist greatly heightens their anxiety, and they may imagine the worst; therefore, the baby should be brought to both parents when they are together as soon after delivery as possible.[40]
- We have arranged for the father to stay with the mother in her room on the maternity division on many occasions. This opportunity to support each other, to cry and curse and talk together, is highly beneficial. We use the process of early crisis intervention, meeting several times with the parents, regardless of whether the father stays in the hospital with the mother. During these discussions we ask the mother how she is doing, how she feels her husband or partner is doing, and how the father feels about the infant. We then reverse the questions and ask the father how he is

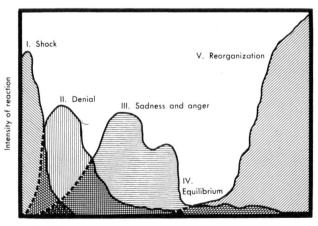

FIGURE 32–4. Hypothetic model of a normal sequence of parental reactions to the birth of a malformed infant. (Modified from Drotar D, et al: The adaptation of parents to the birth of an infant with a congenital malformation: A hypothetical model. Pediatrics 56:710, 1975. Copyright American Academy of Pediatrics, 1975. Reproduced by permission of Pediatrics.)

doing and how he thinks the mother is progressing. The hope is that they will think not only about their own reactions but will begin to consider each other as well.

■ Parents should not be given tranquilizers. These tend to blunt their responses and slow their adaptation to the problem. A small dose of a sedative at night, however, is often helpful.

■ It has been our experience that parents who initially adapt reasonably well often ask many questions and at times appear to be almost overinvolved in clinical care. In our unit we are pleased by this and more concerned about parents who ask few questions or who appear stunned and overwhelmed by the problem.

■ Many anomalies are very frustrating, not only to the parents but also to the physicians and nurses. The physician may be tempted to withdraw from the parents and their infant. The many questions asked by the parent who is trying to understand the problem can be very frustrating for the physician. The parent often appears to forget and asks the same questions repeatedly.

■ Each parent may move through the process of shock, denial, anger, guilt, and adaptation at a different pace, so the two parents may not be synchronized. If they are unable to talk with each other about the baby, their relationship may be severely disrupted. We have found it best to move at the parents' pace. Moving too quickly runs the risk of losing the parents along the way. It is essential to ask the parents how they view their infant.

SUMMARY

Because the newborn baby completely depends on the parents for survival and optimum development, it is essential to understand the process of bonding as it develops from the first moments after the child is born. Although we have only begun to understand this complex phenomenon, those responsible for the care of mothers and infants should re-evaluate hospital procedures that interfere with early, sustained mother-infant contact. They should consider measures that promote a mother's contact with her infant and help her appreciate the wide range of sensory and motor responses of her neonate.

■ REFERENCES

1. Als H, et al: Individualized developmental care for the very low birthweight preterm infant. JAMA 272:853, 1994.
2. Anisfeld E, et al: Early contact, social support and mother-infant bonding. Pediatrics 72:79, 1983.
3. Barnett CR, et al: Neonatal separation: The maternal side of interactional deprivation. Pediatrics 45:197, 1970.
4. Benfield DG, et al: Grief response of parents following referral of the critically ill newborn. N Engl J Med 194:975, 1976.
5. Bibring G: Some considerations of the psychological processes in pregnancy. Psychoanal Study Child 14:113, 1959.
6. Bowlby J: Nature of a child's tie to his mother. Int J Psychoanal 39:350, 1958.
7. Brazelton TB: Effect of maternal expectations on early infant behavior. Early Child Dev Care 2:259, 1973.
8. Brazelton TB, et al: The Earliest Relationship. Reading, Mass, Addison-Wesley Publishing Co, Inc, 1990.
9. Buranasin B, et al: The effects of rooming-in on the success of breast-feeding and the decline in abandonment of children. Asia Pac J Public Health 5:217, 1991.
10. Christenssohn K, et al: Temperature, metabolic adaptation, and crying in healthy fullterm infants cared for skin to skin or in a cot. Acta Paediatr 81:488, 1992.
11. Cohen RL: Some maladaptive syndromes of pregnancy and the puerperium. Obstet Gynecol 25:562, 1966.
12. DeCasper A, et al: Newborns prefer their mothers' voices. Science 208:1174, 1980.
13. Drotar D, et al: The adaptation of parents to the birth of an infant with a congenital malformation: A hypothetical model. Pediatrics 56:710, 1975.
14. Emde R, et al: Human wakefulness and biologic rhythms after birth. Arch Gen Psychiatry 32:780, 1973.
15. Engel GL, et al: Monica: Infant feeding behavior of a mother gastric fistula fed as an infant: A 30 year longitudinal study of enduring effects. In Anthony EJ, Pollack GH (eds): Parental Influences in Health & Disease. Boston, Little, Brown & Co, Inc, 1985, p 29.
16. Enkin M, et al: A Guide to Effective Care in Pregnancy and Childbirth. Oxford, Oxford University Press, 1995, p 347.
17. Fanaroff AA, et al: Follow-up of low birth-weight infants: The predictive value of maternal visiting pattern. Pediatrics 49:288, 1972.
18. Field T: Effects of early separation, interactive deficits and experimental manipulations on infant-mother face-to-face interaction. Child Dev 48:763, 1977.
19. Field T, et al: Tactile kinesthetic stimulation effects on preterm neonates. Pediatrics 77(5):654, 1986.
20. Gottfried AW, Gaiter J (eds): Infant Stress Under Intensive Care: Environmental Neonatology. Baltimore, University Park Press, 1985.
20a. Green M, Solnit A: Reactions to the threatened loss of a child: A vulnerable child syndrome. Pediatrics 34:58, 1964.
21. Harper RG, et al: Observations on unrestricted parental contact with infants in the neonatal intensive care unit. J Pediatr 89:441, 1976.
22. Hodnett ED, et al: Caregiver support for women during childbirth [review]. Cochrane Database Syst Rev 2:CD000199, 2000.
23. Kaitz M, et al: Mothers' recognition of their olfactory cues. Dev Psychobiol 20(6):587, 1987.
24. Kaitz M, et al: Postpartum women can recognize their infants by touch. Dev Psychol 23:35, 1992.
25. Keller WD, et al: Effects of extended father-infant contact during the newborn period. Infant Behav Dev 8:337, 1985.
26. Kennell JH, et al: Discussing problems in newborn babies with their parents. Pediatrics 27:832, 1960.
27. Kennell JH, et al: Continuous emotional support during labor in a U.S. hospital: A randomized controlled trial. JAMA 265:2197, 1991.
28. Keverne EB, et al: Maternal behavior in sheep and its neuro-endocrine regulation. Acta Paediatr Scand 83:47, 1994.
29. Klaus MH, et al: Bonding: Building the Foundations of Secure Attachment and Independence. Cambridge, Mass, Perseus, 1995.
30. Klaus MH, et al: Maternal attachment: Importance of the first post-partum days. N Engl J Med 286:460, 1972.
31. Klaus MH, et al: Effects of social support during parturition on maternal and infant morbidity. Br Med J 293:585, 1986.
32. Klaus MH, et al: Mothering the Mother. Cambridge, Mass, Perseus, 1993.
33. Klaus MH, et al: Your Amazing Newborn. Cambridge, Mass, Perseus, 1998.
34. Lind J, et al: The effect of cry stimulus on the temperature of the lactating breast primipara: A thermographic study. In Morris N (ed): Psychosomatic Medicine in Obstetrics and Gynaecology. S Karger, Basel, Switzerland, 1973.
35. MacFarlane JA, et al: The relationship between mother and neonate. In Kitzinger S, et al (eds): The Place of Birth. New York, Oxford University Press, 1978.

36. Mann NP, et al: Effect of night and day on preterm infants in a newborn nursery: A randomised trial. Br Med J 293(6557):1265, 1986.
37. Mason EA: A method of predicting crisis outcome for mothers of premature babies. Public Health Rep 78:1031, 1963.
38. Minde K, et al: Mother-child relationships in the premature nursery: An observational study. Pediatrics 61:373, 1978.
39. Minde K, et al: Self-help groups in a premature nursery: A controlled evaluation. J Pediatr 96:933, 1980.
40. National Association for Mental Health Working Party: The birth of an abnormal child: Telling the parents. Lancet 2:1075, 1971.
41. Nissen E, et al: Elevation of oxytocin levels postpartum in women. Acta Obstet Gynecol Scand 74:530, 1995.
42. O'Connor S, et al: Reduced incidence of parenting inadequacy following rooming-in. Pediatrics 66:176, 1980.
43. Olshansky S: Chronic sorrow: A response to having a mentally defective child. Social Casework 43:190, 1962.
44. Parke RD: Fatherhood. Cambridge, Mass, Harvard University Press, 1996.
45. Pascoe J, et al: Development of positive feeling in primiparous mothers toward their normal newborn. Clin Pediatr 28(10):452, 1989.
46. Righard L, et al: Effect of delivery room routines on success of first breast-feed. Lancet 336:1105, 1990.
47. Robson K, et al: Delayed onset of maternal affection after childbirth. Br J Psychiatry 136:347, 1980.
48. Rödholm M: Effects of father-infant postpartum contact on their interaction 3 months after birth. Early Hum Dev 5:79, 1981.
49. Rose J, et al: The evidence for a syndrome of "mothering disability" consequent to threats to the survival of neonates: A design for hypothesis testing including prevention in a prospective study. Am J Dis Child 100:776, 1960.
50. Roskies E: Abnormality and normality: The mothering of thalidomide children. New York, Cornell University Press, 1972.
51. Scott KD, et al: A comparison of intermittent and continuous support during labor: A meta-analysis. Am J Obstet Gynecol 180:1054, 1999.
52. Siegel E, et al: Hospital and home support during infancy: Impact on maternal attachment, child abuse and neglect, and health care utilization. Pediatrics 66:183, 1980.
53. Solnit AJ, et al: Mourning and the birth of a defective child. Psychoanal Study Child 16:523, 1961.
54. Sosa R, et al: The effect of a supportive companion on perinatal problems, length of labor, and mother-infant interaction. N Engl J Med 303:597, 1980.
55. Thoman EB, et al: Premature infants seek rhythmic stimulation, and the experience stimulates neurobehavioral development. Journal of Behavioral Pediatrics 12(1):11, 1991.
56. Trevarthen C: Descriptive analysis of infant communicative behavior. In Schaffer HR (ed): Studies in Mother-Infant Interaction. New York, Academic Press, Inc, 1977.
57. Varendi H, et al: Attractiveness of amniotic fluid odor: Evidence of prenatal learning? Acta Paediatrica 85:1223, 1996.
58. Whitelaw A: Kangaroo baby care: Just a nice experience or an important advance for preterm infants? Pediatrics 85:604, 1990.
59. Widström AM, et al: Gastric suction in healthy infants: Effects on circulation and developing feeding behavior. Acta Paediatr Scand 76(4):566, 1987.
60. Widström AM, et al: Short term effects of early suckling and touch of the nipple on maternal behavior. Early Hum Dev 21:153, 1990.
61. Winnicott DW: Collected Papers: Through Paediatrics to Psycho-Analysis. New York, Basic Books, 1958.
62. Winnicott DW: Playing and Reality. London, Tavistock Publications, Ltd, 1971.

Nutrition and Metabolism in the High-Risk Neonate

part one
ENTERAL NUTRITION

Scott C. Denne,
Brenda B. Poindexter,
Catherine A. Leitch,
Judith A. Ernst,
Pamela K. Lemons, and
James A. Lemons

There is accumulating evidence that early nutritional inadequacies have long-term consequences.[96] Providing appropriate nutritional support remains a significant challenge in premature infants, especially in infants with extremely low birth weights (less than 1000 gm). Currently, nearly all such infants experience significant growth retardation during their stay in the neonatal intensive care unit.[87]

Achieving full and consistent enteral nutrition in infants with extremely low birth weights is particularly challenging, given the inherent problems of immature gut motility and function. Data about enteral feeding in this population are limited; most of the information has been obtained from larger, more mature, more stable premature infants. In addition, premature formulas and human milk fortifiers have been designed primarily for this more mature population. This chapter reviews the available evidence on enteral feeding, concentrating on high-risk infants. Recommendations regarding infants with extremely low birth weights are largely extrapolated from data obtained in larger premature infants.

There is reasonable but not universal consensus that growth and body composition in premature infants ideally should mirror that of a fetus of comparable gestational age. It must be noted that fetal growth is not uniform throughout gestation. The fetus gains approximately 5 gm/day at 16 weeks of gestation, 10 gm/day at 21 weeks, and 20 gm/day at 29 weeks; at 37 weeks it reaches a peak daily weight gain of 35 gm.[159] The body composition changes drastically throughout gestation (Table 33–1). The percentages of body water, extracellular water, and sodium and chloride decline progressively; conversely, on a per kilogram basis, the fetus retains progressively more intracellular water, protein, fat, calcium, phosphorus, iron, and magnesium. Between 24 and 40 weeks' gestation, water content declines from approximately 87% to 71%, protein rises from 8.8% to 12%, and fat from 1% to 13.1%. Glycogen represents 1% or less of body weight throughout gestation; the hepatic stores are about 10 to 18 mg/gm of liver until 36 weeks of gestation and increase to about 50 mg/gm of liver by 40 weeks.

ENERGY REQUIREMENTS AND PARTITION OF ENERGY METABOLISM IN THE ENTERALLY FED INFANT

ENERGY BALANCE

Energy balance is a delicate equilibrium between energy intake and energy loss plus storage. Energy loss is the sum of energy expenditure plus excretion of energy-containing substances in urine and feces. Positive energy balance is achieved when exogenous metabolizable energy intake is greater than energy expenditure. Growth is then possible, with the excess energy stored as new tissue, usually fat. If exogenous energy intake is less than expenditure, energy balance is negative, and body energy stores must be mobilized to meet ongoing needs. During the acute phase of disease, the primary goal is not growth but avoidance of catabolism. This is difficult for infants with very low birth weights owing to their higher maintenance energy requirements, lower energy stores, and often reduced intake.

The estimate of caloric needs (Table 33–2) is based on the assumption that postnatal growth should approximate in utero growth of a normal fetus of the same postconceptional age. These needs do not take into account the increased caloric requirements of sick premature infants.

TABLE 33–1 BODY COMPOSITION OF AVERAGE APPROPRIATE FOR GESTATIONAL AGE
FETUS OR NEONATE WEIGHING 750, 1000, 2000, AND 3500 GM

	750 GM	**1000 GM**	**2000 GM**	**3500 GM**
Gestational age (wk)	24–25	27	33	40
Water (%/gm)	87/653	85.4/854	79.8/1596	71/2485
Fat (%/gm)	1/7.5	2.3	6.5/130	13.1/460
Glycogen (%/gm)	1/7.5	1/10	1/20	1/35
Nonprotein energy (kcal)	98	248	1252	4284
(kcal/kg)*	131	248	626	1224
Minerals				
Calcium (mmol per kg/total)	140/105	145/145	170/340	210/735
Chloride (mmol per kg/total)	69/52	66/66	60/120	48/170
Copper (mg per kg/total)	3.6/2.7	3.8/3.8	4/8.1	4.1/14.3
Iron (mg per kg/total)	62/46	64/64	70/141	81/283
Magnesium (mml per kg/total)	7.7/5.8	8/8	8.2/16.5	8.7/30
Phosphorus (mmol per kg/total)	105/80	115/115	130/260	160/560
Potassium (mmol per kg/total)	42/32	42/42	42/85	42/150
Sodium (mmol per kg/total)	95/71	90/90	82/164	79/275
Zinc (mg per kg/total)	17.7/13.3	17.6/3.8	16.9/33.8	15.3/53.6

*Assuming 4.1 kcal/gm of glycogen and 9 kcal/gm of fat.
Modified from Usher RM, et al: Intrauterine growth of live-born Caucasian infants at sea level: Standards obtained from measurements in 7 dimensions of infants born between 25 and 44 weeks of gestation. J Pediatr 74:901, 1969; Widdowson EM: Changes in body proportion and composition during growth. In Davis JA (ed): Committee on Nutrition of the Preterm Infant, European Society of Paediatric Gastroenterology and Nutrition. Oxford, Blackwell Scientific, 1987; and Ziegler EE, et al: Acta Paediatr Scand 299(suppl):90, 1982.

ENERGY LOSSES

Energy is lost either by excretion or by expenditure. The energy in excreta is lost mainly as fecal fat and increases as energy intake increases. The magnitude of this factor can be altered by changing the type of dietary fat.

Usual measurements of total energy expenditure include the energy used to maintain basal metabolic rate (BMR), as well as the postprandial increase in energy expenditure (thermic effect of food or diet-induced thermogenesis), physical activity, and energy for the synthesis of new tissue.[66]

BMR is the largest component of energy expenditure and includes energy requirements for basic cellular and tissue processes. In a critically ill patient, it also includes a "disease factor." Little is known about this component in neonates, but it probably contributes significantly to the BMR in neonates with fever, sepsis, and chronic hypoxia. Because BMR can be measured only after overnight fasting, which is ethically unacceptable for neonates, resting metabolic rate (RMR) has been accepted as an alternative. Absolute metabolic rate increases as the fetus grows. However, on a weight-normalized basis, the metabolic rate decreases.[162] Thus, the RMR of preterm infants on a per kilogram basis is higher than that of term infants, and the nutritional requirements on a per kilogram basis are correspondingly greater. The energy required for thermoregulation and activity can be minimized by keeping the infant in a thermoneutral environment and limiting stimulation. For example, energy requirements for thermoregulation are negligible under thermoneutral conditions, but routine nursing procedures can increase oxygen consumption or energy expenditure by as much as 10% in stable preterm infants. Both of these components might be of considerable magnitude in a critically ill infant. The estimated BMR of infants with low birth weights, including an irreducible amount of physical activity in a thermoneutral environment, is lower immediately after birth than later, and by 2 to 3 weeks of age, approximately 50 to 60 kcal/kg per day is needed to maintain weight.[111] Energy expenditure ranging from 40 to greater than 70 kcal/kg per day has been reported in growing infants with very low birth weights.[46, 100, 111, 128, 130] Estimates of BMR for healthy term infants range from 43 to 60 kcal/kg per day.[14]

The level of energy intake and diet composition determine the magnitude of diet-induced thermogenesis, which represents the energy required for transport, metabolism, and conversion of nutrients into stored energy. Continuous enteral feedings are slightly (4%) more energy efficient than intermittent feedings,[51] because premature infants have higher rates of energy expenditure and diet-induced thermo-

TABLE 33–2 ESTIMATED ENERGY
REQUIREMENTS FOR
GROWING PRETERM
INFANTS

FACTOR	KCAL/KG/DAY
Energy expenditure	
Resting metabolic rate	40–60
Activity	0–5
Thermoregulation	0–5
Synthesis/energy cost of growth	15
Energy stored	20–30
Energy excreted	15
Estimated total energy requirement	90–120

genesis during intermittent feedings than during continuous feedings. Continuous enteral feedings also allow larger intake volumes.

Because neonates sleep 80% to 90% of the time, the energy expended in physical activity is a smaller component of energy expenditure in neonates compared with adults. Nevertheless, activity influences energy expenditure in neonates in measurable ways. For example, differences in energy expenditure have been demonstrated between active (rapid eye movement) and quiet (non–rapid eye movement) sleep in both term and preterm infants.[139, 149] It has been estimated that activity contributes approximately 10% (range, 3% to 17%) to total energy expenditure in the neonatal period.[133] One study[151] directly measured the energy expended in physical activity in preterm infants through the use of long-period respiratory calorimetry to measure total energy expenditure and a force platform to measure work output. The energy expended in physical activity was found to constitute approximately 3.5% of total energy expenditure in a group of 24 stable preterm infants. Although the average magnitude of this component is small, it may have a significant impact on growth in irritable infants with poor responses to nursing care and interventions.

The energy expenditure for growth includes both the energy content of the new tissue deposited (energy stored) and the energy required for the formation of that tissue (metabolic cost of growth) and is therefore largely determined by the composition of the tissue synthesized. The cost of tissue synthesis varies considerably. The cost of depositing absorbed dietary fat into adipose tissue is much less than that of synthesizing new protein. The cost of synthesizing fat from carbohydrate or protein also is considerably greater than that of simply depositing absorbed dietary fat. During growth, a mixture of fat and protein is deposited simultaneously. The total cost of growth has been estimated at 4 to 6 kcal/gm,[14] of which 1 kcal/gm is oxidized for tissue synthesis.

Total energy expenditure is affected by several factors, assuming a thermoneutral environment and minimal interference from nursing procedures. Increases in metabolic rate with postnatal age are influenced primarily by energy intake and weight gain. Energy expenditure increases with increases in metabolizable energy intake, indicating increased substrate oxidation or tissue synthesis. Van Aerde[160] observed that about one fourth of each additional kilocalorie absorbed is expended. If the preterm infant is growing at the same rate as the fetus during the third trimester—that is, gaining approximately 15 gm/kg per day—then about 15% of the total energy intake is used for synthesis of new tissue.

ENERGY STORAGE

Energy storage is a linear function of metabolizable intake, as demonstrated by several investigators. Reichman and colleagues[128] demonstrated that the accretion rate for energy is related more to the level of metabolizable energy intake than to diet composition. Energy requirements for energy storage are difficult to predict. The increase in tissue mass during growth includes the energy stored as protein, carbohydrate (usually less than 1% of body weight), and fat.[111, 162] Therefore, the energy stored can be assumed to equal the sum of the cost of protein plus fat gain. The energy storage component of the energy balance equation is a function of the composition of weight gain, which in turn is a function of protein and energy intake and is likely to be quite variable. Therefore, the energy intake required to produce a specific rate of weight gain cannot be predicted without specifying the composition of that weight gain. From the point of view of energy storage, protein is a poor material, because a small quantity of energy is stored per gram of weight gain. Approximately the same amount of energy is deposited in 1 gm of fat tissue as in about 8 gm of lean tissue.

Most studies of enterally fed preterm infants receiving either human milk or formula report a higher rate of energy storage per gram of weight gain than that estimated for the fetus.[25, 26, 46, 128] This may reflect an adaptation to extrauterine life, and if so, it may also be inappropriate to simulate rates of intrauterine energy and fat accretion. However, the effect of a large amount of weight gained as fat and the optimal rate of weight gain for these infants are presently unknown.[67, 84, 123]

ENERGY INTAKE

Caloric requirements for healthy, growing neonates were initially established by Sinclair[146] and are based on measurements of minimal metabolic rates and on theoretical estimates of caloric needs for normal physiologic functions. These studies revealed that the total daily energy requirements for full-term infants increase sharply from fetal levels during the first 48 hours of life and continue to increase at a lower rate until the end of the second week of life, reaching a value of 100 to 120 kcal/kg per day. Unlike that for full-term infants, the optimal caloric requirement for infants with very or extremely low birth weights is more difficult to define and is still to be determined for those infants and for critically ill neonates.

Low total body energy stores and metabolic requirements of an infant with a very low birth weight enable the infant to live ex utero for only about 4 days after birth without any support. In contrast, a full-term infant can theoretically live for as long as 40 days.[67, 123] Therefore, providing adequate early energy resources is more crucial for preterm neonates than for full-term infants, even without considering their greater normalized rate of in utero growth. Lacking a better standard, nutritionists have adopted the concept that the in utero growth and accretion rate is ideal. Absolute weight gain increases progressively over the second half of gestation; however, the weight-normalized weight gain decreases during this period. Thus, nutritional requirements for fetal growth, when estimated from the specific weight of the fetus, are actually much higher at 24 to 28 weeks' gestation than they are at term.[63] Furthermore, actual weight gain is an underestimate of nutritional requirements, because changes in body composition during this period are not considered. The total water content of the fetus decreases from 90% at 20 weeks to 75% at term, and the size and number of cells increase during this period. Higher weight-normalized nutrient intakes are necessary to produce growth in infants with extremely low birth weights compared with older, more mature infants. Prenatal growth rate and body composition also may influence postnatal nutritional requirements. Greater weight-specific growth rates of 10th percentile infants who are small for gestational age compared with those of 90th percentile infants who are large for gestational age have been shown, suggesting that infants who are small for gestational age may require more nutrient intake per kilogram of body weight than larger infants.[63]

According to the energy balance equation, the energy requirement for maintenance of existing weight and body composition is equal to energy expenditure. Individual infants vary in their activity, in their ease of achieving basal energy expenditure at thermoneutrality, and in their efficiency of nutrient absorption. Enteral intakes of 120 or 130 kcal/kg per day have been recommended, as this allows most infants with low birth weights to grow at 15 to 20 gm/day, similar to growth rates achieved in utero.[131, 133] Increasing the energy intake to 140 to 150 kcal/kg per day has been shown to increase weight gain and triceps-subscapular skinfold thickness but has no effect on gain in length or head circumference or in nitrogen retention.[114, 165] Long-term effects of energy supplementation have not been studied. Positive nitrogen balance without weight gain usually can be achieved at 60 kcal/kg per day with approximately 2.5 gm/kg of protein per day.[4] Owing to inevitable losses, the energy intake necessary to provide this requirement is somewhat higher.[66] The bulk of this additional intake is stored, but some is expended as a result of the greater thermic effect of food and the energy cost of new tissue synthesis. Most preterm infants achieve acceptable weight gain at these levels of energy intake. Infants who are small for gestational age or infants with diseases that increase energy requirements may need higher intakes to achieve the same growth rates.[131] Newborn infants with growth retardation often require an increased caloric intake for growth because of both higher maintenance energy needs and higher energy costs of new tissue synthesis.

The European Society for Paediatric Gastroenterology and Nutrition (ESPGAN)[40–42] has recommended an average intake of 130 kcal/kg per day. The American Academy of Pediatrics[1] and the Canadian Paediatric Society[116] recommend 105 to 130 kcal/kg per day. At present, no valid recommendations can be made with regard to the optimal energy requirements for infants with extremely low birth weights or critically ill infants, except that their energy requirements are most likely higher than those for stable, growing infants with very low birth weights.

CARBOHYDRATES IN THE ENTERALLY FED INFANT

Lactose is the predominant carbohydrate in human milk (6.2 to 7.2 gm/dL) and supplies 40% to 50% of the caloric content. Lactose is hydrolyzed to glucose and galactose in the small intestine by β-galactosidase (lactase). Intestinal lactase activities in premature infants at 34 weeks' gestational age are approximately 30% of those of term infants.[78] Despite low lactase activities in premature infants, lactose is well tolerated by premature infants, and stable isotope data suggest efficient lactose digestion.[78] However, most premature infant formulas include glucose polymers as a significant source of carbohydrate; these glucose polymers are digested by α-glucosidases, which achieve 70% of adult activity between 26 and 34 weeks' gestation. In addition, salivary and mammary amylases may contribute to glucose polymer digestion. Glucose polymers have the advantage of increased caloric density without a rise in osmolality, and they may also enhance gastric emptying.

PROTEIN REQUIREMENTS IN THE ENTERALLY FED INFANT

The protein content and composition of human milk change throughout lactation; the concentration diminishes from about 2 gm/dL at birth to about 1 gm/dL for mature milk. Qualitative changes also occur during lactation, resulting in a whey-casein ratio of 80:20 at the beginning of lactation, changing to 55:45 in mature milk. Indeed, whereas the levels of casein, α-lactalbumin, albumin, and lysozyme remain constant, the levels of secretory immunoglobulin A and lactoferrin decrease; because these different protein fractions have different amino acid profiles, the content of the individual amino acids also is affected.[71, 124] Finally, about 25% of the total nitrogen in human milk is nonprotein nitrogen, the major fractions being urea and free amino acids.

Infant formula has much more protein than human milk. A report by the Life Sciences Research Office recommends that formulas for term infants contain 1.7 to 3.4 gm of protein per 100 kcal[90]; ESPGAN recommends a protein content of 1.8 to 2.8 gm/100 kcal.[42] In practice, most commercially available standard term formulas in the United States contain between 2.1 and 2.4 gm of protein per 100 kcal, which provides infants 2 to 2.5 gm/kg per day for the first month of life. For preterm infants with birth weights between 1200 and 1800 gm, the protein requirement is somewhere between 2.7 and 3.5 gm/kg per day; standard preterm formulas containing between 2.5 and 3 gm of protein per 100 kcal can meet those requirements if fluid intake is not restricted. Infants weighing less than 1200 gm may require more protein, based on Ziegler's factorial approach. The nutrition committee of the Canadian Pediatric Society recommends that infants weighing less than 1000 gm receive 3.5 to 4 gm/kg per day of protein, although there is a paucity of clinical data supporting this recommendation.[116] However, preliminary studies suggest that higher protein intakes in infants less than 1200 gm may improve growth.[21, 35]

Casein-predominant cow's milk formulas have the same whey-casein ratio as cow's milk—that is, 18:82. Whey-predominant formulas are made by adding bovine whey, such that the whey-casein ratio becomes similar to that of human milk (60:40). Nevertheless, the protein and amino acid profile remains very different from that of human milk. Compared with human milk, whey-predominant formulas have higher levels of methionine, threonine, lysine, and branched amino acids, whereas casein-predominant formulas have higher levels of methionine, tyrosine, and branched amino acids.[71, 74]

Plasma amino acid profiles reflect protein intake and the composition of the milk proteins. In that respect, term infants receiving a casein-predominant formula have higher plasma levels of tyrosine, methionine, and phenylalanine compared with human milk–fed infants. Whey-predominant formulas usually produce higher concentrations of threonine.[125] These differences in amino acid concentrations have not resulted in any apparent clinical consequences.

For protein metabolism in a preterm infant, there is discussion whether amino acid concentrations from cord blood or those obtained in breast-fed infants should serve as the reference. Raiha and colleagues suggested that the optimal protein intake in infants with very low birth weights should produce a growth rate similar to that in utero and plasma amino acid profiles and metabolic parameters of protein metabolism similar to those of breast-fed infants.[124] Polberger and colleagues reported that these criteria can be fulfilled with a caloric intake of 120 kcal/kg per day and 3 gm/kg per day of protein, assuming sufficient provision of minerals.[122] Similarly, other studies reported that metabolic indexes, energy balance, and body composition of weight gain were better when feeding 115 kcal/kg per day and 3.6 gm/kg per day of protein than when feeding either 115 kcal/kg per day with 2.24 gm of protein or 149 kcal/kg per day with 3.5 gm of protein.[75, 140] Therefore, with a caloric intake of 115 to 120 kcal/kg per day, the enteral protein requirement of infants with very low birth weights is 3 to 3.6 gm/kg per day. Most of these studies have been done in infants with birth weights between 1000 and 1500 gm; consequently, the requirements of smaller neonates are uncertain. As in term infants, there is no difference in growth, nitrogen retention, and blood urea nitrogen (BUN) between infants fed a whey-predominant formula and those fed a casein-predominant formula; the plasma amino acid levels are different, however, and reflect the dietary protein composition.[9, 74]

Because taurine is a conditionally essential amino acid in humans, it is discussed in this section. Taurine is synthesized endogenously from cysteine and is not part of structural protein.[47] The highest concentrations are present in the retina and brain of the fetus, reaching a peak concentration at birth. Furthermore, tau-

rine plays a role in liver function, growth, and fat absorption. Free taurine is found in human milk in higher concentrations than in maternal plasma, resulting in higher plasma and urine levels in breast-fed infants than in neonates fed unsupplemented formula. Taurine conjugates with bile acids, and infants fed human milk or taurine-supplemented formula have predominantly taurine-conjugated bile acids compared with infants fed a taurine-free diet.[47] When newborn nonhuman primates are fed taurine-deficient formula, growth is depressed,[65] but this is not so for human preterm infants, despite declining plasma and urine taurine levels.[72] Whereas reversible abnormalities were found in the retinograms of children receiving taurine-free, long-term total parenteral nutrition (TPN), the retinograms of preterm infants fed a taurine-free infant formula remained normal.[47] There is some evidence that taurine supplementation in infants weighing less than 1300 gm allows development of more mature auditory brainstem evoked responses than in nonsupplemented infants at 37 weeks' postmenstrual age.[153] Although it remains unclear whether supplemental taurine is necessary, almost all term and preterm formulas contain taurine at a level similar to that in breast milk.

LIPID REQUIREMENTS IN THE ENTERALLY FED INFANT

FACTORS AFFECTING FAT DIGESTION AND ABSORPTION

Fat provides the major source of energy for growing preterm infants. Cow's milk fat is predominantly saturated and is poorly absorbed by preterm infants. Commercial formulas therefore contain medium-chain triglycerides (MCTs) and predominantly unsaturated long-chain triglycerides (LCTs) from vegetable oils. These triglycerides must be broken down by lipases and emulsified by bile salts. At birth, the digestive function of premature infants is not fully developed; preterm infants have decreased gut absorption of lipids because of low levels of pancreatic lipase, bile acids, and lingual lipase.[62, 64] The fact that term and preterm infants absorb fat reasonably well is due to the development of alternative mechanisms for the digestion of dietary fat. One important mechanism is intragastric lipolysis, in which lingual and gastric lipases compensate for the low pancreatic lipase concentration.[60] By 25 weeks' gestation, lingual lipase is secreted by the serous glands of the tongue, and gastric lipase is secreted from gastric glands. The fatty acids and monoglycerides resulting from intragastric lipolysis compensate for low bile acid concentration by emulsifying lipid mixtures. Lingual lipase can also penetrate the core of the human milk lipid globule and hydrolyze the triglyceride core without disrupting the globule membrane. Human milk provides another heterogeneous group of lipases—lipoprotein lipase, bile salt stimulated esterase, and nonactivated lipase—which continue, in the intestine, the lipolysis begun in the stomach.

Lipid digestion and absorption are also affected by the dietary fat composition. Fatty acid absorption increases with decreasing chain length and with the degree of unsaturation, meaning that MCTs with chain lengths of 6 to 12 carbons are hydrolyzed more readily than LCTs and that fatty acids with more double bonds are absorbed more efficiently. To increase the fat absorption of premature infants, the fat in commercial formulas contains relatively high levels of MCTs that can be absorbed without the need for lipase or bile salts. MCT oil has been used for three decades in the production of formulas for infants with low birth weights who do not absorb long-chain fatty acids efficiently and thus lose energy as unabsorbed dietary fat. Standard commercial formulas for healthy term infants do not contain MCTs, and human milk typically contains 8% to 12% of fat as MCTs.[73] Unlike LCTs, MCTs are readily hydrolyzed in the gut, and the released fatty acids are transported across the gut barrier without the need for bile acids. MCTs are then transported directly to the liver via the portal vein as nonesterified fatty acids. In addition, MCTs can enter mitochondria and be oxidized without the need for carnitine-mediated transport through mitochondrial membranes. However, inclusion of MCTs in infant formula remains controversial, because the available data do not support the assertion of improved fat absorption or improved growth in preterm infants.[22, 163]

LIPID COMPONENTS IN HUMAN MILK AND THEIR COMPOSITION

Human Milk Globules

Fat is transported in globules consisting of a membrane composed of a polar mixture of proteins, phospholipids, triglycerides, cholesterol, glycoproteins, and enzymes surrounding a triglyceride core containing 98% of the fat in milk. The milk fat globules are among the largest structural components of milk, having a diameter of 4 μm in mature milk. The size of the globules increases with both length of lactation and length of gestation, with colostrum having smaller globules (especially in milk of women who deliver prematurely) than mature milk. As the total fat content of human milk increases postnatally, the percentage of cholesterol and phospholipids, both of which reside primarily in the milk fat globule membrane, decreases; in addition, the total phospholipid content decreases as lactation progresses. During the first weeks of lactation, preterm milk is also richer in membranous material compared with term or mature milk, resulting in a higher content of cholesterol, phospholipids, and very-long-chain polyunsaturated fatty acids (PUFAs) with chain lengths of 20 to 22 carbons (C20–C22). Because these membranes act as emulsifiers that allow fat dispersion in an aqueous phase and limit lipolysis and oxidation, heat treatment or addition of fortifiers and supplements might disrupt this emulsion.

Total Lipid Content in Human Milk

The milk fat content and nutritional value of human milk vary with time, and it does not always provide a complete source of nutrients for infants with very low birth weights. Its composition and energy content may vary in a pumping session and during subsequent changes throughout lactation.[91] The total fat content of human milk at 3 days' lactation is approximately 2 gm/dL; the fat content of mature milk is approximately 4 to 5 gm/dL, with large individual variations possible.[12] The triglyceride of human milk is its most variable component, changing with gestational and postnatal age, time of day, duration of individual feeds, and maternal diet. Shifts in the dietary practices of a population result in changes in the fatty acid composition of human milk, because the type and amount of fat in the maternal diet affect the composition of milk fat. Maternal diets low in fat and high in carbohydrate lead to de novo synthesis of fatty acids within the mammary gland, which results in high concentrations of fatty acids of less than 16 carbons. Therefore, although the total amount of fat present in the milk remains in the normal range, the fat is more saturated. The protein content of breast milk decreases from about 2 to 3 gm/dL in early lactation to 1 gm/dL in mature milk. Although a more consistent final composition can be obtained by pooling pumped milk, even pooled breast milk cannot provide sufficient sodium, calcium, phosphorus, iron, and vitamins B_2, B_6, C, D, E, and folic acid to meet the needs of infants with very low birth weights. Several studies have shown that such infants have higher rates of weight, length, and head circumference increases when fed fortified preterm human milk compared with those fed only mature human milk.[76, 112]

Fatty Acid Content and Requirements

Fatty acids represent about 85% of the triglycerides and therefore are the principal component of human milk lipids. Fatty acids in human milk are derived from the maternal diet, de novo synthesis by the mammary gland, and mobilization from fat stores. Hachey and colleagues[57] found that medium-chain fatty acids synthesized in the mammary gland accounted for 10% to 12% of milk total lipid, dietary fatty acids accounted for 29%, and adipose tissue and tissue synthesis for 59%. The fatty acid composition of human milk fat reflects the fatty acid composition of the maternal diet. The long-chain polyunsaturated fatty acid (LCP) composition of the milk of women in the United States, Europe, and Africa is quite similar, with the exception of higher amounts of n-3 LCP in the milk of women whose diets contain a large quantity of fish.[82] The dominant fatty acids of mature human milk in the United States are oleic acid (36%), palmitic acid (22%), linoleic acid (16%), stearic acid (8%), and C8–C14 fatty acids (12%).[69] Medium-chain fatty acids (C8–C10) do not normally account for more than 2% of the fats, even in milk from women who have delivered preterm. Arachidonic acid (C20:4n–6) is the main LCP, and eicosapentaenoic acid (C20:5n–3) is found in small quantities in human milk.[12] Docosahexaenoic acid (C22:6n–3) is the main LCP of the n-3 series.

Fatty acid composition changes with progressing lactation and with gestational age. Most striking is the higher content of C8–C14 fatty acids and of LCPs in preterm milk as compared with term milk; the content of LCP decreases with increasing postnatal age. This is an advantage for preterm infants, because shorter fatty acids are easier to digest, and LCPs are essential for brain and retinal development.

There is considerable controversy about the role of trans–fatty acids in atherogenesis and carcinogenesis. These isomers are derived either from the diet or from triglycerides stored in adipose tissue. The main source of exogenous trans-isomers of unsaturated fatty acids is partially hydrogenated vegetable oils. The amount of trans–fatty acids in milk of mothers consuming a western diet ranges between 2.1% and 4.7% of total fatty acids.[32] Trans-isomers have no known nutritional benefits and may be associated with deleterious effects, including impairment of cholesterol and linoleic and linolenic fatty acid metabolism.[16]

LCPs play an important role in the development of the infant's brain during the last trimester of pregnancy and also during the first months of life.[28, 154] The precursor C18 fatty acids for the n-6 and n-3 LCP series are linoleic acid (C18:2n–6) and α-linolenic acid (C18:3n–3). Both are recognized as essential dietary nutrients.[158] These are further elongated and desaturated to form other fatty acids, of which arachidonic acid (AA) and docosahexaenoic acid (DHA) are essential for normal growth and development. Although the capacity for endogenous synthesis of LCP from precursor fatty acids in preterm and term infants was thought to be limited, stable isotope studies demonstrated that both term and preterm infants have the capacity to synthesize DHA and AA.[23, 134] However, it remains unclear whether DHA and AA can be biosynthesized in quantities sufficient to meet the needs of these infants. In utero, LCPs are supplied to the fetus across the placenta. After birth, breast-fed infants receive sufficient preformed dietary LCP with human milk. In contrast, most current infant formulas have little or no LCP. These formulas are modeled after human milk only in the content of saturated fatty acids and of mono- and polyunsaturated fatty acids with a chain length up to 18 carbon atoms; the content of linoleic acid and α-linolenic acid in many commercial formulas is similar to that in human milk.[135] Several investigators have shown that preterm and term infants fed formulas containing linolenic acid but no DHA develop rapid LCP depletion of plasma and tissue lipids relative to cord blood concentrations at birth and in preterm infants fed human milk, despite the availability of the precursor essential fatty acids.[61, 81]

Because DHA is absent in infant formulas yet is necessary for retinal function and brain development,

several investigators studied the effect of diet on infant development. Studies by Carlson, Innis, and Uauy and their colleagues found that reduced visual acuity of formula-fed infants compared with infants receiving human milk was related to lower levels of DHA in the formula-fed groups[17, 70, 156]; however, Carlson and associates reported that improved visual acuity in breast-fed infants may be a short-term phenomenon.[20] Lucas and colleagues noted higher IQ scores at school age of preterm infants fed human milk[96, 97]; however, a relationship between neurodevelopment and higher brain concentrations of DHA in breast-fed as compared with formula-fed infants has not been proved.[99] Deposition of essential fatty acids is required not only in the brain but also for growth of other tissues. Carlson and colleagues showed that the strong relationship between growth and AA levels that exists prenatally continues postnatally.[18] Although visual acuity is higher in infants fed marine oil–supplemented rather than unsupplemented formula, AA status in preterm infants is positively correlated with growth and cognition into the first year of life.[19] This research area remains highly active; comprehensive reviews are available.[145, 155]

Cholesterol

Cholesterol is a major component of cell membranes and a precursor in the synthesis of bile acids and some hormones. It is present in human milk in concentrations ranging from 10 to 15 mg/dL, although commercial formulas contain only trace amounts of cholesterol (approximately 1 to 2 mg/dL).[115] The high cholesterol content of breast milk relative to formula is maintained at this level regardless of maternal diet. Thus, breast-fed infants receive a cholesterol intake 10 to 20 times greater than those fed formulas and, if expressed per unit of body weight, 4 to 5 times higher than the American Heart Association maximum recommended intake. The very low cholesterol content of commercial formulas may be inadequate for infants with very low birth weights, whose ability to produce cholesterol may not be fully developed. Little is known about the rate of cholesterol synthesis in preterm infants and whether cholesterol should be a component of infant formula. Breast-fed infants have higher plasma total cholesterol levels than do formula-fed infants, reflecting the higher cholesterol content of their diet. At present, it is unknown whether early cholesterol intake is important for the human infant's ability to regulate cholesterol synthesis in the face of later dietary cholesterol challenges. Some epidemiologic data have shown that death rates from ischemic heart disease, total cholesterol levels, and lipoprotein levels at 59 to 70 years of age were influenced by birth weight, type of feeding during infancy, weight at 1 year of age, and time of weaning.[44] Currently there are no recommendations regarding the cholesterol content of infant formulas.

Carnitine

Carnitine mediates the transport of long-chain fatty acids into mitochondria for oxidation and the removal of short-chain fatty acids that accumulate in mitochondria. Preterm infants are considered to be at risk for carnitine deficiency,[109, 164] because they are heavily dependent on lipids as an energy source and because the plasma carnitine concentration of preterm infants is low, owing to limited endogenous synthetic ability.[138] Low concentrations of carnitine leading to limited fatty acid oxidation in the fetus may promote accretion of large amounts of fat during the later part of gestation.[63] In preterm infants not receiving supplemental carnitine, plasma and tissue carnitine levels fall even in the presence of adequate precursor amino acid concentrations.[119] Carnitine is found in high concentrations in human milk and has been added to many formulas, although soy-based formulas contain no carnitine.[109]

Lipid Content and Composition of Infant Formula

Recommendations for fat content and composition of term infant formulas have recently been outlined in the comprehensive Life Sciences Research Office report; a minimum fat content of 4.4 gm/100 kcal (40% of total energy) and a maximum of 6.4 gm/100 kcal (57% of total energy) were recommended.[90] This report also recommended a minimum of 350 mg/100 kcal of linoleic acid (about 3% of calories) and a minimum of 77 mg/100 kcal of α-linolenic acid (about 0.7% of calories). The report did not recommend the addition of AA or DHA to term infant formulas. However, some formula manufacturers in Europe and Japan have added DHA or DHA plus AA.

Infants with very low birth weights are susceptible to essential fatty acid deficiency because they were deprived of fat accretion during late pregnancy and must obtain their nutritional requirements from their diet. Human milk provides preterm infants with fatty acids comparable to those obtained during intrauterine nutrition.[27, 68, 157] The American Academy of Pediatrics recommends a minimum of 4.5 gm/100 kcal (40% of calories) and a maximum of 6 gm/100 kcal (54% of calories) for the fat content of premature infant formulas. Recommendations from the Canadian Pediatric Society and ESPGAN are similar, with slightly lower minimums and higher maximums.[40] The recommended content of linoleic acid is 5% of total calories, and for α-linolenic acid it is 1% of calories. Although neither the American Academy of Pediatrics nor the Canadian Pediatric Society currently recommends the addition of DHA and AA to preterm formulas, ESPGAN recommends that 1% of total calories come from C20 and C22 n-6 fatty acids (which includes AA) and that 0.5% of total calories come from C20 and C22 n-3 fatty acids (which includes DHA) in formulas for infants with low birth weights.

ORAL VITAMIN REQUIREMENTS AND SUPPLEMENTS

Vitamins are organic compounds that are essential for metabolic reactions but are not synthesized by the body. They are therefore needed in trace amounts from enteral or parenteral sources. Higher amounts of select vitamins are required by preterm infants, who may have greater needs for growth or because of immature metabolic or excretory function. A comprehensive review of vitamin metabolism and requirements in extremely premature infants is available.[55]

The recommended oral intakes of vitamins for infants are compared in Table 33–3. For some vitamins, the 1993 recommendations for infants with very low birth weights—a consensus of international experts and researchers—differ considerably from those of the American Academy of Pediatrics' Committee on Nutrition in 1998,[1] ESPGAN's Committee on Nutrition in 1987,[41] and the recommended dietary allowances (RDAs) for term newborn infants.[150]

Vitamins are classified as water soluble or fat soluble, based on the biochemical structure and function of the compound. Water-soluble vitamins include the B complex vitamins and vitamin C. They serve as prosthetic groups for enzymes involved in amino acid metabolism, energy production, and nucleic acid synthesis. Needs are considered relative to dietary intake of calories and protein, as well as the rate of energy use. Water-soluble vitamins cannot be formed by precursors (with the exception of niacin from tryptophan) and do not accumulate in the body (with the exception of vitamin B_{12}). Therefore, daily intake is required to prevent deficiency. Excretion occurs in the urine and bile. Most water-soluble vitamins cross the placenta by active transport; vitamin C crosses by facilitated diffusion. Levels of water-soluble vitamins generally are higher in fetal than in maternal blood and are relatively independent of concentrations in the circulation of a nourished mother.[8] Preterm infants and infants of undernourished mothers have lower blood levels of water-soluble vitamins at birth.

Altered urinary losses due to renal immaturity during the first week of life predispose a preterm infant to vitamin deficiency or excess. The need for vitamin C may be greater in a preterm infant who experiences increased urinary losses and lacks p-hydroxyphenylpyruvic acid oxidase, an enzyme that catabolizes tyrosine and is stimulated by vitamin C. Transient neonatal tyrosinemia, however, has not been shown to be detrimental to infants. A limited riboflavin intake (less than 300 μg/100 kcal) may be necessary in the first 3 weeks of life in an infant whose birth weight was below 750 gm and who demonstrates decreased urinary excretion and increased serum levels of riboflavin.[7, 52] The 1993 recommendation for vitamin B_6 (125 to 175 μg/100 kcal) is greater than that of the American Academy of Pediatrics (35 μg/100 kcal), reflective of the increased protein needs of infants with very low birth weights, and lower than the upper limit of ESPGAN (250 μg/100 kcal), reflective of elevated plasma concentrations (approximately six times that of cord blood) in infants receiving this amount.[52]

Fat-soluble vitamins include vitamins A, D, E, and K. These vitamins function physiologically on the

TABLE 33–3 RECOMMENDED ORAL INTAKE OF VITAMINS FOR INFANTS

VITAMIN (AMOUNT PER 100 KCAL)	AAPCON RECOMMENDATIONS FOR PREMATURE INFANTS (1998)	CONSENSUS RECOMMENDATIONS FOR INFANTS WITH VLBW (1993)	ESPGAN-CON RECOMMENDATIONS FOR INFANTS WITH VLBW (1987)	RDA FOR INFANTS FROM BIRTH TO 6 MOS (1989)
Fat Soluble				
Vitamin A (IU)	75–225	583–1250	270–450	1400
With lung disease	—	1250–2333	—	—
Vitamin D (IU)	270	125–333	800–1600 IU/day	300
Vitamin E (IU)	>1.1	5–10	0.6–10	3
Vitamin K (μg)	4	6.66–8.33	4–15	5
Water Soluble				
Vitamin B_6 (μg)	>35*	125–175	35–250	300
Vitamin B_{12} (μg)	>0.15	0.25	>0.15	0.3
Vitamin C (mg)	35	15–20	7–40	30
Biotin (μg)	>1.5	3–5	>1.5	10
Folic acid (μg)	33	21–42	>60	25
Niacin (mg)	>0.25	3–4	0.8–5	5
Pantothenate (mg)	0.3	1–1.5	>0.3	2
Riboflavin (μg)	>60	200–300	60–600	400
Thiamin (μg)	>40	150–200	20–250	300

*Assuming a vitamin B_6–protein ratio of 15 μg/gm.
AAPCON, American Academy of Pediatrics, Committee on Nutrition; ESPGAN-CON, European Society of Paediatric Gastroenterology and Nutrition, Committee on Nutrition of the Preterm Infant; RDA, recommended dietary allowance; VLBW, very low birth weight.
From American Academy of Pediatrics, Committee on Nutrition: Pediatric Nutrition Handbook. Elk Grove Village, Ill, American Academy of Pediatrics, 1998; Tsang RC, et al (eds): Nutritional Needs of the Preterm Infant: Scientific Basis and Practical Guidelines. Baltimore, Williams & Wilkins, 1993; ESPGAN Committee on Nutrition of the Preterm Infant: Guidelines on infant nutrition. Acta Paediatr Scand Suppl 262:1, 1987; Subcommittee on the Tenth Edition of the RDAs, Food and Nutrition Board, Commission of Life Sciences, National Research Council: Recommended Dietary Allowances, 10th ed. Washington, DC, National Academy Press, 1989.

conformation and function of complex molecules and membranes and are important for the development and function of highly specialized tissues. They can be built from precursors, are excreted with difficulty, and accumulate in the body, and therefore they can produce toxicity. They are not required daily, and deficiency states develop slowly. Fat-soluble vitamins require carrier systems, usually lipoproteins, for solubility in blood, and intestinal absorption depends on fat absorption. They cross the placenta by simple or facilitated diffusion. Accumulation takes place throughout pregnancy and depends on maternal blood levels. Therefore, blood concentrations and body stores at birth are lower than normal in preterm infants and in infants of poorly nourished mothers.[8]

The 1993 recommendation for vitamin A for preterm infants is higher than that of the American Academy of Pediatrics and ESPGAN and includes increased intakes for infants with lung disease.[142] These higher intakes are considered safe and may promote regenerative healing from lung injury, possibly reducing the incidence and severity of bronchopulmonary dysplasia.

The recommendations for vitamin D for preterm infants differ significantly throughout the world, with an upper limit as high as 1600 IU/day.[43] Multiple studies have not demonstrated any advantage of high vitamin D intakes, and 400 IU/day appears to be adequate for preterm infants, particularly those who have generous mineral intakes.[29, 83]

Vitamin E in formula, required as 0.6 mg/gm of PUFAs, provides adequate amounts to prevent hemolysis of red blood cell membranes when iron intake is not excessive.[1, 110] The recommended total intake is 3 to 4 IU/day for term infants. Recommendations are somewhat higher for preterm infants; however, pharmacologic supplementation of 100 mg/kg per day of vitamin E is not recommended to reduce the incidence or severity of retinopathy of prematurity, bronchopulmonary dysplasia, and intraventricular hemorrhage.[1, 45] High plasma levels of vitamin E caused by pharmacologic intakes may increase the risk of sepsis and necrotizing enterocolitis; therefore, supplementation in infants with very low birth weights should not exceed 25 IU/kg per day.[56, 113]

An adequate intake of vitamin K to prevent bleeding in the first week of life when enteral intakes are low is recommended as a 1-mg IM injection at birth in both term and preterm neonates over 1000 gm birth weight.[1] For premature infants less than 1000 gm, 0.3 mg is recommended.[1, 54] Term infants can be given 2 mg orally as an alternative. Thereafter, 2 to 3 μg/kg per day or 5 to 10 μg daily is recommended in all babies.

ELECTROLYTES, MINERALS, AND TRACE ELEMENTS

SODIUM, POTASSIUM, AND CHLORIDE

From calculations based on measurements of renal function and from reported data, a sodium intake between 3 and 5 mmol/kg per day (equivalent to between 3 and 5 mEq/kg per day) is usually sufficient to allow growth in orally fed infants weighing less than 1500 gm and of less than 34 weeks' gestation during the first 4 to 6 weeks of life. Sodium concentrations should generally be maintained in the 135 to 140 mEq/L range. The sodium content of human milk is low, and the plasma sodium concentration must be monitored. Supplementation of 2 to 4 mmol/kg per day as sodium chloride may be necessary. For infants who weigh less than 1000 gm, sodium and other electrolytes should be measured frequently to determine their needs accurately during the first 2 weeks of life; sodium supplements of 4 to 8 mmol/kg per day may be required. Premature formulas and fortified human milk provide only 2 to 3 mmol/kg per day at full enteral intake. Between 34 and 40 weeks, the requirements fall to about 1.5 to 2.5 mmol/kg per day. Recommendations for sodium, potassium, and chloride are listed in Table 33–4.

CALCIUM, PHOSPHORUS, AND MAGNESIUM

The peak of fetal accretion of minerals occurs primarily after 34 weeks' gestation, and preterm infants fed low mineral intakes develop poorly mineralized bones. The advisable intakes range from 70 to 200 mg calcium/100 kcal, 50 to 117 mg phosphorus/100 kcal, and 6 to 12 mg magnesium/100 kcal (see Table 33–4). These recommended intakes are 3 to 4.5 times higher for calcium, 5 to 6 times higher for phosphorus, and 1.5 to 3 times higher for magnesium compared with the composition of human milk. Mineral concentra-

tions have been increased in preterm formulas and human milk supplements designed for feeding premature infants in an attempt to meet requirements. Significant increases in calcium and phosphorus content may affect magnesium retention.[48] Several studies have shown improvement of mineral retention or bone mineralization in preterm infants who receive higher calcium and phosphorus intakes compared with their unsupplemented peers.

Consumption of unfortified human milk by infants with very low birth weights after hospital discharge resulted in bone mineral deficits that persisted through 52 weeks postnatally, indicating the need for additional minerals after discharge. Supplemental bioavailable calcium and phosphorus salts may be required by breast-fed, preterm infants until their weight reaches term (3 to 3.5 kg).[58, 83, 126]

IRON

Preterm infants are at increased risk for the development of iron deficiency anemia because they deplete their stores from birth in half the time of a term infant (at about 2 months of age).[117] Infants with very low birth weights or sick infants who are medically managed with frequent blood sampling lose much of the iron present in the circulating hemoglobin, which is then unavailable for erythropoiesis. The American Academy of Pediatrics, the Canadian Paediatric Society, and ESPGAN agree on a recommendation of 2 to 3 mg/kg per day of dietary elemental iron, begun no later than 2 months of age in preterm infants and continued throughout the first year of life.[1, 42, 116] Iron

TABLE 33–4   RECOMMENDED ORAL INTAKE OF MINERAL AND TRACE ELEMENTS FOR PRETERM INFANTS

MINERAL/ELEMENT (AMOUNT PER 100 KCAL)	AAPCON RECOMMENDATIONS (1998)	CONSENSUS RECOMMENDATIONS FOR INFANTS WITH VLBW (1993)	ESPGAN-CON RECOMMENDATIONS (1987)	CPS RECOMMENDATIONS (1989)
Mineral				
Calcium (mg)	175	100–192	70–140	130–200
Chloride (mEq)	—	1.7–2.5	1.6–2.5	2.1–3.3
Magnesium (mg)	—	6.6–12.5	6–12	4–8
Phosphorus (mg)	91.5	50–117	50–90	65–99
Potassium (mEq)	1.6–2.4	1.7–2.6	2.3–3.9	2.1–2.9
Sodium (mEq)	2.1–2.9	1.7–2.5	1–2.3	2.1–2.9
Iron (mg)	1.7–2.5	1.7	1.5	
Trace Elements				
Chromium (μg)	—	0.083–0.42	—	0.043–0.082
Copper (μg)	90	100–125	90	58–100
Fluoride (μg/day)	—	—	—	—
Iodine (μg)	5	25–50	10–45	—
Manganese (μg)	>5	6.3	1.5–7.5	5
Molybdenum (μg)	—	0.25	—	—
Selenium (μg)	—	1.08–2.5	—	—
Zinc (μg)	>500	833	550–1100	420–670

AAPCON, American Academy of Pediatrics, Committee on Nutrition; CPS, Canadian Paediatric Society; ESPGAN-CON, European Society of Paediatric Gastroenterology and Nutrition, Committee on Nutrition of the Preterm Infant; VLBW, very low birth weight.

From American Academy of Pediatrics, Committee on Nutrition: Pediatric Nutrition Handbook. Elk Grove Village, Ill, American Academy of Pediatrics, 1988; Tsang RC, et al (eds): Nutritional Needs of the Preterm Infant: Scientific Basis and Practical Guidelines. Baltimore, Williams & Wilkins, 1993; Canadian Paediatric Society, Nutrition Committee: Nutrient needs and feeding of premature infants. Can Med Assoc J 152:1765, 1995.

intakes of 2 mg/kg per day begun at 2 weeks of age were shown to safely augment ferritin stores in infants with low birth weights without risk of vitamin E deficiency hemolytic anemia.[98] This is achieved with standard iron-containing preterm formulas at full enteral intake. Premature infants receiving human milk require iron supplementation with ferrous sulfate. Higher intakes of 3 and 4 mg/kg per day begun by 1 month of age and continued through age 12 months are suggested for infants who weigh less than 1500 and 1000 gm at birth, respectively.[38]

OTHER TRACE ELEMENTS

Trace elements contribute less than 0.01% of total body weight. They function as constituents of metalloenzymes, cofactors for metal ion activated enzymes, or components of vitamins, hormones, and proteins. The fetus accumulates stores of trace elements primarily during the last trimester of pregnancy. Therefore, the premature infant has low stores at birth and is at risk for trace mineral deficiencies if intakes are not adequate to support requirements for growth. Immature homeostatic control of trace element metabolism also increases the risk of deficiency. Trace minerals that have established physiologic importance in humans include zinc, copper, selenium, manganese, chromium, molybdenum, fluoride, and iodine. The recommended oral intakes for infants are listed in Table 33–4.[1, 59] The trace minerals that are potentially toxic in pediatric patients are lead and aluminum.[129]

HUMAN MILK AND FORMULA

HUMAN MILK

Human milk is the optimal food for term infants because it provides immunologic and antibacterial factors, hormones, enzymes, and opioid peptides not present in alternative infant food sources.[5, 120] The benefits of human milk for gastrointestinal function, host defense, and possibly neurodevelopmental outcome have been well documented.[1]

There is general consensus that human milk is also the optimal primary nutritional source for premature infants. The strongest evidence of the benefit of human milk for premature infants is the reduced incidence of necrotizing enterocolitis.[136] Other benefits include improved gastric emptying, reduced infections, and possibly better neurocognitive development.[5]

The milk from mothers of preterm infants contains more protein and electrolytes than does milk from mothers of term infants. However, these concentrations decline and approach the composition of term human milk in several weeks. Human milk does not completely meet the nutritional needs of premature infants; insufficient protein, calcium, phosphorus, sodium, zinc, vitamins, and possibly energy are provided by human milk to optimally support most premature infants. Human milk fortifiers have been developed and tested and address many of these inadequacies (Table 33–5). Premature infants fed fortified human milk may have growth rates slightly lower than those of infants fed formula, but they may also achieve earlier discharge.[136] Human milk fortifiers should be used in premature infants with birth weights less than 1500 gm and should be considered in those with birth weights less than 2000 gm.

PRETERM FORMULAS

Formulas for premature infants have been developed to meet the nutritional needs of growing preterm infants and have been in use for over 20 years. It must be noted that the design and testing of these formulas did not specifically include extremely premature (less than 1000 gm) infants. Premature formulas contain a reduced amount of lactose (40% to 50%) because intestinal lactase activity may be low in premature infants. The remainder of the carbohydrate content is in the form of glucose polymers, which maintain low osmolality of the formula (300 mOsm or less with a caloric density of 80 kcal/dL). The fat blends of preterm formulas are 20% to 50% MCTs, which is designed to compensate for low intestinal lipase and bile salts. The protein content of preterm formulas is higher than that of term formulas (2.7 to 3 gm/100 kcal), which promotes a rate of weight gain and body composition similar to the reference fetus. Premature formulas are whey predominant, which reduces the risk of lactobezoar formation and may provide a more optimal amino acid intake. Calcium and phosphorus content is also higher in preterm formulas, which results in improved mineral retention and bone mineral content. The vitamin levels of premature formulas vary, and some may require vitamin supplementation. The composition of a number of preterm formulas is shown in Table 33–6.

SPECIALIZED FORMULAS

Occasionally, infants do not tolerate feedings and require formulas specifically designed for conditions of malabsorption or other types of formula intolerance. These formulas are free of lactose and cow's milk protein and provide alternative sources of protein (soy, casein hydrolysates, free amino acids) and carbohydrate (sucrose, corn syrup solids, tapioca starch, cornstarch). Some provide a significant percentage of the fat as MCTs. Specialized formulas are somewhat higher in protein and mineral content but similar in vitamin composition compared with formulas designed for term babies. The vitamin and mineral contents are therefore lower compared with formulas and human milk supplements designed for preterm infants. Multivitamin and mineral supplementation of specialized formulas is generally necessary to provide the recommended intakes for premature infants. Specialized formulas have not been tested in premature infants and therefore are used only temporarily, when necessary. Routine feedings for preterm infants are reinstituted as tolerated.

TABLE 33–5 NUTRIENT COMPOSITION OF HUMAN MILK AND HUMAN MILK SUPPLEMENTS (PER 100 KCAL)

		HUMAN MILK (HM)			ENFAMIL HUMAN MILK FORTIFIER POWDER 1 pkt: 25 mL MATURE PTHM (MEAD JOHNSON)	SIMILAC HUMAN MILK FORTIFIER POWDER 1 pkt: 25 mL MATURE PTHM (ROSS LABORATORIES)	SIMILAC NATURAL CARE (SNC) FORTIFIER LIQUID 1/2 SNC + 1/2 MATURE PTHM (ROSS LABORATORIES)
		Term: Mature*	Preterm: 0–2 wks†	Preterm: Mature‡			
Volume	(mL)	147–161	149–150	149–150	124	124	136
Protein							
Content		1.5	2.4–3.1	2.1	3.12	2.97	2.44
% energy		6	9.6–12	8.4	12.0	11.9	9.8
Whey-casein ratio		80:20	80:20	80:20	73:27	72:28	70:30
Lipid							
Content		5.2	4.9–6.3	5.8	5.6	5.24	5.6
% energy		46.5	42–55	52	50	47.1	50
Source medium-chain triglycerides	(%)	—	—	—	3.1	2.4	25
Coconut	(%)	—	—	—	—	—	10
Soybean	(%)	—	—	—	—	—	15
Oleic	(%)	—	—	—	—	—	—
Oleo	(%)	—	—	—	—	—	—
Composition							
Saturated	(%)	43	41–47		38–43	43–49	54–57
Monosaturated	(%)	42	39–40		39–40	38–39	26–27
Polyunsaturated	(%)	15	13–15		13–15	11–13	17–18
Carbohydrate							
Content		11.9	8–9.8	9.9	9.52	10.41	10.29
% energy		47.7	31–38	40	38.0	41.0	41.2
Lactose	(%)	100	100	100	86	82	75
Glucose polymers	(%)				14	18	25
Minerals and Trace Elements							
Calcium	(mg)	45	31–40	37	145	180	132
	(mmol)	1.1	0.73–0.95	0.9	3.6	4.3	3.2
Chloride	(mg)	63	76–127	82	79	114	81
	(mmol)	1.8	2.1–3.6	2.3	2.3	3.3	2.3
Copper	(µg)	58	107–111	96	134	289	181
Iodine	(µg)	Variable					
Iron	(mg)	0.06	0.13–0.14	0.18	1.93	0.58	0.28
Magnesium	(mg)	4.8	4.3–4.7	4.6	5.04	12.45	8.67
	(mmol)	0.2	0.17–0.2	0.19	0.21	0.52	0.36
Manganese	(µg)	0.65	—	1.0	13.22	11.94	7.05
Phosphorus	(mg)	22.6	20–23	19	72	98	72
	(mmol)	0.73	0.6–0.7	0.61	2.4	3.2	2.3
Potassium	(mg)	72.5	81–93	85	95	70	109.5
	(mmol)	1.86	2.1–2.4	2.2	2.4	1.79	2.8
Sodium	(mg)	22.5	44–77	37	44	50	41
	(mmol)	0.98	1.9–3.3	1.6	1.93	2.17	1.79
Zinc	(mg)	0.38	0.61–0.69	0.51	1.3	1.7	1.1
Vitamins							
Fat soluble							
Vitamin A	(IU)	319	413–497	581	1670	1246	949
Vitamin D	(IU)	3	0.6–1.9	3.0	191	151	84
Vitamin E	(IU)	0.4	0.7–12	1.6	7	5	3
Vitamin K	(µg)	0.3	0.29–3	0.3	5.7	10.5	6.7
Water soluble							
Vitamin B_6	(µg)	133	9–129	22	157	279	147
Vitamin B_{12}	(µg)	0.04	0.01–0.07	0.07	0.31	0.85	0.33
Vitamin C	(mg)	6	6.3–7.4	16	28	44	28
Biotin	(µg)	0.9	0.01–1.2	0.9	4.1	33	21
Folic acid	(µg)	12	5–8.6	5	35	32	23
Niacin	(mg)	0.21	0.2–0.25	0.22	3.9	4.59	2.85
Pantothenic acid	(mg)	0.26	0.33	0.27	1.12	2.07	1.17
Riboflavin	(µg)	50	14–79	72	332	574	373
Thiamin	(µg)	30	1.4–31	31	212	313	151
Other							
Carnitine	(mg)	1.04	n/a	n/a	4.33	0.9§	0.5§
Choline	(mg)	13.4	10–13	10–13	8.4–10.9	8.4–10.9	10–11.5
Inositol	(mg)	22.2–83.5	22	22	17.9	17.9	13.4
Taurine	(mg)	6	8.6	8.6	7.2	7.2	7.7
Osmolality (mOsmol/kg H_2O)		286	290	290	350	385	280

*Fomon SJ: Nutrition of Normal Infants. St. Louis, Mosby–Year Book, 1993, p 410; Lawrence RA: Breastfeeding: A Guide for the Medical Profession, 5th ed. St. Louis, Mosby–Year Book, 2000, p 738; Ogasa K, et al: The content of free and bound inositol in human and cow's milk. J Nutr Sci Vitaminol 21:129, 1975.

†From Anderson DM, et al: Length of gestation and nutritional composition of human milk. Am J Clin Nutr 37:810, 1983; Gross DJ, et al: Nutritional composition of milk produced by mothers delivering preterm. J Pediatr 96:641, 1980; Lemons JA, et al: Differences in the composition of preterm and term human milk during early lactation. Pediatr Res 16:113, 1982.

‡From Meeting the Special Nutrient Needs of Low-Birth-Weight and Premature Infants in the Hospital (AB100). Columbus, Ohio, Ross Products Division, Abbott Laboratories, January 1998, p 56.

§Value for term human milk used.

n/a, not available; PTHM, preterm human milk.

TABLE 33–6 NUTRIENT COMPOSITION OF PREMATURE FORMULAS* (PER 100 KCAL)

		SIMILAC SPEC CARE 20 (ROSS)	SIMILAC SPEC CARE 24 (ROSS)	SIMILAC‡ NEOSURE (ROSS)	ENFAMIL (ENFALAC) PREM FORM 20 (MEAD JOHNSON)	ENFAMIL (ENFALAC) PREM FORM 24 (MEAD JOHNSON)	ENFALAC SPECIAL 24 (MEAD JOHNSON)	ENFAMIL† ENFACARE (MEAD JOHNSON)
Volume	(mL)	148	124	134	148	124	124	136
Protein								
Content	(gm)	2.71	2.71	2.6	3.0	3.0	2.5	2.8
% energy		11	11	10	12	12	10	11
Whey-casein ratio		60:40	60:40	50:50	60:40	60:40	60:40	60:40
Lipid								
Content	(gm)	5.43	5.43	5.5	5.1	5.1	5.05	5.3
% energy		47	47	49	45	45	45	47
Source								
Medium-chain triglycerides	(%)	50	50	25	40	40	40	20
Coconut	(%)	20	20	30‡	20	20	20	15
Soybean	(%)	30	30	45‡	40	40	40	30
Oleic	(%)	0	0	0	0	0	0	35
Oleo	(%)	0	0	0	0	0	0	0
Composition								
Saturated	(%)	66	66	50‡	61	61	42	
Monosaturated	(%)	13	13	28‡	15	15	37	
Polyunsaturated	(%)	21	21	22‡	24	24	21	
Carbohydrate								
Content	(gm)	10.6	10.6	10.3	11.1	11.1	11.2	10.7
% energy		42	42	41	44	44	45	42
Lactose	(%)	50	50	50	40	40	36	40
Glucose polymers	(%)	50	50	50	60	60	64	60
Minerals and Trace Elements								
Calcium	(mg)	180	180	105	165/163/120	165/163/120	135	120
	(mmol)	4.5	4.5	2.6	4.1/4.1/3.0	4.1/4.1/3.0	3.4	3.0
Chloride	(mg)	81	81	88	85/36/85	85/36/85	71	78
	(mmol)	2.3	2.3	2.5	2.4/2.5/2.4	2.4/2.5/2.4	2.0	2.2
Copper	(µg)	0.25	0.25	0.12	0.125/0.120/0.120	0.125/0.120/0.120	0.1	120
Iodine	(µg)	6	6	15	25/7.4/15	25/7.4/15	6.2	15
Iron	(mg)	0.37§ (1.8)	0.37§ (1.8)	1.8	0.25§(1.8)/0.25§/0.2§	0.25§(1.8)/0.25§/0.2§	0.25§(1.8)/0.25§/0.2§	1.8

Phosphorus	(mg)	100	100	83/81/66	83/81/66	66	68	66
	(mmol)	3.2	3.2	2.7/2.6/2.1	2.7/2.6/2.1	2.1	2.2	2.1
Potassium	(mg)	129	129	103/100/129	103/100/129	142	83	105
	(mmol)	3.3	3.3	2.6/2.6/3.3	2.6/2.6/3.3	3.6	2.1	2.7
Magnesium	(mg)	12	12	6.8/7.4/12	6.8/7.4/12	9	6.2	8
	(mmol)	0.5	0.5	0.28/0.31/0.5	0.28/0.31/0.5	0.37	0.26	0.33
Manganese	(µg)	12	12	6.3/12.3/37	6.3/12.3/37	10	10.2	15
Selenium	(µg)	1.8	1.8	1.8/—/—	1.8/—/—	2.3	—	2.3
Sodium	(mg)	43	43	39/40/48	39/40/48	33	34	35
	(mmol)	1.9	1.9	1.7/1.7/2.1	1.7/1.7/2.1	1.4	1.5	1.52
Zinc	(mg)	1.5	1.5	1.5/1/1	1.5/1/1	1.2	0.83	1.25
Vitamins								
Fat soluble								
Vitamin A	(IU)	1250	1250	1250/430/390	1250/430/390	460	370	450
Vitamin D	(IU)	150	150	270/68/62.5	270/68/62.5	70	57	80
Vitamin E	(IU)	4	4	6.3/4.6/2.5	6.3/4.6/2.5	3.6	3.8	4
Vitamin K	(µg)	12	12	8/13/9	8/13/9	11	11	8
Water soluble								
Vitamin B$_6$	(µg)	250	250	150/250/75	150/250/75	100	210	100
Vitamin B$_{12}$	(µg)	0.55	0.55	0.25/0.56/0.5	0.25/0.56/0.5	0.4	0.47	0.3
Vitamin C	(mg)	37	37	20/37/19	20/37/19	15	31	16
Biotin	(µg)	37	37	4/3.7/3	4/3.7/3	9	3.1	6
Folic acid	(µg)	37	37	35/37/36	35/37/36	25	31	26
Niacin	(mg)	5	5	4/4.9/1.2	4/4.9/1.2	1.9	4.1	2.0
Pantothenic acid	(mg)	1.9	1.95	1.2/1.85/0.46	1.2/1.85/0.46	0.8	1.54	0.85
Riboflavin	(µg)	620	620	300/620/160	300/620/160	150	520	200
Thiamin	(µg)	250	250	200/250/79	200/250/79	220	210	200
Other								
Carnitine	(mg)	5.9	5.9	2/2/—	2/2/—	5.9	1.7	2
Choline	(mg)	10	10	12/15.7/12	12/15.7/12	16	13.1	15
Inositol	(mg)	6	6	17/28.2/6	17/25/6	6	25	30
Taurine	(mg)	6.7	6.7	6/5.9/5	6/5.9/5	6.7	4.9	6
Osmolality (mOsmol/kg H$_2$O)		235	280	260/240	310/284	250¶	273	240§

*Trade names and compositions might be different for different countries. Where three numbers are given, the left number is the U.S. value, the center number is the Canadian value, and the right number is the international value.

†Designed to support the growth of premature infants at and after discharge.

‡Ready to feed; NeoSure powder contains 20% coconut oil, 28% soy oil, and 27% safflower oil; 59% saturated, 13% monosaturated, and 28% polyunsaturated fats.

¶Osmolality at 22 kcal/oz.

§Low-iron infant formula.

PRETERM DISCHARGE FORMULAS

It was common practice in the past to feed premature infants premature formula until discharge and then switch to term formula. However, most premature infants are discharged at far below term weight and may have ongoing and catch-up requirements that may not be met by term formulas. A number of studies support this contention, demonstrating improved weight gain, linear growth, and bone mineral content in premature infants fed enriched formulas after discharge.[13, 30, 93] Only one of these studies used an actual preterm discharge formula, which had a nutrient density between preterm and standard term formulas.[93] Although the data regarding the use of preterm discharge formulas are limited, there does seem to be an overall benefit, and the use of such formulas should be strongly considered. Premature infants with chronic lung disease may also benefit from enriched nutrient intakes, especially additional protein, calcium, phosphorus, and zinc.[13]

SUPPLEMENTATION OF INFANT FEEDINGS

Term Infants

Supplementation for healthy, term, breast-fed infants is usually not necessary. However, infants who receive inadequate exposure to sunlight are at risk for vitamin D deficiency, and an intake of 200 to 400 IU/day has been recommended.[1, 148]

Breast-fed infants usually require an additional iron source after 4 to 6 months of age.[1] Standard infant formulas that are iron fortified (1.8 mg iron/100 kcal) provide adequate iron for term infants. Current recommendations are for fluoride supplementation only after 6 months of age.[1]

No vitamin supplements are necessary for term, formula-fed infants who consume at least 750 mL of infant formula daily. Term infants with chronic diseases that result in intake of formula or human milk less than 750 mL/day may require additional supplementation of vitamins and minerals to meet the RDAs.[39]

Infants who experience abnormal gastrointestinal losses (persistent diarrhea or excessive ileostomy drainage) often require supplementation with zinc and electrolytes.[129]

Preterm Infants

Daily multivitamin or mineral preparations may be necessary for preterm infants once enteral feedings have been established. Preterm formulas and human milk fortifiers differ in the amounts of vitamins and minerals they contain (see Tables 33–5 and 33–6); therefore, the need for supplementation varies for infants with very low birth weights.

Preterm infants who require specialized formulas or receive standard infant formulas designed to meet the vitamin and mineral needs of term infants able to consume 750 mL/day require supplementation with vitamins and minerals to provide the recommended intakes. Multivitamin supplements that contain the equivalent of the RDAs for term infants can be given (see Table 33–3). Liquid multivitamin drops do not contain folic acid because of its lack of stability, but it can be added or given separately. Calcium, phosphorus, zinc, and iron supplementation also may be needed.[38, 83, 129]

Breast-fed infants who weigh less than 3.5 kg do not consume enough human milk to acquire the recommended intakes of some vitamins and minerals. Therefore, supplementation with a multivitamin, folic acid, calcium, phosphorus, zinc, and iron may be necessary.

MINIMAL ENTERAL FEEDING

The diversity of approaches to feeding preterm infants underlines the need for studies to dispel myths and find reasonable solutions to the problem of what feeding route to use, which has plagued pediatricians and neonatologists for years. Once suitable TPN solutions for neonates were available, many physicians chose to use strictly parenteral nutrition in sick preterm infants because of concerns about necrotizing enterocolitis. TPN was thought to be a logical continuation of the transplacental nutrition the infants would have received in utero. However, this view discounts any role that swallowed amniotic fluid may play in nutrition and in the development of the gastrointestinal tract. In fact, by the end of the third trimester, amniotic fluid provides the fetus with the same enteral volume intake and approximately 25% of the enteral protein intake of a term breast-fed infant.[92]

Over the past 10 years, investigators have been looking at the utility of minimal enteral feedings. Minimal enteral feedings involve hypocaloric, low-volume enteral nutrition that does not contain sufficient calories to sustain somatic growth. Proposed benefits include maturation of the preterm intestine (both structurally and functionally), reduced liver dysfunction, and improved feeding tolerance. There is direct and indirect evidence of a benefit from minimal enteral feedings without an increase in the incidence of necrotizing enterocolitis.

Animal studies have been done to evaluate some of the anatomic, histologic, and enzymatic differences between enteral and parenteral feeding. Levine and coworkers compared rats receiving IV TPN with those receiving the same solution enterally. After 1 week, they found a decrease in gut weight (22%), mucosal weight (28%), mucosal protein (35%), DNA (25%), disaccharide activity, and mucosal height in the fasted rats.[89] Other investigators confirmed these findings.[24, 37, 132] Thus it appears that enteral feedings may be necessary to maintain the integrity and enhance the maturation of the gastrointestinal tract.

Studies of preterm infants have evaluated gut hormone levels and the maturation of gastrointestinal motility in response to minimal enteral nutrition. Lucas and colleagues evaluated enteroglucagon, gastrin, gastric inhibitory peptide, motilin, and neurotensin in premature infants; these hormones are thought to be important in producing changes in function or growth of the gastrointestinal tract. In response to small volumes of enteral feedings in these premature infants, significant elevations of all these hormones were demonstrated.[50, 94, 95] Berseth and associates used low-compliance perfusion manometry to evaluate the maturation of motility and found that infants who received nutrient feedings (as opposed to sterile water) displayed significant changes in intestinal motor activity in response to feeding. Furthermore, these infants achieved full enteral feedings and full nipple feedings earlier than did their counterparts who were fed sterile water.[10, 11] Shulman and coworkers demonstrated that premature infants who received early feeding had decreased intestinal permeability and increased lactase activity at 10 days of age compared with late-fed controls.[143, 144]

Supported by these animal and physiologic studies, 10 clinical trials evaluating minimal enteral feeding have been performed.* Although eight of these trials were relatively small (60 patients or fewer), the two most recent studies included 100 patients or more. In total, 537 subjects were included in these studies of minimal enteral feeding, which are summarized in Table 33–7. Although study protocols varied significantly, mean birth weight was generally 1000 gm and gestational age 28 weeks, and most subjects required mechanical ventilation. Early feedings were begun about 3 days of age and consisted of human milk or formula at 12 to 24 mL/kg per day. The results of these studies were heterogeneous, but three or more studies measured a reduction in hospital stay, days to full feedings, and feeding intolerance in the early feeding group. Other benefits less consistently observed included improved gastrointestinal motility, increased calcium and phosphorus absorption, and reduced sepsis and sepsis evaluations. Adverse effects of early feeding were not observed in any of the studies, and the incidence of necrotizing enterocolitis, in particular, was no different between early- and late-fed premature infants. Combining all studies, necrotizing enterocolitis occurred in 29 early-fed subjects and 31 late-fed subjects.

In summary, the data from these studies support physiologic and clinical benefit from early minimal enteral feeding, without an increased risk of necrotizing enterocolitis. Although a large multicenter trial that more clearly evaluates early feeding may be desirable, such a trial appears unlikely. Based on the available evidence, strong consideration should be given to initiating early feeding.[79]

METHODS OF FEEDING HIGH-RISK INFANTS

Gavage feeding is appropriate for infants who demonstrate an immature suck and swallowing reflex or a clinical condition that precludes nipple feeding.

Therefore, most infants fed by gavage are younger than 34 weeks' gestational age; however, some more mature infants are unable to nipple feed. Infants who have an increased respiratory rate (over 60 respirations/minute), oral-facial anomalies, central nervous system insults, or other medical complications that prevent feedings by nipple receive feedings through an oral or nasal tube or a tube surgically placed in the stomach, jejunum, or duodenum.

The appropriateness of orogastric versus nasogastric versus transpyloric placement has been debated in the past, with current practice favoring orogastric tube placement. In a 1990 study comparing infants weighing more than and less than 2 kg, smaller infants with nasal placement of a 5 Fr feeding tube demonstrated a decrease in minute ventilation and an increase in pulmonary resistance.[53] Nasal tube placement resulted in partial nasal obstruction and secondary hypoventilation; interestingly, the respiratory changes did not appear clinically significant to the caretaker. Infants weighing more than 2 kg tolerated both orogastric and nasogastric tube placement without difficulty. Placement of an anchored orogastric tube is therefore recommended in smaller infants, with transition to nasogastric intubation when the infant's weight exceeds 2 kg. Transpyloric feedings provide no improvement in energy intake or growth and carry significant risks. Transpyloric feedings should be undertaken only if standard feeding procedures have failed, and gastric feeding should be resumed as soon as possible.

The optimal rate of feeding delivery in tube-fed infants has also been a matter of controversy and may reflect regional differences as well as differences in interpretation of the scientific data. Infants appear to tolerate feedings better if rapid gastric distention is avoided. However, continuous drip feedings that deliver milk very slowly have their own potential hazards. Contamination of the drip with bacteria from the caretakers' hands poses a risk of infection to infants who may be immunocompromised already.[161] Continuous drip feedings may be even more hazardous to infants receiving breast milk, because colonization of expressed milk is universal, and logarithmic growth of bacteria occurs in milk left at room temperature for more than 6 hours.[88] Another disadvantage of continuous drip breast milk feedings is the potential loss of nutrient delivery (up to 34% of the expressed milk fat). Moreover, a recent large randomized study demonstrated increased feeding intolerance and decreased growth in premature infants fed continuously compared with those fed by bolus.[137] Although some premature infants may require continuous feedings, bolus feedings over 20 to 25 minutes are generally recommended as a first approach. Bolus feedings are usually delivered in equal volumes every 3 to 4 hours for term infants, every 3 hours for infants less than 2500 gm, and every 2 to 3 hours for infants less than 1500 gm; most infants less than 1000 gm require feedings every 2 hours. Gastric emptying may be a clinical problem but is enhanced with human milk feedings and when infants are in the prone or

---

*References 10, 11, 34, 36, 103, 105, 118, 137, 147, 152.

TABLE 33–7 STUDIES ON MINIMAL ENTERAL FEEDING IN PREMATURE INFANTS

	AUTHOR AND YEAR OF STUDY		
	Troche 1990[153]	**Dunn 1984–1988[36]**	**Berseth 1992[10]**
Number of Patients	28 (16 E vs 12 L)	39 (19 E vs 20 L)	27 (14 E vs 13 L)
Birth weight (gm)	Unknown	950 (500–1500, stratified)	1241–1550
Gestational age (wk)	25–31	27 (26.8 ± 2.8)	32 (28–32)
Study day	<24 hrs vs when stable	<48 hrs vs 9 days	3–5 vs 10–14
Ventilation req'd	+	+	+
UAL	Unknown	+	Unknown
Feedings			
Types	Unknown	Half-strength EPF	Similiac 20
Volume	1 mL/kg/hr	15–20 mL/kg/day → FS	24 mL/kg/day
Duration	Variable (when acute illness over)	7 days	10 days
Route	NG continuous	NG q2–3 hrs	NG
Outcomes			
Bilirubin	NS	↓ Phototherapy in E	Unknown
Days to full feeds	NS	↓ in E (31 days vs 47 days)	↓ in E (18 days vs 31 days)
Feeding intolerance	NS	Unknown	↓ in E
Days to regain birth weight	Unknown	Unknown	Unknown
Weight gain	E > L at day 30 (223 vs 95 gm)	NS	Unknown
Hospital stay	Unknown	Unknown	38 E vs 55 L
NEC	NS (0/16 E vs 2/12 L)	Unknown	Unknown
Miscellaneous	Weekly serum diamine oxidase and somatomedin-C not studied	↓ Alkaline phosphatase in E at 6 wks IVH grade III–IV = 6/19 E vs 3/20 L	Nipple feedings earlier in E Improved GI maturity in E

	AUTHOR AND YEAR OF STUDY			
	Davey 1991–1992[34]	**Ostertag 1983–1984[118]**	**Meetze 1989–1990[105]**	**Slagle 1985–1986[147]**
Number of Patients	60 (29 E vs 31 L)	34 (17 E vs 17 L)	40 (19 E vs 21 L)	46 (22 E vs 24 L)
Birth weight (gm)	1143 (<2000)	1000 (700–1450)	940 (500–1250, stratified)	1000 (500–1500)
Gestational age (wk)	28.5 (28.6 ± 2.7 SD)	28 (26–32)	28 (25–32)	27 (≤32)
Study day	2 vs 5	1 vs 7	3 vs 15	8 vs 18
Ventilation req'd	+	+	+	+
UAL	+	+	Unknown	+
Feedings				
Types	Human milk or dilute formula	H_2O → Portagen	FS EPF	Human milk, SimSC
Volume	Advance as tolerated	1 mL/kg/hr	2.5 mL/kg/day × 10 days	12 mL/kg/day × 10 days
Duration	Unknown	Advance volume after 7 days	Advance every other day to 22.5 mL/kg/day	Advance 15 mL/kg/day to 180
Route	Unknown	NG	NG	NG q2 hrs
Outcomes				
Bilirubin	NS	Unknown	NS	NS
Days to full feeds	Unknown	Unknown	Unknown	NS
Feeding intolerance	↓ in E	↓ in E	↓ in E	↓ in E by 50%
Days to regain birth weight	NS	Unknown	Unknown	NS
Weight gain	NS	Unknown	NS at day 30 (E = 264 gm vs L = 213 gm)	NS
Hospital stay	NS	Unknown	NS	Unknown
NEC	NS (2/29 E vs 4/31 L)	NS (5/17 E vs 6/17 L)	NS (3/19 E vs 4/21 L)	NS (2/22 E vs 2/24 L)
Miscellaneous	↓ Sepsis evaluations ↓ CVL and ↓ days HA in E IVH grade III–IV: 3 E vs 0 L	E had greater energy and protein intake by week 2	↑ Gastrin E ↑ Triglycerides in L at day 10	

TABLE 33-7 STUDIES ON MINIMAL ENTERAL FEEDING IN PREMATURE INFANTS *Continued*

	AUTHOR AND YEAR OF STUDY		
	Berseth 1993[11]	**McClure 1999[103]**	**Schanler 1999[137]**
Number of Patients	32 (16 E vs 16 L)	100	171
Birth weight (gm)	1450 (1400 ± 115)	1000 (800–1300)	1000
Gestational age (wk)	31 (26–33)	28 (27–30)	28
Study day	7 vs 17	3 vs off mechanical vent	6 vs 16
Ventilation req'd	Unknown	+	+
UAL	Unknown	Unknown	+
Feedings			
Types	E = Similac, L = H₂O	Human milk, FS formula	Human milk, half-strength formula
Volume	24 mL/kg/day	12–24 mL/kg/day	20 mL/kg/day
Duration	By day 17, all start on formula	14 days (mean)	14 days
Route	NG	NG q1 hr bolus	NG, randomized to q3 hr bolus or continuous
Outcomes			
Bilirubin	Unknown	NS	NS
Days to full feeds	↓ in E	↓ in E (25 vs 36)	NS
Feeding intolerance	Unknown	NS	↓ in E
Days to regain birth weight	↓ in E	Unknown	NS
Weight gain	Unknown	↑ in E at 6 wks	NS
Hospital stay	↓ in E	NS; ↓ in E (70 vs 94 days)	NS
NEC	Unknown	NS (1 E vs 2 L)	NS (13 E vs 10 L)
Miscellaneous	GI motility improved earlier in E	E had ↓ episodes of culture-proven sepsis	↑ Calcium, phosphorus, copper retention in E at 6 wks ↑ Intestinal transit time in E at 6 wks

CVL, central venous line; E, early feeding; EPF, Enfamil premature formula; FS, full strength; GI, gastrointestinal; IVH, intraventricular hemorrhage; L, late feeding; NEC, necrotizing enterocolitis; NG, nasogastric; NS, not significant; UAL, umbilical arterial line.

right-sided position. Gastric emptying is prolonged by increasing feeding density.

The substrate used to initiate feedings and the rate of advancement are controversial topics without a great deal of data. There is general consensus that given the advantages of breast milk (including tolerance), it should be the first choice and can be used undiluted. If premature formula is used, it is often given initially at half strength; one study showed reduced feeding intolerance and more rapid achievement of full feeding with half-strength formula compared with full-strength premature formula.[33] In another study, intestinal motor activity in response to first feeding in premature infants was better with 20 kcal/oz premature formula than with 24 kcal/oz premature formula. There is therefore some rationale for initiating feedings with 12 to 20 kcal/oz of enteral substrate, although supporting data, especially in infants less than 1000 gm, remain sparse.

The rate at which enteral feedings should be advanced in infants with very low birth weights is also unclear from available data. A number of retrospective studies suggested that rapid advancement of feedings (greater than 25 mL/kg per day) may increase the risk of necrotizing enterocolitis.[2, 31, 49, 84, 104] Two randomized trials compared advancing feedings at 15 to 20 mL/kg per day and 30 to 35 mL/kg per day; no difference in necrotizing enterocolitis was observed between the two groups in either study.[15, 127] However, because necrotizing enterocolitis is relatively infrequent, it is difficult to be completely confident that the higher rates of advancement are safe. While we await additional data, a rate of advancement of 20 mL/kg per day is a practical guideline.

PROGRESSION TO ORAL FEEDING

Non-nutritive sucking, though having no effect on weight gain or gastric motility, may facilitate the transition to oral feeding.[121] In particular, clinical observation of non-nutritive sucking can help the caregiver assess an infant's readiness for oral feeding. It is standard practice to offer a pacifier during tube feedings to see whether the infant demonstrates autonomic stability and attempts to suck during or between feedings. The infant initially may suck on the tongue or make feeble attempts to place the hand to the mouth, which prompts the offering of an artificial nipple. As the infant begins to suck on the pacifier, a mild baseline elevation of the heart rate generally occurs, followed by a change in the respiratory pattern. As the infant continues to suck, a rhythmic pattern of sucks interspersed with pauses (respirations) usually is established. Swallowing of oral secretions may accompany the sucking bursts and may be heard by cervical auscultation. These are reassuring signs; however, the ominous signals of tachycardia, bradycardia, and apnea indicate that the infant is not ready for oral feedings.

Positioning the infant correctly for the feeding is critical to success. The infant should be held relatively upright, rather than reclined, with care taken to support the back in straight alignment. The head should be supported in the midline, with the shoulders in forward flexion. Premature infants need help maintaining this gentle flexion posture because their movements are usually dominated by extension (a more primitive response). Bundling the infant in a receiving blanket is helpful and allows the infant to pay closer attention to the fine motor task of feeding.[141] In healthy term infants, this feeding posture is assumed without difficulty and is the hallmark of the infant's potent hunger cue.

In the past, feedings were viewed as a procedure involving the transfer of milk from one location to another, with speed and volume the goals. Feeding might better be viewed as a process that involves the active participation of both parties, with successful feeding being redefined as autonomic stability and a feeling of satisfaction. This change in emphasis allows the infant to advance feedings with minimal risk. Routine use of pliable, high-flow-rate nipples is universally cautioned against, because they may be associated with respiratory compromise.[102] A small volumetric container is preferable, because dead space is minimized and a vacuum more easily established. Infants should be allowed to establish their own pace for feeding and should not be prodded by jiggling the nipple or frequently changing the body position. The heart and respiratory rates must be observed closely to detect subtle changes that usually precede apnea and bradycardia.[101] Transcutaneous monitoring is useful in infants who are in transition to oral feedings, but it does not replace careful observation of behavioral cues. State and motor changes are sensitive indicators of the infant's ability to integrate sucking, swallowing, and breathing and routinely are present before more obvious signs of distress.

Sucking and swallowing may be facilitated if the caretaker places a finger halfway between the infant's chin and neck, offering support to the base of the tongue. This gentle, even pressure helps the infant maintain intraoral pressure by stabilizing the jaw, thus creating effective use of the baby's musculature. Some infants also are aided by support of the cheeks, to promote a good seal around the nipple. It is vital that the feeder be aware that the infant may purposely break the seal to catch up on respiratory demands and that he or she is attempting to increase breathing by letting air pass around the nipple. An overzealous feeder may increase the pressure on the cheeks and tongue base as the infant attempts to breathe around the nipple, exacerbating the infant's distress until he or she is pushed into the all too frequently seen apnea and bradycardia.

The nasogastric tube need not be removed for early feedings, because the infant can nipple feed with it in place. The feeding should be terminated promptly if cardiopulmonary compromise appears, with the remainder of the bolus given by tube. Satiety at the end of the feeding leads to a general reduction in muscle tone, with extension replacing flexion, and is often accompanied by sleep.

ESTABLISHING LACTATION

The mother's milk supply is directly related to the response of prolactin and oxytocin to breast stimulation. Because a preterm infant often cannot be placed at the breast, mechanical pumping is frequently elected. The larger automatic pumps are designed to cycle 40 to 50 times per minute and require a minimum of breast manipulation. Because these models are favored by mothers and associated with the highest compliance rates, they are often recommended.[6] Double collection kits can be obtained for simultaneous pumping of both breasts, which halves the collection time and prompts increased prolactin surges, enhancing the total milk yield. Specific instructions on rental of breast pumps should be available to mothers in the nurseries where their infants are housed. Third-party reimbursement can be obtained by prescription or by submitting a letter of medical necessity, so that the cost does not interfere with the mother's desire to initiate lactation.

Emptying the breasts with the pump should be attempted 8 to 10 times daily. If a double collection kit is used, pumping takes 10 minutes. Milk collected should be poured into a container large enough to hold the entire expression, and aliquots should be poured individually according to the infant's requirement. Sterile bottle liners were used in the past for this purpose, but milk is easily contaminated when the feeding is poured out. Volufeed containers may be more appropriate and can be supplied to the mother for milk storage. Banked pasteurized milk has substantial disadvantages, including a marked decrease in many nutritional components.[1] Unpasteurized donor milk is contraindicated because of the potential for transmission of infection (e.g., human immunodeficiency virus).

Freshly expressed milk can be fed to infants immediately, which is the preferred method of delivery. If milk is refrigerated, it should be discarded 24 to 48 hours after collection. Milk that is frozen should be thawed by running it under tepid water until it is room temperature. A microwave should not be used for thawing, to ensure maximum preservation of the host defenses. If the breast milk is fortified, this is best accomplished when the milk is at body temperature and just before administration. All thawed milk left over from a feeding should be discarded. Frozen milk is best stored in a refrigerator that is not self-defrosting, because the cyclic change in temperature may allow the milk lipase to partly denature the milk fat, leading to a change in milk composition.[85]

EARLY BREAST-FEEDING EXPERIENCES

It is suggested that early skin-to-skin contact between mothers and their preterm infants is advantageous for a variety of reasons. Nearly continuous skin contact may be elected for infants in underdeveloped countries where economic constraints preclude intensive care nurseries.[3] Infants born as young as 32 weeks' gestation have demonstrated the ability to coordinate sucking with swallowing and breathing when offered a breast feeding. These same infants, when bottle-fed, showed difficulty with respiratory control and frequently demonstrated "cyanotic attacks."[106] Transcutaneous oxygen monitoring showed rapid desaturation at the onset of the feed, a response that was greater in the bottle-fed infants. The smaller infants showed the most difficulty with oxygen decline, differing from the breast-fed infants both during and after the feeding. Oral feedings are usually offered once daily, with supplementation by orogastric tube, until the infant reaches the equivalent of 34 weeks' gestation. Supplementation by bottle, if desired, can begin then.

Maternal readiness for breast feeding includes an adequate milk supply, operational let-down, projectile and nontender nipples, and the desire to commence. Mothers prefer to offer breast feedings out of the intensive care unit in an adjacent room, if possible, with the infant left on cardiopulmonary monitoring. They do not wish to be left alone and are very appreciative of help from a specialist in infant feeding.[107] Enhancing the distensibility of the nipples by 1 to 2 minutes of electric pumping may encourage easier nipple latch-on. If the nipples are not problematic, it is better to let the infant begin to suck non-nutritively, so that he or she is better prepared for the milk let-down. Reverse holds are an excellent choice for small premature infants, because the upright posture and firm, one-handed support facilitate sucking and swallowing. In this position, the mother can easily visualize the infant's mouth when he or she roots toward the nipple and can be aware of the tongue position. The mother should elicit the rooting reflex by gently stroking the perioral area with her nipple and bring the infant forward as he or she opens the mouth and turns toward the stimulus. Touching the infant's face with anything but the nipple confuses the infant. The mother should compress the skin behind her areola, with her thumb on top of the breast and the other fingers supporting the breast from the underside. This scissors the nipple forward and makes grasping the nipple less difficult. It is advantageous to hold the nipple in this manner throughout the feeding, because the infant may not be able to maintain good position without help. The thumb should be parallel to the infant's mouth, so that the nipple and areola are evenly compressed, allowing for good filling of the lactiferous sinus when the infant drops the jaw between sucks.

The infant can be allowed to establish his or her own pace of sucking without interference. If the post–let-down flow rate is too high, the infant may let go of the nipple or let milk flow out around it. The infant should be repositioned when he or she recovers and allowed to resume the feeding. The clinician should listen for sounds of swallowing during feeding and point them out to the mother, because infant feeding noises are highly reinforcing.

First feeding experiences often involve only one breast and may be brief. A successful feeding is one that both the infant and the mother enjoy and should not be measured by the volume consumed. The volume will rise as the mother's and infant's performances improve over time. It is difficult to clinically assess the volume suckled at a feeding. Estimates of intake can be made by weighing the infant just before and immediately after breast feeding.[108] In the days of mechanical scales, weighing was an unreliable assessment and very stressful to mothers. Electronic scale measurements are much more accurate, and most mothers are happy to know the infant's actual intake to ensure appropriate supplementation. The infant need not be unclothed for this procedure, because he or she can be weighed in clothes and blanket both before and after breast feeding. The weight difference in grams estimates the milliliters consumed.[77] Mothers should be cautioned to pump on their regular schedules while the infant is being weaned to the breast, because their supply will diminish if they interrupt mechanical emptying. If nipple soreness is a problem, drying the breasts with a hand-held blow dryer on the low setting is recommended. Routine mechanical expression can be reduced when the infant feeds vigorously, nurses from both breasts at each feeding, and is gaining weight steadily (15 to 40 gm/day).

PRACTICAL APPROACH TO ENTERAL FEEDING IN THE INFANT WITH EXTREMELY LOW BIRTH WEIGHT

This chapter provides guidelines, theoretical background, and rationale for enteral feeding of the high-risk infant. Nonetheless, many questions remain partly or completely unanswered.

Should intrauterine body composition and growth rates be the reasonable expectation, or even the theoretical goal, for infants with very or extremely low birth weights postnatally?

Are specific components of human milk important in the functional maturation of the newborn infant and, in particular, the neural system?

Are currently available premature formulas optimal for feeding infants with very or extremely low birth weights?

How quickly should enteral feeding be advanced in premature infants, and in what manner (volume and concentration)?

How should feeding protocols be altered by specific factors (e.g., gestational age, respiratory distress, sepsis)?

Despite our lack of adequate and specific answers to some of these fundamental questions, it is important to develop a reasoned approach to nutritional support of the high-risk infant. Considerable flexibility must be incorporated into such guidelines. Clearly, the relative risks insofar as they are known must be carefully weighed against benefit. When sufficient data are not available to address the relative risk versus the benefit, we must use our clinical judgment until adequate studies have been performed.

The following general guidelines represent one approach to enteral feeding of the infant with extremely low birth weight. As discussed in Part Two of this chapter, parenteral nutrition should begin early and continue until full enteral feedings are reached; parenteral nutrition should also be reinitiated without delay when enteral feedings are interrupted.

As IV parenteral nutrition is being provided and advanced, minimal early enteral intake for the infant with extremely low birth weight should be strongly considered, beginning at day 2 or 3 of life. The requirement for mechanical ventilation or the presence of an umbilical arterial line should not prevent initiating minimal enteral feeding. Breast milk from the infant's mother is the preferred enteral substrate; it is usually provided undiluted and ultimately fortified with a standard breast milk fortifier when the infant has achieved full-volume feeds. If breast milk is unavailable, premature formulas are often provided in diluted form, although it is not clear whether such a practice is necessary. Small aliquots of human milk or diluted formula may be provided by the orogastric route on a regular intermittent schedule (1 to 2 mL/kg every 2 hours). Evidence suggests that such minimal intake is well tolerated and may reduce or prevent intestinal atrophy in this high-risk population.[84] Early minimal enteral intake is not intended to provide significant nutrition to the infant; rather, it is thought to serve as a priming nutrient source for the intestine, sustaining continued functional maturation postnatally.

The appropriate pathway to achieving full enteral feedings in premature newborns is an area that often generates strong opinions based on limited or incomplete data. One approach is to advance feedings by 20 mL/kg per day if the infant tolerated the previous 24 hours of feeding; this typically results in full enteral feeding (150 mL/kg per day) in 7 to 10 days. This slow rate of advancement is based on several retrospective studies that examined the risk factors associated with necrotizing enterocolitis.[2, 31, 49, 104] If diluted formula is used, advancements to full volume are made first, and then the concentration is increased. Throughout the process of advancing feeds, adjustments are made if signs and symptoms of feeding intolerance are observed (e.g., residuals, abdominal distention, occult blood in stools, increased respiratory distress). However, because most of these signs and symptoms are nonspecific, it often is less than clear what the optimal clinical response should be. Studies evaluating motility patterns in premature infants during feeding may ultimately help resolve some of these clinical questions.[80, 86]

Although techniques for providing nutrition through peripherally or centrally placed IV catheters have enhanced our ability to support these infants nutritionally, the risks of catheter-related complications (thrombosis, infection) must be considered. Every effort should be undertaken to make a safe transition from IV to orogastric feedings. At this time, we lack appropriate and specific markers by which to monitor the safety or risk of various approaches. Nonetheless, in view of the lack of adequate data, we should avoid dogmatic approaches to the nutritional care of these infants and encourage additional clinical trials of adequate size to address these fundamental issues.

part two
PARENTERAL NUTRITION

Scott C. Denne,
Brenda B. Poindexter, and
Catherine A. Leitch

The nutritional support of infants with extremely low birth weights, especially in early postnatal life, is almost entirely dependent on the parenteral route. In practice, the nutritional requirements of these infants are rarely met, and they lose a great deal of ground in the first 2 weeks after birth.[175] Growth failure in infants with extremely low birth weights is nearly universal,[258] but there is growing evidence that early use of parenteral nutrition may minimize losses and improve growth outcomes.[278, 302, 307] Wilson and colleagues demonstrated in infants with very low birth weights that early, aggressive parenteral nutrition combined with early enteral feeding reduced growth failure without an increased incidence of adverse clinical consequences or metabolic derangement.[307] Parenteral nutrition solutions, although still evolving, have improved markedly from the early days of use, and complications are less common. This part reviews parenteral nutrition, component by component, and provides some practical guidelines for use.

ENERGY REQUIREMENTS IN THE PARENTERALLY FED INFANT

The initial goal of parenteral nutrition is to provide sufficient energy and nitrogen to prevent catabolism and to achieve a positive nitrogen balance. As discussed in Part One of this chapter, energy must be supplied by nutrient intake to cover two major components: energy expenditure and growth. The calories in parenteral nutrition solutions are provided primarily by carbohydrate and fat. The parenteral nutrition solution should provide sufficient amino acids for protein turnover and tissue growth.[242]

Preterm infants have very low energy reserves due to low amounts of body fat as well as low glycogen stores in the liver. Maintaining these limited energy stores requires an energy intake that approximates energy expenditure. Energy expenditure in premature infants is thought to be in the 50 to 60 kcal/kg per day range, but it must be noted that data in ventilated infants and infants with extremely low birth weights are limited.[239] It has long been appreciated that thermal stresses can substantially increase energy expenditure; under extreme environmental conditions, energy expenditure can increase by nearly 100%.[239] Although thermal stresses can theoretically be minimized, in practice, they are likely to be a significant contributor to energy expenditure. Conversely, activity contributes relatively little ((3.5%) to energy expenditure in premature infants.[298]

The energy cost of growth in these infants has been estimated at about 5 kcal/gm.[275] To achieve the equivalent of the estimated third-trimester in utero weight gain of 14 gm/kg per day, theoretically, an additional energy intake of about 70 kcal/kg per day is necessary. However, several studies have shown that nitrogen accretion and growth rates similar to those achieved in utero can be sustained in preterm infants with a parenteral intake of 80 kcal/kg per day if an appropriate amount of nitrogen is provided.[187, 313]

A caloric intake of 50 to 60 kcal/kg per day approximates energy expenditure and therefore is a reasonable value for the maintenance requirements of premature infants for the first few days after birth; these maintenance requirements often are provided by glucose alone. To support normal rates of growth during parenteral nutrition, 90 to 100 kcal/kg per day are required, with most of these calories supplied by lipid and glucose. Parenteral energy requirements are less than those required for enteral nutrition because there is no energy lost in the stools. It is important to point out that these recommendations are based largely on data from larger, relatively stable premature infants. Energy requirements, both for maintenance and for growth, may be higher in infants with extremely low birth weights.[185]

INTRAVENOUS CARBOHYDRATE REQUIREMENTS

Glucose is the most widely used IV carbohydrate for neonates, partly because it is readily available to the brain, which does not require insulin for intracellular uptake. The monohydrate form of dextrose is used in IV solutions; each gram provides 3.4 kcal upon complete oxidation. In other words, a 10% dextrose solution (10 gm dextrose per 100 mL) provides 34 kcal/kg per day if 100 mL/kg per day is infused. As the solution concentration increases, so does osmolarity, ranging from approximately 255 mOsm/L for a 5% solution to 1010 mOsm/L for a 20% solution.[196]

Many other nonglucose carbohydrates have been tried, but with limited success. Galactose, in particular, has been advocated for IV use in neonates because it does not require insulin, nor does it stimulate insulin release. A mixture of glucose and galactose has been evaluated as a means of preventing hyperglycemia in the first days of life. Although no toxicity was noted, the plasma concentration of galactose was substantially higher than that of milk-fed neonates.[295] Fructose, sorbitol, xylitol, and ethyl alcohol have been proposed for IV use as well, but significant toxicities and untoward effects have been reported.[305]

Because the supply of glucose to the fetus depends solely on maternal glucose, cord clamping at the time of birth requires that a number of events occur in order to maintain glucose homeostasis in the newborn. Fetal glucose use in utero matches umbilical glucose uptake, implying that glycogenolysis and gluconeogenesis are minimal in the fetus. Several factors promote glycogen deposition in utero: blunted pancreatic B cell regulation of insulin secretion, high insulin receptor density, and relative glucagon resistance. In late gestation, the fetus begins to prepare for the transition to postnatal life by increasing hepatic glycogen stores and brown fat deposits. Hepatic glycogen synthesis increases in response to increases in adrenal corticosteroid production, also characteristic of late gestation. At the time of delivery, glucagon levels rise, and insulin levels fall. Higher levels of plasma catecholamines, both epinephrine and norepinephrine, directly stimulate increases in hepatic glucose output. The increased levels of epinephrine and glucagon stimulate lipolysis and the activity of phosphorylase, a key enzyme in glycolysis. The increased level of glucagon also results in increased activity of phosphoenolpyruvate carboxykinase, a rate-limiting enzyme in gluconeogenesis. The newborn must be able to initiate gluconeogenesis, because glycogen stores can sustain glucose production only for several hours after birth. All these changes together act to preserve glucose homeostasis after the infant's maternal source of glucose is removed with cord clamping.[255] In addition, the newborn must acclimate to periods of feeding and intermittent fasting, as opposed to the constant glucose supply delivered in utero.

Rates of glucose production and use have been quantified in term and preterm infants using stable isotope methodologies. Because neural tissue makes up a greater proportion of body weight, newborns have higher rates of glucose oxidation than adults, with glucose being the primary energy substrate for the brain. The glucose production rate in term newborns is approximately 3 to 5 mg/kg per minute,[199] whereas premature infants have somewhat higher rates of basal glucose production (and use), at 7.7 to 7.9 mg/kg per minute. Both an increased ratio of brain weight to body weight and decreased fat stores probably contribute to this higher rate of glucose production in infants with extremely low birth weights.[226]

Because a preterm infant has a higher rate of basal glucose use, as well as factors such as hypothermia and respiratory distress, which also increase glucose demand, early administration of parenteral glucose is critical. Although the definition of neonatal hypoglycemia remains controversial, it seems prudent to intervene for a plasma glucose level less than 40 mg/dL, particularly in a premature infant in the first few days of life. No definitive conclusions or prospective studies have established a correlation between hypoglycemia and neurodevelopmental outcomes, particularly in infants with extremely low birth weights,[194, 195] although Koh and colleagues reported neural dysfunction associated with blood glucose of less than 47 mg/dL.[233]

Infants with extremely low birth weights are even more susceptible to hyperglycemia, particularly in the first few days of life, when feedings are almost entirely parenteral. Factors such as sepsis, respiratory distress, and hypoxia may also contribute. Historically, glucose intolerance in infants with extremely low birth weights was attributed to persistent endogenous hepatic glucose production in the face of increased exogenous supply, insufficient insulin production, or tissue insensitivity to insulin. However, Hertz and colleagues demonstrated that clinically stable infants with extremely low birth weights are able to suppress endogenous glucose production when given parenteral glucose. In this study, infants given a glucose infusion at a rate of 9 mg/kg per minute were able to suppress endogenous glucose production to nearly zero, demonstrating that there is no inherent immaturity in this process in extremely premature infants.[226] From a practical standpoint, understanding rates of endogenous glucose production is important to avoid iatrogenic hyperglycemia. In infants with extremely low birth weights, a reasonable approach is to start the glucose infusion rate at 6 mg/kg per minute, gradually advancing to 10 to 12 mg/kg per minute as long as hyperglycemia does not develop.

The definition of hyperglycemia also varies but is generally set at a plasma level above 150 mg/dL (8.3 mmol/L). Each 1 mmol/L (18 mg/dL) rise in the blood glucose concentration produces an increase in serum osmolarity of 1 mOsm/L; this can result in osmotic diuresis and subsequent dehydration with values above 300 mOsm/L and has been associated with higher mortality and a higher rate of intracranial hemorrhage. Hyperglycemia is detected early through frequent glucose monitoring. Plasma glucose levels below 200 mg/dL usually do not require intervention. Reducing the fluid needs and insensible water loss can reduce the glucose intake. Alternatively, a lower concentration of dextrose solution can be used, although less than 2.5% solutions should be avoided.[264] Sterile water can be given enterally to decrease parenteral glucose intake without compromising total fluid intake. Lipid infusions have been shown to increase plasma glucose concentrations in premature infants when given at high infusion rates.[306, 308] However, such high infusion rates are not routinely used in clinical practice. The mechanism most likely involves a change in glucose utilization.[308] Although Yunis and colleagues demonstrated a statistically significant increase in plasma glucose (from 73 to 90 mg/dL) in premature infants given IV lipids,[308] it is unlikely that such an increase would be of clinical significance. Consequently, IV lipids probably contribute little to the hyperglycemia commonly seen in infants with extremely low birth weights. Discontinuing IV lipids only reduces the caloric intake and increases the risk

of essential fatty acid deficiency in this particularly vulnerable population.

A continuous infusion of insulin is occasionally needed to treat hyperglycemia in infants with extremely low birth weights. Doses range from 0.05 to 0.1 U/kg per hour. Some have advocated the use of insulin to "promote growth," using insulin to facilitate tolerance of added parenteral calories.[230, 254] Binder and colleagues found that insulin infusions improve glucose tolerance in infants with very low birth weights and allow provision of an adequate caloric intake to hyperglycemic infants.[176] Collins and colleagues additionally concluded that infants receiving continuous insulin infusions had enhanced weight gain.[191] Using stable isotope methodology, Poindexter and colleagues measured glucose and protein kinetics in response to euglycemic hyperinsulinemia in extremely premature (26 weeks' gestation, birth weight 890 gm), mechanically ventilated newborns. In response to a greater than 10-fold increase in insulin concentrations (from 7 to 79 μU/mL), protein breakdown was reduced by 20%. However, utilization of phenylalanine for protein synthesis also decreased by a similar magnitude, resulting in no net protein gain. In addition, serum lactate concentrations increased nearly threefold during the study period, with an accompanying metabolic acidosis.[269] Therefore, although this level of hyperinsulinemia was successful in reducing protein breakdown in extremely premature infants, the reduction in protein synthesis and the substantial increase in lactic acid concentrations argue against the routine use of exogenous insulin in this population. The potential anabolic effects of insulin during amino acid administration remain unclear.

INTRAVENOUS PROTEIN AND AMINO ACID REQUIREMENTS

When fetal life is interrupted by premature birth, duplicating rates of in utero protein accretion remains a difficult clinical challenge. Failure to provide adequate protein, either in quantity or in quality, can significantly impact the long-term outcome of extremely premature infants. At 26 weeks' gestation, the human fetus accretes approximately 1.8 to 2.2 gm of body protein per day, with the placenta supplying about 3.5 gm/kg per day of amino acids to the developing fetus.[310] In contrast, infants with extremely low birth weights who receive glucose alone lose approximately 1.2 gm/kg of protein each day they do not receive amino acids.[200, 231] This corresponds to a daily loss of 1% to 2% of their total endogenous body protein stores (Fig. 33–1). In just a few days, the gap between what would have been protein accretion in utero and what is now postnatal protein loss widens considerably. As will be discussed in more detail later, early provision of parenteral amino acids can offset this deficit, even if total caloric intake is low.

A variety of methods have been used to quantitate protein requirements in human infants: measurement

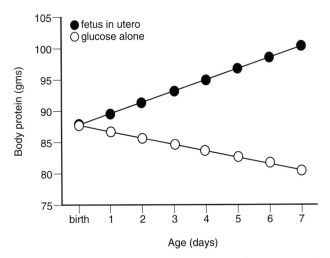

FIGURE 33–1. Change in body protein in human fetus at approximately 26 weeks' gestation (rate of in utero gain is modified from Ziegler[310]) and theoretical loss in 26- to 27-week, 1000-gm birth weight infants receiving glucose alone. (Modified from Denne SC, et al: Proteolysis and phenylalanine hydroxylation in response to parenteral nutrition in extremely premature and normal newborns. J Clin Invest 97:746, 1996.)

of breast milk intake and protein content, fetal accretion rate, nitrogen balance studies, serum amino acid levels, and stable isotope studies investigating the kinetics of labeled amino acids. Clearly, the gold standard needs to be that which safely optimizes growth and development.

Normal human fetal development is characterized by rapid rates of growth and protein accretion. In utero, the placenta supplies amino acids to the fetus far in excess of requirements for protein accretion. The excess amino acids are oxidized by the fetus, contributing significantly to fetal energy production. High rates of protein turnover are required to support protein synthesis, tissue remodeling, and growth. Analysis of fetal body composition indicates that at 28 weeks' gestation, the fetus accretes approximately 350 mg of nitrogen per kilogram per day (protein values in milligrams can be found by multiplying nitrogen values in milligrams by 6.25). At term, nitrogen accretion declines to about 150 mg/kg per day. Postnatal nitrogen loss decreases with gestational age as well, from 180 mg/kg per day at 27 to 28 weeks to 120 mg/kg per day for a full-term infant.[231] Consequently, protein requirements extrapolated from fetal nitrogen accretion rates and postnatal losses have been estimated at 2.5 to 3.5 gm/kg per day for preterm infants and 1.9 to 2.5 gm/kg per day for term infants. As protein losses are inversely related to gestational age, protein requirements are likely to be even higher in extremely premature infants.

EFFICACY OF EARLY PARENTERAL AMINO ACIDS

Several studies have evaluated the efficacy of early parenteral amino acid administration in premature infants.[169, 231, 278, 283, 304] Using nitrogen balance techniques, each study demonstrated the ability of early

parenteral amino acids to reverse the negative nitrogen balance seen in premature infants receiving glucose alone. Saini and colleagues compared infants with extremely low birth weights who received amino acids on the first day of life (1.8 gm/kg per day of Vamin 9) to those not receiving any amino acids until they were older than 72 hours of age and confirmed that positive nitrogen balance can be achieved in sick, ventilator-dependent infants as early as the first day of life.[283] In the study by Van Goudoever and colleagues, positive nitrogen balance was remarkably achieved with only 1.15 gm/kg per day of amino acids and less than 30 kcal/kg per day.[302] A summary of the results obtained from these studies is shown in Table 33–8. It is important to point out that each of these studies used a different amino acid solution. Despite these differences in the composition of the solutions used, all studies demonstrated positive nitrogen balance in infants receiving early parenteral amino acids despite low total caloric intake (~50 kcal/kg per day). Consequently, the initial goal of limiting catabolism and preserving endogenous protein stores can be easily accomplished if parenteral amino acids are initiated on the first day of life in infants with extremely low birth weights.

Stable isotope techniques have also been used to evaluate the effect of amino acids on protein metabolism in premature infants. In these studies, stable isotope tracers of one or more essential amino acids are used to reflect whole body protein kinetics. In addition to demonstrating positive nitrogen balance, Rivera and colleagues found that administration of amino acids (1.5 gm/kg per day of Aminosyn-PF with cysteine added) beginning on the first day of life improves protein balance as a result of increased protein synthesis (as reflected by leucine kinetics).[278] Denne and colleagues demonstrated that provision of 2.5 gm/kg per day of amino acids as part of a complete parenteral nutrition solution acutely reverses the negative protein balance (as reflected by phenylalanine kinetics) seen in response to glucose alone from a 1.5 gm/kg per day loss to a net 0.5 gm/kg per day gain.[200]

Safety is often cited as a reason to delay initiation of amino acids, particularly in the sickest, most immature infants. However, many investigators have demonstrated the safety of early provision of IV amino acids to premature infants. Normal plasma amino acid concentrations have been reported using TrophAmine.[223] Rivera and colleagues studied infants with very low birth weights given amino acids in the first days of life and found no abnormal elevations of plasma amino acids, BUN, or ammonia.[279] Paisley and colleagues conducted a randomized trial of low (1 gm/kg per day) versus high (3 gm/kg per day) amino acid intake in infants with extremely low birth weights immediately after birth. Using BUN and plasma aminograms as indicators of acute amino acid toxicity, they concluded that 3 gm/kg per day of amino acids was as safe as the lower intake.[256] As mentioned earlier, a significant proportion of the amino acids supplied to the developing fetus are oxi-

TABLE 33–8 SUMMARY OF STUDIES OF EARLY AMINO ACID ADMINISTRATION IN INFANTS WITH LOW BIRTH WEIGHTS

STUDY	SUBJECTS	AMINO ACID SOLUTION	ENERGY INTAKE (kcal/kg/day)	INTAKE Nitrogen mg/kg/day	Amino Acids gm/kg/day	BALANCE Nitrogen mg/kg/day	Amino Acids gm/kg/day
Anderson[169]	27–36 wks	Aminosyn	60	0	0	−132	−0.8
	~1600 gm		60	400	2.5	178	1.1
Saini[283]	28 wks	Vamin-9	36	0	0	−132	−0.8
	1000 gm		45	286	1.8	122	0.76
Van Lingen[304]	30 wks	Aminovenous	47	0	0	−96	−0.6
	1500 gm		48	368	2.3	224	1.4
Rivera[278]	28 wks	Aminosyn-PF	50	0	0	−135	−0.8
	1000 gm		50	250	1.5	88*	0.6
Kashyap[231]		TrophAmine	30	0	0	−183	−1.1
	~1000 gm		50	315	2.0	114	0.7
Van Goudoever[302]	29 wks	Primene	26	0	0	−110	−0.7
	1400 gm		29	184	1 .15	10	0.06

*Some of the infants in this group received cysteine supplementation and others did not. Nitrogen balance shown is that of the total group; nitrogen balance in the subgroup that received cysteine was 115 ± 41 mg/kg/day vs 42 ± 42 mg/kg/day in the subgroup that did not receive cysteine.

dized and serve as a significant energy source for the fetus. Urea production is a by-product of amino acid oxidation. In premature infants, rates of urea production are higher than in term neonates and adults, consistent with high rates of protein turnover and oxidation. Some investigators have even suggested that azotemia might be evidence of effective utilization of amino acids as an energy supply rather than protein intolerance. In addition, because the secretion of insulin is thought to depend on adequate plasma concentrations of certain amino acids, such as arginine and leucine, some investigators believe that early administration of amino acids postnatally may help reduce the incidence of hyperglycemia in infants with very low birth weights.

Although the initial goal of parenteral nutrition in premature infants may be to limit catabolism and maintain endogenous protein stores, ultimately, sufficient energy and protein intake to support growth must be provided. This is true regardless of whether parenteral nutrition is used exclusively or as a bridge to full enteral feedings. Multiple investigators have evaluated the influence of nitrogen and energy intake on nitrogen retention. In infants who receive an adequate amount of energy to maintain growth (~70 to 80 kcal/kg per day IV), nitrogen retention increases with increasing nitrogen intake.[202, 266, 273, 287, 313] Even at a protein intake as high as 4 gm/kg per day, retention still increases linearly. This response is in marked contrast to that in adults; their nitrogen retention levels off slightly above zero balance when excess dietary nitrogen is provided.

Zlotkin and colleagues studied the effect of nitrogen intake at two levels of nonprotein energy intake on nitrogen balance and weight gain in parenterally fed neonates.[313] One group of infants received 50 kcal/kg per day and a nitrogen intake of either 480 or 640 mg/kg per day, equal to 3 or 4 gm/kg per day of amino acid intake, respectively. At this low caloric intake, there was no improvement in the rate of nitrogen retention or weight gain with greater nitrogen intake. At higher energy intake (80 kcal/kg per day), increasing the amino acid intake from 2 to 3 gm/kg per day resulted in a significant increase in the rate of weight gain and nitrogen retention. At the higher caloric intake, providing 3 gm/kg per day of amino acids resulted in weight gain (15 gm/kg per day) and nitrogen accretion (approximately 300 mg/kg per day) equal to intrauterine rates. Further increasing protein intake to 4 gm/kg per day at the higher caloric intake resulted in an even higher rate of nitrogen retention, but no further increase in weight gain. Duffy and colleagues also found improved nitrogen retention with a higher caloric intake and demonstrated nitrogen retention similar to the fetal accretion rate when premature infants (birth weight less than 1600 gm) were given 85 kcal/kg per day and 2.9 gm/kg per day of amino acids.[202] Based on these studies, a reasonable estimate of protein requirements for growth in premature infants would be 2.5 to 3.5 gm/kg per day; the requirements of infants with extremely low birth weights may be even higher. In term infants, Zlotkin determined the IV nitrogen requirements to be 280 mg/kg per day (equivalent to 1.8 gm/kg per day of protein).[313]

Many conditions and interventions commonly encountered in extremely premature infants are known to increase protein requirements. Superimposed catabolic conditions such as sepsis or surgical stress increase catabolism. The use of dexamethasone is known to increase protein catabolism by increasing protein oxidation and proteolysis, resulting in decreased accretion of protein.[182, 303]

INTRAVENOUS AMINO ACID MIXTURES

The first parenteral amino acid solutions used in neonates were hydrolysates of fibrin or casein. Concerns about these first-generation solutions included high concentrations of glycine, glutamate, and aspartate; the presence of unwanted peptides; and high acidity. Reports of hyperammonemia and acidosis in the early 1970s were associated with the use of these first-generation solutions in neonates. Although amino acid solutions have been significantly modified (see later), the perceived risks associated with the protein hydrolysates linger, contributing to some clinicians' hesitancy to administer early parenteral amino acids.

The second generation of amino acid solutions consisted of crystalline amino acid mixtures (FreAmine III, Travasol, Aminosyn). The amino acid pattern of these mixtures reflects that of high-quality dietary proteins with large amounts of glycine and alanine, absence of glutamate and aspartate, and absence or poor solubility of tyrosine and cysteine.

The newest solutions include modifications of crystalline amino acids for use in pediatric patients (TrophAmine, Aminosyn-PF, Primene; Table 33–9). Aminosyn-PF (Abbott) and TrophAmine (B. Braun) are the two parenteral amino acid solutions commercially available in the United States that are recommended for use in neonates. The manufacturing of TrophAmine is the result of complicated calculations. Factors taken into account included plasma amino acid concentrations in infants receiving a variety of IV mixtures[168]; 2-hour postprandial plasma concentrations of healthy, 30-day-old, breast-fed, term infants; and three cycles of the experimental mixtures readjusted as necessary. Primene, manufactured in Europe, has an amino acid pattern closely resembling

that of TrophAmine, although Primene's composition was derived from fetal or neonatal cord blood amino acid concentrations. There is no clear evidence that one amino acid mixture is superior to another in promoting nitrogen retention. The exception is a single study in which nitrogen retention was 78% with TrophAmine, versus 66% with a standard amino acid mixture.[223] The pediatric mixtures result in closer to normal plasma amino patterns than do the standard mixtures. During Neopham feeding (2 gm/kg per day), plasma amino acid levels are closer to those of orally fed infants than after Travasol feeding. Except for slightly lower tyrosine and higher phenylalanine levels during TrophAmine feeding (1.9 to 2.4 gm/kg per day) in infants weighing 750 to 1750 gm, plasma amino acid levels are within the 95% confidence limit of the concentrations of normal, growing, preterm infants fed their own mothers' milk. A Primene intake of more than 2.5 gm/kg per day results in elevated aspartate, glycine, and ornithine levels compared with cord samples, whereas an intake of less than 2.5 gm/kg per day does not result in elevated glycine levels. No data are available on Aminosyn-PF.[221, 277]

It is no surprise that the ideal composition of IV amino acid mixtures is unknown. Investigators disagree on the basis for determining optimal plasma amino acid levels. Some advocate using values of breast-fed infants; others suggest using cord plasma levels. The source of nonprotein energy might affect plasma amino acid levels. There is even controversy over the optimal sampling site. To optimize nutrition and growth, particularly in a premature infant, the requirements for specific amino acids need to be more precisely defined. Several amino acids are "conditionally essential" in premature infants. That is, the infant's ability to synthesize these amino acids de novo is less than functional metabolic demands. Cysteine, tyrosine, arginine, glycine, and histidine are generally considered essential amino acids for premature infants.[300] Glutamine may also be conditionally essential for some infants.

Tyrosine is widely regarded as an essential amino acid in preterm infants yet is not present in appreciable amounts in currently available amino acid solutions, owing to its low solubility. Snyderman found lower rates of weight gain, nitrogen retention, and plasma concentrations of tyrosine in premature infants given a tyrosine-deficient diet.[292] Tyrosine is synthesized endogenously from phenylalanine by phenylalanine hydroxylase. The activity of this enzyme in premature infants was thought to be inadequate for growth and nitrogen retention without tyrosine supplements. However, stable isotope studies have demonstrated active phenylalanine hydroxylation in very premature (26 weeks) and premature (32 weeks) infants.[189, 200] Therefore, in the strictest sense, tyrosine is not an essential amino acid. However, it remains unclear whether enough tyrosine can be endogenously produced from phenylalanine in premature infants to support normal rates of protein accretion. N-acetyl tyrosine, although currently added to TrophAmine, is not highly bioavailable. Nonetheless,

TABLE 33–9 COMPOSITION OF COMMERCIAL PARENTERAL AMINO ACID SOLUTIONS*

	AMINOSYN-PF (ABBOTT)	TROPHAMINE (B. BRAUN)	PRIMENE (BAXTER)
Histidine	312	480	380
Isoleucine	760	820	670
Leucine	1200	1400	1000
Lysine	677	820	1100
Methionine	180	340	240
Phenylalanine	427	480	420
Threonine	512	420	370
Tryptophan	180	200	200
Valine	673	780	760
Alanine	698	540	800
Arginine	1227	1200	840
Proline	812	680	300
Serine	495	380	400
Taurine	70	25	60
Tyrosine	44	240†	45
Glycine	385	360	400
Cysteine	—	<16	189
Glutamic acid	820	500	1000
Aspartic acid	527	320	600

*Amino acid concentration in mg/dL; all amino acid mixtures shown are 10% solutions.
†Mixture of L-tyrosine and N-acetyl-tyrosine.
From the American Hospital Formulary Service: Drug Information. Bethesda, Md, 2000, and Drug Product Database.

several studies provide indirect evidence that *N*-acetyl tyrosine improves protein accretion in preterm infants.[219, 220] In addition, it is unclear whether premature infants can adequately catabolize tyrosine via oxidation by the enzymes tyrosine aminotransferase and 4-hydroxyphenylpyruvate dioxygenase. Inability to catabolize tyrosine can lead to transient neonatal tyrosinemia. Further studies are needed to better define premature infants' ability to catabolize tyrosine and to determine whether an alternative source of tyrosine is needed in parenteral amino acid solutions.

Histidine is necessary for normal growth and protein synthesis in the newborn, but the exact requirement is still unclear.[286]

The high glycine content of TPN solutions induces not only hyperglycinemia but also hyperammonemia. Solutions with a high methionine content cause hypermethioninemia, yet it is an essential sulfur-containing amino acid that may be converted into cysteine or cystine and taurine.

Cysteine also is considered an essential amino acid for preterm infants, but it is not soluble in current amino acid solutions.[260] Some studies have shown that fetal liver lacks the enzymatic system to convert methionine into cysteine and that infants on a cysteine-free diet demonstrate impaired growth and low plasma cysteine levels.[297] Other studies have shown that there is enough cystathionase in extrahepatic tissues of the fetus and preterm infant to synthesize cysteine when an adequate amount of methionine is provided. The previously mentioned study by Rivera and colleagues found improved nitrogen retention in a subgroup that received cysteine supplementation (115 ± 41 mg/kg per day versus 42 ± 42 mg/kg per day in the subgroup that received no cysteine). Stable isotope studies have also suggested improved protein retention with cysteine supplementation.[268] Cysteine hydrochloride supplements can be added to parenteral nutrition, but they can cause metabolic acidosis[245, 311, 312, 314] unless appropriately buffered with acetate. The addition of cysteine hydrochloride improves the solubility of calcium and phosphorus in parenteral nutrition solutions.

Glutamine is one of the most abundant amino acids in both plasma and human milk,[183, 280, 291] yet it is not supplied by currently available amino acid solutions because glutamine is unstable in aqueous solution. Glutamine is a major energy substrate for small intestinal mucosa, as proved by a high glutamine uptake from the lumen and from arterial blood during the newborn period in rats. Adding glutamine to the TPN solutions of animals prevents atrophy of small intestinal mucosa and smooth muscle, improves the gut immune function, and reduces the incidence of fatty infiltration of the liver. A small randomized trial conducted by Lacey and colleagues demonstrated the safety of parenteral glutamine supplementation in premature infants. In the subgroup weighing less than 800 gm, they also found that infants receiving glutamine required fewer days on parenteral nutrition (13 versus 21 days), needed a shorter time to achieve full enteral feedings (8 versus 14 days), and

needed less time on the ventilator (38 versus 47 days).[237] A large, multicenter, randomized clinical trial of parenteral glutamine supplementation in infants with extremely low birth weights is currently under way.

Finally, taurine is synthesized endogenously from cysteine and is not part of structural protein. It is present in large concentrations in the retina and brain of the fetus, reaching a peak concentration at birth. When newborn nonhuman primates are fed taurine-deficient formula, growth is depressed,[218] but this does not occur in human preterm infants, despite declining plasma and urine taurine levels.[229] Whereas Geggel and colleagues found reversible abnormalities in the retinograms of children receiving long-term taurine-free TPN, the retinograms of preterm infants receiving a taurine-free formula orally were found to be normal by Tyson and colleagues.[206, 299] One should keep in mind that the composition of IV amino acid mixtures has changed since Geggel's study and that the study may have been too brief to demonstrate changes. Indeed, the smallest preterm infants that are fed intravenously are at highest risk of depletion of body stores and also have renal limitation of taurine conservation.[309] Nevertheless, there is some limited evidence that taurine supplementation might influence auditory brainstem evoked responses (see also Part One of this chapter). Several pediatric IV amino acid solutions (TrophAmine, Primene, Aminosyn-PF) contain one to three times the amount of taurine found in breast milk; in some cases, this might lower the incidence of TPN-induced cholestasis.[201]

In summary, the importance of early amino acid administration cannot be overemphasized. Although it has been the practice of many neonatal intensive care units to delay administration of IV amino acids for several days, we believe that a minimum of 1 to 1.5 gm/kg per day, and preferably 2 to 2.5 gm/kg per day, of amino acids be initiated in the first hours after birth in infants with extremely low birth weights. As none of the currently used amino acid solutions was designed specifically to meet the needs of extremely premature infants, future research efforts should be directed at designing a fourth generation of amino acid solutions to optimize parenteral nutrition given to these infants.

INTRAVENOUS LIPID EMULSIONS

Lipid is provided in parenteral nutrition solutions as a major nonprotein energy source and a source of essential fatty acids. Similar nitrogen-sparing effects have been shown for glucose and lipid in parenterally fed infants under steady-state conditions.[265, 301]

CHARACTERISTICS, CLEARANCE, AND METABOLISM

The commercial IV lipid emulsions are aqueous suspensions containing neutral triglycerides derived from soybean, safflower, and MCT oil or combinations thereof; egg yolk phospholipids to emulsify; and glycerin to adjust the tonicity. The size of the fat particles is similar to that of naturally occurring chylomicrons and ranges between 0.1 and 1 μm, averaging 0.25 μm. Particles of IV lipid emulsions behave to some extent like chylomicrons carrying exogenous triglycerides. The emulsion particles contain less protein and cholesterol and more phospholipids and triglycerides than the chylomicrons synthesized by the small intestine. Triglycerides and cholesterol esters form the hydrophobic core of the lipoproteins, whereas the phospholipids, cholesterol, and small amounts of free fatty acids combine with apoproteins to form the surface film.

Infants with very low birth weights have a limited amount of adipose tissue and diminished levels of lipoprotein lipase, resulting in slower clearance of lipids.[180] Infants whose gestational age is younger than 26 weeks show a marked decrease in lipoprotein lipase activity, whereas those born at 27 to 28 weeks have variable lipoprotein lipase activity.[248] Both hepatic and lipoprotein lipase act on the triglyceride core. Hydrolysis of triglyceride results in the formation of free fatty acids and remnant particles. The free fatty acids can circulate and be used as an energy source, or they can enter adipose tissue, where they are re-esterified to form triglycerides. The remnant particles behave in a similar fashion to natural chylomicron remnants and are rapidly removed by the liver. Lecithin cholesterol acyltransferase (LCAT) acts specifically on the lipid components of the surface film, where it catalyzes the first step in the catabolism of lecithin, a major component of all IV lipid emulsions. Serum cholesterol and phospholipids increase during lipid infusion in neonates. Because LCAT activity is particularly low in infants with very low birth weights, infusion of phospholipids in excess of the infant's clearing ability results in the accumulation of a specific low-density protein, lipoprotein-X. Finally, for fatty acid oxidation to occur, carnitine and acyl-CoA carnitine transferases are essential for permitting transmembranous transport into mitochondria; carnitine synthesis and storage are limited at birth, particularly in infants with very low birth weights.

HEPARIN AND LIPID CLEARANCE IN THE NEWBORN

The clearance of lipid emulsion from the blood occurs similarly to that of natural chylomicrons and is dependent on the activity of lipoprotein lipase.[214, 263] Mature newborns are better able to clear IV lipid emulsions than are preterm neonates. Heparin releases endothelial lipoprotein lipase and hepatic lipase into the circulation. Heparin can increase the activity of lipoprotein lipase, and when it is given in high doses (137 units/day), the increased lipoprotein lipase activity produces high levels of free fatty acids.[296] These results suggest that the heparin-stimulated intravascular lypolysis might exceed a premature infant's ability to clear free fatty acids. Therefore, the use of high-dose heparin in premature infants to stimulate intravascular lipolysis is not recommended.

LIPID EMULSIONS OF 20% VERSUS 10%

The availability of 20% lipid emulsions allows a reduction in the total amount of fluid administered without a reduction in the amount of energy supplied to the infant. The 20% solutions have lower phospholipid-to-triglyceride ratios and liposomal contents than the 10% solutions and have been shown to result in lower plasma triglyceride, cholesterol, and phospholipid concentrations.[216, 217] Given the documented advantages of 20% solutions, they are clearly preferred over 10% solutions.[272]

EMULSIONS CONTAINING MEDIUM-CHAIN TRIGLYCERIDES AND OTHER ALTERNATIVES

The only IV lipid emulsions available in North America are made from soybean oil or a combination with safflower oil. Emulsions using safflower oil as the only oil source are no longer used because of the development of omega-3 fatty acid deficiency, particularly in infants with very low birth weights. However, emulsions containing MCTs are being used elsewhere around the world.[241] There are several theoretical advantages for using IV MCTs. MCTs are hydrolyzed more rapidly by lipoprotein lipase, and the medium-chain fatty acids undergo more rapid oxidation.[198] These solutions have been shown to be well tolerated by infants and result in lower serum cholesterol.[241, 281] However, a study in preterm infants demonstrated that MCT-containing lipid emulsions may not be as effective as LCT-containing emulsions in promoting protein accretion.[240] The composition of IV lipid emulsions is provided in Table 33–10.

In the future, IV lipid emulsions might even contain other types of triglycerides. The addition of short-chain fatty acids seems to reduce small intestinal mucosal atrophy associated with TPN after massive bowel resection.[235, 236] The infusion of very-long-chain fatty acids might prevent TPN-induced liver cholestasis and provide additional protection against oxygen toxicity. Another reason for adjusting the composition of IV lipid emulsions for preterm neonates is the high linoleic acid content, which is known to cause abnormalities in phospholipid composition in the liver and brain of human neonates[247] and has been shown to reduce desaturation and elongation of essential fatty acids in rats.[228]

CARNITINE

Carnitine acts primarily in the transport of long-chain fatty acids across the mitochondrial membrane, where they can be further metabolized. The high free fatty acid levels associated with improved triglyceride hydrolysis probably reflect the limited capacity of preterm infants to oxidize fatty acids due to relative carnitine deficiency. Because preterm infants have low carnitine depots and limited ability to synthesize carnitine, administration of carnitine-free TPN results in low plasma and tissue carnitine levels,[178, 224] and these concentrations decline with postnatal age.[178, 288] Sev-

TABLE 33–10 COMPARISON OF COMMERCIAL (20%) INTRAVENOUS LIPID EMULSIONS AND HUMAN MILK

	INTRALIPID	LIPOSYN-II	MEDIALIPID	CLINOLEIC	HUMAN MILK
TG (gm/L)	200	200	200	200	40
PL (gm/L)	12	12	12	12	0.3
Glycerol (gm/L)	22	25	25	22.5	—
Fatty acids (%)					
Palmitic acid C16:0	10	9	4.5	10.7	22
Stearic acid C18:0	3	3	1.5	3	7
Oleic acid C18:1	25	18	13	65	30
Linoleic acid C18:2	54	66	27	17	15
Linolenic acid C18:3	8	4	4	0.3	0.5

PL, phospholipids; TG, triglycerides.

eral short-term studies showed inconclusive results for carnitine supplementation of TPN solutions.[178, 193, 253] However, carnitine supplementation has been shown to improve fat utilization in infants on long-term parenteral nutrition[225] and is recommended for infants receiving TPN for longer than 4 weeks.[188]

INTRODUCING, ADMINISTERING, AND MONITORING LIPID INFUSIONS

There is much controversy over the early introduction of IV lipid emulsions, particularly in sick infants with very low birth weights. Early studies found an increase in the incidence and severity of chronic lung disease in infants with very low birth weights started on IV lipids in the first week of life. However, more recent studies demonstrated that fat is well tolerated with no adverse effects, including chronic lung disease, even if introduced on the first day of life.[181, 208, 294] Additional concerns regarding parenteral lipids include free fatty acids displacing bilirubin from albumin binding sites and impairment of oxygenation. These issues have been discussed in detail and can be addressed by limiting the rate of infusion by providing lipid over a 24-hour period.[272]

Minimal parenteral fat intake prevents essential fatty acid deficiency and provides additional energy to meet metabolic needs. Essential fatty acid deficiency can develop in infants with extremely low birth weights in less than 72 hours if exogenous fat is not administered.[205] Essential fatty acid deficiency can be avoided through provision of 0.5 to 1 gm/kg per day of IV lipid.[192, 238] The maximum parenteral lipid intake in infants with extremely low birth weights is limited by their inability to remove plasma lipids and by possible side effects; these difficulties can be minimized by infusing lipids over a 24-hour period. The maximum value above that required to prevent essential fatty acid deficiency remains controversial. Several sources recommend a gradual intake of lipid with a maximum fat intake of 2 to 3 gm/kg per day in preterm infants and 3 to 4 gm/kg per day in term infants.

Routine monitoring of serum triglyceride is necessary as lipids are being advanced. Recommendations for plasma triglyceride levels range from less than 150 mg/dL to 200 mg/dL or less.[167, 186]

ELECTROLYTES, MINERALS, AND TRACE ELEMENTS IN PARENTERAL NUTRITION

SODIUM, POTASSIUM, AND CHLORIDE

Sodium can be given as chloride, lactate, acetate, or phosphate salts. Potassium can be provided as chloride, acetate, or phosphate salts. Infants who receive electrolytes solely as chloride salts may develop hyperchloremic metabolic acidosis. A randomized trial demonstrated the utility of acetate in parenteral nutrition solutions.[259]

During the first week of life, infants of less than 28 weeks' gestation often have larger water losses than sodium losses. To prevent hyperosmolar hypernatremia, some have suggested that the sodium intake during the first week of life not exceed 3 mmol/kg per day (equivalent to 3 mEq/kg per day); others have recommended completely excluding sodium for infants with extremely low birth weights. Frequent monitoring of serum sodium and water-sodium balance is mandatory. After the second week of life, sodium requirements are estimated at 3 to 6 mmol/kg per day.[170, 210, 285]

The daily chloride maintenance intake must not be less than 1 mmol/kg per day (the recommended intake is 2 to 3 mmol/kg per day), and in general it should be given as sodium chloride. Also, chloride should not be forgotten when sodium bicarbonate or acetate is given to correct metabolic acidosis.[170]

Hyperkalemia in infants weighing less than 1000 gm is due to a combination of the high rate of cell protein metabolism, potassium shift between the intracellular and extracellular compartments, and immature renal distal tubular function. Serum levels must be monitored closely.[170, 213] After the first week of life, a maintenance dose of 1 to 3 mmol/kg per day prevents hypokalemia.[170] Further discussion of IV electrolyte requirements can be found elsewhere.[184]

CALCIUM, PHOSPHORUS, AND MAGNESIUM

Inadequate calcium and phosphorus intakes have been associated with diminished bone mineralization (osteopenia) in premature infants who are supported with parenteral nutrition. Calcium and phosphorus cannot be provided in the same parenteral solution at concentrations needed to support in utero accretion because of precipitation.[210, 271, 285] The solubility of calcium and phosphorus in parenteral solutions depends on temperature, type and concentration of amino acid, dextrose concentration, pH, type of calcium salt, sequence of addition of calcium and phosphorus to the solution, the calcium-to-phosphorus ratio, and the presence of lipid.[210, 215, 234, 257] Adding cysteine to the parenteral nutrition lowers the pH, which improves calcium and phosphorus solubility. To achieve tissue accumulation of calcium and phosphorus with a minimum of side effects, current recommendations are to use parenteral nutrition solutions containing 50 to 60 mg/dL of calcium, 40 to 50 mg/dL of phosphorus, and 3.6 to 4.8 mg/dL of magnesium, with a calcium-to-phosphorus ratio of 1.7:1 to 1.3:1 by weight and 1.3:1 to 1:1 by molar ratio.[234] Calcium-to-phosphorus ratios of 1.7:1 (by weight) appear to be optimal.[257]

TRACE ELEMENTS

Recommended amounts of trace metals for term and preterm infants are listed in Table 33–11. The 1993 consensus recommendations for preterm infants are defined as transitional (within the first 2 weeks of life) and stable (after 2 weeks of age) and are similar to the American Society for Clinical Nutrition (ASCN) guidelines from 1988.[210, 285] Both agree that zinc should be included in parenteral solutions from day 1 and

that the other trace elements probably are not needed within the first 2 weeks of life.

Zinc and copper are available in the sulfate form and can be added separately to parenteral solutions. Several pediatric trace metal solutions are available that contain zinc, copper, manganese, and chromium in varying proportions. When trace metal solutions are added in amounts that provide the recommended levels for copper, manganese, and chromium, additional zinc is needed to provide the recommended intake for premature infants and those younger than 3 months of age. Because preterm infants can become selenium deficient after 3 weeks of IV feeding, supplementation is suggested after 2 weeks of age.[243, 276] Copper and manganese are discontinued in solutions administered to infants with cholestasis, and chromium and selenium are used with caution and in smaller amounts when renal output is low.[210, 276] Parenteral iron is required only when parenteral nutrition is fed exclusive of an iron-supplemented enteral intake to premature infants for the first 2 months of life or if iron deficiency develops.[204, 210]

INTRAVENOUS VITAMINS IN PARENTERAL NUTRITION

Guidelines for multivitamin administration are listed in Table 33–12. These recommendations are largely based on vitamin concentrations measured in term and preterm infants who received various amounts of the different vitamins.[210]

The delivery of vitamins from parenteral solutions

TABLE 33–11 RECOMMENDED PARENTERAL INTAKE OF TRACE ELEMENTS FOR TERM AND PRETERM INFANTS

| | TERM (μg/kg/day) | PRETERM (μg/kg/day) | | |
| | | Consensus Recommendations (1993) | | |
TRACE ELEMENT	ASCN (1988)	Transitional (first 2 wks of life)	Stable (>2 wks old)	ASCN (1988)
Chromium*	0.20	0–0.05	0.05–0.2	0.2
Copper†	20	0–20	20	20
Iron‡	—	0–0.2	0.1–0.2	—
Fluoride§	—	—	—	—
Iodide	1	1	1	1
Manganese†	1	0–0.75	1	1
Molybdenum	0.25	0	0.25	0.25
Selenium*	2	0–1.3	1.5–2	2
Zinc‖	250	150	400	400

*Renal dysfunction can cause toxicity.

†Impaired biliary excretion can cause toxicity.

‡Recommendation is made with caution because of very limited experience with IV iron in infants and lack of a safe, acceptable IV preparation (estimated daily IV requirement is 100 μg/kg for term infants and 200 μg/kg for preterm infants).

§Because of a lack of information on the compatibility of fluoride in TPN and on the contamination level of fluoride in TPN, firm recommendations cannot be made; with long-term TPN (longer than 3 mos), a dosage of 500 μg/day may be important in preterm infants, who already have a higher incidence of dental caries.

‖The only trace element recommended on day 1 of parenteral nutrition. If the infant requires TPN for longer than 3 mos, the dosage must be reduced to 100 μg/kg/day.

ASCN, American Society for Clinical Nutrition; TPN, total parenteral nutrition.

From the American Society for Clinical Nutrition, Subcommittee on Pediatric Parenteral Nutrient Requirements, from the Committee on Clinical Practice Issues, 1988; and Tsang RC, et al (eds): Nutritional Needs of the Preterm Infant: Scientific Basis and Practical Guidelines. Baltimore, Williams & Wilkins, 1993.

TABLE 33–12 RECOMMENDED PARENTERAL INTAKE OF VITAMINS FOR TERM AND PRETERM INFANTS

VITAMIN	TERM (Daily Dose)		PRETERM (dose/kg/day)*		
	ASCN (1998)	MVI-Pediatric (1 vial; 5 mL)	Consensus Recommendations (1993)	ASCN (1998)	MVI-Pediatric (40% of vial; 2 mL/kg/day)
Fat Soluble					
Vitamin A (IU)	2300	2300	700–1500	1640	920
With lung disease	—	—	1500–2800	—	—
Vitamin D (IU)	400	400	40–160	160	160
Vitamin E (IU)	7	7	3.5 (max = 7)	2.8	2.8
Vitamin K (μg)	200	200	8–10 (300 at birth)	80†	80
Water Soluble					
Vitamin B$_6$ (μg)	1000	1000	150–200	180	400
Vitamin B$_{12}$ (μg)	1	1	0.3	0.3	0.4
Vitamin C (mg)	80	80	15–25	25	32
Biotin (μg)	20	20	5–8	6	8
Folic acid (μg)	140	140	56	56	56
Niacin (mg)	17	17	4–6.8	6.8	6.8
Pantothenate (mg)	5	5	1–2	2	2
Riboflavin (μg)	1400	1400	150–200	150	560
Thiamin (μg)	1200	1200	200–350	350	480

The consensus recommendations (1993) and the American Society for Clinical Nutrition (ASCN) recommendations (1988) are currently not achievable because no ideal IV vitamin preparation is available for preterm infants; 40% of a vial (2 mL/kg/day) of MVI-Pediatric (Armor, USA; Rorer, Canada) is the closest intake that can be achieved at this time.

*Maximum not to exceed dosage for term infant.

†This does not include the 0.5 to 1 mg of vitamin K to be given at birth, as recommended by the American Academy of Pediatrics.

From the American Society for Clinical Nutrition, Subcommittee on Pediatric Parenteral Nutrient Requirements, from the Committee on Clinical Practice Issues, 1988; Tsang RC, et al (ed): Nutritional Needs of the Preterm Infant: Scientific Basis and Practical Guidelines. Baltimore, Williams & Wilkins, 1993; American Medical Association, Department of Food and Nutrition: JPEN J Parenter Enteral Nutr 3:258, 1979.

can be lower than intended. Fat-soluble vitamins may adsorb into the storage bag and delivery tubing; as much as 80% of available vitamin A has been shown to be lost to adsorption.[211, 289] Delivery of the fat-soluble vitamins, particularly vitamin A, may be significantly enhanced if they are infused with separate IV lipid solutions or with admixtures of lipid and amino acid–dextrose solutions.[171] Many of the vitamins are subject to alteration when exposed to light, oxygen, and heat. Therefore, significant destruction may occur within the newborn intensive care unit environment, where higher environmental temperatures and light levels are commonplace.[222]

These studies and recommendations were directed at infants greater than 1000 gm birth weight; the specific vitamin needs of infants with extremely low birth weights remain uncertain.[212] The recommended parenteral intake can be approximated but not precisely delivered with the only available multivitamin preparation. At the standard dosage (2 mL/gm per day), lower amounts of vitamin A and higher amounts of most of the B vitamins are provided.

COMPLICATIONS OF PARENTERAL NUTRITION

Although myriad complications of parenteral nutrition have been reported from the early days of its use, most of these are now rare with the use of present parenteral formulations. Some of the complications

(electrolyte imbalance, hypoglycemia, hyperglycemia, hypocalcemia, hypercalcemia, hypophosphatemia) can be prevented or corrected by manipulating the constituents of the infusate. The primary complications of parenteral nutrition as currently used are cholestasis and complications related to the line.

Hepatic dysfunction has long been recognized as an important complication of parenteral nutrition; this dysfunction is manifested primarily as cholestatic jaundice. The initial lesion seen histologically is cholestasis, both intracellular and intracanalicular, followed by portal inflammation and progressing to bile duct proliferation after several weeks of TPN. With prolonged administration, portal fibrosis and ultimately cirrhosis may develop.

Beale and coworkers reported an incidence of TPN-associated cholestasis of 50% in infants whose birth weight was less than 1000 gm after 2 weeks of hyperalimentation, 18% in those with a birth weight between 1000 and 1499 gm, and 7% in those with a birth weight of 1500 to 2000 gm. The incidence of cholestasis in infants receiving TPN for longer than 90 days is over 90% regardless of birth weight.[172] Similar trends have been reported by other authors, suggesting that those at greatest risk for this complication are premature infants receiving only TPN for prolonged periods.[258, 270]

The precise cause of the cholestasis is unknown and most likely multifactorial. This is expected, considering that the patients at greatest risk are critically ill premature infants who are susceptible to multiple insults, such as hypoxia, hemodynamic instability, and sepsis. A higher incidence of sepsis has been reported in infants affected by cholestasis.[179, 246, 258] Perhaps an equally if not more important factor in the development of cholestasis is the prolonged lack of enteral nutrition; there is expanding evidence that enteral feedings, even at low caloric intakes, can reduce the incidence of cholestasis.[232]

Early studies of parenteral nutrition suggested a possible relationship between the quantity of amino acids and hepatic dysfunction.[177] More recent studies, using historical controls, suggest that the newer amino acid solutions may result in less cholestasis.[221] The specific role of the quantity and composition of parenteral amino acids in the cause of cholestatic jaundice in premature infants remains unclear.

An infant with TPN-associated cholestasis develops a direct hyperbilirubinemia and jaundice, although histologic changes in the liver begin occurring before this is clinically apparent.[174, 190, 270] The earliest detectable biochemical marker, although not routinely measured, is an increase in serum bile acids.[177, 293] In addition to direct hyperbilirubinemia, another sensitive but nonspecific indicator of early cholestatic change is an elevation of γ-glutamyl transpeptidase.[177, 250] Elevation of hepatic transaminases (SGOT and SGPT) is a late finding.[174, 177, 270] The clinical evidence of cholestasis usually resolves with discontinuation of TPN and initiation of enteral feedings. There are reports of advanced liver disease and hepatic failure in infants on TPN[227, 258, 270]; however, severe changes resulting in irreversible liver failure are thought to occur only after several months of use.

As previously noted, normal bile flow usually returns when parenteral nutrition is stopped and enteral feeding is begun. In infants with TPN-associated cholestasis who require continued parenteral nutrition, the use of hypocaloric enteral feeding in combination with parenteral nutrition may stabilize or improve hepatic function. Use of phenobarbital and ursodeoxycholic acid has been shown to be beneficial in some cholestatic states in older children and adults; however, the information on neonates is inadequate to recommend their use.

Indwelling venous catheters used to deliver TPN also may be the source of complications. Both peripheral and central venous routes have been used to deliver TPN, but central delivery allows use of more concentrated formulations. The complications associated with venous catheters are usually the result of improper insertion or placement, bacterial or fungal colonization of the catheter, or vessel irritation or thrombosis.

Peripheral venous access usually is accomplished with Teflon catheters, which may infiltrate within a short time; however, the inclusion of fat emulsion in the infusate may delay the time until infiltration.[261, 262, 267] Peripheral Teflon catheters also may become colonized with bacteria at a rate of over 30% in catheters that have been in place longer than 3 days; peripheral venous catheters placed in the extremities are twice as likely to become colonized as those placed in scalp veins.[197]

Central venous catheters provide the advantage of a lower incidence of infiltration and an ability to deliver higher concentrations of infusate. However, they are not without potential disadvantages. Broviac catheters, in particular, are less than optimal for use in neonates because of the high incidence of infection, ranging from less than 5% to more than 60%, and thrombosis associated with their use in this population.[249, 282] Long-line, small-bore catheters that can be introduced percutaneously or surgically are available for use in the neonatal population.[203, 209] These catheters are composed of either silicone or polyurethane. The incidence of sepsis (less than 10% in all series) and thrombosis with either silicone or polyurethane lines is much lower than with the Broviac catheter.[203, 209] The incidence of line sepsis is not affected by whether these lines are placed percutaneously or surgically; however, there is a lower incidence of both infection and mechanical complication if these lines originate in a distal vein (scalp, arm, hand) rather than a proximal one.[209] Pericardial tamponade, arguably the most serious complication, has been reported to occur with catheters made of both materials.[166, 207, 209] Similarly, vascular perforation, another potentially serious complication, has been reported to occur with both types of catheters; however, in each case, involvement was limited to the extracorporeal portion of the catheter.[209] Thrombosis in these small-bore catheters can be minimized by adding heparin to the infusate in a 1:1 ratio.[203]

Infection is probably the most frequent serious complication associated with peripheral and central catheters. Two of the most commonly implicated bacterial agents are *Staphylococcus epidermidis* and *Staphylococcus aureus*[173, 197]; *Candida albicans* and *Malassezia furfur* (a lipophilic skin flora yeast)[251, 290] are the fungal agents most often implicated. The incidence of sepsis as a complication of TPN increases as gestational age decreases and the duration of TPN increases.[173] The predisposition to develop sepsis in these infants probably is multifactorial. As noted earlier, the incidence of sepsis increases in infants who have developed cholestasis.[179, 246, 258] There is also some evidence that the infusate per se may predispose these infants to nosocomial sepsis. An association has been reported between the use of IV lipid and coagulase-negative staphylococcal bacteremia. Similarly, there are numerous reports of *M. furfur* fungemia in infants receiving IV lipid.[244, 274] In both cases, the incidence increases when lipid is added to the infusate, suggesting that the lipid may provide a rich growth medium for skin flora that have colonized indwelling catheters.

PRACTICAL APPROACH TO ADMINISTRATION OF PARENTERAL NUTRITION

As advances in neonatal care enable increasingly premature and tiny babies to survive, the need for maximizing nutritional support in this population cannot be overemphasized. In 1998, infants with extremely low birth weights (401 to 1000 gm) born at centers participating in the NICHD Neonatal Research Network who survived longer than 72 hours received parenteral nutrition for an average of 27 days (1998 Generic Data Base, NICHD Neonatal Research Network). In addition, many term infants have medical and surgical disorders that preclude enteral feeding in the first several days to weeks of life. Infants who will not receive full-volume enteral feeds for more than several days are likely to benefit from parenteral nutrition.

Early provision of parenteral nutrition, particularly to an infant with extremely low birth weight, is important for a variety of reasons. Glucose solutions alone, with or without electrolyte and mineral additives, cannot prevent protein catabolism or maintain in utero rates of growth and protein accretion. In fact, infants who receive glucose alone obligatorily lose at least 1% of their endogenous nitrogen stores daily. To maximize protein accretion in a newborn infant, an appropriate balance of nonprotein substrate and amino acids must be provided. In addition, exogenous lipids are crucial both for increasing caloric intake and for preventing essential fatty acid deficiency.

The following are practical guidelines for administering parenteral nutrition to term and preterm infants. These recommendations are intended to present a reasonable approach to parenteral nutrition based on the available data.

Parenteral nutrition may be delivered by peripheral IV catheters, central venous catheters, or percutaneous central venous catheters. The decision as to which route is used should be individualized and based on an estimate of how long the infant will be unable to tolerate enteral feedings. In general, a peripheral IV is likely to be adequate to maintain nutritional stores over 1 to 2 weeks, whereas a central line will support growth when a baby is expected to require parenteral nutrition for more than 2 weeks. Percutaneous central venous catheters are being used with increasing frequency in the neonatal intensive care unit, because they allow delivery of a more concentrated nutrient infusate and typically can be maintained longer than a single peripheral IV line. Percutaneous central venous catheters are reasonably safe, although complications have been reported.

Glucose should be provided in the parenteral nutrition solution to maintain normal plasma glucose concentrations and to meet the demand for glucose use. As discussed earlier in this chapter, the glucose production and utilization rates in a term infant are approximately 3 to 4 mg/kg per minute, whereas a premature infant has a much greater need, 6 to 8 mg/kg per minute. Infants who weigh 1000 gm or more usually tolerate a 10% glucose solution initially, whereas infants weighing less than 1000 gm probably need to be started on a 5% glucose solution, given their higher total fluid requirements and predisposition toward hyperglycemia.

Lipids can be started as early as the first day of life. Starting concentrations of 0.5 to 1 gm/kg per day,

infused over 24 hours using a 20% emulsion, should be well tolerated, even by an infant with very low birth weight. Recent studies have demonstrated the safety and efficacy of this approach. Lipid concentrations can gradually be advanced to a maximum of 3 gm/kg per day while normal serum triglyceride levels are monitored and maintained. Many newborn intensive care units routinely employ this slow, stepwise increase for both lipids and amino acids, but there is no compelling evidence that this practice is absolutely necessary.

The appropriate balance of glucose and lipid in parenteral nutrition is critical for achieving maximal nutritional benefit. In fact, nutrient and protein retention is maximal if the nonprotein caloric balance between carbohydrate and lipid is approximately 60:40.[252, 294] This more closely mimics the fat content of breast milk and minimizes excess energy expenditure, which can occur if a disproportionate amount of nonprotein calories is given as glucose. Even at higher protein intakes, a parenterally fed infant with extremely low birth weight may need 80 to 90 kcal/kg per day for nonprotein energy supplies. The caloric requirements of a parenterally fed neonate are much lower than those fed enterally. It is important to realize that providing excessive calories via parenteral nutrition does not correlate with higher rates of growth. In addition, it should be emphasized that it is not difficult to provide adequate nonprotein energy, and it can be done without using highly concentrated glucose solutions (Box 33–1).

This considered, glucose concentrations above 12.5% should be required only on rare occasions. In addition, glucose concentrations above 10% to 12.5% should be reserved for use with central venous access.

As discussed previously, amino acids should be started as early as possible. A pediatric crystalline amino acid mixture should be used, because these mixtures are more likely to approximate plasma amino acid patterns of normal, breast-feeding, term infants. The addition of cysteine to the amino acid solution is supported by currently available information. A reasonable goal would be to include 1.5 to 2 gm/kg per day of amino acids in the first 24 hours of life to supply maintenance protein. One approach to this goal, particularly in an infant with extremely low birth weight and rapidly changing fluid and electrolyte needs, is to give the amino acids in a volume of 80 to 100 mL/kg per day. Additional fluids plus electrolytes can then be "Y'd in" and adjusted as needed, depending on the infant's changing needs. To meet growth requirements, 2.5 to 3.5 gm/kg per day of amino acids and appropriate caloric supplies (at least 80 kcal/kg per day) should be provided to infants with extremely low birth weights.[313] As with the advancement of IV lipids, there are no data supporting the need to advance amino acid intake slowly, as has been the routine practice in many nurseries.

Electrolytes, minerals, and vitamins also should be included in the standard parenteral nutrition solution. Parenteral nutrition, once initiated, probably should be continued until enteral feedings constitute the in-

---

■ **BOX 33-1**

CALCULATING THE CALORIC VALUE OF PARENTERAL NUTRITION*

Example: Fluids at 140 mL/kg/day

$D_{12.5}W$	→17.5 gm/kg dextrose	= 60 kcal/kg	61% of total
Amino acids	→3 gm/kg	= 12 kcal/kg	12%
20% lipid	→3 gm/kg	= 27 kcal/kg	27%
		Total 99 kcal/kg	

Example: Fluids at 110 mL/kg/day

$D_{12.5}W$	→14 gm/kg dextrose	= 47 kcal/kg	55% of total
Amino acids	→3 gm/kg	= 12 kcal/kg	14%
20% lipid	→3 gm/kg	= 27 kcal/kg	31%
		Total 86 kcal/kg	

*Dextrose = 3.4 kcal/gm; protein = 4 kcal/gm; lipid = 9 kcal/gm.

---

fant's minimal fluid requirements. Understanding the optimal means of providing nutrition to neonates is an ongoing process. As survival of premature infants continues to improve, research efforts must focus on maximizing nutritional support.

ACKNOWLEDGMENT

We gratefully acknowledge the contribution of Dr. John Van Aerde to previous versions of this chapter. Some sections required only minor changes.

■ REFERENCES

Part One: Enteral Nutrition

1. American Academy of Pediatrics: Pediatric Nutrition Handbook. Elk Grove Village, Ill, American Academy of Pediatrics, 1998.
2. Anderson DM, et al: The relationship of neonatal alimentation practices to the occurrence of endemic necrotizing enterocolitis. Am J Perinatol 8:62, 1991.
3. Anderson GC, et al: Kangaroo care for premature infants. Am J Nurs 86:807, 1986.
4. Anderson TL, et al: A controlled trial of glucose versus glucose and amino acids in premature infants. J Pediatr 94:947, 1979.
5. Atkinson S: Human milk feeding of the micropremie. Clin Perinatol 27:235, 2000.
6. Auerbach KG, et al: When the mother of a premature infant uses a breast pump: What every NICU nurse needs to know. Neonatal Network 13:23, 1994.
7. Baeckert PA, et al: Vitamin concentrations in very low birth weight infants given vitamins intravenously in a lipid emulsion: Measurement of vitamins A, D, and E and riboflavin. J Pediatr 113:1057, 1988.
8. Bell EF: Upper limit of vitamin E in infant formulas. J Nutr 119:1829, 1989.
9. Bernbaum JC, et al: Growth and metabolic response of premature infants fed whey- or casein-dominant formulas after hospital discharge. J Pediatr 115:652, 1989.
10. Berseth CL: Effect of early feeding on maturation of the preterm infant's small intestine. J Pediatr 120:947, 1992.
11. Berseth CL, et al: Enteral nutrients promote postnatal maturation of intestinal motor activity in preterm infants. Am J Physiol 264:G1046, 1993.
12. Bitman J, et al: Comparison of the lipid composition of breast milk from mothers of term and preterm infants. Am J Clin Nutr 38:300, 1983.
13. Brunton J, et al: Growth and body composition in infants with bronchopulmonary dysplasia up to 3 months corrected age: A randomized trial of a high-energy nutrient-enriched formula fed after hospital discharge. J Pediatr 133:340, 1998.
14. Butte N: Energy requirements during infancy. In Tsang R, et al (eds): Nutrition during Infancy. Philadelphia, Hanley & Belfus, 1988, p 86.
15. Caple J, et al: The effect of feeding volume on the clinical outcome in premature infants. Pediatr Res 41:1359A, 1997.
16. Carlson S, et al: Trans fatty acids: Infant and fetal development. Am J Clin Nutr 66:715S, 1997.
17. Carlson S, et al: Docosahexaenoic acid status of preterm infants at birth and following feeding with human milk or formula. Am J Clin Nutr 44:798, 1986.
18. Carlson S, et al: Arachidonic acid status correlates with first year growth in preterm infants. Proc Natl Acad Sci U S A 90:1073, 1992.
19. Carlson SE, et al: First year growth of preterm infants fed standard compared to marine oil n-3 supplemented formula. Lipids 27:901, 1992.
20. Carlson SE, et al: Visual-acuity development in healthy preterm infants: Effect of marine-oil supplementation. Am J Clin Nutr 58:35, 1993.
21. Carlson SJ, et al: Higher protein intake improves growth of VLBW infants fed fortified breast milk. Pediatr Res 45:278A, 1999.
22. Carnielli V, et al: Medium-chain triacylglycerols in formulas for preterm infants: Effect on plasma lipids, circulating concentrations of medium-chain fatty acids, and essential fatty acids. Am J Clin Nutr 64:152, 1996.
23. Carnielli V, et al: The very low birth weight premature infant is capable of synthesizing arachidonic and docosahexaenoic acids from linoleic and linolenic acids. Pediatr Res 40:169, 1996.
24. Castillo RO, et al: Intestinal maturation in the rat: The role of enteral nutrients. JPEN J Parenter Enteral Nutr 12:490, 1988.
25. Catzeflis C, et al: Whole body protein synthesis and energy expenditure in very low birth weight infants. Pediatr Res 19:679, 1985.
26. Cauderay M, et al: Energy-nitrogen balances and protein turnover in small and appropriate for gestational age low birthweight infants. Eur J Clin Nutr 42:125, 1988.
27. Clandinin M, et al: Fatty acid utilization in perinatal de novo synthesis of tissues. Early Hum Dev 5:355, 1981.
28. Clandinin M, et al: Requirements of newborn infants for long chain polyunsaturated fatty acids. Acta Paediatr Scand Suppl 351:63, 1989.
29. Cooke R, et al: Vitamin D and mineral metabolism in the very low birth weight infant receiving 400 IU of vitamin D. J Pediatr 116:423, 1990.
30. Cooke RJ, et al: Feeding preterm infants after hospital discharge: Effect of dietary manipulation on nutrient intake and growth. Pediatr Res 43:355, 1998.
31. Covert RF, et al: Factors associated with age of onset of necrotizing enterocolitis. Am J Perinatol 6:455, 1989.

32. Craig-Schmidt MC, et al: The effect of hydrogenated fat in the diet of nursing mothers on lipid composition and prostaglandin content of human milk. Am J Clin Nutr 39:778, 1984.

33. Currao W, et al: Diluted formula for beginning the feeding of premature infants. Am J Dis Child 142:730, 1988.

34. Davey AM, et al: Feeding premature infants while low umbilical artery catheters are in place: A prospective, randomized trial. J Pediatr 124:795, 1994.

35. Ditzenberger G, et al: The effect of protein supplementation on the growth of premature infants <1500 grams. Pediatr Res 47:286A, 2000.

36. Dunn L, et al: Beneficial effects of early hypocaloric enteral feeding on neonatal gastrointestinal function: Preliminary report of a randomized trial. J Pediatr 112:622, 1988.

37. Dworkin LD, et al: Small intestinal mass of the rat is partially determined by indirect effects of intraluminal nutrition. Gastroenterology 71:626, 1976.

38. Ehrenkranz RA: Iron, folic acid, and vitamin B_{12}. In Tsang RC, et al (eds): Nutritional Needs of the Preterm Infant: Scientific Basis and Practical Guidelines. Baltimore, Williams & Wilkins, 1993, p 177.

39. Ernst JA, et al: Types and methods of feeding for infants. In Polin RA, et al (eds): Fetal and Neonatal Physiology. Philadelphia, WB Saunders Co, 1992, p 239.

40. ESPGAN: Committee report: Comment on the content and composition of lipids in infant formulas. Acta Paediatr Scand 80:887, 1991.

41. ESPGAN: Guidelines on infant nutrition. Acta Paediatr Scand Suppl 262:1, 1987.

42. ESPGAN: Nutrition and feeding of preterm infants. Acta Paediatr Scand Suppl 336:1, 1987.

43. Evans JR, et al: Effect of high-dose vitamin D supplementation on radiographically detectable bone disease of very low birth weight infants. J Pediatr 115:779, 1989.

44. Fall CHD, et al: Relation of infant feeding to adult serum cholesterol concentration and death from ischaemic heart disease. BMJ 304:801, 1992.

45. Fish WH, et al: Effect of intramuscular vitamin E on mortality and intracranial hemorrhage in neonates of 1000 grams or less. Pediatrics 85:578, 1990.

46. Freymond D, et al: Energy balance, physical activity, and thermogenic effect of feeding in premature infants. Pediatr Res 20:638, 1986.

47. Gaull GE: Taurine in pediatric nutrition: Review and update. Pediatrics 83:433, 1989.

48. Giles MM, et al: Magnesium metabolism in preterm infants: Effects of calcium, magnesium, and phosphorus, and of postnatal and gestational age. J Pediatr 117:147, 1990.

49. Goldman HI: Feeding and necrotizing enterocolitis. Am J Dis Child 134:553, 1980.

50. Gounaris A, et al: Minimal enteral feeding, nasojejunal feeding and gastrin levels in premature infants. Acta Paediatr Scand 79:226, 1990.

51. Grant J, et al: Effect of intermittent versus continuous enteral feeding on energy expenditure in premature infants. J Pediatr 118:928, 1991.

52. Greene HL, et al: Water-soluble vitamins: C, B_1, B_2, B_6, niacin, pantothenic acid, and biotin. In Tsang RC, et al (eds): Nutritional Needs of the Preterm Infant: Scientific Basis and Practical Guidelines. Baltimore, Williams & Wilkins, 1993, p 121.

53. Greenspan JS, et al: Neonatal gastric intubation: Differential respiratory effects between nasogastric and orogastric tubes. Pediatr Pulmonol 8:254, 1990.

54. Greer FR: Vitamin K. In Tsang RC, et al (eds): Nutritional Needs of the Preterm Infant: Scientific Basis and Practical Guidelines. Baltimore, Williams & Wilkins, 1993, p 111.

55. Greer, FR: Vitamin metabolism and requirements in the micropremie. Clin Perinatol 27:95, 2000.

56. Gross S: Vitamin E. In Tsang RC, et al (eds): Nutritional Needs of the Preterm Infant: Scientific Basis and Practical Guidelines. Baltimore, Williams & Wilkins, 1993, p 101.

57. Hachey DL, et al: Human lactation: Maternal transfer of dietary triglycerides labeled with stable isotopes. J Lipid Res 28:1185, 1987.

58. Hall RT, et al: Hypophosphatemia in breast-fed low-birth-weight infants following initial hospital discharge. Am J Dis Child 143:1191, 1989.

59. Hambridge KM: Trace minerals. In Hay WW Jr (ed): Neonatal Nutrition and Metabolism. St. Louis, Mosby, 1991.

60. Hamosh M: Lingual and breast milk lipases. Adv Pediatr 29:33, 1982.

61. Hamosh M: Long chain polyunsaturated fatty acids in neonatal nutrition. J Am Coll Nutr 13:546, 1994.

62. Hamosh M, et al: Fat absorption in premature infants: Medium-chain triglycerides and long-chain triglycerides are absorbed from formula at similar rates. J Pediatr Gastroenterol Nutr 13:143, 1991.

63. Hay WW Jr: Nutritional requirements of extremely low birthweight infants. Acta Paediatr Suppl 402:94, 1994.

64. Hay WW Jr: Nutritional requirements of the extremely-low-birth-weight infant. In Hay WW Jr (ed): Neonatal Nutrition and Metabolism. St. Louis, Mosby Yearbook, 1991, p 361.

65. Hayes KC, et al: Growth depression in taurine-depleted infant monkeys. J Nutr 110:2058, 1980.

66. Heird WC, et al: Protein intake and energy requirements of the infant. Semin Perinatol 15:438, 1991.

67. Heird WC, et al: Practical aspects of achieving positive energy balance in low birth weight infants. J Pediatr 120:S120, 1992.

68. Hoffman D, et al: Effects of supplementation with ω3 long-chain polyunsaturated fatty acids on retinal and cortical development in premature infants. Am J Clin Nutr 57(suppl):807S, 1993.

69. Innis S: Human milk and formula fatty acids. J Pediatr 120:S56, 1992.

70. Innis S: Plasma and red blood cell fatty acid values as indexes of essential fatty acids in the developing organs of infants fed with milk or formulas. J Pediatr 120:S78, 1992.

71. Janas LM, et al: Indices of protein metabolism in term infants fed either human milk or formulas with reduced protein concentration and various whey/casein ratios. J Pediatr 110:838, 1987.

72. Jarvenpaa AL, et al: Feeding the low-birth-weight infant. I. Taurine and cholesterol supplementation of formula does not affect growth and metabolism. Pediatrics 71:171, 1983.

73. Jensen R: The lipids in human milk. Prog Lipid Res 35:53, 1996.

74. Kashyap S, et al: Protein quality in feeding low birth weight infants: A comparison of whey-predominant versus casein-predominant formulas. Pediatrics 79:748, 1987.

75. Kashyap S, et al: Effects of varying protein and energy intakes on growth and metabolic response in low birth weight infants. J Pediatr 108:955, 1986.

76. Kashyap S, et al: Growth, nutrient retention, and metabolic response of low-birth-weight infants fed supplemented and unsupplemented preterm human milk. Am J Clin Nutr 52:254, 1990.

77. Kavanaugh K, et al: Reliability of weighing procedures for preterm infants. Nurs Res 38:178, 1989.

78. Kein C: Digestion, absorption, and fermentation of carbohydrates in the newborn. Clin Perinatol 23:211, 1996.

79. Kliegman R: Experimental validation of neonatal feeding practices. Pediatrics 103:492, 1999.

80. Koenig WJ, et al: Manometrics for preterm and term infants: A new tool for old questions. Pediatrics 95:203, 1995.

81. Koletzko B, et al: Cis- and trans-isomeric fatty acids in plasma lipids of newborn infants and their mothers. Biol Neonate 57:172, 1990.

82. Koletzko B, et al: The fatty acid composition of human milk in Europe and Africa. J Pediatr 120:S62, 1992.

83. Koo WK, et al: Calcium, magnesium, phosphorus, and vitamin D. In Tsang RC, et al (eds): Nutritional Needs of the Preterm Infant: Scientific Basis and Practical Guidelines. Baltimore, Williams & Wilkins, 1993, p 135.

84. La Gamma EF, et al: Feeding practices for infants weighing less than 1500 g at birth and the pathogenesis of necrotizing enterocolitis. Clin Perinatol 21:271, 1994.

85. Lawrence RA (ed): Breast Feeding: A Guide for the Medical Profession. St. Louis, Mosby, 1994.

86. Lebenthal E: Gastrointestinal maturation and motility patterns as indicators for feeding the premature infant. Pediatrics 95:207, 1995.

87. Lemons JA, et al: Very-low-birth-weight outcomes of the NICHD Neonatal Research Network, January 1995 through December 1996. Pediatrics 107:E1, 2001.

88. Lemons P, et al: Breast-feeding the premature infant. Clin Perinatol 13:111, 1986.

89. Levine GM, et al: Role of oral intake in maintenance of gut mass and disaccharide activity. Gastroenterology 67:975, 1974.

90. Life Sciences Research Office Report: Assessment of nutrient requirements for infant formulas. J Nutr 128:2059S, 1998.

91. Lonnerdal B, et al: A longitudinal study of the protein, nitrogen, and lactose contents of human milk from Swedish well-nourished mothers. Am J Clin Nutr 29:1127, 1976.

92. Lucas A: Minimal enteral feeding. Semin Neonatal Nutr Metab 1:2, 1993.

93. Lucas A, et al: Randomised trial of nutrition for preterm infants after discharge. Arch Dis Child 67:324, 1992.

94. Lucas A, et al: Gut hormones and "minimal enteral feeding." Acta Paediatr Scand 75:719, 1986.

95. Lucas A, et al: Metabolic and endocrine consequences of depriving preterm infants of enteral nutrition. Acta Paediatr Scand 72:245, 1983.

96. Lucas A, et al: Early diet in preterm babies and developmental status at 18 months. Lancet 335:1477, 1990.

97. Lucas A, et al: Breast milk and subsequent intelligence quotient in children born preterm. Lancet 339:261, 1992.

98. Lundstrom U, et al: At what age does iron supplementation become necessary in low-birth-weight infants? J Pediatr 91:878, 1977.

99. Makrides M, et al: Fatty acid composition of brain, retina, and erythrocytes in breast- and formula-fed infants. Am J Clin Nutr 60:189, 1994.

100. Marks KH, et al: Day-to-day energy expenditure variability in low birth weight neonates. Pediatr Res 21:66, 1987.

101. Mathew OP: Breathing patterns of preterm infants during bottle feeding: Role of milk flow. J Pediatr 119:960, 1991.

102. Mathew OP: Nipple units for newborn infants: A functional comparison. Pediatrics 81:688, 1988.

103. McClure R, et al: Randomised controlled trial of trophic feeding and gut motility. Arch Dis Child 80:54F, 1999.

104. McKeown RE, et al: Role of delayed feeding and of feeding increments in necrotizing enterocolitis. J Pediatr 121:764, 1992.

105. Meetze WH, et al: Gastrointestinal priming prior to full enteral nutrition in very low birth weight infants. J Pediatr Gastroenterol Nutr 5:163, 1989.

106. Meier P: Bottle- and breast-feeding: Effects on transcutaneous oxygen pressure and temperature in preterm infants. Nurs Res 37:36, 1988.

107. Meier PP, et al: Breastfeeding support services in the neonatal intensive-care unit. J Obstet Gynecol Neonatal Nurs 22:338, 1993.

108. Meier PP, et al: The accuracy of test weighing for preterm infants. J Pediatr Gastroenterol Nutr 10:62, 1990.

109. Melegh B: Carnitine supplementation in the premature. Biol Neonate 58:93, 1990.

110. Melhorn DK, et al: Vitamin E dependent anemia in the premature infant. I. Effects of large doses of medicinal iron. J Pediatr 79:569, 1971.

111. Micheli J-L, et al: Neonatal adaptation of energy and protein metabolism. J Perinat Med 19:87, 1991.

112. Modanlou H, et al: Growth, biochemical status, and mineral metabolism in very-low-birth-weight infants receiving fortified preterm human milk. J Pediatr Gastroenterol Nutr 5:762, 1986.

113. Moran JR, et al: Vitamin requirements. In Polin RA, et al (eds): Fetal and Neonatal Physiology. Philadelphia, WB Saunders Co, 1992, p 248.

114. Moro G, et al: Relationship between protein and energy in the feeding of preterm infants during the first month of life. Acta Paediatr Scand 73:49, 1984.

115. Neu J: The role of dietary cholesterol in infants. Compr Ther 18:35, 1992.

116. Nutrition Committee, Canadian Paediatric Society: Nutrient needs and feeding of premature infants. Can Med Assoc J 152:1765, 1995.

117. Oski FA: Iron requirements of the premature infant. In Tsang RC (ed): Vitamin and Mineral Requirements in Preterm Infants. New York, Marcel Dekker, 1985, p 99.

118. Ostertag SG, et al: Early enteral feeding does not affect the incidence of nectrotizing enterocolitis. Pediatrics 77:275, 1986.

119. Penn D, et al: Effect of nutrition on tissue carnitine concentrations in infants of different gestational ages. Biol Neonate 47:130, 1985.

120. Pierse P, et al: Nutritional value of human milk. Prog Food Nutr Sci 12:421, 1988.

121. Pinelli J, et al: Non-nutritive sucking for promoting physiologic stability and nutrition in preterm infants. Cochrane Database of Systematic Reviews, Issue 4, 2000.

122. Polberger SKT, et al: Growth of very low birth weight infants on varying amounts of human milk protein. Pediatr Res 25:414, 1989.

123. Putet G: Energy. In Tsang RC, et al (eds): Nutritional Needs of the Preterm Infant: Scientific Basis and Practical Guidelines. Baltimore, Williams & Wilkins, 1993, p 15.

124. Raiha N, et al: Milk protein intake in the term infant. I. Metabolic responses and effects on growth. Acta Paediatr Scand 75:881, 1986.

125. Raiha NC: Milk protein quantity and quality in term infants: Intakes and metabolic effects during the first 6 months. Acta Paediatr Scand Suppl 351:24, 1989.

126. Raupp P, et al: Biochemical evidence for the need of long-term mineral supplementation in an extremely low birth weight infant fed own mother's milk exclusively during the first 6 months of life. Eur J Pediatr 149:806, 1990.

127. Rayyis S, et al: Randomized trial of "slow" versus "fast" feed advancements on the incidence of necrotizing enterocolitis in very low birth weight infants. J Pediatr 134:293, 1999.

128. Reichman BL, et al: Diet, fat accretion, and growth in premature infants. N Engl J Med 305:1495, 1981.

129. Reifen RM, et al: Microminerals. In Tsang RC, et al (eds): Nutritional Needs of the Preterm Infant: Scientific Basis and Practical Guidelines. Baltimore, Williams & Wilkins, 1993, p 195.

130. Roberts S, et al: Energetic efficiency and nutrient accretion in preterm infants fed extremes of dietary intake. Clin Nutr 41C:105, 1987.

131. Robertson AF, et al: Feeding preterm infants. Clin Pediatr 32:36, 1993.

132. Rothman D, et al: The effect of short-term starvation on mucosal barrier function in the newborn rabbit. Pediatr Res 19:727, 1985.

133. Sauer PJJ, et al: Longitudinal studies on metabolic rate, heat loss, and energy cost of growth in low birth weight infants. Pediatr Res 18:254, 1984.

134. Sauerwald TU, et al: Intermediates in endogenous synthesis of C22:6w3 and C20:4w6 by term and preterm infants. Pediatr Res 41:183, 1997.

135. Sawatzki G, et al: Pitfalls in the design and manufacture of infant formulae. Acta Paediatr 402(suppl):40, 1994.

136. Schanler R, et al: Feeding strategies for premature infants: Beneficial outcomes of feeding fortified human milk versus preterm formula. Pediatrics 103:1150, 1999.

137. Schanler R, et al: Feeding strategies for premature infants: Randomized trial of gastrointestinal priming and tube-feeding method. Pediatrics 103:434, 1999.

138. Schmidt-Sommerfeld E, et al: Carnitine and total parenteral nutrition of the neonate. Biol Neonate 58:81, 1990.

139. Schulze K, et al: Spontaneous variability in minute ventilation oxygen consumption and heart rate of low birth weight infants. Pediatr Res 15:1111, 1981.

140. Schulze KF, et al: Energy expenditure, energy balance, and composition of weight gain in low birth weight infants fed diets of different protein and energy content. J Pediatr 110:753, 1987.

141. Shaker CS: Nipple feeding premature infants: A different perspective. Neonatal Network 8:9, 1990.

142. Shenai JP: Vitamin A. In Tsang RC, et al (eds): Nutritional Needs of the Preterm Infant: Scientific Basis and Practical Guidelines. Baltimore, Williams & Wilkins, 1993, p 87.

143. Shulman R, et al: Early feeding, antenatal glucocorticoids, and human milk decrease intestinal permeability in preterm infants. Pediatr Res 44:519, 1998.

144. Shulman R, et al: Early feeding, feeding intolerance, and lactase activity in preterm infants. J Pediatr 133:645, 1998.

145. Simmer K: Long chain polyunsaturated fatty acid supplementation in infants born at term. Cochrane Database of Systematic Reviews, Issue 4, 2000.

146. Sinclair LC: Energy needs during infancy. In Fomon S, et al (eds): Energy and Protein Needs during Infancy. Orlando, Fla, Academic Press, 1986, p 41.

147. Slagle TA, et al: Effect of early low-volume enteral substrate on subsequent feeding tolerance in very low birth weight infants. J Pediatr 113:526, 1988.

148. Specker BL, et al: Sunshine exposure and serum 25-hydroxyvitamin D concentrations in exclusively breast-fed infants. J Pediatr 107:372, 1985.

149. Stothers JK, et al: Oxygen consumption and neonatal sleep states. J Physiol 278:435, 1978.

150. Subcommittee on the Tenth Edition of the RDAs, FaNB, Commission of Life Sciences, National Research Council: Recommended dietary allowances. Washington, DC, National Academy Press, 1989.

151. Thureen PJ, et al: Direct measurement of the energy expenditure of physical activity in preterm infants. J Appl Physiol 85:223, 1998.

152. Troche B, et al: Early minimal feedings promote growth in critically ill premature infants. Biol Neonate 67:172, 1995.

153. Tyson JE, et al: Randomized trial of taurine supplementation for infants less than or equal to 1300-gram birth weight: Effect on auditory brainstem-evoked responses. Pediatrics 83:406, 1989.

154. Uauy R: Are ω-3 fatty acids required for normal eye and brain development in the human? J Pediatr Gastroenterol Nutr 11:296, 1990.

155. Uauy R, et al: Essential fat requirements of preterm infants. Am J Clin Nutr 71(suppl):245S, 2000.

156. Uauy R, et al: Safety and efficacy of omega-3 fatty acids in the nutrition of very low birth weight infants: Soy oil and marine oil supplementation of formula. J Pediatr 124:612, 1994.

157. Uauy R, et al: Essential fatty acid metabolism and requirements during development. Semin Perinatol 13:118, 1989.

158. Uauy RD, et al: Effect of dietary omega-3 fatty acids on retinal function of very-low-birth-weight neonates. Pediatr Res 28:485, 1990.

159. Usher R, et al: Intrauterine growth of live-born Caucasian infants at sea level: Standards obtained from measurements in 7 dimensions of infants born between 25 and 44 weeks of gestation. J Pediatr 74:901, 1969.

160. Van Aerde JEE: Acute respiratory failure and bronchopulmonary dysplasia. In Hay WW (ed): Neonatal Nutrition and Metabolism. Chicago, Yearbook Medical Publishers, 1991, p 476.

161. Walker M: Breastfeeding the premature infant. NAACOGS Clinical Issues in Perinatal and Women's Health Nursing 3:620, 1992.

162. Widdowson EM: Changes in body proportion and composition during growth. In Davis JA, et al (eds): Scientific Foundation of Pediatrics. Philadelphia, WB Saunders Co, 1974, p 73.

163. Wu P, et al: Gastrointestinal tolerance, fat absorption, plasma ketone and urinary dicarboxylic acid levels in low-birth-weight infants fed different amounts of medium-chain triglycerides in formula. J Pediatr Gastroenterol Nutr 17:145, 1993.

164. Yeh Y, et al: Impairment of lipid emulsion metabolism associated with carnitine insufficiency in premature infants. J Pediatr Gastroenterol Nutr 4:795, 1985.

165. Yu V: Enteral feeding in the preterm infant. Early Hum Dev 56:89, 1999.

Part Two: Parenteral Nutrition

166. Aiken G, et al: Cardiac tamponade from a fine silastic central venous catheter in a premature infant. J Paediatr Child Health 28:325, 1992.

167. American Academy of Pediatrics: Pediatric Nutrition Handbook. Elk Grove Village, Ill, American Academy of Pediatrics, 1998.

168. Anderson GH, et al: Dose-response relationships between amino acid intake and blood levels in newborn infants. Am J Clin Nutr 30:1110, 1977.

169. Anderson TL, et al: A controlled trial of glucose versus glucose and amino acids in premature infants. J Pediatr 94:947, 1979.

170. Arant BS: Sodium, chloride, and postassium. In Tsang RC, et al (eds): Nutritional Needs of the Preterm Infant: Scientific Basis and Practical Guidelines. Baltimore, Williams & Wilkins, 1993, p 157.

171. Baeckert PA, et al: Vitamin concentrations in very low birth weight infants given vitamins intravenously in a lipid emulsion: Measurement of vitamins A, D, and E and riboflavin. J Pediatr 113:1057, 1988.

172. Beale EF, et al: Intrahepatic cholestasis associated with parenteral nutrition in premature infants. Pediatrics 64:342, 1979.

173. Beganovic N, et al: Total parenteral nutrition and sepsis. Arch Dis Child 63:66, 1988.

174. Benjamin DR: Hepatobiliary dysfunction in infants and children associated with long-term total parenteral nutrition: A clinico-pathologic study. Am J Clin Pathol 76:76, 1981.

175. Berry M, et al: Factors associated with growth of extremely premature infants during initial hospitalization. Pediatrics 100:640, 1997.

176. Binder ND, et al: Insulin infusion with parenteral nutrition in extremely low birth weight infants with hyperglycemia. J Pediatr 114:273, 1989.

177. Black DD, et al: The effect of short-term total parenteral nutrition on hepatic function in the human neonate: A prospective randomized study demonstrating alteration of hepatic canalicular function. J Pediatr 99:445, 1981.

178. Bonner C, et al: Effects of parenteral L-carnitine supplementation on fat metabolism and nutrition in premature neonates. J Pediatr 126:287, 1995.

179. Bos AP, et al: Total parenteral nutrition associated cholestasis: A predisposing factor for sepsis in surgical neonates? Eur J Pediatr 149:351, 1990.

180. Brans YW, et al: Tolerance of fat emulsions in very low birthweight neonates: Effect of birthweight on plasma lipid concentrations. Am J Perinatol 7:114, 1990.

181. Brownlee K, et al: Early or late parenteral nutrition for the sick preterm infant. Arch Dis Child 69:281, 1993.

182. Brownlee KG, et al: Catabolic effect of dexamethasone in the preterm baby. Arch Dis Child 67:1, 1991.

183. Bulus N, et al: Physiologic importance of glutamine. Metabolism 38:1, 1989.

184. Canadian Paediatric Society, Nutrition Committee: Nutrient needs and feeding of premature infants. Can Med Assoc J 152:1765, 1995.

185. Carr B, et al: Total energy expenditure in extremely premature and term infants in early postnatal life. Pediatr Res 47:284A, 2000.

186. Chessex P, et al: Metabolic and clinical consequences of changing from high-glucose to high-fat regimens in parenterally fed newborn infants. J Pediatr 115:992, 1989.

187. Chessex P, et al: Effect of amino acid composition of parenteral solutions on nitrogen retention and metabolic response in very low birth weight infants. J Pediatr 106:111, 1985.

188. Christensen ML, et al: Plasma carnitine concentration and lipid metabolism in infants receiving parenteral nutrition. J Pediatr 115:794, 1989.

189. Clark SE, et al: Parenteral nutrition increases leucine oxidation but not phenylalanine hydroxylation in premature infants. Pediatr Res 41:568, 1997.

190. Cohen C, et al: Pediatric total parenteral nutrition: Liver histopathology. Arch Pathol Lab Med 105:152, 1981.

191. Collins JW, et al: A controlled trial of insulin infusion and parenteral nutrition in extremely low birth weight infants with glucose intolerance. J Pediatr 118:921, 1991.

192. Cooke R, et al: Soybean oil emulsion administration during parenteral nutrition in the preterm infant: Effect on essential fatty acid, lipid, and glucose metabolism. J Pediatr 111:767, 1987.

193. Coran A, et al: The metabolic effects of oral L-carnitine administration in infants receiving total parenteral nutrition with fat. J Pediatr Surg 20:758, 1985.

194. Cornblath M, et al: Hypoglycemia in the neonate. J Pediatr Endocrinol Metab 6:113, 1993.

195. Cornblath M, et al: Hypoglycemia in infancy: The need for a rational definition. Pediatrics 85:834, 1990.

196. Cowett RM: Utilization of glucose during total parenteral nutrition. In Lebenthal E (ed): Total Parenteral Nutrition. New York, Raven Press, 1986, p 123.

197. Cronin WA, et al: Intravascular catheter colonization and related bloodstream infection in critically ill neonates. Infect Control Hosp Epidemiol 11:301, 1990.

198. Deckelbaum R, et al: Medium-chain versus long-chain triacylglycerol emulsion hydrolysis by lipoprotein lipase and hepatic lipase: Implications for the mechanisms of lipase action. Biochemistry 29:1136, 1990.

199. Denne SC, et al: Glucose carbon recycling oxidation in human newborns. Am J Physiol 251:E71, 1986.

200. Denne SC, et al: Proteolysis and phenylalanine hydroxylation in response to parenteral nutrition in extremely premature and normal newborns. J Clin Invest 97:746, 1996.

201. Dorvil NP, et al: Taurine prevents cholestasis induced by lithocholic acid sulfate in guinea pigs. Am J Clin Nutr 37:221, 1983.

202. Duffy B, et al: The effect of varying protein quality and energy intake on the nitrogen metabolism of parenterally fed very low birthweight (<1600 g) infants. Pediatr Res 15:1040, 1981.

203. Durand M, et al: Prospective evaluation of percutaneous central venous Silastic catheters in newborn infants with birth weights of 510 to 3920 grams. Pediatrics 78:245, 1986.

204. Ehrenkranz RA: Iron, folic acid, and vitamin B12. In Tsang RC, et al (eds): Nutritional Needs of the Preterm Infant: Scientific Basis and Practical Guidelines. Baltimore, Williams & Wilkins, 1993, p 177.

205. Foote K, et al: Effect of early introduction of formula vs fat-free parenteral nutrition on essential fatty acid status of preterm infants. Am J Clin Nutr 54:93, 1991.

206. Geggel HS, et al: Nutritional requirement for taurine in patients receiving long-term parenteral nutrition. N Engl J Med 312:142, 1985.

207. Giacoia GP: Cardiac tamponade and hydrothorax as complications of central venous parenteral nutrition in infants. JPEN J Parenter Enteral Nutr 15:110, 1991.

208. Gilbertson N, et al: Introduction of intravenous lipid administration on the first day of life in the very low birth weight neonate. J Pediatr 119:615, 1991.

209. Goutail-Flaud MF, et al: Central venous catheter-related complications in newborns and infants: A 587-case survey. J Pediatr Surg 26:645, 1991.

210. Greene HL, et al: Guidelines for the use of vitamins, trace elements, calcium, magnesium, and phosphorus in infants and children receiving total parenteral nutrition. Am J Clin Nutr 48:1324, 1988.

211. Greene HL, et al: Persistently low blood retinol levels during and after parenteral feeding of very low birth weight infants: Examination of losses into intravenous administration sets and a method of prevention by addition to a lipid emulsion. Pediatrics 79:894, 1987.

212. Greer FR: Vitamin metabolism and requirements in the micropremie. Clin Perinatol 27:95, 2000.

213. Gruskay J, et al: Nonoliguric hyperkalemia in the premature infant weighing less than 1000 grams. J Pediatr 113:381, 1988.

214. Hamosh M: Lipid metabolism in premature infants. Biol Neonate 52:50, 1987.

215. Hanning R, et al: In vitro solubility of calcium glycerophosphate versus conventional mineral salts in pediatric total parenteral nutrition solutions. FASEB J 2:766, 1988.

216. Haumont D, et al: Plasma lipid and plasma lipoprotein concentrations in low birth weight infants given parenteral nutrition with twenty or ten percent lipid emulsion. J Pediatr 115:787, 1989.

217. Haumont D, et al: Effect of liposomal content of lipid emulsions on plasma lipid concentrations in low birth weight infants receiving parenteral nutrition. J Pediatr 121:759, 1992.

218. Hayes KC, et al: Growth depression in taurine-depleted infant monkeys. J Nutr 110:2058, 1980.

219. Heird W, et al: Pediatric parenteral amino acid mixture in low birth weight infants. Pediatrics 81:41, 1988.

220. Heird WC: New solutions for old problems with new solutions. In Cowett R, et al (eds): The Micropremie: The Next Frontier. Columbus, Ohio, Ross Laboratories, 1990, p 71.

221. Heird WC, et al: Amino acid mixture designed to maintain normal plasma amino acid patterns in infants and children requiring parenteral nutrition. Pediatrics 80:401, 1987.

222. Heird WC, et al: Parenteral nutrition. In Tsang RC, et al (eds): Nutritional Needs of the Preterm Infant. Baltimore, Williams & Wilkins, 1993, p 225.

223. Helms RA, et al: Comparison of a pediatric versus standard amino acid formulation in preterm neonates requiring parenteral nutrition. J Pediatr 110:466, 1987.

224. Helms RA, et al: Effect of intravenous L-carnitine on growth parameters and fat metabolism during parenteral nutrition in neonates. JPEN J Parenter Enteral Nutr 14:448, 1990.

225. Helms RA, et al: Enhanced lipid utilization in infants receiving oral L-carnitine during long-term parenteral nutrition. J Pediatr 109:984, 1986.

226. Hertz DE, et al: Intravenous glucose suppresses glucose production but not proteolysis in extremely premature newborns. J Clin Invest 92:1752, 1993.

227. Hodes JE, et al: Hepatic failure in infants on total parenteral nutrition: Clinical and histopathologic observations. J Pediatr Surg 17:463, 1982.

228. Innis SM: Effect of total parenteral nutrition with linoleic acid–rich emulsions on tissue omega 6 and omega 3 fatty acids in the rat. Lipids 21:132, 1986.

229. Jarvenpaa AL, et al: Feeding the low-birth-weight infant. I. Taurine and cholesterol supplementation of formula does not affect growth and metabolism. Pediatrics 71:171, 1983.

230. Kanerek KS, et al: Continuous infusion of insulin in hyperglycemic low-birth-weight infants receiving parenteral nutrition with and without lipid emulsion. JPEN J Parenter Enteral Nutr 15:417, 1991.

231. Kashyap S, et al: Protein requirements of low birthweight, very low birthweight, and small for gestational age infants. In Raiha N (ed): New York, Vevey/Raven Press, 1994, p 133.

232. Kelly D: Liver complications of pediatric parenteral nutrition—epidemiology. Nutrition 14:153, 1998.

233. Koh T, et al: Neural dysfunction during hypoglycemia. Arch Dis Child 63:1353, 1988.

234. Koo WK, et al: Calcium, magnesium, phosphorus, and vitamin D. In Tsang RC, et al (eds): Nutritional Needs of the Preterm Infant: Scientific Basis and Practical Guidelines. Baltimore, Williams & Wilkins, 1993, p 135.

235. Koruda MJ, et al: Parenteral nutrition supplemented with short-chain fatty acids: Effect on the small-bowel mucosa in normal rats. Am J Clin Nutr 51:685, 1990.

236. Kubota A, et al: The effect of metronidazole on TPN-associated liver dysfunction in neonates. J Pediatr Surg 25:18, 1990.

237. Lacey JM, et al: The effects of glutamine-supplemented parenteral nutrition in premature infants. JPEN J Parenter Enteral Nutr 20:74, 1996.

238. Lee EJ, et al: Essential fatty acid deficiency in parenterally fed preterm infants. J Paediatr Child Health 29:51, 1993.

239. Leitch C, et al: Energy expenditure in the extremely low-birth weight infant. Clin Perinatol 27:181, 2000.

240. Liet J-M, et al: Leucine metabolism in preterm infants receiving parenteral nutrition with medium-chain compared with long-chain triacylglycerol emulsions. Am J Clin Nutr 69:539, 1999.

241. Lima L: Neonatal parenteral nutrition with a fat emulsion containing medium chain triglycerides. Acta Pediatr Scand 77:332, 1988.

242. Lloyd DA: Energy requirements of surgical newborn infants receiving parenteral nutrition. Nutrition 14:101, 1998.

243. Lockitch G, et al: Selenium deficiency in low birth weight neonates: An unrecognized problem. J Pediatr 114:865, 1989.

244. Long JG, et al: Catheter-related infection in infants due to an unusual lipophilic yeast—Malassezia furfur. Pediatrics 76:896, 1985.

245. Malloy MH, et al: Total parenteral nutrition in sick preterm infants: Effects of cysteine supplementation with nitrogen intakes of 240 and 400 mg/kg/day. J Pediatr Gastroenterol Nutr 3:239, 1984.

246. Manginello FP, et al: Parenteral nutrition and neonatal cholestasis. J Pediatr 94:296, 1979.

247. Martinez M, et al: Effects of parenteral nutrition with high

doses of linoleate on the developing human liver and brain. Lipids 22:133, 1987.

248. Mitton SG: Amino acids and lipid in total parenteral nutrition for the newborn. J Pediatr Gastroenterol Nutr 18:25, 1994.

249. Mollitt DL, et al: Complications of TPN catheter-induced vena caval thrombosis in children less than one year of age. J Pediatr Surg 18:462, 1983.

250. Nanji AA, et al: Sensitivity and specificity of liver function tests in the detection of parenteral nutrition–associated cholestasis. JPEN J Parenter Enteral Nutr 9:307, 1985.

251. Nicholls JM, et al: *Malassezia furfur* infection in a neonate. Br J Hosp Med 49:425, 1993.

252. Nose O, et al: Effect of the energy source on changes in energy expenditure, respiratory quotient, and nitrogen balance during total parenteral nutrition in children. Pediatr Res 21:538, 1987.

253. Orzali A, et al: Effect of carnitine on lipid metabolism in the newborn. I. Carnitine supplementation during total parenteral nutrition in the first 48 hours of life. Biol Neonate 43:186, 1983.

254. Ostertag SG, et al: Insulin pump therapy in the very low birth weight infant. Pediatrics 78:625, 1986.

255. Padbury JF, et al: Glucose metabolism during the transition to postnatal life. In Polin RA, et al (eds): Fetal and Neonatal Physiology. Philadelphia, WB Saunders Co, 1991, p 402.

256. Paisley JE, et al: Safety and efficacy of low versus high parenteral amino acids in extremely low birth weight neonates immediately after birth. Pediatr Res 47:293A, 2000.

257. Pelegano JF, et al: Simultaneous infusion of calcium and phosphorus in parenteral nutrition for premature infants: Use of physiologic calcium/phosphorus ratio. J Pediatr 114:115, 1989.

258. Pereira GR, et al: Hyperalimentation-induced cholestasis: Increased incidence and severity in premature infants. Am J Dis Child 135:842, 1981.

259. Peters O, et al: Randomised controlled trial of acetate in preterm neonates receiving parenteral nutrition. Arch Dis Child 77:12F, 1997.

260. Pettei MJ, et al: Essential fatty acid deficiency associated with the use of a medium-chain-triglyceride infant formula in pediatric hepatobiliary disease. Am J Clin Nutr 53:1217, 1991.

261. Phelps SJ, et al: Effect of the continuous administration of fat emulsion on the infiltration of intravenous lines in infants receiving peripheral parenteral nutrition solutions. JPEN J Parenter Enteral Nutr 13:628, 1989.

262. Phelps SJ, et al: Risk factors affecting infiltration of peripheral venous lines in infants. J Pediatr 111:384, 1987.

263. Pierro A, et al: Metabolism of intravenous fat emulsion in the surgical newborn. J Pediatr Surg 24:95, 1989.

264. Pildes RS, et al: Hypoglycemia and hyperglycemia in tiny infants. Clin Perinatol 13:351, 1986.

265. Pineault M, et al: Total parenteral nutrition in the newborn: Impact of the quality of infused energy on nitrogen metabolism. Am J Clin Nutr 47:298, 1988.

266. Pineault M, et al: Total parenteral nutrition in the newborn: Amino acids–energy interrelationships. Am J Clin Nutr 48:1065, 1988.

267. Pineault M, et al: Beneficial effect of coinfusing a lipid emulsion on venous patency. JPEN J Parenter Enteral Nutr 13:637, 1989.

268. Poindexter B, et al: The effect of N-acetyl tyrosine and cysteine in parenteral nutrition on protein metabolism in extremely low birth weight neonates. Pediatr Res 47:294A, 2000.

269. Poindexter BB, et al: Exogenous insulin reduces proteolysis and protein synthesis in extremely low birth weight infants. J Pediatr 132:948, 1998.

270. Postuma R, et al: Liver disease in infants receiving total parenteral nutrition. Pediatrics 63:110, 1979.

271. Prestridge LL, et al: Effect of parenteral calcium and phosphorus therapy on mineral retention and bone mineral content in very low birth weight infants. J Pediatr 122:761, 1993.

272. Putet G: Lipid metabolism of the micropremie. Clin Perinatol 27:57, 2000.

273. Putet G, et al: Supplementation of pooled human milk with casein hydrolysate: Energy and nitrogen balance and weight gain composition in very low birth weight infants. Pediatr Res 21:458, 1987.

274. Redline RW, et al: Systemic *Malassezia furfur* infections in patients receiving intralipid therapy. Hum Pathol 16:815, 1985.

275. Reichman BL, et al: Partition of energy metabolism and energy cost of growth in the very low-birth-weight infant. Pediatrics 69:446, 1982.

276. Reifen RM, et al: Microminerals. In Tsang RC, et al (eds): Nutritional Needs of the Preterm Infant: Scientific Basis and Practical Guidelines. Baltimore, Williams & Wilkins, 1993, p 195.

277. Rigo J, et al: A new amino acid solution specially adapted to preterm infants. Clin Nutr 6:105, 1987.

278. Rivera A, et al: Effect of intravenous amino acids on protein metabolism of preterm infants during the first three days of life. Pediatr Res 33:106, 1993.

279. Rivera A Jr, et al: Plasma amino acid profiles during the first three days of life in infants with respiratory distress syndrome: Effect of parenteral amino acid supplementation. J Pediatr 115:465, 1989.

280. Roig JC, et al: Enteral glutamine supplementation for the very low birthweight infant: Plasma amino acid concentrations. J Nutr 126:1115S, 1996.

281. Rubin M, et al: Lipid infusion with different triglyceride cores (long-chain vs medium-chain/long-chain triglycerides): Effect on plasma lipids and bilirubin binding in premature infants. JPEN J Parenter Enteral Nutr 15:642, 1991.

282. Sadiq HF, et al: Broviac catheterization in low birth weight infants: Incidence and treatment of associated complications. Crit Care Med 15:47, 1987.

283. Saini J, et al: Early parenteral feeding of amino acids. Arch Dis Child 64:1362, 1989.

284. Salas-Salvado J, et al: Effect of the quality of infused energy on substrate utilization in the newborn receiving total parenteral nutrition. Pediatr Res 33:112, 1993.

285. Schanler RJ, et al: Parenteral nutrient needs of low birth weight infants. J Pediatr 125:961, 1994.

286. Seashore JH, et al: Urinary 3-methylhistidine/creatinine ratio as a clinical tool: Correlation between 3-methylhistidine excretion and metabolic and clinical states in healthy and stressed premature infants. Metabolism 30:959, 1981.

287. Senterre J: Nitrogen balances and protein requirements of preterm infants. In Visser H (ed): Nutrition and Metabolism of the Fetus and Infant. The Hague, Martinus Nijhoff, 1979.

288. Shenai JP, et al: Tissue carnitine reserves of newborn infants. Pediatr Res 18:679, 1984.

289. Shenai JP, et al: Vitamin A delivery from parenteral alimentation solution. J Pediatr 99:661, 1981.

290. Sheretz RJ, et al: Outbreak of *Candida* bloodstream infections associated with retrograde medication administration in a neonatal intensive care unit. J Pediatr 120:455, 1992.

291. Smith RJ, et al: Glutamine nutrition and requirements. JPEN J Parenter Enteral Nutr 14:237, 1990.

292. Snyderman SE: The protein and amino acid requirements of the premature infant. In Jonxis JH, et al (eds): Nutricia Symposium: Metabolic Processes in the Fetus and Newborn Infant. Leiden, Netherlands, Stenfert Kroese, 1971.

293. Sondheimer JM, et al: Cholestatic tendencies in premature infants on and off parenteral nutrition. Pediatrics 62:984, 1978.

294. Sosenko I, et al: Effect of early initiation of intravenous lipid administration on the incidence and severity of chronic lung disease in premature infants. J Pediatr 123:975, 1993.

295. Sparks JW, et al: Parenteral galactose therapy in the glucose-intolerant premature infant. J Pediatr 100:255, 1982.

296. Spear ML, et al: Effect of heparin dose and infusion rate on lipid clearance and bilirubin binding in premature infants receiving intravenous fat emulsions. J Pediatr 112:94, 1988.

297. Sturman JA, et al: Absence of cystathionase in human fetal liver: Is cystine essential? Science 169:74, 1970.

298. Thureen P, et al: Direct measurement of the energy expenditure of physical activity in preterm infants. J Appl Physiol 85:223, 1998.

299. Tyson JE, et al: Randomized trial of taurine supplementation for infants less than or equal to 1300-gram birth weight: Effect on auditory brainstem-evoked responses. Pediatrics 83:406, 1989.

300. Uauy R, et al: Conditionally essential nutrients: Cysteine, tau-

rine, tyrosine, arginine, glutamine, choline, inositol, and nucleotides. In Tsang RC, et al (eds): Nutritional Needs of the Preterm Infant: Scientific Basis and Practical Guidelines. Baltimore, Williams & Wilkins, 1993, p 267.

301. Van Aerde J, et al: Metabolic consequences of increasing energy intake by adding lipid to parenteral nutrition in full-term infants. Am J Clin Nutr 59:659, 1994.

302. Van Goudoever JB, et al: Immediate commencement of amino acid supplementation in preterm infants: Effect on serum amino acid concentrations and protein kinetics on the first day of life. J Pediatr 127:458, 1995.

303. Van Goudoever JB, et al: Effect of dexamethasone on protein metabolism in infants with bronchopulmonary dysplasia. J Pediatr 124:112, 1994.

304. Van Lingen R, et al: Effects of early amino acid administration during total parenteral nutrition on protein metabolism in pre-term infants. Clin Sci 82:199, 1992.

305. VanEys J: Nonglucose Carbohydrates: Parenteral Nutrition. Philadelphia, WB Saunders Co, 1986.

306. Vileisis RA, et al: Glycemic response to lipid infusion in the premature neonate. J Pediatr 100:108, 1982.

307. Wilson DC, et al: Randomised controlled trial of an aggressive nutritional regimen in sick very low birthweight infants. Arch Dis Child Fetal Neonatal Ed 77:4F, 1997.

308. Yunis KA, et al: Glucose kinetics following administration of an intravenous fat emulsion to low-birth-weight neonates. Am J Physiol 263:E844, 1992.

309. Zelikovic I, et al: Taurine depletion in very low birth weight infants receiving prolonged total parenteral nutrition: Role of renal immaturity. J Pediatr 116:301, 1990.

310. Ziegler E, et al: Body composition of the reference fetus. Growth 40:329, 1976.

311. Zlotkin SH, et al: The development of cystathionase activity during the first year of life. Pediatr Res 16:65, 1982.

312. Zlotkin SH, et al: Sulfur balances in intravenously fed infants: Effects of cysteine supplementation. Am J Clin Nutr 36:862, 1982.

313. Zlotkin SH, et al: Intravenous nitrogen and energy intakes required to duplicate in utero nitrogen accretion in prematurely born human infants. J Pediatr 99:115, 1981.

314. Zlotkin SH, et al: Cysteine supplementation to cysteine-free intravenous feeding regimens in newborn infants. Am J Clin Nutr 34:914, 1981.

34 Fluid, Electrolytes, and Acid-Base Homeostasis

part one
FLUID AND ELECTROLYTE MANAGEMENT

Ira D. Davis and Ellis D. Avner

Fluid and electrolyte management is an important aspect of the care of infants considered to be high risk. It is particularly true for infants with low birth weight because of the frequent need for parenteral fluid administration; the variability of requirements in dictating the quantity and composition of parenteral fluids; the developmental limitations in renal homeostatic mechanisms; and the significant morbidity and mortality of fluid and electrolyte imbalance in the immature infant. In this chapter we discuss the physiologic principles that govern the estimation of fluid and electrolyte requirements for infants, methods of monitoring fluid and electrolyte balance, complications arising from fluid and electrolyte imbalance, and some specific conditions of infants who are at high risk and require special consideration.

BODY FLUID COMPOSITION IN THE FETUS AND THE NEWBORN

At birth, the percentage of body weight represented by water is approximately 75% in term infants and greater in those born prematurely (Fig. 34–1).[18] As gestational age increases, total body water and extracellular water decrease while intracellular fluid content increases. An infant born at 32 weeks' gestation has a total body water and extracellular fluid body weight percentage of approximately 83% and 53%, respectively. During the first week to 10 days of life, all infants experience a reduction in body weight, which in part represents inadequate caloric intake

during this period. However, this physiologic weight loss is largely the result of a reduction in the extracellular compartment of body water.[3, 44–46] The precise mechanism for the postnatal contraction of the extracellular fluid compartment is unclear. However, it has been well documented that infants with low birth weight lose approximately 10% to 15% of the extracellular fluid during the first 5 days of life.[44] This phenomenon is associated with a concurrent diuretic phase resulting in negative fluid and sodium balance.[10, 27]

It is important to recognize that in the first few days of life, physiologic weight loss in an infant with low birth weight represents isotonic contraction of body fluids. The contraction of the extracellular fluid space appears to be part of a normal transitional physiologic process. Perturbations of this normal transitional physiology can lead to imbalances in sodium and water homeostasis. Finally, high fluid intake resulting in a lack of extracellular fluid compart-

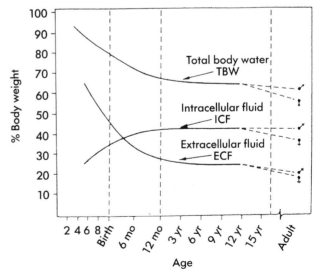

FIGURE 34–1. Change with age in total body water and its major subdivisions. (From Friis-Hansen B: Body water compartments in children: Changes during growth and related changes in body composition. Pediatrics 28:169, 1961. Used with permission of the American Academy of Pediatrics.)

ment contraction may be associated with a higher incidence of symptomatic patent ductus arteriosus[9] and necrotizing enterocolitis.[7]

SODIUM BALANCE IN THE NEWBORN

Renal sodium losses are inversely proportional to gestational age, with fractional excretion of sodium (FENA) as high as 5% to 6% in infants born at 28 weeks' gestation (Fig. 34–2).[47] As a result, preterm infants younger than 35 weeks' gestation may display negative sodium balance and hyponatremia during the initial 2 to 3 weeks of life because of high renal sodium losses and inefficient intestinal sodium absorption.[50] Administration of up to 4 or 5 mEq/kg of sodium per day may be necessary in preterm infants to offset high renal sodium losses during the first few weeks of life. Healthy term neonates have basal sodium handling similar to that of adults, with a FENA of less than 1%, although a transient increase in FENA occurs during the second and third days of life (diuretic phase).[27] Urinary sodium losses may be increased in certain conditions, including hypoxia, respiratory distress, hyperbilirubinemia, acute tubular necrosis, polycythemia, and with increased fluid and salt intake or the use of theophylline and/or diuret-

ics.[22] Pharmacologic agents, such as dopamine, labetalol, propranolol, captopril, and enalaprilat, that affect adrenergic neural pathways in the kidney and the renin-angiotensin axis also may increase urinary sodium losses in the neonate.

The mechanisms responsible for increased urinary sodium losses in the preterm infant are multifactorial. Glomerulotubular imbalance, which occurs when the glomerular filtration rate (GFR) exceeds the reabsorptive capacity of the renal tubules, is due to a preponderance of glomeruli compared to tubular structures, renal tubular immaturity, large extracellular volume, and reduced oxygen availability.[38] Decreased renal nerve activity also may contribute because studies in fetal and newborn sheep demonstrate an inverse relationship between renal nerve stimulation and urine sodium excretion.[38] Finally, fetal and postnatal kidneys exhibit diminished responsiveness to aldosterone in comparison with adult kidneys, resulting in the attenuation of sodium reabsorption.[39]

WATER BALANCE IN THE NEWBORN

THE ROLE OF ANTIDIURETIC HORMONE (ADH)

Water balance is primarily controlled by antidiuretic hormone (ADH), which enables water to be absorbed in the distal nephron collecting duct. ADH secretion is regulated by hypothalamic osmoreceptors that monitor serum osmolality and baroreceptors of the carotid sinus and left atrium that monitor intravascular blood volume. Stimulation of ADH secretion occurs when serum osmolality increases above 285 mOsm/kg or when effective blood volume is diminished. Importantly, intravascular volume has a greater influence on ADH secretion than serum osmolality. Factors that increase ADH secretion also stimulate thirst receptors in the anterior hypothalamus to increase water intake.

Water absorption and excretion is regulated in the distal nephron by the interaction of the vasopressin 2 receptor (V2R) and aquaporin 2 (AQ2) water channels that promote water permeability in water-tight apical membranes of the principal and inner medullary collecting duct cells.[24] Antidiuretic hormone binds to V2R at the basolateral membrane of principal and inner medullary collecting duct cells. Elevated levels of intracellular cyclic adenosine monophosphate (cAMP) mediate the insertion of vesicles containing AQ2 water channels into water-tight apical membranes. The presence of AQ2 water channels on apical membranes allows these membranes to become permeable to water. Withdrawal of ADH stimulates endocytosis of AQ2-containing vesicles, which restores the collecting duct cells to a state of water impermeability.

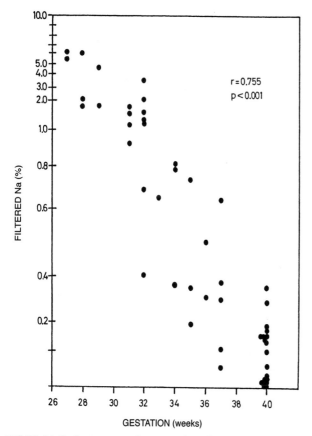

FIGURE 34–2. Scattergram demonstrating the inverse correlation between fractional sodium excretion and gestational age. (From Siegel SR, et al: Renal function as a marker of human renal maturation. Acta Paediatr Scand 65:481, 1976.)

RENAL CONCENTRATING AND DILUTING CAPACITY

Maximal renal concentration and dilution require structural maturity, well-developed tubular transport mechanisms, and an intact hypothalamic-renal vasopressin axis.[36] Renal concentrating and diluting capabilities are less efficient in newborn infants than in adult subjects.[12, 28] In adult subjects, a highly efficient renal concentrating mechanism results in a concentrated urine of up to 1500 mOsm/kg of plasma water, an appropriate defense mechanism against significant fluid restriction. Excessive fluid administration triggers the diluting mechanism of the kidney, with resultant excretion of excess free water with urine osmolality as low as 50 mOsm/kg of plasma water.

In contrast, the neonatal kidney's ability to adjust to fluid perturbations is limited. When challenged, term newborn infants can concentrate up to 800 mOsm/kg of plasma water, whereas preterm infants may concentrate to 600 mOsm/kg of plasma water.[12] Factors that limit renal concentrating capacity include: structural immaturity of the renal medulla, which limits Na, Cl, and urea movement to the interstitium; preferential blood flow through the vasa recta, limiting generation of a medullary gradient; a diminished urea-generated osmotic gradient at the deep corticopapillary tips of the renal medulla; and tubular hyporesponsiveness to vasopressin. Diminished end-organ responsiveness to vasopressin results from diminished transcription and protein synthesis of AQ2 water channels.[15, 53] When challenged with fluid excess, the maximal diluting capacity of the kidney in term infants is approximately 50 mOsm/kg plasma water, whereas the maximal diluting capacity in the preterm infant is 70 mOsm/kg of plasma water.[28, 40]

Although this diluting capacity approximates values seen in adults, newborn infants exhibit a reduced diluting capacity owing to a reduction in GFR and decreased activity of transporters in the early distal tubule (diluting segment).[48] Therefore, excessive fluid restriction places newborns, and particularly preterm infants, at risk for dehydration, and generous fluid intake poses the risk of intravascular volume overload. These facts underscore the importance of careful calculation of fluid and electrolyte requirements and close monitoring of fluid balance in newborn infants who are high risk.

CALCULATION OF FLUID AND ELECTROLYTE REQUIREMENTS

Calculation of fluid and electrolyte requirements in the newborn is based on consideration of mainte-nance needs, deficits, and ongoing losses. Critical factors that govern the fluid and electrolyte requirements of the neonate include gestational age, renal function, ambient air temperature, ventilator dependence, presence of drainage tubes, and gastrointestinal losses.

MAINTENANCE FLUIDS AND ELECTROLYTES

Maintenance fluid requirements refer to fluid quantities that are required to preserve neutral water balance in the newborn. The total amount of fluid required for maintenance is the difference between obligatory losses such as urine production, insensible losses from skin and lungs, and stool losses and the gain in body fluid from water of oxidation. A summary of maintenance fluid requirements during the first month of life for full-term and preterm infants is listed in Table 34–1. *It should be emphasized that the figures in Table 34–1 are only guidelines; they are to be used as a starting point for prescribing maintenance fluid for infants with low birth weight during the first week of life. Further adjustments must be based on evaluation of critical feedback from the infant, as noted later.*

INSENSIBLE LOSSES

Insensible water requirements are based on evaporative losses via the skin and respiratory tract. In newborn infants, one third of insensible water loss occurs through the respiratory tract, and the remaining two thirds occurs through the skin.[21] Because of various physiologic, environmental, and therapeutic factors, insensible water loss represents the most variable component of the basal fluid requirements in newborn infants. Table 34–2 shows the various factors that influence insensible water loss in newborn infants. The most important variable is the maturity of the infant because insensible water loss in a neutral thermal environment with moderately high relative humidity is inversely related to body weight.[17, 52]

Transepidermal water loss accounts for the increased insensible losses of the premature infant (Fig. 34–3).[20] This loss in the premature infant is due to greater water permeability through a relatively immature epithelial layer of skin, a higher surface area–to–body weight ratio, and increased skin vascularity than that of the full-term newborn.

TABLE 34–1 MAINTENANCE FLUID REQUIREMENTS DURING THE FIRST MONTH OF LIFE

BIRTH WEIGHT (gm)	INSENSIBLE WATER LOSS (mL/kg/day)	WATER REQUIREMENTS (mL/kg/day) BY AGE		
		Day 1–2	Day 3–7	Day 8–30
<750	100–200	100–200 +	150–200 +	120–180
750–1000	60–70	80–150	100–150	120–180
1001–1500	30–65	60–100	80–150	120–180
>1500	15–30	60–80	100–150	120–180

Adapted from Veille JC: AGA infants in a thermoneutral environment during the first week of life. Clin Perinatol 15:863, 1988; Taeusch W, Ballard RA (eds): Schaffer and Avery's Diseases of the Newborn, 6th ed. Philadelphia, WB Saunders, 1991; Lorenz J, et al: Phases of fluid and electrolyte homeostasis in the extremely low birth weight infant. Pediatrics 96:484, 1995.

TABLE 34–2 FACTORS AFFECTING INSENSIBLE WATER LOSS IN NEWBORN INFANTS

FACTOR	EFFECT ON INSENSIBLE WATER LOSS
Level of maturity	Inversely proportional to birth weight and gestational age (see Fig. 34–3)
Environmental temperature above neutral thermal zone	Increased in proportion to increment in temperature
Elevated body temperature	Increased by up to 300% at rectal temperature above 37.2°C
High ambient or inspired humidity	Reduced by 30% if ambient or respiratory vapor pressure equals skin or respiratory tract vapor pressure
Skin breakdown (e.g., burn)	Increased; magnitude depends on extent of lesion
Congenital skin defects (e.g., large omphalocele)	Increased; magnitude depends on size of defects
Radiant warmer	Increased by about 50% above values obtained in incubator setting with moderate relative humidity and neutral thermal environment
Phototherapy	Increased by up to 50%
Double-walled isolette or plastic heat shield	Reduced by 10% to 30%

Ambient temperature and relative humidity also play an important role in influencing insensible water losses.[5, 6, 8] A rise in ambient temperature results in an increased insensible water loss. Although a decrease in ambient temperature increases energy expenditure on the basis of cold stress, it has no effect on insensible water loss. Relative humidity of the environment also has a significant influence on insensible water loss.[20] With constant ambient temperature but lower relative humidity, water evaporation from the skin increases secondary to the increased vapor pressure on the skin surface compared with the ambient vapor pressure. In the presence of high relative humidity, the water evaporation is less. Placing an infant under a radiant warmer increases insensible water loss by 50% above the values obtained in an incubator with neutral thermal environment and moderately high relative humidity.[51] Phototherapy also may increase insensible water losses by up to 50%, whereas the use of a double-walled isolette or plastic heat shield reduces insensible water losses by 10% to 30%.[32] (See also Chapter 29.)

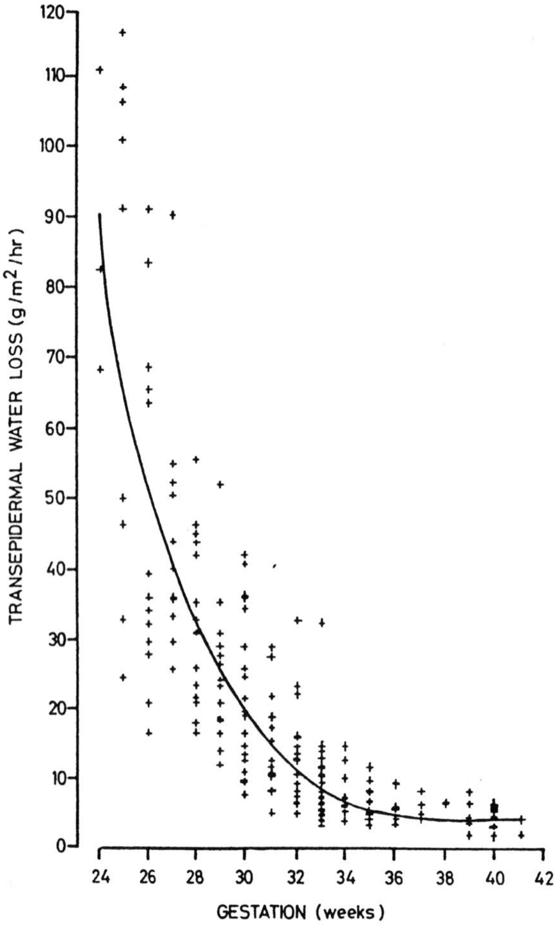

Infants on mechanical ventilation, which provides a humidified oxygen delivery system, have reduced water evaporation from the respiratory tract. Other factors that might increase insensible water losses include the breakdown of skin surface (i.e., burns and conditions associated with large skin defects such as congenital omphaloceles).

URINARY LOSSES

Another component of maintenance fluids is the amount of water required for the formation of urine. The quantity of renal water is dependent on two major factors: status of renal function and renal solute load. Under normal conditions, a major determinant of renal water requirement is renal solute load. Renal solute load is derived from exogenous and endogenous sources. During the first day or two of life, the exogenous solute load of infants with low birth weight is minimal because the infants usually do not receive electrolytes or protein. These infants often have inadequate caloric intake because they generally are not enterally fed and because the amount of calories that can be provided by the parenteral route, using glucose as the sole source of nutrient, is insufficient to meet the basal energy need. The basal energy

FIGURE 34–3. The effects of gestation on transepidermal water loss. Measurements were made from abdominal skin and carried out in the first few days of life. (From Hammarlund K, et al: Transepidermal water loss in newborn infants. III. Relation to gestational age. Acta Paediatr Scand 68:795, 1979.)

requirement for infants with low birth weight is approximately 50 kcal/kg body weight. If these infants are given 70 to 90 mL/kg per day in the first day or two of life using a 5% or 10% glucose solution as the substrate, the caloric intake would be 15 to 35 kcal/kg per day; therefore, these infants derive the remaining mandatory energy requirement from an endogenous source, catabolism. This catabolic state produces approximately 6 mOsm/kg per day of an endogenous solute load presented to the kidney. Therefore, a minimum of 10 mL/kg per day of free water is required to excrete this solute load based on a maximal urinary concentration of 600 mOsm/kg of plasma water. As the infant ages, exogenous intake (parenterally, enterally, or both) and caloric intake increase. Beyond the first few weeks of life, the exogenous solute load increases while the endogenous solute load decreases. It has been estimated that by about 2 or 3 weeks of age, an infant consuming 80 to 120 kcal/kg per day has a total solute load of approximately 15 to 20 mOsm/kg per day, which requires a minimum of 20 to 25 mL/kg per day of free water for excretion of these solutes based on a maximal urinary concentration of 800 mOsm/kg of plasma water.

OTHER FLUIDS

The amount of water loss through the gastrointestinal tract in the form of stool is minimal during the first few days of life, particularly in infants with low birth weight. Once enteral feeds begin, the amount of water lost in the stool is 5 to 10 mL/kg per day. In a growing infant, the amount of water required for the formation of new tissue also should be considered in the calculation of maintenance fluid requirements. Because infants grow at the rate of 10 to 20 gm/kg per day and new tissue contains 70% water, the amount of fluid required for maintenance requirements should provide a net water balance of 10 to 15 mL/kg per day.

ELECTROLYTE REQUIREMENTS

Maintenance sodium or chloride generally are not provided during the first day or two of life due to the relatively high content of sodium and chloride in body fluids. Similarly, potassium is not provided in parenteral fluid until urinary flow has been established and normal renal function is ensured. From days 3 to 7 postnatally, maintenance sodium, potassium, and chloride requirements are approximately 1 to 2 mEq/kg per day. Beyond the first week of life, 2 to 3 mEq/kg per day or more of sodium and chloride are required to maintain the positive electrolyte balance that is necessary for the formation of new tissue.

REPLACEMENT OF DEFICITS AND ONGOING LOSSES

Many clinical conditions require careful evaluation in terms of replacement of deficit and attention to ongoing losses: diarrhea and dehydration, chest tube drainage, surgical wound drainage, and excessive uri-

TABLE 34–3 ELECTROLYTE CONTENT OF BODY FLUIDS

FLUID SOURCE	Na (mmol/L)	K (mmol/L)	Cl (mmol/L)
Stomach	20–80	5–20	100–150
Small intestine	100–140	5–15	90–120
Bile	120–140	5–15	90–120
Ileostomy	45–135	3–15	20–120
Diarrheal stool	10–90	10–80	10–110

Cl, chloride; K, potassium; Na, sodium.

nary losses from osmotic diuresis. The most important principle in replacing these losses is the accurate measurement of the volume and composition of the abnormal fluid losses to guide appropriate replacement. Electrolyte losses can be calculated by multiplying the volume of losses by the known electrolyte contents of respective body fluids (Table 34–3).

Calculations for replacement of abnormal fluid and electrolyte losses can be difficult in infants with accumulation of fluid and electrolytes in static body fluid compartments. This phenomenon is commonly referred to as "third spacing," which occurs in several conditions including sepsis, hydrops fetalis, hypoalbuminemia, intra-abdominal infections and following abdominal or cardiac surgery. For example, an infant with necrotizing enterocolitis often accumulates fluid in the small and large intestinal mucosal and submucosal tissues as well as the peritoneal cavity. Under these circumstances, there may be a large amount of leakage of fluid, electrolytes, and protein into the interstitial tissue that is difficult to quantify and replace. Furthermore, fluid loss into these tissue spaces represents a component of the body fluid that does not contribute to effective arterial plasma volume and circulatory balance of these patients. The most appropriate strategic approach in the management of these infants is to replenish the extracellular fluid compartments with colloid and crystalloid.

MONITORING FLUID AND ELECTROLYTE BALANCE

Interpretation of key clinical feedback is a critical part of successful fluid and electrolyte management strategies in newborns. Fluid and electrolyte balance can be achieved by using a meticulous and organized system that obtains pertinent data and applies the physiologic principles outlined in the beginning of this chapter. A careful clinical assessment of heart rate, blood pressure, skin turgor, capillary refill, oral mucosa integrity, and fullness of the anterior fontanelle is essential. Other pertinent data that must be monitored include body weight, fluid intake, urine and stool output, serum electrolytes, and urine osmolarity or specific gravity.

During the first few days of life, appropriate fluid and electrolyte balance is reflected by a urine output of approximately 1 to 3 mL/kg per hour, a urine-specific gravity of approximately 1.008 to 1.012, and a weight loss of approximately 5% to 15% in term infants and those with very low birth weight, respectively.[45] Microsampling of serum electrolytes can be done at 8- to 24-hour intervals, depending on illness severity, gestational age, and fluid-electrolyte balance. Extracellular volume depletion is manifested by excessive weight loss, dry oral mucosa, sunken anterior fontanelle, capillary refill greater than 3 seconds, diminished skin turgor, increased heart rate, low blood pressure, elevated or diminished serum sodium level, elevated blood urea nitrogen, or metabolic acidosis. Bedside monitoring of growth is essential for the sick newborn infant to monitor adequacy of fluid and caloric intake. Beyond the first week of life, appropriate growth is reflected by a weight gain of 20 to 30 gm per day.

HYPONATREMIA AND HYPERNATREMIA

HYPONATREMIC STATES

Clinical disorders of renal diluting capacity in the newborn result in hyponatremic states defined as a serum sodium less than 130 mmol/L. This condition may result from continued secretion of ADH in the presence of serum hypo-osmolality or when effective blood volume is diminished. Hyponatremia also may occur as a result of a decrease in glomerular filtration rate or an increase in proximal tubular fluid and sodium reabsorption, which diminish delivery of fluid to the distal nephron diluting segments. Finally, defects in sodium chloride transport in the cortical and medullary ascending limb of the loop of Henle, which are water-impermeable regions, also limit the diluting capacity of the nephron.

Early-onset Hyponatremia

Hyponatremia in the newborn infant may occur early during the first week of life or in the latter half of the first month of life. The early-onset form of hyponatremia usually reflects free water excess owing to either increased maternal free water intake or perinatal nonosmotic release of vasopressin.[36] Increased vasopressin release may be seen in conditions such as perinatal asphyxia, respiratory distress, bilateral pneumothoraces, and intraventricular hemorrhage.[35] It also may be seen with various medications, including morphine, barbiturates, or carbamazepine. Early-onset hyponatremia may also occur from excess free water intake or suboptimal sodium intake in formula or IV fluids.

Late-onset Hyponatremia

Late-onset hyponatremia is most commonly due to negative sodium balance. This may occur from either inadequate sodium intake or excessive renal losses owing to a high fractional excretion of sodium, particularly in preterm infants younger than 28 weeks' gestation.[47]

Uncommonly, free water retention from excessive ADH release, renal failure, or edematous disorders also may contribute to late-onset hyponatremia. Water restriction is necessary in treating hyponatremia when these conditions are present.

Congenital Adrenal Hyperplasia

(See also Chapter 47, Part Four.)

The most common form of congenital adrenal hyperplasia is complete absence of 21-hydroxylase activity, which results in severe renal sodium wasting owing to deficient aldosterone production and inhibition of sodium absorption in the distal nephron. Affected females have ambiguous genitalia at birth owing to excess adrenal androgens. These patients typically present with severe hyponatremia, hyperkalemia, and metabolic acidosis at 1 to 3 weeks of age as a result of a salt-losing crisis. Additional laboratory abnormalities in this disorder include elevations of plasma 17-hydroxyprogesterone, progesterone, and androstenedione, increased urinary 17-ketosteroids, elevated plasma renin activity, elevated adrenocorticotropic hormone (ACTH) levels, and undetectable serum cortisol levels. Initial treatment is directed at correcting the electrolyte abnormalities. Normal saline or 3% saline should be used to correct the serum sodium to at least 125 mmol/L, and glucose (0.5 gm/kg) and insulin (0.1 units/kg) should be given for serum potassium values exceeding 7 mEq/L. Bicarbonate at a dose of 1 or 2 mEq/kg also is necessary for treatment of acidosis. Once the electrolyte abnormalities have been successfully managed, glucocorticoid replacement therapy should be instituted. Sodium supplements may be necessary for a prolonged period of time.

Pseudohypoaldosteronism

Aldosterone, a steroid hormone produced in the adrenal cortex, promotes sodium reabsorption and secretion of H^+ and K^+ in the distal nephron through its action on apical Na^+ channels and basolateral Na^+-K^+-ATPase activity.[42] Pseudohypoaldosteronism refers to a group of disorders characterized by an apparent renal tubular unresponsiveness to aldosterone reflected by hyponatremia associated with renal sodium wasting, hyperkalemia, metabolic acidosis, and elevated levels of plasma renin and aldosterone.

Several forms of pseudohypoaldosteronism may present in the neonatal period or during early infancy. Type I primary pseudohypoaldosteronism has two subtypes: renal or multiple target-organ defects. Renal type I pseudohypoaldosteronism is the most common form of type I pseudohypoaldosteronism and is inherited in an autosomal dominant pattern with variable expression.[26] These patients usually present during early infancy with failure to thrive, weight loss, vomiting, dehydration, or shock. Polyhydramnios also may be present during fetal life owing to excess renal salt wasting and polyuria. Sweat and salivary electrolytes are normal in this form of type I pseudohypoaldosteronism. The pathogenesis of the apparent mineralocorticoid resistance of this disease is unknown. Treatment involves administration of large quantities of sodium chloride, 10 to 15 mEq/kg per day. Although the defect in salt handling appears to be lifelong, serum sodium levels typically become easier to control by 1 or 2 years of age because of an increase in dietary sodium intake, maturation of proximal tubular transport of sodium, and improvement in the renal tubular response to mineralocorticoids.[43]

Multiple type I pseudohypoaldosteronism is inherited as an autosomal recessive disorder and often presents in the newborn period with severe salt wasting as a result of losses from the kidney, sweat glands, salivary glands, and colon. Patients with multiple type I pseudohypoaldosteronism have a poorer outcome compared with those with the renal form of type I pseudohypoaldosteronism. The pathogenesis of this form of pseudohypoaldosteronism is defective sodium transport in the amiloride-sensitive epithelial sodium channel.[13] Sodium chloride supplementation often is inadequate in controlling hyperkalemia and metabolic acidosis in patients with multiple type I pseudohypoaldosteronism. Dietary restriction of potassium intake and use of rectal sodium polystyrene sulfonate resin to exchange potassium for sodium often is required. Indomethacin or hydrochlorothiazide also may be necessary to control the hyperkalemia and acidosis. These therapies must be continued throughout the child's lifetime because improvement with age usually does not occur.

Secondary forms of type I pseudohypoaldosteronism are unusual. Partial tubular insensitivity to aldosterone may be seen in the presence of unilateral renal vein thrombosis, neonatal medullary necrosis, or urinary tract malformations.

HYPERNATREMIC STATES

Disturbances in the ability to maximally concentrate the urine result in hypernatremic states, defined as a serum sodium greater than 150 mmol/L. These disorders may arise from low levels of circulating ADH (i.e., central diabetes insipidus) or impaired renal response to ADH (i.e., nephrogenic diabetes insipidus).

Early-onset and Late-onset Hypernatremia

Hypernatremia occurring during the first week of life is typically due to excess sodium intake that commonly occurs following resuscitation with sodium bicarbonate or high insensible losses in infants with very low birth weight.[14] Onset of hypernatremia later in the first month of life usually is due to either excess sodium supplementation or inadequate free water intake.

Diabetes Insipidus

Another cause of hypernatremia in the neonate is diabetes insipidus (DI). Newborns with this disorder present with polyuria, polydipsia, chronic dehydration, irritability, poor feeding, and growth restriction.

Nephrogenic DI is characterized by the inability of the kidney to concentrate urine in response to ADH. This disorder may present during the first week of life owing to either a congenital structural disorder such as obstructive uropathy or nephronophthisis, chronic renal failure, hypercalcemia, or hypokalemia. Nephrogenic DI also may present as a sporadic disorder or as an X-linked recessive or autosomal dominant disorder.[25] These disorders are due to mutations in the V2R and AQ2 water channel genes.[25] Treatment of these disorders includes placement on a low sodium formula to reduce solute intake. Thiazide diuretics, such as chlorothiazide (Diuril) at a dose of 20 to 30 mg/kg per day, also are used to reduce extracellular sodium content, which enhances sodium reabsorption in the proximal tubule and diminishes sodium and water delivery to the distal nephron. Amiloride (0.6 mg/kg per day) may also be necessary to reduce urinary potassium losses that may occur with the use of thiazide diuretics. Although prostaglandin inhibitors have been successfully used to treat nephrogenic DI, long-term use of these agents is not recommended because of gastrointestinal, hematopoietic, and renal complications.

Central DI may be due to midline central nervous system malformations, anoxic encephalopathy, cerebral edema, or trauma. Although some ADH secretion may be present in central DI, levels are insufficient for promoting appropriate amounts of water absorption in the distal nephron. Intranasal desmopressin acetate (DDAVP) at a dose of 5 to 30 μg per day is effective therapy for this condition.

PRENATAL GLUCOCORTICOID THERAPY IN NEONATES WITH VERY LOW BIRTH WEIGHT

Prenatal use of glucocorticoids in conjunction with surfactant replacement therapy has been associated with significant improvements in the survival of infants with extremely low birth weight. In addition to reducing the severity of pulmonary disease and intraventricular hemorrhage and stabilizing blood pressure, prenatal glucocorticoids enhance maturation of the epidermis. Prenatal glucocorticoids also have been associated with the maturation of several ion channels of the proximal renal tubular epithelium, including the Na^+/H^+ exchanger and Na^+/HCO_3^-, as well as with increases in urinary flow rate and fractional excretion of sodium.[1, 4]

Omar and colleagues assessed the effect of prenatal doses of either dexamethasone (6 mg × 4 doses) or betamethasone (12 mg × 2 doses) on sodium and water balance in 16 neonates appropriate for gestational age who weighed less than 1000 gm and were born within 24 hours of the last dose of prenatal steroid dose.[33] These neonates were compared with a similar group of 14 premature newborns who did not have prenatal exposure to steroids. At 7 days of life, prenatal steroid treatment was associated with lower insensible water loss, a decreased incidence of hypernatremia, and a lower fluid intake. Diuresis and natriuresis also occurred earlier in the treated infants. These studies suggest that the beneficial effect of prenatal steroid therapy on water and sodium balance in infants with extremely low birth weight is mediated by maturation of the skin epithelial barrier and the renal epithelial transport systems controlling fluid and electrolyte homeostasis.

FLUID AND ELECTROLYTE THERAPY IN COMMON NEONATAL CONDITIONS

PERINATAL ASPHYXIA

Renal parenchymal injury from perinatal asphyxia frequently results in acute tubular necrosis (ATN), which is commonly accompanied by oliguria or anuria (see Chapter 49 for a more detailed discussion). In the presence of acute renal failure, fluid restriction to amounts equal to urine output and insensible losses is critical in order to avoid volume excess. If urine volume is minimal, maintenance fluids are needed to balance insensible water losses. In a term infant, insensible water loss requirement is approximately 20 to 25 mL/kg per day and stool loss is minimal. Therefore, maintenance fluid requirement during the first day of life in an anuric term infant is approximately 30 mL/kg per day. An anuric preterm infant's insensible losses may be as much as 80 mL/kg per day, depending on gestational age. Fluid restriction is often difficult to accomplish when relatively large volumes of IV drugs are necessary. Furthermore, high caloric density parenteral nutrition often is necessary when fluid restriction is critical in order to avoid fluid overload and water intoxication. Once urine production normalizes, fluid intake can be liberalized to reflect urine output and insensible losses.

If the cause of oliguria or anuria is unclear and the infant is felt to be intravascularly depleted, a test dose of 10 mL/kg body weight of crystalloid or colloid can be given. During the oliguric or anuric phase of ATN, potassium should not be given to avoid hyperkalemia. During the recovery phase of ATN, small infants may experience large urinary sodium and potassium losses, which should be quantitated and replaced.[16]

In severe perinatal asphyxia, the renal parenchymal injury may be severe enough to produce renal failure lasting for several days to weeks or may be permanent in cases with cortical necrosis. In the presence of hyperkalemia, defined as a serum potassium in excess of 7 mEq/L, the cardiac rhythm of the infant should be monitored by continuous electrocardiogram to detect any cardiac arrhythmia. Management options include calcium chloride or calcium gluconate infusion to antagonize the toxic effects of hyperkalemia on the cardiac membrane when an arrhythmia is present, a combination of insulin and glucose infusion, sodium polystyrene sulfonate resin (e.g., Kayexalate), sodium bicarbonate in the presence of a metabolic acidosis, and peritoneal dialysis (see Chapter 49).

SYMPTOMATIC PATENT DUCTUS ARTERIOSUS

(See also Chapter 43.)

Patent ductus arteriosus (PDA) with left-to-right shunt and pulmonary edema is a common cause of morbidity in preterm infants, particularly those with respiratory distress syndrome in the first few days of life. Fluid overload during this period is associated with an increased incidence of symptomatic PDA.[9] Although the reason for the association between fluid overload and risk of PDA is still unclear, it has been shown that fluid overload is associated with the lack of isotonic contraction of body fluids in this group of infants. To prevent the occurrence of a symptomatic PDA, it is important to monitor fluid and electrolyte balance in infants with very low birth weight to ensure that physiologic isotonic body fluid contraction does occur. Prior to the advent of surfactant therapy, occurrence of a diuretic phase was related to improvement in respiratory status.[10, 19, 30]

IV indomethacin currently is the drug of choice to treat a PDA medically. The efficacy of this treatment is well demonstrated. IV indomethacin given during the first 6 hours of life and repeated twice at 12-hour intervals is associated with a significant increase in the rate of ductal closure by the fifth day of life.[29] Renal insufficiency owing to vasoconstriction of the renal microvasculature and thrombocytopenia are potential complications of indomethacin and may be dose related; therefore, urine output should be monitored closely during the course of IV indomethacin therapy, and the lowest possible effective doses of indomethacin should be used.

CHRONIC LUNG DISEASE

(See also Chapter 42, Part Seven.)

Bronchopulmonary dysplasia (BPD) is another common disorder in infants with low birth weight, particularly those weighing less than 1500 gm at birth and requiring assisted ventilation and/or prolonged oxygen administration. These infants exhibit oxygen dependence beyond 36 weeks' postconceptual age, and they may have variable chest x-ray findings that suggest chronic lung injury.[2, 31]

With regard to fluid and electrolyte management, infants with chronic lung disease present complex challenges. First, these infants have a higher basal metabolic rate.[49] In order to meet caloric requirements, caloric density or the volume of parenteral and/or enteral feedings needs to be maximized. Care must be taken to provide optimal fluid and nutrient intake without incurring volume overload and worsening pulmonary disease. Also, these infants often are treated with diuretics such as furosemide or Aldactone, which have significant effects on fluid and electrolyte balance.[23] Furosemide is a potent diuretic agent that results in a marked increase in urinary sodium, potassium, and hydrogen ion leading to hypokalemic metabolic alkalosis (see Part Two of this chapter).[34] Chronic use of this diuretic agent also may result in enhanced urinary excretion of calcium leading to osteopenia of prematurity, urolithiasis, or nephrocalcinosis.[41] Strategies used to avoid these complications include minimizing diuretic usage, frequent serum electrolyte determinations to detect electrolyte imbalance, monitoring urinary calcium excretion, and calcium supplementation to prevent osteopenia of prematurity.

part two
ACID-BASE PHYSIOLOGY AND DISORDERS IN THE NEONATE

Ira D. Davis, John E. Stork, and Ellis D. Avner

Normal metabolism of the neonate occurs within a tightly controlled extracellular pH ranging from 7.35 to 7.43, which corresponds to a hydrogen ion concentration between 44.7 and 37.2 nmol/L. Normal growth and development are critically dependent on this homeostasis, which is threatened in the critically ill newborn and premature infant. This chapter reviews the mechanisms involved in maintaining normal acid-base homeostasis in the neonate.

MAINTENANCE OF ACID-BASE BALANCE

It is convenient to consider the maintenance of the hydrogen ion concentration in terms of compensatory mechanisms that respond rapidly to acute change and systems that chronically maintain the overall balance between acid-base intake, production, excretion, and metabolism.

ACUTE COMPENSATION: BODY BUFFER SYSTEMS

Cellular and extracellular buffers minimize the effects of the acute addition of either acid or base to the body. Bicarbonate, phosphates, and plasma proteins are the major extracellular buffers, and proteins such as hemoglobin, organic phosphates, and bone hydroxyapatite are the major cellular buffers.[58] To gain access to these cellular buffers, $H+$ crosses the cell membrane in exchange for either Na^+ or K^+. In addition, HCO_3^- may cross the cell membrane in exchange for Cl^-. Therefore, acute acidosis may result in hyperkalemia, whereas alkalosis can significantly

lower extracellular potassium. Intracellular buffering accounts for about 47% of an acute acid load, and can reach even higher levels during more prolonged episodes of acidosis. Much of this buffering capacity is in bone, where chronic acidosis results in increased bone resorption and loss of bone sodium, potassium, calcium, and carbonate. These effects on bone partially explain the invariable association of growth failure with acidosis, a factor of major importance in the neonate.[58]

The major buffer system in the extracellular fluid is the carbonic acid–bicarbonate pair. The buffer equation is as follows:

$$H^+ + HCO_3^- \rightleftarrows H_2CO_3 \rightleftarrows H_2O + CO_2 \uparrow$$

Regulation of CO_2 excretion by the respiratory system markedly improves the efficiency of the carbonic acid–bicarbonate buffer at physiologic pH. In the presence of the enzyme carbonic anhydrase, H_2CO_3 is in equilibrium with CO_2. Addition or increased production of acid results in consumption of HCO_3^- and increased H_2CO_3 and CO_2. CO_2 can cross the blood-brain barrier, resulting in a drop in pH. This action stimulates central nervous system chemoreceptors, leading to increased respiration and decreased CO_2 concentration within 12 to 24 hours. Similar respiratory compensation occurs in response to alkali, which leads to increased HCO_3^- concentration resulting in hypoventilation and accumulation of CO_2. The Henderson-Hasselbach equation expresses the relationship of pH, PCO_2, and HCO_3^-:

$$pH = 6.1 + \log [HCO_3^- / (0.03 \times PCO_2)]$$

where 6.1 is the pKa of the carbonic acid–bicarbonate buffer.[66] It is important to note that respiratory compensation does not completely normalize the pH in the presence of a metabolic acidosis. For example, PCO_2 decreases by 1.25 mm Hg for each 1 mEq/L decrease in HCO_3^-, which limits the decrease in pH to 0.005 units. In metabolic alkalosis PCO_2 increases by 0.2 to 0.9 mm Hg for every 1 mEq/L increase in HCO_3^-, limiting the pH change to 0.016 to 0.008 units.

CHRONIC MAINTENANCE OF ACID-BASE BALANCE

Chronic maintenance of hydrogen ion concentration depends on the balance between the production or intake of acid and its metabolism or excretion. Foodstuffs contain a small amount of preformed acid, but most of the daily acid load is a product of metabolism. A large proportion consists of CO_2, which is carried to the lung as bicarbonate and carbamino groups bound to hemoglobin and ultimately excreted through respiration. This is termed *volatile* acid. Hypoventilation or hyperventilation leads to either retention or enhanced excretion of CO_2 and results in acidosis or alkalosis respectively. Metabolic activity also produces approximately 1 mEq/kg per day of nonvolatile acid. Most of this consists of sulfuric acid, which results from metabolism of the sulfur-containing amino acids, methionine and cysteine. The remainder consists primarily of incompletely oxidized organic acids, phosphoric acid and hydrochloric acid.[71, 72] Successful maintenance of acid-base balance depends on renal excretion of this nonvolatile acid.

The role of the kidney in acid-base balance is three-fold:

1. Excretion of the daily production of nonvolatile acid
2. Reabsorption of the total amount of filtered HCO_3^-
3. Compensation for changes in P_{CO_2} as a result of respiratory aberrations by increases or decreases in HCO_3^- excretion, thereby minimizing changes in pH.

The kidney fulfills these roles by urinary acidification, which occurs in two regions of the kidney. Of the filtered bicarbonate, 60% to 80% is reabsorbed in the proximal tubule. This reabsorption is dependent on Na^+ reabsorption and occurs through the exchange of Na^+ for H^+ mechanism in the luminal membrane of proximal tubular cells (Fig. 34–4). As shown, excreted H^+ titrates filtered HCO_3^-, producing H_2CO_3, which is then dehydrated rapidly to CO_2 through the actions of carbonic anhydrase in the cellular brush border. CO_2 crosses into the cell, where HCO_3^- is regenerated and reabsorbed across the basal cell membrane in exchange for C^-. At the terminal portion of the proximal convoluted tubule, the pH of the tubular fluid is reduced to 6.7. A second function of the proximal tubule is production of ammonia by deamination of glutamine. This NH_3 is secreted into the lumen, where it is "trapped" as NH_4^+ because of the decreased pH.

The loop of Henle and the distal tubule play little role in urinary acidification. The loop concentrates HCO_3^- via water extraction, thereby increasing the pH of the tubular fluid to 7.39. At this pH, NH_4^+ loses its proton to become NH_3, which crosses into the interstitium where it is available to the medullary collecting duct.

The remainder of urinary acidification occurs in the cortical and medullary collecting tubule. Hydrogen ion secretion in this region is sufficient to titrate the residual HCO_3^- and filtered buffer anions, such as sulfate, thereby producing *titratable acid* (TA) (Fig. 34–5). The primary mechanism is electrogenic secretion of H^+. This occurs against an increasing pH gradient with a minimum urinary pH of 4.5 to 5. The collecting tubule also takes up ammonia from the medullary interstitium and secretes it into the urine where it is trapped as NH_4^+. This action is important because anions such as Cl^- and SO_4^- will not be protonated at a urine pH of 4.5 to 5.0. Urinary NH_4^+ is excreted with these anions, which prevents loss of cations such as Na^+, Ca^{++}, and K^+. Luminal and peritubular pH, distal salt delivery, and aldosterone control distal nephron H^+ secretion.

Total acid excretion by the kidney can then be measured in the urine as:

$$TA + NH_4^+ - HCO_3^-$$

During a steady state, total acid secretion will equal the production of acid from diet and metabolism. In addition to this basal control, the kidney has the capacity to alter HCO_3^- reabsorption in response to changes in P_{CO_2}, thereby minimizing changes in pH.

DEVELOPMENTAL ASPECTS OF ACID-BASE PHYSIOLOGY

Although nephron formation is complete by 34 weeks' gestation, maturation and functional changes of the nephron continue during the first year of life. This relative immaturity of the kidney, which is more pronounced in the preterm infant, affects basal acid-base status and the response to additional acid and alkali loads.[75] As a result, young infants demonstrate imbalances in acid-base homeostasis that are reflected by a lower blood HCO_3^- concentration (15 to 21 mEq/L) in the neonate compared to that of the adult (Fig. 34–6). During the initial 24 to 48 hours of life, acid-base balance is influenced by the degree of perinatal stress and environmental factors such as temperature and diet.[83] Between 7 and 21 days of life, neonates are in a state of mild metabolic acidosis. In some infants, blood pH may drop below 7.25 or base deficit may exceed 8 mEq/L.[80]

Causes for mild acidosis in the neonate are multifactorial. They include low glomerular filtration rate (GFR), which is more pronounced in the premature or stressed neonate, reduced tubular secretory surface for organic acid secretion, diminished number of organic acid transport sites per unit area of renal tubular surface, and diminished energy available for organic acid transport. Neonates also demonstrate a low threshold for proximal tubular reabsorption of bicar-

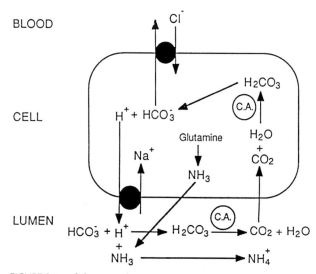

FIGURE 34–4. Schematic drawing of proximal tubular HCO_3^- reabsorption and ammonia generation. See text for explanation. CA, carbonic anhydrase.

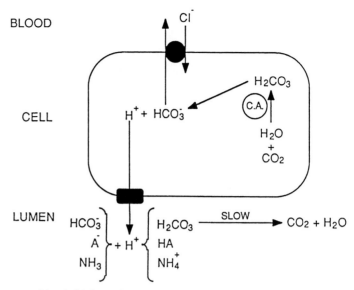

FIGURE 34–5. Schematic drawing of distal methods of urinary acidification, with definition of net acid excretion. See text for explanation. A, acid anion; HA, neutral acid.

Net Acid Excretion =
Titratable Acid + Ammonia − Bicarbonate

bonate and reduced ammonia generation. Finally, low titratable acid secretion secondary to diminished availability of phosphate and other urinary buffers account for this acid-base imbalance.

Premature infants are unable to maximally acidify their urine at birth, exhibiting a minimal urine pH of 6, in contrast to full-term neonates and adults whose urine pH may reach 4.5. The ability of premature infants to maximally acidify their urine and to excrete an acid load correlates with gestational age. By 6 weeks of age, the capacity of premature and term infants to excrete hydrogen ions matures to permit maximal acidification.[84]

In summary, HCO_3^- conservation and net acid excretion are diminished in neonates due to immaturity of the kidney, which is particularly true in premature infants less than 34 weeks' gestation, owing to incomplete nephrogenesis. These limitations not only are

responsible for decreased basal blood HCO_3^- but they also limit the ability of the neonate to respond to additional stresses, particularly acid loading. Renal control of acid-base homeostasis appears to reach adult levels of function by 2 years of age.

DIAGNOSTIC APPROACH TO DISORDERS OF ACID-BASE BALANCE

Altered respiration and abnormal excretion of CO_2 cause either a respiratory acidosis or respiratory alkalosis. Similarly, abnormal production or excretion of acid leads to either a metabolic acidosis or metabolic alkalosis. Acid-base disorders may exist as simple isolated respiratory or metabolic disorders, or they may coexist, producing combined disorders.

The nomogram presented in Figure 34–7 can aid in the diagnosis of simple and combined acid-base disorders. This nomogram describes the 95% confidence limits of the expected compensatory response to a primary abnormality in either P_{CO_2} or HCO_3^-. If the compensatory change in either P_{CO_2} or HCO_3^- falls beyond these limits, a combined disorder is present. A proper diagnosis also can be made using the expected compensatory response values presented in Table 34–4. For example, consider a newborn with pH 7.17, P_{CO_2} 34 mm Hg, and HCO_3^- 12 mEq/L. This is a clear example of an acidosis with a metabolic component, as demonstrated by the low HCO_3^-. It represents a decrease in HCO_3^- of 10 mEq/L from the normal neonatal value of 22 mEq/L. Respiratory compensation should result in a 12.5 mm Hg decrease in P_{CO_2} to 21.5 mm Hg. Therefore, this patient has a respiratory acidosis superimposed on a metabolic acidosis because the P_{CO_2} is elevated above the expected value. Compensation is either renal or respiratory. Absence of compensation is due to temporal

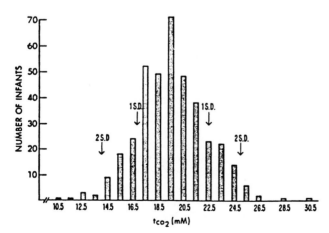

FIGURE 34–6. Frequency distribution of tCO_2 (total CO_2) in 114 infants with low birth weight. Note that the mean is 19.5 mM. 2 SD (standard deviations) includes values as low as 14.5 mM. See text for explanation.

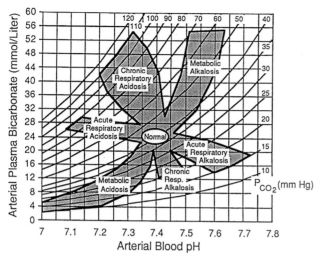

FIGURE 34-7. Acid-base map showing 95% confidence limits for compensatory responses. (From Cogan MG, et al. In Brenner BM, et al: The Kidney. Philadelphia, WB Saunders, 1986, p 462.)

factors, such as acute respiratory acidosis, or superimposed disorder.

BASIC PRINCIPLES OF THERAPY

METABOLIC ACIDOSIS

Metabolic acidosis is a common problem in the critically ill neonate that results from either excess acid production or increased loss of base. Table 34-5 lists common causes of metabolic acidosis in the neonate. Calculation of the anion gap allows differentiation into two groups. An increased anion gap metabolic acidosis, owing to unmeasured acidic anions, results from the addition, increased production, or retention of strong acid. This type of metabolic acidosis is associated with a normal serum chloride. In contrast, a normal anion gap metabolic acidosis is due to either bicarbonate loss or addition of chloride-containing acids and is associated with an elevated serum chloride. Bicarbonate loss may occur in urine or stool.

Correction of the underlying cause is the most important therapeutic measure in the management of metabolic acidosis. The dose of alkali required to treat

TABLE 34-5   COMMON CAUSES OF
METABOLIC ACIDOSIS IN
THE NEONATE

INCREASED ANION GAP

Lactic acidosis
    Hypoxemia, shock, sepsis
    Inborn errors of carbohydrate or pyruvate metabolism
        pyruvate dehydrogenase deficiency
        pyruvate carboxylase deficiency
        mitochondrial respiratory chain defects
Renal failure
Ketoacidosis
    Glycogen storage disease (type I)
    Inborn errors of amino acid or organic acid
        metabolism

NORMAL ANION GAP

Bicarbonate loss:
    acute diarrhea, drainage from small bowel, biliary,
        or pancreatic tube; fistula drainage; bowel
        augmentation cystoplasty; ureteral diversion with
        bowel
Renal tubular acidosis
Mineralocorticoid deficiency
Administration of Cl^--containing compounds:
    arginine HCl, HCl, $CaCl_2$, $MgCl_2$, NH_4Cl
        hyperalimentation, high-protein formula
Carbonic anhydrase inhibitors
Dilution of extracellular fluid compartment

Adapted from Brewer E: Disorders of acid-base balance. Pediatr Clin North Am 37:429, 1990.

metabolic acidosis in newborns ranges from 1 mEq/kg per day for mild base deficits to 5 to 8 mEq/kg per day for more severe base deficits as seen in proximal renal tubular acidosis. Dialysis may be required when acid production is severe during profound states of lactic acidosis or renal failure.[76]

Administration of alkali, such as bicarbonate, has several potential adverse effects. These include volume overload, hypernatremia, decreased oxygen delivery to the brain secondary to shifts in the hemoglobin dissociation curve, increased PCO_2, and a paradoxical intracellular acidosis owing to diffusion of CO_2 into cells.[54, 56, 79] Bicarbonate administration should be reserved for severe acidosis with a pH less than 7.2 because studies demonstrate that cardiac output is compromised at this level.[54, 62] Aggressive alkali therapy is necessary in cases of renal tubular acidosis in order to prevent growth failure.

METABOLIC ALKALOSIS

Metabolic alkalosis is generated from loss of body acid, ingestion of base, or contraction of the extracellular volume, with loss of fluid containing more chloride than bicarbonate. Table 34-6 lists common causes of metabolic alkalosis in the neonate.[58]

Although the kidney is usually very effective in excreting excess alkali, several situations impair excretion, helping to maintain an alkalosis. Extracellular volume contraction limits bicarbonate excretion by

TABLE 34-4   EXPECTED COMPENSATION
IN ACID-BASE DISORDERS

RESPIRATORY	ΔPCO_2		ΔHCO_3^-
Acute acidosis	1 mm Hg ↑	→	↑ 0.1 mEq/L
Acute alkalosis	1 mm Hg ↓	→	↓ 0.25 mEq/L
Chronic acidosis	1 mm Hg ↑	→	↑ 0.5 mEq/L
Chronic alkalosis	1 mm Hg ↓	→	↓ 0.5 mEq/L

METABOLIC	ΔHCO_3^-		ΔPCO_2
Acidosis	1.0 mEq/L ↓	→	↓ 1.25 mm Hg
Alkalosis	1.0 mEq/L ↑	→	↑ 0.2-0.9 mm Hg

TABLE 34-6   COMMON CAUSES OF
METABOLIC ALKALOSIS IN
THE NEONATE

Acid loss: vomiting (e.g., pyloric stenosis), nasogastric
 suction
Diuretics
Chloride deficiency: chronic chloride-losing diarrhea,
 Bartter syndrome, low-chloride formula, loss via skin
 secondary to cystic fibrosis
Administration of alkali: bicarbonate, lactate, acetate,
 citrate

reducing the filtered load of bicarbonate through a decrease in the GFR and stimulation of proximal renal tubular absorption of sodium and bicarbonate. Volume depletion also stimulates renin-angiotensin system-mediated release of aldosterone, which leads to an increase in distal renal tubular absorption of sodium and excretion of both hydrogen ion and potassium. Increased mineralocorticoid activity as a result of volume contraction, excess production of endogenous mineralocorticoids, or exogenous steroids leads to enhanced distal renal tubular excretion of hydrogen ion and potassium. Potassium depletion increases proximal renal tubular sodium absorption, hydrogen ion secretion in the distal renal tubule, and renal ammoniagenesis. Chloride depletion or increased PCO_2 also can maintain a metabolic alkalosis.

Therapy of metabolic alkalosis consists of correction of the underlying disorder. Alkalosis owing to volume contraction typically requires saline administration and potassium repletion. Agents such as arginine hydrochloride, ammonium hydrochloride, and dilute hydrochloric acid should be used only in rare situations because life-threatening complications may occur, such as severe acidosis or a paradoxical intracellular alkalosis. Patients with chronic contraction alkalosis, which is commonly seen in infants with bronchopulmonary dysplasia or congenital heart disease, typically have significant deficits of potassium and chloride. These deficits should be replaced with potassium chloride because serum potassium levels may underestimate significantly the intracellular deficit of potassium. Limits in the rate of administration of potassium, which should not be infused faster than 0.5 to 1.0 mEq/kg per hour, are a result of the slow equilibration rate between the extracellular and intracellular pools of potassium, and they may impede efficient and timely repletion of total body levels of potassium.

Chronic diuretic therapy is a common cause of severe contraction alkalosis in patients with bronchopulmonary dysplasia. Although the long-term complications related to alkalosis are unknown, prolonged pH greater than 7.6 may increase the risk for sensorineural hearing loss.[73]

RESPIRATORY ACIDOSIS AND ALKALOSIS

Respiratory acidosis results from any disorder with decreased alveolar ventilation, resulting in retention of CO_2. This most commonly results from either neonatal respiratory distress syndrome, meconium aspiration syndrome, pulmonary infections, or congenital diaphragmatic hernia. Correction of the underlying cause for respiratory acidosis is essential and frequently requires the use of assisted ventilation to increase excretion of volatile acid (CO_2). For example, respiratory distress syndrome is characterized by diminished alveolar ventilation and retention of CO_2, which typically requires assisted ventilation because alkali administration would further increase the PCO_2 and worsen the respiratory acidosis.

Respiratory alkalosis is rare in the neonate; however, it may occur during excessive assisted ventilation or during central hyperventilation owing to serious central nervous system disease such as intraventricular hemorrhage. Patients with respiratory alkalosis who are dependent on ventilators are treated easily by adjusting the assisted ventilation settings. A search for underlying causes of central hyperventilation is necessary in other patients.

BRIEF CONSIDERATIONS OF SPECIFIC DISORDERS

RENAL TUBULAR ACIDOSIS

Renal tubular acidosis (RTA) disorders are a common cause of normal anion gap metabolic acidosis and result from deficient renal tubular H^+ secretion or HCO_3^- reabsorption.[57, 59] Several types of RTA exist; they are summarized in Table 34-7.

Type I RTA, or distal RTA (classic RTA), results from diminished distal H^+ secretion. Patients with distal RTA often present in the newborn period or during early infancy with lethargy, polyuria, vomiting, dehydration, and failure to thrive. These patients also may have excess urinary sodium and bicarbonate losses as well as hypokalemia. Nephrocalcinosis and urolithiasis may develop when hypercalciuria and hypocitraturia are present. This disorder may occur alone or in association with other acquired or genetic disorders. Patients with distal RTA are unable to acidify their urine and commonly have a urinary pH greater than 6.2.

Type II RTA, or proximal RTA, results from a decrease in the proximal tubule Tm (tubular maximum) for HCO_3^- reabsorption to 14 to 15 mEq/L, resulting in HCO_3^- wastage. The loss of HCO_3^- is often large because 60% to 85% of the filtered HCO_3^- is normally reabsorbed in the proximal tubule. Distal urinary acidification is normal and is associated with a urine pH less than 5.5 when plasma HCO_3^- levels are below 14 to 15 mEq/L. An increase in plasma HCO_3^- beyond the capacity of the proximal tubule results in HCO_3^- wastage and an alkaline urine pH of 7.6 or greater. Proximal RTA often presents in combination with Fanconi syndrome, characterized by proximal tubular wasting of sodium, potassium, glucose, phosphorus, and generalized aminoaciduria. Often 5 to 10 mEq/kg per day of alkali are required to treat proximal RTA because of excessive HCO_3^- wastage.

TABLE 34–7 CLASSIFICATION OF RENAL
TUBULAR ACIDOSIS

TYPE I (DISTAL)

Primary (autosomal dominant or recessive; sporadic)
Associated with other renal disorders
 Obstructive uropathy
 Hypercalciuria/nephrocalcinosis
Associated with acquired or other hereditary diseases
 Osteopetrosis
 Sickle cell anemia
 Hereditary elliptocytosis
 Marfan syndrome
 Primary biliary cirrhosis
Associated with drugs or toxins (amphotericin B)

TYPE II (PROXIMAL)

Primary (familial or sporadic)
Fanconi syndrome
 Primary
 Cystinosis
 Tyrosinemia
 Oculocerebral renal syndrome (Lowe syndrome)
 Hereditary fructose intolerance
 Wilson disease
 Medullary cystic disease
 Focal segmental glomerulosclerosis

TYPE IV (HYPERKALEMIC)

Pseudohypoaldosteronism
 Renal immaturity
 Obstructive uropathy
 Potassium-sparing diuretics
Chloride shunt
Hyporenin hypoaldosteronism
Cyclosporine

Adapted from Brewer E: Disorders of acid-base balance. Pediatr Clin
North Am 37:429, 1990.

As previously discussed, neonates display a mild degree of proximal RTA owing to immaturity of proximal tubular HCO_3^- reabsorption, with maintenance of plasma HCO_3^- from 17 to 21 mEq/L. Over the first year of life, the Tm for HCO_3^- increases to adult levels as the proximal tubule elongates and transport function matures. Some infants demonstrate delayed maturation that results in a persistent proximal RTA, which usually resolves by age 5 or 6.

Measurement of the urine-to-blood P_{CO_2} gradient can be used to assess distal tubular urinary acidification after bicarbonate loading. Following bicarbonate loading in the presence of normal distal tubular acidification, P_{CO_2} should be at least 20 mm Hg greater than the blood P_{CO_2}. With normal function, secreted hydrogen ion combines with bicarbonate to form carbonic acid and ultimately CO_2, leading to a gradient in P_{CO_2} between urine and blood. In distal RTA, this gradient is diminished due to diminished hydrogen ion secretion.[74] Failure to thrive and hypokalemia are the most common presentations in infants. Therapy consists of alkali typically at a dose of 3 mEq/kg per day.

Type IV RTA, or hyperkalemic RTA, results from abnormalities in aldosterone production or from al-tered tubular sensitivity to aldosterone. Therapy for type IV RTA consists of mineralocorticoid supplementation in conditions characterized by a deficiency of aldosterone. Alkali supplementation is required in patients with end-organ resistance to aldosterone. The need for such supplementation seems to diminish by age 5, possibly because of further maturation of the kidney.

LATE METABOLIC ACIDOSIS OF PREMATURITY

In 1964, Kildeberg first used the term *late metabolic acidosis of prematurity* to describe a group of otherwise healthy premature infants between 1 and 3 weeks of age who were characterized by mild to moderate acidosis and decreased growth.[70] All infants were receiving cow's milk formula, which provided 3 to 4 gm of protein per kg of body weight per day.[84] It is interesting that net acid excretion was increased in these infants compared with that of the normal control group. This observation suggests that excessive protein content of cow's milk formula results in endogenous acid production beyond the excretory capacity of the premature kidney, which is limited owing to bicarbonate loss in the urine and reduced phosphate excretion.

Kalhoff and colleagues also described an increase in renal net acid excretion in infants with low birth weight.[68, 69] When randomly assigned to control or bicarbonate therapy groups, infants in the control group with persistent urine pH less than 5.4 for 7 days showed a significant decrease in weight gain and a tendency to decreased nitrogen assimilation. Other studies suggest that alkali therapy may not benefit growth in this situation.[60]

In recent years, metabolic acidosis appears to be less common, which may be explained by a lower protein intake in premature infants. When metabolic acidosis occurs, it is often self-limited and resolves with further renal maturation; nevertheless, alkali therapy may be of benefit in a select group of infants with low birth weight who have a persistently low pH and show evidence of slow weight gain.

NEONATAL BARTTER SYNDROME

In 1962, Bartter and colleagues described a syndrome characterized by hypokalemia, hypochloremic metabolic alkalosis, normal blood pressure, and hyperaldosteronism associated with hyperplasia of the juxtaglomerular complex.[55] Currently, three distinct variants of this syndrome exist.[61] The antenatal variant presents in the neonatal period with dehydration, a history of polyhydramnios, and dysmorphic facies characterized by triangular facies, protruding ears, strabismus, and a drooping mouth. These patients typically have elevated urinary calcium excretion, elevated urinary prostaglandin E levels, nephrocalcinosis, and normal serum magnesium levels. This form of Bartter syndrome is inherited in an autosomal recessive pattern and results from defective transepithelial transport of sodium chloride in the thick as-tion of suspected abnormalities. The following points should be considered:

1. Exposure. This is a subjective evaluation and is represented by the degree of blackening of the film. In general, details of the thoracic spine should be visible through the cardiothymic silhouette.
2. Motion. This causes obvious blurring of the images and results in decreased definition of structures such as the pulmonary vessels and diaphragm.
3. Positioning. Rotation increases magnification of the structures closest to the beam. For example, in the supine position, rotation of the patient to the right causes magnification of the left ribs and left hilum. Also, the heart is projected within the right hemithorax. A simple method of assessing rotation is to compare the relative positions of the anterior ends of the ribs.
4. Extraneous objects. A large portion of the chest of a small premature infant can be completely obscured by electrocardiogram (EKG) electrodes, transcutaneous oxygen monitors, and other equipment. When possible, these and other opaque densities, such as warming mattresses and respirator tubing, should be removed before radiography.
5. Inspiration. The chest x-ray should be exposed at the end of inspiration, which is difficult in neonates with rapid respiratory rates. In some, the tidal volume is so small that there is little difference in the degree of lung aeration during the respiratory cycle. In others, it is difficult to determine whether the resultant increase in lung opacity is caused by expiration or a pathologic decrease in lung volume. As a general rule, on a good inspiratory film, the right diaphragmatic dome should be projected at about the level of the anterior end of the sixth rib.

METHODS OF EXAMINATION

Except for special studies, most radiography of the chest can be accomplished in the newborn nursery using modern portable x-ray equipment. These units employ a single-phase generator capable of exposure times of less than 5 msec at the relatively low kilovoltage required for these infants. In almost every case, blurring because of respiratory motion can be prevented. Further decreases in exposure time have been achieved by using rare-earth screens, although there is some loss of detail with an increase in graininess or mottle because of increased quantum "noise."

Within the radiology department, most chest radiography is done at a distance of 72 inches. This must be reduced to approximately 40 inches when using portable equipment. Although in a larger patient this results in considerable distortion of structures because of magnification, no important degradation of the image occurs with small infants.

Portable x-ray examinations of the chest consist of an anteroposterior (AP) view made with a vertical beam and frequently a lateral view made with a horizontal beam. Careful positioning, which is often undertaken by nursery personnel, is extremely important in obtaining a high-quality radiograph. The AP view is made with the patient lying supine, and proper positioning is facilitated by extending the patient's arms above the head and immobilizing the thighs. For the lateral view, the x-ray tube can be moved so that the x-ray beam is directed horizontally; the patient need not be turned, as would be the case with a vertical-beam view. Occasionally, a lateral decubitus view is necessary, particularly for the evaluation of a pneumothorax. This also is made with a horizontal x-ray beam. The patient is turned so that the unaffected side is dependent.

Ultrasonography, magnetic resonance imaging (MRI), angiography, computed tomography (CT), and radionuclide lung scanning are other imaging techniques that are available for specific diagnostic problems.

Barium esophagrams frequently are indicated in neonates with feeding problems, signs of airway obstruction, and apnea.[18] During this examination, swallowing function and esophageal peristalsis are monitored. Extrinsic lesions compressing the trachea and esophagus, such as vascular rings resulting from aortic arch abnormalities, vascular slings (aberrant left pulmonary artery), and bronchogenic cysts, may be identified. Gastroesophageal reflux[46] frequently is sought in patients being investigated for acute life-threatening episodes (Fig. 35–1).

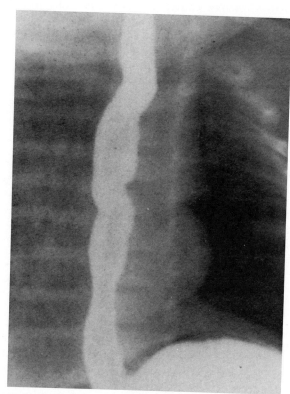

FIGURE 35–1. Massive gastroesophageal reflux and abnormal esophageal peristalsis in a 3-week-old infant with apnea.

cending loop of Henle through the rectifying potassium channel (ROMK) and the sodium-potassium-2-chloride cotransporter (NKCC2) channel.[63, 64, 67, 81]

Treatment of the antenatal form of Bartter syndrome includes the use of indomethacin to inhibit prostaglandin production and aldosterone production, potassium supplementation, and maintenance of adequate intravascular volume. Persistent hypokalemia and nephrocalcinosis rarely leads to chronic renal insufficiency as a result of progressive tubulointerstitial disease.[79]

■ REFERENCES

Part One: Fluid and Electrolyte Management

1. Ali R, et al: Glucocorticoids enhance the expression of the basolateral Na$^+$: HCO$_3^-$ cotransporter in renal proximal tubules. Kidney Int 57:1063, 2000.
2. Bancalari E, et al: Bronchopulmonary dysplasia. Pediatr Clin North Am 33:1, 1986.
3. Bauer K, et al: Effect of intrauterine growth retardation on postnatal weight change in preterm infants. J Pediatr 123:301, 1993.
4. Baum M, et al: Glucocorticoids regulate NHE-3 transcription in OKP cells. Am J Physiol 270:F164, 1996.
5. Baumgart S: Radiant energy and insensible water loss in the premature newborn infant nursed under a radiant warmer. Clin Perinatol 9:483, 1982.
6. Bell EF, et al: Combined effect of radiant warmer and phototherapy on insensible water loss in low birth weight infants. J Pediatr 94:810, 1979.
7. Bell EF, et al: High volume fluid intake predisposes premature infants to necrotizing enterocolitis. Lancet 2:90, 1979.
8. Bell EF, et al: The effects of thermal environment on heat balance and insensible water loss in low birth weight infants. J Pediatr 96:452, 1980.
9. Bell EF, et al: Effect of fluid administration on the development of symptomatic patent ductus arteriosus and congestive heart failure in premature infants. N Engl J Med 302:598, 1980.
10. Bidiwala KS, et al: Renal function correlates of postnatal diuresis in preterm infants. Pediatrics 82:50, 1988.
11. Brosius KK, et al: Postnatal growth curve of the infant with extremely low birth weight who was fed enterally. Pediatrics 74:778, 1984.
12. Calcagno PL, et al: Studies on the renal concentrating and diluting mechanisms in the premature infant. J Clin Invest 33:91, 1954.
13. Chang S, et al: Mutations of the epithelial sodium channel cause salt wasting with hyperkalemic acidosis, pseudohypoaldosteronism type 1. Nat Genet 12:248, 1996.
14. Costarino AT, et al: Sodium restriction versus daily maintenance replacement in very low birth weight premature neonates: A randomized, blind therapeutic trial. J Pediatr 120:99, 1992.
15. Devuyst O, et al: Expression of aquaporins-1 and -2 during nephrogenesis and in autosomal dominant polycystic kidney disease. Am J Physiol 271:F169, 1996.
16. Engelke SC, et al: Sodium balance in very low birth weight infants. J Pediatr 93:837, 1978.
17. Fanaroff AA, et al: Insensible water loss in low birth weight infants. Pediatrics 50:236, 1972.
18. Friis-Hansen B: Body water compartments in children: Changes during growth and related changes in body composition. Pediatrics 28:169, 1961.
19. Guignard JP, et al: Renal function in respiratory distress syndrome. J Pediatr 88:845, 1976.
20. Hammarlund K, et al: Transepidermal water loss in newborn infants. III. Relation to gestational age. Acta Paediatr Scand 68:795, 1979.
21. Hey EN, et al: Evaporative water loss in the newborn baby. J Physiol 200:605, 1969.
22. Jose PA: Neonatal renal function and physiology. Curr Opin Pediatr 6:172, 1994.
23. Kao L, et al: Effect of oral furosemide on pulmonary mechanics in infants with chronic BPD: Results of a double-blind crossover sequential trial. Pediatrics 74:37, 1984.
24. Knepper MA: Molecular physiology of urinary concentrating mechansim: Regulation of aquaporin water channels by vasopressin. Am J Physiol 272:F3, 1997.
25. Knoers N, et al: Nephrogenic diabetes insipidus. Sem Nephrol 19:344, 1999.
26. Kuhnle U, et al: Familial pseudohypoaldosteronism: A review on the heterogeneity of the syndrome. Steroids 60:157, 1995.
27. Lorenz J, et al: Phases of fluid and electrolyte homeostasis in the extremely low birth weight infant. Pediatrics 96:484, 1995.
28. McCance RA, et al: The renal response of infants to a large dose of water. Arch Dis Child 29:104, 1954.
29. Ment LR, et al: Low-dose indomethacin and prevention of intraventricular hemorrhage: A multicenter randomized trial. Pediatrics 93:543, 1994.
30. Mercier CE, et al: Clinical trials of natural surfactant extract in respiratory distress syndrome. Clin Perinatol 20:711, 1993.
31. Northway WH Jr, et al: Pulmonary disease following respirator therapy of hyaline-membrane disease: Bronchopulmonary dysplasia. N Engl J Med 276:357, 1967.
32. Oh W, et al: Phototherapy and insensible water loss in the newborn infant. Am J Dis Child 124:230, 1972.
33. Omar SA, et al: Effects of prenatal steroids on water and sodium homeostasis in extremely low birth weight neonates. Pediatrics 104:482, 1999.
34. Rastogi A, et al: Nebulized furosemide in infants with bronchopulmonary dysplasia. J Pediatr 125:976, 1994.
35. Rees L, et al: Hyponatremia in the first week of life in preterm infants. I. Arginine vasopressin secretion. Arch Dis Child 59:414, 1984.
36. Rees L, et al: Hyponatremia in the first week of life in preterm infants. II. Sodium and water balance. Arch Dis Child 59:423, 1984.
37. Robillard JE, et al: Renal function during fetal life. In Barratt TM, et al (eds): Pediatric Nephrology, 4th ed. Baltimore, Lippincott, Williams & Wilkins, 1998, p 21.
38. Robillard JE, et al: Regulation of sodium metabolism and extracellular fluid volume during development. Clin Perinatol 19:15, 1992.
39. Robillard J, et al: Mechanisms regulating renal sodium excretion during development. Pediatr Nephrol 6:205, 1992.
40. Rodriguez-Soriano J, et al: Renal handling of water and sodium in infancy and childhood: A study using clearance methods during saline diuresis. Kidney Int 20:700, 1981.
41. Ross BS, et al: The pharmacologic effects of furosemide therapy in the low birth weight infant. J Pediatr 92:149, 1978.
42. Rossier B, et al: Mechanisms of aldosterone action on sodium and potassium transport. In Seldin DW, Giebisch G (eds): The Kidney: Physiology and Pathophysiology. New York, Raven Press, 1992, p 1373.
43. Rossler A: The natural history of salt-wasting disorders of adrenal and renal origin. J Clin Endocrinol Metab 59:689, 1984.
44. Shaffer SG, et al: Extracellular fluid volume changes in very low birth weight infants during first 2 postnatal months. J Pediatr 111:125, 1987.
45. Shaffer SG, et al: Postnatal weight changes in low birth weight infants. Pediatrics 79:702, 1987.
46. Shaffer SG, et al: Sodium balance and extracellular volume regulation in very low birth weight infants. J Pediatr 115:285, 1989.
47. Siegel SR, et al: Renal function as a marker of human renal maturation. Acta Paediatr Scand 65:481, 1976.
48. Simpson J, et al: Regulation of extracellular volume in neonates. Early Hum Dev 34:179, 1993.
49. Weinstein MR, et al: Oxygen consumption in infants with bronchopulmonary dysplasia. J Pediatr 99:958, 1981.
50. Wilkins B: Renal function in sick very low birthweight infants. Sodium, potassium, and water excretion. Arch Dis Child 67:1154, 1992.
51. Williams PR, et al: Effects of radiant warmer on insensible water loss in newborn infants. Am J Dis Child 128:511, 1974.

52. Wu PYK, et al: Insensible water loss in preterm infants: Changes with postnatal development and non-ionizing radiant energy. Pediatrics 54:704, 1974.
53. Yamamoto T, et al: Expression of AQP family in rat kidneys during development and maturation. Am J Physiol 272:F198, 1997.

Part Two: Acid-Base Physiology and Disorders in the Neonate

54. Ayus JC: Effect of bicarbonate administration on cardiac function. Am J Med 87:5, 1989.
55. Bartter FC, et al: Hyperplasia of the juxtaglomerular complex with hyperaldosteronism and hypokalemic alkalosis: A new syndrome. Am J Med 33:811, 1962.
56. Baum JD, et al: Immediate effects of alkaline infusion in infants with respiratory distress syndrome. J Pediatr 87:255, 1975.
57. Brewer E: Disorders of acid-base balance. Pediatr Clin North Am 37:429, 1990.
58. Chan JCM: Acid-base disorders and the kidney. Adv Pediatr 30:401, 1983.
59. Chan JCM: Renal tubular acidosis. J Pediatr 102:237, 1983.
60. Corbet AJ, et al: Controlled trial of bicarbonate therapy in high-risk premature newborn infants. J Pediatr 91:771, 1977.
61. Dell KD, et al: Inherited tubular transport disorders. Sem Nephrol 19:364, 1999.
62. Fanconi S, et al: Hemodynamic effects of sodium bicarbonate in critically ill neonates. Intensive Care Med 19:65, 1993.
63. Gill JR Jr: The role of chloride transport in the thick ascending limb in the pathogenesis of Bartter's syndrome. Klin Wochenschr 60:1212, 1982.
64. Gill JR Jr, et al: Evidence for a prostaglandin independent defect in chloride reabsorption in the loop of Henle as a proximal cause of Bartter's syndrome. Am J Med 65:766, 1978.
65. Goodlin RC, et al: The neonate with unexpected acidemia. J Reprod Med 39:97, 1994.
66. Henderson LJ: Das Gleichgewicht zwischen Basen and Sauren in tierschen Organismus. Ergeb Physiol 8:254, 1909.
67. International Collaborative Study Group for Bartter-like Syndromes: Mutations in the gene encoding the inwardly-rectifying renal potassium channel, ROMK, cause the antenatal variant of Bartter syndrome: Evidence for genetic heterogeneity. Hum Mol Genet 6:17, 1997.
68. Kalhoff H, et al: Decreased growth rate of low-birth weight infants with prolonged maximum renal acid stimulation. Acta Paediatr 82:522, 1993.
69. Kalhoff H, et al: Increased renal net acid excretion in prematures below 1600 g body weight compared with prematures and small-for-date newborns above 2100 g on alimentation with a commercial preterm formula. Biol Neonate 66:10, 1994.
70. Kildeberg P: Disturbances of hydrogen ion balance occurring in premature infants. II. Late metabolic acidosis. Acta Paediatr Scan 53:517, 1964.
71. Kildeberg P, et al: Balance of net acid in growing infants. Acta Paediatr Scand 58:321, 1969.
72. Kildeberg P, et al: Balance of net acid: concept, measurement and applications. Adv Pediatr 25:349, 1978.
73. Leslie GI, et al: Risk factors for sensorineural hearing loss in extremely premature infants. J Paediatr Child Health 31:312, 1995.
74. Lin JY, et al: Use of the urine-to-blood carbon dioxide tension gradient as a measurement of impaired distal tubular hydrogen ion secretion among neonates. J Pediatr 126:114, 1995.
75. Lindquist B, et al: Acid-base homeostasis of low birth weight and full term infants in early life. J Pediatr Gastroenterol Nutr 2:S99, 1983.
76. Nash MA, et al: Neonatal lactic acidosis and renal failure: The role of peritoneal dialysis. J Pediatr 91:101, 1977.
77. Oh WH: Renal functions and clinical disorders in the neonate. Clin Perinatol 8:215, 1981.
78. Ritter JM, et al: Paradoxical effect of bicarbonate on cytoplasmic pH. Lancet 335:1243, 1990.
79. Rodriguez-Soriano J: Bartter and related syndromes: The puzzle is almost solved. Pediatr Nephrol 12:315, 1998.
80. Schwartz GJ, et al: Late metabolic acidosis: A reassessment of the definition. J Pediatr 95:102, 1979.
81. Simon DB, et al: Bartter's syndrome, hypokalemic alkalosis with hypercalciuria, is caused by mutations in the Na-K-2Cl cotransporter NKCC2. Nat Genet 13:183, 1996.
82. Stonestreet BS, et al: Renal response in low birth weight neonates: Results of prolonged intake of two different amounts of fluid and sodium. Am J Dis Child 137:215, 1983.
83. Sulyok E, et al: The influence of maturity on renal control of acidosis in newborn infants. Biol Neonate 21:418, 1972.
84. Svenningsen NW, et al: Postnatal development of renal hydrogen ion excretion capacity in relation to age and protein intake. Acta Paediatr Scand 63:721, 1974.

35 Diagnostic Imaging

Stuart C. Morriso

In any attempt to present a subject as broad as neonatal imaging within the confines of a single chapter, many important aspects of the discipline must be omitted and others mentioned only briefly. This chapter discusses the indications and the basic methodology of commonly used imaging methods. Imaging of specific disorders that affect neonates is covered elsewhere in this book.

PATIENT PROTECTION

Prolonged survival of premature infants has resulted in larger numbers of radiographs being taken, thus increasing radiation exposure. Consequently, radiologists have become more concerned with the possible long-term effects of low-dosage diagnostic radiation. Increased life expectancy of many premature infants means that there is more time for radiation-induced cancers to appear. Neonates and children also show an increased radiosensitivity of their tissues compared with adults. The reproductive lives of these exposed infants are ahead of them, and they are unable to give informed consent.

Long-term effects are extremely difficult to measure, because most data must be obtained from laboratory experiments or after accidental human exposure to high doses of radiation. Investigations show a small increased risk for the development of leukemia in children exposed to diagnostic x-rays in utero. An increased incidence of breast carcinoma also has been reported after exposure of the female breast to ionizing radiation. This has been reported both in Japanese survivors of the atomic bomb and after radiation in infancy to treat an enlarged thymus.[22] The radiation dose received by neonates less than 750 gm birth weight is small compared with doses used for risk estimates for cancer.[55]

Certain practical steps can be taken to prevent unnecessary radiation exposure. These include a thorough evaluation of the indications for the radiographic examination, careful collimation of the x-ray beam to the field of interest, gonadal shielding, and avoidance of overexposure and repeat examinations by paying meticulous attention to technical details. High-speed radiographic films combined with rare-earth intensifying screens can markedly decrease radiation exposure and reduce the likelihood of motion artifacts.[50] When such equipment is used in the nursery, however, state-of-the-art portable x-ray units are necessary to realize these benefits.

Exposure of personnel to ionizing radiation from scattered x-rays is a constant source of concern. The most significant way to reduce radiation exposure is to increase the distance from the x-ray tube during any x-ray procedure. Lead aprons and gloves should always be worn by personnel restraining an infant. The radiation dose from scattered radiation, however, is minuscule. Nurses who wore radiation badges for a year in a neonatal intensive care unit did not show any increased exposure above the natural background radiation level.[44] Although all efforts must be made to reduce the amount of radiation exposure to the infant and to the staff in neonatal units, it is important to keep the risks in perspective. The radiation received by staff is generally negligible.[43] If there is a proper clinical indication for an examination to be performed, there should be no hesitation in carrying it out.

Digital computed radiographic imaging[26] has the potential to reduce dosage dramatically and eliminate the problem of lost films. Images can be transferred from the neonatal nursery to the radiology department by the technique of teleradiology.

CHEST

(See also Chapter 42.)

Chest radiographs account for the majority of radiographic studies in newborn infants. Most of these are required because of respiratory distress in premature infants. Radiographic techniques for neonates differ from those used in older infants and children because of the small size and rapid respiratory rates of newborns. Radiologists, neonatologists, and nursery personnel must understand the special requirements for proper radiographic examination of these patients.

ASSESSMENT OF AN OPTIMAL EXAMINATION

A simple check of several technical aspects of the film greatly increases the likelihood of proper interpreta-

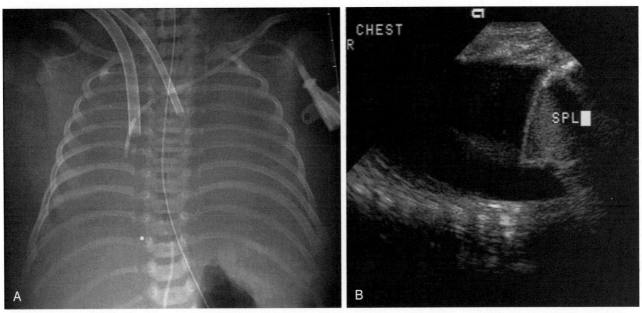

FIGURE 35–2. *A,* Opaque thorax of a neonate treated with extracorporeal membrane oxygenation (ECMO). Note the venous and arterial ECMO catheters. Surgery had been performed earlier for a large left diaphragmatic hernia. *B,* Ultrasound study of the left thorax shows a large pleural fluid collection. SPL, spleen.

Ultrasonography is less useful for chest diagnosis than for abdominal diagnosis because of reduced transmission of sound waves in air. However, if an appropriate "window" can be found, it can be very useful in further characterizing intrathoracic masses and fluid collections. This modality is particularly helpful in differentiating cystic masses from solid masses. Ultrasonography also is a useful method of evaluating diaphragmatic motion and diagnosing pleural effusion. Neonates on extracorporeal membrane oxygenation (ECMO) are particularly suitable for ultrasound examination to distinguish pleural fluid from a collapsed lung (Fig. 35–2). A wide variety of abnormalities can now be diagnosed prenatally (see Chapter 8), which has facilitated the imaging and management of these neonates after birth (Fig. 35–3).

CT with image acquisition time of 5 seconds or less is capable of producing exquisite anatomic detail of intrathoracic structures even in rapidly breathing newborns. The indications for CT in newborn chest diagnosis are usually limited to the evaluation of masses and air-containing or fluid-containing cysts.

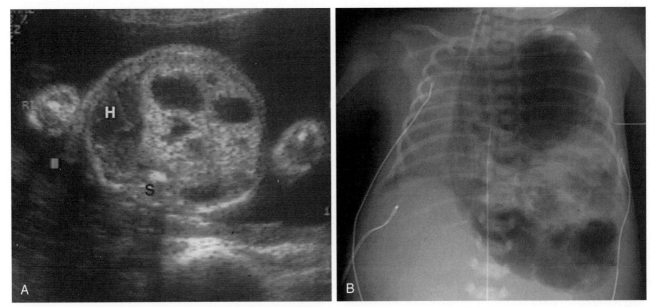

FIGURE 35–3. *A,* Obstetric ultrasound study with a transverse view of the fetal thorax. The fetal spine (S) is posterior. The heart (H) is displaced to the right by a large mass that is solid but also has several large cysts. *B,* Chest x-ray after birth confirms a huge left-sided cystic adenomatoid malformation of the lung.

The CT scan also is an excellent method of evaluating the upper airway for abnormalities such as choanal atresia[49] and choanal stenosis. An obvious disadvantage of this method is the need to transport the infant to the scanner and remove the patient from the protective environment during the scan. With the improvement in scan times, sedation is rarely needed for CT scanning.

These disadvantages also apply to MRI. Although MRI is capable of producing excellent images with a wider range of contrast than CT, and exposure to ionizing radiation is avoided, imaging time is longer. Sedation is frequently necessary, because studies take a minimum of 45 minutes to perform. In neonates, MRI's greatest use is in evaluating the development of the brain, because it is capable of tracking myelinization there and in the spine. Used with EKG-gated techniques, MRI is capable of imaging the neonatal cardiovascular structures (Fig. 35–4), mediastinum, and airway.

Nuclear medicine ventilation scans have shown an interesting reversal of ventilation of the lungs compared with the adult pattern. In neonates, ventilation is preferentially distributed away from the dependent lung; the opposite occurs in adults.[9] This has important implications for therapy of unilateral lung disease.

NORMAL CHEST

The appearance of the normal chest varies throughout the first few days of life. The lungs may be slightly opaque because of retained lung liquid in the early newborn period. The lungs eventually become radiolucent, except for well-defined pulmonary vessels branching from the hila. The minor fissure of the right lung is frequently seen as a fine horizontal line in the midportion. The cardiophrenic and costophrenic angles should be clear. The heart borders, except for the portions adjacent to the hila, should be distinct, and the diaphragmatic pleura should be clearly outlined against the lungs, except for the portion of the left hemidiaphragm that is contiguous to the heart.

The cardiothoracic ratio should be no greater than 0.6. In the first few days of life, a rounded opacity may be seen in the left upper mediastinum, resulting from a normal "ductus bump" associated with the closing of the ductus arteriosus. The tracheal air shadow should curve gently to the right around the left aortic arch (see Fig. 35–4). Displacement of the trachea to the left is abnormal and suggests a mediastinal mass or right aortic arch. The descending thoracic aorta is rarely visible in the newborn.

The *thymus* is often prominent in the newborn, and because of its variable configuration, its appearance causes frequent confusion. The thymus overlies the anterior aspect of the pericardium, obscuring much of the cardiac silhouette; thus, it may simulate a large heart. It is frequently asymmetric and more prominent on the right, sometimes producing a sail-like appearance. Wavelike undulations of its lateral border may be seen because of pressure of the costal cartilages. Aside from these fairly characteristic normal features, the thymus can generally be identified by its homogeneous density, anterior location, lack of associated compression of the trachea, and sharp definition of its edges. A lateral view often excludes cardiomegaly by demonstrating an absence of posterior enlargement of the heart. If concern about a wide mediastinum persists, ultrasonography is an excellent method to confirm the presence of a normal thymus.[17] Normal thymus has an ultrasonographic appearance similar to that of normal liver or spleen. The ratio between the transverse diameter of the cardiothymic image and that of the thoracic cage tends to be slightly larger in infants with respiratory distress syndrome (RDS) than in those with normal lungs.

RADIOGRAPHIC SIGNS OF PULMONARY ABNORMALITIES

Pulmonary Consolidation and Pneumonia

The term *consolidation* indicates a process that causes the alveoli to be filled with a substance having the density of water. The most frequent cause is pneumonia, but hemorrhage, pus, and edema are other possible causes. Varying degrees of opacification of the lungs are the result of consolidation. The densities may be localized or diffuse and are frequently "patchy." The edges of the consolidation are indistinct, and there is frequently an "air bronchogram," with visualization of the relatively radiolucent bronchi within the involved area of the lung.

As opposed to a process in which the airspaces are opacified, involvement of the interstitial tissues of the lung may predominate. In this case, a diffuse reticular or nodular pattern results. Peribronchial disease results in small ring shadows when the smaller, more

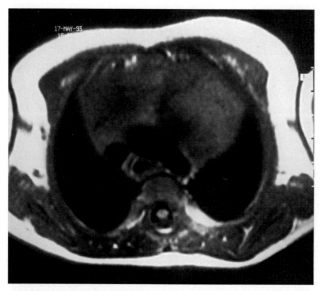

FIGURE 35–4. Axial magnetic resonance imaging scan of a neonate. Note the size of the normal thymus. The left aortic arch displaces the trachea to the right, a similar finding in the normal neonatal chest x-ray.

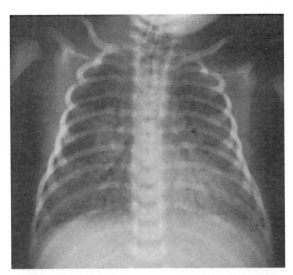

FIGURE 35–5. Diffuse bilateral pulmonary consolidation due to pneumococcal pneumonia in a newborn. Note the prominent "air bronchograms" and reticular pattern resembling respiratory distress syndrome (RDS). The lungs have increased volume, an uncommon finding in RDS.

peripheral bronchi are seen in cross section, but air bronchograms are not seen.

Generalized pulmonary hyperinflation frequently accompanies diffuse pneumonia and is particularly apparent in meconium aspiration pneumonitis. Completely airless, consolidated lobes and segment of lung tend to be less voluminous than when they are filled with air.

Group B streptococcal pneumonia deserves special mention, because some small premature infants may have a lung pattern[19] that closely resembles that seen in RDS (see Chapter 42). This pattern, once thought to be specific for RDS, consists of diffuse bilateral reticulogranularity with exaggerated air bronchograms. We have noted this pattern in neonatal pneumonias of other causes as well (Fig. 35–5). The identification of pleural fluid suggests neonatal pneumonia, as it is never seen with RDS.

Chlamydia pneumonia typically results in coarse, bilateral, interstitial infiltrates in afebrile infants 2 weeks to 3 months of age.[39] Pulmonary candidiasis should be considered in small premature infants with bronchopulmonary dysplasia who develop extensive airspace consolidation.

Atelectasis

As in consolidation, atelectasis also causes an increase in lung density. Furthermore, until the gas is completely resorbed from the bronchi, an air bronchogram may be present. Lobar atelectasis is manifested primarily as changes in position of the fissure. For example, with lower lobe collapse, the major fissure moves posteromedially. In middle lobe collapse, the minor fissure is depressed, whereas right upper lobe collapse causes elevation of the minor fissure.

Atelectasis also results in a shift of the mediastinum toward the side of the collapse. This is most notable in lower lobe atelectasis, but in newborn infants, the compliant mediastinal structure also shifts slightly toward the side of the upper lobe collapse. In addition, lower lobe atelectasis results in elevation of the ipsilateral hemidiaphragm. Narrowing of the intercostal spaces is a frequent secondary sign. Compensatory hyperinflation of uninvolved portions of lung or of the opposite lung also occur and must be differentiated from a primary increase in lung volume, such as occurs in congenital lobar emphysema.

In neonates, the most frequent site of lobar atelectasis is the right upper lobe. This may be because of occlusion of the right upper lobe bronchus associated with faulty positioning of an endotracheal tube, but it is also a frequent finding after extubation, probably because of mucus accumulation and decreased ciliary activity.

Diffuse atelectasis occurs in premature infants who have unstable alveoli resulting from surfactant deficiency. The radiographic hallmark of RDS is a diffuse symmetric reticulogranular pattern (Fig. 35–6). This is the result of microatelectases interspersed with dilated airspaces. In more severe RDS, a radiographic "whiteout" may result from generalized atelectasis. A similar appearance may occur with sudden collapse of both lungs in babies who have been breathing high concentrations of oxygen if they become apneic or develop airway obstruction. Surfactant treatment has been shown to improve the radiographic signs of RDS.[7] Occasionally, the clearing occurs only centrally or in the right lung. This asymmetric pattern is thought to be caused by inadequate distribution of surfactant through the airway. (See Chapter 42.)

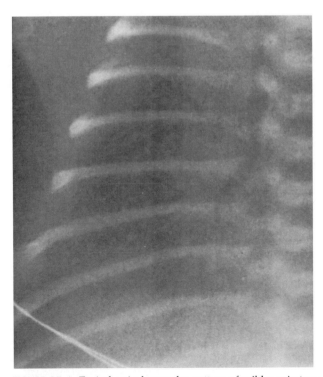

FIGURE 35–6. Typical reticulogranular pattern of mild respiratory distress syndrome.

Distinguishing between diffuse bilateral consolidation and increased lung density because of expiration is sometimes difficult. In general, however, expiration results in constricted, centralized air bronchograms, whereas airspace disease is associated with peripheral extension of air bronchograms.

Pulmonary Hypoplasia and Agenesis

(See also Chapter 42.)

In the absence of a diaphragmatic hernia, unilateral agenesis or pulmonary hypoplasia may be indistinguishable from atelectasis on neonatal chest radiographs. The presence of associated vertebral anomalies or esophageal atresia, however, suggests a pulmonary malformation rather than atelectasis. Bilateral pulmonary hypoplasia is suggested by a small, bell-shaped thorax and the presence of an air leak, such as pneumothorax or pneumomediastinum (Fig. 35–7). These findings often are associated with maternal oligohydramnios, in which case ultrasonographic investigation of possible renal malformations is recommended. The thorax also may appear bell shaped in the presence of various neuromuscular abnormalities (including trisomy 21), as well as in infants requiring therapeutic neuromuscular paralysis for assisted ventilation. In the latter situation, there is often decreased bowel gas and body wall soft tissue edema.

Air Leak

Extravasation of alveolar air has become a less frequent complication of ventilatory failure since the introduction of surfactant therapy. The extravasated air travels from the alveolus, dissects through the

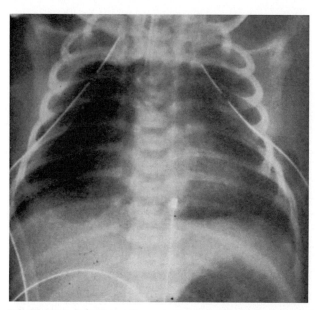

FIGURE 35–7. Infant's small, somewhat bell-shaped chest caused by severe renal malformations and maternal oligohydramnios. Bilateral thoracostomy tubes were inserted for the treatment of pneumothoraces. There is still a large pneumomediastinum elevating the thymus.

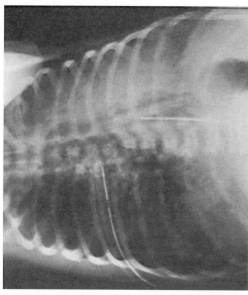

FIGURE 35–8. Lateral decubitus film shows a residual right pneumothorax in spite of the presence of a chest tube. Part of the intrapleural gas is trapped medial to the right lung.

interstitium of the lungs, and enters the mediastinum. Alternatively, air dissecting via the pulmonary lymphatics may perforate the visceral pleura and cause a pneumothorax. Pneumopericardium and pneumoperitoneum are less common manifestations of extraventilatory air.

Pneumothorax in a newborn infant is generally readily recognizable when the gas in the pleural space clearly outlines the visceral pleura. In addition, there is usually considerable mediastinal shift toward the contralateral side and a varying amount of collapse of both lungs. Occasionally, even fairly large pneumothoraces may not be obvious. This is because the air in the supine neonate's thorax tends to assume a position anterior and medial to the lung. The only sign may be enlargement and increased lucency of the affected hemithorax (Fig. 35–8). In this case, a lateral decubitus film, made with the normal side dependent, demonstrates air adjacent to the visceral pleura of the costal surface of the involved lung.

In *pneumomediastinum,* a halo of air may be recognizable on either side of the mediastinum. The hallmark, however, is displacement of the thymus away from the parietal pericardium, the so-called spinnaker sail sign (Fig. 35–9). Air dissection into the soft tissues of the neck is less common in neonates than it is in older infants and children with pneumomediastinum. Unlike mediastinal emphysema, which is limited inferiorly by the central tendon of the diaphragm, a pneumopericardium completely surrounds the heart and origins of the great vessels (Fig. 35–10).

Pulmonary interstitial emphysema may be diffuse, bilateral, or localized to a single lung or lobe. The interstitial gas appears as multiple well-defined circular or elongated lucencies contrasted against the collapsed lung parenchyma. In addition, there is a marked increase in volume of the involved portion

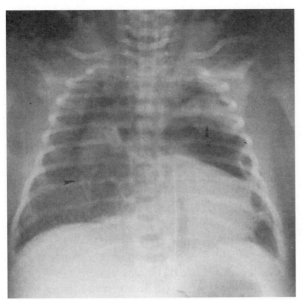

FIGURE 35–9. Separation of the thymic lobes (*arrowheads*) from the pericardial surface resulting from a large pneumomediastinum. There is also a large amount of air in the neck and soft tissues of the chest wall, which occurs less commonly in newborns than in older children.

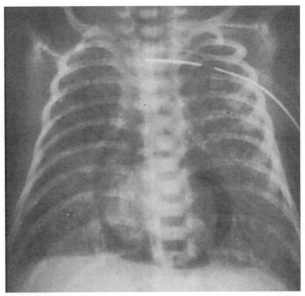

FIGURE 35–10. A pneumopericardium completely surrounds the heart.

of lung. The "bubbly" pattern of diffuse interstitial emphysema can usually be distinguished from focal emphysema associated with bronchopulmonary dysplasia by its rapid onset and the uniform appearance of the bubbles, which typically radiate from the hila. Occasionally, continued expansion of the interstitial gas collections results in localized pulmonary overdistention resembling lobar emphysema.

RADIOGRAPHIC SIGNS OF CARDIOVASCULAR ABNORMALITIES

Large Heart on Chest X-ray

(See also Chapter 43.)

Most causes of cardiomegaly in the neonate do not involve congenital heart disease. Analysis of specific chamber enlargements is not possible with the chest x-ray, and an echocardiogram is necessary for a more specific diagnosis. Metabolic causes of a large heart include hypoglycemia, hypocalcemia, and severe anemia. Infants of diabetic mothers also may have large hearts with associated congestive heart failure (see Chapter 47, Part One). Neonatal asphyxia produces reversible ischemia to the myocardium, again resulting in a large heart. In preterm infants, congestive failure and resultant cardiomegaly are frequent consequences of left-to-right shunt through a patent ductus arteriosus. Other causes include arrhythmias (most commonly paroxysmal atrial tachycardia), myocarditis, and tumors (usually rhabdomyoma). Peripheral arteriovenous malformations, such as vein of Galen aneurysm and hepatic hemangioendothelioma, are other rare causes.

Congenital heart disease may produce a large heart associated with the hypoplastic left heart syndrome

and heart failure (Fig. 35–11). This spectrum of obstruction on the left side of the circulation extends anatomically from the pulmonary vein to the aortic arch and coarctation. It is impossible to distinguish on the chest x-ray where the obstruction has occurred. These infants present in severe heart failure early in the newborn period. Hypoplastic right heart shows decreased pulmonary vascularity from right-to-left shunting, usually at the atrial level. Valvular regurgitation also can produce a large heart, and this is seen with birth asphyxia, congenital tricuspid insufficiency, and Ebstein anomaly. Left-to-right shunts through a ventricular septal defect or atrial septal defect do not produce a large heart in the newborn period.

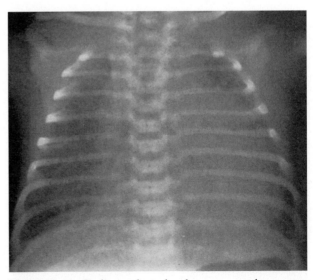

FIGURE 35–11. Cardiomegaly and pulmonary vascular engorgement in an infant with hypoplastic left heart. Pulmonary vascularity is indistinct because of pulmonary venous engorgement from congestive heart failure.

Congestive Heart Failure

In a mature infant, the heart is considered to be enlarged when the cardiothymic-thoracic ratio is greater than 0.6. In preterm infants, the normal ratio is smaller, and the cardiomegaly is often less obvious. Pulmonary venous congestion is manifested by engorgement and increase in size of the pulmonary veins. As pulmonary venous pressure rises, interstitial edema occurs. This is observed as a decrease in the definition of the lung vasculature and by Kerley lines, which are produced by leakage of fluid into the interlobular septa. Kerley B lines are seen as short, horizontal, linear densities in the lung and extending to the pleural surface. They are typically found above the costophrenic angles but may be seen to better advantage in infants in the retrosternal portion of the lungs on lateral views. Kerley A lines are longer linear densities radiating from the hila. Edema of the subpleural alveolar tissue and pleural effusions are more easily seen in small infants than are Kerley lines.

Cyanotic Congenital Heart Disease

The size of the heart may range from relatively normal, as in transposition of the great arteries, to huge, as in Ebstein anomaly. In most cases, the caliber of the pulmonary vessels is reduced. The hila are consequently small, and the lungs appear relatively lucent. In addition, the thymus tends to be involuted because of stress, and the lungs are often hyperinflated. Pulmonary vascular engorgement, rather than oligemia, accompanies cyanosis in patients with D-transposition of the great arteries, resulting from incomplete mixing of systemic and pulmonary blood. Cyanosis with congestive heart failure and radiographic signs of pulmonary edema with a normal cardiothymic silhouette (an appearance that may resemble RDS) suggest the diagnosis of obstructive total anomalous pulmonary venous drainage (Fig. 35–12), which is almost always subdiaphragmatic into the portal vein, hepatic vein, or inferior vena cava.

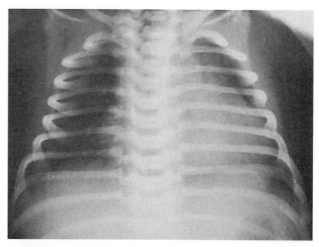

FIGURE 35–13. Marked enlargement of the cardiothymic silhouette and diminished caliber of the pulmonary vessels in a patient with the syndrome of persistent pulmonary hypertension, simulating cyanotic congenital heart disease.

Persistent pulmonary hypertension also may mimic cyanotic congenital heart disease on chest radiographs, because there may be cardiomegaly and pulmonary oligemia (Fig. 35–13). In other cases, congestive heart failure or pulmonary disease such as meconium aspiration may be present. Severe cases of persistent fetal circulation refractory to conventional therapy can be treated with ECMO (see Chapter 42). Diffuse pulmonary opacification is present on the chest x-ray film during this treatment.[52] Ultrasonography is especially helpful in distinguishing this opacification from pleural fluid (see Fig. 35–2) in neonates who are anticoagulated with heparin.[15] The ECMO catheter position must be carefully monitored on repeat films.

Vascular Ring

Vascular rings should be suspected in neonates with respiratory difficulty presenting as an inspiratory stridor. The neonatal trachea is quite mobile, and the normal left aortic arch is inferred by displacement of the trachea to the right (see Fig. 35–4). The aortic arch usually cannot be identified on the chest x-ray film as a separate structure because of the thymus. A barium esophagram is still recommended for the diagnosis of a vascular ring. Echocardiography or MRI may be needed for further anatomic information before surgery (Fig. 35–14).

GASTROINTESTINAL TRACT

(See also Chapter 45.)

METHODS OF EXAMINATION

Initial plain film examination usually consists of an AP supine film made with a vertical beam. As with

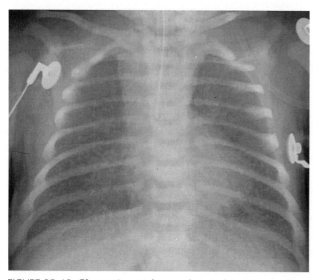

FIGURE 35–12. Obstructive total anomalous pulmonary venous return. Note the pulmonary venous congestion with a normal-sized heart.

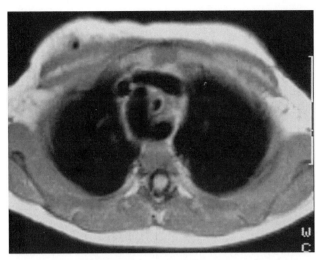

FIGURE 35–14. Vascular ring on magnetic resonance imaging scan. Note the right aortic arch with an aberrant left subclavian artery behind the trachea. Tracheal stenosis due to complete tracheal rings is also present. Compare with Figure 35–4.

chest radiography, additional lateral and decubitus views are made with a horizontally directed x-ray beam. These films can be made without removing the infant from the incubator, allow visualization of air-filled levels, and permit more precise demonstration of free intraperitoneal air (Fig. 35–15). A horizontal-beam lateral view of the abdomen with the infant prone is an aid in demonstrating gas in the rectum and sigmoid colon when distal intestinal obstruction is suspected. Radiographs made with the infant erect or inverted are not recommended; they are stressful to the patient and present considerable technical difficulties.

Ultrasonography is being used more commonly for the diagnosis of gastrointestinal problems and is now the accepted method of diagnosing *hypertrophic pyloric*

stenosis. The elongated and narrowed pyloric channel can be seen surrounded by hypoechoic, thickened muscle (Fig. 35–16). Ultrasonography has the advantage of being noninvasive, but it is technically demanding. If the characteristic ultrasonographic findings of hypertrophic pyloric stenosis are not demonstrated, a fluoroscopic procedure may be required to identify other possible causes of vomiting. Gastric outlet obstruction has been described as a rare complication of prolonged prostaglandin E therapy in neonates with congenital heart disease who are ductus dependent.

CONTRAST MEDIA

Air is a satisfactory contrast medium that can be used to demonstrate the site of bowel obstruction (Fig. 35–17). When it is necessary to opacify the stomach or bowel, barium sulfate is usually the medium of choice because it is relatively inert, readily available, and inexpensive. Water-soluble, iodine-containing contrast media are useful when perforation of the gut is suspected, as they are readily absorbed from the peritoneal surface.

Contrast enemas must be carried out under fluoroscopic control in the radiology department. They are performed using a flexible infant feeding tube that is taped in place. Preparation of the bowel is not necessary and is especially contraindicated when there is *Hirschsprung disease.* Upper gastrointestinal studies also are preferably done fluoroscopically, but if this is contraindicated because of the clinical condition of the infant, the contrast medium can be monitored during its course through the gastrointestinal tract using portable equipment.

A contrast enema is indicated in neonates with suspected Hirschsprung disease.[42] A transition zone, usually involving the sigmoid, between the distal aganglionic bowel and proximal ganglionic bowel,

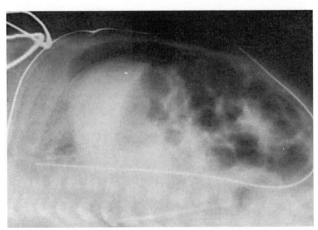

FIGURE 35–15. Horizontal-beam lateral view of the abdomen with the infant supine demonstrates intraperitoneal gas anterior to the liver and adjacent to the anterior abdominal wall. Several examples of the double-wall sign, with the inner wall of the bowel outlined by intraluminal air and the outer wall outlined by intraperitoneal air, are visible anteriorly.

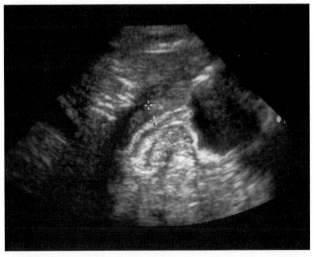

FIGURE 35–16. Ultrasound diagnosis of hypertrophic pyloric stenosis. Longitudinal view shows the thickened and elongated pylorus with fluid in the stomach. Greatly thickened pyloric muscle is measured between electronic cursors.

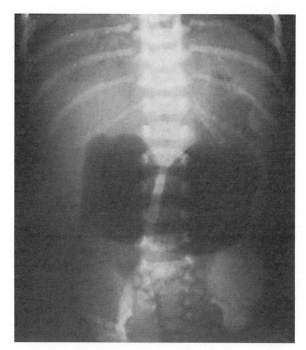

FIGURE 35–17. Anteroposterior recumbent film of the abdomen demonstrating the "double bubble" resulting from gaseous distention of the stomach and first portion of the duodenum caused by duodenal atresia. Note the complete absence of gas distal to the duodenum.

may not always be apparent in neonates. In this situation, rectal suction biopsy is indicated for a definitive diagnosis.[51]

Low-osmolality water-soluble iodine-containing contrast materials (e.g., iohexol and iopamidol) are available and afford a greater degree of safety because they can be prepared in an isotonic solution. They permit more prolonged visualization of the gut and are rapidly absorbed from the peritoneum of patients with gastrointestinal perforation. Experience with these relatively expensive materials suggests that they provide greater safety than do other contrast media.[8] Recommendations for their use include necrotizing enterocolitis, risk of leakage of contrast agent from the gastrointestinal tract, or risk of entry into the lung or mediastinum.

Gastrografin is a high-osmolality water-soluble contrast medium containing a 76% solution of sodium methylglucamine diatrozoate with 37% bound iodine. The major disadvantage of this contrast medium is its high osmolarity (1900 mOsm/L), which causes a shift of water and electrolytes into the lumen of the bowel. This limits its use to the diagnosis and treatment of meconium ileus and meconium plugs. The therapeutic benefits are caused by osmosis of water into the lumen of the bowel and resultant softening of the meconium. Careful monitoring of these infants is essential, because dehydration and electrolyte imbalance can occur.

NORMAL FINDINGS

Air is swallowed immediately after birth and reaches the small bowel about 3 hours later. After approxi-

mately 6 to 8 hours of postnatal life, gas is present throughout the large and small bowels, reaching the rectum by 24 hours. Mild generalized gaseous distention often occurs because of air swallowing. A more generalized bowel distention can occur secondary to nasal continuous positive airway pressure.[23] Newborn infants present a special diagnostic problem because of the similarity in appearance and caliber of the large and small bowels.

GASTROINTESTINAL DISTENTION AND OBSTRUCTION

An increase in the amount of intestinal gas does not necessarily indicate obstruction, because it may occur in a variety of conditions, including septicemia, necrotizing enterocolitis, tracheoesophageal fistula, maternal drug therapy, hypothyroidism, and hypermagnesemia. In these disorders, the gas is distributed throughout the small and large bowels. Obstruction also may be mimicked by excess air swallowing resulting from respiratory distress.

Mechanical bowel obstruction produces gaseous intestinal distention, frequently with air-fluid levels proximal to the site of obstruction. Distal to the obstruction, the intraluminal gas may be diminished or absent. A different pattern is often seen, however, in obstruction resulting from *meconium ileus*. In this disorder, the bowel loops vary in size, are unevenly distributed, and contain few air-fluid levels. The inspissated meconium in the small bowel becomes mixed with air, producing a bubbly appearance (Fig. 35–18). The thick, echogenic meconium seen in meconium ileus should be distinguished from the fluid-

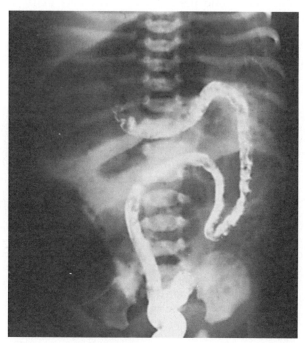

FIGURE 35–18. Anteroposterior recumbent film of the abdomen in an infant with meconium ileus. Note the distended bowel loops of varying sizes and the bubbly appearance of the intestinal contents, particularly in the left flank. The distal ileal obstruction is reflected by the marked diminution in caliber of the colon (microcolon).

filled loops of bowel seen in ileal atresia, and this can be appreciated by ultrasonography.[36]

Duodenal obstruction is usually easily recognizable on plain films because of distention of the stomach and proximal duodenum, which produces the classic "double bubble" appearance. These structures often contain air-fluid levels, and the amount of gas distal to the obstruction varies with the degree of obstruction. The most common entities that produce a double bubble are duodenal stenosis or atresia, annular pancreas, and malrotation with peritoneal bands and midgut volvulus (see Fig. 35–17).

Contrast examinations are often indicated when duodenal obstruction is suspected clinically or is demonstrated on plain films. These studies are particularly urgent because of the importance of recognizing and promptly treating malrotation and midgut volvulus with associated mesenteric vascular insufficiency. When the degree of obstruction appears to be incomplete, the volvulus can be diagnosed by introducing barium into the stomach. If there is an associated malrotation of the midgut, the duodenojejunal junction is displaced medially and inferiorly from its normal position in the left upper abdominal quadrant, and the duodenum and proximal jejunum have a corkscrew or Z-shaped configuration[1] (Fig. 35–19). Midgut volvulus can be diagnosed with color Doppler ultrasonography,[48] but for the diagnosis of malrotation in a neonate with bilious emesis, the contrast upper gastrointestinal study is necessary.

The caliber of the colon is another important observation made on contrast enemas. A ribbon-like unused or *microcolon* occurs when there is lack of normal distention by intestinal contents, resulting from exclusion of succus entericus from the colon during fetal life (see Fig. 35–18). The diminished colonic caliber usually indicates some type of distal ileal obstruction, such as meconium ileus or ileal atresia. In contrast, the caliber of the colon is predicted to be normal in the presence of duodenal or high jejunal obstruction. Exceptions to this rule may occur, however. If the distal ileal atresia occurs late in fetal life, the caliber of the colon may be normal. The caliber of the colon is decreased in nearly 40% of patients with total colonic aganglionosis, presumably because of functional small intestine obstruction. A localized decrease in the caliber of the left colon occurs in Hirschsprung disease, meconium plug syndrome, and the neonatal small left colon syndrome (Fig. 35–20).

PNEUMOPERITONEUM

Early diagnosis of pneumoperitoneum often depends on its recognition on routine AP supine views. Because the air rises anteriorly, a lucency can be seen overlying the liver adjacent to the inferior surface of the diaphragm. A large collection of air causes generalized abdominal distention, and structures not usually visible, such as the falciform ligament (Fig. 35–21), umbilical arteries, or a persistent urachus, may be outlined by the air. Perhaps the most valuable indicator of small amounts of free air is the double-wall sign, in which the mucosal surface of the bowel is outlined by intraluminal air and the serosal surface by intraperitoneal air. The intraperitoneal air is best demonstrated on films made with a horizontal beam and the patient in the supine or decubitus position, which show collections of gas adjacent to the anterior abdominal wall or flanks (see Fig. 35–15).

Although the most important cause of pneumoperitoneum is perforation of the bowel, the possibility of extension of gas from a pneumomediastinum into the peritoneal cavity must be considered in infants with respiratory distress. An air-fluid level in the peritoneal cavity almost certainly indicates bowel perforation, but absence of an air-fluid level is not a com-

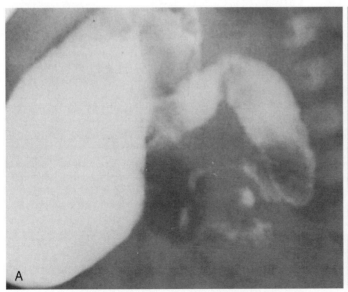
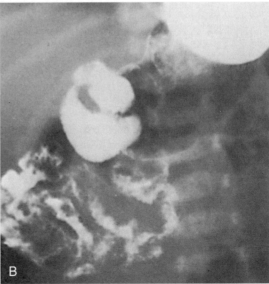

FIGURE 35–19. Partial duodenal obstruction resulting from midgut malrotation with volvulus. *A*, With the patient in a steep oblique position, the distal duodenum and proximal jejunum have a "corkscrew" appearance, and the duodenojejunal junction is not identifiable. *B*, The proximal small bowel is to the right of the midline.

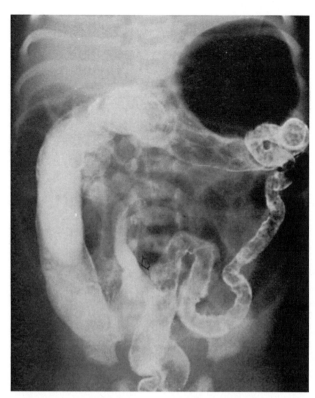

FIGURE 35-20. Barium enema demonstrates the decreased caliber of the left side of the colon with an apparent transition zone at the splenic flexure. The bowel contains a moderate amount of meconium. Besides appearing in cases of Hirschsprung disease, these findings can occur in infants of diabetic mothers with the neonatal small left colon syndrome and in those with meconium plug syndrome.

pletely reliable sign of an intact gastrointestinal tract.[31] The presence of perforation can be confirmed by instilling a small amount of isotonic water-soluble contrast medium through a nasogastric tube and observing its passage into the peritoneal cavity.

PNEUMATOSIS INTESTINALIS

The most common cause of pneumatosis intestinalis is necrotizing enterocolitis, although bowel ischemia secondary to intestinal obstruction is an occasional cause. The intramural gas that collects beneath the serosa or in the submucosa of the intestine may be either localized or diffusely distributed throughout the bowel and appears as small linear or bubbly lucencies (Fig. 35–22). In patients with necrotizing enterocolitis, there also may be intestinal distention with air-fluid levels, intraperitoneal fluid, portal venous gas (Fig. 35–23), or pneumoperitoneum.[35]

It is important to emphasize that clinical features of necrotizing enterocolitis may occur in the absence of pneumatosis.[25] In these patients, a disturbed bowel gas pattern consisting of elongation, dilation, and separation of bowel loops may be seen. Pneumoperitoneum is typically an indication for surgical intervention. Subsequent strictures from healing with fibrosis develop most often in the large bowel (80%).[24]

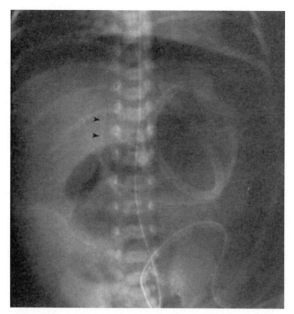

FIGURE 35–21. Anteroposterior recumbent film of the abdomen demonstrates a large pneumoperitoneum, with free air inferior to the diaphragm and outlining the falciform ligament (*arrowheads*).

INTRAVASCULAR GAS

In necrotizing enterocolitis, the intramural gas may dissect into the portal venous system and be seen radiating into the liver from the hilus. Ultrasonography demonstrates portal venous gas in infants with necrotizing enterocolitis before abnormalities are apparent on abdominal films.[32] In the absence of necrotizing enterocolitis, portal vein gas may be introduced through umbilical venous catheters.

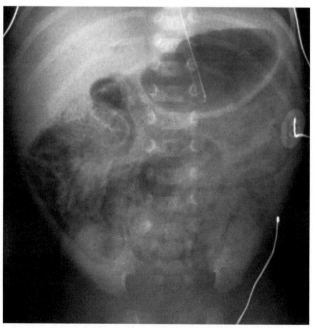

FIGURE 35–22. Necrotizing enterocolitis. Note the linear and bubbly pattern of pneumatosis intestinalis.

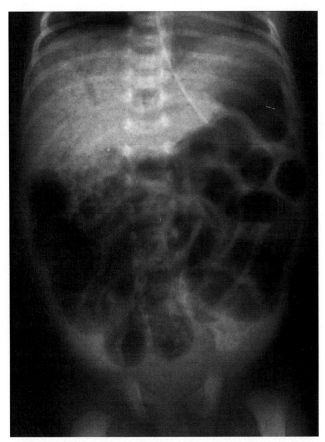

FIGURE 35–23. Portal vein gas is identified as branching radiolucencies overlying the liver in this case of necrotizing enterocolitis.

Pulmonary gas embolism is another cause of intravascular gas and is unrelated to gastrointestinal disease. The embolism occurs when alveolar gas ruptures into the pulmonary vascular bed. The gas is then rapidly distributed throughout the systemic vessels, usually resulting in sudden death. The gas is often particularly prominent within the hepatic veins. The radiographic findings may be mimicked by postmortem accumulations of gas.

INTRA-ABDOMINAL CALCIFICATIONS

In the fetus and the newborn, *intra-abdominal calcifications* can occur within a few days. Calcifications of the peritoneum, intestinal wall, or even intraluminal contents are occasional but important clues to intestinal disorders.

The most frequently recognized calcifications involve the peritoneum and are caused by sterile meconium peritonitis resulting from an intrauterine bowel perforation. The calcifications are usually streaky or plaquelike and often occur over the liver, over the abdominal surface of the diaphragm, or along the flanks (Fig. 35–24). Rarely, these calcifications can occur in the scrotum, as communication with the peritoneal cavity is normal in utero.

Calcifications of intraluminal meconium appear as small, rounded densities that follow the course of the small or large bowel. Within the colon, they have been seen in association with imperforate anus. Small intestinal calcifications have been documented in cases of ileal stenosis, atresia, and total colonic aganglionosis. Rarely, calcification of the bowel wall may occur in patients with intestinal volvulus or atresia. Neuroblastoma and retroperitoneal teratoma commonly contain calcium, and intrahepatic calcifications have been observed in neonates because of transplacental infections and neoplastic lesions (e.g., hemangioma and hepatoblastoma).

BILIARY ABNORMALITIES

(See also Chapter 46.)

The biliary tract in the neonate is best imaged by a combination of ultrasonography, which may detect anatomic lesions such as a choledochal cyst, and biliary scintigraphy using technetium-labeled iminodiacetic acid (IDA) derivatives (Fig. 35–25) to demonstrate the function of the bile ducts. Oral phenobarbital increases the sensitivity of IDA scans. These procedures are most frequently employed in the evaluation of jaundice. Passage of the radionuclide from the liver to the gut indicates patency of the biliary tree and excludes a diagnosis of biliary atresia. Biliary atresia is likely in the absence of excretion of IDA into the bowel from bile ducts, and surgical exploration with an operative cholangiogram is recommended. MRI can now be used to identify the biliary tree and pancreatic duct with the magnetic resonance cholangiopancreatogram.[12]

Cholelithiasis is occasionally seen in newborn infants and may be related to total parenteral nutrition. Spontaneous resolution of gallstones in this age group has rarely been reported. The natural history of neonatal gallstones is unknown, and the clinical presentation ranges from incidental findings on abdominal imaging to acute cholecystitis.[47]

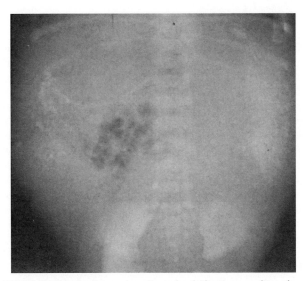

FIGURE 35–24. Ascites and peritoneal calcification resulting from meconium peritonitis.

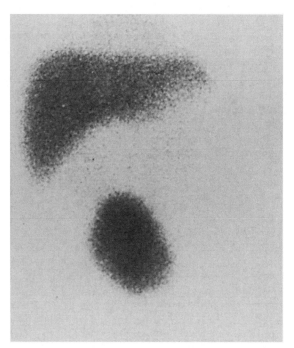

FIGURE 35–25. Technetium-labeled iminodiacetic acid radionuclide study in a patient with biliary atresia. No activity is noted in the gut 90 minutes after injection of the radiopharmaceutical agent. Renal excretion has resulted in radioactivity within the urinary bladder.

URINARY TRACT

(See also Chapter 49.)

A number of different choices are available to image the urinary tract and retroperitoneum. When anatomic information is required, sonographic examination is now the method of choice. Radioisotope studies are more valuable indicators of renal function than of renal structure. The lower urinary tract and vesicoureteral reflux are best evaluated by means of voiding cystourethrography. This can be performed fluoroscopically or with a radioisotope.

ULTRASONOGRAPHY

As indicated in Chapter 8, sound waves are produced by a transducer that, employing the piezoelectric effect, changes electrical energy to mechanical sound waves. Typical frequencies used for these transducers are between 5 and 10 MHz. Sound waves travel from the transducer, which is in contact with the infant's skin, and are reflected at interfaces in which differences in acoustic properties are present. The reflected sound waves, or echoes, are "heard" by the transducer and converted into electrical signals, which produce the image. Because interfaces between soft tissues and bone and between soft tissues and air produce virtually no echoes, the bony skeleton, lungs, and gas-filled loops of bowel are not usually appreciated by ultrasonography. Ultrasonography does not produce ionization and, as far as we know, is biologically safe at the energy levels used. Moreover, no contrast material or IV injections are used. Sedation and preparation are not necessary, and portable ultrasonographic equipment can easily be transferred to the nursery. Doppler ultrasonography can be applied to examine the vasculature. Duplex images of the vessels can be viewed in color or as spectral waves to give information about the direction of flow and the velocity of the blood in the vessel.

Examination of the neonatal genitourinary system should include identification of both kidneys, both adrenal glands, and the bladder. Fluid in the peritoneal cavity, such as urinary ascites, can be easily identified by ultrasonography, and the position of catheters inserted into the umbilical artery and vein should be checked as part of a complete study. Doppler ultrasonography of the renal vessels may detect venous or arterial thromboses.

NUCLEAR IMAGING

Renal scintigraphy provides important functional information about the kidneys that cannot be obtained by other imaging modalities. Renal blood flow and function can be estimated by employing IV injections of technetium-tagged diethylenetriaminepentaacetic acid (DTPA). This radiopharmaceutical is excreted purely by glomerular filtration, and images of the collecting systems can therefore be obtained. Unfortunately, nuclear imaging of neonatal kidneys is limited by their small size, which approaches the limits of resolution of the gamma camera. Computer analysis of the uptake and excretion of the radionuclide can be used to generate a renogram curve. The time taken for 50% of the maximal uptake of radionuclide on the renogram curve to be excreted is called the half-time ($t_{1/2}$). This measurement, together with a provocative test with the diuretic furosemide, can help distinguish obstructed from nonobstructed dilated collecting systems. These measurements also can help monitor therapy and surgery. Technetium-tagged glucoheptonate is another commonly used radiopharmaceutical. Its excretion is by a combination of glomerular filtration and tubular secretion. Therefore, it gives slightly different information, providing visualization of both the collecting system and the renal parenchyma. Dimercaptosuccinic acid (DMSA) is a renal cortical imaging agent that best demonstrates acute pyelonephritis and renal scars.

The radionuclide voiding cystogram gives the patient a much smaller radiation dose than the fluoroscopic voiding cystogram. For this reason, it is recommended as the initial study for reflux in girls and for follow-up studies in both boys and girls. It also has been proposed as a screening test for siblings of children who demonstrate reflux.

VOIDING CYSTOURETHROGRAPHY

In neonates, voiding cystourethrography is useful in the evaluation of vesicoureteral reflux, posterior urethral valves in the male urethra, ambiguous genitalia, and anorectal malformations. The bladder is filled until the patient voids, during which time rapid serial

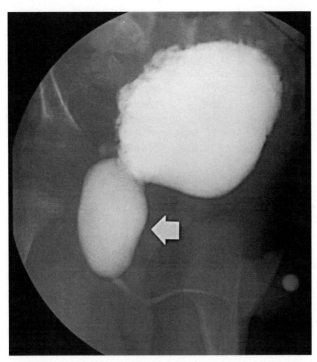

FIGURE 35–26. Voiding cystourethrogram in a male neonate identifies posterior urethral valves. Note the large posterior urethra (*arrowhead*) with a narrow anterior urethra. The bladder is trabeculated posteriorly.

imaging is carried out. A steep oblique position is necessary for visualization of the bladder neck and the entire length of the urethra. Normally, the contour of the bladder is symmetric and smooth. Trabeculation and diverticula suggest outlet obstruction or a neurogenic bladder. An ectopic ureterocele may cause a smooth, rounded intraluminal filling defect. This may be missed if the contrast medium is too dense. Radiographic evaluation of the female urethra is usually unrewarding. Radiographic evaluation of the male urethra, however, is essential to demonstrate anatomic abnormalities such as posterior urethral valves (Fig. 35–26).

The presence or absence of vesicoureteral reflux is an extremely important observation and is the most common diagnosis in neonates with the antenatal finding of hydronephrosis.[56] Because reflux can be identified only during voiding, careful filming must be carried out at this time. Vesicoureteral reflux also allows morphologic assessment of the ureters and collecting systems in infants with reduced or absent renal function.

EXCRETORY UROGRAPHY

In today's practice, indications for a neonatal urogram are rare. Anatomic structures can be visualized by ultrasonography, and physiologic information is provided by nuclear imaging. Because reactions to the injection of contrast materials and other complications, including pulmonary edema and hemorrhage, have been reported even at the usual doses,[2] this study should not be performed in infants with low birth weights (less than 1500 gm) or in infants who are sick or hypotensive. If the study is thought to be essential, waiting until the child is older and bigger is prudent, at which time more satisfactory urograms may be performed.

THE NORMAL NEONATAL KIDNEY

On a sonogram, normal neonatal kidneys differ from those of older children and adults in important ways. They display a relatively echogenic renal cortex[16] and a lack of renal sinus fat. The resistive index, as identified with Doppler ultrasonography, is higher in the first year of life, indicating a higher resistance to flow in the normal infant kidney.[4]

The increased cortical echo pattern of the renal cortex approaches that of the adjacent liver. This is a normal neonatal pattern and should not be mistaken for renal parenchymal disease. It is found in all full-term and premature infants. By 17 weeks of age, this pattern is replaced by one with decreased echoes that persists throughout life. Approximately 50% of infants have already changed to this adult-type pattern by 8 weeks of age. Explanations for the increased echogenicity of the normal neonatal kidney include a greater number of glomeruli, greater cellular content of the glomerular tuft, and presence of loops of Henle within the cortex. These histologic variations result in numerous cellular interfaces in the renal cortex and therefore greater echogenicity.

Both the renal artery and the renal vein can be seen and thromboses in either vessel documented with a color Doppler examination. The lack of perirenal fat is a normal finding in neonates and is one reason why CT scanning, which relies on the natural contrast material produced by fat around abdominal organs, is often unsatisfactory in these infants. The neonatal adrenal glands are relatively large, and both can usually be identified. The adrenal cortex is sonolucent or anechoic, whereas the adrenal medulla is echogenic. The adrenal gland can be identified as a V- or Y-shaped structure, with the right adrenal gland usually easier to identify than the left one.

RENAL MASSES

The most common masses in the newborn period are caused by multicystic dysplasia and hydronephrosis. These entities can be identified and differentiated by ultrasonography,[45] which should be the initial examination of choice (Fig. 35–27). For confirmation, nuclear imaging demonstrates lack of function (Fig. 35–28) in multicystic kidneys; delayed function is noted in hydronephrosis. On ultrasonography, a multicystic dysplastic kidney shows many noncommunicating cysts of various sizes. With hydronephrosis, the fluid collections communicate with the enlarged renal pelvis. Renal parenchyma is usually identified in hydronephrosis but not in multicystic dysplastic kidney. During the last decade, there has been a dramatic increase in neonates with hydronephrosis. This can

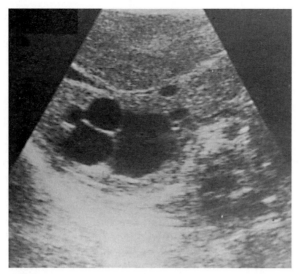

FIGURE 35-27. Ultrasound study of multicystic dysplastic kidney. Transverse view of the upper abdomen shows several cystic collections in the region of the right renal fossa. These do not communicate and are of various sizes.

be explained by the widespread use of obstetric sonography, which is now detecting the true incidence of congenital anomalies of the urinary tract. Before this time, only symptomatic renal masses were diagnosed in the newborn period. Optimal timing for ultrasonographic imaging of a hydronephrosis demonstrated in utero is important. During the first 24 hours of life, a physiologic state of dehydration exists, and hydronephrosis may not always be detected by ultrasonographic screening. It is therefore recommended that postpartum ultrasonographic examination be delayed for several days after delivery in neonates diagnosed with intrauterine hydronephrosis.[30]

Autosomal recessive infantile *polycystic disease* produces bilaterally large kidneys that are very echogenic. There is also a loss of the normal distinction between cortex and medulla. Increased echogenicity of the cysts seems paradoxical but can be explained by the small size of the cysts, which cannot be identified separately. The many tiny cysts produce a multitude of acoustic interfaces, each of which produces echoes. Other renal masses are rare in the newborn period. A solitary solid mass of the kidney often indicates a benign mesoblastic nephroma. Wilms tumor is less common in this age group and cannot be distinguished from mesoblastic nephroma by ultrasonography alone.

Ultrasonography also is helpful in the diagnosis of pelvic masses. Hydrocolpos and hydrometrocolpos can be identified and distinguished from other pelvic masses, such as a distended bladder, anterior meningocele, presacral teratoma, neuroblastoma, and ovarian cyst. With the increased use of obstetric ultrasonography, ovarian cysts are being recognized more frequently. Many of these simple ovarian cysts resolve spontaneously, without the need for surgery. Neonatal ovarian cysts can be followed expectantly with serial ultrasonography,[37] but more complex cysts should be removed surgically, because they often represent an ovarian torsion. Finally, *nephrocalcinosis,* with the potential for subsequent renal calculi in neonates receiving long-term furosemide therapy, is identified and monitored with ultrasonography (Fig. 35-29).

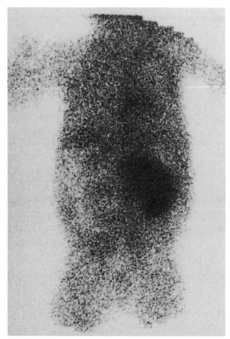

FIGURE 35-28. Radionuclide study of multicystic dysplastic kidney. The right multicystic kidney shows up as an area of decreased function. The normal-functioning kidney is on the left side.

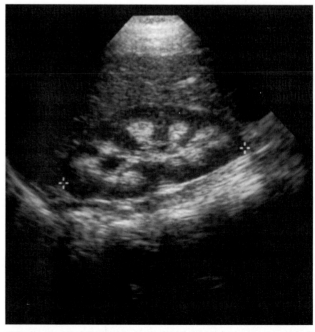

FIGURE 35-29. Nephrocalcinosis. The normal sonolucent (*black*) pyramids of the kidneys have been replaced by echogenic (*white*) diffuse calcification related to long-term furosemide therapy.

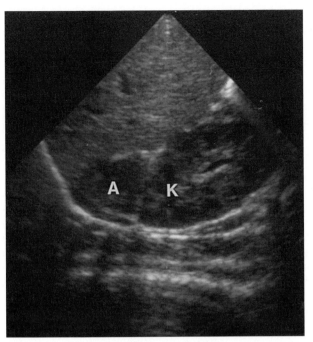

FIGURE 35–30. Ultrasound study of adrenal hemorrhage. Longitudinal view of the right upper quadrant shows a mass (A) above the right kidney (K) and beneath the liver. This represents an adrenal hemorrhage.

ADRENAL HEMORRHAGE

Adrenal hemorrhage is seen on ultrasonography as a mass that replaces the normal adrenal gland (Fig. 35–30). Usually the mass has a mixed echo pattern that changes as the hemorrhage resolves (Fig. 35–31). Follow-up ultrasonographic studies are recommended to confirm a decrease in the size of the mass and to exclude the incidental finding of a neuro-

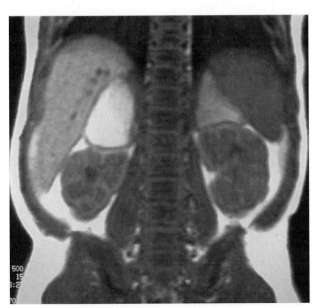

FIGURE 35–31. Bilateral adrenal hemorrhages. Coronal T1-weighted magnetic resonance imaging scan shows the enlarged adrenals with different blood products above each kidney.

blastoma. Occasionally on follow-up abdominal x-rays, calcification can be identified in the region of an earlier adrenal hemorrhage.

SKELETAL SYSTEM

No attempt will be made to describe all the numerous bone abnormalities that can exist in neonates. However, important observations can be made from the bones visible on films of the chest and abdomen, which reflect physiologic and pathologic changes.

The bones of a gestationally mature infant are normally dense. During the first 4 to 6 weeks of life, this density diminishes as bone growth accelerates. By approximately 1 to 2 months of age, physiologic periosteal new bone formation may be seen along the shafts of long bones in rapidly growing healthy infants. This growth usually can be differentiated from abnormal periosteal reaction by its symmetry and lack of underlying osseous lesions. In contrast, the bones of a premature infant appear less well mineralized than normal, and the cortices are relatively thin.

On radiographs of the chest and abdomen, the proximal metaphyses of the humeri or femurs are almost always visible. Abnormalities of these bony structures may reflect either intrauterine disorders or postnatal disorders.

ANTENATAL DISORDERS

Intrauterine infections (see Chapters 22 and 37) frequently cause metaphyseal abnormalities. In *rubella* and *cytomegalovirus* infections, the metaphyses typically are rarefied and contain dense, vertical striations that resemble a celery stalk. *Syphilis* also causes metaphyseal irregularity (osteochondritis), proximal to which is a zone of radiolucency. Syphilis also may produce a periosteal reaction (Fig. 35–32). The value of routine long-bone films in serologically positive neonates has been questioned,[14] but they are still recommended by the Centers for Disease Control and Prevention.[6] Intrauterine insults may rarely produce a horizontal band of increased density in the metaphysis because of growth arrest.

POSTNATAL DISORDERS

Osteomyelitis in the newborn is usually caused by *Staphylococcus, Streptococcus,* or *Candida* organisms. These organisms produce focal lucent metaphyseal areas of bone destruction with or without associated septic arthritis (Fig. 35–33).

The efficacy of bone scans in the diagnosis of osteomyelitis is less firmly established in neonates than in older children. Although radionuclide bone scans may not offer additional information when radiographs are positive, they may reveal lesions when radiographs are normal.[34] These lesions are sometimes clinically silent and found incidentally on films done for other purposes. Because neonatal osteomyelitis is

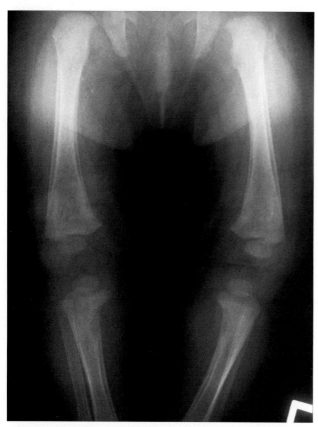

FIGURE 35–32. Congenital syphilis in a neonate. Note the periosteal reaction together with bony destruction of the medial proximal tibial metaphysis (Wimberger sign).

often multifocal, a complete skeletal survey should be done when a single lesion is discovered.

Serial films of chronically ill premature infants, especially those receiving IV alimentation, should be observed closely for signs of *rickets*. In this disorder, the metaphysis is abnormally lucent, and there is a loss of the zone of provisional calcification, which is the dense line at the metaphyseal end of the bone adjacent to the epiphyseal cartilage plate. Rickets is accompanied by metaphyseal fraying and cupping. The metaphyses of the knees and wrists are particularly sensitive indicators of rickets, as are anterior rib ends, which may show a rachitic rosary (Fig. 35–34). Rib fractures are common in these infants, and this observation on the chest x-ray of a premature infant may be the first clue to the diagnosis.

SPINE, PELVIS, AND HIPS

Because the neural arches of the neonatal and infant spine are not ossified, ultrasonography employing high-frequency transducers is capable of demonstrating the spinal cord and subarachnoid space (Fig. 35–35). Ultrasonography is the primary imaging modality for suspected congenital anomalies.[40] The position of the spinal cord can be identified with respect to the adjacent bony structures, as can anomalies such as a tethered cord (Fig. 35–36), lipoma, or other evi-

dence of spinal dysraphism. Sinus tracts, hemangiomata, and hairy patches over the back are indications for spinal ultrasonography. Simple midline dimples have a low risk for spinal dysraphism.[28]

The bony vertebrae are visible on routine chest and abdominal films of the neonate. Common anomalies of vertebral segmentation, such as sagittally cleft (butterfly) vertebrae and *hemivertebrae,* may be incidental radiographic findings or accompany other congenital anomalies, such as esophageal atresia, imperforate anus, agenesis of the lung, and bronchopulmonary foregut malformations. *Spinal dysraphism* is manifested on AP views as an increase in the interpediculate distance of the involved portion of the vertebral column, which indicates a widening of the spinal canal. Varying degrees of caudal regression with agenesis of the lumbosacral spine may be found in infants of diabetic mothers (see Chapter 47, Part One). A thorough evaluation of the genitourinary tract should be performed in all patients with spinal anomalies.

Developmental Dysplasia of the Hip

(See also Chapter 52.)

This condition was previously called congenital dislocation of the hip, but it is now recognized that apart from the rare teratologic hip dislocation, the hip is not dislocated at birth; rather, this disorder is acquired during early infancy. The potential for subluxation and finally dislocation exists in a small number of infants with a shallow acetabulum. Envi-

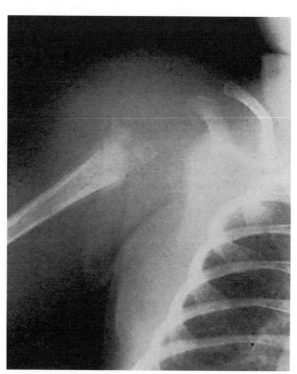

FIGURE 35–33. Osteomyelitis with septic arthritis. Note the severe soft tissue swelling, metaphyseal destruction, and periosteal new bone formation of the proximal humerus.

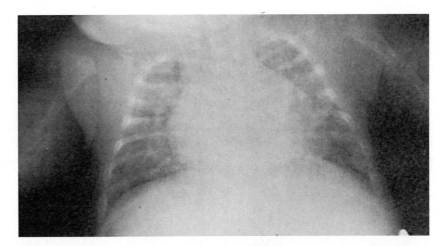

FIGURE 35–34. Infant with chronic lung disease who has severe osteopenia, flaring and rarefaction of the metaphyses, and expansion of the anterior ends of the lower ribs resulting from rickets. There also were multiple long-bone fractures. An alimentation catheter extends into the superior vena cava.

ronmental factors such as breech presentation, female gender, and race (which may be partially explained by different neonatal positioning of the lower limbs) also play a part. Developmental dysplasia is far more common on the left side.

Hip dislocation and acetabular dysplasia can be diagnosed sonographically,[20] and ultrasonography has been proposed both for diagnosis (Fig. 35–37) and as a method of population screening for hip abnormalities. Ultrasonography can also be performed to monitor treatment in the Pavlick harness. An additional advantage is the demonstration of normal vascularity to the femoral head by Doppler examination, potentially preventing the problem of avascular necrosis. The major drawbacks are the expense of population screening and the need for suitably trained personnel.[41] A combination dynamic hip ultrasonographic examination (which duplicates in many ways the physical examination) and static measurement of angles is the proposed standard protocol.

The femoral heads are never ossified in the early newborn period. This limits the value of x-rays, because the cartilaginous femoral head is an important landmark in the diagnosis of developmental dysplasia of the hip. In the absence of femoral head ossification, this diagnosis is recognized by superolateral displacement of the proximal femoral metaphysis and associated acetabular dysplasia. Septic arthritis causes rapid subluxation or dislocation of the hips in the absence of acetabular dysplasia.

ESTIMATION OF GESTATIONAL AGE

Traditionally, ossification of the epiphyseal centers of the knee has been used for radiographic assessment of gestational age, although the appearance of these centers is quite variable. In addition, the humeral heads are readily visible on chest radiographs. They are rarely ossified before 38 weeks' gestation and, if visible, indicate gestational maturity. Although their presence is not diagnostic of postmaturity, infants with respiratory distress in whom these centers are

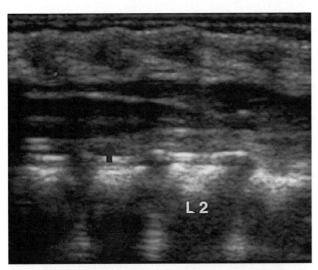

FIGURE 35–35. Normal spinal cord in a neonate. Longitudinal ultrasound examination of the lumbar spinal canal shows a normal spinal cord (*arrow*) within the bony spinal canal. The spinal cord terminates at the second lumbar vertebral body (L2).

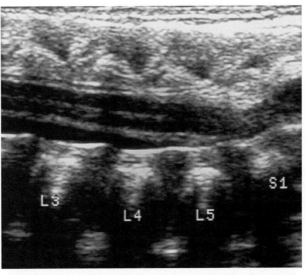

FIGURE 35–36. Tethered cord. Ultrasonography clearly demonstrates the low position of the spinal cord. Compare this with a normal cord (see Fig. 35–35).

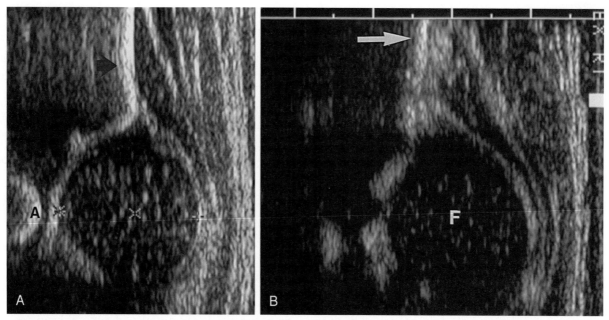

FIGURE 35–37. *A*, Normal neonatal ultrasound study of the hip. Orientation is similar to an x-ray of the left hip. Coronal view of a normal left hip demonstrates the speckled cartilage of the femoral head lying within the acetabulum (A). Iliac bone is shown by the arrow. *B*, Coronal ultrasound study in a neonate with developmental dysplasia of the hip iliac bone (*arrow*). Note the shallow acetabulum in comparison to the normal hip in *A*. F, femoral head.

ossified have a statistically high chance of having meconium aspiration syndrome.

The lower deciduous molar teeth are reliable indicators of gestational age[29] and are frequently included on chest radiographs. Mineralization of the first deciduous molar indicates at least 33 weeks of gestation, whereas mineralization of the second molar indicates at least 36 weeks.

SKULL AND BRAIN

(See also Chapter 38.)

ULTRASONOGRAPHY

Although bone is usually a barrier to the transmission of ultrasound, the infant brain can be studied by placing a transducer on the anterior fontanelle. With variation in the angle of the transducer, the brain can be scanned in any projection. Standard views include the coronal, sagittal, and axial projections. The posterior fontanelle and posterolateral fontanelle can also be used to image the posterior fossa and brainstem. The study can be performed with portable equipment at the crib side. No sedation, contrast material, or ionizing radiation is used.

Pulsations of the normal intracranial arteries and veins (including the venous sinuses) can be identified, and Doppler ultrasonography can be performed to assess flow direction and velocity.[33] Ultrasonography, however, cannot distinguish between gray matter and white matter or appreciate subarachnoid hemorrhage.

COMPUTED TOMOGRAPHY SCANNING

The advantages of CT scanning are that it can identify subarachnoid, subdural, and intraparenchymal hemorrhage that may not be demonstrated on ultrasonography. It is capable of detecting calcification (Fig. 35–38), which is not readily visible by MRI. Identification of bony structures, including the calvarium (Fig. 35–39), paranasal sinuses, mastoid air cells, and inner ear structures, is best accomplished with CT. Contrast material is rarely needed in young infants, and with the newer, faster helical scanners, sedation is usually not needed.

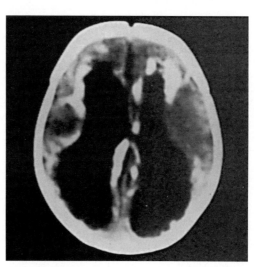

FIGURE 35–38. In utero cytomegaloviral infection shown by computed tomography scan of the head. Note the dilated lateral ventricles with periventricular calcification.

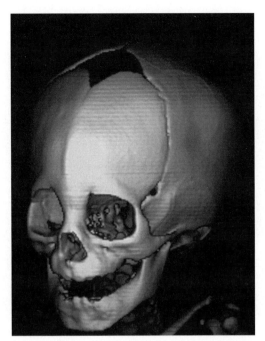

FIGURE 35–39. Metopic suture synostosis. Three-dimensional computed tomography reconstruction outlines the bony bridge of the fused metopic suture in the middle of the frontal bone.

MAGNETIC RESONANCE IMAGING

With MRI, no ionizing radiation is used, and presumably no biologically harmful effects occur. Ferromagnetic materials, such as certain surgical clips and pacemakers, are the only biologic contraindications to these scans. Exquisite anatomic detail can be obtained (Fig. 35–40), with routine differentiation of gray matter and white matter. Anatomy of the brainstem, cerebellum, and basal ganglia can be routinely visualized. Similar anatomic information can be obtained from the spinal cord and adjacent bony structures. Disadvantages include the high cost and need for sedation.

Myelin gives a very high signal on T1-weighted relaxation time images. In fact, on these images, myelin is the brightest structure in the normal neonatal brain, being only slightly less intense than subcutaneous fat. The normal progression of myelination can be followed and staged by T1-weighted images up to 6 to 9 months of age. T2-weighted images are used to follow myelination from ages 8 months to 2 years. Myelination progresses from caudal to cranial; it progresses from dorsal to ventral in the brainstem and from central to peripheral in the brain.

Magnetic resonance angiography can provide detailed anatomic information on intracranial and extracranial arteries and veins without the need for contrast material. Magnetic resonance spectroscopy allows measurement of tissue levels for various metabolites, such as creatinine, glutamine, and lactate. This information has proved helpful in the diagnosis of various metabolic diseases,[54] for example, the localization of lactic acidosis with Leigh disease.

INTRACRANIAL HEMORRHAGE IN THE PREMATURE INFANT

Ultrasonography has proved to be extremely accurate for the diagnosis of germinal matrix hemorrhage in premature infants. Most hemorrhages occur within the first week of life, with the vast majority occurring within 3 days.[10] Because clinical predictions of intracranial bleeding are unreliable, all infants born at less than 32 weeks' gestation or weighing less than 1500 gm should be routinely scanned by ultrasonography. A proposed protocol[38] suggests that the first scan to identify a hemorrhage should be obtained between the third and seventh day of life. A second scan to identify early ventricular dilation can be obtained on day 14 of life. A third scan to identify any delayed ventricular dilation is obtained at 3 months. This proposed timing of head ultrasonographic examinations is for asymptomatic infants to identify hemorrhage and ventricular dilation. If an abnormality is identified on ultrasonography or clinical deterioration occurs, scans should be obtained more frequently.

The normal germinal matrix is not visible by ultrasound examination. It lies between the caudate nucleus and the ependymal lining of the lateral ventricle. Germinal matrix hemorrhages originate in the groove between the thalamus and the head of the caudate nucleus; they are identified on ultrasonography as an echogenic area (Fig. 35–41). This subependymal bleeding may be confined to the germinal matrix or rupture through the ependymal lining into the adjacent lateral ventricle. Further bleeding may cause enlargement of the lateral ventricle (Fig. 35–42). The

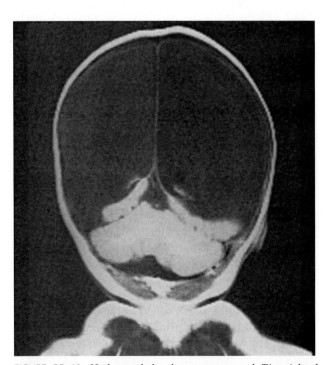

FIGURE 35–40. Hydrancephaly shown on coronal T1-weighted magnetic resonance imaging scan. Note an intact falx with virtually the entire brain above the tentorium having a low-intensity signal characteristic of water.

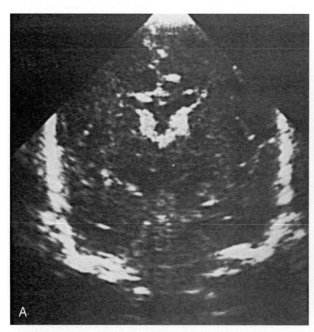
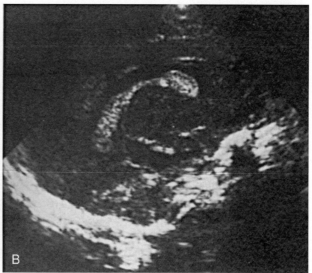

FIGURE 35–41. *A*, Coronal ultrasound examination shows bilateral grade I germinal matrix hemorrhage. *B*, Grade I germinal matrix hemorrhage. Sagittal ultrasonography reveals an echogenic bleed. Normal echogenic choroid plexus outlines the floor of the lateral ventricle.

blood remains echogenic for weeks and occasionally even months. A central sonolucency eventually develops because of the change in the physical properties of the blood, and the clots often retract in size.

Intraparenchymal hemorrhage usually occurs in conjunction with the germinal matrix hemorrhage (see Chapter 38, Part Five). The germinal matrix hemorrhage causes compression of medullary veins, leading to venous hemorrhagic infarction in the adjacent brain parenchyma.[53] Initially identified on ultrasonography as a large echogenic area, with time, this liquefies and can eventually communicate with the adjacent lateral ventricle as a porencephalic cyst (Fig. 35–43). A commonly used grading system[5] that has some prognostic value is as follows:

Grade I: Subependymal germinal matrix hemorrhage
Grade II: Hemorrhage extending into normal-sized lateral ventricles
Grade III: Hemorrhage extending into the lateral ventricles, which are now enlarged
Grade IV: Intraparenchymal hemorrhage; periventricular hemorrhagic infarct

Infants with grade I or II hemorrhages have a relatively good prognosis, probably with no difference in outcome from other infants of similar gestational age. Infants with higher grades, however, do less well, and infants with periventricular hemorrhagic infarcts have significant mortality and morbidity. Persistent ventriculomegaly predicts a poor outcome for grade III hemorrhage.

PERIVENTRICULAR LEUKOMALACIA

(See also Chapter 38, Part Five.)

Periventricular leukomalacia is an ischemic infarct at a watershed area of the white matter located around the lateral ventricles and usually occurs in infants of less than 35 weeks' gestation.[11] Unfortunately, ultrasonography is not a sensitive test for the acute event but may initially show an area of increased periventricular echogenicity. Subsequent development of periventricular cysts is well shown by ultrasonography (Fig. 35–44), often with no preceding recognized clinical cause. The cystic stage occurs approximately 3 weeks after the acute event. The cysts disappear in 1 to 3 months, leaving enlarged lateral ventricles with loss of adjacent white matter.

FIGURE 35–42. Grade III hemorrhage. Enlarged lateral ventricle is filled with cast of blood.

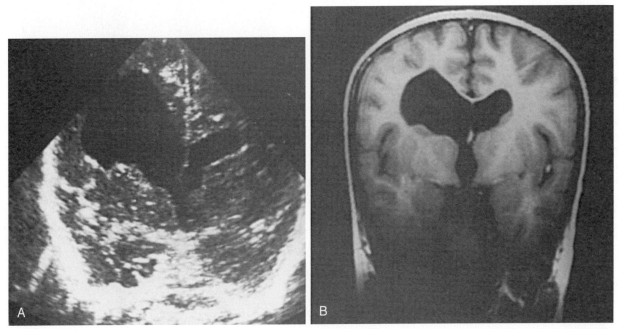

FIGURE 35–43. *A*, Porencephalic cyst. Coronal head ultrasound examination shows a right-sided porencephalic cyst communicating with the right lateral ventricle. The left lateral ventricle is also mildly enlarged. The porencephalic cyst was the site of an earlier intraparenchymal hemorrhage. *B*, Coronal T1-weighted magnetic resonance imaging scan shows a similar porencephalic cyst at the site of a previous periventricular hemorrhagic infarct.

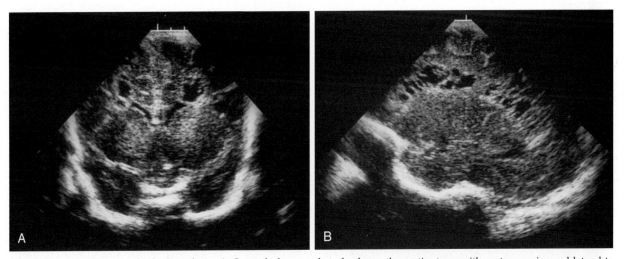

FIGURE 35–44. Periventricular leukomalacia. *A*, Coronal ultrasound study shows the cystic stage, with cysts superior and lateral to the lateral ventricles. *B*, Longitudinal ultrasound study with multiple cysts extending from the frontal lobe into the posterior parietal lobe.

MRI offers further insight into this process by demonstrating a delayed myelination of the brain in many of these infants, who may also show atrophy of the corpus callosum, thalamus, and brainstem. White matter atrophy is also well shown by MRI. Although this study is not practical for the early diagnosis, it can be very helpful in follow-up.

HYPOXIC ISCHEMIC ENCEPHALOPATHY

(See also Chapter 38, Part Three.)

Hypoxic ischemic encephalopathy occurs mainly in full-term infants with birth depression who show other features of ischemia, such as enlargement of the heart and elevation of liver function tests. On ultrasonography, this global ischemia of the brain produces an altered echo pattern of diffusely increased echogenicity, with obliteration of the normal anatomic landmarks such as the sulci and ventricles secondary to the edematous infarcted brain. CT scanning readily shows the diffuse ischemia as areas of low attenuation (Fig. 35–45) and is the preferred imaging test. Follow-up studies may demonstrate diffuse atrophy, enlarged ventricles, calcification of the basal ganglia, and cystic areas of encephalomalacia.

CONGENITAL MALFORMATIONS AND HYDROCEPHALUS

Ultrasonography offers a simple initial imaging technique for the diagnosis and follow-up of cases of ventriculomegaly and hydrocephalus. MRI has now become the optimal test for congenital anomalies of the brain and spine; it alone can show abnormalities of the gyri and sulci, such as lissencephaly (Fig. 35–46), other migrational disorders, and gray matter heterotopias. After the anterior fontanelle is closed, ultra-

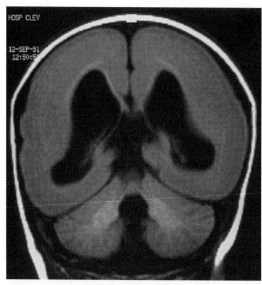

FIGURE 35–46. Lissencephaly. Coronal magnetic resonance imaging scan of the brain demonstrates a smooth surface of the cerebral hemispheres, with no gyri or sulci (compare with Fig. 35–43B). Lateral ventricles are also dilated.

sonography is no longer technically feasible, and MRI or CT must be performed.

MONITORING AND TREATMENT DEVICES

An important aspect of the radiographic examination of the newborn infant is the assessment of the position of various devices, such as endotracheal tubes, nasogastric tubes, umbilical catheters, and IV alimentation catheters. For obvious reasons, these devices must be radiopaque.

The endotracheal tube is visible on most chest radiographs. Its tip should be approximately halfway between the vocal cords and the carina, at approximately the level of the first ribs. In small, premature infants, even slight alterations in the degree of flexion or rotation of the neck cause a remarkable difference in the position of the tube as seen on the AP film.

The position of the nasogastric tube also should be noted on the chest x-ray. Its tip may be displaced inadvertently from the stomach into the lower esophagus. On occasion, the tube is found curled above a previously unsuspected esophageal atresia.

To assess umbilical arterial and venous catheters, a film should be done that includes the chest, abdomen, and pelvis. The umbilical arterial catheter can be seen in the aorta, to the left of the midline after looping into the pelvis to enter the internal iliac artery. Proper position of its tip is either in the thoracic aorta between T8 and T10 (high position) or in the abdominal aorta just above the aortic bifurcation (low position). The umbilical venous catheter ascends toward the porta hepatis to the right of the midline and bypasses the portal system by entering the ductus venosus, which leads to the inferior vena cava. The optimal

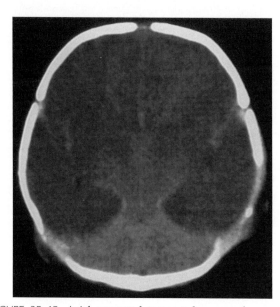

FIGURE 35–45. Axial computed tomography scan of a neonate with hypoxic ischemic encephalopathy. The posterior fossa shows normal attenuation of brain. The ischemic brain of the frontal and temporal lobes, by comparison, shows low attenuation.

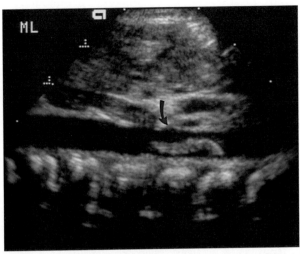

FIGURE 35–47. Abdominal ultrasound study of the aorta with echogenic thrombus (*arrow*) within the lumen.

position of this catheter tip is in the intrathoracic portion of the inferior vena cava or the right atrium.

Catheter position also can be determined by ultrasonography. Although this method requires greater technical expertise, it avoids the use of ionizing radiation and is capable of detecting catheter-related complications, such as thrombi (Fig. 35–47). Aortic thrombus is rarely occlusive, and associated hypertension is managed medically. Any lower extremity ischemic symptoms are usually transient. Other rare complications of catheters include embolus, hematoma of the vessel wall, and even perforation.

Peripherally inserted central venous catheters are usually inserted percutaneously via an upper limb vein; less commonly, the internal or external jugular vein, facial vein, or a lower limb vein is used. Following puncture of the peripheral vein, the catheter is inserted through an introducer sheath and manipulated centrally. It is advanced into the superior vena cava so that the tip lies immediately superior to the right atrium.

Numerous complications of IV alimentation have been reported, including hydrothorax resulting from perforation of the pleural space by the catheter and chylothorax resulting from superior vena cava thrombosis.[27] Venous alimentation and arterial catheters may be responsible for emboli that can disturb growth of the physes of the long bones.

An array of interventional techniques is now available under imaging supervision. These techniques, however, call for very close cooperation with the clinician and the development of special skills on the part of the radiologist. Areas of narrowing can be balloon dilated in a variety of places in the body. These include tracheal and bronchial stenosis[3] and even areas of narrowing in the bowel, such as postoperative esophageal strictures[13] and postinflammatory colonic strictures following necrotizing enterocolitis. Abnormal fluid collections, including abscesses in the abdomen and chest, can be drained or biopsied using imaging techniques without the need for surgery.

■ REFERENCES

1. Ablow RC, et al: Z-shaped, duodenojejunal loop: Sign of mesenteric fixation anomaly and congenital bands. AJR Am J Roentgenol 141:461, 1983.
2. Berdon WE: Pulmonary edema in infants who receive contrast material. Radiology 139:507, 1981.
3. Brown SB, et al: Tracheobronchial stenosis in infants: Successful balloon dilation therapy. Radiology 164:475, 1987.
4. Bude RO, et al: Age dependency of the renal resistive index. Radiology 184:169, 1992.
5. Burstein J, et al: Subependymal germinal matrix and intraventricular hemorrhage in premature infants: Diagnosis by CT. AJR Am J Roentgenol 128:971, 1977.
6. Centers for Disease Control: 1989 sexually transmitted disease treatment guideline. MMWR 38(suppl 8):1, 1989.
7. Clarke EA, et al: Findings on chest radiographs after prophylactic pulmonary surfactant treatment of premature infants. AJR Am J Roentgenol 153:799, 1989.
8. Cohen MD: Choosing contrast media for the evaluation of the gastrointestinal tract of neonates and infants. Radiology 162:447, 1987.
9. Davies H, et al: Regional ventilation in infancy: Reversal of adult pattern. N Engl J Med 313:1626, 1985.
10. Dolfin T, et al: Incidence, severity, and timing of subependymal and intraventricular hemorrhages in preterm infants born in a perinatal unit as detected by serial real-time ultrasound. Pediatrics 71:541, 1983.
11. Fanaroff AA, et al: Periventricular leukomalacia: Prospects for prevention. N Engl J Med 341:1229, 1999.
12. Gibaud L, et al: MR cholangiography in neonates and infants: Feasibility and preliminary applications. AJR Am J Roentgenol 170:27, 1998.
13. Goldthorn JF, et al: Esophageal strictures in children: Treatment by serial balloon catheter dilatation. Radiology 153:655, 1984.
14. Greenberg SB, et al: Are long bone radiographs necessary in neonates suspected of having congenital syphilis? Radiology 182:637, 1992.
15. Gross GW, et al: Thoracic complication of extracorporeal membrane oxygenation: Findings on chest radiographs and sonograms. AJR Am J Roentgenol 158:353, 1992.
16. Haller JO, et al: Increased renal cortical echogenicity: A normal finding in neonates and infants. Radiology 142:173, 1982.
17. Han K, et al: Normal thymus in infancy: Sonographic characteristics. Radiology 170:471, 1989.
18. Haney PJ: Infant apnea: Findings on the barium esophagram. Radiology 148:425, 1983.
19. Haney PJ, et al: Radiographic findings in neonatal pneumonia. AJR Am J Roentgenol 143:26, 1984.
20. Harcke HT, et al: Performing dynamic sonography of the infant hip. AJR Am J Roentgenol 155:837, 1990.
21. Hayden CK Jr, et al: Ultrasonography evaluation of the renal parenchyma in infancy and childhood. Radiology 152:413, 1984.
22. Hildreth NG, et al: The risk of breast cancer after irradiation of the thymus in infancy. N Engl J Med 321:1281, 1989.
23. Jaile JC, et al: Benign gaseous distension of the bowel in premature infants treated with nasal continuous airway pressure: A study of contributing factors. AJR Am J Roentgenol 158:125, 1992.
24. Janik JS, et al: Intestinal stricture after necrotizing enterocolitis. J Pediatr Surg 16:438, 1981.
25. Kliegman RM, et al: Necrotizing enterocolitis. N Engl J Med 310:1093, 1984.
26. Kogutt MS, et al: Low-dose digital computed radiography in pediatric chest imaging. AJR Am J Roentgenol 151:775, 1988.
27. Kramer SS, et al: Lethal chylothoraces due to superior vena cava thrombosis in infants. AJR Am J Roentgenol 137:559, 1981.
28. Kriss VM, et al: Occult spinal dysraphism in neonates: Assessment of high-risk cutaneous stigmata on sonography. AJR Am J Roentgenol 171:1687, 1998.
29. Kuhns LR, et al: Radiological assessment of maturity and size of the newborn infant. CRC Crit Rev Diagn Imaging 13:245, 1980.
30. Laing FC, et al: Postpartum evaluation of fetal hydronephrosis:

Optimal timing for follow-up sonography. Radiology 152:423, 1984.

31. Leonidas JC, et al: Pneumoperitoneum in ventilated newborns. Am J Dis Child 128:677, 1974.

32. Merritt CRB, et al: Sonographic detection of portal venous gas in infants with necrotizing enterocolitis. AJR Am J Roentgenol 143:1059, 1984.

33. Mitchell DG, et al: Neonatal brain: Color Doppler imaging. Part I. Technique and vascular anatomy. Radiology 167:303, 1988.

34. Mok PM, et al: Osteomyelitis in the neonate: Clinical aspects and the role of radiography and scintigraphy in diagnosis and management. Radiology 145:677, 1982.

35. Morrison SC, et al: The radiology of necrotizing enterocolitis. Clin Perinatol 21:347, 1994.

36. Neal M, et al: Neonatal ultrasonography to distinguish between meconium ileus and ileal atresia. J Ultrasound Med 16:263, 1997.

37. Nussbaum AR, et al: Spontaneous resolution of neonatal ovarian cysts. AJR Am J Roentgenol 148:175, 1987.

38. Partridge JC, et al: Optimal timing for diagnostic cranial ultrasound in low-birth-weight infants: Detection of intracranial hemorrhage and intraventricular dilation. J Pediatr 102:281, 1983.

39. Radkowski MA, et al: *Chlamydia* pneumonia in infants: Radiography in 125 cases. AJR Am J Roentgenol 137:703, 1981.

40. Rohrschneider WK, et al: Diagnostic value of spinal US: Comparative study with MR imaging in pediatric patients. Radiology 200:383, 1996.

41. Rosendahl K, et al: Ultrasound screening for developmental dysplasia of the hip in the neonate: The effect on treatment rate and prevalence of late cases. Pediatrics 9:47, 1994.

42. Rosenfield NS, et al: Hirschsprung disease: Accuracy of the barium enema examination. Radiology 150:393, 1984.

43. Russell JGB: Diagnostic radiography in children. Arch Dis Child 63:1005, 1988.

44. Sabau MN, et al: Radiation exposure due to scatter in neonatal radiographic procedures. AJR Am J Roentgenol 144:811, 1985.

45. Sanders RC, et al: The sonographic distinction between neonatal multicystic kidney and hydronephrosis. Radiology 151:621, 1984.

46. Schey WL, et al: Esophageal dysmotility and the sudden infant death syndrome: Clinical experience. Radiology 140:67, 1981.

47. Schirmer WJ, et al: The spectrum of cholelithiasis in the first year of life. J Pediatr Surg 24:1064, 1989.

48. Shimanuki Y, et al: Clockwise whirlpool sign at color Doppler US: An objective and definite sign of midgut volvulus. Radiology 199:261, 1996.

49. Slovis TL, et al: Choanal atresia: Precise CT evaluation. Radiology 155:345, 1985.

50. Smith WL, et al: Selection of optimal screen-film combination for use in the neonatal intensive care unit. AJR Am J Roentgenol 139:1051, 1982.

51. Taxman TL, et al: How useful is the barium enema in the diagnosis of infantile Hirschsprung's disease? Am J Dis Child 140:881, 1986.

52. Taylor GA, et al: Diffuse pulmonary opacification in infants undergoing extracorporeal membrane oxygenation: Clinical and pathologic correlation. Radiology 161:347, 1986.

53. Volpe JJ: Current concepts of brain injury in the premature infant. AJR Am J Roentgenol 152:243, 1989.

54. Wang Z, et al: Proton MR spectroscopy of the brain: Clinically useful information obtained in assessing CNS diseases in children. AJR Am J Roentgenol 167:191, 1996.

55. Wilson-Costello D, et al: Radiation exposure from diagnostic radiographs in extremely low birth weight infants. Pediatrics 97:369, 1996.

56. Zerin JM, et al: Incidental vesicoureteral reflux in neonates with antenatally detected hydronephrosis and other renal abnormalities. Radiology 187:157, 1993.

Infants of Addicted Mothers

36

Tove S. Rosen

David A. Bateman

Abuse of legal and illegal drugs is a major public health problem with high medical and social costs. An estimated 13.6 million Americans used illicit drugs in 1998, with 4.1 million being dependent on them. Patients with conditions related to substance abuse fill half of all occupied hospital beds in the United States. In addition, 75% of murders, assaults, and acts of child abuse are related to drug or alcohol abuse. Women account for approximately 30% of the addicted population, and most female addicts are of childbearing age. A mother's drug abuse may harm her fetus and her child. A recent survey found that 5.5% of women use illicit drugs during pregnancy. As a consequence, these mothers experience an associated increase in obstetric complications, premature labor, syphilis and other sexually transmitted diseases, tuberculosis, hepatitis, human immunodeficiency virus (HIV), and neonatal and long-term complications. These effects are confounded by social and environmental factors such as poor nutrition, poor health care, and suboptimal child-rearing environments and practices.

The popularity trends of illicit and licit drug use change over time and are determined by geographic distribution. Marijuana is the most commonly used illicit drug. There has been a decrease in the use of cocaine and crack but an increase in the use of methamphetamine, heroin, and alcohol since 1995.

The most commonly abused drugs include alcohol, marijuana, cocaine and crack, heroin, amphetamines and methamphetamines, inhalants, and the new club drugs, especially among teenagers and young adults.

HEROIN

There were about 810,000 heroin addicts in the United States in 1995, and this number was most likely an underestimate. The purity of heroin is up, and the price is down. As a result, there has been an increase in the inhalant use of heroin. Smoking and snorting of heroin have become more popular because of the easy availability of high-purity heroin and the fear of

acquired immunodeficiency syndrome (AIDS) associated with IV use.

PATHOLOGY AND PATHOGENESIS

Heroin (diacetylmorphine) is more potent and has a faster action than morphine. Morphine is primarily a μ-opiate receptor agonist. Heroin is deacetylated in the liver to mono-acetyl-morphine and then to morphine and morphine-3-glucuronide.[39] It is highly lipid soluble and crosses easily into the fetus. Once in the fetus, heroin is distributed widely and variably throughout the fetal tissues and body compartments. There appear to be significant differences in its distribution between immature infants and adults. Studies of pregnant animals given morphine showed that the concentration in the fetal brain was two to three times that in the maternal brain, and similar differences in distribution are likely for heroin. Animal studies demonstrated a decrease in nucleic acid and protein synthesis in the fetal brain, with decreased density of cortical neurons and neuronal processes. Alterations in the brain reward system have also been described.

Infants of heroin-addicted women have a higher incidence of being born prematurely, having low birth weights, and being small for gestational age (SGA). Postmortem studies of placentas of heroin-addicted mothers demonstrated that the increased incidence of prematurity may be caused by the high rate of chorioamnionitis or other maternal infections. In addition, autopsies of infants who were SGA and born to narcotic-addicted mothers revealed that their organs were small and consisted of diminished numbers of normal-sized cells. These autopsy results differed from those obtained from malnourished infants born to nonaddicted mothers, whose organs showed a decrease in both the number and the size of their cells. Therefore, it has been postulated that maternal undernutrition is not the only factor responsible for the antenatal growth retardation observed in infants of narcotic addicts; heroin may have a direct growth-inhibiting effect on the fetus.[43, 61, 70, 93]

The incidence of congenital anomalies in infants born to heroin-addicted mothers is no higher than that in the general population. An increased rate of stillbirths has been reported.

CLINICAL MANIFESTATIONS

Signs and symptoms of neonatal narcotic abstinence syndrome (NAS) occur in 50% to 75% of infants born to heroin-addicted mothers and usually begin within the first 24 to 48 hours of life. The incidence of withdrawal has been associated with several factors, such as the dosage of heroin, the duration of maternal addiction, and the time of the last maternal dose. NAS consists of a combination of the following: irritability, jitteriness, coarse tremors, high-pitched cry, fist sucking, sneezing, yawning, tachypnea, poor feeding, regurgitation, vomiting, diarrhea, sweating, hypothermia or hyperthermia, hypertonia, hyperreflexia, myoclonus, and, less often, seizures. In addition, an abnormal sleep cycle, with the absence of quiet sleep and the disturbance of active sleep, has been described in these infants.[29, 92] Furthermore, there is a decrease in both the rate and the intensity of sucking.[29, 73, 92]

Infants born to heroin addicts have a lower incidence of hyperbilirubinemia and respiratory distress syndrome (RDS). The decreased incidence of hyperbilirubinemia may result from induction of the glucuronyl-transferase enzyme system by heroin.[72] The lower incidence of RDS may be caused by a direct effect of heroin on lung maturation, with an accelerated production of surfactant, as suggested by animal studies.[101] Respiratory alkalosis may also occur in these infants. It is believed to be central in origin and may play a role in the decreased incidence of RDS. Thyroid dysfunction has also been described in these infants.

TREATMENT

Therapy for the heroin abstinence syndrome is recommended in the following situations: (1) severe irritability and tremors that interfere with feeding and sleep, (2) vomiting and diarrhea, (3) seizures, (4) hyperthermia or hypothermia, and (5) severe tachypnea interfering with feedings. Other causes of these symptoms must be excluded before initiating treatment.

Many neonatal units use a scoring system to evaluate NAS and determine the necessity of treatment, its efficacy, and its length. Drugs most commonly used for the treatment of NAS include tincture of opium, paregoric, and phenobarbital, singly or in combination (Table 36–1). The choice of medication varies with individual nurseries. The recommendation of the American Academy of Pediatrics Committee on Drugs is to treat NAS with a diluted solution of tincture of opium and to treat other withdrawal syndromes with phenobarbital. Tincture of opium is preferred because paregoric has several toxic effects. Suggested doses are given in Table 36–1. If phenobarbital is chosen, the initial dose should be a loading dose followed by a lower maintenance dosage to allow for an adequate plasma level and rapid clinical response.

TABLE 36–1 DOSAGE SCHEDULE FOR TREATMENT OF INFANTS WITH NARCOTIC ABSTINENCE SYNDROME

Tincture of opium (10 mg/mL)
  Use as 25-fold dilution that contains 0.4 mg/mL morphine equivalent.
  Starting dose is 0.1 mL/kg or 2 drops/kg every 4 hrs with feedings. Dosing may be increased by 2 drops every 4 hrs to control symptoms.
  Continue stabilization dose for 3–5 days and then slowly decrease the dose every 4 hrs without changing the frequency of administration.
Paregoric (0.4 mg/mL of morphine)
  Start with 0.1 mL/kg or 2 drops/kg every 4 hrs with feedings. Dosing can be increased by 2 drops/kg every 3–4 hrs until symptoms are controlled.
  After 3–5 days on stabilizing dose, paregoric can be tapered by decreasing the dosage slowly without changing the frequency of administration.
Phenobarbital
  Start with a 15–20 mg/kg loading dose IM or PO/24 hrs, then 4–6 mg/kg/day maintenance dose every 12 hrs PO.
  Phenobarbital plasma level should be 20–30 mg/mL.
  After stabilization, phenobarbital should be slowly decreased by dose and then by frequency.
Methadone
  Start with 0.05–0.1 mg/kg/day every 6 hrs PO. The dose can be increased by 0.05 mg/kg until symptoms of withdrawal are improved. Maintenance dose should be given every 12–24 hrs.
  Weaning should be slow until dose of 0.05 mg/kg/day is reached, when it can be discontinued because of its long half-life.
Diazepam
  1–2 mg every 8 hrs as needed for control of symptoms.

While maintenance therapy is being given, the plasma drug level should be monitored to prevent toxicity. Once a clinical response has been achieved, the drug should be tapered gradually (every 2 to 3 days) and then discontinued. The duration of treatment in neonatal heroin withdrawal may vary from 4 days to 6 weeks.[73]

The use of naloxone is contraindicated in infants born to narcotic addicts because its use may precipitate severe signs and symptoms of abstinence syndrome and seizures.

PROGNOSIS

With appropriate management in the neonatal period, the morbidity and mortality rates of heroin-addicted infants are comparable to those of other infants with low birth weights or prematurity. Follow-up of these infants is incomplete because of frequent parental moves, missed appointments, and foster care placement. Some reports in children 3 to 6 years of age born to heroin addicts demonstrated continued deficiencies in height, weight, and head circumference; others showed catch-up growth. These children's overall intellectual functioning was not significantly different from that of normal controls, but they exhibited significant difficulties in the general processing of perception and cognition. They also scored significantly lower than controls on tasks requiring attention, concentration, and short-term memory. These children often have behavior problems such as being more aggressive, compulsive, and active than matched controls, and they may have uncontrollable tempers. Neurologic abnormalities in tone, coordination, and balance have also been described. These findings are characteristic of attention deficit hyperactivity disorder. However, these studies were not controlled for confounding variables.[58, 93, 103, 109]

METHADONE

Methadone, a synthetic opiate, has been the therapy of choice for heroin addiction since its introduction for this purpose by Dole and Nyswander in 1965. It blocks the euphoric effects of heroin, thus reducing the craving for the drug. Methadone is metabolized by the liver into two major metabolites and at least five additional metabolites via N-demethylation, aromatic ring hydroxylation, and degradation of both side chains. The metabolites are excreted in the urine, feces, and bile. Methadone itself crosses the placenta. The maternal-cord plasma methadone ratio is 2.7:1, and the maternal-neonatal plasma methadone ratio at about 1 hour of life is 2.2:1, indicating placental limitation of transport of methadone, rapid tissue binding, or both.[87]

INCIDENCE

Mothers on methadone maintenance seem to have better prenatal care and somewhat better lifestyles than those taking heroin. However, there is a high incidence of multiple drug abuse, including cocaine, alcohol, barbiturates, tranquilizers, and other psychoactive drugs; these mothers are often heavy smokers as well. To counteract the high incidence of other drug use, doses of 100 to 125 mg/day of methadone are now being used, compared with the previous doses of 20 to 60 mg/day. The effects of these high doses are not known. The incidence of methadone abstinence syndrome in infants born to mothers on methadone maintenance varies from 70% to 90%, according to most published reports.[86, 103]

CLINICAL MANIFESTATIONS

Infants born to methadone-maintained mothers have higher birth weights than infants of heroin addicts and consequently have a lower incidence of intrauterine growth retardation. It has been shown that the birth weights of these infants correlate with the first-trimester dose of methadone; the higher the methadone dose (at dosages greater than 40 mg/day), the heavier the infant at birth. The mechanism for this trend is unknown. Despite the heavier birth weights,

more methadone-exposed babies have head circumferences less than the third percentile compared with babies who are not drug exposed. The infants with small heads were not necessarily those who were SGA at birth. No increase in the incidence of congenital anomalies has been reported in children born to methadone-maintained mothers.[43, 58, 86, 93, 103]

Thrombocytosis and increased platelet-aggregating activity have been reported in infants born to mothers receiving methadone maintenance with or without other polydrug abuse. The cause of the platelet defects is unknown; they occur after the first week of life, persisting for more than 16 weeks. In addition, abnormal thyroid function (increased triiodothyronine and thyroxine levels) has been described in newborn infants of methadone-treated mothers.

NAS usually occurs within 48 to 72 hours. The signs and symptoms of NAS are more severe and prolonged than the withdrawal symptoms seen in infants of heroin-addicted mothers. The clinical manifestations are similar to those described for heroin withdrawal. The incidence of seizures is higher in infants of methadone-maintained mothers (10% to 20%). When seizures are present, they usually occur between days 7 and 10 of life. These infants have the same disturbances in their sleep cycles as infants of heroin-addicted mothers—very little quiet sleep, and abnormal rapid eye movement (REM) sleep. They also demonstrate abnormal respiratory patterns on pneumograms. The Brazelton Neonatal Behavioral Assessment Scale demonstrated depressed interactive behavior and poor state control, increased tone and tremulousness, and less physical and emotional intimacy.[43, 61] When the infant's NAS produces these physical effects, they may in turn interfere with maternal bonding and care of the infant.

The incidence and severity of abstinence syndrome in infants of methadone-maintained mothers depend on maternal dose, maternal and fetal metabolism, and excretion of the drug. The higher the dose, the more severe the symptoms. The higher the level of methadone in maternal plasma and the more rapid the neonatal metabolism and excretion, the higher the incidence of moderate to severe symptoms and signs of withdrawal. The lower the maternal level of methadone and the slower the neonatal metabolism and excretion of methadone, the less likely it is that the infant will develop manifestations of drug withdrawal. The time of onset of methadone withdrawal symptoms depends on the time of the last maternal dose. For example, in one study, when the last maternal dose was taken within 20 hours of delivery, the onset of withdrawal usually occurred between 24 and 52 hours of life; when the maternal dose of methadone was taken more than 20 hours before delivery, the onset of symptoms occurred before 24 hours of life. In addition, symptomatic infants did not develop the withdrawal syndrome until plasma levels fell below 0.06 μg/mL.[87]

A syndrome of late-onset withdrawal has been described in some infants born to methadone-maintained mothers. This late withdrawal syndrome occurs at 2 to 4 weeks of age, either with or without previously occurring withdrawal manifestations. The symptoms are similar to those of early withdrawal and are often accompanied by a voracious appetite but poor weight gain. The symptoms may continue for several weeks and require continuing treatment. Late withdrawal syndrome may be the result of the strong tissue binding of methadone and the resultant slow excretion, or it may be caused by the discontinuation of other drugs taken by the mother during gestation.[73]

Systolic hypertension has been described in infants of mothers on methadone maintenance. This hypertension occurs at about 2 weeks of age and may persist for 12 weeks. It is not related to the severity of abstinence syndrome. A higher incidence (15 to 20 per 1000 live births) of sudden infant death syndrome (SIDS) also has been reported in these infants. Respiratory and sleeping patterns have been demonstrated to be abnormal.[29, 76, 86]

TREATMENT

Therapy for symptoms of methadone abstinence syndrome includes the same drugs used for heroin withdrawal: tincture of opium, paregoric, phenobarbital, and methadone (see Table 36–1). The duration of treatment for infants of methadone-addicted mothers is usually longer than for infants of heroin-addicted mothers (5 days to 4 months).[73]

PROGNOSIS

The few available follow-up studies of these infants reveal a high incidence of hyperactivity, learning and behavior disorders, and poor social adjustment.[43, 48, 49, 93, 103]

In follow-up, a higher incidence of infection, especially otitis media and candidal infections, was found. A continued higher incidence of head circumference below the third percentile was found. In addition, a higher incidence of neurologic abnormalities such as developmental delays, poor fine and gross motor coordination, balance problems, delayed language development, and lower scores on developmental testing has been described. In follow-up at school age, in general, differences in IQ tests were no longer present. A subgroup of children, however, exhibited persistent abnormal neurologic development such as poor fine motor coordination, balance difficulties, hyperactivity, decreased concentration span, poor task performance, and aggressive behavior. Many of these children demonstrated school problems requiring special attention and referrals.

The outcome for these children appears to depend on many factors, including not only intrauterine drug exposure but also the emotional, familial, and environmental instability that is so frequently associated with the drug culture.

Alternative drugs are being used in the treatment of heroin addiction, such as naltrexone, buprenorphine, and buprenorphine in combination with naloxone. Buprenorphine is a partial morphine agonist and reduces opiate use. It is less toxic than methadone and upon discontinuation causes a milder withdrawal syndrome. In Europe, buprenorphine is being used to treat narcotic addiction; it will soon be used in the United States as well. Studies from Europe showed that infants born to mothers on buprenorphine maintenance did not have an increased incidence of congenital anomalies. They also found a lower incidence of infants who were SGA and a much milder and shorter course of abstinence syndrome.[47, 88]

ALCOHOL

In 1998 there were an estimated 113 million users of alcohol in the United States. About 33 million of these were binge drinkers, and 12.4 million were heavy drinkers. About 20% were women. Approximately 18% to 35% of these heavy to moderate drinkers also had a history of illicit drug use.

Alcohol crosses the placenta readily, and it rapidly reaches the fetus. In studies of mothers receiving alcohol for suppression of labor, blood levels of alcohol in the mother and fetus were similar, with fetal elimination regulated primarily by maternal elimination of ethanol. After birth, blood alcohol levels were higher in the neonate than in the mother and were eliminated more slowly. Acute alcohol withdrawal has been described in neonates born to mothers receiving alcohol for suppression of premature labor. The syndrome consists of the following: an odor of alcohol on the infant's breath for several hours after birth; a 72-hour phase of hyperactivity, tremors, and seizures, followed by a 48-hour phase of lethargy; and finally a return to normal activity and responsiveness.[13, 75]

Much attention has been focused on the effects of chronic in utero alcohol exposure on infants born to mothers who are moderate to heavy alcohol consumers. Alcohol is a physical and behavioral teratogen. Alcohol exposure during pregnancy may result in a spectrum of mild to severe symptoms, from gross morphologic and central nervous system impairments to subtle cognitive and behavioral deficits.*

Alcohol affects many neurochemical and cellular components in the developing brain. It interferes with cellular division, growth, and migration of maturing cells. Animal and human studies of the brain have shown decreased brain weight, decreased number of neurons, and abnormal morphology. Alcohol may also impair several neurotransmitter systems or their receptors. The endocrine environment is affected by alcohol as well. There is a disruption in the thyroid-pituitary axis and the central regulation of the hypothalamic-pituitary-gonadal axis. Alcohol obstructs amino acid transport across the placenta.[42, 55, 85]

The threshold alcohol dose that produces adverse effects varies with the stage of development of the fetus. Factors that play an important role in the outcome of the offspring are quantity and pattern of

---

*References 2, 31, 35, 46, 55, 82.

alcohol consumption, socioeconomic status, maternal age, time of gestation, and individual susceptibility. Moderate drinking has been described as an average of two drinks per day or more than seven drinks per week or three drinks per occasion; heavy drinking is more than two to three drinks per day or five or more drinks per occasion. Abusive drinking is defined as more than 5.4 drinks per day. The number of binge drinking days increases the risk of alcohol-related birth defects.*

Unfortunately, there is no single laboratory test or biochemical marker to detect patients who drink excessively. Screening for alcohol intake depends on a carefully elicited maternal history, which is frequently complicated by the mother's denial. A simple questionnaire has been developed and validated for use in obstetric practice. It is designed to characterize maternal alcohol intake as a function of *tolerance* (T), *annoyance* to others (A), perceived need to *cut down* on drinking (C), and desire for an *eye opener* drink first thing in the morning (E). In addition, the use of maternal biomarkers such as whole blood acetaldehyde, carbohydrate-deficient transferrin, γ-glutamyl transpeptidase, and mean red blood cell volume can help in determining alcohol intake. If two or more markers are positive, alcohol effects are likely to be present. The presence of ethyl linoleate in meconium is an additional sign of moderate to heavy maternal drinking.[10, 97]

Fetal alcohol-related effects (FAE) may express themselves as intrauterine growth retardation; cognitive, behavioral, or psychosocial deficits; or *fetal alcohol syndrome (FAS)*. FAS consists of the following (see Chapters 12 and 28):

1. Central nervous system: microcephaly; withdrawal symptoms, including tremors and irritability (possibly persisting for several months to years, with mild to moderate mental retardation); apnea and seizures; abdominal distention; and opisthotonos.
2. Growth deficiency of perinatal onset, continuing postnatally.
3. Facial characteristics: short palpebral fissures, hypoplastic philtrum, thin upper vermilion, micrognathia, and retrognathia.
4. A variety of anomalies, including cardiac abnormalities (ventricular septal defect, tetralogy of Fallot), joint defects, limitation of motion of elbow and phalangeal joints, hip dysplasia, anomalies of external genitalia, hypoplasia of labia or hypospadias, and skin hemangioma.[35]

The frequency of expression of FAS and FAE has been reported to be 1 or 2 per 1000 to 1 per 300 live births. These alcohol effects depend not only on the amount of alcohol consumed but also on the interaction of quantity, frequency, pattern, type of alcohol, and other drug abuse. Other drugs such as cigarettes, caffeine, and marijuana, as well as poor nutrition, may potentiate the fetal effects of alcohol consump-

tion during gestation. Maternal age also plays a role in FAE. Women older than 30 years of age who are moderate to heavy drinkers have a two to five times higher risk of having impaired infants. Low socioeconomic status is also a contributing factor.[1, 35, 46]

Intrauterine growth retardation has been described as a result of in utero alcohol exposure. If absolute alcohol intake exceeds 1 oz/day before and during pregnancy, there is a high risk of low birth weight, decreased length, and smaller head circumference. This growth retardation may continue through childhood. Studies evaluating human growth hormone, luteinizing hormone, follicle-stimulating hormone, parathyroid hormone, testosterone, thyroxine, and bone age have shown that these are all within normal limits. If alcohol consumption is decreased during the third trimester of pregnancy, the effects on birth weight are minimal. An association has been reported between moderate alcohol intake and renal anomalies such as renal agenesis and hypoplasia.[25, 26, 35, 42, 67]

Follow-up studies of 8- and 12-month-old children of moderate to heavy alcohol users showed persistent growth retardation. This growth retardation was still evident at 10 to 12 years of age.[26, 56] These children's scores on the Bayley Scales of Infant Development at 12 to 26 months of age were significantly lower than those of the control children. Deficits were seen in linguistic representation, spatial and fine motor coordination, and spatial visualization and memory. Follow-up studies of children at ages 6 to 14 years who were exposed in utero to moderate to severe alcohol intake revealed cognitive dysfunction. The mean IQ scores were significantly lower than those of the controls, with difficulties in math, logic, visual perception, spatial relations, and short-range memory and attention. Psychopathologies such as hyperkinesis and sleep and emotional disorders have also been described. No differences were found in the performance of children raised by foster parents compared with those raised by their biologic parents. No correlation existed between dysmorphogenesis and the intelligence score, but a dose-response relationship was present. The low IQ is thought to reflect central nervous system damage secondary to alcohol or its metabolites.[6, 56, 60, 94]

TREATMENT

The treatment of acute alcohol withdrawal includes the same drugs that are used in NAS. Prevention of FAS should center on appropriate management and follow-up of the mother's alcohol intake before and after pregnancy. The recommendation of the National Institute for Alcohol Abuse is not to consume more than two drinks per day during pregnancy (1⅓ oz of absolute alcohol) to prevent any alcohol-associated birth defects or long-term consequences. The American Academy of Pediatrics recommends abstinence from alcohol before and during pregnancy.[35]

MARIJUANA

Marijuana is the most frequently abused drug in the United States among people in their late teens and

---

*References 1, 2, 3, 25, 31, 35, 46.

early 20s. In the past 10 years, there has been a 30-fold increase in the use of marijuana. In 1998 there were an estimated 11 million marijuana users in the United States. Of those 11 million users, an estimated 6.8 million used marijuana more than once a week.

Marijuana, a crude extract from the *Cannabis sativa* plant, contains more than 420 different compounds, many of which are biologically active. Marijuana is quickly absorbed, resulting in a "high" that lasts 2 to 3 hours. Although the high is brief, elimination of a single dose of marijuana may take several days because of its slow rate of metabolism and slow release from fatty tissues. Marijuana (tetrahydrocannabinol, or THC) is hydroxylated to 11-OH-THC, which is biologically active. This metabolite is then further hydroxylated to inactive metabolites that are excreted in urine and feces. The half-life after an acute dose is 56 hours; after chronic use, it is 19 to 28 hours. Accumulation may occur after chronic use. Depression of the hypothalamic neurotransmitters and defects in the immune system have been reported in heavy marijuana users.

In some regions of the United States, marijuana use was found in 5% to 34% of pregnant women. Marijuana crosses the placenta into the fetus. In animal studies, the rate of THC metabolism in the fetus is slow, which may prolong fetal exposure to marijuana. In humans, shortened gestation has been reported, with prolonged and arrested labor. A higher incidence of meconium staining has also been found by some investigators. In the majority of infants, a higher incidence of neonatal complications, structural anomalies, or effects on physical and growth parameters has not been noted. However, those infants born to mothers who are chronic marijuana users have a higher incidence of decreased birth weight. The Brazelton Neonatal Behavioral Assessment Scale revealed a higher incidence of tremors, altered visual responses, and changes in state regulation. Disturbed sleep cycling has also been described.[24] However, other studies have not confirmed these findings.

In follow-up at 6, 12, and 24 months of age, no differences were detected on physical and developmental evaluations in general. A subgroup of infants of heavy marijuana smokers scored lower on the Mental Developmental Index of the Bayley evaluation.[51] Polysomnographs at 3 years of age showed disturbed nocturnal sleep patterns with an increasing number of arousals. Visual evoked potentials performed at 3 to 6 years of age in children of marijuana smokers showed delays in maturation of the visual system compared with control children. The McCarthy subscales produced poorer scores for 4-year-old children on memory and verbal tests compared with those for a control group.[24, 38]

At 6 to 9 years of age, an increase in conduct problems, visual and perceptual deficits, poorer language comprehension, and distractibility were reported. Many of these findings may be related to the home environment and lifestyle to which these children are exposed.[38]

COCAINE

The abuse of cocaine has diminished somewhat from the epidemic levels of the mid-1980s, but it remains a major health problem in the United States. The 1998 National Household Survey on Drug Abuse estimated that 1.8 million Americans (0.8% of the population older than 12 years of age) used cocaine; 595,000 were considered to be heavy users. Cocaine addiction occurred in men and women of all races, ethnicities, and social classes in all areas of the United States. The rate of use among men was double that of women (1.1% versus 0.5%). The rate of cocaine use in the South and West was nearly double the rate in the Northeast and North Central regions (1% versus 0.6%).

Cocaine is administered by snorting, smoking, or inhaling (freebasing) it, or by IV injection. It is frequently used in combination with such drugs as marijuana, alcohol, cigarettes, sedatives, and hypnotics, especially during the "down," hypersomnolent period that follows crack or cocaine binging. Cocaine is well absorbed from all sites of administration. It has local anesthetic effects and is also a powerful stimulant, affecting several neurotransmitters in the central and peripheral nervous systems. Cocaine blocks the presynaptic reuptake of norepinephrine, resulting in tachycardia, elevated blood pressure, and vasoconstriction. Cocaine also interferes with the reuptake of dopamine, producing euphoria, hyperactivity, decreased appetite, and sexual excitement. However, prolonged cocaine use leads to dopamine depletion, dysphoria, depression, and drug craving. Cocaine also disrupts the metabolism of serotonin, leading to increased wakefulness in the sleep-wake cycle.[106]

Cocaine is hydrolyzed by plasma and hepatic cholinesterase and by spontaneous hydrolysis to inactive ecgonine metabolites (principally benzoylecgonine). The half-life of cocaine ranges from 16 to 90 minutes, depending on dose and route. Cocaine is also N-demethylated to norcocaine and transesterified in the presence of ethanol to produce cocaethylene, a potent neurostimulant with a half-life longer than that of cocaine. Both norcocaine and cocaethylene are pharmacologically active metabolites with toxic effects that may exceed those of cocaine. Crack is an inexpensive, alkaloid form of cocaine. Because crack has a lower melting point than cocaine hydrochloride and is highly lipid soluble, it can be smoked. The lung surfaces rapidly absorb crack, resulting in increased plasma levels and a quick high. Because of its short-lived effect (elimination half-life of 10 minutes), crack use becomes more frequent and quickly leads to addiction.[12, 68, 106]

Cocaine is second only to marijuana as the most commonly used illicit drug by women of childbearing age. Data collected in the 1996 National Household Survey on Drug Abuse estimated that 13% of the 2.5 million women pregnant at the time of the survey had used cocaine during their lifetime; 70,000 (2.8%) had used it during the past year. There are data suggesting that pregnancy and childbirth may provide a powerful incentive to curtail cocaine use. The prevalence of cocaine use during pregnancy varies geographically and among different age groups, races, and social classes. The rate of cocaine use among pregnant African-American women was 4.5%, more than 10 times the rate among pregnant white women and six times the rate among pregnant Hispanic women. The rate of cocaine use during pregnancy for women who used alcohol and cigarettes was 9.5%, compared with a rate of 0.1% for nonusers. Cocaine users were more likely to be nonwhite, multiparous, and poor, with no prenatal care. A high incidence of obstetric and neonatal complications has been associated with cocaine and crack abuse. The obstetric findings include a higher incidence of spontaneous abortions, stillbirths, fetal distress, premature labor, and abruptio placentae and placenta previa. A ~~ong~~ association between cocaine use during preg-

~~transmitted~~ diseases, especially ~~ted.~~[91, 111]

~~cholinester-~~

~~ther and~~

~~bolism of~~

~~cocaine. The N-demethylation~~ pathway is more active in pregnancy, resulting in a higher concentration of norcocaine in the urine. Although cocaine crosses the placenta freely, maternal uterine artery vasoconstriction may limit fetal exposure. Fetal cocaine levels are generally lower than maternal levels, with similar elimination half-lives. Cocaine given intravenously to a ewe during the end of gestation caused a dose-dependent increase in blood pressure, a decrease in uterine blood flow, and an increase in uterine vascular resistance. The fetus showed hypoxemia, hypertension, and tachycardia. Direct administration of cocaine to the fetus caused an increase in heart rate and blood pressure but no changes in fetal oxygenation. The added indirect hypoxemic effects related to uterine artery vasoconstriction may make maternal cocaine ingestion more detrimental to fetal health than if the drug were given directly to the fetus.[32, 106, 110]

Cocaine-exposed newborns are about twice as likely to require neonatal intensive care unit stays as their unexposed counterparts. Neonatal effects include a higher incidence of low birth weight, prematurity and its associated complications, and smaller head circumference. On average, cocaine-exposed newborns are born 1 to 2 weeks earlier than unexposed newborns. The earlier delivery may be related to the direct α-adrenergic effect of cocaine, to placental abruption, or to increased rates of maternal infection. The most consistently found fetal effect is growth retardation. Several mechanisms may act in concert to produce growth retardation. These include poor maternal nutritional status and decreased nutrient intake, decreased placental nutrient transfer associated with diminished uterine artery perfusion, interference with placental amino acid transport, and direct inhibition of cell differentiation and proliferation, particularly in the central nervous system. In most studies, the unadjusted magnitude of fetal

growth discrepancy ranges from 300 to 600 gm in birth weight and from 1 to 2 cm in both length and head circumference. After adjustment for maternal demographic factors and the presence of other insults to fetal growth (including maternal sexually transmitted diseases and the use of such substances as alcohol, heroin, and tobacco) only 20% to 50% of these deficits appear attributable to cocaine itself. Growth retardation is usually symmetric, but several studies have found disproportionate deficits in head circumference that may indicate that cocaine exerts a direct neuropathic effect on fetal brain growth. Several animal studies found that cocaine interferes with brain cell differentiation, cell migration, and phenotypic expression. In vitro studies show that cocaine may initiate neuronal apoptosis.*

Some studies have reported a higher incidence of congenital anomalies, particularly of the genitourinary system, in infants of cocaine-using mothers; other studies have failed to find such an association. An association between cocaine exposure and vascular occlusive malformations including intestinal atresia, limb reduction, and abdominal wall defects has been reported but not confirmed. Several studies using cranial ultrasonography and computed tomography scans demonstrated a higher incidence of hemorrhagic infarcts, cystic lesions, intraventricular hemorrhages, and echodensities, particularly in neonates whose mothers were heavy users of cocaine. Increased cerebral arterial blood flow velocity during the first 1 to 2 days of life has been described, which may place the infant at greater risk for intracranial hemorrhage. The risk of intracranial hemorrhage in term or near-term infants born to mothers with light to moderate cocaine use during pregnancy is probably small. Abnormal electroencephalograms (EEGs) and visual evoked potentials have been reported in cocaine-exposed infants. However, follow-up EEGs were within normal limits after 2 to 12 months. Abnormalities of the eye include transient abnormal vascularization of the iris, retinal defects and hemorrhage, and strabismus. An increased incidence of early-onset necrotizing enterocolitis was also reported in association with cocaine exposure. Many of these findings occur infrequently or primarily with heavy exposure and have not been consistently demonstrated or confirmed.†

There have been reports of cocaine intoxication in infants consuming breast milk containing cocaine. The infants exhibited tremors, irritability, seizures, and diarrhea lasting up to 48 hours. Both breast milk and the infants' urine were positive for cocaine and its metabolites. Cocaine enters breast milk readily because of its low molecular weight and high fat solubility and has been detected up to 36 hours after its use. Seizures, tremors, and ataxia have been reported in infants and toddlers apparently intoxicated by passive inhalation of crack smoke in poorly ventilated "crack dens."

---

*References 23, 59, 66, 71, 79, 80, 110, 111.
†References 30, 36, 37, 52, 62, 89.

The incidence of SIDS in infants exposed to cocaine in utero ranges from 4 to 9 deaths per 1000 live births, a rate that is three to seven times higher than normal. However, studies that controlled for other risk factors for SIDS found small or no increases attributable to cocaine. No study has controlled for maternal smoking. Abnormalities of respiratory pattern and abnormal hypoxic arousal responses have been described in several studies of cocaine-exposed infants and newborn animals.[9, 99, 106]

The results of neurobehavioral studies of cocaine-exposed newborns are contradictory and inconclusive. In an early report, investigators using the Brazelton Neonatal Behavioral Assessment Scale demonstrated abnormalities in interactive behavior and organizational response to environmental stimuli; however, other studies using the same assessment tool showed different effects or no effect. A study using the Neonatal Intensive Care Unit Network Neurobehavioral Scale found increased motor tone and activity; more jerks, startles, and tremors; and poorer auditory and visual tracking during the first 2 days of life in cocaine-exposed compared with unexposed newborns. Similar dose-related alterations in tone and an increased incidence of coarse tremors were found in a study that used the Neurologic Exam for Children.[18, 23, 27, 33, 36]

The few available long-term follow-up studies describe catch-up growth by 12 months of age for the majority of infants of cocaine-addicted mothers. Longitudinal neurodevelopmental studies, in constrast, supply ambiguous results, although most indicate some form of long-term negative effects. In several studies, poor developmental outcome was related to the interaction between cocaine exposure and small head circumference. Richardson found that at 3 years of age, intrauterine cocaine exposure was a predictor of both head circumference and composite score on the Stanford-Binet Intelligence Scale. Chasnoff and colleagues reported that at 2 years of age there was still a difference in head size in the cocaine or polydrug group of infants versus a control group. Mean scores for the Bayley Scales of Infant Development were within normal limits and similar to those in the control group. At 3 years of age, the mean scores on the Stanford-Binet test were not statistically different from those of controls. Path analysis showed that head circumference, home environment, and level of perseverance at a task mediated much of the effect of drug exposure on the children's scores. However, the study had a high attrition rate, and only a select population could be followed. Another study of school-aged children (also with many lost to follow-up) found no difference in IQ scores between children with and without prenatal exposure to cocaine; however, mean IQ scores were low in both groups (82.9 versus 82.4). Overall, these studies illustrate that children of cocaine-addicted mothers, particularly those with smaller than expected head size, are at risk for intellectual and developmental problems. Tronick pointed out that the most worrisome finding in most follow-up studies is the overall poor developmental

performance of infants and children, regardless of cocaine exposure status. These infants are usually recruited from low-income backgrounds and may have been subjected to multiple severe medical and psychosocial insults that could overshadow any specific effects of intrauterine cocaine exposure.[7, 22, 84, 102, 107]

PHENCYCLIDINE

Phencyclidine hydrochloride (PCP, or angel dust), a veterinary immobilizing agent, is one of the most dangerous drugs of abuse. PCP can be smoked, snorted, or ingested orally. PCP acts as both a stimulant and a depressant of the central nervous system and may affect muscular coordination and speech and give a feeling of drunkenness. Use of PCP may cause unpredictable, violent, and bizarre behavior, including disorientation, hallucinations, and prolonged schizophrenic-like psychosis. Its use today not widespread, but it is frequently as another drug of ab

PCP is high absorbed. It is ronides into several metabolites. The excretion half-life (1 to 3 days) of PCP depend on urinary pH, with acidic urine enhancing its excretion.[74]

PCP crosses the placenta into the fetus. This has been shown in both animal and human studies. In studies in the rabbit, the fetal PCP level was found to be 10-fold that of maternal plasma. Literature on human neonates is limited. Urine of neonates born to mothers taking PCP has been positive for PCP. PCP has been shown to cause progressive degeneration and death of human fetal cerebral cortical neurons in tissue cultures. These findings may be mediated by the inhibitory effects of PCP on potassium channels. Growth parameters and physical evaluations in general have been within normal limits, except for one study with two patients.[95] One of the neonates was microcephalic, and both neonates exhibited signs and symptoms of withdrawal syndrome requiring treatment. Another study reported sudden outbursts of agitation, flapping, coarse tremors, and facial grimacing with sudden and rapid changes in the level of consciousness. The Brazelton Neonatal Behavioral Assessment Scale demonstrated significant changes in the lability of states and in consolability. At 3 months' follow-up, these same infants were within normal limits in both growth and developmental parameters. The Bayley Scales were in the normal range. No further follow-up is available.[21, 41, 63, 69, 98]

AMPHETAMINES AND METHAMPHETAMINE

Amphetamines are one of the most potent central nervous system stimulants and sympathomimetics and are frequently used by teenagers and young adults as diet inducers or stimulants. The abuse of methamphetamine, or "ice," is a major problem, especially in the midwestern and western United States in both urban and rural settings. It can be smoked or used intravenously, intranasally, or orally. Its mood-elevating effects and addictive potential are similar to those of cocaine or crack. Tolerance develops quickly, requiring higher and more frequent doses. The intensity of its effect depends on the route of administration and dosage. The "high" derived from methamphetamine may last 10 to 24 hours, followed by a "crash" lasting 4 to 5 days. Methamphetamine has more pronounced central effects than amphetamines.

Amphetamines and methamphetamine are well absorbed and quickly localized in tissues, especially the central nervous system. Excretion is pH dependent and is enhanced by acidic urine.

Experiments with methamphetamine in the pregnant ewe demonstrated rapid transfer and distribution in the fetus. The peak concentration was greater in the mother than in the fetus, but elimination from the fetus was slower. Methamphetamine is eliminated via the kidneys. The fetal lung had the highest concentration of methamphetamine. Although the brain and heart had the lowest concentrations, the concentration in those organs was still three to four times that of the plasma. Amniotic fluid, with concentrations higher than maternal and fetal concentrations 2 to 24 hours after administration, may act as a reservoir for the drug. After IV administration, a 50% to 60% increase in maternal blood pressure, an increase in heart rate and cardiac output, increased systemic vascular resistance, and decreased uterine blood flow were found. The fetus demonstrated a 20% to 37% increase in blood pressure, an increase in heart rate, and a decrease in pH, oxygen partial pressure, and oxygen saturation. These findings were dose related.[14, 95]

Abuse of either amphetamine or methamphetamine during pregnancy is generally associated with a higher incidence of perinatal mortality, prematurity, and growth deficits. In a study in Sweden, neonates born to amphetamine addicts exhibited drowsiness, respiratory distress, and jitteriness. On follow-up, these infants remained lethargic for several months, with frequent infections and poor weight gain. Other studies reported a higher incidence of emotional disturbances and delays in gross and fine motor coordination during early childhood. Neonates born to mothers using methamphetamine during gestation were found to be SGA and to exhibit hypersensitivity to sound, abnormal sleeping patterns, and increased tone. Abnormal cranial ultrasound scans demonstrating cystic and echodense areas and hemorrhages were also described, most likely related to the vasoconstrictive properties of methamphetamine. These lesions are similar to those found in cocaine-exposed infants.[57, 60, 96]

Studies in the rat demonstrated that adult rats exposed to methamphetamines in utero have behavior and brain monoamine function changes.[108]

PHENOBARBITAL

Phenobarbital is frequently used in the treatment of seizure disorders and for sedation. It also is a com-

monly abused drug among patients of all socioeconomic classes. Phenobarbital crosses the placenta readily and is distributed rapidly throughout the fetus, with the greatest concentrations in the liver and brain. Infants of phenobarbital-addicted mothers are usually full term and of appropriate weight for gestational age. In addition, their Apgar scores are usually good. The incidence of phenobarbital withdrawal symptoms is not known. When they do occur, symptoms begin at a median age of 7 days (range, 2 to 14 days) and may last 2 to 4 months. Desmond and associates described two stages of phenobarbital withdrawal: an acute stage consisting of irritability, constant crying, sleeplessness, hiccups, and mouthing movements, followed by a subacute stage marked by a voracious appetite, frequent regurgitation and gagging, episodic irritability, hyperacusis, sweating, and a disturbed sleep pattern. The second stage may last from 2 to 4 months. The late onset of phenobarbital withdrawal probably results from its slow metabolism and excretion by the newborn. Treatment consists of swaddling, frequent feedings, and protection from noxious external stimuli. If there is no improvement with these methods, the infants should be given phenobarbital, with the phenobarb slowly withdrawn after control of symptoms.[28]

MISCELLANEOUS DRUGS

Several cases of neonatal withdrawal syndrome have been reported secondary to in utero exposure to pentazocine (alone or combined with tripelennamine), a non-narcotic analgesic that previously was thought to be nonaddictive. These infants were SGA and developed withdrawal symptoms at about 24 hours of age. Symptoms consisted of hypertonia, hyperactivity, tremors, and vomiting. Treatment with phenobarbital for 14 to 17 days was effective.[20, 40]

Other drugs that may cause withdrawal symptoms include codeine, propoxyphene, glutethimide, and short- and long-acting diazepines.* Long-term benzodiazepine use does not increase the overall incidence of congenital malformations. However, late-pregnancy chronic use has resulted in "floppy baby syndrome," consisting of apnea, decreased tone, poor feeding, and poor response to cold stress. These symptoms may last for several hours to months. Withdrawal symptoms similar to narcotic withdrawal have also been described secondary to long-acting diazepines; these occur late because of the drugs' slow metabolism and excretion in neonates. No reports are available concerning withdrawal from chlordiazepoxide (Librium) and meprobamate, but a four-fold increase in the incidence of malformation has been reported in infants whose mothers took these drugs during early pregnancy.[64, 65, 100]

Inhalant abuse is another public health problem, especially in adolescents (12 to 17 years). There are currently 883,000 inhalant abusers, and many of these

---

*References 19, 53, 64, 65, 83, 100, 104.

women become pregnant. The inhalants abused include paint thinners and adhesives containing toluene or 1,1,1-trichloroethane, lighter fluid or butane gas, and nitrous oxide. Case reports of infants born to women abusing inhalants such as paint and glue found a higher incidence of perinatal death, prematurity, and low birth weight. These infants also exhibited a syndrome similar to FAS, with microcephaly, narrow bifrontal diameter, short palpebral fissures, hypoplastic midface, wide nasal bridge, abnormal palmar creases, and blunt fingertips. Follow-up of these children revealed continued growth retardation, microcephaly, and developmental delays.[5, 50, 81]

The use of LSD has reappeared among college-age youths. Ocular malformations, including microphthalmos, intraocular cartilage, cataract, primary persistent hyperplastic vitreous, and retinal dysplasia, have been reported secondary to intrauterine LSD exposure.[16]

Every few years, new drugs of abuse are introduced. The present group of designer or club drugs consists of methylenedioxymethamphetamine (MDMA, ecstasy), gamma hydroxybutyrate (grievous bodily harm, G, date rape drug), ketamine (special K), and Rohypnol (roofies). Ecstasy is similar to amphetamine and mescaline, with stimulant and psychedelic effects that last for 3 to 6 hours. In one study, infants born to mothers abusing ecstasy did not show any increased incidence in abortions or congenital anomalies.[105]

DRUG SCREENING METHODS

Most screening procedures used for pregnant women and their newborns employ a panel of drug-specific assays, with drugs selected according to the frequency of their use, their illegality, and their potential for harm. Typical drug screening panels include tests for opiates (morphine, codeine, heroin, and synthetic derivatives), methadone, amphetamines, cocaine metabolites (benzoylecgonine), marijuana (cannabinoids), phenothiazines, benzodiazepines, and barbiturates. Testing methods include immunoassays (fluorescence polarization immunoassay, radioimmunoassay, and enzyme-linked immunoassay), spectrophotometric assays (ultraviolet and mass spectrophotometry), and chromatographic methods (thin-layer, gas, and gas-liquid chromatography).[12, 90]

Drug screening is usually conducted as a two-tiered procedure, with the initial test performed using a rapid, inexpensive, but sensitive method. Confirmation of positive results (those with drug concentrations exceeding a threshold level) is usually done using a more specific method capable of identifying lower concentrations of the drug. The enzyme-mediated immunoassay technique (EMIT), employing a bacterial antigen-antibody lysosome system, is the simplest and most rapid system available and is often used for initial screening tests. The National Institute of Drug Abuse published guidelines specifying threshold levels for immunoassays of commonly abused drugs, and these have been widely applied to clinical testing. Concern has been raised, however, that the high cutoff values underestimate drug exposure in pregnant women and newborns; the use of lower threshold values would result in higher rates of exposure detection. For example, Casanova and colleagues found that 27% of infants whose urine was found to contain cocaine metabolites at a concentration greater than 5 ng/mL would not have been identified at a threshold level of 300 ng/mL.[15]

Other immunoassays are more sensitive than EMIT (e.g., radioimmunoassay), but because the antibodies used for these tests may cross-react with related compounds, confirmation by an independent method is required. For example, the immunoassay for morphine yields a positive result in the presence of morphine metabolites, codeine, and dihydrocodeine. The technique combining gas chromatography and mass spectrophotometry (GC-MS) is generally used to confirm a positive screening test. GC-MS provides highly specific substance identification at concentrations much lower than immunoassay screening techniques and is capable of identifying unexpected or novel substances, including so-called designer drugs. With proper sample preparation, immunoassays and GC-MS can be applied to a variety of tissues and body fluids, including urine, meconium, amniotic fluid, vernix caseosa, hair, and nails.[12, 78, 90]

Urine toxicologic testing is a reliable, noninvasive, and inexpensive measure of recent drug use or exposure. However, testing maternal or newborn urine as a measure of fetal drug exposure has serious limitations. For example, a newborn urine test for benzoylecgonine collected at delivery reflects, at most, drug use only during the 3 to 4 days before delivery; this interval narrows in proportion to the time elapsed between the mother's last use and delivery. Thus, mothers who test positive at delivery are usually heavy, frequent users of illicit drugs; infrequent or intermittent use is often not detected. The results of newborn urine drug tests are also dependent on the time of specimen collection. A negative urine result for the newborn of a drug-using mother may be due to the mother's abstention from drug use or the inability to collect urine early enough after birth.[12, 33]

The presence of drugs or drug metabolites in meconium or hair provides a long-term, semiquantitative measure of fetal exposure. Drug metabolites in meconium reflect drug intake during the second and third trimesters of pregnancy. During gestation, drug metabolites accumulate in meconium either by direct deposition from bile or by ingestion of metabolites present in amniotic fluid. The meconium can be analyzed for drugs of abuse using immunoassays or chromatographic methods. In one large study of a high-risk urban population, 44% of newborns passed meconium containing metabolites of cocaine, marijuana, or opiates, but only 11% of the mothers admitted to illicit drug use; 52% of their infants had positive urine tests, and 88% had positive meconium drug screens. However, another study found no difference in the rates at which cocaine and metabolites were isolated from urine, meconium, and amniotic fluid, provided the same highly sensitive methodology (GC-MS at 5 ng/mL) was used for all samples.[15, 78]

Maternal or newborn hair can be analyzed for metabolites of drugs of abuse using radioimmunoassay with GC-MS confirmation. Collection of a maternal or newborn hair sample usually requires the informed consent of the mother. Animal studies indicate that drugs and drug metabolites accumulate in hair in proportion to their concentration in the blood nourishing the hair root; in theory, as the hair grows, it should provide a quantitative and temporal register of drug use, particularly during the latter part of pregnancy. In reality, the conditions that lead to deposition of drug or drug metabolites in hair have not been fully worked out, and the results of hair analysis are difficult to interpret. The radioimmunoassay for benzoylecgonine, the major metabolite of cocaine, in hair is highly sensitive and specific. However, benzoylecgonine may be washed out of hair by alkaline hair treatments, or it may accumulate in hair via the spontaneous hydrolysis of cocaine incorporated into hair as a result of environmental exposure to crack fumes. An experiment with human volunteers showed that the quantity of isotopically labeled cocaine incorporated into hair correlated poorly with the actual dose of cocaine. Additionally, labeled cocaine binds to melanin, with higher concentrations accumulating in the hair of dark-haired, dark-skinned persons. These methodologic issues have discouraged the use of hair analysis as a quantitative and forensic measure of exposure.[44, 45]

Where maternal drug use in pregnancy is common, many hospitals have instituted selective newborn drug screening. Infants may be chosen for screening based on risk assessment of the mother or on symptoms present in the mother or newborn. Commonly cited maternal risk factors include inadequate prenatal care, sexually transmitted disease, history of past illegal substance use, referral to the child welfare system for child abuse or neglect, and prostitution. The purpose of such screening is, in part, to identify mothers whose drug use has caused presumptive harm to their newborns. Such mothers are deemed at risk for providing inadequate newborn care. Risk-based screening for any substance should never be undertaken without fully exploring the legal implications of a positive test. Written protocols need to be established that specify the collection, handling, transport, analysis, and reporting of results for newborn screening specimens. Most states require that positive results of newborn drug screening tests be reported to the local child welfare agency. This referral generally leads to an investigation of family circumstances, involvement of the family court, and possibly removal of the newborn to foster care.

■ REFERENCES

1. Abel EL: Fetal alcohol syndrome: The "American paradox." Alcohol Alcohol 33:195, 1998.
2. Abel EL: What really causes FAS? Teratology 59:4, 1999.
3. Abel EL, et al: How do physicians define "light," "moderate," and "heavy" drinking? Alcohol Clin Exp Res 22:979, 1998.
4. Arendt R, et al: Motor development of cocaine-exposed children at age two years. Pediatrics 103:86, 1999.
5. Arnold GL, et al: Toluene embryopathy: Clinical delineation and developmental follow-up. Pediatrics 93:216, 1994.
6. Aronson M, Hagberg B: Neuropsychological disorders in children exposed to alcohol during pregnancy: A follow-up study of 24 children born to alcoholic mothers in Goterborg, Sweden. Alcohol Clin Exp Res 22:321, 1998.
7. Azuma SD, et al: Outcome of children prenatally exposed to cocaine and other drugs: A path analysis of three-year-data. Pediatrics 92:396, 1993.
8. Bateman DA, Hagarty MC: Passive freebase cocaine ("crack") inhalation by infants and toddlers. Am J Dis Child 143:25, 1989.
9. Bauchner H, et al: Risk of sudden infant death syndrome among infants with in utero exposure to cocaine. J Pediatr 113:831, 1988.
10. Bearer CF, et al: Ethyl linoleate in meconium: A biomarker for prenatal ethanol exposure. Alcohol Clin Exp Res 23:487, 1999.
11. Bleyer AW, et al: Barbiturate withdrawal syndrome in a passively addicted infant. JAMA 221:185, 1972.
12. Braithwaite RA, et al: Screening for drugs of abuse. I. Opiates, amphetamines and cocaine. Ann Clin Biochem 32:123, 1995.
13. Brien JF, et al: Disposition of ethanol in maternal blood, fetal blood, and amniotic fluid of third trimester pregnant ewes. Am J Obstet Gynecol 152:583, 1985.
14. Burchfield DJ, et al: Disposition and pharmacodynamics of methamphetamine in pregnant sheep. JAMA 265:1968, 1991.
15. Casanova OQ, et al: Detection of cocaine exposure in the neonate: Analysis of urine, meconium and amniotic fluid from mothers and infants exposed to cocaine. Arch Pathol Lab Med 118:988, 1994.
16. Chan CC, et al: Multiple ocular anomalies associated with maternal LSD ingestion. Arch Ophthalmol 96:282, 1978.
17. Chasnoff IJ, et al: Cocaine intoxication in a breast-fed infant. Pediatrics 80:836, 1987.
18. Chasnoff IJ, et al: Cocaine use in pregnancy. N Engl J Med 313:666, 1985.
19. Chasnoff IJ, et al: Maternal non-narcotic substance abuse during pregnancy: Effects on infant development. Neurobehav Toxicol Teratol 6:277, 1984.
20. Chasnoff IJ, et al: Pentazocine and tripelennamine ("T's and blue's"): Effects on the fetus and neonate. Dev Pharmacol Ther 6:162, 1983.
21. Chasnoff IJ, et al: Phencyclidine: Effects on the fetus and neonate. Dev Pharmacol Ther 6:404, 1983.
22. Chasnoff IJ, et al: Cocaine/polydrug use in pregnancy: Two-year follow-up. Pediatrics 89:284, 1992.
23. Chiriboga CA, et al: Dose-response effect of fetal cocaine exposure on newborn neurologic function. Pediatrics 103:79, 1999.
24. Dahl RE, et al: A longitudinal study of prenatal marijuana use. Arch Pediatr Adolesc Med 149:145, 1995.
25. Day NL, et al: Prenatal exposure to alcohol: Effect on infant growth and morphologic characteristics. Pediatrics 84:536, 1989.
26. Day NL, et al: Prenatal alcohol use and offspring size at 10 years of age. Alcohol Clin Exp Res 23:863, 1999.
27. Delaney-Black V, et al: Prenatal cocaine and neonatal outcome: Evaluation of dose-response relationship. Pediatrics 98:735, 1996.
28. Desmond M, et al: Maternal barbiturate utilization and neonatal withdrawal symptomatology. J Pediatr 80:190, 1972.
29. Dinges DF, et al: Fetal exposure to narcotics: Sleep as a measure of nervous system disturbance. Science 209:619, 1980.
30. Doberczak TM, et al: Neonatal neurologic and electroencephalographic effects of intrauterine cocaine exposure. J Pediatr 113:354, 1988.
31. Eckardt M, et al: Effects of moderate alcohol consumption on the central nervous system. Alcohol Clin Exp Res 22:998, 1998.
32. Evans RT, et al: Longitudinal study of cholinesterase changes in pregnancy. Clin Chem 34:2249, 1988.
33. Eyler FD, et al: Birth outcome from a prospective, matched study of prenatal crack/cocaine use. II. Interactive and dose effects on neurobehavioral assessment. Pediatrics 101:237, 1998.

34. Ferriero DM, et al: Impact of addictive and harmful substances on fetal brain development. Curr Opin Neurol 12:161, 1999.
35. Fetal alcohol syndrome and fetal alcohol effects: Committee on Substance Abuse, American Academy of Pediatrics. Pediatrics 91:1004, 1993.
36. Frank DA, et al: Neonatal neurobehavioral and neuroanatomic correlates of prenatal cocaine exposure: Problems of dose and confounding. Ann N Y Acad Sci 846:40, 1998.
37. Frank DA, et al: Level of in utero cocaine exposure and neonatal ultrasound findings. Pediatrics 104:1101, 1999.
38. Fried PA: Behavioral outcomes in preschool and school-age children exposed prenatally to marijuana: A review and speculative interpretation. NIDA Research Monograph No. 164, October 1999, p 242.
39. Gerdin E, et al: Disposition of morphine-3-glucuronide in the pregnant rhesus monkey. Pharmacol Toxicol 66:185, 1990.
40. Goetz RL, et al: Neonatal withdrawal symptoms associated with maternal use of pentazocine. J Pediatr 84:887, 1974.
41. Goodwin PJ, et al: Phencyclidine effect of chronic administration in the female mouse in gestation, maternal behavior, and the neonates. Psychopharmacology 69:63, 1980.
42. Guerri C: Neuroanatomical and neurophysiological mechanisms involved in central nervous system dysfunctions induced by prenatal alcohol exposure. Alcohol Clin Exp Res 22:304, 1998.
43. Hans SL: Maternal opioid drug use and child development. In Maternal Substance Abuse and Developing Nervous System. Chicago, Academic Press, 1992.
44. Henderson GL, et al: Incorporation of isotopically labeled cocaine and metabolites into human hair. 1. Dose-response relationships. J Anal Toxicol 20:1, 1996.
45. Henderson GL, et al: Incorporation of isotopically labeled cocaine into human hair: Race as a factor. J Anal Toxicol 2:156, 1998.
46. Jacobson JL, et al: Relation of maternal age and pattern of pregnancy drinking to functionally significant cognitive deficit in infancy. Alcohol Clin Exp Res 22:345, 1998.
47. Jernite M, et al: Buprenorphine and pregnancy: Analysis of 24 cases. Arch Pediatr 6:1179, 1999.
48. Johnson HL, et al: Path analysis of variables affecting 36-month outcome on population of multirisk children. Infant Behav Dev 10:451, 1987.
49. Johnson HL, et al: Resilient children: Individual differences in developmental outcome of children born to drug abusers. J Genet Psychol 151:523, 1990.
50. Jones HE, Balster RL: Inhalant abuse in pregnancy. In Sorosky JI: Substance Abuse in Pregnancy. Obstet Gynecol Clin North Am 25:153, 1998.
51. Kaltenbach KA: Prenatal opiate exposure: Developmental effects in infancy and early childhood. OSAP Monograph 11:49, DHHS Publ No. (ADM)92–1814, 1992.
52. King TA, et al: Neurologic manifestations of in utero cocaine exposure in near term and term infants. Pediatrics 96:259, 1995.
53. Klein RB, et al: Probable neonatal propoxyphene withdrawal: A case report. Pediatrics 55:882, 1975.
54. Kolar AF, et al: Children of substance abusers: The life experiences of children of opiate addicts in methadone-maintenance. Am J Drug Alcohol Abuse 20:159, 1994.
55. Konovalov HV, et al: Disorders of brain development in the progeny of mothers who used alcohol during pregnancy. Early Hum Dev 48:153, 1997.
56. Larroque B, Kaminski M: Prenatal alcohol exposure and development at preschool age: Main results of a French study. Alcohol Clin Exp Res 22:295, 1998.
57. Larson G: The amphetamine addicted mother and her child. Acta Paediatr Scand 278:7, 1980.
58. Lifschitz MH, et al: Patterns of growth and development in narcotic-exposed children: NIDA Res Monogr 114:323, 1991.
59. Little BB, et al: Brain growth among fetuses exposed to cocaine in utero: Asymmetrical growth retardation. Obstet Gynecol 77:361, 1991.
60. Little BB, et al: Methamphetamine abuse during pregnancy: Outcome and fetal effects. Obstet Gynecol 72:541, 1988.

61. Little BB, et al: Maternal and fetal effects of heroin addiction during pregnancy. J Reprod Med 35:159, 1990.
62. Lopez SL, et al: Time of onset of necrotizing enterocolitis in newborn infants with known perinatal cocaine exposure. Clin Pediatr 34:429, 1995.
63. Mattson MP, et al: Degenerative and axon outgrowth altering effects of phencyclidine in human fetal cerebral cortical cells. Neuropharmacology 31:279, 1992.
64. McElhatton PR: The effects of diazepine use during pregnancy and lactation. Reprod Toxicol 8:461, 1994.
65. Milkovich BA, et al: Effects of prenatal meprobamate and chlordiazepoxide hydrochloride on human embryonic and fetal development. N Engl J Med 291:1268, 1974.
66. Mirochnick M, et al: Relation between meconium concentration of the cocaine metabolite benzoylecgonine and fetal growth. J Pediatr 126:636, 1995.
67. Moore CA, et al: Does light-to-moderate alcohol consumption during pregnancy increase the risk for renal anomalies among offspring? Pediatrics 99:E11, 1999.
68. Morishima HO, et al: The comparative toxicity of cocaine and its metabolites in conscious rats. Anesthesiology 90:1684, 1999.
69. Mvula MM, et al: Relationship of phencyclidine and pregnancy outcome. J Reprod Med 44:1021, 1999.
70. Naeye RL, et al: Fetal complications of maternal heroin addiction, abnormal growth, infections and episodes of stress. J Pediatr 75:945, 1969.
71. Nassogne MC, et al: Selective direct toxicity of cocaine on fetal mouse neurons: Teratogenic implications of neurite and apoptotic neuronal loss. Ann N Y Acad Sci 846:51, 1998.
72. Nathenson G, et al: The effect of maternal heroin addiction on neonatal jaundice. J Pediatr 81:899, 1972.
73. Neonatal drug withdrawal: Committee on Drugs, AAP. Pediatrics 101:1079, 1998.
74. Nicholas MJ, et al: Phencyclidine: Its transfer across the placenta as well as into breast milk. Am J Obstet Gynecol 143:143, 1982.
75. Nichols MM: Acute alcohol withdrawal syndrome in a newborn. Am J Dis Child 113:714, 1967.
76. Olsen GD, et al: Ventilatory response to carbon dioxide of infants following chronic prenatal methadone exposure. J Pediatr 96:983, 1980.
77. Ornoy A, et al: The developmental outcome of children born to heroin-dependent mothers, raised at home or adopted. Child Abuse Negl 20:385, 1996.
78. Ostrea EM Jr: Testing for exposure to illicit drugs and other agents in the neonate: A review of laboratory methods and the role of meconium analysis. Curr Probl Pediatr 29:37, 1999.
79. Ostrea EM, et al: Drug screening of newborns by meconium analysis: A large-scale, prospective, epidemiologic study. Pediatrics 89:107, 1992.
80. Pastrakuljic A, et al: Maternal cocaine use and cigarette smoking in pregnancy in relation to amino acid transport and fetal growth. Placenta 20:499, 1999.
81. Pearson MA, et al: Toluene embryopathy: Delineation of the phenotype and comparison with fetal alcohol syndrome. Pediatrics 93:211, 1994.
82. Polygenis D, et al: Moderate alcohol consumption during pregnancy and the incidence of fetal malformations: A meta-analysis. Neurotoxicol Teratol 20:61, 1998.
83. Reveri M, et al: Neonatal withdrawal symptoms associated with glutethimide (doriden) addiction in the mother during pregnancy. Clin Pediatr 16:424, 1977.
84. Richardson GA: Prenatal cocaine exposure: A longitudinal study of development. Ann N Y Acad Sci 846:144, 1998.
85. Roebuck TM, et al: A review of the neuroanatomical findings in children with fetal alcohol syndrome or prenatal exposure to alcohol. Alcohol Clin Exp Res 22:339, 1998.
86. Rosen TS, et al: Children of methadone-maintained mothers: Follow-up to 18 months. J Pediatr 101:192, 1982.
87. Rosen TS, et al: Pharmacologic observations on the neonatal withdrawal syndrome. J Pediatr 88:1044, 1976.
88. San L, et al: Follow-up after six-month maintenance period on naltrexone versus placebo in heroin addicts. Br J Addict 86:983, 1991.

89. Silva-Araujo A, et al: Development of the eye after gestational exposure to cocaine: Vascular disruption in the retina of rats and humans. Ann N Y Acad Sci 801:274, 1996.

90. Simpson D, et al: Screening for drugs of abuse. II. Cannabinoids, lysergic acid diethylamide, buprenorphine, methadone, barbiturates, benzodiazepines and other drugs. Ann Clin Biochem 34:460, 1997.

91. Sisson CG, et al: The resurgence of congenital syphilis: A cocaine-related problem. J Pediatr 130:289, 1997.

92. Sisson TRC, et al: Effect of neonatal withdrawal on neonatal sleep patterns. Pediatr Res 8:451, 1974.

93. Soepatmi S: Developmental outcomes of children of mothers dependent on heroin or heroin/methadone during pregnancy. Acta Paediatr Suppl 404:36, 1994.

94. Steinhausen HC, Spohr HL: Long-term outcome of children with fetal alcohol syndrome: Psychopathology, behavior and intelligence. Alcohol Clin Exp Res 22:334, 1998.

95. Stek AM, et al: Maternal and fetal cardiovascular responses to methamphetamine in the pregnant sheep. Am J Obstet Gynecol 169:888, 1993.

96. Stewart JL, Meeker JE: Fetal and infant deaths associated with maternal methamphetamine abuse. J Anal Toxicol 21:515, 1997.

97. Stoler JM, et al: The prenatal detection of significant alcohol exposure with maternal blood markers. J Pediatr 133:346, 1998.

98. Strauss AA, et al: Neonatal manifestation of maternal phencyclidine (PCP) abuse. Pediatrics 68:550, 1981.

99. Suguihara C, et al: Decreased ventilatory response to hypoxia in sedated newborn piglets prenatally exposed to cocaine. J Pediatr 128:389, 1996.

100. Sutton LR, Hinderliter SA: Diazepam abuse in pregnant women on methadone maintenance. Clin Pediatr 29:108, 1990.

101. Taeusch HW Jr, et al: Heroin induction of lung maturation and growth retardation in fetal rabbits. J Pediatr 82:869, 1972.

102. Tronick EZ, Beeghly M: Prenatal cocaine exposure, child development, and the compromising effects of cumulative risk. Clin Perinatol 26:151, 1999.

103. Van Baar AL, et al: Development after prenatal exposure to cocaine, heroin, methadone. Acta Paediatr Suppl 404:40, 1994.

104. Van Leeuwen G, et al: Narcotic withdrawal reaction in a newborn infant due to codeine. Pediatrics 36:635, 1965.

105. Van Tonningen-van Driel MM, et al: Pregnancy outcome after ecstasy use: 43 cases followed by the Teratology Information Service of the National Institute for Public Health and Environment. Ned Tijdschr Geneeskd 143:27, 1999.

106. Volpe JJ, Epstein HJ: Effect of cocaine use on the fetus. N Engl J Med 327:399, 1992.

107. Wasserman GA, et al: Prenatal cocaine exposure and school-age intelligence. Drug Alcohol Depend 50:203, 1998.

108. Weissman AD, et al: In utero methamphetamine effects. I. Behavior and monoamine uptake sites in adult offspring. Synapse 13:241, 1993.

109. Wilson GS, et al: The development of preschool children of heroin addicted mothers: A controlled study. Pediatrics 63:135, 1979.

110. Woods JR: Maternal and transplacental effects of cocaine. Ann N Y Acad Sci 846:1, 1998.

111. Zuckerman B, et al: Effects of maternal marijuana and cocaine use on fetal growth. N Engl J Med 320:762, 1989.